SALEM HEALTH
MAGILL'S MEDICAL GUIDE

SALEM HEALTH

MAGILL'S MEDICAL GUIDE

Eighth Edition

Volume 1

Abdomen – Conception

Medical Editors

Bryan C. Auday, Ph.D.
Gordon College

Michael A. Buratovich, Ph.D.
Spring Arbor University

Geraldine F. Marrocco, Ed.D., APRN, CNS, ANP-BC
Yale University School of Nursing

Paul Moglia, Ph.D.
South Nassau Communities Hospital

SALEM PRESS
A Division of EBSCO Information Services, Inc.
Ipswich, Massachusetts

GREY HOUSE PUBLISHING

Magill's Medical Guide: Health and Illness, 1995
Supplement, 1996
Magill's Medical Guide, revised edition, 1998
Second revised edition, 2002
Third revised edition, 2005
Fourth revised edition, 2008
Sixth edition, 2011
Seventh edition, 2014
Eighth edition, 2018

∞ The paper used in these volumes conforms to the American National Standard for Permanence of Paper for Printed Library Materials, Z39.48 1992 (R2009).

Note to Readers

The material presented in *Magill's Medical Guide* is intended for broad informational and educational purposes. Readers who suspect that they suffer from any of the physical or psychological disorders, diseases, or conditions described in this set should contact a physician without delay; this work should not be used as a substitute for professional medical diagnosis or treatment. This set is not to be considered definitive on the covered topics, and readers should remember that the field of health care is characterized by a diversity of medical opinions and constant expansion in knowledge and understanding.

Publisher's Cataloging-in-Publication Data
(Prepared by The Donohue Group, Inc.)

Names: Auday, Bryan C., editor.
Title: Magill's medical guide / medical editors: Bryan C. Auday, Ph.D., Gordon College [and three others].
Other Titles: Salem health (Pasadena, Calif.)
Description: Eighth Edition. | Ipswich, Massachusetts : Salem Press, a division of EBSCO Information Services, Inc. ; Amenia, NY : Grey House Publishing, 2018. | Includes bibliographical references and index. | Contents: Volume 1. Abdomen-Chronic wasting disease -- Volume 2. Chyme-Gram staining -- Volume 3. Growth-Nervous system -- Volume 4. Neuralgia, neuritis, and neuropathy-Shingles -- Volume 5. Shock-Zoonoses, Appendixes, Indexes.
Identifiers: ISBN 9781682176313 (set) | ISBN 9781682176320 (v.1) | ISBN 9781682176337 (v.2) | ISBN 9781682176344 (v.3) | ISBN 9781682176351 (v.4) | ISBN 9781682176368 (v.5)
Subjects: LCSH: Medicine--Encyclopedias.
Classification: LCC RC41 .M345 2018 | DDC 610.3--dc23

First Printing

printed in the United States of America

Publisher's Note

Since 1995, *Magill's Medical Guide* has been acclaimed by every major reference reviewer, and it has become a staple in high school, college, medical school, and public libraries. Designed for laymen and written for health care consumers, the *Medical Guide* is a perfect mix of accessibility and depth, providing general readers with an authoritative reference source that helps bridge the gap between medical encyclopedias for professionals and popular self-help guides. It is an up-to-date and easy-to-use compendium of medical information suitable for student research as well as use by general readers, including patients and caregivers. This *Eighth Edition* continues to build on this value.

Purchase of the printed set entitles the buyer to free online access to the *Medical Guide's* content. This online version is made available through the Salem Press online platform. Users can search the full text by performing keyword searches and browse the complete list of contents for quick and easy access to the desired topic. Information about how to activate online access can be found at the end of this Publisher's Note.

Scope of Coverage

The 1,289 entries in this encyclopedia (128 more than the previous edition) describe major diseases and disorders of the human body, the basics of human anatomy and physiology, specializations in medical practice, and common surgical and nonsurgical procedures. The *Eighth Edition* offers entries by 400 writers from the fields of life science, medicine, and biopsychology. Every essay is signed by the original author(s), including medical or other advanced degrees, and each updated entry is also signed by the revising author. These writers examine various diseases and disorders, both genetic and acquired, the detailed knowledge of human bodily systems and structures that medical practice requires, and the medical professions and procedures that apply this knowledge. Hundreds of photographs and medical drawings provide invaluable visual context for entries about diseases, research, surgery, and human anatomy. For each disease and disorder, a concise *Information On* box lists causes, symptoms, duration, and treatments, acting as a quick reference tool for the reader.

Readers will find topics that focus on specific disorders, as well as those that survey the range of afflictions attacking a particular system. The majority of entries treat physical disorders:

Other entries consider psychological, emotional, and learning disorders that originate in or have significant impact on the physical health of the body. Some basic conditions that are often the object of medical attention are covered, includ-

- bacterial and viral infections
- cancers of various types
- genetic defects
- heart and circulatory disorders
- abdominal and gastrointestinal disorders
- bone and muscle defects
- brain and nervous system problems
- dental diseases
- eating and nutritional disorders
- endocrine disorders
- immune disorders
- kidney and urinary system disorders
- liver disorders
- reproductive system disorders of both men and women
- respiratory diseases
- sexually transmitted diseases
- skin disorders
- sleep disorders
- trauma-related disorders
- vector-borne diseases
- visual disorders

ing Aging, Pregnancy and Gestation, Childbirth and its complications, Puberty and Adolescence, Menopause, and Sexuality.

Entries on anatomy and biology include overviews of anatomical organs and systems and of biological components and processes. A broad view of medical practice—its areas of specialization and health care provision—is offered by entries on such topics as Emergency Medicine, Nursing, and Orthopedics. Diagnostic and imaging techniques, nonsurgical and surgical procedures, both major and minor, are covered. In addition, other areas of medical science are represented: alternative medicine, medical and neuroethics, genetics, organizations, procedures in the field of psychiatry, general surgical procedures, testing and examinations, and various types of transplantation.

Entry Length and Format

The essays in the *Eighth Edition* are arranged in an encyclopedic format—alphabetically from Abdomen through Zoonoses. The lengths of the entries vary from shorter entries of 500 words to medium-length entries of 1,000 words to full, essay-length treatments of 2,500 to 3,500 words. All entries begin with standard information about the type of entry, the anatomy or bodily system affected, the specialties involved, and a brief definition of the topic. For essays of 1,000 words or more, next comes a list of key terms with brief definitions. Several main subsections of text follow and depend on the type of entry.

Entries on Diseases or Disorders: "Causes and Symptoms" defines the condition and describes its cause and its possible manifestations in patients, and "Treatment and Therapy" explores the various treatments available to alleviate symptoms or effect a cure.

Entries on Anatomy or Biology: "Structure and Functions" defines the physiological or biological system, including its components and role, and "Disorders and Diseases" describes the medical conditions that can result from malfunction of and injury to this physiological system.

Entries on Development: "Physical and Psychological Factors" charts the stages of development and analyzes the underlying physiological and emotional/psychological components, and "Disorders and Effects" addresses the overall impact of the developmental process.

Entries on Procedures: "Indications and Procedures" relates the circumstances under which the procedure is usually performed, identifying the condition it is intended to correct and detailing the basic steps involved, and "Uses and Complications" discusses the various applications and possible risks and complicating factors.

Entries on Specialties: "Science and Profession" addresses the training and responsibilities of various specialists, and "Diagnostic and Treatment Techniques" outlines the means by which they counsel patients, diagnose conditions, perform operations or procedures, and otherwise treat medical problems.

The last section of all longer entries is "Perspective and Prospects," which places the topic in a larger context within medicine—past, present, and future. For example, an entry on a disease may cover the earliest known investigation into the condition, the evolution of its treatment over time, and promising areas of research for a greater understanding of its causes and cure. An entry on a procedure may address the innovations that led to contemporary technology, improvements or changes that have been made in the procedure, and where this medical technique may be headed. Every entry lists the author's byline, and cross-references to other entries of interest in the encyclopedia. All essays conclude with the section "For Further Information," which lists general bibliographic works and relevant websites for the reader to consult; bibliographies for many longer entries provide brief annotations evaluating the features, contents, and value of the sources.

Special Features

Several special features assist readers in locating topics of interest. The "Complete Table of Contents," found at the beginning of each volume, allows the scope of the encyclopedia to be seen in its entirety. Shading behind the entries of each specific volume helps to anchor the user to the contents of the volume they are using.

Volume 1 includes this Publisher's Note, and the Editor's Introduction that details the content changes and additions in this eighth edition. At the back of each volume are "Entries by Specialties and Related Fields" and "Entries by Anatomy or System Affected," which direct the reader to essays by category; for example, a reader looking up "Oncology" on the specialty list will find entries on diseases (such as Cancer, Malignancy and Metastasis, and Sarcoma), specialties (such as Cytology and Pathology), diagnostic procedures (such as Mammography), and treatments (such as Chemotherapy, Radiation Therapy, and Tumor Removal). The back of Volume 5 includes these valuable features:

- Glossary of medical terms;
- Definitions of almost 700 diseases and other medical conditions;
- Appendix detailing training, degrees, and duties of various health care professionals;
- General bibliography arranged by category;
- List of organizations and support groups, with full contact information;
- Symptoms and warning signs of various diseases and conditions;
- Pharmaceutical list;
- Comprehensive index.

Editors and Contributors

The contributors to this work are academicians from a variety of disciplines in the life sciences, as well as health care professionals and faculty members at universities and medical teaching institutions; their names, degrees, and affiliations are listed in the front matter to Volume 1. We thank them for generously sharing their expertise. Special acknowledgment is extended to the panel of Medical Editors for *Salem Health Magill's Medical Guide, Eighth Edition*: Bryan C. Auday, Ph.D., Gordon College (Wenham, MA); Michael Buratovich, Ph.D., Spring Arbor University; Geraldine Marrocco, EdD., APRN, CNS, ANP-BC, Yale University School of Nursing; Paul Moglia, Ph.D., South Nassau Communities Hospital. Their efforts ensured a thorough revision.

Salem Online Database

Activating online access is quick and easy. Volume 1 of every set of *Salem Health Magill's Medical Guide* includes an Activation Number attached to the inside back cover. This number is used to activate your title online. If you already have an active Salem Online account, go to **https://online.salempress.com** and click on **Activate Title/Administrator Login** in the upper right-hand corner of the page. Enter your user name and password and then click **Activate Title** to enter your unique activation code.

Customers opening a new account for the first time should go to **https://online.salempress.com** and click on **Activate Title/Administrator Login** at the top of the page. Click **Register Now** to sign up and enter your activation code. Once this is done, a few simple questions will complete the process.

For additional activation information or for help accessing your account, please call us at (800) 221-1592 and we will be glad to do the activation for you.

Editor's Introduction

Every year, our understanding of the field of medicine and healthcare grows exponentially. As basic research in a variety of scientific disciplines increases, efforts to apply this newly discovered knowledge to disease and illness follow a similar trajectory. One challenge we editors faced in assembling this *Eighth Edition* concerns how to capture and represent the major changes within medicine over the past four years. Several new developments were identified and incorporated into this new edition. For example, advances in medical technology can often stimulate rapid progress in diagnostic and treatment protocols. One response to addressing the use of technology in medicine was to add new entries. These included applications of deep brain stimulation, functional magnetic resonance imaging (fMRI), and transcranial magnetic stimulation (TMS), which today play an important role in treating and aiding our understanding of neurological disorders.

In addition, new entries in this edition fill gaps in the table of contents regarding anatomy, physiology, and diseases. A more comprehensive list of new or revised articles from the rapidly expanding area of neuroscience is included in the *Eighth Edition*. A sampling of these include: Neurorehabilitation, Brain damage, Strokes, Dementias, Parkinson's disease, Brain disorder, Depression, and Asperger's syndrome. Also, numerous entries from the disciplines of neurology, psychiatry, and clinical neuropsychology from previous editions have been revised. These include entries such as Antipsychotic drugs, Addiction, and Traumatic brain injury. Another area that received attention concerns medical ethics. Questions that raise important ethical issues abound concerning the appropriate use of new technologies. Besides updating the previous entry on Ethics, two new entries were added. A new entry on the topic of Brain death discusses the difficulty of determining exactly when death occurs and the importance of addressing end of life discussions with medical specialists. A second new entry addresses Memory erasure procedures that involve the use of pharmaceuticals to diminish emotional content of memories as a means to alleviate people suffering from post-traumatic stress.

The *Eighth Edition* also includes multiple entries addressing issues of the aging population in the United States. Demographic trends clearly indicate that the biopsychosocial needs of Baby Boomers, today's senior citizens, require a new and better way of approaching healthcare. Patient-centered models, using inter-professional, or multidisciplinary-teams, will disseminate the specific aims of Healthy People 2020 and the Affordable Care Act and strengthen programs aimed at disease prevention and health promotion, and promote a climate that protects consumers from unnecessary cost and over utilization of valuable health care dollars.

In the previous edition, we expanded our coverage of genetic concepts and diseases, developmental malformations, and infectious diseases. In this new edition, we have significantly updated articles relating to cancer, infectious diseases, and basic medicine. We have also added new articles that discuss new treatment modalities, such as ASTYM®, Carticel®, hyaluronic acid injection, and drugs not discussed in previous editions, such as anticoagulants, NSAIDs, and opioids. Additionally, we have included new articles about CRISPR, an exciting genomic-editing tool, and tissue engineering, both of which we believe will change how clinical medicine is practiced. Finally, we have included new articles about contentious issues in health care, such as physician-assisted suicide, and the anti-vaccine movement.

The intensive updates throughout have revised the articles for clarity, completeness, relevance and recency. Several articles like Alcoholism, Safety issues for children, and Venous insufficiency have been extensively rewritten. The entry on Antibodies contains an expanded discussion on phagocytosis, polyclonal antibodies, and clinical diagnostic agents. Fractures and dislocations now includes discussion of vertebroplasty and kyphoplasty, new methods that result in improved spine stabilization and health, and medicine's growing focus on nutritional deficiencies in bone health and healing. Steroid abuse is no longer only the purview of professional athletes and the *Eighth Edition*'s update incorporates the key role of psychological factors. Rape and sexual assault includes the latest guidelines for forensic chain of custody protocols now routinely taught in emergency medicine and the available therapeutic interventions that are immediately available to victims seeking help, both new to this edition. The section on Ovaries includes the most recent breakthroughs in understanding gonadotrophies and hormone release during the process of ovulation. Take-home DNA testing kits, unheard of at the time of the *Seventh Edition*'s publication, have democratized accessing genetic information. Genetic engineering also presents the now-available successful treatments of chronic lymphocytic leukemia, x-linked severe combined immunodeficiency gene therapies, and the potential treatment of Parkinson's disease. Bleeding now includes the latest understanding of the key role vitamin K plays in clotting and blood health. And Animal rights updates readers on the more proactive momentum of the century-old antivivisection movement and the resulting controversy. It also includes legal developments in criminalization of animal abuse, intentional harm, and neglect.

This edition also includes *In the News* sidebars that evaluate media stories about ongoing research and experimental treatments. These boxes both highlight the latest information and provide readers with a critical view of popular reports that may (or may not) prove crucial to the future understanding and treatment of certain medical conditions. The topics covered include chemotherapy targeting cancer stem cells, the Accord Trial concerning cardiovascular risks for type 2 diabetes, and new screening methods for Down syndrome.

Our goal is for this new edition of *Magill's Medical Guide* is to provide easy access to the full range of medical and heath care concerns with ample resources for further research. We anticipate that readers will either have experience with one of the topics covered here, or have a loved one who has. To reach our goal, we have reviewed the majority of entries from the previous edition, updated and revised many of them, and added a significant number of new topics. We hope that we have succeeded.

—*Bryan C. Auday, Ph.D.*
Michael A. Buratovich, Ph.D.
Geraldine F. Marrocco, Ed.D., APRN, CNS, ANP-BC
Paul Moglia, Ph.D.

List of Contributors

Erika A. Abrahamsen
Gordon College

Sarah Acker
Yale University

Richard Adler, Ph.D.
University of Michigan-Dearborn

E. Victor Adlin, M.D.
Temple University School of Medicine

Anubhav Agarwal, M.D.
South Nassau Communities Hospital

Patricia A. Ainsa, M.P.H., Ph.D.
University of Texas, El Paso

Saeed Akhter, M.D.
Texas Technological University Health Science Center

Bruce Ambuel, Ph.D.
Medical College of Wisconsin

John J. B. Anderson, Ph.D.
University of North Carolina, Chapel Hill

Wendell Anderson
Northstar Writing & Editing, American Medical Writers Association

Earl R. Andresen, Ph.D.
University of Texas, Arlington

Daruenie Andujar
Gordon College

Walter Appleton
Grosse Pointe Woods, Michigan

Michele Arduengo, Ph.D.
Milton, Wisconsin

Samar Aslam, M.D.
South Nassau Communities Hospital

Bryan C. Auday, Ph.D.
Gordon College

Catherine Avelar, B.S.
Cornell University of Veterinary Medicine

Mihaela Avramut, M.D., Ph.D.
Verlan Medical Communications, American Medical Writers Association

Gloria Reyes Báez, M.D.
University of Puerto Rico School of Medicine

Dana K. Bagwell
Memory Health and Fitness Institute

Jimmy Bajaj, D.O.
South Nassau Communities Hospital

Pamela J. Baker, Ph.D.
Bates College

Anita Baker-Blocker, M.P.H., Ph.D.
Ann Arbor, Michigan

Iona C. Baldridge
Lubbock Christian University

Nancy Banasiak, M.S.N., P.N.P.-B.C., A.P.R.N.
Yale University School of Nursing

Veronica N. Baptista, M.D.
Stanford Medical Group

Adriel Barrios-Anderson
Brown University

Lawrence W. Bassett, M.D.
University of California, Los Angeles, School of Medicine

Robert J. Baumann, M.D.
University of Kentucky

John A. Bavaro, Ed.D., R.N.
Slippery Rock University

Barbara C. Beattie
Sarasota, Florida

Tanja Bekhuis, Ph.D.
TCB Research

Paul F. Bell, Ph.D.
Heritage Valley Health System

Gregory A. Benitz, Psy.D.
San Francisco, California

Alvin K. Benson, Ph.D.
Utah Valley State College

Cynthia Breslin Beres
Glendale, California

Carol D. Berkowitz, M.D.
Harbor-UCLA Medical Center

Leonard Berkowitz, D.O.
South Nassau Communities Hospital

Milton Berman, Ph.D.
University of Rochester

Matthew Berria, Ph.D.
Weber State University

Silvia M. Berry, M.Sc., R.V.T.
Englewood Hospital and Medical Center, New Jersey

Leah M. Betman, M.S., C.G.C.
Centreville, Virginia

Massimo D. Bezoari, M.D.
Huntingdon College

Jigna Bhalla, Pharm.D.
American Medical Writers Association

Anna Binda, Ph.D.
American Medical Writers Association

Jennifer Birkhauser, M.S., M.D.
University of California, Irvine

Virginiae Blackmon
Fort Worth, Texas

Robert W. Block, M.D.
University of Oklahoma

Jane Blood-Siegfried, R.N., D.N.Sc., C.P.N.P.
Duke University School of Nursing

Paul R. Boehlke, Ph.D.
Wisconsin Lutheran College

Prodromos G. Borboroglu, M.D.
Navy Medical Center, San Diego

Wanda Todd Bradshaw, M.S.N., N.N.P., P.N.P., C.C.R.N.
Duke University School of Nursing

Barbara Brennessel, Ph.D.
Wheaton College

Peter N. Bretan, M.D.
University of California Medical Center, San Francisco

Kenneth H. Brown, Ph.D.
Northwestern Oklahoma State University

Thomas L. Brown, Ph.D.
Wright State University School of Medicine

Carolynn Bruno, Ph.D., A.P.R.N., C.N.S., F.N.P.-C.
New York University, Rory Meyers College of Nursing

Mitzie L. Bryant, B.S.N., M.Ed.
St. Louis Board of Education

Faith Hickman Brynie, Ph.D.
Bigfork, Montana

Fred Buchstein
John Carrol University

Suzette Buhr, R.T.R., C.D.A.
American Medical Writers Association

Amy Webb Bull, D.S.N., A.P.N.
Tennessee State University School of Nursing

Michael A. Buratovich, Ph.D.
Spring Arbor University

Edmund C. Burke, M.D.
*University of California Medical Center,
San Francisco*

John T. Burns, Ph.D.
Bethany College

Rosslynn S. Byous, D.P.A., PA-C
*University of Southern California, Keck
School of Medicine*

Jeffrey R. Bytomski, D.O.
Duke University Medical Center

Lauren M. Cagen, Ph.D.
University of Tennessee, Memphis

James J. Campanella, Ph.D.
Montclair State University

Edmund J. Campion, Ph.D.
University of Tennessee

Brian Campos
Brown University

Louis A. Cancellaro, M.D.
*Veterans Affairs Medical Center, Mountain
Home, Tennessee*

Byron D. Cannon, Ph.D.
University of Utah

Shiliang Alice Cao
Brown University

Richard P. Capriccioso, M.D.
University of Phoenix

Mary Allen Carey, Ph.D.
University of Oklahoma

Cheryl Carrao, D.O.
South Nassau Communities Hospital

Christine M. Carroll, R.N., B.S.N.,
M.B.A.
American Medical Writers Association

Culley C. Carson III, M.D.
*University of North Carolina School of
Medicine*

Donatella M. Casirola, Ph.D.
*University of Medicine and Dentistry, New
Jersey Medical School*

Cristina Cesaro, D.O.
South Nassau Communities Hospital

Anne Lynn S. Chang, M.D.
Stanford University

Karen Chapman-Novakofski, R.D.,
L.D.N., Ph.D.
University of Illinois

Kathleen A. Chara, M.S.
Roseville, Minnesota

Paul J. Chara, Jr., Ph.D.
Northwestern College

Kerry L. Cheesman, Ph.D.
Capital University

Richard W. Cheney, Jr., Ph.D.
Christopher Newport University

Derrick Cheng
Brown University

David L. Chesemore, Ph.D.
California State University, Fresno

Valentina Chiarelli, Ph.D.
Università degli Studi di Trieste

Francis P. Chinard, M.D.
New Jersey Medical School

Leland J. Chinn, Ph.D.
Biola University

Ariel Choi
Brown University

Kathleen Chung
Brown University

David A. Clark, M.D.
*Louisiana State University Medical
School, New Orleans*

Nancy Handshaw Clark, Ph.D.
*American University of the Caribbean
School of Medicine/Kingston Hospital,
Surrey, England*

Julien M. Cobert
Duke University

Jaime S. Colomé, Ph.D.
California Polytechnic, San Luis Obispo

Pam Conboy
American Medical Writers Association

Arlene R. Courtney, Ph.D.
Western Oregon State College

Sarah Crawford, Ph.D.
Southern Connecticut State University

James Danckert, Ph.D.
University of Waterloo

Tish Davidson
Fremont, California

LeAnna DeAngelo, Ph.D.
Arizona State University

Roy L. DeHart, M.D., M.P.H.
University of Oklahoma

Anna Delamerced
Brown University

Patrick J. DeLuca, Ph.D.
Mount St. Mary College

Cynthia L. De Vine
American Medical Writers Association

Thomas E. DeWolfe, Ph.D.
Hampden-Sydney College

Shawkat Dhanani, M.D., M.P.H.
*VA Greater Los Angeles Healthcare
System*

Jackie Dial, Ph.D.
MedicaLink, LLC

Mary Dietmann, Ed.D., A.P.R.N.,
C.N.S.
*Sacred Heart University College of
Nursing*

Kenneth Dill, M.D.
South Nassau Communities Hospital

Stephen DiMaria
Brown University

Sandra Ripley Distelhorst
Vashon, Washington

Matthew Doiron, B.A.
Spaulding Rehabilitation Hospital

Katherine Hoffman Doman
Greene County, Tennessee

Mark R. Doman, M.D.
*Veterans Affairs Medical Center, Mountain
Home, Tennessee*

Lillian Dominguez
Brown University

Desiree Dreeuws
Sunland, California

Cherie H. Dunphy, M.D.
University of North Carolina, Chapel Hill

Allison Dussault, RN
Yale University

Patricia Stanfill Edens, Ph.D., R.N.,
F.A.C.H.E.
The Oncology Group, LLC

Miriam Ehrenberg, Ph.D.
*City University of New York, John Jay
College*

Ebrahim Elahi, M.D.
Mount Sinai School of Medicine

Ophelia Empleo-Frazier, M.S.N.,
G.N.P.-B.C., W.C.C, D.C.P.
Yale University School of Nursing

Benjamin Estrada, M.D.
University of South Alabama

Elicia Estrella, M.S., C.G.C., L.G.C.
Children's Hospital, Boston

Renée Euchner, R.N.
American Medical Writers Association

C. Richard Falcon
Roberts and Raymond Associates, Philadelphia

L. Fleming Fallon, Jr., M.D., Ph.D., M.P.H.
Bowling Green State University

Meika A. Fang, M.D.
Veterans Affairs Medical Center, West Los Angeles

Phillip A. Farber, Ph.D.
Bloomsburg University

Elizabeth Farrington, A.G.P.C.N.P.-B.C.
Yale University

Frank J. Fedel
Henry Ford Hospital, Detroit

Nicholas Feo
South Nassau Communities Hospital

Caroline Taylor Ferguson
International Neuroethics Society

Marisela Fermin-Schon, R.N.
Yale University

Mary C. Fields, M.D.
Collin County Community College

K. Thomas Finley, Ph.D.
State University of New York, Brockport

Jesse Fishman, Pharm.D.
Children's Healthcare of Atlanta

M. A. Foote, Ph.D.
M. A. Foote Associates

Kimberly Y. Z. Forrest, Ph.D.
Slippery Rock University of Pennsylvania

Ronald B. France, Ph.D.
LDS Hospital, Salt Lake City

Katherine B. Frederich, Ph.D.
Eastern Nazarene College

Paul Freudigman, Jr., M.D.
Pennsylvania State University, Hershey Medical Center

Paul J. Frisch
Nanuet, New York

Joanne R. Gambosi, B.S.N., M.A.
Gold Canyon, Arizona

Christi N. Gandham, D.O.
Oceanside, New York

Laura Garasimowicz, M.S.
Prenatal Diagnosis of Northern California

Bianca Garcia, M.D.
South Nassau Communities Hospital

Frances García, M.D.
Universidad Central del Caribe School of Medicine

Keith Garebian, Ph.D.
Mississauga, Ontario

Jason Georges
Glendale, California

Soraya Ghayourmanesh, Ph.D.
City University of New York

Joseph T. Giacino, Ph.D.
Spaulding Rehabilitation Hospital, Massachusetts

Jennifer L. Gibson, Pharm.D.
Marietta, Georgia

Lenela Glass-Godwin, M.WS.
Texas A&M University

Wallace A. Gleason, Jr., M.D.
University of Texas, Houston

James S. Godde, Ph.D.
Monmouth College

Amanda Grannis, B.A.
Binghamton University

Daniel G. Graetzer, Ph.D.
University of Montana

Hans G. Graetzer, Ph.D.
South Dakota State University

James E. Grant, M.P.H.
Michigan Department of Community Health, Lansing, MI

Carly A. Gray
Yale University

David A. Gremse, M.D.
University of South Alabama College of Medicine

Frank Guerra, M.D.
University of Colorado School of Medicine

Yelena Guller, Ph.D.
Spaulding Rehabilitation Hospital, Massachusetts

Lonnie J. Guralnick, Ph.D.
Western Oregon State College

L. Kevin Hamberger, Ph.D.
Medical College of Wisconsin

Ronald C. Hamdy, M.D.
James H. Quillen College of Medicine

Emad Hanna, M.D., M.Sc.
South Nassau Communities Hospital

Beth M. Hannan, M.S., C.G.C.
Albany Medical Center

Robert J. Harmon, M.D.
University of Colorado School of Medicine

Linda Hart, M.S., M.A.
University of Wisconsin-Madison

Peter M. Hartmann, M.D.
York Hospital, Pennsylvania

Robin Hasslen, Ph.D.
St. Cloud State University

H. Bradford Hawley, M.D.
Boonshoft School of Medicine, Wright State University

Robert M. Hawthorne, Jr., Ph.D.
Marlboro, Vermont

Carol A. Heintzelman, D.S.W.
Millersville University of Pennsylvania

Peter B. Heller, Ph.D.
Manhattan College

Collette Bishop Hendler, R.N., M.S., C.I.C.
Abington Memorial Hospital

Diane Andrews Henningfeld, Ph.D.
Adrian College

Stephen Henry, D.O.
South Nassau Communities Hospital

Martha M. Henze, M.S., R.D.
Boulder Community Hospital, Colorado

David Hernandez
Brown University

Margaret Trexler Hessen, M.D.
Drexel University College of Medicine

Jane F. Hill, Ph.D.
Bethesda, Maryland

Trevor Hinshaw
Gordon College

Carl W. Hoagstrom, Ph.D.
Ohio Northern University

David Wason Hollar, Jr., Ph.D.
Rockingham Community College

Carol A. Holloway
Grosse Point Woods, Michigan

Christine G. Holzmueller
Glen Rock, Pennsylvania

Elaine Hong
Gordon College

David Hornung, Ph.D.
St. Lawrence University

Ryan C. Horst
Eastern Mennonite University

Howard L. Hosick, Ph.D.
Washington State University

Katherine H. Houp, Ph.D.
Midway College

Carina Endres Howell, Ph.D.
Lock Haven University of Pennsylvania

Shih-Wen Huang, M.D.
University of Florida

Jason A. Hubbart, M.S.
University of Idaho, Moscow

Larry Hudgins, M.D.
Veterans Affairs Medical Center, Mountain Home, Tennessee

Mary Hurd
East Tennessee State University

Chris Iliades, M.D.
Centerville, Massachusetts

Peter Iltis, Ph.D.
Gordon College

April D. Ingram
Kelowna, British Columbia, Canada

Tracy Irons-Georges
Glendale, California

Vicki J. Isola, Ph.D.
Hope College

Louis B. Jacques, M.D.
Wayne State University School of Medicine

Samar Post Jamali
Yale University

Ilia Jbankov
Yale University

Thomas C. Jefferson, M.D.
University of Arkansas for Medical Sciences

Krystal Jenkins
New York Institute of Technology

Albert C. Jensen, M.S.
Central Florida Community College

Cheryl Pokalo Jones
Townsend, Delaware

Daniel Jones, D.D.S., Ph.D.
Indiana Wesleyan University

Claire Joseph, M.L.S., M.A., A.H.I.P.
South Nassau Communities Hospital

Roushig Grace Kalebjian, M.A., R.N.
Yale University

Karen E. Kalumuck, Ph.D.
The Exploratorium, San Francisco

Ahmad Kamal, M.D.
Stanford University Medical School

Clair Kaplan, A.P.R.N., M.S.N.
Yale University School of Nursing

Susan J. Karcher, Ph.D.
Purdue University

Armand M. Karow, Ph.D.
Xytex Corporation

Laurence Katz, M.D.
University of North Carolina, Chapel Hill

Rupinder P. Kaur, D.O.
South Nassau Communities Hospital

Allee Keener
Gordon College

Mara Kelly-Zukowski, Ph.D.
Felician College

Ing-Wei Khor, Ph.D.
Oceanside, California

Michael R. King, Ph.D.
University of Rochester

Cassandra Kircher, Ph.D.
Elon University

Vernon N. Kisling, Jr., Ph.D.
University of Florida

Samuel V. A. Kisseadoo, Ph.D.
Hampton University

Hillar Klandorf, Ph.D.
West Virginia University

Robert T. Klose, Ph.D.
University College of Bangor

Walter Klyce
Brown University

Jeffrey A. Knight, Ph.D.
Mount Holyoke College

Marylane Wade Koch, R.N., M.S.N.
University of Memphis, Loewenberg School of Nursing

Nicholas Koen
Brown University

Anita P. Kuan, Ph.D.
Woonsocket, Rhode Island

Steven A. Kuhl, Ph.D.
Lander University

Jeanne L. Kuhler, Ph.D.
Auburn University, Montgomery

Joyce W. Lacy, Ph.D.
Azusa Pacific University

David J. Ladouceur, Ph.D.
University of Notre Dame

Joshua Lampert, MS-III
Miami, Florida

Nicholas Lanzieri
Pace University

Jeffrey P. Larson, P.T., A.T.C.
Northern Medical Informatics

Joshua Lampert, MS-III
Miami, Florida

Victor R. Lavis, M.D.
University of Texas, Houston

David M. Lawrence
J. Sargeant Reynolds Community College

Christie Leal, D.O.
Long Beach, New York

Charles T. Leonard, Ph.D., P.T.
University of Montana

Lorraine Lica, Ph.D.
San Diego, California

Lauren Lichten, M.S., C.G.C.
Tufts Medical Center

Stan Liu, M.D.
University of California, Los Angeles, School of Medicine

Martha Oehmke Loustaunau, Ph.D.
New Mexico State University

Eric V. D. Luft, Ph.D., M.L.S.
SUNY, Upstate Medical University

Arthur J. Lurigio, Ph.D.
Loyola University Chicago

Courtney H. Lyder, M.D.
Yale University School of Nursing

Elizabeth Lynn, M.D.
South Nassau Communities Hospital

Maura S. McAuliffe
Austin, Texas

Nancy E. Macdonald, Ph.D.
University of South Carolina, Sumter

Mary Frances McGibbon, D.N.P., R.N., M.S.N., F.N.P.-B.C.
City University of New York

Jeffrey A. McGowan
West Virginia University

Mary Beth McGranaghan
Chestnut Hill College

James P. McKenna, M.D.
Heritage Valley Health System

Wayne R. McKinny, M.D.
University of Hawaii School of Medicine

Marianne M. Madsen, M.S.
University of Utah

Janet Mahoney, R.N., Ph.D., A.P.R.N.
Monmouth University

Laura Gray Malloy, Ph.D.
Bates College

Nancy Farm Mannikko, Ph.D.
Centers for Disease Control and Prevention

Katia Marazova, M.D., Ph.D.
Paris, France

Debra Ellen Margolis, D.O.
St. Joseph's Hospital and Medical Center, Paterson, New Jersey

Bonita L. Marks, Ph.D.
University of North Carolina, Chapel Hill

Geraldine F. Marrocco, Ed.D., A.P.R.N., C.N.S., A.N.P.-B.C.
Yale University School of Nursing

Charles C. Marsh, Pharm.D.
University of Arkansas for Medical Sciences

Robert L. Martone
Wyeth Neuroscience

Amber M. Mathiesen, M.S.
Saint Luke's Boise Medical Center

Maki Matsumura
Yale University

Karen A. Mattern
Visiting Nurse Association Home Health Services

Grace D. Matzen
Molloy College

Mary Frances McGibbon, D.N.P., R.N., M.S.N., F.N.P.-B.C.
City University of New York

Ralph R. Meyer, Ph.D.
University of Cincinnati

Robert D. Meyer, Ph.D.
Chestnut Hill College

Elva B. Miller, O.D.
Harrisonburg, Virginia

George Miller, Jr., M.D.
South Nassau Communities Hospital

Roman J. Miller, Ph.D.
Eastern Mennonite College

Randall L. Milstein, Ph.D.
Oregon State University

Eli C. Minkoff, Ph.D.
Bates College

Vicki J. Miskovsky
Walter Reed Army Medical Center

Nicole Mitchell
Yale University

Briana Moglia
Fort Lauderdale, Florida

Michael Moglia
Glen Cove, New York

Paul Moglia, Ph.D.
South Nassau Communities Hospital

Robin Kamienny Montvilo, R.N., Ph.D.
Rhode Island College

Sharon Moore, M.D.
Veterans Affairs Medical Center, Mountain Home, Tennessee

George A. Morgan, Ph.D.
Colorado State University

Marvin Morris, L.Ac., M.P.A.
American Medical Writers Association

Sheila J. Mosee, M.D.
Howard University

Judy Mouchawar, M.D., M.S.P.H.
University of Colorado Health Sciences Center

Rodney C. Mowbray, Ph.D.
University of Wisconsin, LaCrosse

William L. Muhlach, Ph.D.
Southern Illinois University

Karen M. Nagel, R.Ph., Ph.D.
Midwestern University

John Panos Najarian, Ph.D.
William Patterson College

Donald J. Nash, Ph.D.
Colorado State University

Victor H. Nassar, M.D.
Emory University

Mary A. Nastuk, Ph.D.
Wellesley College

Nicole Negbenebor
Brown University

Elizabeth Marie McGhee Nelson, Ph.D.
Christian Brothers University

Cindy Nesci, D.C.
East Pointe, Michigan

Bryan Ness, Ph.D.
Pacific Union College

Marsha M. Neumyer
Pennsylvania State University College of Medicine

Derek Nhan
University of Colorado, Denver

William D. Niemi, Ph.D.
Russell Sage College

Christopher J. Norman, B.A., B.S.N., R.N.-B.C., B.C.
Yale University

Jane C. Norman, Ph.D., R.N., C.N.E.
Tennessee State University

Kathleen O'Boyle
Wayne State University

Annette O'Connor, Ph.D.
La Salle University

Oladele A. Ogunseitan, Ph.D., M.P.H.
University of California, Irvine

Colm A. Ó'Moráin, M.A., M.D., M.Sc., D.Sc.
University of Dublin, Trinity College

Kristin S. Ondrak, Ph.D.
University of North Carolina at Chapel Hill

Gwenelle S. O'Neal, D.S.W.
Rutgers University

J. Timothy O'Neill, Ph.D.
Uniformed Services University of the Health Sciences

Oliver Oyama, Ph.D.
Duke/Fayetteville Area Health Education Center

Maria Pacheco, Ph.D.
Buffalo State College

Barbara Pahud, M.D., M.P.H.
Children's Mercy Kansas City, University of Missouri, Kansas City, University of Kansas Medical Center

Robert J. Paradowski, Ph.D.
Rochester Institute of Technology

Gowri Parameswaran
Southwest Missouri State University

David Parr
Gordon College

RoseMarie Pasmantier, M.D.
State University of New York Health Science Center, Brooklyn

Paul M. Paulman, M.D.
University of Nebraska Medical Center

Cheryl Pawlowski, Ph.D.
University of Northern Colorado

Joseph G. Pelliccia, Ph.D.
Bates College

Angel Perez, M.D.
South Nassau Communities Hospital

Fortunato Perez-Benavides, M.D.
Texas Tech University

Madeline Pesec
Brown University

Carol Moore Pfaffly, Ph.D.
Fort Collins Family Medicine Center

Kenneth A. Pidcock, Ph.D.
Wilkes University

Heather E. Pierce, L.S.W.
Unison Behavioral Health Group, Toledo, Ohio

Linda L. Pierce, Ph.D, R.N.
Medical College of Ohio

Scott W. Pierce, L.S.W.
Firelands Counseling and Recovery Services, Sandusky, Ohio

Nancy A. Piotrowski, Ph.D.
University of California, Berkeley

Luzanna Plancarte, M.D.
South Nassau Communities Hospital

George R. Plitnik, Ph.D.
Frostburg State University

Connie Pollock
Glendale, California

Melanie Porter, Ph.D.
Macquarie University

Darleen Powars, M.D.
Los Angeles County-USC Medical Center

Frank J. Prerost, Ph.D.
Midwestern University

Layne A. Prest, Ph.D.
University of Nebraska Medical Center

Nancy E. Price, Ph.D.
American Medical Writers Association

Victoria Price, Ph.D.
Lamar University

Cynthia F. Racer, M.A., M.P.H.
American Medical Writers Association

Rashmi Ramasubbaiah, M.D.
Western Kentucky University

Lillian M. Range, Ph.D.
University of Southern Mississippi

Dandamudi V. Rao, Ph.D.
University of Medicine and Dentistry of New Jersey

C. Mervyn Rasmussen, M.D.
Bremerton Naval Hospital, Washington

Diane C. Rein, Ph.D., M.L.S.
Purdue University

Andrew J. Reinhart, M.S.
Washington University School of Medicine

Douglas Reinhart, M.D.
University of Utah

Jerome L. Rekart, Ph.D.
Rivier University

Andrew Ren, M.D.
Kaiser Permanente Los Angeles Medical Center

Wendy E. S. Repovich, Ph.D.
Eastern Washington University

Peter D. Reuman, M.D., M.P.H.
University of Florida

Betty Richardson, Ph.D.
Southern Illinois University, Edwardsville

Alice C. Richer, R.D., M.B.A., L.D.
Norwood, Massachusetts

Brad Rikke, Ph.D.
University of Colorado at Boulder

John L. Rittenhouse
Eastern Mennonite College

Felix Rivera, M.D.
South Nassau Communities Hospital

Connie Rizzo, M.D., Ph.D.
Columbia University

Jeffrey B. Roberts, M.D.
Duke University Medical Center

Larry M. Roberts, J.D.
Pasadena, California

James L. Robinson, Ph.D.
University of Illinois, Urbana-Champaign

Hilda Velez Rodriguez, M.S.
San Juan, Puerto Rico

Ana Maria Rodriguez-Rojas, M.S.
GXP Medical Writing, LLC

Linda Roethel, M.D.
South Nassau Family Medicine

Charles W. Rogers, Ph.D.
Southwestern Oklahoma State University

Eugene J. Rogers, M.D.
Chicago Medical School

John Alan Ross, Ph.D.
Eastern Washington University

Lynne T. Roy
Cedars-Sinai Medical Center, Los Angeles

Nadja Rozovsky, Ph.D.
Somerville, Massachusetts

Irene Struthers Rush
Boise, Idaho

Virginia L. Salmon
Northeast State Community College

Susan L. Sandel, Ph.D.
MidState Behavioral Health System

Robert Sandlin, Ph.D.
San Diego State University

Sarit Sandowski, OMS-II
New York Institute of Technology

Alexander Sandra, M.D.
University of Iowa, Carver College of Medicine

Tulsi B. Saral, Ph.D.
University of Houston, Clear Lake

Andrea Sarchi, OMS-IV
New York Institute of Technology

Lisa M. Sardinia, Ph.D.
Pacific University

David K. Saunders, Ph.D.
Emporia State University

Jacob S. Sawyer, Ph.M.
Columbia University

Zachary Sax
South Nassau Communities Hospital

Elaine M. Schaefer, D.O.
South Nassau Communities Hospital

Elizabeth D. Schafer, Ph.D.
Loachapoka, Alabama

Rosemary Scheirer, Ed.D.
Chestnut Hill College

Steven A. Schonefeld, Ph.D.
Tri-State University

Kathleen Schongar, M.S., M.A.
The May School

John Richard Schrock, Ph.D.
Emporia State University

Jay D. Schvaneveldt, Ph.D.
Utah State University

Jason J. Schwartz, Ph.D., J.D.
Los Angeles, California

Marie Schwartz
Yale University

Miriam E. Schwartz, M.D., M.A., Ph.D.
University of California, Los Angeles

Rebecca Lovell Scott, Ph.D., P.A.-C.
Sandwich, Massachusetts

Rose Secrest
Chattanooga, Tennessee

John J. Seidl, M.D.
Medical College of Wisconsin

Carol A. Selden, R.D.
Allegiance Health, Jackson, Michigan

Sibani Sengupta, Ph.D.
American Medical Writers Association

Thomas L. Sevier, M.D., F.A.C.S.M., F.A.C.P.
Performance Dynamics, Inc., Astym Program

Gregory B. Seymann, M.D.
University of California, San Diego School of Medicine

Frank E. Shafer, M.D.
Allegheny University of the Health Sciences

Uzma Shahzad, M.D.
South Nassau Communities Hospital

Christopher D. Sharp, M.D.
Stanford University School of Medicine

Holly K. Shaw, Ph.D., R.N.
Adelphi University

John M. Shaw
Education Systems

Martha Sherwood-Pike, Ph.D.
University of Oregon

George C. Shields, Ph.D.
Lake Forest College

Sonia Shubert
Yale University

R. Baird Shuman, Ph.D.
University of Illinois, Urbana-Champaign

Mel Siegel, M.A.
Fordham University

Sanford S. Singer, Ph.D.
University of Dayton

Virginia Slaughter, Ph.D.
University of Queensland, Australia

Jane A. Slezak, Ph.D.
Fulton Montgomery Community College

Julie M. Slocum, R.N., M.S., C.D.E.
Women and Infants' Hospital

Genevieve Slomski, Ph.D.
New Britain, Connecticut

Caroline M. Small
Silver Spring, Maryland

Dwight G. Smith, Ph.D.
Southern Connecticut State University

H. David Smith, Ph.D.
University of Michigan

Jane Marie Smith
Butler County Community College

Roger Smith, Ph.D.
Portland, Oregon

Lisa Levin Sobczak, R.N.C.
Santa Barbara, California

Angela Spano
Huntingdon College

Carly Stabb
Yale University

Claire L. Standen, Ph.D.
University of Massachusetts Medical School

Sharon W. Stark, R.N., A.P.R.N., D.N.Sc.
Monmouth University

William D. Stark, D.D.S.
Monrovia, California

Toby R. Stewart, Ph.D.
University of Nebraska Medical Center, Omaha

Glenn Ellen Starr Stilling, M.A., M.L.S.
Appalachian State University

James R. Stubbs, M.D.
University of South Alabama

Wendy L. Stuhldreher, Ph.D, R.D.
Slippery Rock University

Giri Sulur, Ph.D.
University of California, Los Angeles

Pavel Svilenov
Wisconsin Lutheran College

Steven R. Talbot, R.V.T.
University of Utah Vascular Laboratory

Sue Tarjan
Santa Cruz, California

Billie M. Taylor, M.S.E., M.L.S.
Arkadelphia, Arkansas

William F. Taylor
Detroit, Michigan

Gerald T. Terlep, Ph.D.
Wayne State University

Bethany Thivierge, M.P.H., E.L.S.
Technicality Resources

Susan E. Thomas, M.L.S.
Indiana University South Bend

Nicole Thomasian
Brown University

Roberta Tierney, M.S.N., J.D., A.P.N.
Indiana University

Venkat Raghavan Tirumala, M.D., M.H.A.
Western Kentucky University

Leslie V. Tischauser, Ph.D.
Prairie State College

Winona Tse, M.D.
Mount Sinai School of Medicine

Mary S. Tyler, Ph.D.
University of Maine

John V. Urbas, Ph.D.
Kennesaw State College

Maxine M. Urton, Ph.D.
Xavier University

Nicole M. Van Hoey, Pharm.D.
Arlington, Virginia

Anju Varanasi, M.D.
South Nassau Communities Hospital

Mikhail Varshavski, OMS-IV
New York Institute of Technology

Charles L. Vigue, Ph.D.
University of New Haven

James Waddell, Ph.D.
University of Minnesota

Peter J. Waddell, Ph.D.
University of South Carolina

Anthony J. Wagner, Ph.D.
Medical University of South Carolina

Edith K. Wallace, Ph.D.
Heartland Community College

C. J. Walsh, Ph.D.
Mote Marine Laboratory

Peter J. Walsh, Ph.D.
Fairleigh Dickinson University

Marc H. Walters, M.D.
Portland Community College

Annita Marie Ward, Ed.D.
Salem-Teikyo University

John F. Ward, M.D.
Navy Medical Center, San Diego

Marcia Watson-Whitmyre, Ph.D.
University of Delaware

Judith Weinblatt, M.A., M.S.
New York, New York

Marcia J. Weiss, M.A., J.D.
Point Park College

Barry A. Weissman, O.D., Ph.D.
University of California, Los Angeles, School of Medicine

David J. Wells, Jr., Ph.D.
University of South Alabama Medical Center

Zhongqi Weng
Yale University

Mark Wengrovitz, M.D.
Pennsylvania State University, Hershey Medical Center

Althea Williams, M.B.A.
South Nassau Communities Hospital

Beth Williams
Yale University

Lee Williams
New York City, New York

Russell Williams, M.S.W.
University of Arkansas for Medical Sciences

Lindsey L. Wilner, Psy.D.
Gansevoort, New York

Bradley R. A. Wilson, Ph.D.
University of Cincinnati

Michael Windelspecht, Ph.D.
Appalachian State University

Barbara Woldin
American Medical Writers Association

Stephen L. Wolfe, Ph.D.
University of California, Davis

Bonnie L. Wolff
Pacific Coast Cardiac and Vascular Surgeons

Paul Y. K. Wu, M.D.
University of Southern California

Robin L. Wulffson, M.D.
American Medical Writers Association

Geetha Yadav, Ph.D.
Bio-Rad Laboratories Inc.

Lynda J.-S. Yang, M.D., P.D., F.A.A.N.S.
University of Michigan

Daniel L. Yazak, D.E.D.
Montana State University, Billings

Claudine Yee
Brown University

Garry Young, Ph.D.
Nottingham Trent University

Rachel Zahn, M.D.
Solana Beach, California

Kathleen Zanolli, Ph.D.
University of Kansas

W. Michael Zawada, Ph.D.
University of Colorado Health Sciences Center

Mark Zelman, Ph.D.
Aurora University

George D. Zgourides, M.D., Psy.D.
John Peter Smith Hospital

Ming Y. Zheng, Ph.D.
Gordon College

Susan M. Zneimer, Ph.D.
US Labs

Nillofur Zobairi, Ph.D.
Southern Illinois University

Complete Table of Contents

Volume 1

Shading indicates current volume.

Shading indicates current volume.

Shading indicates current volume.

Volume 2

Volume 3

Volume 4

Volume 5

SALEM HEALTH

MAGILL'S MEDICAL GUIDE

Abdomen

Anatomy

Anatomy or system affected: Bladder, gastrointestinal system, intestines, kidneys, liver, reproductive system, stomach, urinary system, uterus

Specialties and related fields: Gastroenterology, gynecology, internal medicine, nephrology, urology

Definition: The cavity in the central portion of the trunk that contains the vital organs most closely associated with the digestive process and the elimination of waste material.

Key terms:

chyme: the semiliquid state of foods that have gone through the first stage of digestion in the stomach

Kupffer cells: specialized cells in the liver that perform the function of removing bacterial debris from the blood that has circulated throughout the body

urea: the major waste product produced in the kidneys that, when gathered in sufficient quantity and liquefied, flows into the bladder for elimination as urine

Structure and Functions

The abdomen is the portion of the body's trunk that begins immediately below the diaphragm, which is the main respiratory muscle in the chest cavity, and extends to the lower pelvic region. The abdominal area is defined by a muscular wall made up of fatty tissue and skin, which determines the general shape of the body from the chest to the lower pelvis. The entire abdominal cavity is lined by a membrane called the peritoneum. This membrane encloses the essential organs of the abdomen: the stomach, small and large intestines, liver, gallbladder, bladder, pancreas, and kidneys. In females, the abdominal casing also contains the uterus, ovaries, and Fallopian tubes. At the front of the abdomen is the navel, essentially a scar which forms following the cutting of the umbilical cord after birth.

Any overview of the abdomen requires a composite view of the functions performed by each of the organs contained in it. With the exception of the female reproductive organs, all the organs contained in the abdominal cavity serve in one way or another in the process of food digestion, the transfer of diverse essential food by-products to the rest of the body, and the disposal of waste products via the urinary tract and the anal passage.

The esophagus is the tube through which all solid and liquid foods enter the stomach, which is the topmost organ in the abdominal cavity. Because it is essentially a bag, the stomach can assume different shapes and adjust in size to accommodate different volumes of food that reach it through the esophagus. In adult humans, the average capacity of the stomach is about one quart. The essential digestive function of the stomach is to convert foods from their original states to a general semiliquid state referred to as *chyme*.

This first stage of digestion is carried out by the chemical action of some thirty-five thousand gastric glands that

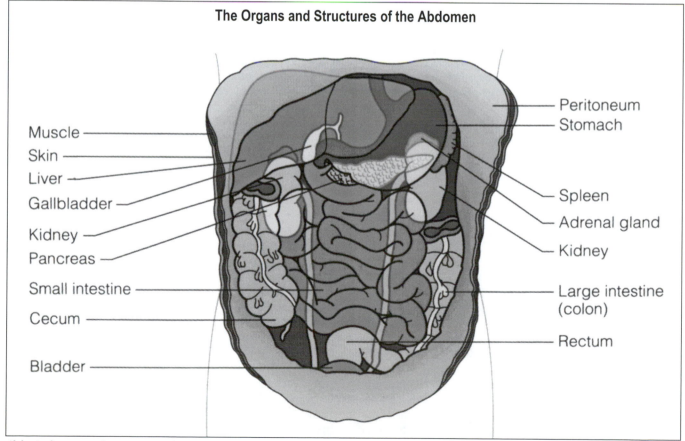

The Organs and Structures of the Abdomen

Muscle
Skin
Liver
Gallbladder
Kidney
Pancreas
Small intestine
Cecum
Bladder

Peritoneum
Stomach
Spleen
Adrenal gland
Kidney
Large intestine (colon)
Rectum

Abdominal organs and structures are those located between the rib cage and the pelvic bone.

make up the inner folds of the inner layer of the stomach, the gastric mucosa. As the gastric glands actively secrete gastric juice, the second layer of the stomach wall, which is muscle tissue, contracts and expands, providing the physical movement that is necessary for the gastric juice and food material to come into full contact.

Gastric juice actually begins to flow from the inner lining of the stomach even before food is present. This may occur when one smells food or even when one imagines the flavor of food. Among the component parts of gastric juice are the enzymes pepsin and rennin, hydrochloric acid, and mucus, the latter of which protects the lining of the stomach from the effects of high acidity. Pepsin and rennin begin to break down different types of proteins when an optimum acid environment (a pH between 1 and 3) exists.

Once the initial stage of digestion has occurred, food passes from the stomach into the upper portion of the small intestine, or duodenum, via the pyloric sphincter. This passageway will not allow food to enter the small intestine until it is suitably modified by the action of the stomach.

In the small and large intestines, partially broken-down food is reduced further by the action of gastric juices that are either secreted into the intestines from other abdominal organs (the pancreas and liver, most notably) or secreted by the mucous membranes of the intestines themselves. It is in the small intestine that most of the breaking-down digestive work of gastric juices takes place. Food particles reach a certain level of decomposition so that they may be absorbed into the bloodstream through the mucous membranes of the intestine. The bulk of what is left is allowed to pass from the small intestine and through a gate-like passageway called the cecum and then to the large intestine or colon.

The function of the colon and the component juices that it contains is to separate out the three essential components that remain following the absorptive work of the small intestine: water, undigested foodstuff, and bacteria. Most of the water passes back into the body through the walls of the colon, while undigested food and bacteria are propelled farther down the gastrointestinal tract for eventual elimination as feces.

The importance of other organs in the abdomen-the liver, kidneys, pancreas, gallbladder, and bladder-is as complex as that of the intestines and in several cases goes beyond the basic function of digestion. Closest to the stomach and the digestive process itself, perhaps, is the action of the pancreas. The pancreas is the glandular organ located directly beneath the stomach. It is connected to the duodenum (the first and shortest segment of the small intestine), to which it provides pancreatic juice containing three digestive enzymes: trypsin, amylase, and lipase. These agents join the secretions of the small intestine, as well as bile flowing from the liver, to complete the digestive process that breaks down proteins, carbohydrates, and fats. They can then be absorbed through the walls of the intestine for the general nourishment of the body. In addition to its role in the digestive process, the pancreas possesses endocrine cells, called the islets of Langerhans, that secrete two hormones, insulin and glucagon, directly into the bloodstream. These two hormones work together to influence the level of sugar in the blood. When the insulin-secreting cells of the pancreas fail to function effectively, then diabetes mellitus may result.

Like the pancreas, the liver, which is the largest glandular organ of the body, shares in the digestive process by producing bile, a fluid essential for the emulsification of fats passing through the small intestine. Bile salts, as they are called, are stored in the gallbladder until they are released into the small intestine. This contribution to the digestive process, however, represents only a minimal part of the liver's functions, many of which have vital effects on body functions far beyond the abdominal cavity. Because blood filled with oxygen flows into the liver from the aorta through the hepatic artery, on one hand, and blood containing digested food enters the liver from the small intestine via the portal vein, on the other, the relationship between "harmonizing" liver functions and the content of the blood is absolutely critical.

The metabolic cells that make up liver tissue, known as hepatic cells, are highly specialized. According to their specialized function, the hepatic cells in the four unequal-sized lobes of the liver may affect several factors: the amount of glycogen (converted and stored glucose) that should be reconverted to glucose and passed (for added energy) into the bloodstream; the conversion of excess carbohydrates and protein into fat; the counteraction of the harmful ammonia by-product of protein breakdown by the production of urea; the production of several essential components of blood, including plasma proteins and blood-clotting agents; the storing of key vitamins and minerals such as vitamins A, D, K, and B-12; and the removal of bacteria and other debris that collect in the blood itself-a function of the phagocytic, or Kupffer, cells in particular.

It is the next pair of vital abdominal organs, the kidneys, that separates many of the waste products associated with the liver's metabolic functions, including urea and mineral salts, out of the blood and removes them from the body in the form of urine. This separation is performed by millions of tiny filtering agents called nephrons. Blood penetrates the interior of the kidney by way of an incoming arteriole that branches off from the main renal artery. After the filtering process has been completed, cleansed blood flows back into the main bloodstream via an outgoing arteriole and a system of blood vessels leading to the main renal vein. Waste materials remain, after filtering, in a tube-like extension of each nephron until they can be concentrated in the form of urine in a chamber in the middle of the kidney called the kidney pelvis. From this chamber, urine is propelled by muscular compression through the ureter tubes leading to the bladder, the last organ (in males) contained within the lower abdominal cavity. In addition to removing waste products from the blood, the kidneys can adjust the level in the blood of other substances-such as sodium, potassium, and calcium-that are needed by the body but that may exist in excess at certain times. Because the two kidneys perform exactly the same functions, it is possible to survive with only one healthy kidney.

Although obviously essential for temporary storage of urine and final elimination of liquid waste through the process of urination, the bladder is the least complicated organ in the abdominal cavity. The bladder is essentially a sac with a liquid capacity of about one pint. Its functions are governed by varied tension in and loosening of muscles in the walls of the sac and the external sphincter. When the pressure of collected urine reaches a certain point, nervous impulses cause the external sphincter to relax. Urine flow out of the bladder into the urethra tube can be controlled, up to a certain point, in humans and most mammals by conscious thought.

Disorders and Diseases

Given the concentration in the abdomen of vital regulatory organs, much medical research has focused on the pathology of this area of the body. Although there are a number of specific diseases that attack individual abdominal organs, the entire region is vulnerable to cancerous tumors. Medical science has tended to associate cancers in certain abdominal organs with dietary habits that are either of recent origin (consumption of highly processed foodstuffs in industrialized Western societies, for example) or geographically or ethnically distinctive-the East Asian, specifically Japanese, vulnerability to certain types of stomach cancer, for example. The latter vulnerability may, however, also be tied to dietary or other environmental considerations that vary in different populated areas of the globe.

Although cancers may strike any of the vital abdominal organs, chances of successful surgical intervention to remove tumors vary greatly according to the location of the cancer. Liver cancer, for example, is essentially untreatable through surgery, while the treatment of cancer of the colon has a significant success rate. This variation is partially attributable to the fact that the vital processes performed by the intestines may not be seriously threatened when a portion of the organ is removed in cancer surgery.

The most important specific diseases associated with the abdomen include peritonitis, hepatitis, and diabetes. Among these diseases, diabetes has received the most attention, both for its widespread impact on all sectors of the population and for the amount of research that has gone into the task of finding a cure. Diabetes occurs when the pancreas fails to produce enough insulin to metabolize the sugar substance glucose. A breakdown in this function impairs proper cell nourishment and results in excessive sugar in the blood and urine. This state, referred to as hyperglycemia, can affect a number of body functions outside the abdominal cavity, leading, for example, to atherosclerosis and vascular degeneration in general. Because many diabetes patients must inject insulin into their bodies to counteract a malfunctioning pancreas, an opposite, equally dangerous side effect, hyperinsulinism, may also occur. The most serious degenerative effect that menaces patients suffering from diabetes, however, occurs when the chemical and hormonal imbalance originating in the pancreas brings negative reactions to the kidneys, causing the latter to fail. Medical science has perfected various technical means for addressing this problem, most of which are connected with the mechanical process called dialysis.

Hepatitis is an inflammation that attacks the liver. The two common forms are hepatitis A (formerly called infectious hepatitis) and hepatitis B (formerly called serum hepatitis). Both are transmitted as a result of unsanitary conditions, the first in food and water supplies and the second when unsterile hypodermic needles or infected blood come into contact with the victim's own bloodstream. Unlike most other diseases associated with the abdominal organs, hepatitis is extremely contagious. Hepatitis B can present dangers in using plasma supplied by donors, as there can be an incubation period from six weeks to six months before external signs of the disease occur.

Perhaps the most common abdominal disease, curable through the use of antibiotics if treated in time, is peritonitis. This is an acute inflammation of the peritoneum, the membrane that lines the entire abdominal cavity. It can occur as a result of direct bacterial invasion from outside the body or as a side effect of ruptures occurring in one of the organs contained in the abdomen. Peritonitis typically develops as a result of complications from appendicitis, bleeding ulcers, or a ruptured gallbladder.

Perspective and Prospects

The history of medical analysis of disorders of the abdominal area goes back as far as written history itself, ranging from simple indigestion and painful (and possibly fatal) gallstones to very serious and only recently understood diseases such as diabetes.

Perhaps the most noteworthy advancement in medical knowledge affecting the organs of the abdominal region has been the development of more sophisticated means to counteract the effects of kidney disorders. While there were some striking advances (but not full levels of success) in organ transplant surgery beginning in the 1970s, a technique called dialysis made remarkable strides. First used shortly after World War II as an effective but costly and physically limiting treatment, dialysis involves the use of a machine that receives blood pumped directly from the patient's heart and processes this blood in place of the kidney. This involves filtering out excretory products, adding essential components that "refresh" blood needs (such as heparin to combat clotting as well as proper amounts of saline fluid), and then returning the blood to resume its vital function within the circulatory system.

Although the essential principles of dialysis did not change drastically in the last quarter of the twentieth century, levels of efficiency in a process that had to be repeated over a ten-hour period several times a week definitely did. Development of much smaller, portable dialysis devices made it possible for patients to follow their doctors' instructions in carrying out their own treatment between hospital or office visits, thus lessening the chances of very dangerous crises at the outset of kidney failure.

The most notable hope for patients afflicted with kidney disorders is successful transplant from a healthy or recently deceased donor. By the early twenty-first century, transplants had also become foreseeable for those suffering from diseases that strike other organs in the abdominal cavity, especially the liver. Thus, healthy organ transplant technology can be said to represent one of the most important domains of future research, involving specialists of all the subsections of medicine relating to the abdominal cavity.

—*Byron D. Cannon, Ph.D.*

See also Abdominal disorders; Adrenalectomy; Amniocentesis; Anatomy; Appendectomy; Appendicitis; Bariatric surgery; Bladder removal; Bypass surgery; Cesarean section; Cholecystectomy; Colitis; Colon; Colon therapy; Colonoscopy and sigmoidoscopy; Colorectal cancer; Colorectal polyp removal; Colorectal surgery; Constipation; Crohn's disease; Dialysis; Diaphragm; Diarrhea and dysentery; Digestion; Diverticulitis and diverticulosis; Endoscopy; Enemas; Fistula repair; Gallbladder; Gallbladder diseases; Gastrectomy; Gastroenterology; Gastroenterology, pediatric; Gastrointestinal disorders; Gastrointestinal system; Gastrostomy; Hernia; Hernia repair; Ileostomy and colostomy; Incontinence; Indigestion; Internal medicine; Intestinal disorders; Intestines; Irritable bowel syndrome (IBS); Kidney transplantation; Kidneys; Laparoscopy; Liposuction; Lithotripsy; Liver; Liver transplantation; Nephrectomy; Nephritis; Nephrology; Nephrology, pediatric; Obstruction; Ovaries; Pancreas; Pancreatitis; Peristalsis; Peritonitis; Pregnancy and gestation; Prostate gland; Reproductive system; Roundworms; Small intestine; Splenectomy; Sterilization; Stomach, intestinal, and pancreatic cancers; Stone removal; Stones; Tubal ligation; Ultrasonography; Urethritis; Urinary disorders; Urinary system; Urology; Urology, pediatric; Uterus; Worms.

For Further Information:

Bernard, Claude. *Memoir on the Pancreas and on the Role of Pancreatic Juice in Digestive Processes.* Translated by John Henderon. New York: Academic Press, 1985.

De Wardener, H. E. *The Kidney: An Outline of Normal and Abnormal Function.* 5th ed. New York: Churchill Livingstone, 1985.

Feldman, Mark, Lawrence S. Friedman, and Lawrence J. Brandt, eds. *Sleisenger and Fordtran's Gastrointestinal and Liver Disease: Pathophysiology, Diagnosis, Management.* 9th ed. Philadelphia: Saunders/Elsevier, 2010.

Marieb, Elaine N. *Essentials of Human Anatomy and Physiology.* 10th ed. San Francisco: Benjamin Cummings, 2012.

Palmer, Melissa. *Dr. Melissa Palmer's Guide to Hepatitis and Liver Disease.* New York: Penguin Group, 2004.

Ronco, Claudio, and Rinaldo Bellomo, eds. *Critical Care Nephrology.* 2d ed. Philadelphia: Saunders/Elsevier, 2009.

Tortora, Gerard J., and Bryan Derrickson. *Principles of Anatomy and Physiology.* 14th ed. Hoboken, N.J.: John Wiley & Sons, 2012.

Voung, Mao Kang, and Jiang Shi Sung. *Liver Disease and Peritonitis.* New York: Nova Biomedical Books, 2012.

Abdominal disorders

Disease/Disorder

Anatomy or system affected: Abdomen, bladder, gastrointestinal system, intestines, kidneys, liver, stomach, urinary system

Specialties and related fields: Emergency medicine, family medicine, gastroenterology, internal medicine

Definition: Disorders affecting the wide range of organs found in the torso of the body, including diseases of the stomach, intestines, liver, and pancreas.

Key terms:

gastrointestinal: referring to the small and large intestines

pathogen: any microorganism that can cause infectious disease, such as bacteria, viruses, fungi, or other parasites

peritoneum: a membrane enclosing most of the organs in the abdomen

Causes and Symptoms

The main trunk, or torso, of the human body includes three major structures: the chest cavity, contained within the ribs and housing the lungs and heart; the abdomen, containing the stomach, kidneys, liver, spleen, pancreas, and intestines; and the pelvic cavity, housing the sexual organs, the organs of elimination, and related structures.

The abdomen is, for the most part, contained within a membrane called the peritoneum. The stomach lies immediately below the chest cavity and connects directly with the small intestine, a long tube. It fills the bulk of the abdominal cavity, winding around and down to the pelvic bones in the hips. The small intestine then connects to the large intestine, which extends upward and crosses the abdomen just below the stomach and then turns down to connect with the rectum. Other vital organs within the abdominal cavity include the liver, kidneys, spleen, pancreas, and adrenal glands. All these structures are subject to infection by viruses, bacteria, and other infective agents; to cancer; and to a wide range of conditions specific to individual organs and systems.

Diseases in the abdominal cavity are usually signaled by pain. Identifying the exact cause of abdominal pain is one of the most difficult and important tasks that the physician faces. The familiar stomachache may be simple indigestion, or it may be caused by spoiled, toxic foods or by infection, inflammation, cancer, obstruction, or tissue erosion, among other causes. It may arise in the stomach, the intestines, or other organs contained within the abdominal cavity. In addition, pain felt in the abdomen may be referred from other sources outside the abdominal cavity. A good example would be a heart attack, which arises in the chest cavity but is often felt by the patient as indigestion. Another example is the abdominal cramping that is often associated with menstruation and premenstrual syndrome (PMS). However, because severe abdominal pain could mean that the patient is in great danger, the physician must decide quickly what is causing the pain and what to do about it.

By far the most common cause of stomach pain is indigestion, but this term is so broad as to be almost meaningless. Indigestion can be brought on by eating too much food or by eating the wrong foods or tainted foods; it can be brought on by alcohol consumption, smoking, poisons, infection, certain medications such as aspirin, and a host of other causes. It may be merely an annoyance, or it may indicate a more serious condition, such as gastritis, gastroenteritis, an ulcer, or cancer.

The stomach contains powerful chemicals to help digest foods. These include hydrochloric acid and chemicals called pepsins (digestive enzymes). To protect itself from being digested, the stomach mounts a defense system that allows the chemical modification of foods while keeping acid and pepsin away from the stomach walls. In certain people, however, the defense mechanisms break down and bring the corrosive stomach chemicals into direct contact with the stomach walls. The result can be irritation of the stomach lining, called gastritis. Gastritis may progress to a peptic ulcer, identified as a gastric ulcer if the inflammation occurs in the stomach wall or a duodenal ulcer if it occurs in the wall of the duodenum, the first section of the small intestine. In most cases, the ulcer is limited to the surface of the tissue. In severe cases, the ulcer can perforate the entire wall and can be life-threatening.

A common cause of stomach pain is the medication used to treat arthritis and rheumatism. These drugs include aspirin and a group of related drugs called nonsteroidal anti-inflammatory drugs (NSAIDs). As part of their activity in reducing bone and joint inflammation and pain, NSAIDs interfere with part of the stomach's network of self-protective devices and allow acids to attack stomach and duodenal walls, sometimes resulting in gastritis or ulceration.

Bacterial and viral infections often result in abdominal distress. Foods that sit too long unrefrigerated provide a good environment for bacteria to grow. These bacteria may be inherent in the food itself (for example, *Salmonella* in poultry and *E. coli* in meats) or they may come from the hands of people who prepare and serve them. The bacteria may cause human infection directly, or they may release toxins into the food. The result can be mere annoyance, debilitating illness, or deadly infection, depending upon the organism involved. *Salmonella* and *Staphylococcus* are two of the many bacteria that can cause food poisoning. Toxin-producing *E. coli* can be acquired from improperly cooked meat and can cause fatal infections. *Clostridium botulinum* toxin, occasionally found in canned or preserved foods, leads to probably the most serious form of food poisoning; victims often do not recover.

Other bacterial and viral infections of the gastrointestinal tract are also common causes of abdominal disease. Some of these viruses and bacteria include noroviruses, rotavirus, and *Shigella*. Viral gastroenteritis is the second most common disease in the United States (after upper respiratory tract infections) and a leading cause of death in infants and the elderly.

Appendicitis (inflammation of the appendix) is frequently seen. The appendix is a tiny organ at the end of the small intestine. It has no known purpose in the physiology of modern humans, but occasionally it becomes infected. If the infection is not treated quickly, the appendix can burst and spread infection throughout the abdominal area, a condition that can be life-threatening.

Diarrhea, with or without accompanying abdominal pain, is a major symptom of gastrointestinal disease. It is commonly associated with bacterial or viral infection but may also be attributable to the antibiotics used to treat bacterial infections, or to noninfectious inflammatory conditions such as Crohn's disease or ulcerative colitis.

Other gastrointestinal diseases are peritonitis (inflammation of the membrane that covers the abdominal organs), diverticulitis, constipation, obstruction, colitis, and the various cancers that can afflict the gastrointestinal system,

---

Information on Abdominal Disorders

Causes: Appendicitis, cancer, cirrhosis, colitis, constipation, Crohn's disease, diabetes mellitus, diverticulitis, food poisoning, gastritis, gastroenteritis, hepatitis, obstruction, pancreatitis, peritonitis, stones, ulcers, etc.
Symptoms: Pain
Duration: Acute or chronic
Treatments: Lifestyle changes, acid-neutralizing drugs, surgery

---

such as stomach and colon cancers. The latter is one of the more common, yet preventable, forms of cancer in the United States.

The liver is the largest internal organ in the human body and perhaps the most complicated; it is subject to a wide range of disorders. It is the body's main chemical workshop, and it is responsible for a large number of activities that are vital to body function. The liver absorbs nutrients from the intestinal tract and metabolizes them; that is, the liver modifies nutrients so that they can be used by the cells. The liver introduces nutrients into the bloodstream, supplying it with glucose, protein, and other substances that the body needs. The liver detoxifies the blood and allows poisons, drugs, and other harmful agents to be eliminated. The liver also manufactures and stores many important substances, such as vitamin A and cholesterol.

Chief among liver disorders are the various forms of hepatitis and cirrhosis. Hepatitis is inflammation of the liver, and it can be caused by a viral infection, alcohol, or drugs. There are many forms of viral hepatitis; the three most significant are hepatitis A, B, and C.

Hepatitis A is the most common form; it is caused by a virus that is transmitted through contaminated food or water. Hepatitis B and C are blood-borne diseases; that is, these viruses are carried in the blood and in other body fluids, such as semen and saliva. They can be transmitted only when infected body fluids are transferred from one person to another. These diseases are commonly spread through the use of contaminated needles and during surgical and dental procedures. Nurses and other staff members in health care facilities can be exposed to hepatitis B and C when taking and handling infected blood samples. A pregnant woman who is infected can pass the disease on to her fetus. In the past, blood transfusions were a common source of infection; however, blood tests for these viruses are now available. Potential blood donors are screened, and those who test positive cannot donate blood.

Cirrhosis develops when the liver is damaged by some substance such as alcohol. Liver cells are destroyed, and as the liver attempts to regenerate, scar tissue is formed. The steady flow of blood through the organ is impeded, as are vital functions such as the removal of waste materials from the blood.

The liver is also subject to a number of cancers. Cancer cells can spread to liver tissue from other parts of the body, or they can originate there as a result of hepatitis B or C or other chronic liver diseases such as cirrhosis.

The gallbladder is a small sac connected to the liver. The liver manufactures bile, a substance that aids in the digestion of fats. Bile is stored in the gallbladder and passes through the bile duct into the small intestine. A common disorder of the gallbladder is the formation of gallstones, crystalline growths that can be as fine as sand or as large as a golf ball. If the stones clog the passage to the bile duct, severe pain may result. Removal of the gallbladder (cholecystectomy) is often necessary.

The pancreas, a vital gland situated near the liver, contains both exocrine tissue (which produces digestive enzymes) and endocrine tissue (which produces the hormone insulin). Both are subject to disease. Dysfunction of the endocrine portion ("Islets of Langerhans") causes diabetes mellitus, a disorder of glucose metabolism. Pancreatitis is a potentially life-threatening inflammation of the pancreas caused most frequently by gallstones or by alcohol and other toxins.

The other major organ system in the abdomen is comprised of the kidneys and the urinary tract. The system includes the two kidneys, which sit in the middle of the back on either side of the spine; the two ureters, which transport urine from the kidneys; the bladder, a pouchlike organ that collects the urine; and the urethra, which expels urine from the body. The kidneys and related organs are subject to several disorders. Infection of the bladder or kidneys is quite common, particularly in young women and in the elderly. Kidney stones are also common and may be familial. Illnesses in other organs and systems may be reflected in the kidneys, and cancer may be primary in the kidney or may spread there from another site. Medications, other drugs, and toxins may cause severe kidney damage as well.

The peritoneum is the membranous lining of the abdominal cavity. When the organs within the cavity become inflamed, and particularly if there is any leakage of their contents, the peritoneum also becomes inflamed, a condition called peritonitis.

Treatment and Therapy

Many abdominal disorders are related to the overproduction of stomach acids, which damage the intestinal walls; the treatment of such conditions is often associated with changes in lifestyle. In treating gastrointestinal reflux disease, or GIRD, in which stomach acid backs up into the throat, physicians may suggest that the patient change habits that may be contributing to the condition, perhaps by stopping smoking, reducing the intake of alcohol, losing weight, and avoiding certain foods and medications. Preparations to neutralize stomach acids are used, as well as drugs that reduce the amount of stomach acid produced. Surgery is rarely indicated.

Hiatal hernia, the protrusion of part of the stomach through the diaphragm, usually produces no symptoms. There may be reflux of stomach acids into the esophagus, which can be treated by the same methods used in treating gastrointestinal reflux disease. Surgery is sometimes indicated.

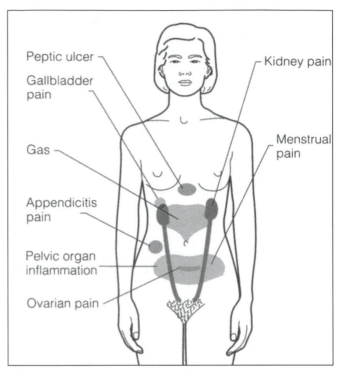

Abdominal disorders are many and varied; some common disorders and their sites are shown here.

Gastritis is commonly treated with agents that neutralize stomach acid or other agents that reduce the production of stomach acid. When gastritis appears to be caused by drugs taken for arthritis or rheumatism (for example, aspirin or NSAIDs), the physician may change the drug or the dosage to reduce stomach irritation.

In treating gastric and duodenal ulcers, the physician seeks to heal the ulcers and prevent their recurrence. Acid-neutralizing agents are sometimes helpful, but more often agents such as histamine (H2) blockers and proton pump inhibitors that reduce the flow of stomach acids are used. It has been suggested that gastritis and ulcers are associated with certain bacteria. Consequently, some physicians add antibiotics to the regimen to destroy the pathogens. Surgery is sometimes required to control bleeding from ulcers.

Bacterial infections in the gastrointestinal tract are, as a rule, self-limiting. They run their course, and the patient recovers. Sometimes, however, appropriate antibiotics are needed. Likewise, little other than supportive therapy can be offered for most viral infections.

Appendicitis is usually treated surgically. Peritonitis, whether resulting from appendicitis or from other causes, is treated with antibiotics following surgical repair of the primary problem.

Most cases of hepatitis A resolve without complication; no specific treatment is available. Bed rest, dietary measures, and general support procedures are the only steps that can be taken. Hepatitis B and C can become chronic and can progress to chronic active hepatitis, which may lead to liver failure, cirrhosis, liver cancer, and death. New treatments with antiviral drugs and immune modulators such as interferon are curative in some patients. Vaccines against both hepatitis A and B are available and recommended for all children and for adults who are at high risk. There is no vaccine for hepatitis C. There is no treatment for cirrhosis, although physicians may be able to treat some of its complications.

Kidney infections are usually readily treated with antibiotics. Kidney stones often require surgical removal or lithotripsy, a procedure in which ultrasonic waves are used to break up the stones. Recurrence is common, but sometimes can be prevented with dietary changes or medication.

Perspective and Prospects

Medical science has made great progress in the treatment of disorders arising in the abdominal cavity, but there is much to be done. Most important is the identification of agents to treat or immunize against various viral diseases, particularly those that occur in the gastrointestinal tract and the liver.

The vaccine against hepatitis B has been in use for years, but the incidence of the disease has remained relatively constant. If immunization is used for children successfully, however, the rate of hepatitis B infection among children should drop.

New treatment modalities are being developed for many of the diseases that occur in the abdominal cavity. One of the most significant successes has been in the treatment of peptic ulcers. The new drugs being used not only neutralize acid in the stomach but also cut off the secretion of acid into the stomach. One of these agents was the most-prescribed drug in the world for many years, indicating the importance of this therapeutic approach.

Innovations are also occurring in the treatment of diabetes mellitus, the disease caused by malfunction in the pancreas. Medications have been found that promise to treat and prevent some of the potentially fatal diseases that diabetes can cause.

Because the abdominal area contains so many vital organ systems, it is the seat of perhaps the widest range of diseases that afflict the human body-and hence, the target for the greatest amount of research and, potentially, the greatest advances in medicine.

—*C. Richard Falcon;*
updated by Margaret Trexler Hessen, M.D.

See also Abdomen; Appendectomy; Appendicitis; Bladder cancer; Bladder removal; Cholecystectomy; Colitis; Colon; Colon therapy; Colonoscopy and sigmoidoscopy; Colorectal cancer; Colorectal polyp removal; Colorectal surgery; Constipation; Crohn's disease; Diabetes mellitus; Dialysis; Diarrhea and dysentery; Digestion; Diverticulitis and diverticulosis; Endoscopy; Gallbladder diseases; Gastroenterology; Gastroenterology, pediatric; Gastrointestinal disorders; Gastrointestinal system; Gastrostomy; Hernia; Hernia repair; Incontinence; Indigestion; Internal medicine; Intestinal disorders; Irritable bowel syndrome (IBS); Kidney cancer; Kidney transplantation; Kidneys; Laparoscopy; Lithotripsy; Liver; Liver transplantation; Nephrectomy; Nephritis; Nephrology; Nephrology, pediatric; Nonalcoholic steatohepatitis (NASH); Obstruction; Peristalsis; Peritonitis; Prostate cancer; Prostate enlargement; Shunts; Small intestine; Splenectomy; Stomach, intestinal, and pancreatic cancers; Stone removal; Stones; Ultrasonography; Urethritis; Urinary disorders; Urinary system; Urology; Urology, pediatric.

For Further Information:
"Abdominal Pain." *MedlinePlus*, Apr. 20, 2013.
American College of Gastroenterology. http://patients.gi.org.
Barrett, Amanda, and Daus Mahnke. "Acute Abdomen." *Health Library*, Oct. 31, 2012.
Guillory, Gerard. *IBS: A Doctor's Plan for Chronic Digestive Disorders*. 3d ed. Point Roberts, Wash.: Hartley & Marks, 2001.
"Hepatitis." *Centers for Disease Control and Prevention*, Mar. 12, 2013.
Kapadia, Cyrus R., James M. Crawford, and Caroline Taylor. *An Atlas of Gastroenterology: A Guide to Diagnosis and Differential Diagnosis*. Boca Raton, Fla.: Parthenon, 2003.
Litin, Scott C., ed. *Mayo Clinic Family Health Book*. 4th ed. New York: HarperResource, 2009.
Runge, Marschall S., and M. Andrew Gregnati, eds. *Netter's Internal Medicine*. 2d ed. Philadelphia: Saunders/Elsevier, 2009.

Abortion

Procedure
Anatomy or system affected: Reproductive system, uterus
Specialties and related fields: Ethics, gynecology
Definition: The induced termination of pregnancy, which usually is legal only before the fetus is viable.
Key terms:
dilation: making something wider or larger
embryo: the unborn young from conception to about eight weeks
fetus: the unborn young from about eight weeks to birth
quickening: the point at which a fetus first begins to move in the uterus
uterus: a hollow, muscular organ located in the pelvic cavity of females, in which a fertilized egg develops
viability: the point at which a fetus is able to survive outside the uterus

The Controversy Surrounding Abortion

Induced abortion is the deliberate ending of a pregnancy before the fetus is viable or capable of surviving outside a female's body. Abortion has been practiced in every culture since the beginning of civilization. It has also been controversial. The first law designating it as a crime dates to ancient Assyria, where, in the fourteenth century BCE, women who were convicted of abortion were impaled on a stake and left to die. Early Hebrew law also condemned abortion, except when necessary to save the woman's life. The Greeks allowed abortion, but the famous physician Hippocrates (ca. 460 BCE-ca. 370 BCE) denounced the procedure and said that it violated a doctor's responsibility to heal. Roman law said that a fetus was part of a woman and that abortion was her decision, although a husband could divorce his wife if she had an abortion without his consent. Most abortions in ancient times seemed to be related to unwanted pregnancies.

The Christian church determined abortion to be a sin in the first century. In the fifth century, however, Saint Augustine argued that the fetus did not have a soul before "quickening," that point during a pregnancy, usually between the fourth and sixth months, at which the woman first senses movement in her womb. Until 1869, abortion until quickening was legal in most of Europe. In that year, however, Roman Catholic pope Pius IX declared abortion at any

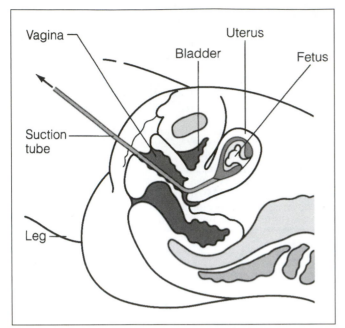

Elective or induced abortions can be performed in the first trimester using a simple suction technique; after the third month, much riskier and more complex methods are required.

point to be murder. This position has been upheld by all subsequent popes.

In Protestant countries, the principle of legality until quickening held true until around 1860. In that year, the British Parliament declared abortion a felony; that law remained on the books for more than one hundred years. In 1968, the Abortion Act passed by Parliament radically reduced the restrictions, allowing abortions in cases in which doctors determined that the pregnancy threatened the physical or mental health of the woman.

In the United States, abortion before quickening was legal until the 1840s. By 1841, ten states had declared abortion to be a criminal act, but punishments were weak and the laws frequently ignored. The movement against abortion was led by the American Medical Association (AMA), founded in 1847. In 1859, the AMA passed a resolution condemning abortion as a criminal act. Within a few years, every state declared abortion a felony. Not until 1950 did the AMA reverse its position, when it began a new campaign to liberalize abortion laws. Many doctors were concerned about the thousands of women suffering from complications and even death from illegal abortions. Consequently, seventeen states, including California, passed laws providing for legal abortions under certain conditions. The remaining states, however, continued to prohibit abortions. In 1973, the US Supreme Court ruled in *Roe v. Wade* that abortions in all states were generally legal. This ruling made abortions in the United States available on the request of the pregnant woman.

About 25 percent of the world's population live in countries that have very restrictive abortion laws. Most other nations authorize abortions under various conditions. The World Health Organization (WHO) estimates that there are approximately 50 million abortions per year throughout the world, and that about 40 to 50 percent of these are considered illegal.

Before 1970, statistics on abortions in the United States were generally not kept or reported, and they can only be estimated. In the nineteenth century, it is believed that there was one abortion for every four live births, a rate only a bit lower than that in the latter part of the twentieth century. The number of abortions in any year varied from five hundred thousand to 1 million, most of them illegal. In 1969, the Centers for Disease Control (CDC), a branch of the US Department of Health and Human Services, began an annual abortion count. Legal abortions in 1970 numbered about two hundred thousand. The number of illegal abortions is unknown. Ten years later, legal abortions reached 1.2 million, and by 1990, they had increased to 1.6 million; they have dropped slightly but steadily since 1990. The CDC estimated that there were about 325 abortions for every one thousand live births in the 1980s, a number consistent with findings for the 1990s. The number of abortions in any year rarely fluctuated by more or less than 3 percent from these figures.

Ireland, which has traditionally had the most stringent abortion laws, passed legislation in 2013 allowing for abortion in cases in which the mother's life is threatened. Eastern European countries, with more abortions than live births, have abortion rates three to four times higher than Western European countries. Nearly 60 percent of all abortions occur in Asia, with Vietnam and China having the highest rates of abortion.

In *Roe v. Wade*, the Supreme Court ruled that abortions are legal under certain conditions. These conditions include the welfare of the woman and the viability of the fetus. During the first three months of pregnancy, according to the Court, the government has no legitimate interest in regulating abortions-with one exception: States can require that abortions be performed by a licensed physician in a "medical setting." These physician-only statutes, enacted by some states, have made it more difficult for nurse practitioners and certified nurse midwives to expand their role to surgical abortion, but in many states they can provide medication abortion. In all other circumstances, the decision to abort is strictly that of the pregnant woman as a constitutional right of privacy.

During the second trimester, abortions are more restricted. They are legal only if the woman's health needs to be protected, and they require the consent of a doctor. The interest of the fetus is protected during the third trimester, when it becomes able to survive on its own outside the woman's body, with or without artificial life support. At this point, states can prohibit abortions except in cases where the life or health of the mother is threatened. In a companion case, *Doe v. Bolton*, "health" was defined as "all factors-physical, emotional, psychological, familial, and the woman's age." This broad definition of health effectively makes it possible for a woman to have an abortion at any time during her pregnancy, circumventing state restrictions. The determination of viability is to be made by doctors, not by legal authorities. This ruling effectively struck down all antiabortion laws across the United States.

In the aftermath of *Roe v. Wade*, abortion became an intensely emotional political issue in the United States. The Hyde Amendment of 1976 eliminated federal funding for abortions, and other legislation blocked foreign aid to family planning programs, which members of Congress who were opposed to abortion saw as "pro-abortion." In *Webster v. Reproductive Health Services* (1989), the Supreme Court upheld its ruling in *Roe v. Wade*, but it also sustained a rule forbidding the use of public facilities or public employees for carrying out abortions. The Court also supported a requirement that a test for viability be done before any late-term abortion and ruled that states could ban funding for abortion counseling. The issue continued to divide North Americans, with opponents arguing that abortion at any point during the pregnancy constituted murder.

A 2004 survey of women who had abortions, conducted by the Alan Guttmacher Institute, revealed the most common reasons for making that decision. Seventy-five percent said that having a baby would interfere with work or going to school. About 75 percent said they could not afford a child. Half of the women said that they did not want to be a single parent. Women beneath the poverty level, regardless of race, religion, or ethnic background, were more likely to have an abortion than were middle-class women. African American women and Latinas had higher rates of abortion than did white women (three and two times as likely, respectively). Fifty-two percent of abortions were performed on women under the age of twenty-five.

Religion appears to be a factor in the decision to seek an abortion: The percentage of Catholic women having abortions was 29 percent higher than the percentage of Protestant women. The lowest percentage of abortions was found among evangelical, "born-again" Christians. Nonreligious women had abortions at four times the rate of religious women. Teenagers under the age of fifteen and women over the age of forty had the highest rates of abortion of any age group. Thirty-three percent of all abortions occur before the fetal period of development. Fifty-five percent of abortions were performed between eight and twelve weeks into the pregnancy. The risk of death associated with abortion increases from one death for every 530,000 abortions at eight weeks or fewer to one death per six thousand abortions performed at twenty-one or more weeks of gestation.

Techniques and Procedures

A variety of techniques can be used to perform abortions. They vary according to the length of the pregnancy, which is usually measured by the number of weeks since the last menstrual period (LMP). Instrumental techniques are usually used very early in a pregnancy. They include a procedure called menstrual extraction, in which the entire contents of the uterus are removed. It can be done as early as fourteen days after the expected onset of a period. A major problem with this method is a high risk of error; the human embryo may still be so small at this age that it can be missed. It is also true that a high proportion of women

undergoing this procedure are in fact not pregnant. Nevertheless, this method is easy and very safe. Death rates from this technique average less than one in one hundred thousand.

The majority of abortions in the United States are done by a procedure known as vacuum aspiration, or suction curettage. This technique can be used up to about fourteen weeks after the LMP. It can be performed with local anesthesia and follows several steps. First, the cervix is expanded with metal rods that are inserted one at a time, with each rod being slightly larger than the previous one. When the cervix is expanded to the right size, a transparent, hollow tube called the vacuum cannula is placed into the uterine cavity. This instrument is attached to a suction device, which looks something like a drinking straw. An electric or hand-operated vacuum pump then empties the uterus of its contents. Finally, a spoon-shaped device called a curette is used to check for any leftover tissue in the uterus. The entire procedure takes less than five minutes. This method, first used in China in 1958, is among the safest procedures in medicine. There are about six times more maternal deaths during regular birth than during vacuum aspiration.

An older method, dilation and curettage (D & C), was common up to the 1970s, but it has largely been replaced by vacuum aspiration. In a D & C, the cervix is expanded or dilated and a curette is used to scrape out the contents of the uterus. The biggest difference is the use of general anesthesia during the process. Since most abortion-related deaths result from complications from anesthesia, a method that requires only local anesthesia, such as aspiration, greatly reduces the dangers of the procedure.

For the period from thirteen to twenty weeks, a method called dilation and evacuation (D & E) is usually preferred. The cervix is expanded with tubes of laminaria (a type of seaweed), and the fetus is removed with the placenta, the part of the uterus by which the fetus is nourished. Forceps, suction, or a sharp curette is sometimes used. The procedure is usually safe, but sometimes if the fetus is large, it must be crushed and dismembered to remove it through the cervix. One variation of this procedure involves delivering the fetus breech, except for the head, and then inserting a suction tube through an incision made in the head. The brain is then sucked out, which collapses the skull, and the fetus is then easily removed. In 2003, legislation banning this procedure, called the Partial-Birth Abortion Ban Act of 2003, was passed by Congress and signed into law by President George W. Bush. The act's constitutionality, which had been challenged, was upheld by the Supreme Court in 2007.

Along with these methods of menstrual extraction, physicians can use "medical induction" techniques when required. Amnioinfusion is an old example of this method that was used on fetuses from sixteen to twenty weeks old. This process has largely been replaced by D & E, which has proven far less dangerous.

Amnioinfusion usually requires hospitalization, local anesthesia, and the insertion of a large needle into the uterus. Between 100 and 200 milliliters of fluid is withdrawn and a similar amount of hypertonic saline solution infused into the uterine cavity. Within ninety minutes, the fetal heart stops. The woman then goes into labor and delivers a dead fetus within twenty-four to seventy-two hours. These kinds of abortions generally have much higher risk of complications than did D & E. On rare occasions, a fetus has been born alive, but the main risks are infection, hemorrhage, and cervical injuries to the woman. The psychological difficulties associated with this procedure can be severe, especially the knowledge that the fetus delivered would be dead.

Another method uses prostaglandins, naturally occurring hormones that cause uterine contractions and expulsion of the fetus, rather than a saline solution. The hormones can be given to the patient in several different ways: intravenously, intramuscularly, through vaginal suppositories, or directly into the amniotic sac. Prostaglandins are used for inducing second-trimester abortions and are as safe as saline solutions. Their major advantage is to reduce the duration of the abortion, but they also have severe side effects. They cause intense stomach cramps and other gastrointestinal discomfort, and about 7 percent of the fetuses expelled show some sign of life.

Surgical techniques for abortion are very rare, although sometimes they prove necessary in special cases. Hysterotomy resembles a cesarean section. An incision is made in the abdomen, and the fetus is removed. Hysterotomy is usually used in the second trimester, but only in cases where other methods have failed. The risk of death is much higher in this procedure than in most others. Even more rare is a hysterectomy, the removal of the uterus. This is done only in cases in which a malignant tumor threatens the life of the pregnant woman.

In the late 1980s, the French "abortion pill," RU-486, was approved for use in many parts of Europe. By the mid-1990s, it had been safely and effectively used in more than fifty thousand abortions. Progesterone is a hormone that causes the uterus to develop the lining that houses a fertilized egg. If the egg is not fertilized, the production of progesterone stops, and the uterine lining is discarded during menstruation. RU-486 contains an antiprogesterone; it prevents the production of progesterone.

The antiprogesterone mifepristone was approved for legal use in the United States in 2000. It is usually used in a regimen in conjunction with misoprostol, which augments the effect of mifepristone by causing the uterus to contract. The regimen begins with the oral administration of mifepristone, followed by at-home administration of misoprostol. It has proved to be highly safe and effective, although a few serious side effects can sometimes occur, the major one being sustained bleeding. Because of this, women are carefully screened to determine if they are candidates for mifepristone use; women with low blood counts are not offered the procedure. Cramps and nausea are also reported in a number of cases, and women are provided medication to relieve these symptoms. There is apparently no effect on subsequent pregnancies.

The drug is administered in the United States mostly under protocols that involve an ultrasound or the testing of serum hormone levels to determine that the pregnancy is in an appropriately early stage. Next comes follow-up care with a physical examination, an ultrasound or test for hormone levels, and contraceptive counseling and provision that meets the woman's needs. Properly done, medication abortion may be up to 95 to 97 percent effective, but women must return for follow-up care to ensure that the procedure was successful.

Because the abortion will take place at home, there is sufficient privacy. To be a candidate for the procedure, however, a woman must be capable of managing her medication and the passage of the fetus, with associated side effects. Various evidence-based protocols are employed in respect to timing the administration of the drug and the number of days of gestation at which the drug will be provided. The drug is intended only for termination of early first-trimester pregnancies. In many states, medication abortion is provided by nurse practitioners and certified nurse midwives, while surgical abortion is provided by physicians.

Perspective and Prospects

Abortion is the most frequently performed surgical procedure in the United States. As long as women have restricted access to contraceptive choice and unwanted pregnancies, that will continue to be the case. Abortion is a very safe procedure, although there can be complications. Generally, the earlier the procedure is performed, the less severe the risk. The lowest chance of medical complications occurs during the first eight weeks of pregnancy. After eight weeks, the risk of complications increases by 30 percent for each week of delay. Nevertheless, the death rate per case is very low, about half that for tonsillectomy. These statistics apply only to those areas of the world where abortion is legal, since women in those places tend to have earlier abortions.

In parts of the world where it remains against the law, abortion is a leading cause of death for women. WHO estimates that as many as five hundred thousand women a year die during abortions. About two hundred thousand of these deaths result from complications following abortions performed by unqualified medical personnel. About half of the total deaths take place in Southeast Asia and Africa. Before the *Roe v. Wade* decision, it was estimated that anywhere from a few hundred to several thousand American women died every year from the procedure. The best estimate was that in the 1960s about 290 women died every year as a result of complications from abortions. In the 1980s, the average was twelve per year, mostly from anesthesia complications. As of 2013, 0.6 deaths result per one hundred thousand legal induced procedures. Safe and legal abortion is an important component of women's health and reproductive freedom.

—Clair Kaplan, A.P.R.N./M.S.N.;
additional material by Leslie V. Tischauser, Ph.D.;
Paul J. Chara, Jr., Ph.D.

See also Amniocentesis; Cervical, ovarian, and uterine cancers; Childbirth; Childbirth complications; Contraception; Embryology; Ethics; Fetal tissue transplantation; Genetic counseling; Genetics and inheritance; Gynecology; Hippocratic oath; Hysterectomy; Law and medicine; Pregnancy and gestation; Reproductive system; Sterilization; Uterus; Women's health.

For Further Information:

Baer, Judith A. *Historical and Multicultural Encyclopedia of Women's Reproductive Rights in the United States*. Westport, Conn.: Greenwood Press, 2002.

Denney, Myron K. *A Matter of Choice: An Essential Guide to Every Aspect of Abortion*. New York: Simon & Schuster, 1983.

Foster, A. M., and L. L. Wynn. *Emergency Contraception: The Story of a Global Reproductive Health Technology*. New York: Palgrave Macmillan, 2012.

Goldman Marlene B., Rebecca Troisi, and Kathryn M. Rexrode. *Women and Health*. Boston: Elsevier/Academic, 2013.

Greer, Germaine. *Sex and Destiny: The Politics of Human Fertility*. New York: Harper & Row, 1984.

Higgins, Melissa, and Joseph W. Dellapenna. *Roe v. Wade: Abortion and a Woman's Right to Privacy*. Minneapolis: ABDO, 2013.

Hull, N. E. H., and Peter Charles Hoffer. *Roe v. Wade: The Abortion Rights Controversy in American History*. Lawrence: University Press of Kansas, 2001.

Lowdermilk, Deitra Leonard, et al. *Maternity and Women's Health Care*. St. Louis, Mo.: Mosby, 2012.

McFarlane, Deborah R. *The Politics of Fertility Control: Family Planning and Abortion Policies in the American States*. New York: Chatham House, 2001.

Mohr, James C. *Abortion in America: The Origins and Evolution of National Policy, 1800-1900*. New York: Oxford University Press, 1979.

National Right to Life Organization. http://www.nrlc.org.

Planned Parenthood. http://www.plannedparenthood.org.

Riddle, John M. *Contraception and Abortion from the Ancient World to the Renaissance*. Cambridge, Mass.: Harvard University Press, 1994.

Sciarra, John J., et al. *Gynecology and Obstetrics*. Vol. 6. Philadelphia: Harper & Row, 1991.

United Nations, Department of Economic and Social Affairs, Population Division. *World Abortion Policies 2013*. New York: Author, 2013.

World Health Organization. *Safe Abortion: Technical and Policy Guidance for Health Systems*. Geneva: Author, 2012.

Abscess drainage

Procedure

Anatomy or system affected: Brain, breasts, gallbladder, glands, gums, kidneys, liver, lungs, nervous system, pancreas, respiratory system, skin, spleen, stomach, urinary system

Specialties and related fields: Dermatology, emergency medicine, family medicine, general surgery

Definition: The removal of a collection of pus in tissue through an opening in the skin.

Indications and Procedures

When bacteria infect tissue, the body's defense systems attempt to isolate them and destroy the infective agents. An abscess develops when the bacteria become walled off from surrounding noninfected tissues and white blood cells enter the area to rid the body of the pathogens. The ensuing battle between the white blood cells and bacteria causes the death of these cells as well as of surrounding tissue. These dead cells form pus.

Staphylococci bacteria are the most common pathogens that cause abscesses to form, resulting in pain, swelling, and fever. If the abscess is near the skin, it is easily detected. The presence of abscesses in deeper tissues, however, may need to be confirmed using computed tomography (CT) scanning or magnetic resonance imaging (MRI).

The physician will usually prescribe antibiotics to help destroy the bacteria. Unfortunately, the antibiotics may not have access to the site of infection because the abscess is usually encapsulated by tissue. If this is the case, the physician must drain the abscess cavity. He or she will make an incision into the cavity to allow the pus to drain. Occasionally, a tube will be inserted to maintain the opening for continued drainage of the cavity. The tube can be removed once the infection is gone.

The patient will be asked to watch for signs of recurrent infection after the abscess is removed, because some bacteria may remain. The abscess can reappear if these bacteria are not destroyed by the body's immune system or by antibiotics.

Uses and Complications

Abscesses can develop in any organ. Common sites, however, are under the skin, in the breasts, and around the teeth and gums. In rare cases, abscesses are found in the liver or brain. Fungi and protozoans are important pathogens in liver abscesses.

Most abscesses dissipate after they are drained and/or the patient is treated with antibiotics. Occasionally, antibiotic treatment alone will cause the abscess to subside. The rapid detection and treatment of abscesses in the liver and brain are critical because the damage to these vital organs is irreparable.

—Matthew Berria, Ph.D., and Douglas Reinhart, M.D.

See also Abscesses; Antibiotics; Bacterial infections; Biopsy; Breast biopsy; Breast disorders; Breasts, female; Culdocentesis; Cyst removal; Cysts; Cytology; Cytopathology; Dermatology; Ganglion removal; Hydroceles; Infection; Otorhinolaryngology; Periodontal surgery; Periodontitis; Pus; Quinsy; Root canal treatment; Skin; Skin disorders; Staphylococcal infections; Testicular surgery.

For Further Information:

Ariel, Irving M., and Kirk K. Kazarian. *Diagnosis and Treatment of Abdominal Abscesses*. Baltimore: Williams & Wilkins, 1971.

Balasegaram, M. *Management of Hepatic Abscess*. Chicago: Year Book Medical, 1981.

Hau, T., J. R. Haaga, and M. I. Aeder. *Pathophysiology, Diagnosis, and Treatment of Abdominal Abscesses*. Chicago: Year Book Medical, 1984.

Icon Health. *Abscess: A Medical Dictionary, Bibliography, and Annotated Research Guide to Internet References*. San Diego, Calif.: Icon, 2004.

McDermott, Shaunagh, Diane A. Levis, and Ronald S. Arellano. "Approaches to the Difficult Drainage and Biopsy." *Seminars in Interventional Radiology* 29, no. 4 (December, 2012): 256-263.

Neff, Deanna M. "Incision and Drainage of a Skin Abscess." *Health Library*, November 26, 2012.

"Percutaneous Abscess Drainage." *Radiological Society of North America*, August 10, 2012.

Abscesses

Disease/Disorder

Anatomy or system affected: All

Specialties and related fields: All
Definition: Any enclosed collection of pus, whether sterile or infected.

Causes and Symptoms

When bacteria enter the body's tissue, white blood cells migrate to the site to fight infection. As they fight off the bacteria, they subsequently die. These dead white blood cells, and the enzymes that they produce as they decay, accumulate as fluid. It is this fluid that forms what is commonly known as pus. An enclosed collection of pus is called an abscess. Abscesses may occur at various sites within the body. Because bacteria often enter the body through the skin, abscesses commonly occur at sites just under the skin. Perhaps the most common abscesses are staph infections, which are caused by the bacterium *Staphylococcus aureus*.

Abscesses can occur in the abdomen, pelvis, kidneys, spleen, pancreas, liver, or prostate gland, or in the area behind the abdominal cavity (the retroperitoneal space). Abscesses can also occur in the head, neck, or hands, or in any of the muscles throughout the body. Throat abscesses are more likely to develop in children than in adults, often as a result of an infection such as strep throat. Though most commonly under the skin, where they are readily discernible, abscesses can also form deep within the body, where

> **Information on Abscesses**
> **Causes:** An enclosed collection of pus following bacterial infection
> **Symptoms:** Heat, swelling, tenderness, redness at the site; when systemic, fever or weight loss
> **Duration:** Acute
> **Treatments:** Drainage

they are undetectable unless a diagnostic procedure such as computed tomography> (CT) scanning or magnetic resonance imaging (MRI) is used. Signs aiding in the diagnosis of an abscess include heat, swelling, tenderness, and redness at the site. Bodywide, or systemic, symptoms such as fever or weight loss can also accompany abscesses, often when they are deeper.

Because people with weakened immune systems have a decreased ability to ward off infection, they are more likely to develop abscesses than are people with healthy immune systems. Abscess formation is frequently seen in patients with diabetes, sickle cell disease, and acquired immunodeficiency syndrome (AIDS), or in patients on steroid therapy.

Abscesses can foster processes that infect the blood, causing sepsis, which can spread infection to distant sites

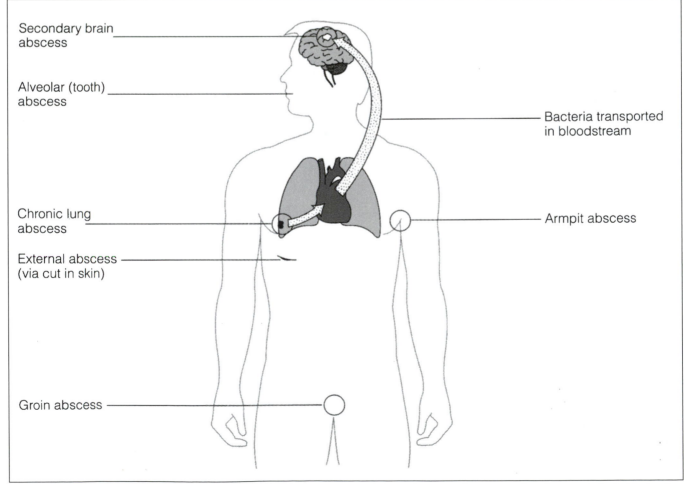

Secondary brain abscess

Alveolar (tooth) abscess

Chronic lung abscess

External abscess (via cut in skin)

Groin abscess

Bacteria transported in bloodstream

Armpit abscess

Abscesses are commonly located in soft tissues and near lymph nodes but may appear in internal organs and may cause other abscesses via bacterial migration.

within the body. A locally spread abscess can cause bleeding in nearby vessels or impair the functioning of a major organ.

Treatment and Therapy

Patients often will not seek medical attention for an abscess until it has become painful or inconvenient. The abscess may come to a point, or "head," and rupture spontaneously. If the abscess does not rupture, then it may require drainage. The site is numbed with an anesthetic; the abscess is cut open and drained. The pus is manually expressed. When the abscess is large enough, packing may be inserted to minimize bleeding and to help prevent the reaccumulation of pus. The packing is often removed the following day. Usually, antibiotics are not needed, but they may be prescribed to prevent reinfection. Deep abscesses sometimes require CT-guided drainage. Analyzing the pus in a laboratory can often help to guide treatment.

Prompt treatment of infections will often prevent the development of abscesses. Patients should be instructed to take care of injuries of any type, particularly bites and puncture wounds. The prognosis after treatment is good, as most abscesses should heal well.

—*Leonard Berkowitz, D.O.,*
and Paul Moglia, Ph.D.

See also Abscess drainage; Acne; Bacterial infections; Cyst removal; Cysts; Hydroceles; Infection; Lymphatic system; Pus; Quinsy; Septicemia; Skin; Skin disorders; Staphylococcal infections; Tumor removal; Tumors; Wounds.

For Further Information:

"Abscess." In *Ferri's Clinical Advisor: Instant Diagnosis and Treatment*, edited by Fred F. Ferri. St. Louis, Mo.: Mosby, 2011.

"Abscess." *MedlinePlus*, Apr. 17, 2013.

"Abscesses." In *The Merck Manual Home Health Handbook*, edited by Robert S. Porter, et al. 3rd ed. Whitehouse Station, N.J.: Merck Research Laboratories, 2009.

Amini, Richard, Srikar Adhikari, and Michael Blaivas. "Cutaneous Abscesses: Current Review of Microbiology, Sonographic Diagnosis, and Management." *Current Medial Literature: Dermatology* 18,1 (Feb. 2013): 1-9.

Calvagna, Mary,and Peter Lucas. "Boil." *Health Library*, Jan. 14, 2013.

Hau, T., J. R. Haaga, and M. I. Aeder. *Pathophysiology, Diagnosis, and Treatment of Abdominal Abscesses*. Chicago: Year Book Medical, 1984.

Icon Health. *Abscess: A Medical Dictionary, Bibliography, and Annotated Research Guide to Internet References*. San Diego, Calif.: Author, 2004.

Abuse of the elderly

Anatomy or system affected: All systems potentially affected

Specialties and related fields: Mental/behavioral health, psychology, sociology

Definition: A single, or repeated act, or lack of appropriate action, occurring within any relationship where there is an expectation of trust which causes harm or distress to an older person.

Overview

Lack of agreement regarding the definition of elder abuse and its parameters has made the assessment of prevalence and incidence problematic. The definition of "elder" may also vary depending on culture and location across the world. In North America and Europe, the cut off is 65 years; the United Nations uses 60 years or greater to describe "old"; and in some societies "old" is when you become a grandparent. Mysyuk, Westendorp, and Lindenberg studied the history and definitions of elder abuse and found the definition to be related to phrases such as: granny battering, elder mistreatment, battered elder syndrome, old age abuse. See Table 1 for details of each phrase.

The incidents of elder abuse are increasing as the general population is aging around the world. Elder abuse has not been recognized in the public until recently, and it is still under recognized and underreported across societies. Abuse of the elder can have devastating consequences for the victim including poor quality of life, psychological distress, loss of property, and security. It can occur at all levels of socioeconomic status, all parts of the world, and in multiple settings.

Types of Abuse

There are five divided types of abuse: physical abuse, psychological/emotional abuse, financial/material abuse, sexual abuse, and neglect. See Table 2 for characteristics and examples of the five types of abuse. Sooryanarayana et. al. conducted a review of 1,831 articles on elder abuse from 1990 to 2011, and found that psychological abuse is the most common form of elder abuse, suggesting that abuse may not be identified exclusively on physical examination.

Screening

Several tools have been created, almost exclusively for North America, but few are accepted for wide application because they are regarded as not accurate, specific, or sensitive enough to be reliable. Tools include the Hwalek-Sengstock Elder Abuse Screening Test (HSEAST), the Brief Abuse Screen for the Elderly (BASE), the Caregiver Abuse Screen (CASE), the Indicators of Abuse Screen (IOA), and the Elder Abuse Suspicion Index (EASI). Screening for elder abuse should be considered in the context of cultural norms. For example, some rituals that take place in one culture may be offensive and considered abuse in another. The general approach for detecting elder abuse is through identifying high risk factors including: social isolation, frailty of the victim including functional disability and cognitive impairment, pathology of the abuser (such as alcohol or other substance abuse, cognitive impairment or mental health problems), caregiver stress/anger, dependence of abuser on victim (specifically in financial abuse), and also the degree of reliance of the victim on the abuser. Once abuse is identified, the clinician must play an important role to keep the patient safe and provide patient advocacy.

	Table 1. Definitions of Elder Abuse			
Definitions	**Properties**			**General Developments**
	Rational	**Forms**	**Circumstances**	
Granny battering (Bakker;Burston)	• "Ill treatment" of older people • Parallel with "baby battering"	Physical assault	• Family crisis • Stresses caring daughter • Vulnerable women • Ageist, negative assumptions	1975-1977 Females and physical abuse
Elder abuse (O'Malley et al.)		Physical pain, mental anguish	• Dependence of older person • Intention of harm by caregiver • Deprivation by caretaker of service • Relationship caregiver-caretaker	
Elder mistreatment (Beachler)				1979-1982 Risk factors and widening of actions
Battered elder syndrome (Block & Sinnott)	• "Labeling": syndrome, disease • Powerless and sick older people	Physical, economic, and psychological		
Granny battering (Eastman)	• "Systemic: physical abuse of an elder person by relative"		• Importance of the quality of relationships, females	
Old age abuse (Eastman)	• Applies to older people, not just grannies • A new term "maltreatment" • Narrowing the setting		• Caregiving relative	1984 Widening of victims
Elder mistreatment (Comijis)			• Acts or lack of actions • Personal or professional settings	1998 Widening of perpetrators
Elder abuse (WHO)	• Excludes random acts of violence or criminal behavior • Reduces specifically but increases the territory covered by the problem		• Focus on trust relationship	2002-2003 Widening of context
Elder mistreatment (Bonnie & Wallace)	• Excludes cases of self-neglect, and victimization of elders by strangers • Ambiguous terms "harm," "trust relationships" • Intentional actions		• Vulnerable elder caregiver	

Source: Mysyuk, Westendorp, and Lindenberg, 2013

	Table 2. Types of Abuse	
Types of Elder Abuse	**Characteristics**	**Examples**
Physical Abuse	The infliction of pain or injury	Slapping, hitting, kicking, force-feeding, restraining, striking with objects
Psychological/Emotional Abuse	Infliction of mental anguish	Verbal aggression or threat, threats of institutionalization, social isolation, humiliating statements
Financial/Material Abuse	Illegal or improper exploitation and/or use of funds or resources	Theft of money, coercion to deprive the older person of his or her assets, such as forcible transfer of property
Sexual Abuse	Nonconsensual contact of any kind with an older person	Suggestive talk, forced sexual activity, touching, fondling with a nonconsenting competent or incompetent person
Neglect	Intention or unintentional refusal or failure of designated caregiver to meet needs required for older person's well-being	Failure to provide adequate food, clothing, shelter, medical care, hygiene, or social stimulation

Source: Perel-Levin, 2008

Reporting

As stated by the World Health Organization, "Although the extent of elder mistreatment is unknown, its social and moral significance is obvious; therefore, it demands a global multifaceted response, one which focuses on protecting the rights of older persons." If you are concerned or suspicious that elder abuse is occurring close to you, please contact 1-800-677-1116 (for United States only), and a trained operator will help lead you to a near-by agency. More information can be found through the Department of Health and Human Services: National Center on Elder Abuse (http://www.ncea. aoa.gov/index.aspx).

—*Sonia Shubert*

See also Adult protective services; Assisted living; Elderly care; Institutional abuse.

For Further Information:

Department of Health and Human Services. National Center on Elder Abuse: Administration on Aging. Retrieved October 8, 2013, from http://www.ncea.aoa.gov/index.aspx.

"Elder Abuse." World Health Organization. Retrieved October 8, 2013, from http://www.who.int/ageing/projects/elder_abuse/en/.

Mysyuk, Y., R. Westendorp, and J. Lindenberg. "Added Value of Elder Abuse Definitions: A Review." *Ageing Research Review* 12, no. 1 (2013): 50-57.

Perel-Levin, Silvia. *Discussing Screening for Elder Abuse: A Primary Health Care Level.* Geneva, Switzerland World Health Organization, 2008.

Sooryanarayana, M.D., W. Choo, and N. Hairi. "A Review on the Prevalence and Measurement of Elder Abuse in the Community." *Trauma, Violence & Abuse* 14, no. 4 (2013), 316-325.

Abusive relationships

Biopsychosocial

Anatomy or system affected: Physical, emotional, financial

Specialties and related fields: Medical, nursing, psychiatry, social work, psychology, legal

Definition: Abusive relationships are patterns of abusive and coercive behaviors used to maintain power and control over another person. Abuse can be emotional, financial, sexual or physical and can include threats, isolation, and intimidation.

Abusive relationships, also known as Intimate Partner Violence (IPV) is a serious, preventable public health problem affecting more than 32 million Americans. In countries around the world, 10 to 69 percent of women report physical assault by an intimate partner at some time in their life.

The term "intimate partner violence" describes actual or threatened psychological, physical, or sexual harm by a current or former partner or spouse. IPV can occur among heterosexual or same-sex couples and does not require sexual intimacy.

Abusive behaviors are those in which one partner inflicts a pattern of violence, coercion, neglect, emotional manipulation, sexual abuse, and/or financial domination to control the other partner's feelings or behavior. The abuser often uses isolation, threats, and intimidation to gain power. Abusive behavior tends to escalate steadily over time.

Overview

Dating relationships most often begin positively, with physical attraction and compatibility. Most couples plan for the future, compromise, trust each other, and give each other space when necessary. Individuals normally have friends outside the relationship, as well as interaction with their families. However, when one partner tries to control the other with verbal put-downs, isolation, threats, sexual abuse, or violence, the relationship has become abusive.

Abuse occurs when a person wants to control an intimate partner. A person might become an abuser for several reasons. He or she might be naturally aggressive or may have learned aggression from family, friends, or negative role models in society. People who come from a home in which one parent abused the other may consider this behavior normal and emulate what they have seen. Other individuals may have difficulty controlling their temper or feel disrespected if their partner does not obey them.

Contributing factors include financial difficulties, unemployment, and family upheaval. While sometimes blamed on alcohol or drug use, abuse always has underlying causes. However, the use of substances may lower an abuser's inhibitions or cloud his or her reasoning, contributing to the abuse.

For the victim's part, he or she might also have learned such behavior at home or may not know what to expect from a relationship and consider the behavior normal. Many victims have low self-esteem and rely on their connection to their partner. They may believe the partner's put-downs are true. Once the abuse becomes physical, they may feel responsible for the abuser's anger and deserving of the punishment they receive.

Physical violence is the intentional use of physical force with the potential to cause harm, injury, disability, or death. Physical violence includes scratching, pushing, shoving, throwing, grabbing, biting, strangulating, shaking, slapping, punching, or burning. It may also include using a weapon, restraints, or one's size or strength against another person.

Physical violence varies in frequency and severity, ranging from one hit to chronic severe battering.

Physical abuse is more common than most people realize. More than one-third of all women have been physically assaulted during their lives. About one-fourth of these women have been severely battered and one-tenth have been raped by their partner. Among teens surveyed in New York who were in a relationship, one-third were afraid of being physically harmed by a boyfriend or girlfriend and one-fifth had actually been physically attacked. Among men, one in fourteen had been physically abused by a partner, and the majority of attacks occurred in same-sex relationships.

At the beginning of an unhealthy relationship, an aggressive, controlling person often comes on strong; he or she declares love quickly and wants to spend all of his or her time with the new partner. The aggressor often uses guilt to begin gaining control by making statements such as "If you loved me, you would do what I ask." The aggressor may call or text the partner with increasing frequency to keep tabs on his or her whereabouts and activities.

Once the abuser establishes control in the relationship, he or she uses guilt, shame, and fear to continue dominating the victim. The abuser may try to isolate the victim, both physically and emotionally, from friends and family. The abuser might move the partner to a new location and try to cut off the partner's ability to maintain ties by preventing employment, removing access to money, and making threats.

Most physical abuse is not continuous but occurs in a cycle of anger, violence, remorse, and promises. It is then followed by a period of more normal behavior. In some relationships, these cycles last a year or more while in others they are repeated more frequently. A couple's relationship may be relatively normal for months, even if the abuser maintains control through threats and occasional displays of temper. However, as stress and anger build up in the individual, a violent incident becomes more likely. Sometimes the abuser sets up the victim before the violence begins. For example, Rick sends his girlfriend Olivia on an errand that he decides should take 20 minutes to complete. Olivia is aware that Rick's stress is building and tries to hurry back, but it takes her 30 minutes to return. Rick becomes furious and accuses her of meeting someone, and, feeling justified, calls her names and hits her. Later Rick apologizes, brings Olivia flowers, and promises never to hurt her again. The relationship returns to its normal state until Rick's anger bursts through again.

The effects of abuse on the victim are not only physical, but also emotional. The victim suffers from varying degrees of depression, stress, sleeplessness, anger, fear, and shame depending on the frequency and severity of the abuse. The victim may be estranged from family and friends and feel that there is nowhere to turn for help. While terminating (leaving)the relationship may seem like the obvious solution, the victim may have been made to feel worthless, have no money, and be afraid of what the abuser will do in retaliation. The abuser may have threatened to harm the victim or his or her family in the event of an escape. These are not idle threats, either. The risk of injury or even death rises dramatically after an abused partner leaves the relationship. With the help of a shelter, family support, and sometimes the law, victims can make a plan for a safe escape, but it can be a long process before they can transition back to a normal life.

—Nancy Comstock;
updated by Geraldine Marrocco

For Further Information:

"About Domestic Violence." *Georgia Coalition Against Domestic Violence.* GCADV, n.d. Web. 16 May 2016.
Borrello, Antonio. "Warning: 6 Early Signs of an Abusive Relationship." *Huffpost Women.* TheHuffingtonPost.com, 1 Sept. 2015. Web. 16 May 2016.
Cory, Jill, and Karen McAndless-Davis. *When Love Hurts: A Woman's Guide to Underrstanding Abuse in Relationships.* New York: Penguin, 2016. Print.
"Domestic Violence and Abuse." *Helpguide.* Helpguide.org, Apr. 2016. Web. 16 May 2016.
Mouradian, Vera E. "Abuse in Intimate Relationships: Defining the Multiple Dimensions and Terms." *National Violence Against Women Prevention Research Center.* Natl. Violence Against Women Prevention Research Ctr., 2000. Web. 16 May 2016.
Sanchez, Crystal. "8 Steps That Explain Why Women Stay in Abusive Relationships." *Ms. Magazine.* Liberty Media, 11 May 2016. Web. 16 May 2016.
"Teen Dating Violence." *Office for the Prevention of Domestic Violence.* NYS Office for the Prevention of Domestic Violence, 2014. Web. 16 May 2016.
Tjaden P, Thoennes N. Extent, nature, and consequences of intimate partner violence: findings from the National Violence Against Women Survey. Publication No. NCJ-181867, US Department of Justice, Washington, DC 2000.
The World Health Organization. World report on violence and health. Chapter 4. Violence by intimate partners.tp://www.who.int/violence_injury_prevention/violence/global_campaign/en/chap4.pdf (Accessed on August 07, 2011).

Accidents

Disease/Disorder
Anatomy or system affected: All
Specialties and related fields: All
Definition: An occurrence in a sequence of events that produces unintended injury, death, or property damage. "Accident" refers to the event, not the result of the event. "Unintentional injury" refers to the result of an accident and is the preferred term in the health community for accidental injury.
Key terms:
autograft: a thin layer of skin taken from an unburned area on the patient's body and placed over the burned area
comminuted fracture: a bone broken into fragments
compound fracture: a bone break that breaks the skin
compression fracture: a break of a short bone in which its soft tissue is damaged
computed tomography (CT) scanning: a technique for producing cross-sectional images of the body in which X rays pass through at different angles and are computer analyzed
concussion: disturbance of electrical activity in the brain due to a blow to the head or neck
contusion: a bruise; injury to tissue without breaking the skin
corrosives: having a burning (caustic) and locally destructive effect
emetic: something that causes vomiting (emesis)
magnetic resonance imaging (MRI): a technique that uses magnetic fields and radio waves to create high-quality cross-sectional images without using radiation
mucous membrane: the soft, pink layer of cells that produce mucus to keep body structures lubricated; found in eyelids and respiratory and urinary tracts
whiplash injury: injury to the ligaments, joints, and soft tissues of the neck region of the spine due to a sudden, violent jerking motion

Causes and Symptoms

Unintentional injury continued to be the fifth leading cause of death in the United States as of 2000, exceeded by heart disease, cancer, stroke, and chronic obstructive pulmonary diseases (asthma, pneumonia, and influenza). In 2000, injuries had a financial impact on the average American household of approximately $4,600. Individuals and households sustain this loss by paying higher prices for goods and services and higher taxes or through direct, out-of-pocket loss. The leading cause of unintentional injury and death remains motor vehicle accidents, followed by poisoning, falls, drowning, and burns. Other injuries and deaths result from air transportation accidents, weather, and major disasters.

As of 2000, motor vehicle unintentional injuries, including those from automobile and motorcycle accidents, remained the leading cause of injury and death in the United States in individuals aged one to thirty-eight. Males between fifteen and twenty-one accounted for 60 percent of the deaths from automobile crashes. Not wearing seat belts in automobiles and not wearing helmets while operating other vehicles can lead to serious head trauma and death.

Children and adults should wear helmets to guard against head injuries when cycling, even with stable vehicles such as tricycles. (PhotoDisc)

Falls are a serious problem for seniors and the leading cause of death in people sixty-five and older.

Broken bones, cuts, bruises, and whiplash are the most common injuries in accidents involving one or more vehicles. More serious injuries from vehicles, sports, and falls include trauma to the head and neck; spinal cord injuries; knee injuries; eye injuries and blindness; comminuted, compression, and compound fractures; hip fractures; severed limbs; and severe burns.

Vehicle accidents are those caused by automobiles and motorcycles and cause more serious injuries, such as head trauma, spinal cord injuries, blindness, and burns. Self-propelled vehicles, bicycles, scooters, skateboards, and in-line skates are also included in this group and produce less serious injuries, such as cuts, bruises, and simple fractures.

Head injuries are always considered serious. They cause more deaths and disabilities than any other neurologic condition before the age of fifty and occur in 70 percent of all unintentional injuries. They are the leading cause of death in men and boys up to thirty-five years of age. Motorcycle head injuries are most serious in those who do not wear helmets. Upon impact, the rider is thrown toward the ground at accelerated speeds, causing severe blunt force trauma, especially to the head.

The brain fits loosely within the skull so that blunt force to the skull or violent shaking of the head back and forth causes the brain to bounce off the skull. This violent brain movement causes bruising, tearing, and bleeding between the brain tissue and the skull.

There are two types of brain injury, diffuse and focal. Diffuse is most common and includes concussion. One-third of those who die from brain injury die from diffuse brain injury. An injury victim can have a concussion without losing consciousness and have no visible signs of trauma on the head, such as a bump or cut. If signs of amnesia, impaired attention, distractibility, and changes in cognitive functioning (knowing information such as one's immediate location) are temporary after concussion, this may imply the patient has had no structural damage. This does not, however, indicate the severity of the injury. A CT (computed tomography) scan or MRI (magnetic resonance imaging) is used to diagnose the extent of diffuse and focal brain injuries. Careful examination by a neurosurgeon is necessary.

Focal brain injury involves a specific area of the brain. This includes brain contusions that occur from a direct blow to the head (and are similar to other external bruises); ischemia, which is damage to the brain tissue due to a reduction in the flow of blood to the brain; infarction, which causes affected brain tissue to die from lack of blood supply; and pressure which is caused by the brain tissue swelling from the trauma.

A direct blow to the head can cause an epidural hematoma, which is bleeding between the skull and the brain membranes. This occurs quickly and causes unconsciousness at the time of injury, perhaps a lucid interval, and then coma. Subdural hematomas cause bleeding that occurs slowly within the brain tissue, are frequently complicated by contusions of the brain tissue, and carry a significant risk of death even with surgery. A favorable outcome with any brain injury depends on rapid and careful transportation to a hospital for diagnosis and treatment.

Bicycle, scooter, skateboard, and in-line skate injuries are sustained in falls. About half of these occur to hands and arms, one-third to head and face, and one-third to legs and feet, including fractures and dislocations. Other injuries include lacerations requiring stitches, cuts and bruises, and strains and sprains. Fatalities may occur when a victim collides with an automobile.

Sports injuries are generally to ligaments, muscles, and joints. More serious sports injuries include concussions, broken bones, and spinal cord injuries. Knee injuries can be sustained in vehicular and sports accidents and falls. Most severe knee injuries occur in competitive sports accidents, particularly football. The most common are ligament or cartilage tears and traumatic arthritis. A "blown out knee" is a tear of the anterior cruciate ligament, one of four principal ligaments in the knee and most important for stability of the knee.

Unintentional injuries from falls are most common in patients aged fifty-five to seventy-five and are the primary cause of fatal injury for people aged sixty-five and older. Approximately 60 percent of fatal falls occur in the home, 30 percent in public places, and 10 percent in institutions. Hip fractures are the most serious injury sustained from falls. The impact on the injured individual's quality of life can be devastating. Most patients cannot return home or live independently after a hip fracture. A seriously injured patient requires a caregiver on duty twenty-four hours a day, which can be costly. Lack of mobility causes severe depression, especially for someone who had been active. Climbing to reach an object is not the cause of most falls in older adults, but rather vision problems, poor lighting, slippery surfaces, wearing house shoes with soft soles, balance problems resulting from disease or medication, and clutter such as papers or magazines on the floor.

Poison is any substance that produces disease conditions or tissue injury, or otherwise interrupts natural life processes when in contact with or absorbed into the body. Most poisons taken in sufficient quantity are lethal. A poison, depending on the type, may attack the surface of the body or, more seriously, internal organs or the central nervous system.

Poisoning is a leading cause of accidents resulting in unintentional injury and death. These agents include illicit drugs (street drugs and those not prescribed by a physician), medicines (over-the-counter and prescribed drugs), mushrooms, eggs, shellfish, and gases or vapors. Poisons are usually classified by effects as corrosives, irritants, or systemic or nerve poisons (narcotics).

The American Association of Poison Control Centers estimates that 2.5 million poison cases, fatal and nonfatal, were reported during 2000. These incidents have nearly tripled in the last thirty years. This may be due to the increase in the use of illegal street drugs.

Common results of poisoning include burns to the skin or eye tissue, or to mucous membranes of the mouth, throat, esophagus, stomach, and other parts of the body with which a caustic poison might come in contact when swallowed or inhaled; central nervous stimulation or depression; cerebral edema; renal (kidney) and/or hepatic (liver) failure; brain damage; and death.

Corrosives are strong acids or alkalies that, when swallowed, burn the skin or lining of the mouth, throat, and stomach, causing bloody vomiting. Ammonia is an example of a common household corrosive. Irritants (such as iodine, arsenic, and laxatives) act directly on the mucous membrane, causing inflammation and gastrointestinal upset with pain and vomiting. Irritants can be absorbed slowly and become cumulative until they take effect suddenly, causing serious illness or death. Central nervous system poisons (narcotics) affect the heart, liver, lungs, and kidneys, as well as the respiratory and circulatory systems. Examples of household narcotics include alcohol, turpentine, cyanide, and strychnine (found in some pesticides). Botulin toxin, the bacteria that causes botulism (food poisoning), is one of the most dangerous poisons known and is included in this group. Asphyxiants include gas poisons such as carbon monoxide. Gases, when inhaled, get into the bloodstream and prohibit the body from properly absorbing oxygen. Blood poisoning, or septicemia, is included in this category. Microorganisms get into the bloodstream through a wound or infection, also preventing, in advanced stages, proper oxygen absorption. Smoke from house fires is an asphyxiant and causes most fire-related deaths.

Deaths from residential fires are second only to those occurring as the result of automobile accidents. In 2000 alone, five thousand people were killed in house fires. Most accidents causing burns can be avoided by preventing the cause. Burns are the most devastating of all unintentional injuries, causing red and painful areas on skin with blisters, scarring, contractions of skin resulting in a decrease in motion, dehydration, shock, damage to lungs from inhalation of smoke and hot air, and loss of skin that can be traumatic and life-threatening.

Treatment and Therapy

Simple fractures, those bones broken with little or no displacement, can be set in the hospital emergency room or clinic by a general or orthopedic surgeon. A cast is applied to hold the bones in place until they grow together again. The patient is usually asked to come back in six weeks for new X rays and probable cast removal. Comminuted fractures (bone broken into fragments), compression fractures (damage to soft tissue at site), and compound fractures (bone protruding through skin) require surgery. These fractures may cause deformity of the limbs if extensive and if surgical intervention cannot return the bone fragments to proper alignment. In some compression or comminuted fractures, a steel plate is attached with screws through healthy bone above and below the fractured area, and a cast is applied. Traction may be required and the patient kept hospitalized and immobile for several weeks. Physical therapy may be required to regain strength and mobility in the legs or motion in the joints of the upper extremities.

Skull fractures are easier to diagnose and treat. A simple linear skull fracture, depending on the location, often requires no intervention except hospitalization for observation. A skull fracture that goes deeper than the thickness of the skull requires surgical evaluation.

Any foreign objects or objects impaled in a victim's head will be removed only in the operating room by a neurosurgeon, with the patient being kept for at least a twenty-four-hour observation. Patients who have had severe head wounds often require extensive physical and psychological therapy. Personality changes can occur, causing the patient to exhibit agitated behaviors, anger, and the inability to cope with everyday activities. Relearning normal bodily functions, such as speech, walking, and writing, becomes a series of frustrating, monumental tasks. Behaviors can be so uncontrolled that confinement is necessary so that there is no danger to the patient or others. Medications combined with psychotherapy and physical therapy can typify the long road back to normalcy. Some patients never fully recover.

Repair to an injured knee is done under general anesthesia. Instruments are inserted into the knee joint through several small punctures. While viewing the ligaments through the arthroscope, the surgeon can repair or remove damaged tissue. If torn, the anterior cruciate ligament can be rebuilt. Most arthroscopic surgery is performed on an outpatient basis. Meniscal cartilages are the "shock absorbers" between the femur (thighbone) and the tibia (large leg bone) at the knee joint. A tear in the meniscal cartilage is the most common knee injury requiring surgical intervention. Arthroscopic surgery is done on an outpatient basis, and the patient is allowed to walk on the affected leg as soon as it feels comfortable. Physical therapy may be recommended for both anterior cruciate ligament and meniscal cartilage tears. Chances of returning to competitive sports are quite good, even for those who play professionally.

Poisoning should be treated immediately but with the direction of a health care professional. Most poison cases can be handled in the home after consulting a poison control center. In most cases of poisoning, ingestion of large quantities of water or milk (dilution) is called for. Sometimes an emetic is administered. Some common household emetics include a tablespoon of salt dissolved in warm water or two tablespoons of mustard dissolved in a pint of warm water. Vomiting must never be induced in a person who has swallowed a corrosive poison. An antidote is given for ingestion of corrosives, which neutralizes the chemical, absorbs it, or prevents it from being absorbed. Transport to a local hospital is always necessary.

The first forty-eight hours are important in burn treatment. When admitted to the hospital for severe burns, patients require stabilization of breathing and replacement of fluids to prevent dehydration and shock. Wounds are debrided in surgery to promote blood flow to healthy tissue underneath the wound. Grafts may be required. Surgical dressings soaked in antibiotics are applied to prevent infection. Many surgeries may be required until the grafts cover all the burned areas. Medical staff work to develop pain management strategies specific to each person's suffering. Physical and occupational therapy, though painful, must not be avoided. Burn injury places the patient at risk for severe loss of motion. Exercise, nutrition, and emotional support are important factors in helping the burn patient to heal.

Perspective and Prospects

There are three major ways to prevent accidents: education, making the home and workplace safer, and banning dangerous activities and equipment. Air bags have helped tremendously to eliminate many types of injuries in automobiles, and many lives have been saved. Whiplash, head and neck trauma, and eye injuries have been less serious since air bags have been installed in automobiles. With bicycle riders especially, wearing a helmet is the single most effective safety device available to reduce fatal injury to the brain and disfiguring injury to the face from crashes. The best investment against bicycle, scooter, skateboard, and in-line skate injuries is protective gear.

New technologies and advanced training in sports medicine for health care professionals have greatly advanced complete recovery for unintentional injuries received in competitive sports. Artificial turf, though easier to care for, causes many knee and back injuries from slipping. Biotechnology has made great advances in providing safer equipment for sports participants, more effective imaging technology (such as magnetic resonance imaging, or MRI, and computed tomography, or CT, scanning equipment) for diagnosing all injuries, and physical therapy techniques and equipment to help those who have disabling injuries such as those involving the spinal cord. New materials and designs for limb prostheses are aiding those who have lost limbs to lead normal lives, even in competitive sports. There have been several examples of runners being competitive despite a leg or foot prosthesis. Pharmaceutical research is making advances in medications that can control pain without being addictive, for those with behavior problems and depression resulting from severe head trauma.

For seniors, a simple screening test can accurately identify those who are most likely to fall. Constant review and adjustment of medications by a physician are musts for preventing side effects such as dizziness, drowsiness, or disorientation. Installing grab bars in the shower and around the toilet, installing rails on both sides of the stairs, increasing lighting throughout the home and encouraging its use, and removing tripping hazards have been very effective in preventing falls. Most important for seniors is the encouragement of regular exercise to improve strength and balance.

Measures to prevent poisoning include labeling of household products, elimination of lead from gasoline, use of carbon monoxide detectors, and improved monitoring of exposure to toxic elements within industry and throughout the environment. The telephone number of a poison control center should be posted at home and in the workplace. More than 50 percent of accidental poisonings in 2000 happened in the home and involved such products as aspirin, barbiturates, insecticides, and cosmetics. Awareness, safety, and education are the keys to preventing accidents involving poisons.

Improvements in burn care have resulted in fewer deaths and better infection control. Technological advances in the provision of skin substitutes, improved monitoring techniques, surgical instrumentation, and better understanding of the underlying metabolic changes have all contributed to successful therapy.

—Virginiae Blackmon

See also Asphyxiation; Balance disorders; Bleeding; Brain damage; Brain disorders; Bruises; Burns and scalds; Casts and splints; Choking; Coma; Concussion; Critical care; Critical care, pediatric; Death and dying; Drowning; Electrical shock; Emergency medicine; Emergency medicine, pediatric; Emergency rooms; First aid; Food poisoning; Fracture and dislocation; Fracture repair; Frostbite; Hip fracture repair; Hip replacement; Hyperbaric oxygen therapy; Intensive care unit (ICU); Laceration repair; Lead poisoning; Mercury poisoning; Paramedics; Poisoning; Poisonous plants; Prostheses; Radiation sickness; Resuscitation; Safety issues for children; Safety issues for the elderly; Shock; Snakebites; Spinal cord disorders; Sunburn; Unconsciousness; Whiplash; Wounds; Zoonoses.

For Further Information:

Beers, Mark H., et al., eds. *The Merck Manual of Diagnosis and Therapy.* 18th ed. Whitehouse Station, N.J.: Merck Research Laboratories, 2006. The sections on burns, poisoning, and bites and stings are very complete and informative resources for the lay reader, if a bit technical. Includes pictures, charts, and graphs.

English, Peter. *Old Paint: A Medical History of Childhood Lead-Paint Poisoning in the United States to 1980.* New Brunswick, N.J.: Rutgers University Press, 2001. Chapters include "Lead Poisoning Before 1920," "The Scientific Study of the American Workplace," "Peeling and Flaking Paint: A 1950s Transformation," and "New Therapies: Industry and Public Health Responses."

Gronwall, Dorothy, Philip Wrightson, and Peter Waddell. *Head Injury: The Facts-A Guide for Families and Care-Givers.* 2d ed. New York: Oxford University Press, 1998. Examines common wounds and injuries of the brain and the process of rehabilitation.

Matthews, Dawn D., ed. *Household Safety Sourcebook: Basic Consumer Health Information About Household Safety.* Detroit, Mich.: Omnigraphics, 2002. A comprehensive and accessible handbook detailing the prevention and treatment of common household accidents, including those caused by fire, chemicals, water, electricity, and home equipment and appliances.

Monafo, W. W. "Initial Management of Burns." *New England Journal of Medicine* 335 (1996): 1581-1586. A technical article but accessible to the lay reader with some medical knowledge.

National Center for Emergency Medicine Informatics. http://ncemi.org. Site provides Web links, frequently asked questions, bibliographies, and articles.

National Safety Council. *Injury Facts 2005-2006.* Itasca, Ill.: Author, 2006. Complete injury statistics without much text, offering good facts and topic organization.

Nestle, Marion. *Safe Food: The Politics of Food Safety.* Updated ed. Berkeley: University of California Press, 2010. Examines food-borne microbial illnesses that plague American consumers as part of its range of topics, arguing that the food industry acts in its own economic self-interest rather than out of concern for the public welfare.

Roberts, Anthony H. N. "Burn Prevention: Where Now?" *Burns* 26, no. 6 (August, 2000). Accessible to general readers and includes applicable information.

Accountable care organizations (ACOs)
Health care system

An Accountable Care Organization (ACO) is a network of providers who assume medical and financial responsibility for a group of patients in an effort to coordinate care, decrease duplication of services, enhance quality and control costs. The Centers for Medicare and Medicaid Services (CMS) led early initiatives and defines Accountable Care Organizations (ACOs) as groups of healthcare providers, hospitals, and doctors, voluntarily working together to provide high quality care to their Medicare patients.

ACOs may be initiated with private insurers and CMS. Quality metric reporting (numeric values assigned to specific aspects of care that are deemed samples of and indicators the quality of care the ACOs provide) is required, including care delivered and outcomes. Payments to the ACO reflect cost of care and allow providers to share in any savings it achieves for the payer on a percentage basis.

The network principle of ACOs removes the need for patients to assume responsibility for coordinating their own health care. For example, many diseases require multiple specialists to provide care and often specialists do not coordinate that care on a routine basis increasing costs through redundant tests and unnecessary treatments and drugs. The result is more costly care for both the patient and the payer with outcomes that may be less than optimal.

Overview

First proposed as a theoretical model for improving health care as a way to combat rising health care costs, the concept of the ACO was made an integral part of the 2010 Patient Protection and Affordable Care Act, known popularly as either the Affordable Care Act (ACA) or Obamacare. Under the ACA, ACOs must manage the care of at least 5,000 Medicare patients for a minimum of three years, in addition to their other patients.

The ACO model was touted as a way to both improve health care and bring down costs. The Centers for Medicare and Medicaid Services reported that according to 2014 quality and financial performance results, 353 Medicare ACOs in two different programs, the Pioneer Model and Medicare Shared Savings Program, generated a total savings of $411 million and that 97 of the ACOs qualified for shared savings payments of more than $422 million. However, the ACO programs caused the Medicare trust fund to accrue a net loss of $2.6 million. By the first quarter of 2015, the total number of ACOs had grown to 744, covering a total of 23.5 million individuals.

As the model matured, private payers developed ACOs in conjunction with large health systems and multispecialty physician groups. Humana, Aetna and UnitedHealth, all large payers, have developed ACOs. While not responsible for medical care, payers felt that attention to quality and outcome would lower costs and, like government ACOs, share cost savings with the providers on a percentage basis.

Opponents of the model suggest that ACOs may eliminate choice in health care by driving provider consolidation and moving doctors who prefer to remain independent providers out of the market. There remains skepticism about the cost savings ACOs will provide over time. The ultimate goal will be for provider networks to accept full financial responsibility for a group of patients.

—*Patricia Stanfill Edens, PhD, RN, LFACHE*

For Further Information:

Accountable Care Organizations. Centers for Medicare and Medicaid Services. Downloaded August 10, 2017 from https://www.cms.gov/Medicare/Medicare-Fee-for-Service-Payment/ACO/index.html

"Are Medicare ACOs Working? Experts Disagree." *Kaiser Health News.* Kaiser Family Foundation, 21 Oct. 2015. Web. 11 Aug. 2016.

Crosson, Francis J. "The Accountable Care Organization: Whatever Its Growing Pains, the Concept Is Too Vitally Important to Fail." *Health Affairs* 30.7 (2011): 1250-55. Digital file.

Gold, Jenny. "Accountable Care Organizations, Explained." *Kaiser Health News.* Kaiser Family Foundation, Downloaded on August 10, 2017 from http://khn.org/news/ aco-accountable-care-organization-faq/.

Japsen, Bruce. *Inside Obamacare: The Fix for America's Ailing Health Care System.* New York: Forbes Media, 2014. Print.

King, Raymond C., et al. *The ABCs of ACOs: A Practical Handbook on Accountable Care Organizations.* Chicago: American Bar, 2015. Digital file.

McClellan, Mark. "A National Strategy to Put Accountable Care into Practice." *Health Affairs* 29.5 (2010): 982-90. Digital file.

Rittenhouse, D., et al. "Primary Care and Accountable Care—Two Essential Elements of Delivery-System Reform." *New England Journal of Medicine* 36 (2009): 2301-3. Digital file.

Acetaminophen

Biology

Also known as: Paracetamol and commercially as Tylenol and Panadol

Anatomy or system affected: Muscular system, nervous system

Specialties and related fields: Pain mediation, neurophysiology

Definition: An analgesic or pain relief drug for general aches and pains and also used for fever reduction

Key terms:

analgesic: a substance that reduces pain

antipyretic: a substance that lowers body temperature

non-steroidal anti-inflammatory drugs: drugs that do not have the steroid structure and reduce inflammation

methemoglobinemia: a condition where there is an elevated blood level of methhemoglobin where the iron is in a state which cannot carry oxygen

cyclooxygenase(COX): an enzyme in the synthesis of prostaglandins and thromboxanes

Structure and Functions

Acetaminophen is a non-steroidal anti-inflammatory drug (NSAID) that is a mild analgesic and antipyretic used to alleviate pain and reduce fever. It is the most widely used non-prescription drug in the general treatment of minor to moderate pain and fever reduction and is increasingly used to reduce osteoarthritic pain. For severe pain, acetaminophen is often used in combination with an opiate such as codeine.

Although the mechanism of action of acetaminophen is unclear, it may reduce the cyclooxygenase (COX) enzymes, COX-1 and COX-2, enzymes that synthesize prostaglandins and thromboxanes, within the central nervous system but not outside the central nervous system explaining its analgesic and antipyretic effect and non-effect on inflammation. Prostaglandins and thromboxanes have many physiological effects. Acetaminophen is not a direct inhibitor of either COX-1 or COX-2 but seems to reduce their amounts by inhibiting their oxidation to the active forms. Whether acetaminophen inhibits COX-3 is the subject of debate.

The therapeutic and inhibitory effect of acetaminophen toward the prevention of cataracts is currently under investigation.

Acetaminophen is increasingly used as treatment for osteoarthritis and has managed to maintain low gastrointestinal toxicity effects even at over-the-counter (OTC) doses. The widespread availability of the drug increased reports of self-overdosing and reports of severe liver damage and skin reactions. These complications are often seen when acetaminophen is used with alcohol, fasting, other drugs, and diet. The concerns of overdosing have continued to increase. The Food and Drug Administration has attempted to strengthen its messaging about the dangers of overdosing and limit the dose/tablet or capsule. Label warnings concerning liver damage and rare skin reactions were required in 2011, and further refinement was suggested in 2017. Acetaminophen is currently the leading NSAID with no significant contradictory reports to hinder consumers from continuing its use.

Perspective and Prospects

During the Middle Ages, typical antipyretic agents were derived from cinchona bark and white willow bark, more commonly known as the chemical family of salicins. The scarcity of the cinchona tree fueled the need for an alternative source for antipyretic agents. Harmon Northrop Morse first acetaminophen in 1877 at the Johns Hopkins University through the reduction of *p*-nitrophenol with tin in the presence of glacial acetic acid. Joseph von Mering first used acetaminophen in humans in 1887 and reported in 1893 that acetaminophen caused methemoglobinemia stimulating its discontinuation as a drug in humans. By 1948, scientists had demonstrated that acetaminophen is not toxic in humans and is an effective analgesic. The rediscovery of acetaminophen sparked public interest in the United States and was subsequently introduced to the market in 1950 as Triogesic, a combination with aspirin and caffeine. However, fears of agranulocytosis side effects, where the deficiency of white blood cells increases the vulnerability to infections, led to withdrawal of the drug from the market until it was reintroduced as a prescription drug in 1953 and as a single non-prescription analgesic in 1959. By the 1960s, acetaminophen proved its safety and reliability among its predecessors, particularly acetanilide and phenacetin, whose side effects included gastrointestinal ulceration and hemorrhage, among others.

—*Pamela Rose V. Samonte and Rhea U. Vallente, PhD; updated by Charles L. Vigue, PhD*

For Further Information:

"Acetaminophen." Drugs, Herbs and Supplements. U.S. National Library of Medicine. American Society of Health-System Pharmacists, Inc. 8 Aug. 2014. Web. 25 Nov. 2015. https://www.nlm.nih.gov/medlineplus/druginfo/meds/a681004.html.

"Acetaminophen Information." U.S. Food and Drug Administration, 4 Dec. 2015. Web. 25 Nov. 2015. http://www.fda.gov/Drugs/DrugSafety/InformationbyDrugClass/ ucm165107.htm.

Javaherian, Atash (Author and Editor) and Pasha Latifpour (Editor). Acetaminophen: Properties, Clinical Uses and Adverse Effects (Pharmacology - Research, Safety Testing and Regulation; Public Health in the 21st Century). Hauppauge, NY: Nova Science Publishers, 2012. Print.

Liew, Zeyan, et al. "Acetaminophen Use During Pregnancy, Behavioral Problems, and Hyperkinetic Disorders." *JAMA Pediatrics* 168.4 (2014): 313-20. Print.

"Acetaminophen (Tylenol, Tylenol Arthritis Pain, Tylenol Ext, Little Fevers, Children's Fever/Pain)." MedicineNet.com. http://www.medicinenet.com/acetaminophen/article.htm

Prescott, L. F. "Paracetamol: Past, Present, and Future." Am J Ther. 7.2 (2000): 143-7. Print.

"Use Only as Directed" . ProPublica. https://www.propublica.org/article/tylenol-mcneil-fda-use-only-as-directed.

Achalasia

Disease/Disorder

Also known as: Esophageal achalasia, achalasia cardiae, cardiospasm, esophageal aperistalsis

Anatomy or system affected: Chest, gastrointestinal system

Specialties and related fields: Gastroenterology, general surgery, radiology

Definition: A swallowing disorder that prevents the movement of food from the esophagus to the stomach.

Key terms:

esophagus: the muscular tube that connects the pharynx with the stomach

GERD: gastroesophageal reflux disease or acid efflux disease; regurgitation of stomach acid into the esophagus

peristalsis: The successive waves of contraction and relaxation that pass along the muscular wall of the gastrointestinal tract

sphincter: a circular band of voluntary or involuntary muscle that encircles an orifice of the body or one of its hollow organs

Causes and Symptoms

The muscular tube called the esophagus has three parts: (1) the upper esophageal sphincter, a ring of muscle that separates the esophagus from the throat; (2) the middle esophagus (about 8 inches long); and (3) the lower esophageal sphincter, another specialized ring of muscle at the junction

---

Information on Achalasia

Causes: Degeneration of the inhibitory nerves that innervate the esophagus

Symptoms: Difficulty swallowing, chest pain, regurgitation of swallowed food, hiccups, weight loss, heartburn, sensation of fullness or a lump in the throat

Duration: Arises at any age and remains for a lifetime although certain treatments can alleviate symptoms

Treatments: Nitrates and calcium channel blockers, balloon dilation, Botox injection, surgery

---

of the esophagus with the stomach. Both of these sphincters remain closed to prevent food from backing up either into the throat or from the stomach into the esophagus. Upon swallowing, the upper sphincter relaxes and opens to allow the passage of food and then contracts and propels the food into the esophagus. This wave of muscle contraction progresses down the esophagus (peristalsis), driving the food to the lower esophageal sphincter. When the wave of esophageal muscle contractions reaches the lower esophageal sphincter (LES), the LES relaxes and opens to allow passage of the food to the stomach.

In people with achalasia, the inhibitory nerves that innervate the esophagus (myenteric plexus) degenerate for unknown reasons. Consequently, the LES cannot effectively relax and open to allow food to pass into the stomach and the muscles that line the esophagus do not contract, preventing the movement of food through the esophagus to the stomach. As the disease progresses, the muscles of the esophagus begin to degenerate and, over time, the esophagus stretches and dilates. Achalasia affects approximately 1 in 100,000 people per year.

The most common symptoms of achalasia include difficulty swallowing (dysphagia) and the sensation that swallowed materials get stuck in the chest. Other symptoms include regurgitation of swallowed food and liquids, chest pain, heartburn, hiccups, a sensation of a lump or fullness in the throat, and weight loss.

The routine regurgitation of food may lead to the aspiration of food into the lungs, and aspiration pneumonia. Also the irritating effects of pooling food and liquids in the esophagus may cause chronic inflammation of the esophagus (esophagitis). Constant irritation of the esophagus increases the risk of esophageal cancer.

Because other conditions can produce similar symptoms (hiatus hernia and GERD), confirming an achalasia diagnosis requires other tests. A barium swallow test involves swallowing a thick, chalky-tasting barium solution while X-rays are taken. The barium outlines the esophagus on the X-ray and reveals an esophagus dilated above a constricted region. Esophageal manometry or esophageal motility studies examine the pressure in the esophagus. In this test a pressure sensor is inserted through the mouth or nose into the esophagus. To confirm a diagnosis of achalasia, the LES should show high pressure at rest, a failure to relax after swallowing, and the lower esophagus should show no peristaltic contractions. Endoscopy uses a thin, lighted, flexible tube (endoscope) that is inserted through the mouth to view the inside of the gastrointestinal tract. Patients with achalasia have a dilated esophagus that retains food with small erosions or ulcers on the inner surface.

Two different diseases, Chagas disease and esophageal cancer, can mimic achalasia. Endoscopy can detect esophageal cancer, but Chagas disease, caused by infection with the parasite Trypanosoma cruzi, can affect any portion of the gastrointestinal tract.

Treatment and Therapy

Two classes of drugs, organic nitrates and calcium channel blockers can relieve achalasia symptoms. Unfortunately, these agents have undesirable side effects and lose effectiveness over time.

Balloon dilation requires that the patient swallow a small, collapsed balloon. An X-ray machine is used to guide the balloon, and once positioned at the LES, the balloon is inflated to stretch the lower esophagus. Although patients may require more than one balloon dilation treatment, about 60 percent of patients show relief of symptoms one year after this procedure and 25 percent five years after.

Boxtox injections utilize a modified version of a toxin made by the bacterium Clostridium botulinum. Endoscopic injections of botulinum toxin (Botox) into the esophageal muscles relax it and relieve obstruction. Botox injections work well in older patients.

Surgery that cuts the muscles of the esophagus (myotomy) can also relieve symptoms long term. Surgeons also wrap part of the stomach around the esophagus (fundoplication) to prevent the reflux of stomach contents into the esophagus. Patients who have Botox injections, myotomies or balloon dilations have an increased risk of GERD after the surgery and might need to take proton-pump inhibitors (e.g., omeprazole, lansoprazole, rabeprazole, and others) after surgery.

Procedures and Prospects

The first description of achalasia dates from Sir Thomas Willis in 1672. In 1913, Ernest Heller performed the first successful surgical myotomy to treat achalasia. For this reason, the myotomy procedure used to treat achalasia is called a Heller myotomy. In 1929, Hurt and Rake discovered that the inability of the LES to relax caused the symptoms of "cardiospasm," as it was known then, and they renamed the condition "achalasia," which means "failure to relax."

New developments in achalasia treatment involve reducing the trauma of myotomy and improving its outcomes. Laparoscopic myotomies insert small instruments and a fiber optic camera into the abdomen through a small incision and greatly shorten the patient's recovery time and reduce complications. An even less invasive procedure called peroral endoscopic myotomy inserts all surgical instruments into the esophagus through the mouth by means of an endoscope. Since peroral endoscopic myotomy does not require an incision, it further shortens the recovery time and decreases the rate of complications.

—*Michael A. Buratovich, Ph.D.*

See also Food Allergies; Gastroenterology; Hiccups; Neurology

For Further Information:
Moonen, An J., and Guy E. Boekxstaens, "Management of Achalasia." *Gastroenterology of North America* 42, no. 1 (2013): 45-55.
Sayadi, Roya, and Joel Herskowitz, *Swallow Safely: How Swallowing Problems Threaten the Elderly and Others.* Natick, Mass.: Inside/Outside Press, 2010.
Stavropoulos, Stavros N., Rani Modayil, and David Friedel. "Achalasia." *Gastrointestinal Endoscopy Clinics of North America* 23, no. 1 (2013): 53-75.

Acid-base chemistry

Biology

Anatomy or system affected: Cells
Specialties and related fields: Biochemistry, cytology, hematology, pharmacology
Definition: The interaction between acids and bases in the cells of the body, the proper functioning of which is crucial in digestive metabolism, respiration, and the buffering capacity of body fluids.

Key terms:

acidosis: condition of high blood carbon dioxide levels and low pH that results from such diseases as emphysema and pneumonia

alkalosis: a condition of abnormally low carbon dioxide levels that results from hyperventilation (rapid breathing)

Brønsted-Lowry definition (of an acid and a base): an acid is a substance that can donate protons, while a base is a proton acceptor

buffer: a solution which contains components that enable a solution to resist large changes in pH when small quantities of acids and bases are added

cellular respiration: the chemical utilization of oxygen and the production of carbon dioxide in the cell itself

extracellular respiration: the process of oxygen transport from the lungs to the cells and carbon dioxide transport from cells back to the lungs

general acid (or base) catalysis: the process in which a partial transfer of a proton from a Brønsted acid (or partial proton abstraction by a Brønsted base) lowers the free energy of a reaction's transition state

pH: a measure of acidity in a solution, which is equal to the negative logarithm of the hydrogen ion concentration; a neutral solution has a pH of 7, an acidic solution has a pH less than 7, and a basic solution has a pH greater than 7

Structure and Functions

The existence of acids and bases is critical to the functioning of the human body. An acid is a compound that contains hydrogen, can accept unshared electron pairs, has a pH that is less than 7, and is water-soluble. A base is a compound that contains a hydroxyl (OH) group, can give up unshared pairs of electrons, can accept protons, has a pH that is greater than 7, and is water-soluble. An acid and a base can react together to form a salt.

Both acids and bases can be classified further as either "hard" or "soft." Bases are classified as soft if they have high polarizability and low electronegativity, are easily oxidized, or have low-energy, empty orbitals. Opposite properties tend to classify them as hard bases. Hard acids are those that have low polarizability, small size, and a high oxidation state (valence) and that do not have easily removed outer electrons. Soft acids possess reversed properties. Generally, a hard acid always reacts with a hard base and a soft acid always reacts with a soft base. The reaction of a hard acid (or base) with a soft base (or acid) is always unfavorable (absorbs energy). The hard-and-soft concept of acids and bases is used only as a way to classify and predict reactions. In the acid-base reactions of a living being, however, one must consider acids as proton donors and bases as proton acceptors.

A neutral solution is defined as one whose proton (hydrogen ion) and hydroxyl concentrations are equal. A solution that has more protons than hydroxyl groups is acidic, while a solution with more hydroxyl ions than protons is basic. Expressing the hydrogen ion concentration in moles per liter is rather complex. Instead, the pH of a solution is used. The pH is the negative logarithm of the hydrogen ion concentration. Neutral solutions have a pH of 7, acidic solutions have a pH that is less than 7, and basic solutions have a pH that is higher than 7. Thus, a pH of zero is strongly acidic and a pH of 14 is strongly basic.

Buffers are solutions whose contents allow very small changes in pH upon the addition of small quantities of acids and bases. Usually, buffers are solutions of a weak acid and one of its salts, or they are solutions of a weak base and one of its salts. A buffer becomes ineffective when there are no more anions (if a weak acid is part of the buffer) or cations (if a weak base is involved). At this point, the buffer capacity of the solution is said to be exceeded.

General acid catalysis is a process in which partial proton transfer from an acid lowers the free energy of a reaction's transition state. A reaction can also be accomplished by a general base catalysis, in which a base enhances the rate by partially stealing a proton. Such reactions often have such a high activation energy that they cannot take place unless the specific catalysis is involved.

Many well-known substances encountered in everyday life are weak acids or bases. Aspirin (acetylsalicylic acid, a headache remedy), phenobarbital (a sedative), niacin (nicotinic acid, vitamin B), and saccharin (an artificial sweetener) are weak acids. The majority of drugs and narcotics (such as heroin, cocaine, and morphine) in their free-base states are weak bases. Among the components of deoxyribonucleic acid (DNA), which is a polymer of deoxyribonucleotide units, are nitrogenous bases, the purines and pyrimidines. An amino acid is either neutral, acidic, or basic, depending on the chemical group found in its side chain.

The normal metabolic processes of the body result in the continuous production of acids, such as carbonic acid (H_2CO_3), phosphoric acid (H_3PO_4), lactic acid, and pyruvic acid. In cellular oxidations, the main acid end product is carbonic acid, with 10 to 20 moles formed per day. In terms of acidity, this amount is equivalent to 1 to 2 liters of concentrated hydrochloric acid. Although some alkaline end products are also formed, the acid type predominates, and the body is faced with the necessity of continually removing the large quantities of acids that are formed within cells. The greatest restriction is that these products should be transported to the organs of excretion (via the extracellular fluids) with a minimal change in the hydrogen ion concentration.

Most biochemical processes are extremely sensitive to the level of hydrogen ions. The enzymes and other proteins involved in biological reactions, as well as many of the smaller molecules, are weak electrolytes whose state of ionization is a function of the hydrogen ion concentration. Most enzymes are active only within a narrow pH range, usually from 5 to 9. At a pH other than the optimum one, the binding of substrates to enzymes, the catalytic activity of enzymes, and changes in protein structure are seriously affected. Since the catalytic properties of enzymes are dependent on their state of ionization, it is not surprising that living cells cannot tolerate more than very minor changes in hydrogen ion levels. As a result, biological fluids are in general strongly buffered, so that their pH is maintained within narrow limits under physiological conditions.

Blood is buffered by plasma proteins and by hemoglobin, which can either accept or donate protons. The role of buffers can be understood by the following example. The addition of 0.01 mole hydrochloric acid in 1 liter of blood lowers the pH only from 7.4 to 7.2. When added to an isotonic saline (sodium chloride) solution, the same amount of hydrochloric acid lowers the pH from 7.0 to 2.0, since the saline solution has no buffering capacity. Another example of the effectiveness of the blood plasma indicates that 1.3 liters of concentrated hydrochloric acid are needed to drop the pH of the whole 5.5 liters of blood of an average human being from 7.4 to 7.0.

Metabolism in tissues leads to the production of carbon dioxide (CO_2), which, when dissolved in water, forms carbonic acid and the following equilibrium:

$$CO_2 + H_2O \rightleftharpoons H_2CO_3 \rightleftharpoons H^+ + HCO_3^-$$

carbon dioxide   water   carbonic acid   bicarbonate anion

Carbon dioxide enters the bloodstream from tissues and is exchanged in the lungs for oxygen, which is then transported throughout the body by the hemoglobin in the blood. The fact that the ratio of bicarbonate to carbonic acid is relatively high (10:1) seems to put this buffer well outside its maximum capacity. Nevertheless, the system is appropriate because the need to neutralize excess acid (such as lactic acid, which is produced during exercise) is much greater than the need to neutralize excess base. The excess bicarbonate serves this purpose. Strenuous exercise also leads to an increased formation of carbon dioxide by body tissues, which is accumulated in the air spaces of the lungs. Under normal circumstances, the bicarbonate in the blood buffer will lead to a shifting in the equilibrium toward the optimum 7.4 value. Should excess alkalinity take place, carbon dioxide from the lungs can be reabsorbed to form carbonic acid, which will help the neutralization process.

Many biochemically important reactions take place because of either acid or base catalysis, including the hydrolysis of peptides and esters, the reactions of phosphate groups, tautomerizations (keto-enol equilibria), and condensations of carbonyl groups. Sometimes, the side chains of several amino acid residues in aspartic acid, glutamic acid, histidine, cysteine, tyrosine, and lysine act in the enzymatic capacity of general acid and/or base catalysis.

The kidneys, which are usually seen as the organs of excretion, also act as regulators in water, electrolyte, and acid-base balance. Acid-base balance takes place in the tubules of the kidneys through the exchange of sodium ions and hydrogen ions. It is regulated by the pH of blood plasma and the ability of the tubular cells to acidify the urine through proton and ammonia formation. The glomerular filtrate contains the electrolytes, acids, and bases present in the blood plasma. The cations are mostly sodium ions, while the anions are either chloride, phosphate, or bicarbonate. At a pH of 7.4, 95 percent of the carbon dioxide is in the form of sodium bicarbonate, while 83 percent of the phosphate is disodium hydrogen phosphate. Normally, most of the sodium ions are taken up by the tubular cells in exchange for the protons formed there. The sodium ions are then returned to the plasma after associating with the bicarbonate anions. The role of the kidneys is to stabilize the bicarbonate concentration and to neutralize the nonvolatile sulfuric and phosphoric acids. Base conservation by the kidneys takes place with the aid of ammonia formed by the decomposition of glutamine (via the enzyme glutaminase) and the amino acids (via amino acid oxidase).

Disorders and Diseases

Acids and bases are among the most important chemicals of the living being. Life depends on pH and acid-base reactions. The presence of buffers is also important for the optimum function of enzymes. Thus, in metabolic reactions enzymes have pH optima that allow the maximum catalysis of the substrate reactions. The means of maintaining a steady pH of 7.4 in the blood involve a mechanism for the regulation of acid-base balance, which includes water and electrolyte balance, hemoglobin, and blood buffers, as well as the action of lungs and kidneys.

The pH of different body fluids in human beings varies greatly. For example, the pH range of gastric juices is 1 to 2, while that of intestinal juices is 8 to 9. If the blood plasma pH of 7.4 for a healthy individual varies by 0.2 or more units, then serious medical conditions arise; if not corrected, they may lead to death. Such reactions occur primarily because the functioning of enzymes is sharply pH-dependent.

Life can be described as a continuous fight against pH change. Nature has equipped the body with the buffers and the various mechanisms that keep organs functioning. The kidneys, lungs, and skin all share the common role of controlling the ionic balance of the organism and thus controlling the bicarbonate concentration and pH. Cell pH regulation is complicated, however, because of the heterogeneous nature of the cell contents. For example, mitochondrial fluid is more alkaline than that of the cytoplasm, which allows the establishing of a hydrogen ion gradient between these two compartments of the cell. Basic functions such as oxidative phosphorylation, which is the transfer of metabolic energy to adenosine triphosphate (ATP), are believed to depend on this hydrogen ion gradient.

When the blood pH is lower than 7.4, acidosis results. Most forms of acidosis are metabolic or respiratory in origin. Metabolic acidosis is caused by a decrease in bicarbonate and occurs with uncontrolled diabetes mellitus (as a result of ketosis, the excessive production of ketone bodies such as acetone), with certain kidney diseases, with poisoning by an acid salt, and in cases of vomiting when nonacid fluids are lost. Respiratory acidosis may occur with diseases that impair respiration, such as emphysema, asthma, and pneumonia. Under these conditions, carbon dioxide is not properly expired and, as a result, carbonic acid levels increase relative to those of bicarbonate.

Alkalosis results when bicarbonate becomes favored in the buffer ratio. Metabolic alkalosis is observed when excessive vomiting (loss of acid, in the form of hydrochloric acid) takes place, while respiratory alkalosis occurs with hyperventilation (such as that brought on by a high altitude). Mountain climbers reaching the summit of Mount Everest without supplemental oxygen were found to have pH increases to 7.7 or 7.8.

The chief cause of dental decay is lactic acid, which is formed in the mouth by the action of specific bacteria, such as *Streptococcus mutans*, on the carbohydrates (and their by-products) that are attached to tooth surfaces in a sticky plaque. The normal pH of plaque is 6.8, but lactic acid lowers it to 5.5 or less, which speeds up the corrosion of enamel and leads to tooth decay. The application of fluoride-containing substances directly to the teeth or the drinking of fluoride-containing water changes the composition of teeth and forms a new substance called fluorapatite, which forms a new enamel that is much more resistant to acidity.

Perspective and Prospects

Acids and bases have been known to human beings since ancient times. The word *acid* is derived from the Latin *acidus* (sour) and has been redefined several times over the centuries. Alchemists have considered an acid as a substance with a sour taste, that dissolves many metals, and that reacts with alkalies to form salts. The French scientist Antoine-Laurent Lavoisier (1743-94) insisted that an acid should involve the presence of oxygen. In 1810, the English chemist Sir Humphry Davy (1778-1829) showed that hydrogen is the element that all acids have in common. In 1840, German Justus von Liebig (1803-73) redefined an acid as a compound that contains hydrogen and produces hydrogen gas upon reaction with metals. His definition coincided with the theories postulated separately by the Swedish chemist Svante A. Arrhenius (1859-1927) and the German chemist Carl W. Ostwald (1883-1943), who also pointed out that bases were substances that carried a hydroxyl group.

In 1909, the Danish chemist Søren Peter Lauritz

Sørensen (1868-1939) proposed the pH system, which has become the standard measure of acidity. In separate works announced in 1923, Johannes N. Brønsted (1879-1947) and Thomas M. Lowry supported the Arrhenius-Ostwald theory and went further to postulate that the hydrogen ion is never found in the free state but instead exists in combination with another base (for example with water when the hydrogen is in an aqueous solution). As a result, their work broadened the definition of a base, which according to them would include any compound that was a proton (hydrogen ion) acceptor. In 1938, American Gilbert N. Lewis (1875-1946) broadened the acid-base concept even further: An acid is an electron pair acceptor, while a base is an electron pair donor. In 1963, Ralph Gottfrid Pearson proposed the simple and effective way of classifying acids and bases as hard or soft.

—*Soraya Ghayourmanesh, Ph.D.*

See also Acidosis; Cells; Cytology; Enzymes; Fluids and electrolytes; Food biochemistry; Kidneys; Metabolism; Respiration.

For Further Information:

Berg, Jeremy M., John L. Tymoczko, and Lubert Stryer. *Biochemistry.* 7th ed. New York: W. H. Freeman, 2012.

Bishop, Michael L., Edward P. Fody, and Larry Schoeff, eds. *Clinical Chemistry: Principles, Procedures, Correlations.* 6th ed. Philadelphia: Lippincott Williams & Wilkins, 2009.

Caret, Robert L., Joseph J. Topping, and Katherine J. Denniston. *Principles and Applications of Organic and Biological Chemistry.* 2d ed. Dubuque, Iowa: Wm. C. Brown, 1997.

Karinen, H. M., et al. "Prediction of Acute Mountain Sickness by Monitoring Arterial Oxygen Saturation During Ascent." *High Altitude Medicine and Biology* 11, no. 4 (Winter 2010): 325-332.

Petrucci, Ralph H., William S. Harwood, and F. Geoffrey Herring. *General Chemistry: Principles and Modern Applications.* 10th ed. Toronto, Ont.: Pearson Canada, 2011.

Sackheim, George I., and Dennis D. Lehman. *Chemistry for the Health Sciences.* 8th ed. Upper Saddle River, N.J.: Pearson/Prentice Hall, 2009.

Thibodeau, Gary A., Kevin T. Patton, and Catherine Parker Anthony. *Structure and Function of the Body.* 14th ed. St. Louis: Elsevier, 2012.

Voet, Donald, and Judith G. Voet. *Biochemistry.* 4th ed. Hoboken, N.J.: John Wiley & Sons, 2011.

Acid reflux disease

Disease/Disorder

Also known as: Gastroesophageal reflux disease (GERD)

Anatomy or system affected: Gastrointestinal system, mouth, stomach, throat

Specialties and related fields: Gastroenterology

Definition: A chronic digestive disorder in which the lower esophageal sphincter (LES), which keeps digestive juices in the stomach, relaxes and permits gastric acid to rise into the esophagus, causing a burning sensation.

Key terms:

barium study: a medical procedure in which the patient drinks a liquid barium sulfate mixture prior to undergoing an X-ray examination of the chest and abdomen; used to identify problems in the upper gastrointestinal tract

esophagus: the gullet and beginning of the digestive tract

heartburn: a burning sensation generally felt in the chest and below the breastbone, often extending from the neck into the chest, in which acid and pepsin rise from the stomach into the esophagus

hiatal hernia: a condition in which a portion of the stomach protrudes into the chest cavity through an opening in the diaphragm

upper endoscopy: a medical procedure in which the physician inserts a flexible tube down the throat to inspect and examine the lining of the esophagus, stomach, and small intestine; to assess injuries; and to take biopsies (tissue samples)

Causes and Symptoms

Approximately one-third of Americans experience heartburn at least once a month, and 10 percent experience the sensation daily. Heartburn reportedly affects sufferers during the day and at night, impacting their job performance as well as their sleep. Heartburn is the major symptom of acid reflux disease, also called gastroesophageal reflux disease (GERD). A burning sensation radiating up through the middle of the chest behind the sternum (breastbone) characterizes heartburn, which can be aggravated by a variety of foods; alcohol; emotions such as anger, fear, or stress; and even particular positions such as reclining, lifting, or bending forward. Abdominal exercises, girdles, and tight belts can increase abdominal pressure and trigger reflux. Many women experience heartburn during pregnancy, especially in the later stages. Overweight people and smokers are also commonly affected.

Common foods and beverages implicated in acid reflux disease include coffee, tea, cocoa, cola drinks, mints, chocolate, fried and fatty foods, onions, garlic, citrus fruits, tomato products, and spicy foods. This list is not exhaustive, and certain people may be troubled by substances not included. Medications can exacerbate heartburn and reflux, including, but not limited to, oral contraceptives; aspirin; medications used to treat asthma, rheumatoid arthritis, and osteoporosis; antidepressants; and tranquilizers. Additionally, medical conditions such as asthma, diabetes, peptic ulcers, and some cancers may contribute to acid reflux disease, as can treatments such as chemotherapy or narcotic use for pain management.

The lower esophageal sphincter (LES), which connects the esophagus to the stomach, acts as a barrier to protect the esophagus from the backflow of acid from the stomach. Normally, it works like a dam, opening to allow food to pass into the stomach and closing to prevent food and acid from flowing back into the esophagus. If the sphincter weakens or relaxes, the contents of the stomach flow up into the esophagus. The reason for this occurrence is uncertain, but it is known that sphincter function can be impaired by diet, medications, and nervous system factors. Other factors that can also contribute to acid reflux disease include impaired stomach motility or an inability of the stomach muscles to contract normally, resulting in a delayed emptying of the contents. The acid remains at the top of the stomach near the LES rather than moving downward, creating pressure and reflux. Failure of contractions to clear the acid or a shortage of saliva to neutralize the acid may also contribute to heartburn.

Information on Acid Reflux Disease

Causes: Relaxation of the lower esophageal sphincter, allowing gastric acid into the esophagus; aggravated by some foods, alcohol, some medications, stress, certain positions, late-stage pregnancy
Symptoms: Burning sensation in chest and throat
Duration: Chronic, with acute episodes
Treatments: Diet and lifestyle changes (smaller meals, avoidance of some foods, etc.), antacids, histamine blockers, acid-pump inhibitors, surgery

Hiatal hernia, a condition in which a portion of the stomach protrudes into the chest cavity through an opening (hiatus) in the diaphragm (the muscle separating the chest and abdomen), exists to some degree in about 30 percent of Americans. In cases of hiatal hernias so large that they risk strangulation (becoming twisted and cutting off blood supply), complicated by severe GERD or esophagitis, surgery may be performed. Otherwise, medication in the form of a histamine blocker, which suppresses the secretion of stomach acids, is used.

Treatment and Therapy

Medical tests often used to evaluate the presence and severity of acid reflux disease include barium studies and upper endoscopy. Other tests performed less frequently include pH monitoring (to measure reflux over a twenty-four-hour period), the Bernstein test, and esophageal manometry. In the Bernstein test, which is used to evaluate the cause of chest pain after heart problems have been ruled out, saline and diluted hydrochloric acid are infused into the esophagus. If this reproduces the patient's symptoms, it can be inferred that reflux is the cause. Esophageal manometry measures pressure in the esophagus and LES.

Counseling patients to modify their diet and lifestyle is the basic treatment for reflux symptoms. Generally, patients should eat smaller meals more often and more slowly, avoiding spicy foods and those that increase acid production. They should not have bedtime snacks. Patients should relax both while eating and between meals. They should remain upright after eating and should not bend, strain, or lift for the following three hours. Those who are overweight should lose excess pounds, and patients should not smoke or chew gum. They should exercise on an empty stomach and avoid tight, constricting clothing, which may put pressure on the stomach. Patients with GERD should elevate the head of their beds by placing blocks under the bed's legs.

Over-the-counter antacids (Tums, Rolaids, and Mylanta, for example) can be effective in reducing or neutralizing acid in mild cases of heartburn. In chronic cases, however, histamine blockers may be prescribed. These medications act directly on the acid-secreting cells in the stomach to stop them from producing hydrochloric acid that can wash into the esophagus. Several of these medications (Tagamet, Zantac, and Pepcid) are available over the counter. Prokinetics or gastrokinetics are a group of medications that increase the speed at which the stomach empties food, acid, and fluids. In severe cases of GERD, they may be used instead of histamine blockers. Another class of medication is the proton-pump inhibitor or acid-pump inhibitor, which suppresses acid secretion in the stomach by inactivating the enzyme responsible for acid release in the stomach. These medications include Prevacid, Aciphex, Protonix, Nexium, and Prilosec (the latter is available over the counter). Additionally, chamomile, ginger, licorice, catnip, papaya, pineapple, marshmallow root, and fennel have all been said to aid in digestion.

Approximately 95 percent of GERD cases are controlled by medication; the remainder require surgery (fundoplication) to tighten the LES. Another technique is radiofrequency ablation, which applies controlled radiofrequency energy to the LES and upper part of the stomach, causing the lining to expand slightly as the valve tightens. The Bard endoscopic suturing system places stitches on either side of the sphincter; as the physician ties the sutures together, the valve tightens.

—*Marcia J. Weiss, M.A., J.D.*

See also Gastroenterology; Gastroenterology, pediatric; Gastrointestinal disorders; Gastrointestinal system; Heartburn; Hernia; Hernia repair; Indigestion; Over-the-counter medications; Stress; Stress reduction; Vagotomy.

For Further Information:

"GERD." *MedlinePlus*, Apr. 8, 2013.
Lasalandra, Michael, and Lawrence S. Friedman. *The Sensitive Gut.* New York: Fireside, 2001.
Rosenthal, M. Sara. *Fifty Ways to Relieve Heartburn, Reflux, and Ulcers.* Chicago: Contemporary Books, 2001.
Sachar, David B., Jerome D. Waye, and Blair S. Lewis, eds. *Pocket Guide to Gastroenterology.* Baltimore: Williams & Wilkins, 1991.
Udall, Kate Gilbert. *Managing Acid Reflux.* Orem, Utah: Woodland, 2007.
Wood, Debra, and Daus Mahnke. "Heartburn-Overview." *Health Library*, Sept. 27, 2012.

Acidosis

Disease/Disorder
Also known as: Acidemia
Anatomy or system affected: Brain, gastrointestinal system, heart, intestines, muscles, respiratory system
Specialties and related fields: Alternative medicine, anesthesiology, biochemistry, critical care, emergency medicine, environmental health, exercise physiology, gastroenterology, hematology, internal medicine, nursing, occupational health, osteopathic medicine, pharmacology, preventive medicine, sports medicine, toxicology, vascular medicine
Definition: A state of excess acidity in the body's fluids; metabolic acidosis involves the kidneys, while respiratory acidosis involves the lungs.
Key terms:

acid-base balance: the ratio of carbonic acid to base bicarbonate, with a pH between 7.35 and 7.45
acids: water-soluble compounds with a pH between 0 and 6.9 that contain hydrogen and can donate hydrogen ions (protons) to other substances
bases: water-soluble compounds with a pH between 7.1

and 14.0 that contain a hydroxyl group and can accept hydrogen ions (protons) from acids; can combine with acids to form salts and water and turns litmus blue

bicarbonate: an incompletely neutralized carbonic acid lacking one hydrogen atom

buffer: in this context, a substance that maintains the proper pH ratio of carbonic acid to base bicarbonate

ion: an atom with a positive or negative electrical charge

metabolize: to break down carbohydrates, fats, and proteins for energy or repair while eliminating wastes

oxidation-reduction: the transfer of electron(s) from one now-positive substance (oxidation) to one now-negative (reduction)

pH: standing for p(otential of) H(ydrogen), a measure of the balance between acid-forming, positively charged ions and alkaline-forming, negatively charged ions; a pH of 7.0 is neutral, anything less is acid, and anything greater is alkaline (normal pH for body fluids is slightly alkaline at 7.35 to 7.45)

Causes and Symptoms

Acidosis is a state of excess acidity in the body's fluids. For metabolism to function normally and oxygen to be delivered properly to tissues and organs, blood pH must remain within a narrow, slightly alkaline range between 7.35 and 7.45. Acids and bases (alkalies) in bodily fluids kindle the chemical reactions that support living. The organs that largely regulate the acid-base balance are the kidneys and lungs.

Acidosis arises from either a decrease of base bicarbonate (bicarbonate combined with such minerals as calcium, magnesium, or phosphorous-a base) or an increase of carbonic acid (combined carbon dioxide and water-an acid). Medicine recognizes both metabolic and respiratory acidosis, although clinically the two are often intertwined. Metabolic acidosis involves the kidneys, which metabolize, neutralize, or excrete any acid but carbon dioxide. Respiratory acidosis involves the ability of the lungs to exhale carbon dioxide, which is a gas but readily combines with water to form carbonic acid. Acidosis can be verified through an analysis of arterial blood gases.

Metabolic acidosis occurs when metabolism is impaired, sometimes by ingestion of a substance that exceeds the capacity of the kidneys to buffer. Acidifying ingestibles include wood alcohol (methanol), antifreeze (ethylene glycol), and salicylates such as aspirin in large doses. Certain infections can cause metabolic acidosis. Poorly controlled type 1 diabetes mellitus causes metabolic acidosis when inadequate insulin levels enable ketone bodies from fat breakdown to acidify the blood. When overexertion exceeds the ability of the blood to supply muscles, lactic acid is produced; the same thing occurs when poor blood supply exceeds normal oxidative metabolism. To remedy acidic blood, the body leeches buffering minerals such as calcium, magnesium, sodium, and potassium from organs and bones.

Respiratory acidosis occurs when the lungs cannot expel enough carbon dioxide. It is often caused by diseases such as emphysema, chronic bronchitis, advanced pneumonia,

> ## Information on Acidosis
> **Causes:** Excess acid in blood (metabolic type); excess carbon dioxide in lungs (respiratory type)
> **Symptoms:** Range from none in mild cases to nausea, vomiting, and fatigue with deeper and faster breathing (metabolic type); headache and drowsiness with slowed breathing (respiratory type)
> **Duration:** Acute or chronic
> **Treatments:** Dependent on cause; buffer the acidifying agent to regain normal pH (metabolic type); improve or mechanically augment lung function (respiratory type)

pulmonary edema, or asthma, all of which damage the lungs or bronchi. It can also occur with diseases of the nerves or muscles that move the chest or diaphragm. Apnea that interrupts sleep breathing or hyperventilation can cause respiratory acidosis. It can also result from oversedation with narcotic opioids or strong sedatives that slow breathing. In cardiac arrest, metabolic and respiratory acidoses are concurrent.

Acidosis can be chronic or acute. Its symptoms can range from unnoticed to vague and unspecific to disturbing or life-threatening. Because their causes differ, metabolic and respiratory acidosis also vary in their symptoms. Symptoms of metabolic acidosis include nausea, vomiting, and fatigue from blood-borne acids and a tendency (which may be absent in infants) to breathe quickly and deeply as the body attempts to expel more carbon dioxide. Respiratory acidosis can cause headache, confusion, and breathing that is shallow, slow, or both in the effort to expel carbon dioxide.

Treatment and Therapy

Metabolic acidosis is treated by determining the cause and correcting the imbalance. The acidic substance in the blood must be removed or buffered, although this may prove difficult. Treatments vary for metabolic acidosis caused by kidney disease, shock, cancer, poisoning, diabetes, and cardiac arrest. In mild cases, acidosis may be corrected by giving intravenous fluids. In severe cases, bicarbonate can be given intravenously. This provides only temporary relief, however, and may create further problems with excessive sodium.

Respiratory acidosis is generally controlled by improving lung function. Diseases such as asthma or emphysema may respond to bronchodilators, which open the airways. Children under five years of age may develop simultaneous metabolic and respiratory acidosis from salicylate poisoning; vomiting can then be induced with ipecac syrup. Whenever breathing is impaired sufficiently to prevent the exchange of carbon dioxide and oxygen, mechanical ventilation may be required.

Perspective and Prospects

Properly functioning bodily processes require oxygen. The more acidic the blood, however, the less oxygen it can carry. The simple process of living produces quantities of metabolic and respiratory acids that, in health, the body continually and silently buffers. In the Western world, people further challenge the acid-base balance through diet, with animal products such as meat, eggs, and dairy as well as with processed foods such as white four and sugar and beverages such as coffee and soft drinks. Many common drugs are acid-forming, as are artificial sweeteners. As long as they function normally, the lungs and kidneys oppose the tendencies of bodily fluids to exceed normal pH parameters. Having healthy lung and kidney function, and avoiding or balancing acid in the diet, can help maintain optimal internal chemistry.

—Jackie Dial, Ph.D.

See also Acid-base chemistry; Fluids and electrolytes; Metabolism; Respiration.

For Further Information:

"Acidosis." *MedlinePlus*, Mar. 22, 2013.

Gennari, F. John, et al., eds. *Acid-Base Disorders and Their Treatment*. Boca Raton, Fla.: Taylor & Francis, 2005.

Hogan, Mary Ann, et al. *Fluids, Electrolytes, and Acid-Base Balance*. 2d ed. Upper Saddle River, N.J.: Pearson/Prentice Hall, 2007.

Lewis, James L., III. "Acidosis." In *The Merck Manual Home Health Handbook: Third Home Edition*, edited by Robert S. Porter. Whitehouse Station, N.J.: Merck Research Laboratories, 2009.

"Metabolic Acidosis." *MedlinePlus*, Mar. 22, 2013.

"Respiratory Acidosis." *MedlinePlus*, Mar. 22, 2013.

Acne

Disease/Disorder

Anatomy or system affected: Skin

Specialties and related fields: Dermatology, family medicine, pediatrics

Definition: A group of skin disorders, the most common of which, acne vulgaris, usually affects teenagers; another form, acne rosacea, usually afflicts older people.

Key terms:

acne rosacea: a skin eruption that usually appears between the ages of thirty and fifty; unlike acne vulgaris, it is not characterized by comedones

acne vulgaris: a skin eruption that usually occurs in puberty and is characterized by the development of comedones, which may be inflamed

comedo (pl. comedos, comedones): the major lesion in acne vulgaris; it occurs when a hair follicle fills with keratin, sebum, and other matter, and may become infected

pilosebaceous: referring to hair follicles and the sebaceous glands

sebaceous glands: glands in the skin that usually open into the hair follicles

sebum: a semifluid, fatty substance secreted by the sebaceous glands into the hair follicles

testosterone: the most potent male hormone, which exists in both sexes; it starts the chain of events that leads to acne vulgaris

Causes and Symptoms

Many skin disorders are grouped together as acne. The two most common are acne vulgaris and acne rosacea. Other acne diseases include neonatal acne and infantile acne, seen respectively in newborn babies and infants. Drug acne is a consequence of the administration of such medications as corticosteroids, iodides, bromides, anticonvulsants, lithium preparations, and oral contraceptives, to name some of the more common agents that are sometimes involved in acne outbreaks. Pomade acne and acne cosmetica are associated with the use of greasy or sensitizing substances on the skin, such as hair oil, suntan lotions, cosmetics, soap, and shampoo. They may be the sole cause of acne in some individuals or may aggravate existing outbreaks of acne vulgaris. Occupational acne, as the name implies, is associated with exposure to skin irritants in the workplace. Chemicals, waxes, greases, and other substances may be involved. Acné excoriée des jeunes filles, or acne in young girls, is thought to be associated with emotional distress. In spite of the name, it can occur in boys as well. Two forms of acne are seen in young women. One is pyoderma faciale, a skin eruption that always occurs on the face. The other is perioral dermatitis (*peri*, around; *ora*, the mouth), characterized by redness, pimples, and pustules. Acne conglobata is a rare but severe skin disorder that is seen in men between the ages of eighteen and thirty.

In acne vulgaris, a disruption occurs in the normal activity of the pilosebaceous units of the dermis, the layer of the skin that contains the blood vessels, nerves and nerve endings, glands, and hair follicles. Ordinarily, the sebaceous glands secrete sebum into the hair follicles, where it travels up hair shafts and onto the outer surface of the skin, to maintain proper hydration of the hair and skin and prevent loss of moisture. In acne vulgaris, the amount of sebum increases greatly, and the hair shaft that allows it to escape becomes plugged, holding in the sebum.

Acne vulgaris usually occurs during puberty and is the result of some of the hormones released at that time to help the child become an adult. One of the major hormones is testosterone, an androgen (*andros*, man or manhood; *gen*, generating or causing), so called because it brings about bodily changes that convert a boy into a man. In boys, testosterone and other male hormones cause sexual organs to mature. Hair begins to grow on the chest and face and in pubic areas and armpits. Musculature is increased, and the larynx (voice box) is enlarged, so the voice deepens. In males, testosterone and other male hormones are produced primarily in the testicles. In girls, estrogens and other female hormones are released during puberty, directing the passage of the child from girlhood to womanhood. Testosterone is also produced, mostly in the ovaries and the adrenal glands.

In both sexes during puberty, testosterone is taken up by the pilosebaceous glands and converted to dihydrotestosterone, a substance that causes an increase in the size of the glands and increased secretion of the fatty substance sebum into hair follicles. At the same time, a process occurs that closes off the hair follicle, allowing sebum, keratin, and other matter to collect. This process is called intrafollicular hyperkeratosis (from *intra*, inside, *follicular*, referring to the follicle, *hyper*, excessive, and *keratosis*, production of keratin). Keratin buildup creates a plug that blocks the follicle opening and permits the accumulation of sebum, causing the formation of a closed comedo. As more and more material collects, the comedo becomes visible as a white-capped pimple, or whitehead. Closed comedones are the precursors of the papules, pustules, nodules, and cysts characteristic of acne vulgaris. *Papula* means "pimple," a pustule is a pimple containing pus, *nodus* means a small knot, and the word "cyst" comes from *kystis*, meaning "bladder," or in this case a sac filled with semisolid material. Sometimes cysts are referred to generically as sebaceous cysts, but the material inside is usually keratin.

Another lesion in acne vulgaris, called an open comedo, occurs when a sac in the outer layer of the skin fills with keratin, sebum, and other matter. Unlike the closed comedo, it is open to the surface of the skin and the material inside appears black-hence the term "blackhead." Blackheads are unsightly, make the skin look dirty, and suggest that they are caused by bad hygienic habits. This is not true, but exactly why the material in the sac turns black is not fully understood. Some believe that the natural skin pigment melanin is involved.

Blackheads are usually easily managed and rarely become inflamed. It is the closed comedo, or whitehead, that causes the disfiguring lesions of acne vulgaris. As the closed comedo fills with keratin and sebum, colonies of bacteria, usually *Propionibacterium acnes*, develop at the site. The bacteria secrete enzymes that break down the sebum, forming free fatty acids that inflame and irritate the follicle wall. With inflammation, white blood cells are drawn to the area to fight off the bacteria.

The comedo enlarges with further accumulation of white blood cells, keratin, and sebum until the follicle wall ruptures, spreading inflammation. If the inflammation is close to the surface of the skin, the lesion will usually be a pustule. If the inflammation is deeper, a larger papule, nodule, or cyst may form.

Clothing, cosmetics, and other factors may exacerbate acne vulgaris. Headbands, chin straps, and other items can cause trauma that ruptures closed comedones and spreads infection. Ingredients in cosmetics, soaps, and other preparations used on the skin can contribute to the formation of comedones in acne vulgaris. Lanolin, petrolatum, laurel alcohol, and oleic acid are among the chemicals commonly found in skin creams, cosmetics, soaps, shampoos, and other preparations applied to the skin. They have been shown to aggravate existing acne in some people and to bring on acne eruptions in others.

It was long thought that fatty foods-such as chocolate, ice cream, desserts, and peanut butter-contributed to acne, perhaps because teenagers eat so much of them. This theory has been largely discarded. Except for specific allergic sensitivities, foods do not appear to cause or in any other way affect the eruptions of acne vulgaris.

Cases of acne vulgaris are classified as mild, moderate, or severe. In mild and moderate acne vulgaris, the number of lesions ranges from a few to many, appearing regularly or sporadically and occurring mostly in the top layer of the skin. Consequently, these cases are sometimes called "su-

---

Information on Acne

Causes: Medications, greasy substances or irritants, hormones

Symptoms: Skin lesions, inflammation

Duration: Often chronic

Treatments: Drying agents (resorcinol, salicylic acid, sulfur); vitamin A acid (Retin A, tretinoin); topical antibiotics (benzoyl peroxide, tetracycline, clindamycin, erythromycin); oral antibiotics (tetracycline)

---

perficial acne." In severe cases, the acne lesions are deep, extending down into the skin, and characterized by inflamed papules and pustules.

Superficial acne, or mild-to-moderate acne vulgaris, is easily managed with the therapies available. The teenager goes through a year to two dealing with "zits." The problem may be irritating and may cause inconvenience and discomfort, but it is common among teenagers, and little lasting harm is done. With time and treatment, the skin clears and the problem is over.

With deep or severe acne, however, the condition can be devastating, physically and psychologically. In these cases, the lesions may come in massive eruptions that cover the face and extend to the neck, chest, and back. The lesions can be large and deep, frequently causing disfiguring pits and craters that become lifelong scars. The victims of severe acne can suffer profound psychological damage. The disease strikes at a time when most teenagers are especially concerned with being gregarious, popular, and well liked. The chronic, constant disfigurement effectively isolates the individual, however, often making him or her unwilling to risk social contact.

The other common form of acne is acne rosacea, so called because of the "rosy" color that appears on the face. Unlike acne vulgaris, it rarely strikes people under thirty years of age and is not characterized by comedones, although papules and pustules are common. It is predominantly seen in women, although its most serious manifestations are seen in men. The cause of acne rosacea is unknown, but it is more likely to strike people with fair complexions. It is usually limited to the center of the face, but eruptions may occur on other parts of the body.

Acne rosacea is progressive; that is, it gets worse as the patient grows older. It seems to occur most often in people who have a tendency to redden or blush easily. The blushing, whether it is caused by emotional distress, such as shame or embarrassment, or by heat, food, or drink, may be the precursor of acne rosacea. The individual finds that episodes of blushing last longer and longer until, eventually, the redness becomes permanent. Papules and pustules break out, and surface blood vessels become dilated, causing further redness. As the disease progresses, tissue overgrowth may cause the nose to swell and become red and bulbous. Inflammation may develop in and around the eyes and threaten vision. These severe symptoms occur more often in men than in women.

Treatment and Therapy

The majority of acne patients are treated at home with over-the-counter preparations applied topically (that is, on the skin). For years, many of the agents recommended for acne contained sulfur, and some still do. Sulfur is useful for reducing comedones, but it has been suggested that sulfur by itself may also cause comedones; however, sulfur compounds, such as zinc sulfate, are not suspected of causing comedones. Resorcinol and salicylic acid are commonly included in topical over-the-counter preparations to promote scaling and reduce comedones. Sometimes sulfur, resorcinol, and salicylic acid are used singly, sometimes together, and sometimes combined with topical antiseptics or other agents.

While most patients will be helped by the available over-the-counter agents, many will not respond adequately to such home therapy. These patients must be seen by a doctor, such as a family practitioner or dermatologist. The physician attempts to eliminate existing lesions, prevent the formation of new lesions, destroy microorganisms, relieve inflammation, and prevent the occurrence of cysts, papules, and pustules. If the patient's skin is oily, the physician may advise washing the face and other affected areas several times a day. This has little effect on the development of comedones, but it may improve the patient's appearance and self-esteem. The physician will also use medications that are similar to over-the-counter antiacne agents but more powerful. These include drying agents, topical antibiotic preparations, and agents to abrade the skin, such as exfoliants or desquamating (scale-removing) agents.

Various topical antibiotics have been developed for use in acne vulgaris, such as topical tetracycline, clindamycin, and erythromycin. One that is often used is benzoyl peroxide, a topical antibiotic that can penetrate the skin and reach the sites of infection in the hair follicles. It is also a powerful irritant that increases the growth rate of epithelial cells and promotes sloughing, which helps clear the surface of the skin. It is effective in resolving comedones and seems to suppress the release of sebum. Because it has a high potential for skin irritation, benzoyl peroxide must be used carefully. Physicians generally start with the weaker formulations of the drug and increase the strength as tolerance develops.

Vitamin A has been given orally to patients with acne vulgaris in the hope of preventing the formation of comedones. The effective oral dose of the vitamin for this purpose is so high, however, that it could be toxic. Therefore, a topical form of vitamin A was developed called vitamin A acid, retinoic acid, or tretinoin (marketed as Retin A). Applied directly to the skin, it has proved highly beneficial in the treatment of acne vulgaris. It clears comedones from the hair follicles and suppresses the formation of new comedones. It reduces inflammation and facilitates the transdermal (through-the-skin) penetration of medications such as benzoyl peroxide and other topical antibiotics. Like benzoyl peroxide, vitamin A acid can be irritating to the skin, so it must be used carefully. When benzoyl peroxide and vitamin A acid are used in combination in the treatment

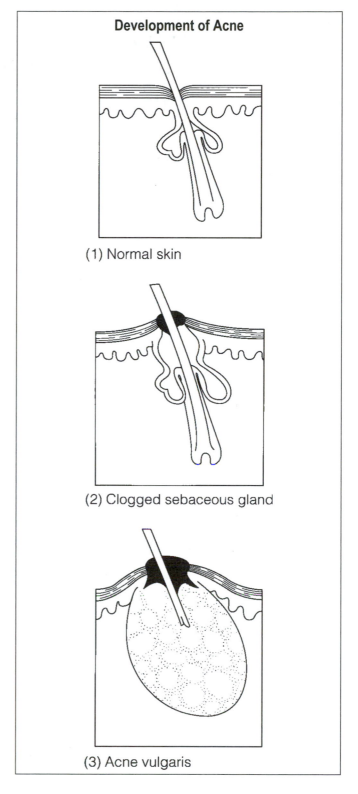

Development of Acne

(1) Normal skin

(2) Clogged sebaceous gland

(3) Acne vulgaris

of acne vulgaris, their therapeutic effectiveness is significantly increased. The physician generally prescribes a morning application of one and an evening application of the other.

When large comedones, pustules, or cysts form, the physician may elect to remove them surgically. The procedure is quite effective in improving appearance, but it does nothing to affect the course of the disease. Furthermore, it demands great skill on the part of the physician to avoid causing damage and irritating the surrounding skin, rupturing the comedo wall, and allowing inflammation to spread. The patient should be advised not to try to duplicate the process at home: Picking at pimples could create open lesions that may take weeks to heal and may produce deep scars. Sometimes, the physician will insert a needle into a deep lesion in order to drain the material from it. Sometimes, the physician tries to avoid surgery by injecting a minute quantity of corticosteroid, such as triamcinolone acetonide, into a deep lesion to reduce its size.

The physician may wish to add the benefits of sunlight to medical therapy. Sunlight helps dry the skin and promotes scaling and clearing of the skin, which is probably why acne improves in summer. The physician may suggest sunbathing, but an overzealous patient could become sunburned or chronically overexposed to the sun, thereby risking skin cancer. The beneficial effects of natural sunlight are not necessarily achievable with a sunlamp and, over a long period of exposure, the ultraviolet light produced by some lamps may actually increase sebum production and promote intrafollicular hyperkeratosis.

About 12 percent of patients with acne vulgaris develop severe or deep acne. In devising a treatment regime for these cases, the physician has many options to help clear the patient's skin, reduce the number and occurrence of lesions, and prevent the scarring that can disfigure the patient for life. Both the topical medications benzoyl peroxide and vitamin A acid are used, singly and in combination, as well as many other topical preparations. Nevertheless, these patients often also require oral antibiotics to fight their infection from within.

It may take weeks for oral antibiotic therapy to achieve results, and it may even be necessary for the patient to continue the therapy for years. Therefore, the physician looks for an antibiotic that is effective and safe for long-term use. Oral tetracycline is often the physician's choice because it has been proven effective against *Propionibacterium acnes*, and it seems to suppress the formation of comedones. Oral tetracycline is usually safe for long-term therapy, and it is economical. Other oral antibiotics used to treat acne vulgaris are erythromycin, clindamycin, and minocycline.

Yet in long-term therapy with any broad-spectrum antibiotic, there is always the possibility that the agent being used will not only kill the offending organism but also destroy "friendly" bacteria that aid in bodily processes and help protect the body from other microorganisms. When this happens, disease-causing pathogens may be allowed to flourish and cause infection. For example, prolonged use of antibiotics in women may allow the growth of a yeastlike

---

In the News:
Registry for Women Using Accutane

On March 1, 2006, the Food and Drug Administration (FDA) started iPLEDGE, a mandatory registry designed to control use of the powerful acne medicine isotretinoin, sold under the brand names Accutane, Amnestreem, Claravis, and Sotret. The registry had been recommended by FDA advisory committees in 2000 and 2004 to help prevent birth defects in children born to women using isotretinoin and to collect information on the incidence of suicide among users. The manufacturer of Accutane, Roche Pharmaceuticals, had always strongly warned women of the dangers that use during pregnancy posed for developing fetuses. Even so, Roche reported that between 1982, when the FDA first approved sale of isotretinoin, and 2000 there had been 383 live births among women taking the drug; 162 infants (42 percent) were born with brain or heart defects or mental retardation. (In June, 2009, Roche stopped selling Accutane in the United States, but the generic version is still available.)

Women who plan to become pregnant and who seek a prescription for isotretinoin must register with iPLEDGE and must submit two negative pregnancy tests before receiving a prescription; they also must be tested before each monthly refill, and they must agree to take two forms of birth control while using the drug—or else promise to abstain from sex for one month before treatment, while under treatment, and for one month afterward. Women have to sign a document acknowledging that they understand isotretinoin increases the risk of birth defects, depression, and suicide. Men desiring the drug are required to sign the document as well, to ensure that they knew why they should not share pills with women. Physicians prescribing isotretinoin and wholesalers and pharmacists who distribute it are also required to register with iPLEDGE and to agree to enforce the restrictions.

Many dermatologists are uncomfortable with the iPLEDGE regulations. They consider isotretinoin indispensable in treating severe cases of acne resistant to less powerful medications and fear that onerous conditions for access to the drug might discourage patients.

—*Milton Berman, Ph.D.*

---

fungus, *Candida*, which can cause vaginitis. Prolonged use of clindamycin may allow the proliferation of *Clostridium difficile*, which could result in ulcerative colitis, a severe disorder of the lower gastrointestinal tract.

If, for any reason, the physician believes that oral antibiotics are not working or must be discontinued, there are other therapeutic agents and other procedures that may be helpful in treating severe, deep acne vulgaris. One medication that is highly effective, but also potentially very harmful, is isotretinoin. As the name implies, isotretinoin (meaning "similar to tretinoin") is derived from vitamin A, but it is both more effective and more difficult to use. Unlike the topical vitamin A acid preparations, isotretinoin is taken orally. It is highly effective in inhibiting the function of sebaceous glands and preventing the formation of closed comedones by reducing keratinization, but isotretinoin also produces a wide range of side effects. The majority of these are skin disorders, but the bones and joints, the eyes, and other organs can be affected. Perhaps the most serious adverse effect of isotretinoin is that it can cause severe abnormalities in the fetuses of pregnant women. Therefore, pregnancy is an absolute contraindication for isotretinoin. Before they take this drug, women of childbearing age are checked to ensure that they are not pregnant. They are advised to use strict contraceptive measures one month before therapy, during the entire course of therapy, and for at least one month after therapy has been discontinued.

Estrogens, female hormones, have been used to treat severe acne in girls and women who are more than sixteen years of age. The aim of this therapy is to counteract the sebum-stimulating activity of circulating testosterone and to reduce the formation of comedones by reducing the amount of sebum produced. Estrogens cannot be used in males because the dose required to reduce sebum production could produce feminizing side effects.

Persistent lesions can be treated with cryotherapy. In this procedure, an extremely cold substance such as dry ice or liquid nitrogen is carefully applied to the lesion. This technique is effective in reducing both small pustules and deeper cysts. For patients whose skin has been deeply scarred by acne, a procedure called dermabrasion, in which the top layer of skin is removed, may help improve the appearance.

Although its cause is unknown, acne rosacea can be treated. The topical antiparasitic drug metronidazole, applied in a cream, and oral broad-spectrum antibiotics such as tetracycline have been found effective. It may be necessary to continue antibiotic therapy for a long period of time, but the treatment is usually effective. Surgery may be required to correct the bulbous nose that sometimes occurs with this condition.

Perspective and Prospects

Most acne vulgaris (about 60 percent) is treated at home. There has been significant improvement in the treatment of mild-to-moderate acne vulgaris, so for most of these patients, the condition can be limited to an annoyance or an inconvenience of the teen years. Only recalcitrant cases of acne vulgaris are seen by physicians. Of those cases treated by doctors, the majority are seen by family physicians, general practitioners, and other primary care workers. Severe acne is usually referred to the dermatologist, who is skilled in the use of the more serious medications and the more exacting techniques that are required in treatment.

For at least 85 percent of those experiencing puberty, acne vulgaris is a fact of life. It is a natural consequence of the hormonal changes that occur at this time. It is not likely that any drugs or techniques will be found to avoid acne in the teenage years, as this would involve tampering with a fundamental growth process. It can be expected, however, that in this condition, as in so many others, progress will continue to be made, and newer, more effective, and safer agents will be developed.

—C. Richard Falcon

See also Abscesses; Blisters; Boils; Cysts; Dermatology; Puberty and adolescence; Rosacea; Skin disorders.

For Further Information:

"Acne." *MedlinePlus*, Mar. 27, 2013.

Ceaser, Jennifer. *Everything You Need to Know About Acne*. Rev. ed. New York: Rosen, 2003.

Chu, Anthony C., and Anne Lovell. *The Good Skin Doctor: A Leading Dermatologist's Guide to Beating Acne*. New York: HarperCollins, 1999.

Goldberg, David J. *Acne and Rosacea: Epidemiology, Diagnosis, and Treatment*. London: Manson, 2012.

Hellwig, Jennifer, and Purvee S. Shah. "Acne." *Health Library*, Sept. 10, 2012.

Litin, Scott C., ed. *Mayo Clinic Family Health Book*. 4th ed. New York: HarperResource, 2009.

Parker, James N., and Philip M. Parker, eds. *The Official Patient's Sourcebook on Acne Rosacea*. San Diego, Calif.: Icon Health, 2002.

Webster, Guy F., and Anthony V. Rawlings, eds. *Acne and Its Therapy*. New York: Informa Healthcare, 2007.

Acquired immunodeficiency syndrome (AIDS)

Disease/Disorder

Anatomy or system affected: Blood, brain, eyes, gastrointestinal system, immune system, intestines, liver, lungs, lymphatic system, mouth, psychic-emotional system, reproductive system, respiratory system, skin, throat

Specialties and related fields: Bacteriology, dermatology, epidemiology, gastroenterology, gynecology, hematology, immunology, internal medicine, microbiology, neurology, oncology, ophthalmology, osteopathic medicine, otorhinolaryngology, pathology, pharmacology, proctology, psychiatry, public health, pulmonary medicine, virology

Definition: A disease state caused by infection with human immunodeficiency virus (HIV), leading to a progressive deterioration of the immune system and characterized by development of any of a large number of opportunistic infections.

Key terms:

highly active antiretroviral therapy (HAART): the use of a combination of three or four anti-HIV drugs in an HIV-positive individual to suppress replication of new HIV particles and slow the progression to full-blown AIDS

Kaposi's sarcoma: a form of blood vessel tumor that produces pink to purple splotches or plaques on the skin in about 25 percent of persons with AIDS and may also affect internal organs; caused by sexual transmission of human herpes virus 8 (HHV8)

lentivirus: a classification of retroviruses characterized by a very long incubation period (ten to twenty years) before symptoms of a disease appear

opportunistic infection: an infection caused by any type of pathogen in individuals who have an impaired immune system

Pneumocystis pneumonia: a form of pneumonia caused by the fungus *Pneumocystis carinii* and commonly seen in persons with AIDS

protease inhibitors: any of a number of drugs that inhibit the assembly of HIV

retrovirus: a virus with ribonucleic acid (RNA) as its genetic material that produces a deoxyribonucleic acid (DNA) copy of the RNA to be integrated into a chromosome of the host cell, from which it will make new infectious copies of the RNA during the viral life cycle

seroconversion: the detection of anti-HIV antibodies in the blood of an HIV-infected person, who is then said to be HIV-positive

syndrome: a collection of symptoms associated with a particular disease state; an individual patient may show some, but not necessarily all, of these symptoms

T4 cells: also called CD4 cells or T-helper cells; a specific type of white blood cell (lymphocyte) which regulates the entire immune system and is the preferred target for HIV infection, resulting in immunodeficiency

viral load: a measurement of the amount of HIV present in the blood; often used to monitor the effectiveness of anti-HIV therapy

Causes and Symptoms

Acquired immunodeficiency syndrome (AIDS) is caused by the human immunodeficiency virus (HIV), a member of the lentivirus family of retroviruses. This virus is thought to have arisen in Africa in the early to mid-twentieth century from related viruses in the chimpanzee and the sooty mangabey monkey. The virus cannot survive long in the air and cannot be transmitted by casual contact. Individuals can be infected only by the exchange of certain body fluids, including semen, vaginal fluid, blood, and human milk. Other body fluids such as sweat, tears, saliva, urine, and feces may contain HIV, but the virus exists in such low concentrations that these fluids are completely ineffective in transmitting an infection. The most common mode of transmission is through sexual contact in which semen or vaginal fluid is exchanged. The presence of another sexually transmitted disease (STD), such as gonorrhea, syphilis, chlamydia, genital herpes, or human papillomavirus, increases dramatically the risk of acquiring an HIV infection through sexual contact.

The second most common mode of transmission is through the sharing of needles contaminated with HIV-positive blood by intravenous (IV) drug users. A pregnant HIV-positive woman may transmit the virus to her child in utero, or more commonly during childbirth. Mother-to-child transmission may also occur through breast-feeding in which the virus is present in the milk. Early in the AIDS epidemic and before a blood test for HIV was available, blood and blood products from blood banks were sometimes contaminated with HIV that subsequently infected recipients. Indeed, more than 90 percent of hemophiliacs became HIV-positive through injections of HIV-contaminated clotting factor VIII. Because of the development of a heat treatment for clotting factor VIII and the screening of the blood supply, hemophiliacs are no longer at high risk for HIV infection. Although the blood supply is relatively safe today, a very low probability of acquiring HIV through a transfusion of contaminated blood still exists, as a recently infected donor may not yet test positive for HIV.

Although HIV can infect virtually all cells of the body, it has a strong affinity for cells of the immune system. The virus uses a cell surface receptor called CD4 to bind to the membrane of a cell. The CD4 receptor is found on many cells in the body but is in relatively high concentrations on the surface of a class of T lymphocytes called T4 or CD4 cells. The virus uses a coreceptor called CXCKR4, also found on the membrane, that promotes the fusion of the membrane of the virus particle with the membrane of the cell, thereby allowing entry of the virus. Persons who lack the co-receptor on their cells appear to resist infection by

---

Information on Acquired Immunodeficiency Syndrome (AIDS)

Causes: HIV infection through the exchange of certain body fluids, then destruction of T lymphocytes of the immune system

Symptoms: Initially, flulike or mononucleosis-like symptoms, then none until opportunistic infections (candidiasis, cytomegalovirus, ulcers, *Pneumocyctis carinii* pneumonia, histoplasmosis, toxoplasmosis) and cancers (Kaposi's sarcoma, Burkitt's lymphoma) become common

Duration: Chronic, eventually fatal

Treatments: Surgery, chemotherapy, and radiation for cancers; antibiotics for bacterial and fungal infections; anti-HIV drugs (nucleoside analogues, reverse transcriptase inhibitors, protease inhibitors, fusion inhibitors)

---

the virus. The T4 cells are also known as T-helper cells, as they produce a series of chemical signals called lymphokines that are needed for the development and maintenance of the entire immune system. While the body constantly makes new T4 cells, HIV has a very small edge in the rate at which these T4 cells are infected and destroyed. Thus, there is a slow but progressive decrease in T4 lymphocytes in the body and loss of immune function. This process may take ten or more years.

The clinical course of infection occurs in three stages. Initially upon infection, HIV produces an acute retroviral syndrome referred to as the prodromal stage, beginning about three to four weeks after initial infection and lasting for two to three weeks. During a retroviral syndrome, the patient experiences flulike or mononucleosis-like symptoms. The patient will believe that he or she simply has a moderate-to-severe case of influenza or, if the symptoms are prolonged, mononucleosis. During this period, HIV is rapidly proliferating, disseminating throughout the body and infecting lymphoid tissues. Viral load is high at this stage, and the patient is highly infectious. At the same time, the T4 cell count, which normally is about 1,000 per cubic millimeter, drops by about half. The patient's immune system will mount an antibody response against HIV, but these antibodies are ineffective in stopping the infection. When such antibodies are detectable, the patient is then said to have seroconverted. Anti-HIV antibody detection by a simple blood test is the basis for assigning HIV-positive status. In most cases, seroconversion occurs between six to eighteen weeks after initial infection, although, in rare cases, antibodies may not be detectable until later. By three months, 95 percent of patients will have seroconverted; by six months, more than 99 percent will have detectable circulating antibodies to HIV.

The second stage is called the clinical latency period or asymptomatic stage. Without anti-HIV therapy, this period may last ten or more years. It is during this time that the patient usually has no AIDS symptoms. Early in the latent period, T4 cell counts usually recover somewhat during the first year of infection, averaging approximately 700 per cubic millimeter. After that, there is a very slow decline. In the meantime, viral loads, which were high during the acute retroviral syndrome stage, drop by several orders of magnitude as the T4 count rises. At about one year into the infection, the viral load very slowly increases as the latent period progresses.

The third phase is full-blown AIDS. This usually occurs when the T4 count drops below 200 per cubic millimeter. Opportunistic infections and cancers become common, and patients may have several infections simultaneously. Many of these diseases are rare in healthy individuals. Most common is *Pneumocystis carinii* pneumonia, a form caused by a fungus that is virtually unseen in individuals with a normal immune system. Indeed, the fungus is present in a majority of the population yet almost never causes pneumonia unless the immune system is compromised. As one of the functions of the immune system is to destroy cancer cells when they arise, immune impairment leads to development of cancer in about 40 percent of those with AIDS. One of these cancers is Kaposi's sarcoma, a normally very rare tumor of blood vessels characterized by pink to purple spots or slightly raised areas on the skin. These lesions may also arise on internal organs, where they can impair function. Kaposi's sarcoma is caused by human herpes virus 8 (HHV8) and is sexually transmitted. It is primarily found in gay men with AIDS and not often seen in IV drug users or in girls and women with AIDS. The other cancer commonly associated with AIDS is non-Hodgkin's lymphoma, often in the brain.

In 1987, the Centers for Disease Control (CDC) published the criteria for the diagnosis of AIDS, including the appearance of one or more opportunistic infections or cancers. Twenty-three different conditions were listed in the definition: candidiasis of the bronchi, trachea, or lungs; esophageal candidiasis; disseminated or extrapulmonary coccidiomycosis; extrapulmonary cryptococcosis; chronic intestinal cryptosporidosis (greater than one month in duration); cytomegalovirus disease (other than liver, spleen, or lymph nodes); cytomegalovirus retinitis (with loss of vision); HIV encephalopathy; herpes simplex causing chronic ulcers (greater than one month in duration) or bronchitis, pneumonitis, or esophagitis; disseminated or extrapulmonary histoplasmosis; chronic intestinal isosporiasis (greater than one month in duration); Kaposi's sarcoma; Burkitt's lymphoma; immunoblastic lymphoma; primary lymphoma of the brain; *Mycobacterium avium* complex or *M. kansasii*; extrapulmonary infection due to *Mycobacterium tuberculosis*; other or unidentified *Mycobacterium* species; *Pneumocystis jiroveci* pneumonia; progressive multifocal leukoencephalopathy (PML); recurrent *Salmonella* septicemia; toxoplasmosis of the brain; and wasting syndrome caused by HIV. In 1993, three conditions were added to the criteria: pulmonary tuberculosis, recurrent pneumonia, and invasive cervical carcinoma. Moreover, the definition was expanded to include any HIV-positive person whose T4 count had dropped to 200 per cubic millimeter or lower or whose level of T4 lymphocytes had fallen to 14 percent or less of total lymphocytes.

Treatment and Therapy

As of 2013, no effective vaccine had been developed to prevent HIV infection. While a number of candidate vaccines have been under development and in clinical trials, none has proven successful. The usual strategies used with most antiviral vaccines in the past, immunization with attenuated or inactivated viruses, have so far proven ineffective for HIV given its significant rate of mutation. Control of the epidemic has shifted significantly toward preventing exposure and decreasing infectivity by treating to reduce viral load, a measure of the number of viruses in blood and in body fluids.

AIDS treatment and therapy fall into two categories: prophylaxis and treatment of opportunistic infections to slow progression to full-blown AIDS. Treatment of opportunistic infections must follow established guidelines for the individual disease. Thus, in the treatment of Kaposi's sarcoma, surgery, chemotherapy, and radiation treatment singly or in combination are utilized. Bacterial and yeast or other fungal infections are treated with antibiotics or antifungal agents. Although some medications may reduce the severity of viral infections, such infections are not easily treated. Because a person with AIDS might suffer from more than one opportunistic infection and/or cancer at the same time, simultaneous treatments often take a severe toll on the patient. The life expectancy for an individual who has progressed to full-blown AIDS is about two years. Death results from an opportunistic infection or cancer.

The second strategy for HIV treatment involves interfering with the viral life cycle with the aim of slowing viral replication. Anti-HIV drugs target several steps in the life cycle, primarily at the levels of reverse transcription or assembly. In 1987, the first generation of drugs was developed to treat HIV. The first effective treatment utilized zidovudine (ZDV), commonly called azidothymidine (AZT), a drug originally developed for chemotherapy of cancer. ZDV inhibits the viral encoded enzyme, reverse transcriptase, involved in copying the RNA viral genome into a DNA copy. As a result, a nucleoside analogue is inserted into the growing DNA, which stops further synthesis of the DNA copy. Other nucleoside analogues that have a similar effect include ddI, ddC, d4T, 3TC, emtricitabine, and abacavir. In a similar manner, the nucleotide analogue tenofovir blocks DNA replication. Nevirapine, delaviridine, and efavirenz are non-nucleoside drugs that bind directly to and inhibit reverse transcriptase. Although this group of drugs inhibits reverse transcriptase, their mode of action is different from nucleoside or nucleotide analogues.

The final step in HIV replication involves the cleavage of a large precursor protein into smaller structural proteins, an event taking place at the cell surface and followed by release of the completed virus. The cleaving enzyme is called a protease and is encoded by the virus. The second generation of anti-HIV drugs, which were developed in the 1990s, were protease inhibitors, drugs that interfere with cleavage of the precursor and prevent viral assembly. As a result, functional virions cannot be made. Saquinavir, ritonavir, indinavir, nefinavir, amprenavir, lopinavir, fosamprenavir, atazanavir, tipranavir, and darunavir are approved drugs in this class. Other types of anti-HIV drugs called fusion inhibitors (for example, enfuvirtide) interfere with entry of the virus into a cell. In addition, integrase inhibitors, a new class of drugs, have been in clinical trials. These drugs prevent the DNA copy of the virus from inserting itself into one of the cell's chromosomes. Thus the anti-HIV arsenal includes drugs that act at different sites or stages in the HIV life cycle.

The HIV reverse transcriptase makes numerous mutations during the synthesis of DNA. Consequently, resistance to individual anti-HIV drugs arises easily and frequently. Beginning in 1995, a new strategy for anti-HIV therapy called highly active antiretroviral therapy (HAART), also known as AIDS cocktail therapy, was developed. HAART consists of using a combination of three or more anti-HIV drugs, including two reverse transcriptase inhibitors and at least one protease inhibitor. HAART therapy is very effective, as it has been estimated that it prolongs the life expectancy of a person with AIDS by three to ten years. Moreover, many patients with full-blown AIDS and in terminal stages of the disease have made remarkable recoveries when placed on HAART. In many cases, viral loads were dramatically reduced, T4 cells made some recovery, and the incidence of opportunistic infections was reduced. Another advantage of multiple drug therapy is that the probability of HIV developing simultaneous resistance to three or four different drugs is very low, extending the useful therapeutic life of the individual drugs.

The long-term effectiveness of HAART is underscored by an examination of the AIDS deaths in the United States. In 1981, the CDC began to track the number of AIDS deaths. Each year, the number of deaths climbed steadily, reaching a peak of 50,610 in 1995. In 1996, the first full year of widespread HAART therapy, AIDS deaths dropped by 25 percent, and they have continued to drop every year since. In 2011, an estimated 1.7 million people died of the disease worldwide, down from approximately 2.3 milllion in 2005. While these statistics are encouraging, about half of all persons with AIDS cannot tolerate the drugs. Moreover, those taking anti-HIV drugs often experience mild-to-serious side effects.

Perspective and Prospects

AIDS was first recognized as a new disease in the United States in late 1980. Michael Gottlieb at the University of California, Los Angeles (UCLA) diagnosed gay men with *Pneumocystis carinii* pneumonia and Kaposi's sarcoma, diseases that in the past were extremely rare. In June, 1981, the CDC alerted doctors in a report on this new epidemic for the first time in the *CDC Weekly Morbidity and Mortality Report*. Shortly thereafter, the *New York Times* reported on the new "gay cancer." At first, the disease was called gay-related immunodeficiency (GRID). The name was changed to acquired immunodeficiency syndrome, or

AIDS, in an August 8, 1982, article in the *New York Times*, representing the first time that the term was used in a publication. The change reflected the fact that this new disease was not restricted to gay men; cases involving intravenous drug users, hemophiliacs, and infants were being diagnosed. In January 1983, Luc Montagnier and colleagues at the Pasteur Institute in Paris were the first to isolate the virus causing AIDS. It was given the name human immunodeficiency virus, or HIV, in 1985; previously, the virus had been given several names by different researchers. With the isolation of the virus, a blood test could be developed.

Testing of blood and blood products started in March 1985. A test called enzyme-linked immunosorbent assay (ELISA) screens for the presence of anti-HIV antibodies. Results once took weeks, but the test is now automated and is performed in less than four hours at a cost of less than ten dollars at publicly supported laboratories.

HIV has been confirmed in the United States since at least 1969. At that time, a physician in St. Louis, Missouri, had a young male patient with a variety of AIDS symptoms. After the patient died, the pathologist took samples of his tissues and froze them. Later, when tests to detect HIV became available, the tissue samples were tested and found positive for HIV. The oldest positively identified HIV sample came from blood collected from a male patient by a Belgian physician in Kinshasa, Democratic Republic of the Congo. The doctor had saved many blood samples taken between 1959 and 1982; thus, the earliest confirmation of HIV infection in Africa dates from 1959. The virus has probably been present in the human population for much longer, but without blood or tissue samples, this cannot be confirmed.

Two major classes of HIV have been identified: HIV-1, which arose in Central Africa, and HIV-2, which arose in Western Africa. HIV-1 and HIV-2 have long been known to be genetically similar to viruses know as simian immunodeficiency viruses (SIV) in chimpanzees (SIVcmp) and the sooty mangabey monkey (SIVsm). In 2006, scientists determined that in all likelihood, HIV-1 originated in chimpanzees from regions of the nation of Cameroon; as many as one-third of chimpanzees from some colonies were found to carry SIV. The first confirmed human infection was that of a man from the nearby Congo, who developed AIDS in 1959. However, evidence suggests that HIV may have emerged in humans as early as 1930.

The statistics associated with the AIDS epidemic are startling. In the United States at the end of 2007, an estimated 1.1 million persons were living with AIDS; approximately 14,000 persons died from AIDS during the year. Worldwide numbers only begin to illustrate the extent of the epidemic. The World Health Organization (WHO) estimates that in 2011, more than 2.5 million persons became infected with the virus, with nearly 2 million deaths. Over 3 million of newly infected persons are undert the age of fifteen. Nearly 34 million persons worldwide were estimated to be living with AIDS. In the absence of effective treatment, most of those persons will die, often after infecting others with the virus, and leave behind a generation of orphans.

It is hoped that several new medications in development will enlarge the arsenal of anti-HIV drugs. The success of HAART promises to extend the life of persons with AIDS by many years. Current studies are testing whether it is better to start HAART therapy early after infection or to wait until T4 counts are declining. Additional studies will determine whether the therapy may be interrupted for varying periods of time. A significant issue is the high financial burden of such therapy. A typical HAART regimen may cost $1,500 to $2,000 per month. Although many people in affluent countries can purchase these drugs through insurance providers or government subsidy, this financial burden precludes the use of HAART or indeed almost any anti-HIV drug in the developing world, where HIV prevalence is so high. Thus, effective prevention of HIV infections, through vigorous public education about HIV and AIDS, is absolutely critical. Such a program in Uganda dramatically reduced the incidence of HIV infections, showing the effectiveness of public education campaigns. In 2009, WHO reported that since the 2001 United Nations Declaration of Commitment on HIV/AIDS, treatment and education have reduced the rate of new infections by 17 percent worldwide. In 2011, the UN General Assembly adopted a new declaration, setting new targets in the global fight against HIV/AIDS.

—Ralph R. Meyer, Ph.D.;
updated by Richard Adler, Ph.D.

See also Epidemics and pandemics; Epidemiology; Gates Foundation; Human immunodeficiency virus (HIV); Immune system; Immunodeficiency disorders; Immunology; Kaposi's sarcoma; Opportunistic infections; Retroviruses; Sexually transmitted diseases (STDs); Terminally ill: Extended care; Viral infections.

For Further Information:
Behrman, Greg. *The Invisible People: How the U.S. Has Slept Through the Global AIDS Pandemic, the Greatest Humanitarian Catastrophe of Our Time.* New York: Free Press, 2004.
Cichocki, Mark. *Living with HIV: A Patient's Guide.* Jefferson, N.C.: McFarland, 2009.
Ezzell, Carol. "Hope in a Vial: Will There Be an AIDS Vaccine Anytime Soon?" *Scientific American* 186 (June, 2002): 38-45.
Fan, Hung Y., Ross F. Conner, and Luis P. Villarreal. *AIDS: Science and Society.* 5th ed. Sudbury, Mass.: Jones and Bartlett, 2007.
Friedman-Kien, Alvin, and Clay J. Cockerell. *Color Atlas of AIDS.* 2d ed. Philadelphia: Elsevier Health Sciences, 1996.
Matthews, Dawn D., ed. *AIDS Sourcebook.* 3d ed. Detroit, Mich.: Omnigraphics, 2003.
U.S. Department of Health and Human Services. *AIDSInfo,* 2013.
MedlinePlus. "HIV/AIDS." MedlinePlus, 30 Apr, 2013

Acupressure

Treatment
Also known as: Shiatsu
Anatomy or system affected: Muscles, musculoskeletal system, nervous system, skin
Specialties and related fields: Alternative medicine, preventive medicine, sports medicine
Definition: A specialized form of massage used to stimulate the body's energy pathways.

Indications and Procedures

Acupressure is an ancient Chinese procedure that uses pressure from the fingertips, knuckles, or a blunt-tipped instrument called a *tei shin* to stimulate points on the body. (The Japanese version is known as shiatsu.) The rhythmic, moderately deep massage is used to treat muscular pain, migraines, insomnia, backaches, and gastrointestinal and gynecological problems. The procedure can be performed by the patient and is beneficial for relieving chronic pain and increasing the range of motion by loosening tight muscles. Practitioners claim that acupressure can alleviate fatigue because it opens blocked energy pathways.

Uses and Complications

Acupressure works on the body's organ, glandular, and muscular systems. Like acupuncture, acupressure targets designated points on the body along lines called meridians. Meridians are not nerve pathways; rather, they correspond to energy pathways through which healthy Chi (pronounced "chee") energy flows. (Chi is comparable to the Western idea of vitality or life force.) These body points are believed to correspond to various organs and body functions. Practitioners believe that when these points are stimulated, the balance of energy in the body is restored and the

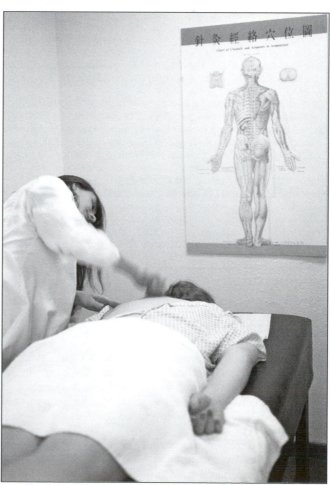

A patient receiving acupressure treatment. (PhotoDisc)

patient finds relief from physical illness or disease.

Muscle tension causes the large muscle groups to contract and so restricts the flow of Chi. The body is then out of balance, and the ability of the patient's body to heal is inhibited. Acupressure massage seeks to increase blood circulation, relieve muscle tension, and unblock energy pathways.

Practitioners of traditional Western medicine believe that acupressure stimulates the release of endorphins, the body's own chemicals that act as pain-blockers. Other benefits of acupressure have been recognized and accepted by traditional medicine. Acupressure is used in sports medicine to relieve muscle spasms and pain. The increased blood flow and muscle relaxation help to minimize possible or further injury to the body. Acupressure is often used in connection with other traditional Western medical treatments because no known risks are associated with the procedure.

—*Virginia L. Salmon*

See also Acupuncture; Alternative medicine; Anxiety; Circulation; Holistic medicine; Massage; Motion sickness; Muscle sprains, spasms, and disorders; Muscles; Pain; Pain management; Sports medicine; Stress; Stress reduction; Touch.

For Further Information:

"Acupressure, Shiatsu, and Other Asian Bodywork." *American Cancer Society*, March 1, 2011.

Bauer, Cathryn. *Acupressure for Everybody: Gentle, Effective Relief for More than One Hundred Common Ailments*. New York: Henry Holt, 1991.

Borimnejad, Leili, et al. "The Effects of Acupressure on Preoperative Anxiety Reduction in School Aged Children." *HealthMed* 6, no. 7 (2012): 2359-2361.

Cross, John R. *Acupressure and Reflextherapy in the Treatment of Medical Conditions*. Boston: Butterworth-Heinemann, 2001.

Gach, Michael R. *Acupressure's Potent Points: A Guide to Self-Care for Common Ailments*. New York: Bantam Books, 1990.

Lee, Jeong-Sook. "Acupressure for Treating Neurological Disorders: A Systematic Review." *International Journal of Neuroscience* 121, no. 8 (August, 2011): 409-414.

Meeus, Cathy. *Secrets of Shiatsu*. New York: Dorling Kindersley, 2001.

Saul, Helen. *Healing with Acupressure*. Chicago: Keats, 2002.

Teeguarden, Iona Marsaa. *A Complete Guide to Acupressure: Jin Shin Do*. Tokyo: Japan Publications, 2002.

Acupuncture

Treatment

Anatomy or system affected: All

Specialties and related fields: Alternative medicine, anesthesiology, preventive medicine

Definition: An ancient therapy developed in China in which designated points on the skin are stimulated by the insertion of needles, the application of heat, massage, or a combination of these techniques in order to treat impaired body functions or to induce anesthesia.

Key terms:

Ch'i: Chinese concept of the vital essence; when Ch'i is unbalanced, disease results

meridians: designated pathways in the body with points that react to acupuncture stimulation

yang: Chinese concept of the positive, male element of the universe

yin: Chinese concept of the negative, female element of the universe

Indications and Procedures

The theory and practice of acupuncture are rooted in the Chinese concept of life-the Chi or qi (both are pronounced "chee"). The belief is that all things, animate and inanimate, have an internal source of energy, the Chi. This energy stabilizes the chemical composition of matter, and when this matter is broken down, energy is released. The practice of acupuncture is thought to stimulate this energy to relieve pain and speed healing.

According to the ancient Chinese system of medicine, two categories of organs are associated with the Chi: the Tsang and the Fou. The Fou is the group of organs that absorb food, digest it, and expel waste. They are all hollow organs such as the stomach, the large and small intestines, the bladder, and the gallbladder. Tsang organs are all associated with the blood-the heart, which circulates the blood around the body; the lungs, which oxygenate the blood; the spleen, which controls the red corpuscles; and the liver and the kidneys. For the flow of energy to remain steady, it must pass unimpeded from one organ to another. If the organ is weak, the resultant energy that is passed on to the next organ is weakened. Acupuncture stimulates specifically designated points found on pathways in the body (called meridians) to correct the problem.

According to the Chinese system, the human "circuit" of energy is made up of twelve meridians, which stretch along the limbs from the toes and the fingers to the face and chest. There are six meridians in the upper limbs and six in the lower. Ten meridians are connected to a main organ by branches from the sympathetic nervous system, and each of these meridians contains the Chi, which varies in strength and is governed by the nerve impulses arising from the organs. The meridians and their attendant vessels contain the flow of energy that enables the body to function efficiently.

The meridian points that proved to be effective for certain ailments were organized, and specific names were given to each. Later, the meridian line concept was hypothesized in order to explain the effectiveness of the points. These meridian points were selected by observing the effects of stimulation on particular signs and symptoms.

According to modern medical concepts, some of these points are thought to be relating points at which the autonomic nervous system is stimulated by a specific visceral disorder. Anatomically, some of the meridian points appear to correspond to areas where a nerve appears to surface from a muscle or areas where vessels and nerves are located relatively superficially, such as areas between a muscle and a bone or between a bone and a joint. These areas are generally composed of connective tissue.

The meridians are stimulated by the insertion of needles. The needles that are commonly used range in size from the diameter of a hair to that of a sewing needle. In China, round and cutting needles are commonly used. In Europe, the needles are slightly shorter and slightly wider in diameter.

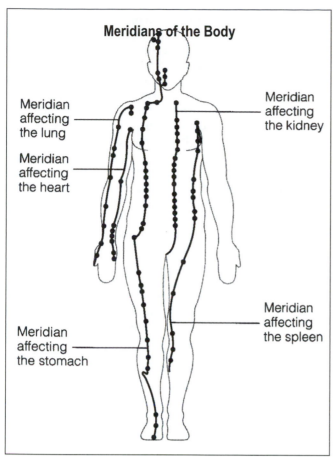

Meridians of the Body

Meridian affecting the lung

Meridian affecting the heart

Meridian affecting the stomach

Meridian affecting the kidney

Meridian affecting the spleen

Acupuncture is an ancient Chinese medical practice based on the concept of meridians, channels in the body through which flows the life force called Ch'i; acupuncture involves the insertion and manipulation of tiny needles along these meridians.

The needles are made of gold, silver, iron, platinum, or stainless steel. Stainless steel needles are most commonly used. Infection caused by needle puncture is said to be extremely rare. This may be the case because the minor injury created by the needle is controlled by biological reaction. It is routine to wipe the skin with alcohol before inserting the sterilized needle. The needle itself may be wiped with alcohol sponges before each insertion on the same patient. Needles are discarded after being used in patients with a history of jaundice or hepatitis.

Insertion of a needle requires great skill and much practice. There are three different angles of penetration into the skin: perpendicular, oblique, and horizontal. These angles correspond to 90 degrees, 45 degrees, and a minimum angle, respectively. The angles may be chosen on the basis of the thickness of the skin and the proximity to muscle or bone at the desired puncture point. The depth of penetration will vary.

Tapping (the tube method) is one method of insertion: When the diameter of the needle is small, this method is extremely effective. The needle is placed into the tube from either direction, and the tube is shorter than the needle. Gentle tapping of the needle handle with the right index finger introduces the needle easily. The tapping finger must be removed from the needle head immediately; otherwise,

it causes pain. The tube is removed gently with the right index finger and thumb.

In the twirling method (the freehand method), the left thumb and index finger make contact at the acupuncture point. The left hand is called the pushing hand. Next, the skin is cut with the needle tip, after which the needle is inserted by pushing and twirling it with the right hand.

The objective of the advancement of the needle and the needle motion is to create a needle feeling in the patient. This is a dull, aching, paralyzing, or compressing feeling or a combination of these sensations that radiates to a distal or proximal portion of the body. When the patient notices the needle feeling, the operator increases the feeling by using various needle motions. Numerous motions are available, such as the single-stick, twirling, vibration, intermittent, and retention motions.

Light skin and muscle massage is recommended in order to prepare the body to accept needle stimulation. Prepuncture massage makes skin cutting easier and helps the patient relax. In addition to these advantages, massage may make it possible to detect pathologies such as nodules, spasms, pain, and depression. Postpuncture massage helps to confirm muscle hypersensitivity and the disappearance of pain or hard nodules that existed before the acupuncture was performed.

The amount of stimulation equals the strength of stimulation multiplied by the number of treatments; this is dependent on the sensitivity of the patient. Gradual increases of stimulation are essential. In general, for acute disease, treatment is usually given once a day for ten days and then terminated for three to seven days. For chronic ailments, treatment is administered once every two to three days for ten treatments and then terminated for seven days. The patient is placed in a supine, sitting, prone, or side position—the position that is most convenient for the patient and physician. A special position, however, may be needed in order to relax the painful area.

One of the most important factors to be considered in effective acupuncture treatment is the accurate selection of acupuncture points. These points must be selected according to the specific ailment. The precise location of acupuncture points is crucial for obtaining the maximum therapeutic effect. This is difficult because of the different sizes and shapes of patients' bodies. Each acupuncture point is considered to be only about 3 millimeters in diameter.

Uses and Complications

Acupuncture, which is one mode of stimulation therapy, works by changing the pattern of passage of stimulation from the peripheral nerves to the central nervous system. Stimulation treatments such as hot soaks and the management of certain pain problems with physical therapy have long been in existence.

The basic approach of modern medicine involves removing the causal factor of disease. In this approach, the pain associated with disease or with a surgical procedure may not be eradicated instantaneously, however, and the management of pain becomes an issue until the disease is cured or until the surgery and recuperation are complete. Controlling chemical receptors and reducing the sensitivity of those receptors is one way of treating pain. Intensive studies of the stimulation that causes pain have indicated that intrinsic chemical substances (polypeptides) such as histamine and serotonin, which stimulate the receptors, are essential for pain. Therefore, an antagonistic drug for these chemicals is often effective in controlling pain.

Although acupuncture is used to treat conditions as diverse as allergies, circulatory disorders, dermatologic disorders, gastrointestinal disorders, genital disorders, musculoskeletal disorders, neurologic disorders, and psychiatric and emotional disorders, the use of acupuncture for pain control (analgesia) can be described as the most basic level of treatment.

The English words "anesthesia" and "analgesia" are misleading when used to describe the freedom from surgical or obstetrical pain that can be produced by acupuncture. If "analgesia" is described as insensibility to pain without loss of consciousness, it is a more appropriate word than "anesthesia," which is described as an insensibility, general or local, induced by anesthetic agents, and a loss of sensation of neurogenic or psychogenic origin.

Acupuncture can produce numbness in any part of the body. The patient under acupuncture analgesia remains able to converse and cooperate with the surgical or obstetrical team. Obstetric patients are aware of uterine contractions and are able to use their muscles to bring forth the fetus. Surgical patients can tell when incisions are made but do not perceive them as painful. There is no loss of memory, as in hypnosis or general anesthesia, and no paresthesia (abnormal sensations) comparable to the sensations following local anesthesia.

Most operating room deaths and cases of cardiac arrest in the United States are caused by chemical anesthesia rather than by surgery. Patients with anesthetic risks because of heart, liver, or kidney disease tolerate acupuncture analgesia well. Acupuncture is contraindicated for children under the age of seven, hemophiliacs, pregnant women, and people who have a fear of needles.

Acupuncture can be used to induce a feeling of well-being and calmness to allay the fear and apprehension most patients feel before surgery. It also appears to reduce both bleeding during surgical procedures and the incidence of shock. Postoperative acupuncture analgesia patients are spared nausea and the difficulties with urinating and defecating that frequently follow chemical anesthesia. Acupuncture analgesia does not mask symptoms as chemical anesthetics and analgesics do. The patient remains aware of his or her symptoms, but acupuncture diminishes those symptoms to a tolerable level.

Postoperative pain does not usually occur for several hours after acupuncture analgesia has been terminated. When it does occur, acupuncture can be used again instead of narcotics, and the treatment seldom needs to be repeated more than once or twice. Some acupuncturists leave small needles superficially inserted for several days to give postoperative pain relief. Others give regular acupuncture treatments, leaving the needles in place for twenty minutes per day for as many days as are necessary.

The main disadvantage of acupuncture analgesia is that it is less reliable than chemical analgesia or anesthesia. In some cases, acupuncture analgesia cannot be induced or becomes inadequate during a surgical procedure. It may not produce the relaxation desirable for some abdominal surgeries. For this reason, backup chemical anesthetics and analgesics are also available in most cases.

The actual induction of acupuncture analgesia takes about twenty minutes-slightly longer than chemical anesthesia. In most cases, electroacupuncture instruments must remain attached to all acupuncture needles during the entire procedure, but these can usually be kept away from the surgical field. The more skilled the acupuncturist, the fewer the needles required. In China, major surgical procedures have been performed with only one acupuncture needle as analgesia and without electric supplementation.

The same type of thin (usually 30-gauge) stainless steel needles that are used for acupuncture treatments are used for acupuncture analgesia. In general, the points that are used to relieve chronic pain in a specific area are the points of choice for analgesia. To obtain sufficient analgesia for surgery, it is usually necessary to heighten the effect of the acupuncture needles by twirling them continually or by attaching electronic instruments to them to deliver a current of about two hundred microamperes, with a pulsating wave at a frequency of two hundred per minute during the entire procedure. The use of electronic instruments will usually increase the depth of analgesia or prolong an analgesic

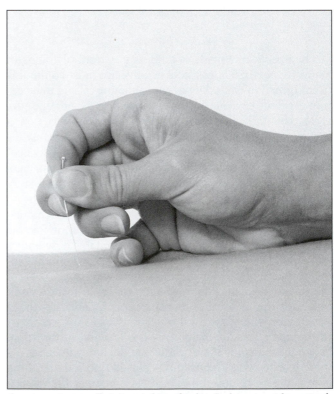

An acupuncture needle is inserted into the skin. Such treatment has gained in acceptance among Western health care providers, and many insurance companies now provide coverage for it. (PhotoDisc)

effect that is beginning to wear off.

Besides the acupuncture points for analgesia of specific areas of the body, points are often used to relieve anxiety and promote a feeling of well-being. Needles are usually inserted for twenty minutes the evening before surgery, as well as for at least twenty minutes before the actual surgery begins.

The theoretical principles of vital energy transmission are used in determining which acupuncture points should be effective for the anticipated surgery. Acupuncture points on meridians passing directly through, or in the vicinity of, the surgical area are usually selected. An attempt is made to use points on these meridians that are as far away from the surgical field as possible.

Perspective and Prospects

According to most reports, acupuncture appears to have been developed in the northernmost area of the middle region of China around 300 BCE. People in this area were primarily nomads, moving from one area to another.

Chinese high priests, who also often served as physicians, observed that men who were wounded in combat often reported the sudden disappearance of illnesses from which they had suffered for years. For example, a wound in a specific area of the foot would reduce blood pressure or relieve a headache or toothache, or an injury on the dorsal aspect of the knee joint would cure a migraine. Over the years, the high priests recorded numerous observations of the phenomenon of a wound in one part of the body curing a long-standing complaint at another point. They discovered that it was the location of the wound that was significant. A pinprick in the correct location was enough to effect relief. It was noted that certain points of the body responded more noticeably to stimulation than other points and that frequently there was a direct correlation between the points that were responsive and a particular ailment. They were subsequently named meridian points.

At a later time, when metal was introduced to the culture, needles were used as an irritant at meridian points, and it was thought that pain from a specific ailment was diverted in a linear fashion through the meridian points to the surface of the body. Thus the concept of the "meridian line" was developed, and thus acupuncture was discovered.

At first, the surgeon-priests used fish bones and sharpened splinters of bamboo to effect the pricks. Later came finely honed needles. Warlords and nobles were treated with needles forged from gold and silver. As the science of acupuncture developed, it was discovered that the needles needed only to be inserted in a point of skin measuring about one-tenth of an inch.

The earliest book describing acupuncture was written in 50 BCE. It described the clinical applications of acupuncture with anatomical physiological references that were based principally on the concept of the meridian lines of the body.

In 1912, Yüan Shih-K'ai, who had trained in a modern Western culture, took office as president of the Republic of China. Under his rule, old Chinese medicine-including acupuncture-that had developed from tradition and experience was unable to survive except in outlying areas of China. In 1949, however, when Mao Zedong formed the People's Republic of China, he tried to repopularize the old methods of Chinese medicine, which had been helpful to him. In the 1930s, when Mao and his followers were retreating to the north, he was forced to depend mainly on these traditional methods for medical treatment.

In 1955, Shyuken, a follower of Mao, stated his belief that acupuncture was effective in the management of illness. He wished to study the ancient Chinese way of medicine more systematically, comparing it to Western medicine, which he believed to be too analytical. Thus, a new medical movement began that united Western and Chinese medical practices.

Stimulation therapy using local heat, massage, and pressure has been known since ancient times. Long periods of observations and analysis by Chinese physicians of the effects of irritation of varying degrees at particular points on the body surface made it possible to relate specific points on the body (meridian points) to specific conditions.

According to ancient Chinese clinical concepts, the meridian points served as peeping holes into the body and passing holes for energy. The total number of meridian points was believed to be 365. Each was named according to its effect, anatomical location, appearance, and relation to the meridian line. These meridian points were selected initially according to measurements based on the patient's own unique anatomical standard (using the length between certain anatomical points; for example, between the shoulders). The exact location of a meridian point was then selected by the examiner, who felt with his or her fingertips the areas chosen by the initial measurement and observed the patient's response.

Acupuncture's popularity, like that of most techniques and discoveries, has waxed and waned throughout the years; for the most part, however, the Chinese have remained faithful to the five-thousand-year-old practice. The laws and methods of acupuncture have endured, although these methods have been increasingly combined with Western medical techniques. Gradually, the practice of acupuncture has spread throughout the world, particularly in France, Russia, Japan, Switzerland, Germany, and the United States.

In 1997, the US National Institutes of Health (NIH) concluded that the efficacy of acupuncture is highly promising and a worthwhile research endeavor, especially in treating postoperative chemotherapy nausea and dental pain. It was noted that acupuncture could be useful in asthma and addiction treatment and in stroke rehabilitation. Research has identified many of the mechanisms of action in acupuncture, most notably the release of opioids and other peptides and the corresponding changes of neuroendocrine functioning.

In 2002, the National Health Interview Survey found that 8.2 million adults in the United States had used acupuncture and that 2.1 million had used it within the last year. Although the number of people who use acupuncture is significant, the Food and Drug Administration (FDA) reports exceedingly few complications.

A review of government-funded research studies on acupuncture found numerous uses being evaluated, including labor stimulation, postsurgical wound healing, control of chemotherapy-induced vomiting, and the treatment of substance abuse, incontinence, autism, cerebral palsy, and depression.

—Genevieve Slomski, Ph.D.;
updated by LeAnna DeAngelo, Ph.D.

See also Acupressure; Addiction; Alternative medicine; Anesthesia; Anesthesiology; Anxiety; Circulation; Holistic medicine; Motion sickness; Muscle sprains, spasms, and disorders; Muscles; Pain; Pain management; Sports medicine; Stress; Stress reduction.

For Further Information:

"Acupuncture." *Mayo Clinic*, January 25, 2012.
"Acupuncture: An Introduction." *National Center for Complementary and Alternative Medicine*, August 2011.
Cassidy, Claire Monod. *Contemporary Chinese Medicine and Acupuncture*. New York: Churchill Livingstone, 2002.
Ernst, Edzard, and Adrian White, eds. *Acupuncture: A Scientific Appraisal*. Boston: Butterworth-Heinemann, 2000.
Kidson, Ruth. *Acupuncture for Everyone: What It Is, Why It Works, and How It Can Help You*. Rochester, Vt.: Inner Traditions International, 2001.
Manaka, Yoshio, Kazuko Itaya, and Stephen Birch. *Chasing the Dragon's Tail: The Theory and Practice of Acupuncture in the Work of Yoshio Manaka*. Brookline, Mass.: Paradigm, 1997.
Molassiotis, A., et al. "A Randomized, Controlled Trial of Acupuncture Self-Needling as Maintenance Therapy for Cancer-Related Fatigue after Therapist-Delivered Acupuncture." *Annals of Oncology* 24, no. 6 (June, 2013): 1645-1652.
Mann, Felix. *Reinventing Acupuncture: A New Concept of Ancient Medicine*. Boston: Butterworth-Heinemann, 2000.
Stux, Gabriel, and Bruce Pomeranz. *Basics of Acupuncture*. 5th ed. New York: Springer, 2003.

Acute respiratory distress syndrome (ARDS)

Disease/Disorder

Also known as: Respiratory distress syndrome (RDS), adult respiratory distress syndrome

Anatomy or system affected: Circulatory system, lungs, respiratory system

Specialties and related fields: Cardiology, public health, pulmonary medicine

Definition: Respiratory failure caused by filling of the lungs with fluid from the capillaries, leading to a shortage of oxygen in the body that can eventually lead to death if not treated.

Key terms:

aspiration: the breathing of material into the lungs (such as vomit or food particles)

sepsis: overwhelming infection in the bloodstream, which blocks blood flow; the body's immune system is affected and organ failure can result

tachypnea: rapid breathing

Causes and Symptoms

During acute respiratory distress syndrome (ARDS), the lungs lose their ability to fill with air because they are filling with fluid from the capillaries (small blood vessels) instead. Damage to the vascular endothelium can cause

---

> **Information on**
> **Acute Respiratory Distress Syndrome (ARDS)**
>
> **Causes:** Lung injury, sepsis, drug overdose, blood-borne infection, transfusion, acute pancreatitis, pneumonia, trauma, aspiration, long-term illnesses
> **Symptoms:** Difficulty breathing, low blood pressure, shock, organ failure
> **Duration:** Symptoms develop within twenty-four to forty-eight hours; syndrome can last up to six months
> **Treatments:** Mechanical ventilation, air pressure release ventilation (APRV), positive end-expiratory pressure (PEEP), corticosteroids, nitric oxide

sepsis, while damage to the alveolar epithelium can cause the aspiration of gastric (stomach) contents. Either sepsis or aspiration of gastric contents can lead to ARDS because they both cause inflammation of the alveoli, the sacs within the lungs that normally fill with air when a person breathes. Inflammation of these alveoli causes them to fill with liquid instead. The liquid comes from the capillaries located within the walls of the alveoli that transport oxygen from the alveoli to the bloodstream. The buildup of fluid (edema) in the alveoli causes them to collapse, thus ending the transport of oxygen in the body.

The ratio of arterial partial oxygen tension, called PaO_2, to FiO_2, which is the fraction of inspired oxygen, is used to quantitatively describe the occurrence and severity of ARDS. The oxygen pressure of this ratio, expressed as $PaO_2:FiO_2$, indicates that the initial acute lung injury condition has occurred if its value is less than 300 millimeters of mercury (mmHg). If the oxygen pressure continues to decrease to a value of less than 200 mmHg for this ratio, then the patient is diagnosed with ARDS.

Death can result if ARDS is untreated because vital organs, such as the brain and kidneys, will stop functioning. If ARDS is diagnosed and treated in time, then death can be avoided, but permanent damage frequently occurs. Diagnosis using a chest X ray or an anteroposterior (AP) portable chest radiograph can facilitate the administration of the treatments. Additional diagnostic tests include sputum cultures and analysis, bronchoscopy, arterial blood gas testing, and blood chemistries testing.

The ratio of arterial partial oxygen tension, called PaO_2, to FiO_2, which is the fraction of inspired oxygen, is used to quantitatively describe the occurrence and severity of ARDS. The oxygen pressure of this ratio, expressed as $PaO_2:FiO_2$, indicates that the initial acute lung injury condition has occurred if its value is less than 300 millimeters of mercury (mmHg). If the oxygen pressure continues to decrease to a value of less than 200 mmHg for this ratio, then the patient is diagnosed with ARDS.

Death can result if ARDS is untreated because vital organs, such as the brain and kidneys, will stop functioning. If ARDS is diagnosed and treated in time, then death can be avoided, but permanent damage frequently occurs. Diagnosis using a chest X ray or an anteroposterior (AP) portable chest radiograph can facilitate the administration of the

---

In the News: Patient Positioning Has No Effect on ARDS Treatment

Italian researchers have reported that the previously advocated face-down positioning of patients being treated for acute respiratory distress syndrome (ARDS) does not increase the survival rate. Luciano Gattinoni and Paolo Taccone reported their results in the November 11, 2009, issue of the *JAMA: The Journal of the American Medical Association*. ARDS is characterized by a shortness of breath as a result of lung damage. Eventually the alveoli (sacs) in the lungs fill with fluid, preventing the transport of oxygen and leading to the condition of hypoxemia. Hypoxemia refers to low levels of oxygen in the blood; it can be further described as severe, with a PaO_2:FiO_2 ratio of less than 100 millimeters of mercury (mmHg), or as moderate, with a PaO_2:FiO_2 ratio between 100 and 200 mmHg. In this ratio, PaO_2 describes the patient's arterial partial oxygen tension and FiO_2 is the fraction of inspired oxygen. Severe hypoxemia often leads to organ failure and death.

Mechanical ventilation is used to provide oxygen in the lungs, and in 1976 it was reported that positioning a patient face-down (prone) was more successful with mechanical ventilation than was the face-up (supine) position. It was believed that this prone position allowed the lung to be exposed to less strain than did the supine position, thus leading to a positive oxygenation effect for patients. However, there had been no randomized clinical trials to support this treatment.

The 2009 study was a randomized, controlled clinical trial conducted at twenty-three centers in Italy and two centers in Spain involving 342 patients receiving treatment on mechanical ventilation with cases of moderate and severe ARDS. During this study, conducted between 2004 and 2008, supine positioning was randomly chosen for 174 patients and prone positioning was randomly chosen for 168 patients. The mortality rates were similar, approximately 30 percent, for patients with severe and moderate hypoxemia no matter which position was chosen. Furthermore, patients in the prone position actually experienced higher rates for complications, at 94.6 percent, while patients in the supine position experienced a 76.4 percent rate for complications. Thus, prolonged prone positioning should not be applied to patients, although the role of prone positioning for patients with the most severe cases of hypoxemia will be investigated further.

—Jeanne L. Kuhler, Ph.D.

---

treatments. Additional diagnostic tests include sputum cultures and analysis, bronchoscopy, arterial blood gas testing, and blood chemistries testing.

Treatment and Therapy

Mechanical ventilation, the traditional treatment for ARDS, is a type of assisted breathing used when a patient has so much difficulty with breathing that death could otherwise result. After several days on a mechanical ventilator, however, the patient can develop pneumonia with a 50 percent mortality rate. Therefore, alternative treatments are being developed and optimized to decrease the dependence on mechanical ventilation.

One of these alternative treatments, air pressure release ventilation (APRV), has been shown to be more effective at promoting spontaneous breathing with increased cardiac and organ responses. Because of this increased effectiveness, APRV requires a patient to spend less time on the ventilator, leading to decreased rates of pneumonia.

Positive end-expiratory pressure (PEEP) decreases the collapse of the alveoli. Ventilators plot a pressure-volume curve of the lung in order to determine the minimum PEEP to apply to a patient. This collection of pressure-volume data is crucial because the PEEP must match the surface tension of the alveoli. If the PEEP is too high, then the flow of blood to the heart will be negatively impacted.

Corticosteroids can be a helpful treatment because they suppress the inflammation during the early phase of ARDS, when the alveoli are just beginning to fill with fluid. However, this treatment is very limited in scope. Doses of more than 2 milligrams per kilograms (mg/kg) per day are not beneficial, and these doses must be administered within the first three to five days. After that, it is too late for corticosteroids to be effective.

Nitric oxide can bind to hemoglobin and function as a selective pulmonary vasodilator. However, its effects are small and vary widely from patient to patient.

Perspective and Prospects

It was in 1994 that the American-European Consensus Conference (AECC) first defined the specific symptoms and possible causes of ARDS to facilitate the study of the pathogenesis of this syndrome and to develop treatments. Although ARDS has been recognized since World War I as a potentially fatal respiratory failure, the specific term "acute respiratory distress syndrome" was not adopted until 1967.

The results of a study by the National Institutes of Health (NIH) conducted in the 1970s indicated the incidence of ARDS to be seventy-five cases per 100,000 persons. After the formal definition was proposed in 1994 by the AECC, a study conducted from 1999 to 2000 indicated a frequency of eighty-six cases per 100,000 persons. Although ARDS can affect both males and females with equal probability at any age, there is an increase in the occurrence of ARDS with increasing age, with 306 per 100,000 for the seventy-five to eighty-four-year-old age group. In 2004, 1,736 deaths occurred in the United States as a result of 190,000 cases of ARDS.

—Jeanne L. Kuhler, Ph.D.

See also Critical care; Emergency medicine; Hyperventilation; Lungs; Oxygen therapy; Pneumonia; Pulmonary diseases; Pulmonary medicine; Respiration; Severe acute respiratory syndrome (SARS).

For Further Information:

"Acute Respiratory Distress Syndrome (ARDS)."Â *bmc.org*. American Lung Association. Web. 21 May 2013.

Irwin, Richard S., and James M. Rippe, eds. *Irwin and Rippe's Intensive Care Medicine*. 6th ed. Philadelphia: Wolters Kluwer Health/ Lippincott Williams & Wilkins, 2008.

Marino, Paul L. *The ICU Book*. 3d ed. Philadelphia: Lippincott Williams & Wilkins, 2007.

Wae, L., et al. "The Acute Respiratory Distress Syndrome." *New England Journal of Medicine* 342 (2000): 1334-1349.

Addiction

Disease/Disorder

Anatomy or system affected: Brain, nervous system, psychic-emotional system

Specialties and related fields: Psychiatry, psychology

Definition: A process whereby an organism comes to depend on a substance psychologically and/or physiologically. Physiological dependence is marked tolerance and/or withdrawal from the specific substance.

Key terms:

abstinence: complete refrainment from the use of a substance of abuse

compulsion: a persistent, irresistible urge to perform a stereotyped behavior or irrational act, often accompanied by repetitious thoughts (obsessions) about the behavior

pharmacodynamics: changes in tissue sensitivity or physiologic systems in response to pharmacological substances

pharmacokinetics: the action of pharmacological substances within a biological system; pharmacologic substance absorption, distribution, metabolism, and elimination by an organism

physiological dependence: a state of tissue adaptation to a substance of abuse marked by tolerance and/or withdrawal

psychological dependence: need for a substance provided by its reinforcing properties, causing persistent desire to cut down or control use, use across varied situations to the exclusion of other behavior, use despite other worsening physical or psychological conditions, and/or great amounts of time spent finding, using, or recovering from substance effects

reinforcement: a process that increases the frequency or probability of a response

substance abuse: the continued use of a psychoactive substance despite repeated impairment, within a twelve-month period, of social, occupational, or legal functioning or continued exposure to physical hazards

tolerance: a condition in which the same dose achieves a lesser effect, or in which successively greater doses of a substance are required to achieve the same desired effect

withdrawal: a physical and mental condition following decreased intake of an abusable substance, with symptoms ranging from anxiety to convulsions and seizures

Causes and Symptoms

Addiction is a disorder that can affect any animal and may result from the use of a variety of psychoactive substances. Typically, addiction involves psychological or physiological dependence, or both.

Tolerance involves pharmacokinetics, pharmacodynamics, and environmental or behavioral conditioning. Pharmacokinetics refers to the way in which a biological system, such as a human body, processes a drug. Substances are subject to adsorption into the bloodstream, dis-

---

Information on Addiction

Causes: Repeated use of psychoactive substances

Symptoms: Tolerance; withdrawal (anxiety, convulsions, seizures); associated health risks (heart attacks, breathing difficulties, coma, cancer, cirrhosis, ulcers)

Duration: Chronic

Treatments: Cognitive and behavioral therapies; replacement drugs (methadone for heroin, nicotine patches for smoking); antagonists (naltrexone for opiates); metabolic inhibitors (Antabuse for alcohol)

---

tribution to different organs (such as the brain and liver), metabolization by these organs, and then elimination. Over time, the processes of distribution and metabolism may change, such that the body eliminates the substance more efficiently. Thus, the substance has less opportunity to affect the system than it did initially, reducing any desired effects. As a result, dose increases are needed to achieve the initial or desired effect.

Pharmacodynamics refer to changes in the body as a result of a pharmacologic agent being present. Tissue within the body responds differently to the substance at the primary sites of action. For example, changes in sensitivity may occur at specific sites within the brain, with direct or indirect impact on the primary action site. Direct changes at the primary sites of action denote tissue sensitivity. An example might be an increase in the number of receptors in the brain for that particular substance. Indirect changes in tissue remote from the primary action sites denote tissue tolerance, or functional tolerance. In functional tolerance, physiologic systems that oppose the action of the drug compensate by increasing their effect. Once either type of tolerance develops, the only way for the desired effect to be achieved is for the dose of the substance to be increased.

Finally, environmental or behavioral conditioning is involved in the development of tolerance. Organisms associate the reinforcing properties of substances with the contexts in which the drugs are experienced. Such contexts may be physical environments, such as places, or emotional contexts, such as when the individual is depressed or anxious. Over the course of repeated administrations in the same context, the tolerance that develops is associated with that specific context. Thus, an organism may experience tolerance to a drug in one situation, but not another. Greater doses of the reinforcing substance would be needed to achieve the same effect in the former situation, but not in the latter.

Tolerance develops differently depending on the type of substance taken, the dose ingested, and the routes of administration used. Larger doses may contribute to quicker development of tolerance. Similarly, routes of administration that produce more rapid and efficient absorption of a substance into the bloodstream tend to increase the likelihood of an escalating pattern of substance use leading to dependence. For many drugs, intravenous injection and in-

A baby born addicted to cocaine is monitored closely; women put their unborn children at risk by using harmful substances during pregnancy. (PhotoDisc)

halation are two of the fastest routes of administration, while oral ingestion is one of the slowest. Other routes include intranasal, transdermal, rectal, sublingual, intramuscular, subcutaneous, and intraocular administration.

For some substances, the development of tolerance also depends on the pattern of substance use. For example, even though two individuals might use the same amount of alcohol, it is possible for tolerance to develop more quickly in one person than in the other. Two individuals might each drink fourteen drinks per week, but they would develop tolerance at different rates if one consumes two drinks on each of seven nights and the other consumes seven drinks on each of two nights in a week. Because of their patterns of use, the first drinker would develop tolerance much more slowly than the second, all other things being equal.

Withdrawal occurs when use of the substance significantly decreases or ceases. Withdrawal varies by the substance of abuse and ranges from being minor or nonexistent with some drugs (such as hallucinogens) to quite pronounced with other drugs (such as alcohol). Mild symptoms include anxiety, tension, restlessness, insomnia, impaired attention, and irritability. Severe symptoms include seizures, convulsions, perceptual distortions, irregular tremors, high blood pressure, and rapid heartbeat. Typi-

cally, withdrawal symptoms can be alleviated or extinguished by readministration of the substance of abuse. Thus, a compounding problem is that the addicted individual often learns to resume drug use in order to avoid the withdrawal symptoms.

Addiction occurs with both legal and illegal drugs. Alcohol and nicotine are two of the most widely abused legal addictive drugs. Over-the-counter drugs, such as sleeping aids and high doses of antihistamines and cough medicines, also have abuse potential. Similarly, prescription drugs, such as tranquilizers (for example, sedative-hypnotics) and antianxiety agents, have abuse and addiction potential. Common illegal addictive drugs include cocaine, marijuana, hallucinogens, heroin, and methamphetamine.

Not everyone who uses these substances will automatically become addicted. In the United States, for example, surveys have shown that approximately 65 percent of adults drink alcohol each year. In contrast, less than 13 percent of the population goes on to develop alcohol problems serious enough to warrant a medical diagnosis of alcohol abuse or dependence. Similarly, despite the fact that large numbers of individuals are prescribed opiates or sedative-hypnotics for pain while hospitalized, roughly 0.7 percent of the adult population is addicted to opiates and 1.1 percent is addicted to sedative-hypnotics or antianxiety drugs.

Thus, the development of addiction often requires repeated substance administration, as well as other biological and environmental factors. This does not mean that anyone is immune to addiction; any person can become addicted to a drug given enough dosage and exposure.

When addiction is present, the consequences are multiple and complex. Substance abuse, for instance, is distinct from substance dependence. Substance abuse involves repeated use in hazardous situations or repeated use resulting in deteriorated performance in social, occupational, or legal functioning. Substance dependence usually involves a pattern of problems that have persisted for a year or longer. These problems are characterized by tolerance, withdrawal, unsuccessful quit attempts or repeated desire to quit, continued use despite psychological or physical problems caused or exacerbated by the substance use, increasing amounts of time spent on the substance, decreasing amounts of time spent on other activities, and loss of control over one's use of the substance. Loss of control occurs when a person uses the substance in greater amounts or for longer periods of time than intended.

In terms of health, there are many acute and chronic effects of addiction. With cocaine, for example, acute cardiac functioning may be affected, such that the risk of heart attacks may be increased. Similarly, individuals addicted to opiates, alcohol, and sedative-hypnotics must contend with such risks as falling into a coma or experiencing depressed respiratory functioning. Finally, the acute effects of any of these drugs can impair judgment and contribute to careless behavior and social problems. As a result, accidents, severe trauma, and habitually dangerous behavior, such as risky sexual behavior, may be associated with substance use disorders such as abuse and dependence.

Chronic health consequences are common. Smoking and exposure to secondhand smoke are associated with cancers of the mouth, throat, and lungs, as well as premature deterioration of the skin. Chew tobacco products have similar associations with cancers of the throat and mouth. Alcohol is associated with cancers of the mouth, throat, and stomach, as well as ulcers and liver problems. General malnutrition is a risk for heroin and alcohol users, since they often fail to eat properly. Injected drugs such as heroin and cocaine are associated with problems such as abscesses, hepatitis, and acquired immunodeficiency syndrome (AIDS), since shared needles may transmit blood-borne diseases. Finally, substance use contributes to health problems during pregnancy. Problems such as low birth weight in the children of smokers, fetal alcohol syndrome in the children of female drinkers, and withdrawal difficulties in children born to other types of substance users are well documented.

An emerging area of "new" addiction has been the phenomenon of Web, or Internet, addiction, which includes the compulsive use of services such as e-mail. Such problems (such as gambling, compulsive sexual behavior, compulsive shopping, eating disorders, and workaholism) share features with other addictive behaviors involving substance use and are often studied together. Additionally, these behaviors may often coexist in persons who use substances of abuse, so there is a clear need to study them simultaneously.

Treatment and Therapy

Because of the potential combination of psychological and physiological addiction processes, dependence is a type of disorder that often demands both psychological and pharmacological treatments. Typically, interventions focus on decreasing or stopping the substance use and reestablishing normal psychological, social, occupational, and physical functioning in the addicted individual. Though the length and type of treatments may vary with the particular addictive drug and the duration of the addiction problem, similar principles are involved in the treatment of all addictions. Similar strategies are used for problems of abuse. Because abuse is limited to problems that are more social in nature, however, pharmacological treatments often are not used for abuse problems alone.

Psychological treatments focus primarily on extinguishing psychological dependence, as well as on facilitating more effective functioning by the addicted individual in other areas of life. Attempts to change the behavior and thinking of the addicted individual usually involve some combination of individual, group, or family therapy. Adjunctive training in new occupational skills and healthier lifestyle habits is also common.

In general, treatment focuses on understanding how the addictive behavior developed, how it was maintained, and how it can be removed from the person's daily life. Assessments of the situations in which the drug was used, the needs for which the drug was used, and alternative means of addressing those needs are primary to this understanding. Once these issues are identified, a therapist then works with the client to break habitual behavior patterns that were contributing to the addiction. For example, a client would learn not to drive through neighborhoods where drugs might be sold, go to business meetings at restaurants that serve alcohol, or maintain relationships with drug-using friends. Concurrently, the therapist helps the client design new behavior patterns that will decrease the odds of continued problems with addiction. Problems related to the drug use would then be addressed in some combination of individual, family, or group therapy. Drug education is also important to help clients and family members learn about the dangers of continued use.

The therapy or therapies selected depend on the problems related to drug use. For example, family therapy might be more appropriate in cases in which family conflicts are related to drug use. In contrast, individual therapy might be more appropriate for someone whose drug use is linked to thinking distortions or mood problems. Similarly, group therapy might be most appropriate for individuals lacking social support to deal with stress, or whose social interactions are contributing to their drug use. Regardless of the type of therapy, however, the basic goal remains: facilitating the client's solving of his or her specific problems. Additionally, the development of new ways of coping with intractable problems, rather than relying on drug use as a means of coping, would be critical.

Cognitive and behavioral therapies have been quite useful for breaking the conditioned effects of addiction. Some psychological dependence, for example, is based on placebo effects. A placebo effect occurs as a result of what people believe a drug is doing for them, rather than from anything that the drug actually has the power to accomplish. In addition, the practice of using addictive drugs within certain contexts is associated with drug tolerance, such that certain situations trigger compulsions leading to drug use. In this way, cognitive therapy can be used to challenge any faulty thinking associations that individuals have made about what the drugs do for them in different situations. This may involve increasing patients' awareness of the negative consequences of their drug use and challenging what they perceive to be its positive consequences. As a complement, such therapies correct distorted thinking that is related to coping with stressful situations or situations in which drug use might be especially tempting. In such situations, individuals might actually have the skill to handle the stress or temptation without using drugs. Without the confidence that they can successfully manage these situations, however, they may not even try, and instead revert to drug use. As such, therapy facilitating realistic thinking about stress and coping abilities can be quite beneficial.

The first nationwide study examining the effects of matching treatments to clients with alcohol problems has concluded its initial phase. The United States-based study, Project MATCH, initiated in 1989, was supported by the National Institute on Alcohol Abuse and Alcoholism. It was designed to examine the effect of matching clients to one of three individual treatment approaches-cognitive-behavioral, twelve-step facilitation, or motivational enhancement-based on the psychosocial characteristics of the participants, such as severity of problems or the presence of other mental health problems. Results of this and following studies have suggested that all clients gain benefits from participating in treatment. Assessment is also beneficial to clients. Additionally, clients without other severe psychiatric symptoms tend to do better in treatment, relative to clients with other severe psychiatric symptoms. Clients with other severe psychiatric symptoms usually require additional or somewhat different treatment approaches related to having co-occurring disorders.

Similarly, behavioral therapies are used to break down conditioned associations between situations and drug use. For example, smokers are sometimes made to smoke not in accordance with their desire to smoke, but according to a schedule over which they have no control. As a result, they are made to smoke at times or in situations where it is inconvenient, leading to an association between unpleasant feelings and smoking. While such assigned drug use would not be used with illegal drugs, the basic principles of increasing negative or unpleasant feelings with drug use in specific situations can be used. Rewarding abstinence has also been a successful approach to treatment. In this way, positive reinforcement is associated with abstinence and may contribute to behaviors related to abstinence being more common than behaviors related to drug use.

Pharmacological treatments concentrate on decreasing physical dependence on the substance of abuse. They rely on behavioral principles and on five primary strategies. The first strategy, based on positive reinforcement, is pharmacological replacement. Prescribed drugs with effects at the sites of action similar to those of the addictive drug are used. These prescribed drugs, however, usually fail to have reinforcing properties as powerful as the addictive drug and focus mainly on preventing the occurrence of withdrawal symptoms. Nicotine patches for smokers and methadone for heroin users are examples of replacement therapies.

A second strategy involves the use of both reinforcement and extinction, the behavioral process of decreasing and eventually extinguishing the drug-taking behavior. Partially reinforcing and partially antagonistic drugs are prescribed. The net effect is that the prescribed drug staves off withdrawal symptoms but yields less reinforcement than drug replacement therapy, serving to facilitate the process of extinction for the drug taking.

Antagonists, or drugs that completely block the receptors responsible for the reinforcing effects of the drug action, are prescribed alone as a third strategy. With this strategy, extinction is the primary behavioral principle in effect. The prescribed drug blocks the primary receptor sites and does not yield positively reinforcing drug effects. Even if the addictive drug is taken in addition to the antagonist, no positively reinforcing effects are experienced. Thus, without reinforcement, drug-taking behavior should eventually cease. Naltrexone, typically used for opiate addiction, is a good example of this strategy.

Punishment is another behavioral principle used in pharmacological therapy. Metabolic inhibitors, or drugs that make the effects of the addictive substance more toxic, are often used to discourage drug use. Antabuse, a drug often given for problems with alcohol, is such a substance. When metabolic inhibitors are prescribed, individuals using these drugs in combination with their substance of abuse experience toxic and unpleasant effects. Thus, they begin to associate use of the addictive substance with very noxious results and are discouraged from continuing their drug use.

Symptomatic treatment of withdrawal effects is used as a fifth strategy. Based on reinforcement, this strategy simply encourages the use of drugs likely to reduce withdrawal effects. Unfortunately, these drugs may also have abuse potential. For example, when benzodiazepines are given to individuals with alcohol or opiate dependence, one dependency may be traded for another. As such, symptomatic treatment is helpful but is not a treatment of choice by itself. In fact, none of these pharmacological treatments is recommended for use in isolation; they are recommended for use with complementary psychological treatments.

An exciting development has been the discovery of the utility of naltrexone, a drug commonly used in the treatment of opioid addiction, in the early phases of successful response to treatment for alcohol dependence when it is combined with psychosocial therapies. In addition, investigators have been studying how alternative medicine might be of use for substance use problems. Examples are the use of acupuncture and massage in the treatment of illicit substance use, such as stimulant use. While results in this area are promising, it is important to note that none of these treatments should be used alone but rather as an adjunct to traditional treatment approaches.

Finally, vaccines are being designed to help immunize people against addiction to such drugs as amphetamines, cocaine, nicotine, and phencyclidine (PCP). Vaccines are designed to create antibodies that attack the drug once it is inside the body but before it has reached the brain; proteins bind to the drug and prevent it from having its effects. The benefit is that it prevents individuals who use the drug from feeling the drug's effects, thereby decreasing the cravings for the drug.

Perspective and Prospects

The use of substances to alter the mind or bodily experiences is a practice that has been a part of human cultures for centuries. Time and again, even through legislated acts such as Prohibition, drug and alcohol use have persisted. The continued use of drugs for recreational and medicinal practices seems virtually inevitable, and it is unlikely that substance abuse and dependence will disappear from the world's societies. Consequently, an understanding of substance use, how it leads to addiction, ways to minimize the development of addiction problems, and strategies for improving addiction treatments will be critical.

At different times in history, addiction has been viewed as strictly a moral, medical, spiritual, or behavioral problem. As the science of understanding and treating addiction has progressed, the variety of ways in which these aspects of addiction combine has been noted. Modern treatments and theories no longer view addiction from one strict point of view, but instead recognize the heterogeneity of paths leading to addiction. Such an approach has been helpful not only in treating addiction but also in preventing it. Efforts to curb the biological, social, and environmental forces contributing to addiction have become increasingly important.

Addiction remains a disorder with no completely effective treatment. Of individuals seeking treatment across all addictive disorders, fewer than 20 percent succeed the first time that they attempt to achieve long-term abstinence. As a result, individuals suffering from addiction often undergo multiple treatments over several occasions, with some individuals experiencing significant problems throughout their lives. Many people, however, do make gains in treatment, so treatment should be pursued.

While no 100 percent effective treatment exists for addiction, researchers have made important strides in understanding some of its biological underpinnings. For example, in studies on cocaine addiction, it has been shown that hormonal fluctuations play an important role in women's responses to drugs. It appears that women have decreased sensitivity to cocaine, relative to men, and that this effect varies depending on a woman's stage of her menstrual cycle.

Researchers are also examining whether circadian rhythms may also be related to addiction. Moreover, since fruit flies and humans share genetic similarities, the flies are often used for the study of human conditions, such as addiction. New research on fruit flies suggests that sensitivity to cocaine appears to be related to the genes that control what is commonly called the "biological clock." In experiments using flies missing several biological clock genes, the flies did not become sensitized to cocaine. This suggests that biological clocks may be related to the development or maintenance of addiction to cocaine.

In this context, the challenges ahead are not to prevent all substance use, but rather to decrease the odds that a person will abuse substances or become addicted and to reduce harm for those already experiencing problems by getting them to treatment. Improved pharmacological and psychological treatments will be important. Finding new ways of tailoring treatment for addiction to the needs and backgrounds of the different individuals affected will be one critical task for health professionals, particularly as ethnic, racial, and cultural differences are better understood. Continued exploration of new pharmacological treatments to combat withdrawal, decrease cravings, and facilitate abstinence is necessary. Additionally, further research into the relationship among use, abuse, and dependence will be helpful in making diagnoses in this area of work even more useful.

—*Nancy A. Piotrowski, Ph.D.*

See also Alcoholism; Caffeine; Club drugs; Eating disorders; Ergogenic aids; Marijuana; Mouth and throat cancer; Narcotics; Nicotine; Obsessive-compulsive disorder; Prescription drug abuse; Psychiatry; Psychology; Steroid abuse; Stress; Substance abuse; Weight loss medications.

For Further Information:

American Psychiatric Association. *Diagnostic and Statistical Manual of Mental Disorders: DSM-IV-TR*. 4th ed. Arlington, Va.: Author, 2000. This manual provides detailed descriptions of the behaviors and types of symptoms used to describe and diagnose different addictive disorders. It is written by mental health professionals from psychiatric, psychological, and social work backgrounds.

Block, Jerald J. "Issues for DSM-V: Internet Addiction." *American Journal of Psychiatry* 165 (March, 2008): 306-307. Results of a case study that concludes that "Internet addiction appears to be a common disorder that merits inclusion" in updated editions of the *Diagnostic and Statistical Manual of Mental Disorders*.

Brickman, Philip, et al. "Models of Helping and Coping." *American Psychologist* 37 (April, 1982): 368-384. This article describes a four-model perspective on helping and coping with problems related to addiction. A classic in the addiction field, providing a good review of historical factors influencing different treatment models.

Dupont, Robert L. *The Selfish Brain: Learning from Addiction*. Center City, Minn.: Hazelton, 2000. Discusses the commonalities across different types of addiction in an easy-to-understand manner.

Julien, Robert M. *A Primer of Drug Action: A Concise, Nontechnical Guide to the Actions, Uses, and Side Effects of Psychoactive Drugs*. 11th ed. New York: Freeman, 2008. A nontechnical guide to drugs, written by a medical professional. Describes the different classes of drugs, their actions in the body, their uses, and their side effects. Basic pharmacologic principles, classifications, and terms are defined and discussed.

Miller, William R., and Nick Heather, eds. *Treating Addictive Behaviors*. 2d ed. New York: Plenum Press, 2004. This book, written by medical and psychological scientists, is an overview of treatment strategies for problems ranging from nicotine to opiate addiction. Psychological, behavioral, interpersonal, familial, and medical approaches are outlined and discussed.

Sussman, Steven, and Susan L. Ames. *Drug Abuse: Concepts, Prevention, and Cessation*. New York: Cambridge University Press, 2008. A comprehensive overview of issues and concerns related to preventing problems related to drug use; focuses especially on teenagers.

Weil, Andrew, and Winifred Rosen. *From Chocolate to Morphine: Everything You Need to Know About Mind-Altering Drugs*. Rev. and updated ed. Boston: Houghton Mifflin, 2004. This book on psychoactive substances provides basic information to the general reader. Psychoactive substances are identified and defined. Also outlines the relationships between different types of drugs, the motivations to use drugs, and associated problems. As the title suggests, the discussion ranges from legal, caffeinated substances to illegal and prescription drugs.

Addison's disease

Disease/Disorder

Also known as: Chronic adrenal insufficiency, hypoadreno-corticism

Anatomy or system affected: Endocrine system, glands, kidneys

Specialties and related fields: Endocrinology, nephrology

Definition: A failure of adrenal cortex function in which production of any or all of the hormones synthesized by the cortex is decreased.

Key terms:

adrenal cortex: the outer portion of the adrenal gland; produces a wide variety of regulatory hormones

adrenal gland: the gland located on top of each of the kidneys

androgenic hormones: any of several hormones that regulate the expression of male characteristics

corticosteroid: an adrenal cortex hormone that controls processes such as protein and carbohydrate metabolism and electrolyte balance

cortisol: a steroid hormone that regulates inflammation

glucocorticoid: an adrenal cortex hormone that regulates a variety of bodily functions, such as inflammation and the mobilization of fat

mineralocorticoid: an adrenal cortex hormone that regulates the retention of minerals such as potassium and sodium

Causes and Symptoms

Anything that results in damage to the adrenal gland has the potential to cause the development of Addison's disease. Most commonly, the disorder is the result of an autoimmune malfunction, in which the body begins to react against its own tissue. The disorder may also result from adrenal cancers or infections. The prevalence rate is approximately 1 per 100,000 people.

The specific cause of the adrenal insufficiency may be either primary or secondary. In the case of primary adrenal insufficiency, the disorder arises directly within the outer region of the adrenal gland, called the adrenal cortex. Most of the time, the disorder is associated with an autoimmune

---

Information on Addison's Disease

Causes: Lack of hormone production by adrenal cortex from autoimmune dysfunction, cancer, or infection; abnormal regulation of adrenal hormone production by pituitary gland

Symptoms: Extreme fatigue, low blood pressure, appetite loss, fainting, severe diarrhea and vomiting, craving of salty foods, skin darkening

Duration: Chronic, with acute episodes (Addisonian crises)

Treatments: Hormone replacement, dietary changes (such as increased salt content)

---

dysfunction in which the body produces antibodies against adrenal tissue. Over time, the adrenal cortex is destroyed and the secretion of glucorticoid, mineralocorticoid, and adrenogenic hormones, the products of the adrenal cortex, ceases. Another cause of primary adrenal insufficiency is bacterial infections, particularly those associated with tuberculosis. The first identification of the disease, described by Thomas Addison in 1855, was associated with a tuberculosis infection in his patient. Other less common causes include fungal infections and malignancies.

Secondary adrenal insufficiency does not originate with the adrenal glands but rather is associated with abnormal regulation of adrenal hormone production, a function of the pituitary gland. Among the hormones produced within the pituitary gland is adrenocorticotropic hormone (ACTH), which stimulates glucocorticoid production by the adrenal cortex. Insufficient ACTH production results in a decrease in corticoid secretion. Any damage to the pituitary (or the hypothalamus, which actually regulates ACTH production by the pituitary) has the potential to affect ACTH production indirectly.

With Addison's disease, the onset of symptoms is gradual and can easily be overlooked or misdiagnosed during the early stages of the disease. Initially, the person may exhibit extreme fatigue, low blood pressure, and loss of appetite. The person may faint upon standing. Severe diarrhea and vomiting are also common. As a result of salt loss, the person may crave salty foods. Severe expression of such symptoms is referred to as an Addisonian crisis; if untreated, it may be life-threatening. Because the production of ACTH itself is regulated by corticosteroid production in a feedback mechanism, reduced adrenal function results in increased levels of ACTH. This in turn can produce skin changes, particularly a darkening which mimics that of deep tanning. The presence of darkening equally over both exposed and unexposed skin can be indicative of Addison's disease, particularly if other symptoms are also present.

A definitive diagnosis of Addison's disease is based upon a series of blood and urine tests. Patients may exhibit abnormally high levels of potassium, a potentially life-threatening situation, or a low level of sodium. More definitive tests measure the concentration of corticol hormones in the urine. Because ACTH production is controlled by corticosteroid concentrations, an increase in blood ACTH may also be observed. The definitive test begins with the intravenous injection of ACTH. Cortisol levels in the blood are then measured over a one-hour period. If cortisol levels do not change, this result is indicative of a likely adrenal insufficiency.

Treatment and Therapy

The treatment of Addison's disease generally involves replacing the hormones that the adrenal cortex is no longer manufacturing. Oral medication is available for most of these hormones, though dietary changes may also be necessary. For example, if the mineralocorticoid aldosterone is insufficient, resulting in a salt imbalance, then patients taking aldosterone supplements may also be advised to increase the salt content of their food.

Other forms of treatment may be symptomatic. If the patient suffers from low blood pressure or severe salt imbalances, conditions that are potentially life-threatening, then intravenous medication may be necessary.

As the monitoring of potassium and sodium levels is critical, it is generally recommended that patients routinely visit their physicians. It is important that a patient exhibiting symptoms of an Addisonian crisis (vomiting, diarrhea) receive immediate salt replacement and probably hydrocortisone as well.

Because secondary adrenal deficiency most often originates in the pituitary gland, the primary result is a decrease in ACTH production. In turn, the adrenal cortex is deficient only in the production of cortisol. Treatment generally involves the oral replacement of cortisol, often in the form of synthetic prednisone.

Perspective and Prospects

Addison's disease is a lifelong, chronic condition. While in the past it was often a life-threatening disorder, proper monitoring and hormone replacement can allow most people with the disease to live relatively normal lives with no restrictions. Because in most individuals the immediate cause is an autoimmune disorder, it is possible that eventually stem cell research, along with improved methods of controlling autoimmune phenomena, will provide a means for replacing adrenal tissue.

—*Richard Adler, Ph.D.*

See also Adrenalectomy; Autoimmune disorders; Corticosteroids; Endocrine disorders; Endocrinology; Endocrinology, pediatric; Glands; Hormones.

For Further Information:

Bar, Robert, ed. *Early Diagnosis and Treatment of Endocrine Disorders*. Totowa, N.J.: Humana Press, 2003.

Besser, G. Michael, and Michael Thorner, eds. *Clinical Endocrinology*. 2d ed. St. Louis, Mo.: Gower-Mosby, 1994.

Greenspan, Francis S., Dolores M. Shoback, and David G. Gardner, eds. *Greenspan's Basic and Clinical Endocrinology*. 8th ed. New York: McGraw-Hill, 2007.

Kronenberg, Henry M., et al., eds. *Williams Textbook of Endocrinology*. 11th ed. Philadelphia: Saunders/Elsevier, 2008.

MedlinePlus. "Addison Disease." *MedlinePlus*, Apr. 8, 2013 (reviewed May 2, 2012).

Parker, James N., and Philip M. Parker, eds. *The Official Patient's Sourcebook on Addison's Disease*. San Diego, Calif.: Icon Health, 2002.

Rennert, Nancy J., MD. "Addison's Disease." *MedlinePlus*, Dec. 11, 2011.

Adenoid removal. *See* Tonsillectomy and adenoid removal.

Adenoids

Anatomy

Also known as: Pharyngeal tonsils, nasopharyngeal tonsils

Anatomy or system affected: Ears, immune system, lymphatic system, mouth, nose, throat

Specialties and related fields: General surgery, immunology, internal medicine, otorhinolaryngology, speech pathology

Definition: A type of tonsil, part of the lymphatic system.

Structure and Functions

The nasopharyngeal tonsils, usually referred to as adenoids when swollen, are a mass of soft tissue in the nose-mouth area. Along with the palatine tonsil and the lingual tonsil, they belong to the lymphatic system, part of the body's immune system. Adenoids lie in the back of the nasal passage and above the pharynx, which is the uppermost part of the throat.

Much like lymph nodes, the lymphoid tissue of the adenoids wards off infection and are part of the body's first line of defense against bacteria that enter through the mouth and nose. They are largest in children, particularly those of three to four years of age, which is the period when humans are most susceptible to respiratory infection. Afterward, the adenoids slowly shrink and may even disappear.

Disorders and Diseases

In the process of fighting infection, the adenoids can become enlarged, sometimes with a diameter of greater than 40 millimeters (1.5 inches). This condition is called adenoid hypertrophy. In such cases, the mass may prevent breathing through the nose, obstruct the eustachian tube, and cause snoring, soreness, change in the voice, and sleep apnea. Excessive mouth breathing, in turn, can lead to changes in the facial structure of children (called adenoid facies), such as an elongated face and pinched nostrils. The enlarged adenoids may also harbor chronic infection, or adenoiditis, that fosters recurrent sinusitis and ear infections. In rare cases, cancer may cause the adenoids to swell.

Physicians may treat infected adenoids with a penicillin-derived drug. In the case of penicillin allergy or intractable infection, the adenoids can be removed surgically in an adenoidectomy, which is usually concurrent with the removal of the other tonsils in a tonsillectomy. Lasting about thirty minutes, it is usually an outpatient procedure and leaves patients with a sore throat for about a week.

Perspective and Prospects

Adenoidectomies were once routine, but that began to change in the 1980s. Pediatricians worried that removal of the adenoids could retard development of a child's immune system, and so the procedure came to be reserved for severe cases of adenoiditis.

—*Roger Smith, Ph.D.*

See also Lymphatic system; Otorhinolaryngology; Pediatrics; Tonsillectomy and adenoid removal; Tonsillitis.

For Further Information:

Beers, Mark H., ed. *The Merck Manual of Medical Information: Home Edition*. 17th ed. Whitehouse Station, N.J.: Merck Research Laboratories, 2008.

Hallberg, Anne C. *Tonsillar Disorders: Etiology, Diagnosis, and Treatment*. Hauppauge, N.Y.: Nova Science, 2011.

Munir, Nazia, and Ray Clarke. *Ear, Nose, and Throat at a Glance*. Hoboken, N.J.: John Wiley & Sons, 2013.

Parker, Steve. *The Human Body Book*. New York: Dorling Kindersley, 2013.

Parthasarathy, A., et al., eds. *Atlas of Pediatric Infectious Diseases*. London: J. P. Medical Limited, 2013.

Thibodeau, Gary A., and Kevin T. Patton. *Structure and Function of the Body*. 14th ed. St. Louis: Mosby Elsevier, 2012.

Adenoviruses

Disease/Disorder

Anatomy or system affected: Eyes, gastrointestinal system, immune system, intestines, lungs, nervous system, respiratory system, skin, stomach, urinary system

Specialties and related fields: Gastroenterology, immunology, ophthalmology, public health, urology, virology

Definition: Medium-sized viruses that can cause respiratory infections and diarrhea by infecting the epithelial linings of the respiratory, gastrointestinal, and urinary tracts, and the eyes.

Causes: Direct contact, fecal-oral transmission, insufficient chlorination of swimming pools

Symptoms: Bronchitis, common cold syndrome, conjunctivitis, croup, diarrhea, gastroenteritis, pneumonia, skin rashes

Duration: Days to months, or even years, depending on the infected host

Treatments: None; alleviation of symptoms

Key terms:

capsid: the protein shell of a virus

conjunctivitis: inflammation or infection of the eyelid membrane

croup: a respiratory disease that causes severe coughing

cystitis: inflammation of the urinary bladder

gastroenteritis: inflammation involving the stomach and small intestine

genus: a unit used to classify living organisms and fossils

icosahedral: characterized by having sixty rotational symmetries

virus: a small infectious agent that must enter a host cell to reproduce

Causes and Symptoms

Adenoviruses are members of the *Adenoviridae* family of viruses, which is divided into several genera whose

---

Information on Adenoviruses

Causes: Direct contact, fecal-oral transmission, insufficient chlorination of swimming pools

Symptoms: Bronchitis, common cold syndrome, conjunctivitis, croup, diarrhea, gastroenteritis, pneumonia, skin rashes

Duration: Days to months, or even years, depending on the infected host

Treatments: None; alleviation of symptoms

---

members can cause infections in a wide range of vertebrates, including humans and birds. Birds are commonly infected by members of the *Aviadenovirus* genus and the *Siadenovirus* genus. Examples of these viruses include *Fowl AdenovirusA* from the *Aviadenovirus* genus and *Turkey adenovirusB* from the *Siadenovirus* genus.

Humans can become infected by any of the subgroups labeled A through F of the *Mastadenovirus* genus. These six subgroups of *Mastadenovirus* that consist of more than fifty-two distinct human adenovirus serotypes. Members of subgroups C, D, E, and F can cause bronchitis, common cold syndrome, conjunctivitis, croup, cystitis, diarrhea, gastroenteritis, pneumonia, and skin rashes. While they do not cause cancer, adenovirus members of subgroups A and B have been shown to cause tumor growth in mice.

Exposure to the virus in insufficiently chlorinated swimming pools and drinking water can lead primarily to conjunctivitis, diarrhea, gastroenteritis, and skin rashes. Direct contact or fecal-oral transmission can cause any of the aforementioned conditions in addition to respiratory infections, such as the common cold, bronchitis, and pneumonia. Poorly disinfected surfaces in public areas or crowded locations such as schools and hospitals increase the likelihood of becoming infected.

A computed-generated rendering of an adenovirus. (© Pseudolongino/Dreamstime.com)

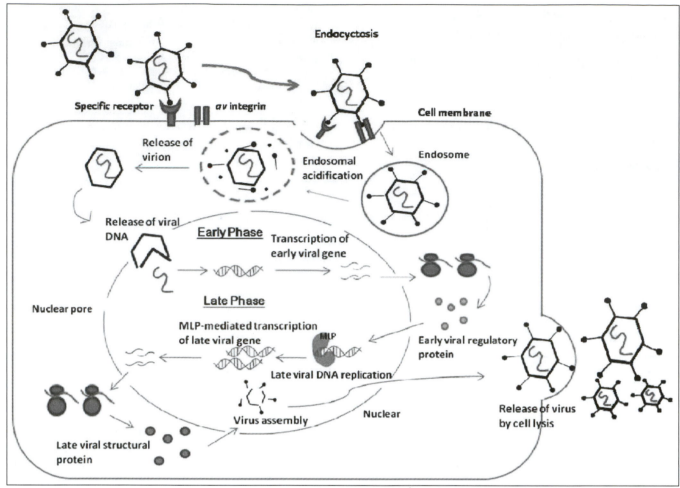

Adenovirus life cycle

Each adenovirus particle has an overall icosahedral shape, with a diameter of 60 to 90 nanometers. This particle shape is composed of three general types of proteins: capsid, minor, and core proteins. The exact function of each of the minor proteins, labeled as the IIIA, VI, VIII, and IX proteins, is not known precisely and is still under investigation. The IIIA protein is believed to assist with penetration of the virus into a host cell, while proteins VI, VIII, and IX are believed to assist with overall stabilization and assembly of the virus particle. Six proteins are classified as the core proteins. They are designated as proteins V, VII, Mu, TP (Terminal Protein), IV2a, and protease. Proteins V and VII have histone-like functions, while the Mu, TP, and IV2a proteins assist with genome replication and packaging processes. Protease is believed to facilitate growth and maturation processes.

Considerably more detail is known about the behavior and structure of the capsid proteins located on the exterior of the adenovirus particle, because of electron microscopy and X-ray crystallography. The capsid proteins include a hexon monomer that provides the greatest influence on the overall shape; the penton base proteins serve the function of penetration into the host cell (human or bird cells); and the fiber proteins extend outward from the pentons, allowing them to interact with specific cellular receptors, including the coxsackievirus-adenovirus receptor, on a host. Once the globular domain at the end of each fiber protein binds to the appropriate cellular receptor (cellular integrins), the virus enters the host cell. Adenovirus replication occurs in two phases, described as the early phase and the late phase, during which deoxyribonucleic acid (DNA) replication begins. All adenoviruses contain double-stranded DNA genomes, and adenovirus replication occurs in the nucleus of the host cell.

Treatment and Therapy

Although outbreaks of adenovirus infection occur most often in winter, spring, and early summer, adenovirus infections can occur anytime during the year. Some adenoviruses are endemic to those parts of the world with especially unsanitary conditions, making outbreaks common in these areas. Young children are infected by adenoviruses with the greatest frequency, and most people have been infected by at least one adenovirus by the age of ten. Generally, the symptoms are treated, but no treatment specifically targets the adenovirus itself. Antiviral medications (ganciclovir, vidarabine ribavirin, and cidofovir) have been used to treat immunocompromised individuals with varying degrees of success.

In the News:
Mutation in Adenovirus Responsible for Fatalities

An adenovirus causing fatal respiratory infection has been identified at military bases in Texas, Washington, Oregon, South Carolina, and New York, according to John Su of the Centers for Disease Control and Prevention (CDC). Although adenoviruses of various types have been causing numerous illnesses since being identified in the 1950s, they have typically not caused the deaths of patients so quickly. Most adenoviruses cause pneumonia, conjunctivitis, and gastrointestinal disease as a result of insufficient use of disinfectants. Only a small percentage of cases have required hospitalization, and deaths have been rare.

However, adenovirus serotype 14 (Ad14), one of the first adenovirus strains to be identified in 1955, has developed a mutation that causes it to be much more lethal. Seven of the thirty hospitalized patients died within days of the first symptoms. Infectious disease expert Dr. David N. Gilbert discovered this mutated Ad14. Samples from all five states were analyzed and found to have exactly the same sequence data of genes, and each had the same mutation, according to polymerase chain reaction (PCR) and immunofluorescence studies.

According to Oregon health investigator Paul Lewis, Ad14 has increased dramatically from rarely occurring a few years ago to now being the cause of more than 50 percent of all adenovirus infections in Oregon. This Ad14 can survive on surfaces for weeks, thus making it even more crucial for people to adhere to good hand-washing habits and to seek out medical treatment at the occurrence of escalating flulike symptoms to prevent the development of pneumonia.

—Jeanne L. Kuhler, Ph.D.

Some adenoviruses can survive for days outside of the body because of their stability to both acidic and basic conditions. Therefore, the best treatment continues to be prevention through frequent hand washing and avoidance of the fecal-oral transmission that can occur with poor quality drinking water or direct contact with the water of small lakes, as well as transmission via insufficiently chlorinated swimming pools.

Perspective and Prospects

A live attenuated oral vaccine exists against type-4 and type-17 adenoviruses. It is administered as two tablets. These two adenoviruses can cause respiratory disease with influenza-like symptoms, eye and other infections, which may rarely lead to pneumonia or other serious complications. In the United States, adenovirus vaccine is approved only for military personnel ages 17 to 50. Its use varies among different branches of the military. Most often, it is given to new recruits because of the potential for viral diseases to spread widely due to dormitory-style living conditions. Side effects include mild respiratory and gastrointestinal discomfort. About one percent of recruits develop a fever. There is no indication that the adenovirus vaccines will be extended to a civilian population, as symptoms of adenovirus infection are generally mild.

—Jeanne L. Kuhler, PhD;
updated by Tish Davidson, A.M.

See also: Bronchitis; Childhood infectious diseases; Common cold; Conjunctivitis; Croup; Diarrhea and dysentery; Gastroenteritis; Infection; Influenza; Noroviruses; Pneumonia; Pulmonary diseases; Rashes; Rotavirus; Viral infections.

For Further Information:

"Adenovirus" In: Davidson, Tish. *Vaccines: History, Issues, and Science.* Santa Barbara, CA: Greenwood, 2017; 122-23.

"Adenoviruses." U.S. Centers for Disease Control and Prevention May 23, 2017. https://www.cdc.gov/adenovirus/ index.html (accessed July 30, 3017). *Official government information on shinglesfrom the National Center for Immunizationand Respiratory Diseases.*

"Adenovirus Infections." In: Kimberlin DW, Brady MT, Jackson MA, Long SS eds. 2015 *Red Book: Report of the Committee on Infectious Diseases.* 30th ed. Elk Grove Village, IL: American Academy of Pediatrics; 2015: 226-8.

Gompf, Sandra. "Adenoviruses." *Medscape.com* May 18, 2017. http://emedicine.medscape.com/article/211738-overview (accessed July 30, 2017).

Pringle, Craig R. "Adenovirus Infections." In: *Merck Manual Professional Edition Online* 2017. http://www. merckmanuals.com/professional/infectious-diseases/respiratory-viruses/adenovirus-infections (accessed July 30, 2017).

Adipose tissue

Anatomy

Anatomy or system affected: Systemic

Specialties and related fields: Medicine, nursing, nutrition, exercise physiology

Definition: Adipose tissue is connective tissue in which fat is stored and the cells distended by droplets of fat

Adipose tissue is the anatomical name for body fat found in humans and other mammals. Adipose tissue is composed of a loose collection of adipocytes, or cells specially designed to provide storage for lipids and triglycerides. Lipids and triglycerides are naturally occurring, non-water soluble molecules that store energy for the body's future use. These fat reserves help insulate and protect the body. They provide a source of energy when food is unavailable. When more energy is consumed than the body needs, the quantity of adipose tissue grows, leading to obesity.

For many years, scientists believed that adipose tissue functioned simply as a storage container, holding energy in fat for future use. Twenty-first-century research has shown that it takes an active role in a number of key body functions, including regulating appetite, body weight, immunity, reproduction, and the way the body uses insulin and ingested fats. Although too much body fat can be a bad thing, adipose tissue plays an essential role in overall health.

Background

The two main forms of adipose tissue are white and brown. The center of most white adipocytes is a vacuole, or a sack surrounded by a membrane, filled with lipids. The remainder of the cell components surround the vacuole, giving the adipocyte a ring-like appearance. In brown adipocytes, lipids are dispersed in smaller drops throughout the cell. Brown adipocyte cells have a larger blood supply to help promote the provision of heat to the body. Adipocytes may be as small as 30 microns or larger than 230 microns. Brown cells are generally smaller than white cells. They are loosely held together by collagen fibers to form the third layer of the body under the skin.

White and brown adipose tissue are similar in composition but have some key differences. White adipose tissue stores energy and helps regulate other functions of the body. In addition, white adipose tissue is a poor conductor of heat, making it a very effective form of insulation for the body. This type is far more common and is the type people usually are referring to when they speak of body fat.

Brown adipose tissue is found more commonly in small mammals, such as mice and rats, and in human infants. The main function of brown adipose is to maintain body heat. Therefore, it is more common in small mammals, which are more vulnerable to cold because of their size. Human infants are generally unable to generate body heat by shivering, so the presence of a larger percentage of brown adipose tissue functions as an additional heat source.

As babies grow, brown adipose tissue disappears, and it is rarely present in adults. However, some individuals can develop so-called "beige" fat cells. This type of adipose tissue has been found in mice and in some people who exercise heavily. Exercise prompts skeletal muscles to release a protein called irisin, which in turn acts on white adipose cells to make them function like brown cells. An athlete's lean body can then compensate for the lack of insulating body fat by generating heat from the transformed white adipose tissue as if it were brown adipose tissue.

The number and type of adipose fat cells changes over an individual's lifetime. Each adipocyte has a life span of about ten years, after which it is replaced by a new cell. In humans, brown cells diminish, and white cells become more predominant. People have a tendency to gain weight with age, which is known to be the result of individual adipocytes growing in size. It is unclear, however, whether the body continues to increase the number of adipocytes it produces once an individual reaches adulthood or simply replaces worn out cells.

In addition to helping to regulate the body's temperature through insulation or heat generation, adipose tissue functions as an unofficial part of the endocrine system. The endocrine system regulates most of the body's important functions through the release of hormones from the thyroid, pancreas, pituitary gland, adrenal glands, and other glandular organs. Adipose tissue releases more than fifty adipokines, or substances that act like hormones, even though it is not technically part of the endocrine system.

Two of the more important adipokines produced by adipose tissue are adiponectin and leptin. Adiponectin affects how the body metabolizes fats and sugar; with more adiponectin, fats and sugars are more efficiently processed through the bloodstream. Among the more important results of this are increased glucose tolerance and decreased insulin resistance, leading to lower risk of diabetes. Leptin helps the hypothalamus regulate appetite; when leptin levels are low, individuals are more likely to overeat and become obese. In addition, a relationship exists between the amount of adipose tissue and the effectiveness of the adipokines, and researchers continue to study this relationship as a potential means to reduce the incidence of weight-related illnesses such as diabetes.

Topic Today

The role of adipose tissue in overall health is thought to be related to inflammation. Inflammation is the body's response to something harmful. Researchers have determined that high levels of adipose tissue—obesity—create a low level of persistent inflammation in a body, which affects the immune system and makes the body more susceptible to attack in the form of illnesses, including cancer. Adipose tissue has also been found to affect the function of the reproductive system, including the levels of the hormones necessary for fertility. The presence of either too much or too little adipose tissue can negatively affect fertility and reproduction.

Scientists continue to work to understand the complex interactions between adipose tissue and other body systems in the hopes of reducing or eliminating diseases such as type 2 diabetes and other weight-related conditions. They also are considering the unique aspects of adipose tissue to help find treatments for other conditions. For example, among the materials that make up adipocytes are stem cells, which are generally more abundant in and more easily harvested from adipose tissue than stem cells from bone marrow and other sources. These cells may help to treat bones that resist healing after breaks and other conditions.

—*Janine Ungvarsky;*
updated by Geraldine Marrocco

For Further Information:

Bartelt, Alexander, and Joerg Heeren. "Adipose Tissue Browning and Metabolic Health." *Nature Reviews Endocrinology*, vol. 10, 2014, pp. 24-36, www.nature.com/nrendo/ journal/v10/n1/full/nrendo.2013.204.html. Accessed 5 Oct. 2016.

Blamire, John. "Adipose Tissue." *BIOdotEDU*. Brooklyn College, 2005, www.brooklyn.cuny.edu/bc/ahp/LAD/C4d/ C4d_adipose.html. Accessed 3 Oct. 2016.

Bohler, Henry Jr., et al. "Adipose Tissue and Reproduction in Women." *Fertility and Sterility*, vol. 94, no. 3, Aug. 2010, www.fertstert.org/article/S0015-0282(09)00749-3/fulltext. Accessed 3 Oct. 2016.

Catalán, V., et al. "Adipose Tissue Immunity and Cancer." *Frontiers in Physiology*, Oct. 2013, www.ncbi.nlm.nih.gov/pubmed/ 24106481. Accessed 3 Oct. 2016.

Coelho, Marisa, et al. "Biochemistry of Adipose Tissue: An Endocrine Organ." *Archives of Medical Science*, vol. 9, no. 2, 2013, www.ncbi.nlm.nih.gov/pmc/articles/ PMC3648822/. Accessed 3 Oct. 2016.

Corvera, Sylvia, and Olga Gealekman. "Adipose Tissue Angiogenesis: Impact on Obesity and Type-2 Diabetes." *Molecular Basis of Disease*, vol. 1842, no. 3, Mar. 2014, www.science direct.com/science/article/pii/ S0925443913002111. Accessed 3 Oct. 2016.

Greenberg, Andrew S., and Martin S. Obin. "Obesity and the Role of Adipose Tissue in Inflammation and Metabolism." *The American Journal of Clinical Nutrition*, vol. 83, no. 2, Feb. 2006, ajcn.nutrition.org/content/83/2/461S.full. Accessed 3 Oct. 2016.

Tawonsawatruk, T., et al. "Adipose Derived Pericytes Rescue Fractures from a Failure of Healing—Non-union." *Scientific Reports*, vol. 6, 21 Mar. 2016, www.nature.com/articles/srep22779. Accessed 3 Oct. 2016.

Adolescent sexuality

Biology

Anatomy or system affected: Reproductive, endocrine, musculoskeletal systems, psychological development, gender identity

Specialties and related fields: Pediatric medicine, psychiatry, social work, education, epidemiology

Definition: Human sexuality is a broad concept that embodies interaction among anatomy, hormones, and physiology, psychology, interpersonal relationships, and sociocultural influences

Adolescent sexuality is the sexual development, feelings, and behavior of children going through adolescence. It involves several different aspects, including exposure to sex, experimenting, discovering gender identity, and forming romantic relationships. Around twelve years of age, adolescents begin exploring their sexuality. Both boys and girls experiment sexually, such as masturbating. Some adolescents will even engage in sexual acts with others. However, adolescents lack emotional and cognitive maturity, so sexually active adolescents could put themselves at risk for unwanted pregnancies and sexually transmitted diseases (STDs). Parents should, therefore, talk to their children about sex at an early age.

Overview

Sexuality is a major part of adolescent development. As an adolescent hits puberty and begins to mature, he or she will be exposed to sex and will begin experimenting. Adolescents are exposed to sex through the Internet, television, and entertainers and other celebrities. Between the ages of twelve and fifteen, adolescents become curious about their sexuality and begin experimenting. Boys around this age generally show more interest in sex than girls. Usually at twelve or thirteen, adolescents begin reading about sex and viewing sexual images. Such material may include information about sex, drawings in books, and pornographic images and videos. They may find this material in anatomy books, in adult magazines, on television, and on the Internet. Adolescents of this age may also begin *peeping*, or secretly observing someone naked or removing his or her clothes. Typically, adolescents who engage in any of these activities try to avoid getting caught or deny the activities.

Masturbation plays a significant role in adolescents' sexual experimentation, especially for boys. They may experience frequent erections, and some may occur spontaneously. This can be attributed to the chemical and hormonal changes of *puberty*, or the set of changes an adolescent undergoes as he or she develops sexually. Boys often experiment with their erections, frequently engaging in *masturbation*, which is the stimulation of one's own genitals, usually to achieve orgasm. Adolescent girls may experience spontaneous vaginal secretions, either because of sexual arousal or because of hormonal fluctuations during their menstrual cycle. Girls also engage in masturbation, but because girls are generally less aware of their sexual arousal than boys, girls typically do not masturbate as frequently as boys.

Understanding distinctions between gender, sexual orientation, and sexual behavior is a critical concept in adolescent health and is influenced greatly by the culture in which one lives. An individual's impression of gender or sexuality often is conveyed first to him or her by parents during early childhood. Parents or other immediate family members help children define what is male and female and how they express themselves as members of their gender. Some authors argue that social environments after birth may have little or no impact on gender identity or sexual orientation, with prenatal hormones having major effects on organizing developing sexuality.

As children become adolescents, influences broaden with peer, media, and community norms of gender and sexuality impacting their individual value systems. Media exerts a powerful influence on adolescents and their perception of gender roles and sexual behavior. American adolescents are exposed to several hours of media (television, radio, internet) each day, during which they experience significant exposure to sexual content, which often contains implicit and explicit references to intercourse. Electronic media and social networking provide adolescents with even more ways to explore their burgeoning sexuality. Online social networking sites for adolescents frequently mention or feature sex and sexual behaviors. In a national survey of United States teenagers (ages 13 to 19), 20 percent self-reported sending and 48 percent reported receiving sexual messages. Longitudinal research consistently links degree of exposure to sexuality in the media to increased sexual risk taking and adverse outcomes.

Adolescent sexuality occurs in the context of many other aspects of adolescent development and is more complicated for sexual minorities or lesbian, gay, bisexual, transgender, queer, or questioning (LGBTQQ) youth. Regardless of the acronyms and current issues in terminology, the individual youth is the person best suited to describe and define identity and behaviors. Many youth refuse categorization, preferring more diffuse terminology such as gender queer, queer, pansexual, or fluid regarding gender and sexuality. What matters for most youth is that their health care provider asks about their personal perspective, experience, and what terminology best suits their needs.

When adolescents turn fourteen or fifteen, they typically become interested in romantic relationships. They may seek a partner with whom to have such a relationship. These relationships may be short-term or long-term.

At about fifteen or sixteen years of age, girls begin to explore the moral and physical consequences of sex. They may grow concerned about a teen pregnancy. They may also ask themselves what sexual activities are acceptable and under what circumstances sex is okay. Boys around this age are not as concerned about these issues.

Many adolescents between sixteen and eighteen years of age will experience an increase in sexual activity. This may be in the form of masturbation or sexual acts with a partner. The frequency and intensity of this sexual activity may increase. During this time, adolescents also typically seek long-term, committed relationships.

At nineteen to twenty-two years of age, adolescents may show an interest in casual dating and casual sexual encounters. Others may be more interested in committed, monogamous relationships. Adolescents around these ages will generally make wise decisions regarding sex because their emotional and cognitive maturity has improved.

Typically, however, adolescents do not have the necessary emotional and cognitive maturity to make wise decisions regarding sexual activity. Furthermore, they are unable to handle the possible consequences of sex. For instance, many adolescents do not realize the gravity of unprotected sex and may engage in this activity, exposing themselves to an unwanted pregnancy and STDs. Adolescents may also have the misconception that other forms of sexual intercourse, such as oral or anal sex, are safer than penile-vaginal intercourse. These adolescents, however, are still at risk for STDs or even pregnancy.

Because of these risk factors, parents should discuss sex and sexuality with their adolescent children. However, the discussion about sex is often difficult for both parents and adolescents. Parents may have difficulty bringing up the subject, and adolescents may feel embarrassed talking about sex with their parents. Despite the uncomfortable nature of the sex talk, it is an important part of an adolescent's sexual development. Parents should begin talking to their child about sex before he or she hits puberty. This would likely make the parents and adolescent more comfortable talking about sex as the child grows. Parents should share factual information about sex with their child. In particular, they should explain the consequences of having sex and the dangers of unprotected sex, including the possibility of pregnancy and contracting STDs. Parents should also address any questions their child may have regarding sex. Other topics parents should discuss with their child include peer pressure and media pressure associated with sex, values and morals with regard to sex, and sexual orientation.

—*Michael Mazzei;*
updated by Geraldine Marrocco

For Further Information:

Brown, RT. "Adolescent sexuality at the dawn of the 21st century." *Adolesc Med* 2000; 11:19.

Breuner, CC, Mattson G, Committee on Adolescence, Committee on Psychosocial Aspects of Child and Family Health. Sexuality Education for Children and Adolescents. *Pediatrics* 2016; 138.

Ferrell, Keith. "Adolescent Sexuality: Talk the Talk before They Walk the Walk." *Healthy Children.* American Academy of Pediatrics. Winter 2008. Web. 22 Sept. 2014. http://www.healthychildren.org/Documents/Healthy-Children-Magazine/HealthyChildren-08winter.pdf

Oswalt, Angela. "The Development of Adolescent Sexuality." *Seven Counties Services.* Web. 22 Sept. 2014. http://sevencounties.org/poc/view_doc.php?type=doc&id=41180 &cn=1310

Oswalt, Angela. "The Development of Sexual Orientation." *Seven Counties Services.* Web. 22 Sept. 2014. http://sevencounties.org/poc/view_doc.php?type=doc&id=41179&cn=1310

Oswalt, Angela. "Middle to Late Adolescence (Ages 15 to 22): The Age of Romance." *Seven Counties Services.* Seven Counties Services. Web. 22 Sept. 2014. http://sevencounties.org/poc/view_doc.php?type=doc&id=41181&cn=1310

Savic I, Garcia-Falgueras A, Swaab DF. "Sexual differentiation of the human brain in relation to gender identity and sexual orientation." *Prog Brain Res* 2010; 186:41.

Strasburger VC, Jordan AB, Donnerstein E. "Health effects of media on children and adolescents." *Pediatrics* 2010; 125:756.

Adrenal glands

Anatomy

Also known as: Suprarenal glands

Anatomy or system affected: All

Specialties and related fields: Biochemistry, endocrinology, genetics, internal medicine

Definition: A pair of small hormone-producing glands located atop the kidneys. Each adrenal is made up of a complex outer layer of cells (the cortex), which produces steroid hormones, and an inner layer (the medulla), which produces epinephrine and norepinephrine.

Key terms:

cortex: the outer layer of the adrenal gland, the area that produces steroid hormones

hormone: a chemical messenger secreted by one cell type and acting on another type, causing a predictable response; hormones regulate nearly everything in the body, including digestion, sleep, growth, sexual development, and reproductive cycles

medulla: the central portion of the adrenal gland, the area that produces epinephrine (adrenaline)

steroids: a class of fat-soluble chemicals that are structurally related to one another and share the same chemical skeleton; includes hormones, drugs, and other molecules

stress: the body's reaction to a change that requires a physical, mental, or emotional adjustment response

Structure and Functions

The adrenal glands are perched on top of each kidney; they are often referred to as "caps" or "hats" on the kidneys. The name in Latin describes this position well: "adrenal" means "toward the kidney" and "suprarenal" means "on top of the kidney." These ductless glands are triangular or pyramidal in shape and measure roughly 1 to 1.5 centimeters in height and 7 to 8 centimeters in length. Each gland consists of two parts: a medulla (center portion) and the surrounding cortex. Together they are responsible for releasing three different classes of hormones that are critical for normal survival. These hormones control such vital functions as daily metabolism (such as managing blood sugar levels), regulating salt and water balance, regulating inflammation, controlling basic stress responses (the fight-or-flight response), and initiating and controlling the onset of puberty.

The adrenal glands work interactively with both the hypothalamus and the pituitary in the brain. The hypothalamus releases corticotropin-releasing factor (CRF), which stimulates the anterior pituitary to secrete adrenocorticotropic hormone (ACTH). ACTH in turn stimulates the adrenal glands to produce cortisol and other hormones, which then causes the hypothalamus to stop producing CRF.

The cortex (80 to 90 percent of the adrenal gland) is the complex outer layer of cells in the adrenal gland, and it secretes a variety of hormones into the bloodstream. The outermost layer of the cortex is known as the zona glomerulosa; it secretes aldosterone, the primary mineralocorticoid, which regulates salt (sodium) excretion from the body. This in turn causes water to be retained, increasing blood volume and therefore blood pressure. The middle layer is the zona fasciculata, which secretes glucocorticoids such as cortisol and corticosterone. They help control the body's use of carbohydrates, lipids, and proteins for the production of energy needs in the body. They also suppress inflammatory responses in the body and thus have a significant effect on the function of the immune system. The innermost layer (next to the medulla) is the zona reticularis, which secretes androgens that affect the development and maintenance of male characteristics as well as muscle development in both males and females.

The medulla is the inner portion of the adrenal gland, surrounded completely by the cortical layers. Unlike the cortex, it is not essential for life. However, the hormones it secretes are used each day as the body deals with various stressors. The principal hormones of the adrenal medulla are epinephrine and norepinephrine. Epinephrine (also known as adrenaline) causes an increase in heart rate and in the force of heart contractions. It also facilitates increased blood flow to the muscles and brain and causes the relaxation of smooth muscles in the gastrointestinal tract, the reproductive tract, and surrounding small blood vessels. Thus, its net effect is to prepare the body for the sympathetic nervous system response during times of physical activity or stress of various types. Its partner, norepinephrine, also causes contraction of blood vessels and elevation of heart rate and triggers the release of stored glucose into the bloodstream.

Disorders and Diseases

A variety of adrenal disorders are known, including those caused by lack of individual enzymes in the hormone-producing pathways. The three most common disorders are Cushing's syndrome, Addison's disease, and congenital adrenal hyperplasia.

Cushing's syndrome occurs when excess amounts of cortisol are secreted from the adrenal glands. This may be a by-product of adrenal tumors, may be the result of adrenal hyperplasia, or may be caused by various medications. Treatment can include surgery, irradiation, or drugs, depending on the etiology. Adrenalectomy (adrenal gland removal) may be performed if a tumor is present.

Addison's disease (also called adrenal insufficiency or hypocortisolism) occurs when at least 90 percent of the adrenal cortex has been destroyed, and it results in the inability of the body to control stress responses. It is characterized by weight loss, muscle weakness, fatigue, low blood pressure, and occasional darkening of the skin, and it can be fatal. Several conditions, including autoimmunity, polyendocrine deficiency syndrome, and tuberculosis, can lead to this condition. As with insulin-dependent diabetes, Addison's disease requires lifelong hormone replacement therapy.

Congenital adrenal hyperplasia (CAH) is an inborn deficiency in the ability of the adrenal glands to make cortisol.

This is usually caused by an enzyme deficiency or malfunction, resulting in some hormone pathways (such as cortisol) being turned off and others (such as androgens) being turned on more than normal. Treatment usually involves cortisol injections.

Perspective and Prospects

The adrenal glands were first described in humans in 1563 by Italian physiologist Bartolomeo Eustachio. The first studies of their function in the human were published in 1855 by Thomas Addison, who also later described their dysfunction and for whom Addison's disease is named. In 1929 Walter Cannon popularized the concept of the "fight-or-flight" response as the basic function of the adrenal medulla, and in 1936 Hans Selye put forth the idea of the "alarm" reaction for the cortex.

There are a variety of disorders associated with the adrenal glands, and treatment options, from medicine to surgery, vary and depend on the specific adrenal problem being addressed.

—*Kerry L. Cheesman, Ph.D.*

See also Addison's disease; Adrenalectomy; Adrenoleukodistrophy; Brain; Congenital adrenal hyperplasia; Corticosteroids; Cushing's syndrome; Endocrine disorders; Endocrinology; Endocrinology, pediatric; Glands; Hormone therapy; Hormones; Kidneys; Systems and organs.

For Further Information:
Frisch, Lawrence. "Adrenalectomy-Open Surgery." *HealthLibrary*, May 18, 2013.
Garnier, Linda. *My Battle with Cushing's Disease*. Coral Springs, Fla.: Llumina Press, 2003.
Lam, Michael, and Dorine Lam. *Adrenal Fatigue Syndrome*. Loma Linda, Calif.: Adrenal Institute Press, 2012.
Loechner, Karen. "Adrenal Insufficiency and Addison's Disease." *National Endocrine and Metabolic Diseases Information Service.* April 6, 2012.
Hsu, C. Y., and Scott Rivkees. *Congenital Adrenal Hyperplasia: A Parents' Guide*. Bloomington, Ind.: AuthorHouse, 2005.
Pozzilli, Paolo, et al. *Atlas of Endocrine and Metabolic Disease*. Chicester, England: John Wiley and Sons, 2014.
Stewart, P. M. "The Adrenal Cortex." In *Williams Textbook of Endocrinology*, edited by Shlomo Melmed. 12th ed. Philadelphia: Elsevier/Saunders, 2012.
Wilson, James L. *Adrenal Fatigue: The Twenty-first Century Stress Syndrome*. Petaluma, Calif.: Smart Publications, 2001.

Adrenalectomy

Procedure

Anatomy or system affected: Abdomen, endocrine system, glands, kidneys, urinary system

Specialties and related fields: Endocrinology, general surgery

Definition: The surgical removal of one or both of the adrenal glands.

Indications and Procedures

The adrenal glands produce chemical substances which regulate the body's responses to stress, including the fight-or-flight response. Occasionally, if the adrenal glands become diseased (for example, with cancer) or the hormones that they produce aggravate another condition (such as breast cancer), a physician may determine that they must be surgically removed. Benign tumors of the adrenal gland may sometimes produce additional hormones that disrupt body functions. The tumors, and possibly the adrenal glands, must be removed to rectify the condition.

Depending on the type of tumor, adrenalectomy may require a major surgery or a less invasive laparoscopic surgery. Candidates for laparoscopic surgery include patients whose tumors are less than 10 centimeters in diameter and have no malignant characteristics. In the laparoscopic procedure, the surgeon makes three to four small incisions, then inserts small telescopes on long instruments into the abdominal cavity. The abdomen is inflated with gas, and a camera on an instrument displays images on a monitor. The surgeon uses these images to navigate to the tumor and, with fine instruments, ties off blood vessels and disconnects the adrenal gland. The gland is placed into a small plastic bag inserted into the abdomen and then removed through the incision.

An open adrenalectomy is performed on large or cancerous tumors. It requires a large incision under the rib cage along the middle of the abdomen, or along the side of the body. This more invasive procedure allows the surgeon to explore the organs of the abdominal cavity for disease. The colon and a portion of the small intestine are moved to expose the kidneys. After the adrenal veins and arteries are sealed, each gland is dissected from its position at the top of each kidney. Internal organs are replaced, drains are brought out through the incisions, and the incisions are closed. The procedure may also be performed by a posterior approach through the rib cage.

Uses and Complications

Open adrenalectomies require four to five days of hospitalization, whereas laparoscopic procedures require two to three days. Complications of abdominal surgery are possible, including infection and internal bleeding, as are other potential complications of major surgery, including negative reaction to anesthesia. The risks of the surgery are small in comparison to the risk of not removing the adrenal tumor. The patient is monitored closely postsurgery and given oral supplements for the hormones normally provided by the adrenal glands.

—*Karen E. Kalumuck, Ph.D.*

See also Abdomen; Abdominal disorders; Adrenal glands; Cancer; Corticosteroids; Cushing's syndrome; Endocrinology; Glands; Hormones; Kidneys; Nephrectomy; Tumor removal; Tumors.

For Further Information:

"Adrenalectomy." *Medline Plus*, January 29, 2013.
"Adrenalectomy-Laparoscopic Surgery." *Health Library*, May 28, 2013.
"Adrenalectomy-Open Surgery." *Health Library*, May 28, 2013.
Beldegrum, Arie, et al., eds. *Renal and Adrenal Tumors*. New York: Oxford University Press, 2002.
Ernest, Ingrid. *Adrenalectomy in Cushing's Disease: A Long-Term Follow-up*. Copenhagen: Periodica, 1972.
Hunt, Thomas K., et al. *Adrenalectomy*. Boston: Little, Brown, 1978.
Libertino, John A., and Andrew C. Novick, eds. *Adrenal Surgery*. Philadelphia: W. B. Saunders, 1989.

Adrenoleukodystrophy

Disease/Disorder

Also known as: Melanodermic leukodystrophy, Siemerling- Creutzfeldt disease, X-linked ALD

Anatomy or system affected: Brain, ears, endocrine system, eyes, genitals, glands, nervous system, psychic-emotional system, reproductive system, respiratory system, skin

Specialties and related fields: Audiology, dermatology, emergency medicine, endocrinology, genetics, neurology, ophthalmology, pathology, pediatrics, psychiatry, pulmonary medicine

Definition: A variable X-linked genetic disorder with symptoms ranging from adrenal insufficiency to progressive neurological deterioration.

Key terms:

adrenal gland: an endocrine gland that makes steroid hormones in the cortex (outer layer) and stress hormones (epinephrine) in the medulla (inner layer)

adrenocorticotropin (ACTH): a hormone made in the pituitary gland in the brain that stimulates the adrenal cortex to make steroid hormones

demyelination: a loss of the fatty, white substance that coats nerves

peroxisome: a cellular organelle that contains enzymes and metabolizes hydrogen peroxide

Causes and Symptoms

X-linked adrenoleukodystrophy (ALD) is caused by mutations in the *ABCD1* gene. The *ABCD1* gene codes for the ALD protein. This protein is located in the membrane of an essential cellular organelle, the peroxisome, which has a role in cellular metabolism. Very long chain fatty acids (VLCFA) are metabolized in the peroxisome. The buildup of saturated VLCFA in tissues causes the symptoms of X-linked adrenoleukodystrophy. A diagnosis can be made in males by identifying an elevated VLCFA level in body fluids. In females, VLCFA levels are not reliable, and genetic testing is necessary.

The symptoms of X-linked ALD vary from one individual to the next, even within the same family. The gene mutation or level of VLCFA in body fluids is not a predictor of symptom type or age of onset. Because the *ABCD1* gene is located on the X chromosome, the disease presentation is different in males and females. The clinical presentation of X-linked ALD in males can be categorized into three groups. About 35 to 50 percent of males with X-linked

---

Information on Adrenoleukodystrophy

Causes: Mutations in the *ABCD1* gene, inherited in more than 90 percent of cases

Symptoms: Adrenal insufficiency, increased skin pigment, hyperactivity, difficulty swallowing, difficulty talking, seizures, small testes, psychosis, vision loss, hearing loss, paresis (weakness)

Duration: Lifelong

Treatments: Oral steroids, bone marrow transplants

ALD have a childhood cerebral disorder. The age of onset varies from three to ten years but can occur as late as twenty-one years of age. Boys with the cerebral type of X-linked ALD have a progressive loss of the myelin that encloses the nerves in the brain (demyelination). As the condition progresses, characteristic abnormalities can be seen on brain magnetic resonance imaging (MRI). The neurological symptoms may include cognitive disturbances, hyperactivity, seizures, and psychosis. Boys with X-linked ALD may also experience vision and hearing loss. They enter a vegetative state and die within approximately two to four years of the onset of neurological symptoms. Insufficient hormone production from the adrenal gland, also known as Addison's disease, is identified in 90 percent of boys with the childhood cerebral type of X-linked ALD. The symptoms of untreated Addison's disease may include vomiting, fatigue, low blood pressure, weakness, increased skin pigmentation, and coma. Adrenal insufficiency can be detected through identification of an elevated plasma adrenocorticotropin (ACTH).

The second type of X-linked ALD is an adult-onset disorder typically referred to as adrenomyeloneuropathy (AMN). The symptoms of AMN include progressive weakness of the legs, paresis, sphincter disturbance, and sexual dysfunction. Onset of symptoms ranges from the econd to fourth decade but typically occurs in the late twenties. About 70 percent of men with AMN also have Addison's disease.

For approximately 10 percent of males with X-linked ALD, Addison's disease is the only symptom, which usually manifests initially at around age eight but can start in adulthood. Most men with Addison's disease as the only symptom of X-linked ALD will eventually develop neurological involvement. Rarely, males with an *ABCD1* gene mutation are asymptomatic.

Approximately 10 to 50 percent of females with an *ABCD1* gene mutation will have neurological symptoms, which are milder and progress more slowly than in men but are otherwise similar to AMN. The onset of symptoms is typically in a person's thirties.

Treatment and Therapy

The treatment for the adrenal insufficiency identified in most males with X-linked ALD is steroid hormone replacement.

For the childhood cerebral type, management is typically supportive, and stimulants can be helpful for treatment of hyperactivity. However, bone marrow transplantation is a permanent cure. Because it is associated with a high mortality rate of about 20 percent, as of 2009, it is only recommended in the early stages of cerebral involvement, when abnormalities are first noted on brain MRI.

For males with AMN and symptomatic females, treatment is typically supportive, including physical therapy and psychological counseling.

Perspective and Prospects

The first description of symptoms consistent with child-hood cerebral X-linked adrenoleukodystrophy in the medical literature was by Ernst Siemerling and Hans Gerhard Creutzfeldt in 1923. The first adult patient with AMN was described by Herbert Budka in 1976. The incidence of X-linked ALD is now estimated at 1 in 20,000 male births.

The first attempt to cure X-linked ALD was in the 1980s. The proposed treatment was dietary restriction of VLCFA; however, the levels of VLCFA were not lowered in body fluids. The next attempt was a combination of dietary restriction and administration of a dietary supplement called "Lorenzo's oil," a mixture of glyceryl trioleate and glyceryl trierucate. This combination lowers the level of VLCFA in the body fluids. Unfortunately, in symptomatic patients, it does not alter the course of their disease. In presymptomatic patients, some studies have suggested that administration of Lorenzo's oil and dietary restriction of VLCFA reduces the chances of cerebral or neurological involvement. The efficacy of Lorenzo's oil is an area of research. Gene therapy is also an area of research for the treatment of X-linked ALD. A few cases of successful gene therapy in patients with cerebral type X-linked ALD were reported in 2009.

—*Beth M. Hannan, M.S., C.G.C.*

See also Addison's disease; Adrenal glands; Brain; Brain disorders; Endocrine disorders; Endocrinology; Endocrinology, pediatric; Genetic diseases; Glands; Hormones; Leukodystrophy; Metabolic disorders; Metabolism; Nervous system; Neuralgia, neuritis, and neuropathy; Neuroimaging; Neurology; Neurology, pediatric.

For Further Information:
Alan, Rick. "X-linked Adrenoleukodystrophy." *Health Library*, Sept. 30, 2012.
Fernandes, John, et al., eds. *Inborn Metabolic Diseases.* 4th ed. New York: Springer, 2006.
MedlinePlus. "Adrenoleukodystrophy." *MedlinePlus*, Dec. 1, 2011 (updated Mar. 22, 2013).
Rimoin, David, et al., eds. *Emory and Rimoin's Principles and Practice of Medical Genetics.* 5th ed. Philadelphia: Churchill Livingstone, 2007.
Scriver, Charles, et al., eds. *The Metabolic and Molecular Bases of Inherited Disease.* 8th ed. New York: McGraw-Hill, 2001.

Advance directives

Health care system

Specialties and related fields: Emergency medicine, ethics, family medicine, geriatrics and gerontology, public health

Definition: Legal documents that allow an individual to specify in writing the type of medical care they would want in case they are unable to speak or act on their own behalf.

Key terms:

Do not resuscitate/do not intubate order: a document that directs medical staff not to use heroic measures if a patient's heart stops or the patient stops breathing.

Durable power of attorney: a legal document that appoints a proxy to make medical-related decisions for a person if that person becomes unable to make decisions.

living will: A signed legal document that tells what medical treatment a person does or does not want, such as artificial nutrition and hydration, mechanical ventilation, or kidney dialysis..

History

With the advancement of medical technology, questions have arisen surrounding patients' rights to accept or deny care. Specifically, the development of mechanical ventilators and cardiopulmonary resuscitation (CPR) in the 1930s through the 1950s spurred discussions about the use of technology to indefinitely sustain a person's life. A number of state court cases during this time questioned the right of an individual or an incapacitated individual's family to refuse medical care. In 1990, a Supreme Court decision cited the 14th Amendment and established the right of a competent person to refuse unwanted medical treatment. Shortly thereafter, the Patient Self-Determination Act (PSDA) was passed. This Act was the first federal legislation that acknowledged the patient's right to either accept or refuse treatment. The Act mandated that all patients be provided with information regarding their right to establish advance directives, and that it should be documented in the patient's medical record whether or not an advance directive exists.

Types

There are two primary forms of advance directives. A living will is the most common form. This is a document that specifies what kind of healthcare an individual would choose in the case that they are unable to speak for themselves. One specific type of living will is a Do Not Resuscitate/Do Not Intubate order (DNR/DNI), which instructs the health care team not to attempt CPR or insert a breathing tube in the case of cardiac or pulmonary arrest. Additional decisions that might be addressed within a living will include the use of dialysis, tube feeding, and organ or tissue donation. Most states have state-specific documents for advance directives. Some states honor directives from other states, but this may depend on the similarity between the two states' laws. To avoid ambiguity in the case that a state does not have a clear policy regarding out-of-state directives, patients may file state-specific directives in more than one state. An individual is not required to seek medical or legal guidance when preparing a living will, which can sometimes make interpretation difficult. In twenty-six states, a living will is not valid if a woman is pregnant (Emanuel, 2013).

A second form of advance directive is a Durable Power of Attorney for Healthcare (DPAHC). With this directive the individual identifies a proxy who will act as the medical decision maker if they are no longer able to make decisions. This document makes it clear who is in charge of medical decision making, and thereby is a way to avoid conflict and confusion among health care teams and family members. State law varies as to whether the person must be in a vegetative state before the directive becomes active. An alternative proxy may also be named in case the primary proxy is not reachable at the time an incident occurs. If no health care proxy is named, the closest family member is usually deemed legally responsible for health care decisions.

Two additional forms of advance directives exist. A comprehensive advance medical care directive offers in-depth information about what kind of care the patient would desire given various medical scenarios. The last type of directive, termed a Values History, is not recognized by law. It is meant to provide context to decisions specified by other directives, and can be helpful if needed for interpreting decisions arises.

—*Beth Williams*

See also: Cardiopulmonary resuscitation (CPR); Coma; Critical care; Death and dying; Ethics; Euthanasia; Hippocratic oath; Hospice; Law and medicine; Living will; Resuscitation; Terminally ill: Extended care.

For Further Information:
American Association of Retired Persons. *Advance Directives: Planning for the Future.* www.aarp.org. Accessed October 2, 2013.

Brown, B. A. "The History of Advance Directives: A Literature Review." *Journal of Gerontological Nursing* 29, no. 9 (2003): 4.

Emanuel, E., ed. *Legal Aspects of End of Life Care.* Emanuel, L. (Ed), Waltham, Mass.: 2013.

Koch, K. A. "Patient Self-Determination Act." *Journal of the Florida Medical Association* 79, no. 4 (1992): 240.

Meisel, A., L. Snyder, and T. Quill. "Seven Legal Barriers to End-of-Life Care." *JAMA: The Journal of the American Medical Association* 284, no. 19 (2000): 2495-2501.

Silveira, M. J., S.Y. Kim, and K.M. Langa. "Advance Directives and Outcomes of Surrogate Decision Making before Death." *New England Journal of Medicine* 362, no. 13 (2010): 1211-1218.

Aerobics

Biology

Anatomy or system affected: Cardio-vascular, muscle-skeletal

Specialties and related fields: Exercise physiology, sports medicine

Aerobics, from the Greek words for air and life, is a term from the field of biology. It refers to sustained moderate physical activity during a specific period of time that requires an additional effort from the cardiovascular system—that is, heart and lungs—in order to increase the transport of oxygen to the muscles. Aerobic exercise is aimed at improving cardiovascular conditioning and lung function. Since its early days as a dance and exercise routine, aerobics has fueled a multibillion dollar industry and become a vital part of American culture.

Brief History

In biology, the word "aerobic" is used to describe organisms that need oxygen to live. Aerobics exercises, then, stimulate breathing are are designed to improve how the body oxygenates. Aerobics as an exercise discipline began in the postwar years of the twentieth century, when a medical doctor and former military officer, Kenneth H. Cooper, authored the book *Aerobics* (1968). Cooper was already a respected exercise expert because of the studies he performed with the military. He worked not only to improve the physical condition of American soldiers but also to identify their individual limitations.

Cooper soon became known beyond military circles, as he expanded his research to better understand the benefits of intense physical activity called "cardiovascular workout." His research explored not only physical benefits, but also mental benefits. He continued to publish books on his findings, but it wasn't until 1982 that he could actually put into practice the overall techniques described in his work. In the beginning, however, aerobics lacked widespread acceptance. Some of the obstacles it faced in order to become universally popular were lack of adequate spaces to practice it and the tedium of repetitive exercise.

Cooper's first book has sold about 30 million copies worldwide. Nevertheless, the books and workout videos produced by actor Jane Fonda turned aerobics into an unprecedented mass phenomenon. By the 1990s, advances in the fields of biomechanics and physiology brought radical changes to the field of aerobics. These studies reduced the incidence of injuries incurred in doing aerobic exercise and helped increase the benefits to the body.

The addition of music, dance elements, and attractive gear made aerobic exercise more appealing and played a fundamental role in its widespread popularity. Other cardiovascular exercises were added to enhance aerobics, including boxing, martial arts, water exercises, and bicycling. Technology expanded apace, and gadgets meant to measure factors such as cardiovascular workout and calorie loss entered the market. Aerobics is the most practiced exercise worldwide.

Overview

What made aerobics different from other exercise routines, such as calisthenics, is the link to dance music. This novelty and the fact that it is usually practiced in groups increased its popularity. Eventually aerobics became a common household experience, as routines recorded on videocassettes by experts and celebrities, especially Jane Fonda and Richard Simmons, could be played at home. In time, fitness programs became incorporated into many workplaces.

Another factor that popularized aerobics is that practically everybody can practice some type of aerobics without being an athlete. A typical aerobics routine consists of warming and stretching exercises for about 20 to 30 minutes, to raise the cardiac rate to its target level. The appropriate level depends upon age and health conditions. Exercise intensity then decreases. Some exercise programs include a strength sequence for body-sculpting purposes. Merging aerobics with elements of other dance forms or sports has become commonplace, producing jazzercise, zumba, spinning, kickboxing, and many others.

Many social forces came together that helped spread the popularity of fitness by way of aerobic exercise. These included science, such as the studies on the health benefits of fitness, as well as government incentives, commercial interests, and national culture. In the United States, the cultivation of health and fitness had long been a cultural factor. The benefits of a healthy lifestyle had been touted by experts and popular periodicals since the nineteenth century. Nevertheless, prior to World War II, to be overly concerned with physical prowess and health was considered strange.

Decades prior to the success of aerobics trailblazer Jane Fonda, strongman Charles Atlas (1892-1972) and exercise guru Jack LaLanne (1914-2011) ran extremely successful marketing campaigns touting the benefits of proper nutrition and exercise. In 1956, President Dwight Eisenhower created the President's Council on Youth Fitness, with the main objective of raising public awareness across the nation. It developed a plan of action and a nationwide pilot program that studied the fitness level of more than eight thousand children between the ages of 5 and 12. In 1965, under President Lyndon B. Johnson, another nationwide fitness study took place with children ages 10 to 17 years of age.

These government studies highlighted a concern, specific to the Cold War period, with the health and fitness of the young. They heralded not only the eventual popularity of aerobics, but also of other new fitness sports such as jogging, which became a craze in the 1970s. Jogging, however, is a mostly solitary sport, and in the 1980s, a preference for the shared experience of health clubs and gyms prevailed.

In the second decade of the twenty-first century, the revenues from the health and fitness industry reached about $33 billion a year, and with continued expectations for growth. Approximately 45 million Americans spend money on exercise technology and gear, club memberships, and myriad other products related to fitness. The expense and other social factors associated with exercise programs, have been cited as cause for exclusion. According to many social scientists, fitness has become a vital part of American identity, raising questions about who gets left behind from participation in it and why. The fact that there are many who cannot afford gym memberships and gear suggests a link between fitness and issues of social class.

—*Trudy Mercadal, MA, PhD;*
updated by Geraldine Marrocco

For Further Information:

Bishop, Jan Galen. *Fitness through Aerobics*. San Francisco: Cummings, 2013. Print.

Black, Jonathan. *Making the American Body: The Remarkable Saga of the Men and Women Whose Feats, Feuds, and Passions Shaped Fitness History*. Lincoln: U of Nebraska P, 2013. Print.

Cooper, Kenneth H. *Aerobics Program for Total Well-Being: Exercise, Diet and Emotional Balance*. New York: Bantam, 2013. Print.

_____. *Regaining the Power of Youth at Any Age: Startling New Evidence from the Doctor Who Brought Us Aerobics, Controlling Cholesterol, and the Antioxidant Revolution*. Nashville: Nelson, 2005. Print.

Ehrman, Jonathan, Paul Gordon, Paul Visich, and Steven Keteyian. *Clinical Exercise Physiology*, 3rd ed. Champaign: Human Kinetics, 2013. Print.

Malcolm, Dominic. *The Sage Dictionary of Sports Studies*. Thousand Oaks: Sage, 2008. Print.

McKenzie, Shelley. *Getting Physical: The Rise of Fitness Culture in America*. Lawrence: UP of Kansas, 2013. Print.

Zoumbaris, Sharon K., ed. *Encyclopedia of Wellness*. Santa Barbara: Greenwood, 2012. Print.

Aging

Development

Anatomy or system affected: All

Specialties and related fields: Geriatrics, gerontology, psychology

Definition: A series of time-dependent anatomical, physiological, and psychological changes that diminish physiological reserve and functional capacity and that produce emotional transformations. Some changes can also signal positive processes of maturation.

Key terms:

ageism: a negative or prejudiced view of aging endorsed by an individual or society

geriatrics: the medical specialty focusing on the treatment of elderly patients

gerontology: the formal study of the phenomena of aging from maturity to old age

nonnormative aging: significant factors that affect aging that are person-specific

normative age-graded: biological and environmental factors affecting aging that are correlated with chronological age

normative history-graded: events affecting aging that are widely experienced within a particular culture at a given time

primary aging: aging intrinsic to a person as determined by inherent or hereditary influences

secondary aging: changes in a person caused by hostile factors in the environment, which could include trauma, pollution, and acquired disease

Physical and Psychological Factors

Aging takes place over the course of life, and the rate of change varies between individuals and groups. Differences in aging are genetically determined in part, but there is also a substantial environmental component. These environmental factors can include nutrition, lifestyle choices, and toxins in the environment. Primary aging relates to the genetic components of aging, while secondary aging focuses on environmental factors.

Aging is influenced by a number of normative age-graded factors that typically take place at a particular chronological time. These factors can be biological, as reflected in puberty and menopause, as well as environmental, having an impact on the socialization of the individual, such as the changes needed to enter school or to assume a work role. Normative history-graded factors refer to events that are shared by a society and have an impact, either positive or negative, on the aging process. The Great Depression in the 1930s, World War II, and the Vietnam War are examples of normative history-graded events. When a major event has an impact on a single generation in a society, it is known as a cohort effect. When an event affects the entire population, it is termed a period effect. The Great Depression is considered to be a period effect, while the Vietnam War is labeled a cohort effect. Normative age-graded factors are considered to be most important during childhood and in old age, while normative history-graded events are considered to have their greatest impact on aging in the early and middle adulthood periods of life. Nonnormative factors recognize that each individual experiences unique factors that influence the personal aging process. A natural disaster, a divorce, and winning the lottery are considered

Aging and the Brain

Normal brain (third decade)   Aged brain

The human brain shrinks with age as nerve cells are lost and brain tissue atrophies.

to be nonnormative factors.

A multitude of age-related changes are typically benign and permit an individual to function, perform daily functions, and remain active in society. With increasing age, however, a number of biological changes lead to a decline in efficiency of function and performance. Some general signs of bodily aging include decreases in physical stature and loss of bone mineral density. A quantitative loss of cells in the body results in a decrease in overall muscle mass, perhaps as high as 80 percent. A loss of fat beneath the skin results in an increased sensitivity to temperature extremes. In general, the skin of the aging person atrophies with shrinking of the sweat and sebaceous glands, leading to dry and itchy skin. A decline in blood vessels causes a slowing of healing, and a loss of skin elasticity occurs with the breakdown of elastin.

Age-related changes in the cardiovascular system include narrowing of the blood vessels due to the thickening of the endothelial lining and a decline in smooth muscle mass. The blood vessels become rigid and contribute to a gradual elevation of blood pressure. Changes in the heart include thickening of the myocardium, a reduction in size of the ventricular cavities, and a decrease in volume of blood pumped per contraction. Heart rate may slow with age, as the cells in the sinus node can decline up to 90 percent. Consequently, elderly people may show limited heart rate increases when experiencing stress or trying to increase activity level. Changes in the respiratory system show a number of functional declines. Smooth muscle in the bronchi, diaphragm, and chest wall becomes weakened as a result of an increase of collagen deposits, contributing to a diminished work capacity in late life. Reductions in the lung surface area, decreased maximum ventilatory volume of the lungs, and limitations on maximum oxygen utilization can produce senile emphysema. This age-related condition limits the amount of exercise and energy that an older person can expend at any given time. By age sixty-five, an individual cannot fully expand the chest when seated. Secondary aging factors can contribute significantly to the diminished function of the respiratory system, as pollutants in the environment and smoking have been found to exaggerate these changes.

Musculoskeletal changes caused by aging include a loss of muscle mass, with striated musculature diminishing by approximately 50 percent by age eighty. As these cells are lost, they are replaced by fat cells. With age, the mineralization of bone declines for both men and women, but women experience osteoporosis at an accelerated rate after menopause. Both older men and older women are at increasing risk of fractures with age, but women experience this enhanced risk ten years sooner than do men.

In the nervous system, the brain shows a number of normative changes with age. In general, the brain decreases in size, primarily due to loss of mass in the white matter. Gray matter loss contributes significantly to this decrease after age seventy-five. Brain weight also diminishes beginning at age forty. The somatosensory system provides information from nerve endings located in the skin, joints, and muscles. As people age, the ability of the somatosensory system to detect stimuli in the environment and to provide accurate sensory information declines. Older adults have difficulty perceiving joint movement and position; this decline places them at an increased risk for falls.

Significant changes take place in the gastrointestinal system, with impaired gastric acid production in the stomach, slowing of the transit time in the large intestine, and decreased absorptive surface areas in the small intestine. The liver decreases in size and weight and shows a reduction in function. Other significant age-related changes to biological function include decreased renal blood flow; impaired function of the immune system; diminished levels of estrogen, progesterone, and testosterone; and decline in thyroid hormone levels.

Most noticeable to many older adults are the age-related changes to the sensory systems, as visual and auditory losses can routinely have an adverse effect on the performance of daily activities. With age, the lens and cornea of the eye thicken and show a yellowing. The lens is less flexible and increases in opaqueness, making focus more difficult. Production of the aqueous humor, the clear liquid that fills the anterior chamber of the eye, is reduced, leading to the increase in intraocular pressure associated with glaucoma. The ability to track moving objects declines as smooth pursuit eye movements show decrements. With advancing age, the auditory system shows a diminished capacity for sensitivity to higher frequencies, a condition known as presbycusis. According to the National Center for Health Statistics, 25 to 40 percent of adults over age sixty-five report concerns about a decline in speech perception. The problem is worsened in noisy environments. Taste and smell decrease in sensitivity with age to a degree that eating experiences become less pleasurable.

Although one unifying biological theory of aging does not exist, the National Institute on Aging has proposed two categories of aging theories: program theories and error theories. The program theories suggest that aging is due to a switching on and off of specific genes. When defects develop in the switching process, people experience the biological changes and functional declines associated with primary aging. The genetic nature of aging is shown in the maximal life spans that are found in all species. These species-specific differences in life span suggest an underlying genetic basis for aging. Since aging involves a complex array of normative age-related changes, it is expected that many interacting genes are involved in the overall process of growing old. One example of a program theory is the deliberate biological programming theory. This theory evolved from the research of Leonard Hayflick, who identified a limit for cell duplication. The theory holds that within a normal cell is a store of memory that dictates its life expectancy.

In contrast, the error theory approach maintains that aging is due in part to the wear and tear process that takes place over time. This approach posits that important components in the biological makeup of individuals wear out and cannot be repaired or replaced. Toxins in the environment and free radicals may contribute to the reduction in function of various systems as a result of wear and tear. Free radicals are chemical molecules with an odd number of electrons, which makes them highly reactive with other chemical compounds. Free radicals are produced through normal metabolic processes as well as by exposure to ionizing radiation, ozone, and chemical toxins. Research has shown that free radicals are associated with deoxyribonucleic acid (DNA) damage, cross-linkage with collagen to alter the characteristics of connective tissue, and cancer.

Psychological theories of aging usually are concerned with explaining the differences in behavior, changes in behavior, and patterns of action shown among persons of various ages. The psychological theories can be divided into three major categories: stability template, orderly change, and random change. The stability template approach emphasizes that the primary factors associated with development take place during infancy and childhood. It is during the early years of life that one's personality is formed, and this provides a template for all future behaviors. As the aging individual faces new situations or challenges from the environment, behavior can be predicted based on the outcomes of early childhood experiences. From the stability template perspective, the older adult often demonstrates regressive behaviors, acting in childlike fashion, when normative age-related biological changes produce excessive stress. The resulting anxiety causes the older person to seek behaviors that were rewarding or comforting in the past. The theories of Sigmund Freud are an example of the stability template approach and promote the idea that the essentials of personality development are concluded at age five or six.

The orderly change theories suggest that aging takes place in a predictable pattern throughout the life span. This pattern is defined by specific stages that accompany the progression through life. Orderly change theorists believe that each stage of life-adolescence, young adulthood, middle age, and late life-presents specific challenges or tasks that must be completed in order to experience successful aging and avoid negative emotions such as depression. The eight stages of development described by Erik Erikson are an example of an orderly change theory.

The random change perspective emphasizes the nonnormative factors of aging and suggests that development takes place as a result of a variety of events that may or may not have an impact on individuals at different points in life. This approach is highlighted by the work of Paul B. Baltes, who concludes that a wide variation occurs in the behavior of people as they age, which in turn is dependent upon each individual's particular circumstances.

In addition to general developmental theories, the psychological factors of aging focus on the changes in mental processes. Psychology differentiates between fluid intelligence and crystallized intelligence. Fluid intelligence is considered to be the basic abilities and cognitive skills found in a person. It reflects on the quality of one's brain and how quickly information is perceived and processed, how well associations and patterns are recognized, and the efficiency of memory function. This is analogous to a computer's hardware structure. Crystallized intelligence refers to culturally based and acquired cognitive functions. Development is dependent on experience with the world and the formal education system. The computer analogy would be its software. Development of cognitive ability is usually viewed as a stage phenomenon that begins during infancy when the child interacts with the surrounding environment through his or her reflexes and continues throughout life. Exposure to an enriched environment facilitates the development of crystallized intelligence. As a person reaches old age, tests of intelligence requiring speed or reaction time typically show a decline in ability. The developmental theory of Jean Piaget is an example of a well-known and highly researched approach to explain cognitive development from infancy onward.

Another significant approach to explain aging has been through the formation of social theories focusing on activity level throughout the life span. Disengagement theory suggests that aging inevitably requires a process of separating or disengaging oneself from physical, social, and psychological efforts. This disengagement is needed in response to the biological changes associated with old age. Activity theory was designed as an alternative view of aging and holds that normative aging requires remaining active throughout life. High activity levels are seen as positively related to good health, longevity, and life satisfaction. Most recently, continuity theory has been proposed as a compromise position between disengagement and activity theories. The continuity approach promotes the notion that older adults must maintain behavior according to the pattern of life that had been established before old age.

Disorders and Effects

Hutchinson-Gilford progeria syndrome and Werner's syndrome are two forms of accelerated aging called progeria. The person with Hutchinson-Gilford syndrome experiences dwarfism and pseudosenility. Individuals with this genetic form of accelerated aging appear like very old and small humans. They usually die in their teenage years of coronary heart disease. Werner's syndrome, also caused by genetic factors, affects persons in their late twenties and thirties and produces a shortened life span. The afflicted person ages very rapidly and develops a pinched facial expression, cataracts, diabetes, hypogonadism, a beak-like nose, prominent teeth, and a recessive chin.

Dementia is a fairly common condition that increases in frequency with age. It involves deficits in two or more areas of cognition that have a negative impact on daily functioning. Dementia produces impairment of memory and orientation and disruption in the ability to plan, organize, sequence, and make decisions. The majority of persons in old age who experience dementia have Alzheimer's disease. The Alzheimer's Association estimated that in 2012, over five million Americans were living with the disease and that the number of cases of Alzheimer's disease would increase to nine million by the year 2025. The risk for Alzheimer's disease increases by approximately 1 percent with each year of life after age sixty-five. It is a progressive deteriorating disorder that attacks memory first before progressing through wandering, aggressiveness, and confusion of time and space to an eventual loss of self-awareness and a total inability to assume self-care. The characteristic brain pathology of Alzheimer's disease includes cell loss, neurofibrillary tangles, and senile plaques found throughout the neocortex of the brain but concentrated in the hippocampus, frontal, parietal, and temporal lobes. Persons with Alzheimer's disease can experience loss of approximately 40 percent of their brain mass. Four different chromosomes have been identified that heighten risk for the development of Alzheimer's disease. Currently, there is no cure for the disorder and treatment is primarily supportive. Cholinesterase inhibitors and memantine, which improve the naturally occurring neural transmitter acetylcholine in the brain and have been shown to delay the progression of the disease, have been the medications of choice in treatment. Vascular dementia is caused by underlying cerebrovascular disease and has a more abrupt onset compared to Alzheimer's disease.

Many of the age-related changes experienced among older adults have been suggested as contributing to the development of late-life depression. Depression is the most common emotional disturbance found in the elderly population. The prevalence of depression is highest among those older adults experiencing some medical illness or functional impairment. Suicide rates are high among older adults and highest among white men over the age of eighty-five. Many older adults experience "chronic suicide," a slow steady decline in health and function caused by personal neglect of one's needs.

One of the major effects of age-related changes is the

need to compensate for functional declines. For many older adults to live independently, often requires some degree of home care. Impairments are measured in terms of daily living activities, which include eating, bathing, toileting, and moving in and out of chairs and bed. Remaining in the home can take on a significant level of psychological importance, since it is part of an older person's identity and helps to maintain a sense of autonomy and control in one's life.

Perspective and Prospects

Historically, the ancient Greeks provided some of the first writings on aging in discussing how old age brings increased anxiety about death. During the Roman era, Cicero suggested ways for elderly people to make themselves useful in advisory and administrative roles. He emphasized the importance of a developed mind and enhanced character as compensations for physical decline. The first manual to describe the problems associated with aging was published in the fifteenth century. Overall, however, historical writers had little to say about the positive attributes of aging.

Many common beliefs about aging have often resulted in oversimplified and biased stereotypes about older adults. These stereotypes may portray elderly persons as uninterested, weak, unattractive, undesirable, rigid, incapable of sexual activity, conservative, and lacking in intellectual acuity. This perspective encourages discrimination against older persons and is termed *ageism*. Senility is not a medical term but is commonly used in US society. It implies that old people lose the intellectual capacity to make intelligent decisions. As the number of older adults has increased and the importance of scientific investigations of aging has been expanded, positive counterpoints to aging have emerged. A new realistic image of older adults portrays the healthy elderly population as resourceful, optimistic, intelligent, flexible, and sexual beings. The study of aging has increased in importance as the geriatric population continues to grow in number and proportion of the population. According to census conducted in 2010 by the US Census Bureau, the sixty-five and over population in the United States is growing at a faster rater than is the general population. People are living longer as a result of the control of infectious diseases and improvements in health care, sanitation, and nutrition. The segment of the population aged sixty-five and older grew from 5 percent of the population in 1900 to 13 percent in 2010, and it is projected to increase to 22.9 percent by the year 2050. In 2000, there were approximately 35 million Americans over the age of sixty-five; in 2010, there were 40.3 million over the age of sixty-five; and this number is projected to increase to 70 million by 2030. Life expectancy at birth increased from forty-nine years in 1900 to approximately eighty-one years for women and seventy-six years for men in 2010. (Women tend to outlive men because of higher male mortality caused by heart disease, lung cancer, and emphysema.)

Despite the increases in the older population, aging is a relatively new topic of study. Initially, the pioneers in the fields of development focused on describing, explaining, and understanding the infancy and childhood periods of life. Researchers next moved to the study of adolescence, and they considered old age as a period of deterioration with a focus on chronic disease. Gerontology, the formal study of the phenomena of aging from maturity to old age, began producing significant research only in the 1950s. Geriatrics, the medical treatment of elderly patients, was proposed as an academic discipline in 1987 by the National Institute of Medicine.

—*Frank J. Prerost, Ph.D.*

See also Age spots; Aging: Extended care; Alzheimer's disease; Arteriosclerosis; Arthritis; Assisted living facilities; Deafness; Death and dying; Dementias; Depression; Diabetes mellitus; Geriatrics and gerontology; Gray hair; Hearing aids; Hearing loss; Heart disease; Hip replacement; Hormone therapy; Hot flashes; Kyphosis; Memory loss; Menopause; Midlife crisis; Osteoarthritis; Osteoporosis; Parkinson's disease; Polypharmacy; Progeria; Prostate enlargement; Psychiatry, geriatric; Safety issues for the elderly; Sense organs; Stress; Strokes; Supplements; Vitamins and minerals; Wrinkles.

For Further Information:
Arking, Robert. *The Biology of Aging: Observations and Principles.* 3d ed. New York: Oxford University Press, 2006.

Cohen, Gene D. *The Mature Mind: The Positive Power of the Aging Brain.* New York: Basic Books, 2006.

Eaton, William W., ed. *Medical and Psychiatric Comorbidity over the Course of Life.* Washington, D.C.: American Psychiatric Publishing, 2006.

Hill, Robert D. *Positive Aging: A Guide for Mental Health Professionals and Consumers.* New York: W. W. Norton, 2005.

Kunkel, Suzanne R., J. Scott Brown, and Frank Whittington, eds. *Global Aging: Comparative Perspectives on Aging and the Life Course.* New York: Springer Publishing, 2014.

Markut, Lynda A., and Anatole Crane. *Dementia Caregivers Share Their Stories: A Support Group in a Book.* Nashville, Tenn.: Vanderbilt University Press, 2005.

Sugar, Judith A., et al. *Introduction to Aging: A Positive, Interdisciplinary Approach.* New York: Springer Publishing, 2013.

Whitbourne, Susan Krauss, and Martin J. Sliwinski, eds. *The Wiley-Blackwell Handbook of Adulthood and Ageing.* Chichester, England: Blackwell Publishing, 2012.

Aging: Extended care

Specialty

Anatomy or system affected: All

Specialties and related fields: Audiology, cardiology, critical care, dentistry, geriatrics and gerontology, neurology, nursing, nutrition, oncology, ophthalmology, optometry, pharmacology, physical therapy, psychiatry, psychology, public health, rheumatology

Definition: The management of the health, personal care, and social needs of elderly people as they experience decreases in physical, mental, and/or emotional abilities.

Key terms:

ageism: discrimination against individuals based on their age or the overlooking of individuals' abilities to make positive contributions to society because of their age

case management: an interdisciplinary approach to medical care characterized by the inclusion of physical, psychological, social, emotional, familial, financial, and historical data in patient treatment

cognitive functioning: a general term describing mental processes such as awareness, knowing, reasoning, problem solving, judging, and imagining

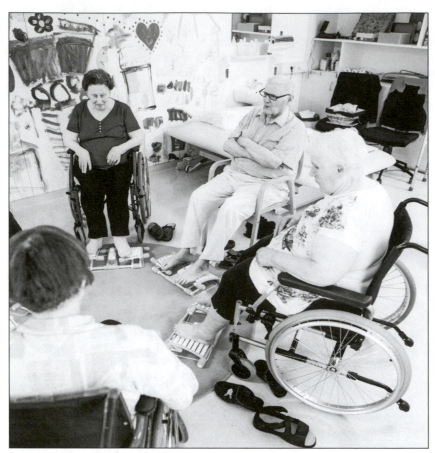

Seniors participating in foot reflexology at a retirement home.

malnutrition: a physical state characterized by an imbalance of dietary proteins, carbohydrates, fats, vitamins, and minerals, given an individual's physical activity and health needs

mental statusexam: a comprehensive evaluation assessing general health, appearance, mood, speech, sociability, cooperativeness, motor activity, orientation to time and reality, memory, general intelligence, and other cognitive functioning

neurocognitive disorder (formerly known as organic brain syndromes: clusters of condition that frequently lead to behavioral and psychological symptoms involving impaired brain function, where etiology is unknown; includes delirium, delusions, amnesia, intoxication, and dementias

organicmental disorders: mental and emotional disturbances from transient or permanent brain dysfunction, with known organic etiology; includes drug or alcohol ingestion, infection, trauma, and cardiovascular disease

psychosocial interventions: treatments that enhance individual psychological and social functioning by assisting with the development of the skills, attitudes, or behaviors necessary to function as independently as possible

The Problems Associated with Aging

The process of aging is inevitable. In the earlier stages of life, aging involves the acquisition and development of new skills and abilities, facilitated by the guidance and assistance of others. Later, the middle stages involve the chal-

lenges of maintaining and applying those skills and abilities in a manner that is primarily self-sufficient. Finally, in the end stages of life, aging involves the deterioration and loss of skills and abilities, with adequate functioning again being somewhat dependent on the assistance of others.

For many individuals, the final stages are brief, allowing them to live independently right up to their time of death. Thus, many experience little loss of their abilities to function independently. Others, however, endure more extended stages of later life and require greater care. For these individuals, losses in physical, emotional, and/or cognitive functioning frequently result in a need for specialized care. Such care involves whatever is necessary so that these individuals may live as comfortably, productively, and independently as possible.

The conditions leading to a need for long-term care are as varied as the elderly themselves are. Special needs for elders requiring extended care often include the management of physical, health, emotional, and cognitive problems. Physical problems dictating lifestyle adjustments include decreased speed, dexterity, and strength, as well as increased fragility. Changes to the five senses are also common. Visual changes include the development of hyperopia (farsightedness) and sometimes decreased visual acuity. Hearing loss is also common, such that softer sounds cannot be heard when background noise is present or sounds need to be louder in order to be perceived. Particularly noteworthy is that paranoia, depression, and social isolation often result as side effects of visual and hearing impairments in elders; they are not always signs of mental deterioration. Similarly, one's sense of touch may also be affected, such that the nerves are either more or less sensitive to changes in temperatures or textures. Consequently, injuries attributable to a lack of awareness of potential hazards or super sensitivities to temperature or texture may result. One example would be an elderly woman overdressing or under dressing for the weather because of an inability to judge the outside temperature properly. Another would be an elderly man cutting or wounding himself out of a lack of awareness of the sharpness of an object. Finally, both taste and smell may change, creating a situation in which subtle tastes and odors become imperceptible or in which tastes and smells that were once pleasant become either bland or unpleasant.

Health problems among the aged often demand increased management as well. Coordination of drug therapies and other medical interventions by a case manager is critical, as a result of increasing sensitivities in elders to physical interventions. Typical health conditions bringing

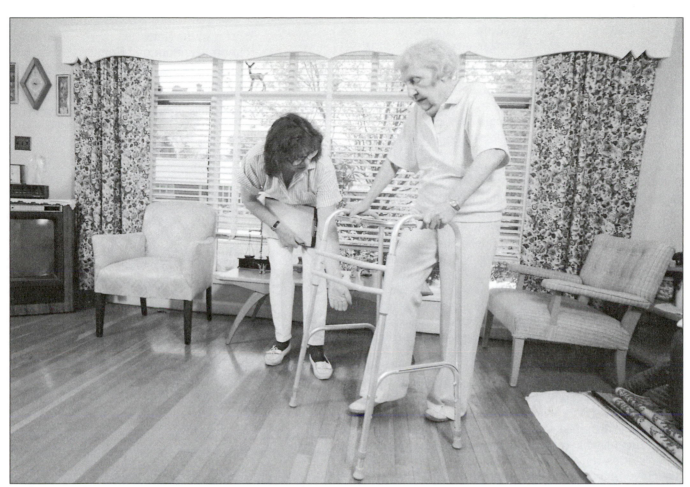

A home care professional helps an elderly woman use a walker for support. Such services allow many older people to have a more active and independent lifestyle. (Digital Stock)

elderly people into long-term care settings may include heart disease and stroke, hypertension, diabetes mellitus, arthritis, osteoporosis, chronic pain, prostate disease, and cancers of the digestive tract and other vital organs. Estimates are that approximately 86 percent of the aged are affected by chronic illnesses. Long-term care addresses both the medical management of these chronic illnesses and their impact on the individual.

An issue related to health and physical problems in the aged is malnutrition. For a variety of reasons, elders often fall victim to malnutrition, which can contribute to additional health problems. For example, Vitamin D deficiency can increase both the severity of heart disease and the likelihood of osteoporosis and tooth loss. Thus, a vicious cycle of medical problems can be put into motion. Factors contributing to malnutrition are multifaceted. Poverty, social isolation, decreased taste sensitivity, and tooth loss combine with lifelong dietary habits that can sometimes predispose certain elders to malnutrition. As such, attention to the maintenance of healthy dietary habits in the elderly is critical to successful long-term care, regardless of the type of setting in which the care is being given.

Along with these physical aspects of aging come emotional and cognitive changes. Depression, anxiety, and paranoia over health concerns, for example, are not uncommon. Additionally, concerns about the threat of losing one's independence, friends, and former lifestyle may contribute to acute or chronic mood disorders. Suicide is a particular danger with the elderly when mood disorders such as depression are present. Elderly people are one of the fastest growing groups among those who commit suicide. The stresses accompanying losing a spouse or enduring a chronic health problem can often be triggers to suicide for depressed elders. One should note, however, that elders are not particularly prone to depression or suicide because of their age but that they are more likely to experience significant stressors that lead to depression.

More common, less lethal problems associated with conditions such as depression, anxiety, and paranoia are weight change, insomnia, and other sleep problems. Distractibility, decreased ability to maintain attention and concentration, and rumination over distressing concerns are also common. Finally, some elders may be observed as socially isolated and prone to avoidance behavior. As a result, some become functionally incapacitated because of distressing emotions.

What is critical to remember, in addition to these signs, is that some elders may not describe their problems as emotional at all, even though that is the primary cause of their discomfort. Individual differences in how people express themselves must be taken into account. Thus, while some elders may report being depressed or anxious, others may instead report feeling tired. Reports of low-level health problems that are vague in nature, such as aches and pains, are also common in elders who are depressed. It is not uncommon for emotional problems to be expressed or described indirectly as physical complaints.

Decreased cognitive functioning may result from more serious problems than depression, such as organic mental syndromes. These typically include problems such as dementias from Alzheimer's disease, Pick's disease, Huntington's disease, alcohol- related deterioration, or stroke related problems. Other causes may be brain tumors or thyroid dysfunction. With all dementias, however, the hallmark signs are a deterioration of intellectual function and emotional response. Memory, judgment, understanding, and the experience and control of emotional responses are affected. Functionally, these conditions reveal themselves as a combination of symptoms, including increased forgetfulness, decreased ability to plan and complete tasks, difficulties finding names or words, decreased abilities for abstract thinking, impaired judgment, inappropriate sexual behavior, and sometimes severe personality changes. In some cases, affected individuals are aware of these difficulties, usually in the earlier stages of the disease processes. Later, however, even though their behavior and abilities may be quite disturbed, they may be completely unaware of the severity of their problems. In these cases, long term care often begins as a result of outside intervention by concerned friends and family members.

Options for Long-Term Care

Extended care for the aged requires an interdisciplinary effort that usually involves a team of nurses, nurse practitioners, physicians, psychologists, , social workers, and other rehabilitative specialists. Depending on the nature of the problems requiring care and management, any of these professionals may take part in the care process. Additionally, the involvement of concerned individuals who are close to the elder needing care is critical. Family members (including the spouse, significant partners, children, and extended family) and close friends are invaluable sources of information and of emotional and instrumental support. Their ability to assist an elder with instrumental tasks such as cooking, housecleaning, shopping, and money and medication management is crucial to the successful implementation of a long-term care plan.

In all cases, long-term care for the aged involves the design of a comprehensive plan to address the multifaceted needs of the elder. Just as younger persons have psychological, social, intellectual, and physical needs, so do elders. As such, thorough assessment of an elder's abilities, goals, expectations, and functioning in each of these areas is required. A mental status exam and a thorough physical exam are usually the primary methods of evaluation. Once needs are identified, a plan can then be designed by the team of health care professionals, family and friends assisting with care, and, whenever possible, the elder. In general, the

---

In the News: Remote Monitoring at Home

Remote monitoring provides real-time health care data while patients are away from their health care providers. Conceivably, a patient could be anywhere in the world while providing his or her doctor with general monitoring data such as blood pressure or feedback from a newly installed pacemaker. Historically, remote monitoring devices have been stand-alone contraptions that involve extensive training to utilize; however, more recent advances include data reporting using the Internet, wireless local area networks, and cell phones.

At least as early as 2002, the Food and Drug Administration (FDA) granted approval for remote monitoring of patients with cardiovascular complications. In November, 2009, the FDA approved a more general health data reporting device that can work in tandem with a cell phone. This streamlining of health care could potentially save hospitals the unnecessary expense of emergency room visits while simultaneously alerting a patient that a hospital visit is needed. Remote monitoring shows particular promise for the aging population, as it can help maintain general health while monitoring chronic conditions. Cell phones and other wireless devices can provide the patient with reminders, alerts, and motivational encouragement to engage in healthy behaviors throughout the day. This daily feedback can alert the patient of small changes in health status, such as informing the patient of high blood pressure, and then provide strategies to compensate. Catching and changing lifestyle factors early could save an untold number of unnecessary procedures yearly.

Noncompliance with a provider's orders is an estimated $100 billion yearly tax on the health care system. Daily feedback would permit providers to track patients who do not adhere to medical regimes. Cell phones with global positioning systems (GPS) could easily monitor a patient's daily activity level. Remote monitoring holds the possibility of improving patient's quality of life, reducing health care costs and enhancing early detection of health changes in those individuals most at risk.

—*Dana K. Bagwell; updated by Geraldine Marrocco*

---

overarching goal is to design a case management plan that maximizes the independent functioning and quality of life of the aged person, given certain physical, psychiatric, social, and other needs.

Specific management strategies are designed for the problems that need to be addressed. Physical, health, nutritional, emotional, and cognitive problems all demand different management settings and strategies. Additionally, care settings may vary depending on the severity of the problems identified. In general, the more severe the problems, the more structured the long-term care setting and the more intense the psychosocial interventions.

For less severe problems, adequate management settings may include the elder's own home, the home of a family member or friend, a shared housing setting, or a seniors' apartment complex. Shared housing is sometimes called group-shared, supportive, or matched housing. Typically, it refers to residences organized by agencies where up to twenty people share a house and its expenses, chores, and management. Ideal candidates for this type of setting include elders who want some daily assistance or companionship but who are still basically independent. Senior apartments, also called retirement housing, are usually "elderly-only" complexes that range from garden-style apartments to high-rises. Ideal candidates for this type of setting include nearly independent elders who want privacy, but who no longer desire or can manage a single-family home. In either of these types of settings, the use of periodic or regular at-home nursing assistance for medical problems, or "home-helpers" for more instrumental tasks, might be a successful adjunct to regular consultation with a case manager or physician.

Problems of moderate severity may demand a more structured setting or a setting in which help is more readily available. Such settings might include continuing care retirement communities or assisted-living facilities. Continuing care retirement communities, also called life-care communities, are large complexes offering lifelong care. Residents are healthy, live independently in apartments, and are able to use cafeteria services as necessary. Additionally, residents have the option of being moved to an assisted-living unit or an skilled level of care as health needs dictate. Assisted-living facilities-also called board-and-care, institutional living, adult foster care, and personal care settings-offer care that is less intense than that received in a medical setting or nursing home. These facilities may be as small as a home where one person cares for a small group of elders or as large as a converted hotel with several caregivers, a nurse, and shared dining facilities. Such settings are ideal for persons needing instrumental care but not round-the-clock skilled medical or nursing care. When more severe conditions such as incontinence, dementia, or an inability to move independently are present, nursing, convalescent, or extended care homes are more appropriate settings. Intense attention is delivered in a hospital like setting where all medical and instrumental needs are addressed. Typical nursing homes serve a hundred clients at a time, utilizing semiprivate rooms for personal living space and providing community areas for social, community, and family activities. Often, the decision to place an elder in this type of facility is difficult to make. The decision, however, is frequently based on the knowledge that these types of facilities provide the best possible setting for the overall care of the elder's medical, health, and social needs. In fact, appropriate use of these facilities discourages the overtaxing of the elder's emotional and familial resources, allowing the elder to gain maximum benefit. An elder's placement into this type of facility does not mean that the family's job is over; rather, it simply changes shape. Incorporation of family resources into long-term care in a nursing home setting is critical to the adjustment of the elder and family members to the elder's increased need for care and attention. Visits and other family involvement in the elder's daily activities remain quite valuable.

Regardless of the management setting, some basic caveats exist with regard to determining management strategies. First and foremost is that the aged individuals should, whenever possible, be encouraged to maintain independent functioning. For example, even though physical deterioration such as decreased visual or hearing abilities may be present, there is no need to take decision-making authority away from the elder. Decreased abilities to hear or see do not necessarily mean a decreased ability to make decisions or think. Second, it is crucial to ask elders to identify their needs and how they might desire assistance. Some elders may wish for help with acquiring basic living supplies from outside the home, such as foods and toiletries, but desire privacy and no assistance within the home. In contrast, others may desire independence outside the home with regard to social matters but need more instrumental assistance within the home. Finally, it is important to recognize that even the smallest amount of assistance can make a significant difference in the lifestyle of the elder. A prime example is availability of transportation. The loss of a driver's license or independent transportation signifies a major loss of independence for any elder. Similarly, the challenges posed by public transit may seem insurmountable because of a lack of familiarity or experience. As such, simple and small interventions such as a ride to a store or a doctor's office may provide great relief for elders by assisting their efforts to meet their own needs.

Special management strategies may be required for specific problem areas. For physical deterioration, adequate assessment of strengths and weaknesses is important, as are referrals to medical, rehabilitative, and home-help professionals. Hearing and visual or other devices to make lifting, mobility, and day-to-day tasks easier are helpful. Similarly, assisting the aged with developing alternative strategies for dealing with diminished sensory abilities can be valuable. Examples would be checking a thermometer for outdoor temperature to determine proper dress, rather than relying purely on sensory information, or having a phone that lights up when it rings. Health conditions also demand particular management strategies, varying greatly with the type of problem experienced. In all cases, however, medical intervention, drug therapies, and behavior modification therapies are commonly employed. Dietary problems (such as malnutrition or diabetes), cardiovascular problems (such as heart attacks), and emotional problems (such as depression) often require all three approaches. Finally, cognitive problems, particularly those related to depression, are sometimes alleviated with drug therapies. Others related to neurocognitive disorders or organic mental disorders require medical interventions and significant behavior modification therapies and/or psychosocial interventions for elders and their families.

Perspective and Prospects

Advances in modern medicine are continually extending the human life span. Cures for dread diseases, improved management of chronic health problems, and new technologies to replace diseased organs are facilitating this evolution. For many, these advances translate into greater longevity, the maintenance of a high quality of life, and fewer obstacles related to ageism. For others, however, the trade-off for longevity is some loss of independence and a need for extended care and management. Thus, the medical field is also affected by the trade-off of extending life, while experiencing an increasing need to improve strategies for long-term care for those who are able to live longer and longer despite health conditions. As a result of this evolution, long-term care for the aged presents special challenges to the medical field. Over time, medicine has been a field specializing in the understanding of particular organ systems and the treatment of related diseases. While an understanding of how each system affects the functioning of the whole body is necessary, health care providers must struggle to understand the complexities in the case management required for high-quality long-term care for the aged. Care must be interdisciplinary, addressing the physical, mental, emotional, social, and familial needs of the aged individual. Failure to address any of these areas may ultimately sabotage the successful long-term management of elderly individuals and of their problems. In this way, medical, psychiatric, social work, and rehabilitative specialists need to work together with elders and their families for the best possible results.

Integrated case management with a team leader is increasingly the trend so that a variety of services can be provided in an orchestrated manner. While specialty providers still play a role, managers (usually primary care nurse practitioners or physicians) ensure that complementary drug therapies as well as psychiatric and other medical treatments are administered. Additionally, they are key in bringing forth family resources for emotional and instrumental support whenever possible, as well as community and social services when needed. What was once viewed as helping a person to die with dignity is now viewed as helping a person to live as long and as productive a life as possible. Increasing awareness that old age is not simply a dying time has facilitated an integrated approach to long-term care. The news that elders can be as social, physical, sexual, intellectual, and productive as their younger counterparts has greatly stimulated improved longterm care strategies. No longer is old age seen as a time for casting elders aside or as a time when a nursing home is an inescapable solution in the face of health problems affecting the aged. Alternatives to care exist and are proliferating, with improved outcomes for both patients and care providers.

—*Nancy A. Piotrowski, PhD;*
updated by Ophelia Empleo-Frazier,
MSN, GNP-BC, WCC, DCP

See also: Aging; Alzheimer's disease; Arthritis; Assisted living facilities; Audiology; Brain; Brain disorders; Critical care; Death and dying; Dementias; Depression; Endocrinology; Ethics; Euthanasia; Geriatrics and gerontology; Hearingloss; Home care; Hospitals; Incontinence; Living will; Malnutrition; Nursing; Nutrition; Ophthalmology; Optometry; Orthopedics; Osteoporosis; Pharmacology; Polypharmacy; Psychiatry, geriatric; Rheumatology; Safety issuesfor the elderly; Sense organs; Terminally ill: Extended care; Visiondisorders.

For Further Information:
American Psychiatric Association. *Diagnostic and Statistical Manualof Mental Disorders: DSM-V* 5th ed. Arlington, Va.2013.
Cassel, Christine K., ed. *Geriatric Medicine*. 4th ed. New York: Springer, 2003.
Foreman, Marquis D., K. Milisen, and Terry T. Fulmer. *Critical Care Nursingof Older Adults: Best Practices*. 3d ed. New York: Springer, 2010.
Ham, Richard, et al., eds. *Primary Care Geriatrics: A Case-Based Approach*. 6th ed. St. Louis, Mo.: Mosby/Elsevier, 2013.
Katz, Paul R., Robert L. Kane, and Mathy D. Mezey. *Advances in Long-Term Care*. Vol. 4. New York: Springer, 2004.
Levin, Mora Jean. *How to Care for Your Parents: A Practical Guide to Eldercare*. New York: W. W. Norton, 1997.
Matthews, J. L. *Long-Term Care: How to Plan and Pay for It*. 11th ed. Berkeley, Calif.: Nolo, 2016.
Miller, Carol A. *Nursingfor Wellness in Older Adults*. 7th ed. Philadelphia: Wolters Kluwer/Lippincott Williams & Wilkins, 2014.
Namazi, Kevan H., and Paul K. Chaftez, eds. *Assisted Living: Current Issues in Facility Management and Resident Care*.Westport, Conn.: Auburn House, 2000.
Nicholl, Claire, and K. Jane Wilson. *ElderlyCare Medicine*. 8th ed. Oxford: Wiley-Blackwell, 2012.
Weisstub, David N. *Aging: Caring for Our Elders*. Boston: Kluwer Academic, 2001.

Agnosia
Disease/Disorder
Also known as: Alexia, amusia, anosognosia, apraxia, astereognosis, cerebral achromatopsia
Anatomy or system affected: Brain, ears, eyes, nerves, nervous system
Specialties and related fields: Genetics, neurology, occupational health, speech pathology
Definition: Inability to identify objects or persons using one or more of the senses, even though the basic sensory modalities are not defective.

Causes and Symptoms

Agnosia is typically caused by brain damage produced by head injury, stroke, infection, or carbon monoxide poisoning that sometimes causes lesions in the parietal and temporal lobes of the brain, significantly impairing an individual's cognitive processes. Agnosia can also result from neurological disorders, especially if the occipitotemporal border of the ventral stream is damaged. The three main types of agnosia are visual agnosia, auditory agnosia, and tactile agnosia. Some types of agnosia have been found to be genetic.

Victims of agnosia may not recognize objects, persons, shapes, sounds, or smells but retain their cognitive abilities in other areas. Sufferers often have difficulty recognizing the geometric features of an object or a face and determining the use of the object or whether the face is familiar. Some patients can see only one object at a time, while others see multiple objects but recognize only one at a time. Some do not consciously perceive the orientation of an object but will reach for it with a correctly oriented grasp.

Treatment and Therapy

Since no specific treatment or direct cure has been found for agnosia, treatment is generally symptomatic and

Information on Agnosia

Causes: Brain damage, dementia, heredity, neurological disorders, stroke
Symptoms: Inability to recognize familiar objects, people, sounds, shapes, smells, and/or stimuli
Duration: Three months to years
Treatments: Symptomatic and supportive, occupational therapy, speech therapy

supportive. Depending on the etiology, some patients with agnosia can be assisted in compensating for disorder deficits through speech or occupational therapy.

In order to treat the specific problems of a particular patient, the primary cause of the disorder must be determined. Physical examination often identifies primary deficits in individual senses or communication that are not related to agnosia. Images of the brain obtained through computed tomography (CT) scanning or magnetic resonance imaging (MRI) are used to characterize any brain lesions and to check for atrophy that may suggest a degenerative disorder.

Perspective and Prospects

Case studies reporting selective inabilities to recognize faces or objects were reported throughout the nineteenth century. Starting in 1947, studies led by Joachim Bodamer, a German neurologist, helped to develop theories about visual agnosia. Different victims show different types and levels of impairment. Evidence indicates that there may be a specific face perception system in the brain. In the early twenty-first century, a form of congenital prosopagnosia, or face blindness, was identified. It is inherited by 2.5 percent of the population. As more research uncovers details about various types of agnosia, medical recognition, effective treatments, and specific therapies will be enhanced.

—*Alvin K. Benson, Ph.D.*

See also Alzheimer's disease; Anosmia; Audiology; Brain; Brain damage; Brain disorders; Dementia; Ears; Eyes; Hearing; Nervous system; Neurology; Sense organs; Smell; Touch; Vision; Vision disorders.

For Further Information:

Brust, John. *Current Diagnosis and Treatment in Neurology.* New York: McGraw-Hill Medical, 2007.
Farah, Martha J. *Visual Agnosia.* 2d ed. Cambridge, Mass.: MIT Press, 2004.
Parker, James N., ed. *The Official Patient's Sourcebook on Agnosia: A Revised and Updated Directory for the Internet Age.* San Diego, Calif.: Icon Health, 2002.
National Institute of Neurological Disorders and Stroke. "NINDS Agnosia Information Page." *National Institute of Neurological Disorders and Stroke*, Oct. 2, 2007.

AIDS. *See* Acquired immunodeficiency syndrome (AIDS).

Alcoholism
Disease/Disorder
Anatomy or system affected: Brain, liver, pancreas, nervous system, psychic-emotional system
Specialties and related fields: Family medicine, internal medicine, psychiatry, psychology
Definition: A condition in which dependence on alcohol harms a person's health, social functioning, or family life.
Key terms:
cirrhosis: chronic liver disease characterized by the loss of normal liver cells and the replacement of normal liver tissue with fibrous tissue
delirium tremens: severe alcohol withdrawal syndrome, with symptoms including confusion, delirium, visual hallucinations, severe tremors, and clinically unstable involuntary body functions
distillation: the use of heat to separate or purify mixtures of liquid chemicals that boil at different temperatures by vaporization and cooling back into the liquid state
Korsakoff's psychosis: mental illness named after Sergei Korsakoff that involves severe confusion and inability to remember recent memories, usually caused by alcoholism
metabolism: the physical and chemical processes involved in growth, production of energy, and elimination of waste material
proof: a designation of beverage alcohol content that is defined as twice the percentage of alcohol by volume
psychosis: a severe mental state characterized by loss of normal social function and being either withdrawn from or unable to accurately perceive reality

Causes and Symptoms

The basis for alcoholism is physical dependence on alcoholic beverages and consequent problems in behavior and health. Problems related to alcohol developed in ancient history after humans discovered that fruit or grain, mashed and suspended in water, fermented into beverages that produced euphoria in users. The first production of fermented beverages was recorded in Biblical, Babylonian, and Egyptian sources.

The active ingredient in fermented beverages is ethyl alcohol (alcohol, CH_3CH_2OH), a flammable, colorless, mild-smelling liquid that boils at 173 degrees Farenheit (78.37 degrees Celcius). Alcohol content in such beverages is indicated as "proof," which is twice the percentage of alcohol by volume. For example, 20-proof wine contains about 10 percent alcohol by volume. In contrast, 80-proof brandy and vodka, beverages known as hard liquors, contain about 40 percent alcohol by volume, because such liquors have been "fortified" by adding pure alcohol prepared via distillation. Other beverages known as hard liquors include whiskey, scotch, and rye. They typically are discussed separately from beer and wine.

Abuse of alcoholic beverages first became epidemic during the Middle Ages, when development of widespread alcohol distillation produced hard liquors and made it easy to attain alcoholic euphoria and stupor. In 2011, almost 52 percent of individuals in the United States ages 18 years and older reported being current regular drinkers. Binge drinking, or drinking five or more drinks in about 2 hours, was reported by 16.7 percent of adults. In 2010, 11.4 percent of persons aged 12 years or older admitted to driving under the influence within the past year. In 2011, alcohol caused 25,692 deaths, excluding accidents and homicides. A subset of 15,990 deaths were attributable specifically to alcoholic liver disease. The overall number of deaths increases substantially when adding alcohol-related accidents and homicides.

Some deaths attributable to alcohol result from alcohol poisoning, which arises from excessive consumption in a short time period. The drug primarily depresses the action of the central nervous system, creating the desired euphoric effects of alcohol consumption. Given a drink or two, a drinker may become relaxed, talkative, and uninhibited. A few more drinks, however, may increase blood alcohol levels above 1 gram per Liter (0.1 percent v/v) and further depress the central nervous system, causing lack of coordination, slurred speech, and overpowering drowsiness. If just a little more alcohol is imbibed before unconsciousness occurs and blood alcohol levels rise much above 3 grams per Liter (0.3 percent v/v), further depression of the central nervous system depresses breathing and may cause death.

People engaged in the problematic use of alcohol are sometimes called alcoholics. Many professionals, however, prefer to refer to these persons as individuals with alcohol use disorders. This is in keeping with the goal of not engendering a cultural stigma that may be associated with the use of other more denigrating terms. While it is true that some persons with alcohol dependence will use alcohol to the point of compulsive use, seriously disrupting their health and ability to survive, others may become physiologically dependent on alcohol and remain functional for a long time. If the problem worsens, however, then they may experience very serious consequences. It is not uncommon, for instance, for persons with severe alcohol dependence to suffer accidents, life-threatening withdrawal and other health problems, violence, and even suicide.

Chronic alcoholism damages many body organs. Best known is liver disease, or cirrhosis of the liver. Another common problem is brain damage. Mental disorders caused by injury to the cerebral hemispheres may include delirium tremens (the "DTs") and Korsakoff's psychosis. Both the DTs, characterized by hallucination and other psychotic symptoms, and Korsakoff's psychosis, which is characterized by short-term memory loss and confabulation, or stories to cover this loss, may be accompanied by severe physical debility requiring hospitalization.

Alcohol dependence can damage the kidneys, the heart, and the pancreas. In fact, a number of diseases of other organs are thought to arise from alcohol dependence. There is much evidence to suggest that a synergism exists between chronic alcohol use and smoking tobacco, which leads to an increased risk of developing various cancers of the head and neck.

Severe effects in the liver occur because most ingested alcohol is metabolized there. In the presence of alcohol, other chemical substances may not be metabolized in a normal fashion. One example has to do with fat, a major di-

---

Information on Alcoholism

Causes: Repeated and excessive use of alcohol

Symptoms: Lack of coordination, slurred speech, impaired judgment, overpowering drowsiness, semiconsciousness, breathing difficulties, unconsciousness; tolerance; withdrawal (confusion, delirium, hallucinations, tremor, clinically unstable involuntary body functions); associated health risks (cirrhosis, pancreatitis, fetal alcohol syndrome, anemia, cancer)

Duration: Chronic

Treatments: Cognitive and behavioral therapies, self-help groups, metabolic inhibitor disulfiram (Antabuse), opioid antagonist naltrexone (ReVia, Vivitrol), GABA-ergic agonist acamprosate (Campral)

---

etary source of energy. The metabolism of alcohol in the liver produces excess energy that is then directed toward the synthesis of fat. Excess fat accumulates in the liver leading to a condition called "fatty liver," which precedes cirrhosis of the liver. Cirrhosis results in the replacement of dead liver cells with nonfunctional fibrous tissue. It should be noted, however, that not all fatty liver disease results from alcohol use. There are other causes, such as nonalcoholic fatty liver disease or nonalcoholic steatohepatitis (NFLD/NASH), which may result from many different types of health conditions.

Another problem that results from excessive alcohol metabolism is that the liver no longer destroys the many other toxic chemicals that are consumed. This defect adds to problems seen in cirrhosis and leads to dissemination of such chemicals through the body, where they can damage other body parts. In addition, resistance to the flow of blood through the cirrhotic liver develops, which can burst blood vessels in the esophagus or cause other potentially dangerous kinds of internal bleeding. As a consequence of these problems, alcoholic liver disease, including cirrhosis, has become a major, worldwide cause of death.

There is no clearly defined physical explanation for the development of alcoholism. It is a condition that varies from individual to individual and also has many different causes. Often, it is viewed as the result of a biological predisposition to addiction and/or social problems and psychological stresses. Those in cultures where consumption of alcoholic beverages is equated with manliness or sophistication may be at greater risk. Those under great psychological or social stress are also at risk, as drinking may be an inexpensive and easy way to experience some relief. Other proposed causes of behaviors that lead to alcoholism include, but are not limited to, habitual drinking, other mental health problems, domineering parents, adolescent peer pressure, exposure to deviant peer groups, personal feelings of inadequacy, loneliness, job pressures, marital discord, and cultural pressures to drink.

The heritability of alcoholism is estimated to be 40 to 60 percent. Research has shown that individuals with relatives affected by alcohol problems have three to four times the risk of having these problems as well, compared to individuals without relatives affected by alcohol problems. The causes for this risk include genetics and stress. However, it is important to realize that some people, such as Southeast Asians, are genetically protected from risk. Genetic variants of alcohol metabolizing enzymes can lead to unpleasant effects such as racing heartbeat, facial flushing, headache, and nausea when alcohol is consumed. The development of unpleasant effects are important in having a distaste for alcohol, which precludes the development of alcoholism in these and some other ethnic and national groups.

Another disease attributable to alcoholism is fetal alcohol syndrome, which occurs in many children of mothers who drank heavily during pregnancy. These children may be hyperactive, mentally retarded, and facially disfigured, and they may exhibit marked growth retardation. Fetal alcohol syndrome is becoming more frequent as alcohol consumption increases worldwide.

Commonly observed symptoms of dependence on alcohol include the need to drink more to feel the same effects (tolerance); drinking the same amount but feeling less effect (tolerance); having physical or psychological symptoms, or both, when not able to drink (withdrawal); not being able to control one's drinking; frequent desire to quit; spending much time getting alcohol, drinking, or recovering from drinking; giving up other activities to drink; the development of physical or psychological problems because of drinking; and the worsening of physical or psychological problems because of drinking. Severe symptoms may include tremors, shakes, memory loss (blackouts), and diminished cognitive abilities such as the inability to understand verbal instructions or to memorize a simple series of numbers. These symptoms are attributable to changes in the central nervous system. Finally, physical effects also might include diminished sexual desire and sexual activity, and a high level of alcohol in the blood appears to cause diminished libido as well as impotence.

Treatment and Therapy

In the mid-1930s, alcoholism, previously viewed as criminal and immoral behavior, was first conceived to be a disease. There is no known immediate cure for alcoholism. Treatments with demonstrated effectiveness for alcohol problems, however, do exist. Treatments involving combined biological, psychological, and social approaches, complete with follow-up, often appear most helpful. For most individuals, however, an important phase-and permanent feature-of treatment involves total abstinence from alcoholic beverages, all medications that contain alcohol, and any other potential sources of alcohol in the diet.

The recognition of alcoholism as a medical problem has led to the establishment of alcohol rehabilitation centers, where psychiatric treatment, medication, and other therapies are used in widely different combinations. The supportive programs of the organization Alcoholics Anonymous (AA) are also viewed as effective deterrents to a return to alcohol problems. Another well-known medical treatment aimed at encouraging sobriety is the drug

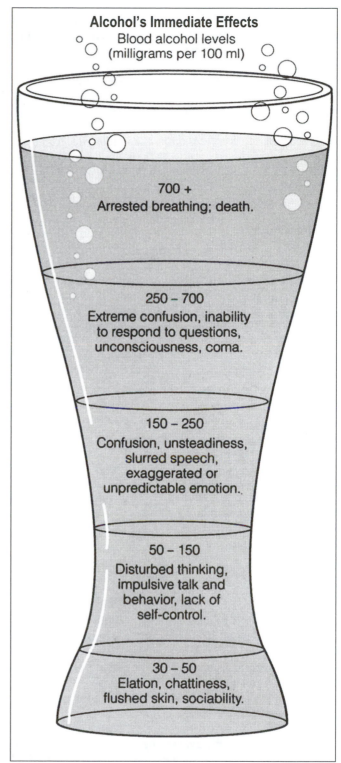

Alcohol's Immediate Effects
Blood alcohol levels
(milligrams per 100 ml)

700 +
Arrested breathing; death.

250 – 700
Extreme confusion, inability to respond to questions, unconsciousness, coma.

150 – 250
Confusion, unsteadiness, slurred speech, exaggerated or unpredictable emotion.

50 – 150
Disturbed thinking, impulsive talk and behavior, lack of self-control.

30 – 50
Elation, chattiness, flushed skin, sociability.

The presence of 30-50 milligrams of alcohol per every 100 milliliters of blood, which represents the effects of an average drink (a glass of beer, wine, or an ounce of hard liquor), has immediate effects; as the amount increases, effects progress toward death.

disulfiram, more popularly known as Antabuse. This drug is given when individuals who wish to avoid all use of alcoholic beverages require a deterrent to drinking in order to achieve this goal. It is important to note, however, that no drug should ever be given secretly to someone by well-meaning family or friends. This is especially important with disulfiram because of the serious physical consequences that will be suffered if the person drinks alcohol.

These dangers are the result of the biochemistry of alcohol metabolism via the two enzymes (biological protein catalysts) alcohol dehydrogenase and aldehyde dehydrogenase. Normally, alcohol dehydrogenase converts alcohol to the toxic chemical acetaldehyde. Aldehyde dehydrogenase quickly converts the acetaldehyde to acetic acid, a metabolic fuel from which the body may derive energy. Disulfiram blocks the activity of aldehyde dehydrogenase and causes acetaldehyde levels to build up in the body when alcohol is consumed. The presence of acetaldehyde in the body then quickly leads to violent headache, great dizziness, heart palpitation, nausea, and vertigo. When the amount of alcohol found in a drink or two (or even the amount taken in cough medicine) is consumed in the presence of disulfiram, these symptoms can escalate to the extent that they become fatal.

An interesting sidelight is the view of many researchers that abstinence from alcohol may be genetically related to the presence of too much alcohol dehydrogenase and/or too little aldehyde dehydrogenase in the body. Either of these unbalanced conditions is thought to produce enough acetaldehyde from a small amount of any alcohol source to cause aversion to all alcohol consumption. This is viewed as particularly relevant in Japan, where about 50 percent of the population lacks aldehyde dehydrogenase, and this lack correlates well with the low predisposition of many Japanese to become alcohol dependent. It must be remembered, however, that no one is immune from developing problems with alcohol. Even someone who belongs to a group known to lack these particular enzymes does not merit a license to use alcohol without care.

As a result of the symptoms of alcohol withdrawal common during detoxification and the presence of other mental health disorders in nearly half of all individuals diagnosed with alcohol dependence, other therapeutic drugs are often used in treatment. Examples include lithium (more often given when certain mood problems are present), major tranquilizers, and sedative hypnotics. The function of these psychoactive drugs is to diminish the discomfort of alcohol withdrawal and stabilize the individual.

Tranquilizers and the related sedative hypnotics must also be used with great care, under close supervision of a physician. Many such drugs are addictive. In addition, some of these drugs have strong additive effects when mixed with alcohol, and such effects can be fatal. Detailed information on the uses and dangers of these different drugs in the treatment of alcohol problems can be found in The Merck Manual of Diagnosis and Therapy.

Naltrexone (Revia, Vivitrol) reduces alcohol cravings and risk of relapse by blocking opioid receptors in the brain. It may be given orally or injected into muscle in a long-acting form for a course of treatment lasting about three months. Naltrexone should not be given at the same time as opioid pain medication due to potential drug interaction. Also, naltrexone should not be used when there is alcoholic liver disease because naltrexone is metabolized through the liver.

Acamprosate (Campral) reduces alcohol cravings by restoring balance between inhibition and excitation of nerve cells in the brain via effects on glutamate and GABA (?-aminobutyric acid). It is excreted from the body by the kidneys and therefore appropriate for use when there is alcoholic liver disease. The dose of acamprosate must be adjusted downward with renal disease. Acomprosate is not used in the presence of renal failure. The recommended course of treatment is one year, after which acamprosate may be discontinued.

It is believed that the advent of AA in 1935 has been crucial to the concept of alcoholism as a disease, rather than as immoral behavior to be condemned. This organization, founded by William Griffith Wilson and Robert Holbrook Smith, operates on the premise that abstinence is the best course of treatment for alcoholism. The methodology of the organization is psychosocial. First, individuals who desire to stop drinking are brought to the realization that they can never use alcoholic beverages without succumbing to serious problems. Then, the need for help from a "higher power" is identified as crucial to abstinence. In addition, the organization develops a support group of people in the same situation. It is this support group feature of AA that is recognized as a valuable milieu for facilitating change.

There are 114,642 AA groups worldwide, including 64,414 groups in the United States and Canada. An estimate of the worldwide membership of AA in 2013 was over 2.1 million. Members, ranging widely in age, achieve results varying from periods of sobriety (lasting longer and longer as membership in the organization continues) to lifelong sobriety. While valuable, it is important to remember that AA is not a formal medical treatment for alcohol problems. It is not necessarily treatment managed by medical, psychiatric, and other formally trained counselors. The results of the operation, however, are viewed by most as beneficial to all parties who seek help from the organization.

Alcohol rehabilitation centers apply varied combinations of drug therapy, psychiatric counseling, and social counseling, depending on the treatment approach for the individual center. Group therapy, however, is the dominant mode of treatment in the United States.

Perspective and Prospects

Modern efforts to deal with alcohol problems are often considered to have begun in the early twentieth century, with the activities of the American temperance movement and the Anti-Saloon League. These activities culminated in the period called Prohibition after Congress passed the 1919 Volstead Act, proposed by Minnesota congressman Andrew J. Volstead. The idea behind the act was that making intoxicating beverages impossible to obtain would force sobriety on Americans. Prohibition turned out to be self-defeating, however, and it increased the incidence of alcohol and related problems. Subsequently, the act was repealed in 1933, ending Prohibition.

The next, and much more useful, effort to combat alcoholism was the founding of AA. Because AA does not reach the majority of individuals with alcohol problems, other efforts have evolved as treatment methodologies. Among these have been psychiatric counseling, alcohol rehabilitation centers, family counseling, and alcohol management programs in the workplace. Treatment efforts have even been established on the. These endeavors, funded by the federal government and private industry, largely from 1970 forward, continue to improve treatment success by identifying problems earlier, encouraging prevention, and making treatment more effective for a broader range of people.

—Sanford S. Singer, Ph.D;
updated by George W. Miller Jr., M.D., FAAFP

See also Addiction; American Indian health; Cirrhosis; Dementias; Fetal alcohol syndrome; Intoxication; Jaundice; Liver disorders; Osteonecrosis; Psychosis; Substance abuse

For Further Information:

Alcoholics Anonymous. http://www.aa.org. A group whose primary purpose is to help members stay sober and help other alcoholics to achieve sobriety.

Alcoholics Anonymous: *The Big Book Online.* 4th ed. http://www.aa.org/bigbookonline/. Offers steps to recovery and personal stories of rehabilitation.

Collins, R. Lorraine, Kenneth E. Leonard, and John R. Searles, eds. *Alcohol and the Family: Research and Clinical Perspectives.* New York: Guilford Press, 1990. Reprinted in 2005, this book addresses genetics, family processes, and family-oriented treatment. Aspects of genetic testing and markers are covered, along with adolescent drinking, children of alcoholics, and alcoholism's effect on a marriage.

Galanter, Marc, and Herbert D. Kleber, eds. *The American Psychiatric Publishing Textbook of Substance Abuse Treatment.* 4th ed. Arlington, Va.: American Psychiatric Press, 2008. Presents authoritative clinical information on alcohol and other drug addictions and their treatment.

Hester, Reid K., and William R. Miller, eds. *Handbook of Alcoholism Treatment Approaches.* 3rd ed. Boston: Allyn & Bacon, 2003. A comprehensive guide to alcohol treatment methods designed for both practitioners and researchers.

Lawson, Ann W., and Gary Lawson, eds. *Alcoholism and the Family: A Guide to Treatment and Prevention.* 2nd ed. Austin, Tex.: Pro-Ed, Inc., 2004. Explores the application of the principles of family therapy to alcoholism treatment.

National Institute for Alcoholism and Alcohol Abuse. http://www.niaaa.nih.gov. A clearinghouse for information on alcohol use disorders and treatment resources.

Porter, Robert S. *The Merck Manual of Diagnosis and Therapy.* 19th ed. Whitehouse Station, N.J.: Merck Research Laboratories, 2011. This book contains a compendium of data on the etiology, diagnosis, and treatment of alcoholism. Contains good cross-references to the psychopathology related to the disease, drug rehabilitation, and Alcoholics Anonymous.

Substance Abuse and Mental Health Services Administration. http://www.samhsa.gov. A resource for information on mental health and substance use disorders.

Allergies

Disease/Disorder

Anatomy or system affected: Gastrointestinal system, immune system, lungs, nose, skin, stomach
Specialties and related fields: Dermatology, family medicine, immunology, internal medicine, otorhinolaryngology, pediatrics, pharmacology
Definition: Exaggerated immune reactions to materials that are intrinsically harmless; the body's release of pharmacologically active chemicals during allergic reactions may result in discomfort, tissue damage, or, in severe responses, death.

Key terms:

allergen: any substance that induces an allergic reaction

anaphylaxis: an immediate immune reaction, triggered by mediators that cause vasodilation and the contraction of smooth muscle

basophil: a type of white blood cell that contains mediators associated with allergic reactions; represents 1 percent or less of total white cells

histamine: a compound released during allergic reactions that causes many of the symptoms of allergies

IgE: a type of antibody associated with the release of granules from basophils and mast cells

mast cell: a tissue cell with granules containing vasoactive mediators such as histamine, serotonin, and bradykinin; the tissue equivalent of basophil

Causes and Symptoms

Allergies represent inappropriate immune responses to intrinsically harmless materials, or antigens. Most allergens are common environmental antigens. Approximately one in every six Americans is allergic to material such as dust, molds, dust mites, animal dander, or pollen. The effects range from a mere nuisance, such as rhinitis, or nasal irritation, associated with hay fever allergies or the itching of poison ivy, to the life-threatening anaphylactic shock that may follow a bee sting. Allergies are most often found in children, but they may affect any age group.

Allergy is one of the hypersensitivity reactions generally classified according to the types of effector molecules that mediate their symptoms and according to the time delay that follows exposure to the allergen. P.G.H. Gell and Robin Coombs defined four types of hypersensitivities. Three of these, types 1 through 3, follow minutes to hours after the exposure to an allergen. Type 4, or delayed-type hypersensitivity (DTH), may occur anywhere from twenty-four to seventy-two hours after exposure. People are most familiar with two of these forms of allergies: type 1, or immediate hypersensitivity, commonly seen as hay fever or asthma; and type 4, most often following an encounter with poison ivy or poison oak.

Type 1 hypersensitivities have much in common with any normal immune response. A foreign material, an allergen, comes in contact with the host's immune system, and an antibody response is the result. The response differs according to the type of molecule produced. A special class of antibody, IgE, is secreted by the B lymphocytes. IgE, when complexed with the specific allergen, is capable of binding to any of several types of mediator cells, mainly basophils and mast cells.

Mast cells are found throughout the skin and tissue. The mucous membranes of the respiratory and gastrointestinal tract in particular have high concentrations of these cells, as

Microscopic pollens, which are responsible for many allergic reactions. (PhotoDisc)

many as ten thousand cells per cubic millimeter. Basophils, the blood cell equivalents of the mast cells, represent 1 percent or less of the total white cell count. Though the cells are not identical, they do possess features related to the role that they play in an allergic response. Both basophils and mast cells contain large numbers of granules composed of pharmacologically active chemicals. Both also contain surface receptors for IgE molecules. The binding of IgE/allergen complexes to these cells triggers the release of the granules.

A large number of common antigens can be associated with allergies. These include plant pollens (as are found in rye grass or ragweed), foods such as nuts or eggs, bee or wasp venom, mold, or animal dander. A square mile of ragweed may produce as much as 16 tons of pollen in a single season. In fact, almost any food or environmental substance could serve as an allergen. The most important defining factor as to whether an individual is allergic to any particular substance is the extent and type of IgE production against that substance.

Type 1 allergic reactions begin as soon as the sensitized person is exposed to the allergen. In the case of hay fever, this results when the person inhales the pollen particle. The shell of the particle is enzymatically dissolved, and the specific allergens are released in the vicinity of the mucous membranes in the respiratory system. If the person has had prior sensitization to the materials, his/her immune system recognizes it as a foreign matter, so IgE molecules are se-

creted by localized lymphocytes, bind to the allergens, and form an antibody/antigen complex.

A sequence of events is set in place when the immune complexes bind to the surface of the mast cell or basophil. The reactions begin with a cross-linking of the IgE receptors on the cell. Such cross-linking is necessary because, in its absence, no granules are released. On the other hand, artificial cross-linking of the receptors in laboratory experiments, even in the absence of IgE, results in the release of vasoactive granules.

Following the activation of the cell surface, a series of biochemical events occurs, the key being an influx of calcium into the cell. Two events rapidly follow: The cell begins production of prostaglandins and leukotrienes, two mediators that play key roles in allergic reactions, and pre-

---

Information on Allergies

Causes: Antigens such as pollen, mold, certain foods (nuts, eggs, seafood), drugs (penicillin), bee or wasp venom, animal dander, dust mites, etc.

Symptoms: Sneezing, runny nose, coughing, itching, breathing difficulties, hives, inflammation, vomiting, diarrhea, shock

Duration: Chronic, with acute episodes

Treatments: Antihistamines, mast cell stabilizers, steroids (cortisone), desensitization existing granules begin moving toward the cell surface. When they reach the cell surface, the granules fuse with the cell membrane, releasing their contents into the tissue.

The contents of the granules mediate the clinical manifestations of allergies. These mediators can be classified as either primary or secondary. Thus, clinical responses are divided into immediate and late-phase reactions. Primary mediators are those found in preexisting granules and released initially following the activities at the cell surface. They include substances such as histamine and serotonin, associated with increased vascular permeability and smooth muscle contraction. Histamine itself may constitute 10 percent of the weight of the granules in these cells. The results are a runny nose, irritated eyes, and bronchial congestion. These substances include the leukotrienes (also called slow reactive substances of anaphylaxis, or SRS-A) and prostaglandins. Pharmacological effects from these chemicals include vasodilation, increased capillary permeability, contraction of smooth muscles in the bronchioles, and, more important, a group of chemotactic activities that attract many different white cells in the site to magnify the inflammatory reaction. This is why an allergic reaction is divided into two phases and the late reaction may last for days.

Foods to which one is allergic may trigger similar reactions in the gut. Mast cells in the gastrointestinal tract also contain receptors for IgE, and contact with food allergens results in the release of mediators similar to those in the respiratory passages. The result may be vomiting or diarrhea. The allergen may also pass from the gut into the circulatory system or other tissues, triggering asthmatic attacks or hives.

In severe allergic reactions, the response may be swift and deadly. The venom released during a bee sting may trigger a systemic response from circulating basophils or mast cells, resulting in the contraction of pulmonary muscles and rapid suffocation, a condition known as anaphylactic shock. The leukotrienes, platelet-activating factor, and prostaglandins play key roles in these reactions.

Delayed-type hypersensitivities, also known as contact dermatitis reactions, are most commonly manifested following the presentation of a topical allergen. These may include the catechol-containing oils of poison oak, the constituents of hair dyes or cosmetics, environmental contaminants such as nickel or turpentine, or any of a wide variety of environmental agents. Rather than being mediated by antibodies, as are the other types of hypersensitivities, DTH is mediated through a specific cellular response. These cells appear to be a special class of T

In the News: Peanut Allergies

In the United States alone, between fifty and one hundred fifty people die each year from serious allergic reactions to peanuts. One and a half million Americans have a demonstrated allergic sensitivity that puts them at risk for life-threatening reactions to peanut protein exposure. Reactions can be so severe to minute amounts of airborne peanut protein that some schoolchildren must eat lunch in peanut-free rooms, and many airlines have stopped serving peanuts to passengers. Because peanuts and peanut oil can be ingredients in a diverse range of food items such as chili, potato chips, and egg rolls, peanut allergy sufferers live under a constant threat of having an adverse reaction despite their best efforts to avoid the allergen.

In the March 13, 2003, issue of the *New England Journal of Medicine*, Hugh A. Sampson and his colleagues of Mount Sinai School of Medicine in New York reported the results of a study that show the first successful preventive treatment for peanut allergy. In a double-blind study, eighty-four volunteers with peanut allergy were given either placebo shots or injections of various doses of the experimental drug TNX-901 once a month over a four-month period. At the end of the study, participants were given capsules of peanut flour in increasing amounts until they exhibited an allergic reaction. The results showed that those given placebos reacted when given the equivalent of half a peanut. People who received low doses of the drug could ingest a bit more before reacting. Those receiving the highest doses could ingest, on average, the equivalent of nine peanuts (and for some, twenty-four peanuts) before developing an allergic response.

TNX-901 is a genetically engineered antibody that prevents allergic response by binding to potentially harmful immune cells that are produced in response to allergen exposure. Binding these immune cells interrupts the series of events that lead to an allergic reaction.

While TNX-901 is not a cure for peanut allergy, its preventive potential makes the required monthly shot appealing to those afflicted with the disorder. Since accidental exposure to peanut protein is estimated to be equivalent to one or two peanuts, TNX-901 could provide sufferers with confidence that accidental peanut exposure would not lead to a life-threatening reaction. Legal disputes have hampered its development, however, and a similar drug called Xolair is being researched. Other researchers are examining oral immunotherapy as a treatment for peanut allergy.

—*Karen E. Kalumuck, Ph.D.*

(for thymus-derived) lymphocytes.

DTH reactions are initiated following the exposure to the appropriate antigen. Antigen-presenting cells in the skin bind and "present" the allergen to the specific T lymphocytes. This results in the secretion by these T cells of a variety of chemicals mediating inflammation. These mediators, or cytokines, include gamma interferon, interleukin-2, and tumor necrosis factor. The result, developing over a period of twenty-four to seventy-two hours, is a significant inflammatory response with subsequent localized damage to tissue.

The other classes of hypersensitivity reactions, types 2 and 3, are less commonly associated with what most people consider to be allergies. Yet they do have much in common with type 1, immediate hypersensitivity. Type 2 reactions are mediated by a type of antibody called igG. Clinical manifestations result from the antibody-mediated destruction of target cells, rather than through the release of mediators. One of the most common forms of reaction is blood transfusion reactions, either against the A or B blood group antigen or as a result of an Rh incompatibility. For example, if a person with type O blood is accidentally transfused with type A, an immune reaction will occur. The eventual

The Body's Response to Allergens

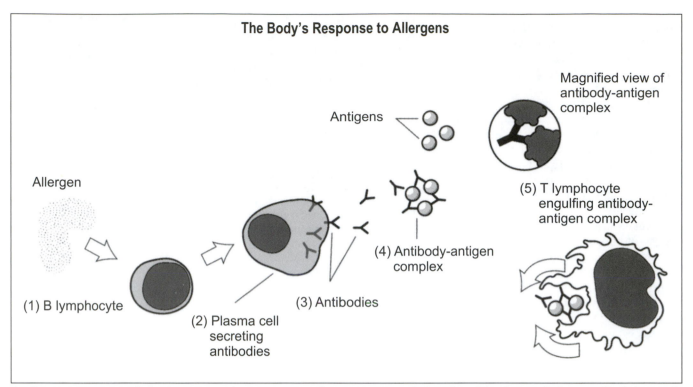

An allergic reaction is caused when foreign material, or antigens, enter the immune system, which produces B lymphocytes (1) that cause blood plasma cells to secrete antibodies (2). The antibodies (3) link with antigens to form antigen-antibody complexes (4), which then are engulfed and destroyed by a T lymphocyte (5).

result is destruction of the incompatible blood cells. Rh incompatibilities are most commonly associated with a pregnant woman who is lacking the Rh protein in her blood (that is, Rh negative) carrying a child who is Rh positive (a blood type obtained from the father's genes). The production of IgG directed against the Rh protein in the child's blood can set in motion events that result in the destruction of the baby's red blood cells, a condition known as erythroblastosis fetalis. This is usually not problematic during a woman's first pregnancy, but becomes a problem in later pregnancies when her immune system is able to recognize the baby's Rh factor as a foreign body.

Type 3 reactions are known as immune complex diseases. In this case, sensitivity to antigens results in formation of IgG/antigen complexes, which can lodge in the kidney or other sites in the body. The complexes activate what is known as the complement system, a series of proteins that include vasoactive chemicals and lipolytic compounds. The result can be a significant inflammation that can lead to kidney damage. Type 3 reactions can include autoimmune diseases such as arthritis or lupus, or drug reactions such as some forms of penicillin allergies (some penicillin allergies are type 1).

It should be kept in mind, however, that none of these reactions is inherently abnormal. Under normal circumstances, these same reactions mediate an inflammatory defense against foreign pathogens. For example, the normal role of IgE appears to be associated with the destruction of parasites such as are found in helminthic infections (such as parasitic worms). The release of mediators under these conditions is important as a defensive reaction leading to the expulsion or destruction of worms. It is only when these same mediators are released inappropriately that one observes the symptoms of allergies.

Most individuals are familiar with immediate hypersensitivity reactions involving a localized area. The most common form of allergy is rhinitis, known as hay fever, which affects approximately 10 percent of the population. When a person inhales an environmental allergen such as ragweed pollen, the result is a release of pharmacologically active mediators from mast cells located in the upper respiratory tract. If the release occurs in the lower respiratory tract, the condition is known as asthma. In both instances, the eyes and nose are subject to inflammation and the release of secretions. In mild cases, the person suffers from watery discharges, coughing, and sneezing. In more severe asthma attacks, the bronchioles may become constricted and obstruct the air passages.

Treatment and Therapy

Three methods for dealing with allergies exist: avoidance of the allergen, palliative treatments, and desensitization. Ideally, one can attempt to avoid the allergen. For example, cow's milk, a common allergen, should not be given to a child at too young an age, and one can stay away from patches of poison ivy or avoid eating strawberries if one is allergic to them.

Avoidance, however, is not always possible or desirable, as the problem may be the fur, for example, from the family cat. Pets are problematic because their bodily secretions, such as urine or saliva, dry on household objects. When an object, such as a pillow, is used, the molecules become disturbed and the airborne molecules create a pool of allergens that are hard to get rid of, since so many household objects are usually contaminated.

It is sometimes difficult to identify the specific substance causing the symptoms. This is particularly true when dealing with foods. Various procedures exist to identify the irritating substance, skin testing being the most common. In this procedure, the patient's skin is exposed to small amounts of suspected allergens. A positive test is indicated by formation of hives or reddening within about twenty to thirty minutes. If the person is hypersensitive to a suspected allergen and finds a skin test too risky, then a blood test, a radioallergosorbent (RAST) test may be substituted. In addition to running a battery of tests, a patient's allergy history (including family history, since allergies are in part genetic) or environment may give clues as to the identity of the culprit.

The most commonly used method of dealing with allergies is a palliative treatment-that is, treatment of the symptoms. Antihistamines act by binding to histamine receptors on target cells, interfering with the binding of histamine. Two types of histamine receptors exist: H-1 and H-2. Histamine binding to H-1 receptors results in contractions of smooth muscles and increased mucus secretion. Binding to H-2 receptors results in increased vasopermeability and swelling. Anti-histamines that act at the level of the H-1 receptor include alkylamines and ethanolamines and are effective in treating symptoms of acute allergies such as hay fever. Histamine II blockers such as cimetidine are used primarily in the treatment of peptic ulcers to control gastric secretions, but they occasionally are used as adjunctive therapy or in the prevention of severe allergic reactions.

Many antihistamines can be obtained without a prescription. If they are not used properly, however, the side effects can be serious. Overuse may result in toxicity, particularly in children; overdoses in children can be fatal. Because antihistamines can depress the central nervous system, side effects include drowsiness, nausea, constipation, and drying of the throat or respiratory passage. This is particularly true of histamine 1 blockers. A new generation of H-1 antihistamines is available on the market. They are long-acting and are free of the sedative effect of other antihistamines.

Other symptomatic treatments include the use of cromolyn sodium, which blocks the influx of calcium into the mast cell, and thus is called a mast cell stabilizer. It acts to block steps leading to degranulation and the release of mediators. In more severe cases, the administration of steroids (cortisone) may prove useful in limiting symptoms of allergies.

Anaphylaxis is the most severe form of immediate hypersensitivity, and unless treated promptly, it may be fatal. It is often triggered in susceptible persons by common environmental substances: bee or wasp venom, drugs such as penicillin, foods such as peanuts and seafood, or latex protein in rubber. Symptoms include labored breathing, rapid loss of blood pressure, itching, hives, and/or loss of bladder control. The symptoms are triggered by a sudden and massive release of mast cell or basophil mediators such as histamine, leukotrienes, or prostaglandin derivatives. Treatment consists of an immediate injection of epinephrine and the maintenance of an open air passage into the lungs. Corticosteroids and antihistamines are also administered. If cardiac arrest occurs, cardiopulmonary resuscitation must be undertaken. Persons in known danger of encountering such a triggering allergen often carry with them an emergency kit containing epinephrine and antihistamines.

Contact dermatitis is a form of delayed-type hypersensitivity, developing several days after exposure to the sensitizing allergen. Rather than resulting from the presence of IgE antibody, the symptoms of contact dermatitis result from a series of chemicals released by sensitized T lymphocytes in the area of the skin on which the allergen (often poison ivy or poison oak) is found. Treatments generally involve the application of topical corticosteroids and soothing or drying agents. In more severe cases, systemic use of corticosteroids may be necessary.

In some persons, the relief of allergy symptoms may be achieved through desensitization. This form of immunotherapy involves the repeated subcutaneous injection of increasing doses of the allergen. In a significant number of persons, such therapy leads to a decrease in symptoms. The idea behind such therapy is that repeated injections of the allergen may lead to production of another class of antibody, the more systemic IgG. These molecules can serve as blocking antibodies, competing with IgE in binding to the allergen. Because IgG/allergen complexes can be phagocytosed (destroyed by phagocytes) and do not bind receptors on mast cells or basophils, they should not trigger the symptoms of allergies. Unfortunately, for reasons that remain unclear, not all persons or all allergies respond to such therapy.

The type 1 immediate hypersensitivity reactions commonly run in families. This is not so surprising if one realizes that the regulation of IgE production is genetically determined. Thus, if both parents have allergies, there is little chance that their offspring will escape the problem. On the other hand, if one or both parents are allergy-free, the odds are at least even that the offspring will also be free from such reactions.

Perspective and Prospects

Though allergies in humans have probably existed since humans first evolved from ancestral primates, it was only in the nineteenth century that an understanding of the process began to develop. Type 1 hypersensitivity reaction was first described in 1839 through experiments in which dogs were repeatedly injected with egg albumin and developed an immediate fatal shock. The term "anaphylaxis" was coined for this phenomenon in 1902, when Paul Portier and Charles Richet observed that dogs repeatedly immunized with extracts of sea anemone tentacles suffered a similar fate. Richet was awarded the 1913 Nobel Prize in Physiology or Medicine for his work on anaphylaxis.

In the 1920s, Sir Henry Dale established that at least some of the phenomena associated with immediate hypersensitivity were caused by the chemical histamine. Dale sensitized guinea pigs against various antigens. He then observed that, when the muscles from the uterus were removed and exposed to the same antigen, histamine was released and the muscles underwent contraction (known as the Schultz-Dale reaction).

The existence of a component in human serum, which mediates hypersensitive reactions, was demonstrated by Otto Prausnitz, a Polish bacteriologist, and Heinz Kustner, a Polish gynecologist, in 1921. Kustner had a strong allergy to fish. Prausnitz removed a sample of serum from his colleague and injected it under his own skin. The next day, Prausnitz injected fish extract in that same region. Hives immediately appeared, indicating that the serum contained components that mediated the allergy. For some time, the Prausnitz-Kustner test, or P-K test, remained a means of testing for allergens under circumstances in which a person could be tested for sensitivity. (It is no longer in use be-

cause of safety concerns.) In this test, a serum sample from the test subject was injected under the skin of a surrogate (usually a relative) and later followed with test allergens. The presence of a wheal and flare reaction (hives) indicated sensitivity to the allergen. The serum component responsible for this sensitivity was later identified as the antibody IgE by K. and T. Ishizaka and S.G.O. Johansson in 1967. The target cells to which the IgE bound were later identified as mast cells and basophils.

The discovery of IgE allowed scientists to develop a blood test called a radioallergosorbent test (RAST) that could measure a specific IgE antibody to an allergic substance. RAST is fully as sensitive as a skin test and thus can be a substitute in some clinical circumstances. Furthermore, discoveries of numerous mediators from mast cells and other white cells such as cytokines, chemokines, interleukins, growth factors, and interferon have helped scientists understand the pathology of allergy at the molecular level. It helps clinically to divide the allergic reaction into immediate reaction (onset within a few minutes after exposure to allergens) and delayed or late-phase reaction (onset hours after exposure to antigens and a reaction that may last for days). The definition of allergy has now expanded from the traditional, immediate allergic reaction to the inclusion of chronic inflammatory processes in the tissues. With a better understanding of how allergies develop, better treatments can be offered to patients who suffer from this disorder.

The eventual goal of research is to understand the molecular defects that result in allergies and ultimately to find a means to eliminate the problem, rather than simply offer palliative measures. For example, it is now known that interleukin-4 (one of the mediators of T cells) raises IgE production, while interferon (another mediator of T cells) lowers IgE production. By understanding the regulation of IgE production, it may become possible to inhibit IgE production in allergic persons selectively, without affecting the desired functions of the immune response.

—*Richard Adler, Ph.D.; updated by Catherine Avelar, B.S.*

See also Antihistamines; Asthma; Autoimmune disorders; Bites and stings; Celiac sprue; Decongestants; Dermatitis; Dermatology; Diaper rash; Food allergies; Food poisoning; Gastroenterology; Gastroenterology, pediatric; Gastrointestinal disorders; Gastrointestinal system; Hay fever; Hives; Host-defense mechanisms; Immune system; Immunization and vaccination; Immunology; Lungs; Mold and mildew; Multiple chemical sensitivity syndrome; Poisonous plants; Pulmonary medicine; Pulmonary medicine, pediatric; Rashes; Shock; Skin; Skin disorders; Sneezing

For Further Information:

Adelman, Daniel C., et al., eds. *Manual of Allergy and Immunology.* 4th ed. Philadelphia, Pa.: Lippincott Williams & Wilkins, 2002. Examines research developments and the clinical diagnosis and treatment of allergies and immune disorders. Topics include asthma, disorders of the eye, diseases of the lung, anaphylaxis, insect allergies, drug allergies, rheumatic diseases, transplantation immunology, and immunization.

Brostoff, Jonathan, and Linda Gamlin. *Food Allergies and Food Intolerance: The Complete Guide to Their Identification and Treatment.* Rochester, Vt.: Inner Traditions, 2000. Examines the role of food allergies in chronic health conditions such as migraines and persistent fatigue and gives a step-by-step process for identifying and treating food allergies.

Cutler, Ellen W. *Winning the War against Asthma and Allergies.* Albany, N.Y.: Delmar, 1998. This clearly written book provides practical information on all aspects of allergies-what they are, their causes, testing, diagnosis, and treatment, including nontraditional therapies. Preventive measures are covered, as are scenarios for various allergy elimination therapies.

Delves, Peter J., et al. *Roitt's Essential Immunology.* 11th ed. Malden, Mass.: Blackwell, 2006. Written by a leading author in the field, the text provides a fine description of immunology. The section on hypersensitivity is clearly presented and profusely illustrated. Though too detailed in places, most of the material can be understood by individuals who have taken high school biology.

Eggleston, P. A., & Wood, R. A. (1992, November). "Management of Allergies to Animals."

In Allergy and Asthma Proceedings (Vol. 13, No. 6, pp. 289-292). OceanSide Publications, Inc.

Joneja, Janice M. V., and Leonard Bielory. *Understanding Allergy, Sensitivity, and Immunity.* New Brunswick, N.J.: Rutgers University Press, 1990. The authors provide extensive discussion of allergies and the roles played by the immune system. They describe the means by which one can learn to cope with allergies and discuss various testing methods for the identification of allergens.

Kindt, Thomas J., Richard A. Goldsby, and Barbara A. Osborne. *Kuby Immunology.* 6th ed. New York: W. H. Freeman, 2007. The section on hypersensitivity in this immunology textbook is well written and includes a mixture of detail and overview of the subject. Particularly useful are discussions of the various types of hypersensitivity reactions. Some knowledge of biology is useful.

Life, Death, and the Immune System. New York: W. H. Freeman, 1994. This comprehensive collection of articles from Scientific American provides basic information and research directions on AIDS, autoimmune disorders, and allergies as well as an excellent discussion of the immune system in general.

Ring, J., Krämer, U., Schäfer, T., and Behrendt, H. "Why Are Allergies Increasing?" *Current Opinion in Immunology* 13, no. 6 (2001): 701-708. This article shows evidence, and gives possible explanations, for the increasing prevalence of allergies in Western countries.

Skoner, D.P. "Allergic Rhinitis: Definition, Epidemiology, Pathophysiology, Detection, and Diagnosis." *Journal of Allergy and Clinical Immunology* 108, no. 1 (2001): S2-S8.

Walsh, William. *The Food Allergy Book.* New York: J. Wiley, 2000. In this excellent guide to one highly prevalent form of allergy, the author presents useful background information on food allergies and a pragmatic guide to identifying and eliminating food allergens from one's diet.

Young, Stuart, Bruce Dobozin, and Margaret Miner. *Allergies.* Rev. ed. New York: Plume, 1999. In addition to discussing the diagnosis and treatment of allergies, the authors evaluate the various remedies on the market at the time of publication. Also useful are lists of organizations to contact for further information.

Allied health

Health care system

Definition: A designation used to describe the services and personnel that support the providers of direct patient care within the larger health care system.

Key terms:

anesthetist: a health care specialist who administers an agent (anesthetic) that makes the patient insensitive to sensation or pain

audiologist: a hearing impairment specialist involved in evaluation, measurement, and rehabilitation

chiropractic: a health care strategy which teaches that disease can be caused by the pinching of spinal nerves, the treatment of which involves spinal adjustment

kinesiotherapist: a health care specialist who provides therapy to a patient's muscles through muscular movement and exercise

nuclear medicine: an area of medicine that uses radioactive nucleotides in diagnostic and treatment procedures

optometry: a specialty that deals with problems in the refractive power of the eyes and with the making of corrective lenses

paramedical: related to the science or practice of medicine

perfusionist: a health care specialist who operates extracorporal circulation equipment when it is necessary to support or replace a patient's circulatory or respiratory function

podiatry: the specialty that deals with the diagnosis and treatment of foot problems, including minor surgery

sonographer: a health care specialist who records and displays the results of an ultrasonic scan which produces a sonogram of a specific anatomical area

Boundaries within Medicine

Allied health refers to a field of health care in which workers participate with physicians and/or nurses in a team effort to promote health and prevent disease in the patient. Allied health occupations may be either professional or technical, depending on the extent and caliber of didactic learning and clinical study as well as on the duties associated with the occupation.

Throughout the evolution of the American health-care system, the role of the physician has remained relatively stable and of primary importance. The American Medical Association (AMA) successfully developed specialty categories to solidify the role of the physician and to protect the doctorate in medicine.

The designation "allied health" appears to be a creation of the AMA to describe those paramedical occupations that developed within the evolving health care system in response to the advancing technology and expanding health care facilities, such as hospitals, clinics, medical centers, and laboratories. The AMA, through its various societies and committees, guided the formation of a variety of occupations to perform tasks that would not or could not be performed by the medical doctor or nurse. These occupations were carefully husbanded by strict job descriptions, educational guidelines, and evaluation criteria. For the most part, allied health professions are those fields that the Committee on Allied Health Education and Accreditation (CAHEA) of the AMA has scrutinized according to essential criteria that have been adopted by the particular profession. These criteria are primarily the standards that are established by a profession as a means to establish education programs that instruct new professionals, to perform a self-study by each program, and to be evaluated by an outside visiting team. A profession is also characterized by the establishment of a society or association by those practitioners of the occupation for the purpose of supporting the research, teaching, and learning of its members. The society sets standards of job performance and evaluation and also establishes a code of ethics to which its members adhere.

Those professions not accredited by the CAHEA are dentistry, optometry, podiatry, chiropractic, veterinary medicine, physical therapy, and nursing. Whether a profession finds the designation "allied health" complimentary or acceptable appears to depend on the status of the profession with respect to its age, the amount of education and responsibility required, and whether autonomy from the AMA is desired. The more autonomous a profession, the more impressive the identity and social status of its practitioners with respect to salary, power, and influence. For example, although a physical therapist can have a private practice rather than be employed in a hospital or another setting that guarantees a certain number of patients, a therapist is not legally allowed to treat a patient without an order from a physician. According to the Bureau of Labor Statistics, In 2011, the median salary for a physical therapist (PT) was about $78,000; those in private practice earned slightly more. To have a private practice, a physical therapist must cultivate a list of local physicians for referrals.

The nursing profession is a good example of a health profession that, to a greater or lesser extent, is not under the allied health umbrella. It is not listed by either the CAHEA or the Association of Schools of Allied Health Professions (ASAHP). Although the US government provided scholarships for nurses in the Allied Health Personnel Training Act of 1966, nursing is excluded from the definition in the Health Professions Education Amendment of 1991. Nursing has been continuously able to maintain its integrity as a profession for a number of reasons: It has always had solidarity provided by the National League of Nursing (NLN), it has continued to develop its education requirements and responsibilities, it requires government licensure, and it has a very visible role in health-care delivery-to some extent more than that of the physician.

The nursing profession continues to develop and is reaching into areas that were traditionally considered to be the domain of the physician. Nurse practitioners are able to take medical histories, read x-rays, order and read tests, and diagnose conditions. They are able to prescribe medications in eighteen states and can be reimbursed for some services by Medicare and Medicaid. Nurse anesthetists can work independently of a doctor in a variety of health-care delivery settings.

According to the 1991 Health Professions Education Amendment, the term "allied health profession" excludes both the nurse and the physician assistant. It includes all those who have had educational training in a science program relating to health services, earning anything from a certificate to a doctorate. It further defines allied health care personnel as individuals who share in the responsibility of the delivery of health-care services or those related to health care. Such services include the identification, evaluation, and prevention of disease and disorders, as well as those related to diet and nutrition, health promotion, rehabilitation, and health systems management.

Those professionals who are excluded from the label of allied health care personnel by the government are doctors of medicine, osteopathy, dentistry, veterinary medicine, optometry, podiatry, pharmacy, chiropractic, and clinical psychology. Also excluded are pharmacists with bachelor's degrees, social workers, and those with graduate degrees in public health and health administration. It is confusing, however, to have physician assistants excluded from allied health by the government and the CAHEA but included in the designation by the ASAHP. Physical therapy is included by the government and the ASAHP but excluded by the CAHEA. The reason for such apparent confusion rests with the various points of view. The government is interested in the service provided by the particular occupation. The ASAHP is interested in promoting allied health education, professional growth, and collaboration between the professions and in influencing public policy as it relates to these factors. The CAHEA has the responsibility of overseeing the allied health education programs that are under the AMA umbrella.

According to the ASAHP, allied health professionals serve in a variety of autonomous and service positions. Therapists and counselors function in private practice and are directly involved with their patients. The medical technologist practices in a laboratory profession at least once removed from patient contact. Allied health care professionals work in every aspect of the health delivery system in a variety of disciplines with a variety of educational experiences. They work throughout the country in a number of physical settings, including hospitals, physicians' office laboratories, clinics, hospices, community programs, schools, and extended-care facilities.

Because of the dynamic state of health care, many allied health care occupations eventually become professions. The expansion of knowledge and evolving technology require increased learning and understanding. The aspiring practitioner of a particular occupation is confronted with a body of information that must be mastered. Those involved with the occupation must organize the information, find new applications, and teach what they know to students interested in the occupation. Essentials or standards are adopted, and a new allied health profession is born. The evolution of the medical technologist or clinical laboratory scientist from the help hired by the pathologist provides a good example of how a profession begins and then sustains itself. The first allied health professions to establish essential criteria and have their education programs evaluated by the AMA were occupational therapy, medical technology, and physical therapy.

Science and Profession

Allied health is a designation that can be understood only in the context of direct health care providers and patients. Direct health care providers are those who are licensed to interact directly with the patient in diagnosis and/or treatment. Examples are medical doctors of various specialties, nurses, dentists, optometrists, chiropractors, and podiatrists. Ancillary activities that support direct care would be described as allied health. Those careers that are involved with these activities are allied health careers or professions.

The ancillary activities to primary care have come about for many reasons. Among them are the advances in technology that have resulted in more sophisticated diagnostic testing. Only the direct caregiver such as a medical doctor (and in some cases, a nurse practitioner) can make a diagnosis. This activity may require data, however, that are provided by the medical technologist, audiologist, diagnostic medical sonographer, or radiologic technologist; some data are provided only after time-consuming and specialized laboratory activity provided by the cytotechnologist or the blood bank technology specialist. Health care often involves specialized equipment and someone specifically trained in running it, such as the perfusionist, the radiation therapy technologist, and the cardiovascular technologist; the more mundane but very important task of medical record keeping is performed by an administrator and technicians; highly specialized areas of therapy have resulted in careers that require a very narrow area of medical understanding or a specialized area that complements the medical activity of the doctor, such as art therapist, music therapist, occupational therapist, physical therapist, and respiratory therapist.

Allied health has become an important aspect of the American health-care system. Sophisticated technology and equipment, new therapeutic techniques, routine record keeping, complex laboratory tests, and specialized therapies have resulted in careers that complement the duties of the direct caregiver. Clinical care can only be as good as the primary-care professionals supported by allied health care professionals. An adequate allied health system depends on the support of allied health educational institutions, professional organizations, and clinical settings that support service delivery, research, and education.

If the designation "allied health" is to be related to those professions whose essential criteria for their education programs are adopted by the CAHEA, then three things must be considered when describing each of the allied health professions: first, the educational background in terms of degree requirements and of didactic and clinical experience; second, the occupational duties to be performed; and third, the association or organization that takes on the responsibility of sponsoring the profession with regard to organizing, developing, teaching, and evaluating.

For a number of allied health occupations, either a bachelor's degree is not required or this requirement varies among programs. Examples of such occupations often use the designation "technician," as in emergency medical technician, histologic technician, medical laboratory technician, medical record technician, and respiratory therapist technician. Others receive very specialized training, such as the diagnostic medical sonographer and the perfusionist. Examples of those allied health professionals in fields whose essential criteria are evaluated and accredited by the CAHEA and that have maintained the bachelor's degree are anesthesiology assistants, athletic trainers, specialists in blood-bank technology, cytotechnologists, medical il-

lustrators, medical records administrators, nuclear medicine technologists, occupational therapists, radiation therapy technologists, radiographers, and respiratory therapists.

Even under the aegis of the AMA, however, CAHEA evaluation and accreditation are not enough to be used to define allied health personnel. The ASAHP lists approximately sixty-five careers that fall under the definition of allied health professions as outlined by the federal government. Among those careers are art therapist, audiologist, dance therapist, dental assistant, dietitian, educational therapist, genetic counselor, health-care administrator, histotechnologist, kinesiotherapist, music therapist, nutritionist, ophthalmic medical technologist, optician, optometric technician, physical therapist, psychiatric technician, recreational therapist, speech/language pathologist, veterinary technician, and vocational rehabilitation counselor. The ASAHP listing of allied health careers demonstrates an allied health view that extends beyond the medical profession into autonomous professional areas such as dentistry, optometry, dietetics, nutrition, physical therapy, and veterinary medicine.

Credentials such as certification, registry, or licensure of an occupation/profession are the final aspect that has an impact on the allied health professions. Certification implies that an individual has met certain ethical criteria and has achieved the minimal standards required to practice a particular occupation. Certification is usually provided by a nongovernment agency. Registry, which is usually provided by a government agency, involves being placed on a government listing. It is usually used with occupations that involve a minimal threat to public safety.

Licensure is an important part of the health care system because it attempts to protect both the public (which must rely on competent care) and the health-care personnel (who must protect the profession to which they belong). Public safety is achieved when a government agency is given the responsibility of overseeing the credentials of a person who attempts to practice a particular occupation or use a particular title. The health-care worker is protected because licensure prevents unqualified practitioners from entering the occupation or profession. It also appears to increase salary benefits and prestige, as well as to provide the profession with greater visibility with respect to legislative government and the public in general.

Probably one of the most important aspects of licensure is that it legally defines the extent of the activities that may be performed in the profession or occupation. For example, medical technologists and respiratory therapists can monitor arterial blood gases and electrolytes. If licensure to perform the tests were given to only one of the occupations, however, it would be illegal for individuals in the unlicensed profession to perform the tests. Licensure is particularly significant to the allied health professions because duties may overlap, especially in the variety of health-care settings that are being developed.

The negative aspects to licensure should also be considered for their impact on allied health and most health-care professions. There is a decrease in mobility when each state has its own licensing commission or agency. Some studies indicate that many rural areas do not have adequate care, and it is believed the licensure of professions not already licensed in some states, such as medical technology, could add to this problem by discouraging the movement of health care workers to these areas.

Finally, licensure affects not only individuals but also the facilities in which health care is practiced. Laboratories and direct-care facilities such as hospitals are usually regulated by government licensure. The movement of health-care treatment from hospitals to the many alternative facilities that now exist may also require that standards be established and evaluated.

Because of the uniformity of the health-care system, there is ease of mobility horizontally (from location to location) for those in allied health occupations. There is consistency of facilities, equipment, job opportunity, job description, operating procedures, and regulations. Yet the very reason for the creation of most allied health occupations or professions-the requirement for specialized knowledge, procedures, or technology-makes them narrow in focus. Consequently, many people agree that there is less vertical mobility within some allied health positions.

Nevertheless, the educational requirements for some allied health occupations, particularly a bachelor's degree in liberal arts, provide greater opportunity for advancement. Job advancement opportunities can also increase with advanced degrees. For example, a bachelor's degree in medical technology or a master's degree in business administration provides an individual with professional opportunities in many of the ancillary industries that support the American health-care system.

Perspective and Prospects

The health-care system in the United States is the product of three major forces: private enterprise, government, and charity. Although each of these forces may have had different objectives, their united goal has been the improved health of the American population. The primary location for the delivery of health care has been the hospital. The health-care professions that evolved within this system and that have, in large part, given direction to its evolution are the medical profession and the nursing profession.

With the establishment of hospitals as the site of health-care delivery, the nursing profession made itself fundamental to the continued evolution of health care. The hospital became the keystone of the entire health care system, as well as the focal point where each of the three forces would exert its influence.

As a result of health care moving from the private home to the public setting of the hospital, the health care of the patient improved, but at the same time it became more technology-oriented and more costly. Since the 1950s, technological advances have had a direct effect on patient care and therefore on the ever-evolving professions of medicine and nursing. During this same time of technological growth and specialized care, new areas of health care have begun to develop that are outside the accepted areas of medicine and nursing but allied to them because their common goal is the health of the patient.

As many as sixty-seven professions can be described as allied health. They complement the activities of not only the physician and nurse but also a variety of direct caregivers such as dentists, optometrists, and clinical psychologists. Allied health activities take place in hospitals, physicians' office laboratories, private laboratories, clinics, schools, extended care facilities, and the variety of other facilities utilized by direct care providers.

Advanced technology, the professions that constitute the health-care team, and the administrative bureaucracy form the nearly $2 trillion health-care industry in the United States. For 2011, the World Bank estimated that health care spending was 17.9 percent of the gross domestic product of the United States. The health-care system also provides one of the most rapidly expanding areas for job opportunities in the American economy.

Allied health occupations and professions are an integral part of the American health care system. Their role is indispensable to those professions responsible for patient diagnosis and treatment. Allied health provides a vast market for scientific products and instrumentation. It is composed of and supported by an array of professional organizations and educational institutions that will provide the impetus for its continued growth and evolution.

—*Patrick J. DeLuca, Ph.D.*

See also American Medical Association (AMA); Anesthesiology; Audiology; Blood banks; Cardiac rehabilitation; Clinics; Cytopathology; Environmental health; Health maintenance organizations (HMOs); Hospice; Hospitals; Imaging and radiology; Laboratory tests; Nuclear radiology; Nursing; Occupational health; Palliative medicine; Paramedics; Physical rehabilitation; Physician assistants; Preventive medicine; Pulmonary medicine; Sports medicine; Surgical technologists.

For Further Information:

American Medical Association. *Health Professions: Education Standards*. Chicago: Author, 1999.

"Best Healthcare Jobs." *U.S. News and World Report*, 2013.

Bishop, V. *Leadership for Nursing and Allied Health Care Professions*. New York: Open University Press, 2009.

Clerc, Jeanne M. *An Introduction to Clinical Laboratory Science*. St. Louis, Mo.: Mosby Year Book, 1992.

Corder, Brice W., ed. *Medical Professions Admission Guide: Strategy for Success*. Champaign, Ill.: National Association of Advisors for the Health Professions, 1998.

Idziak, Janine Marie. *Ethical Dilemmas in Allied Health*. 2d ed. Dubuque, Iowa: Kendall Hunt, 2010.

Miller, Benjamin F., Claire Brackman Keane, and Marie T. O'Toole. *Miller-Keane Encyclopedia and Dictionary of Medicine, Nursing, and Allied Health*. Rev. 7th ed. Philadelphia: Saunders/Elsevier, 2005.

Mosby's Medical Dictionary. 8th ed. St. Louis, Mo.: Mosby/Elsevier, 2009.

Alopecia

Disease/Disorder

Also known as: Hair loss, pattern baldness

Anatomy or system affected: Hair, head

Specialties and related fields: Dermatology

Definition: Temporary or permanent hair loss.
Key terms:

anagen: active growth phase of hair follicles

catagen: transition between growth and resting phases of hair follicles

dihydrotestosterone: male hormone, a derivative of testosterone that plays a key role in androgenic alopecia

keratin: a family of fibrous structural proteins that compose skin, nails, and hair

telogen: the resting phase of hair follicles

terminal hair: thick, pigmented hairs found on the scalp and other parts of the body

vellus: short, fine, unpigmented hair that covers most of the person's body from childhood

---

Information on Alopecia

Causes: Genetics factors, hormones, and inflammation of hair follicles as a result of infection or autoimmunity

Symptoms: Hair loss with or without inflammation of the scalp

Duration: Can arise in the early 20s in men, and as early as the 30s in women, resulting in permanent hair loss

Treatments: Depends on cause, but for nonscarring alopecia: oral finasteride, topical minoxidil, and injections of bimatoprost, or hair transplantation surgery; treatments vary for scarring alopecia

---

Causes and Symptoms

During the ninth week of development, small patches of fetal skin cells aggregate in response to signals sent by the underlying dermis. These small, raised areas (epithelial placodes) grow downward, below the skin and elongate to become hair germs and then hair pegs. As the elongating hair peg grows further into the dermis, cells from the dermis accumulate at the growing end of the hair peg. The hair peg becomes a bulbous peg and outgrowths sprout from the sides to form the sebaceous gland, and connective

tissue cells from surrounding tissue condense to form the arrector pili muscle that attaches to a bulge on the lower part of the bulbous peg. Dermis cells form the dermal papilla, which becomes the hair root and pigment cells (melanocytes) infiltrate the developing hair follicle to convey color to the growing hair shaft.

From about the third month of development, the fetus is covered with lanugo hair (Latin, "lana" meaning wool). The fetus sheds this lanugo hair about four weeks before birth, and begins to form the two types of neonatal hair: unpigmented and short (1-2 centimeters) vellus hairs that lack a sebaceous gland and do not produce another hair in their place, and terminal hairs that grow on the head and other parts of the body, have pigment, and initially appear rather thin and short.

Hair follicles progress through a series of growth and regression phases known as the hair cycle. The hair cycle consists of three phases: (1) an active growth phase called anagen; (2) a regression phase called catagens; and (3) a resting phase known as telogen. The length of time spent in each phase varies with ethnicity and the length of time spent in anagen determines the length of the hair. Anagen normally lasts from two to six years, telogen lasts approximately three months, and catagen lasts about three weeks. Some 85 percent of all hair follicles are in anagen, and 15 percent in telogen. Disruption of the hair cycle often results in alopecia or hair loss.

There are two types of alopecia: nonscarring in which hair loss occurs without scarring of the scalp, and scarring in which hair loss occurs with scarring. Some types of nonscarring alopecia occur as a secondary consequence of particular disorders or diseases. For example, nutritional deficiencies, in particular of iron, can cause alopecia, as can an underactive thyroid gland (hypothyroidism), or syphilis. Other types of nonscarring alopecia include alopecia areata (AA), androgenic alopecia (AGA), telogen effluvium, anagen effluvium, traction alopecia, trichotillomania, and monilethrix. AA occurs when immune cells infiltrate the hair follicle, disrupt the hair cycle and cause programmed cell death of the hair follicle leading to hair loss and smooth, bald skin. Studies of inheritance patterns strongly argue for a genetic component to AA. AGA or male/female pattern hair loss involves the

Source: Paus, Ralf, Iain S. Haslam, Andrey A. Sharov, and Vladimir A. Botchkarev. "Pathobiology of Chemotherapy-Induced Hair Loss." Lancet Oncology 14 (February 2013): e51, Figure 1.

Hair follicle embryogenesis. (www.keratin.com)

miniaturization of the hair follicle as a consequence of transforming the hair from terminal hair to vellus hair. The conversion of the circulating hormone testosterone into a derivative known as dihydrotestosterone or DHT in the hair follicle drives this miniaturization. AGA affects up to 70 percent of men and 40 percent of women in mid-adult life. Inheritance also plays a prominent role in AGA. Telogen effluvium results from physiological stresses such as high fever, severe illness, and drug-induced hair loss. These conditions cause anagen to prematurely stop growing and enter catagen; however, instead of renewing anagen the hair is shed. Environmental insults also cause anagen effluvium, in which the hair follicles enter anagen but do not grow and stay stuck in anagen without ever growing any hair. Hair weaves and ponytails that constantly pull on the hair can cause traction alopecia. Trichotillomania refers to the behavior of pulling one's hair out. Monilethrix results from inherited mutations in genes (KRT81, KRT83, or LFT86) that encode hair structural proteins known as keratins. The hair has a beads-on-a-string appearance and is also fragile.

Scarring or cicatricial alopecia results from inflammation of the hair follicle caused either by an autoimmune response against the hair follicle or by infection of the hair follicle by either fungi (tinea capitis) or bacteria (acne necrotica, folliculitis decalvans). Autoimmune diseases that cause hair loss include discoid systemic lupus erythematosis, dermatomyositis, and sclero- derma. Lichen planopilaris results from abnormalities in fatty acid metabolism that causes a toxic buildup of fatty acids in the hair follicle that damage it, initiate inflammation, and cause hair loss. Central centrifugal cictricial alopecia

causes a band of hair loss down the center of the scalp, and occurs most commonly in African-American females. It seems to result from a combination of particular hair care practices and an inherited propensity for hair follicle inflammation. Perifolliculitis capitis abscedens et suffodiens or dissecting cellulitis mainly occurs in African-American men. Obstruction of the hair follicle causes inflammation and painful nodules on the scalp. Bacterial infection of the hair follicle plays a role in hair loss, but it is unclear if infection causes the condition or it occurs secondarily. Brocq pseudopelade causes scarring alopecia, but its cause remains unknown.

Particular drugs can also cause alopecia (see Table 1), as can cancer. Alopecia mucinosa, for example, results from cancers of particular white blood cells called T-lymphocyte (T-cell lymphomas).

Table 1. Medications that Cause Alopecia	
Associated Medication	**Type of Medicine**
Citalopram	Antidepressant - selective serotonin reuptake inhibitor (SSRI)
Cyclophosphamide	Anticancer drug
Danazol	Synthetic testosterone
Fluoxetine	Antidepressant - SSRI
Fluvoxamine	Antidepressant - SSRI
Gold	Used in dental crowns
Interferon-a	Immune system modulator used to treat virus infections and autoimmune diseases
Mycophenolate mofetil	Immunosuppressant drug
Phenytoin	Antiseizure medicine
Tacrolimus	Immunosuppresant drug
Venlafaxine	Treats major depressive disorder, anxiety, and panic disorder
Methotrexate	Antimetabolite that treats cancers, rheumatoid arthritis, and severe psoriasis
Leflunomide	Treats rheumatoid arthritis, and psoriatic arthritis
Intravenous immunoglobulins	Treats cancers, autoimmune diseases, and infectious diseases

Treatment and Therapy

Alopecia remains a difficult condition to treat. Early intervention works best for both scarring and nonscarring alopecia. For nonscarring alopecia, oral finasteride, topical minoxidil, and injections of bimatoprost have shown some efficacy with some patients, but they must be used indefinitely and may lose effectiveness over time. Patient education and changes in hair care practices can reduce hair loss in people with traction alopecia. Trichotillomania may require psychiatric intervention, but some studies have shown that oral N-acetylcysteine reduces this compulsive behavior.

For scarring alopecia, treatments vary from one condition to the next. For autoimmune diseases that cause alopecia, drugs that suppress the immune response plus retinoids to promote skin health are typically used. For infectious types of scarring alopecia, oral antibiotics and topical corticosteroids help resolve these conditions, but the exact drug combinations vary according to each disease (see Table 2).

For alopecia mucinosa, the underlying cancer must be addressed.

Table 2. Treatment of Scarring Alopecia	
Disease	**Treatment**
Autoimmune diseases	
Discoid systemic lupus erythematosis	• For rapidly progressing disease: hydroxychloroquine with oral prednisone • For slowly progressing disease: • Triamcinolone acetonide with topical corticosteroids • Oral retinoids (acitretin, isotretinoin) have also proven effective
Dermatomyositis	• First line - Oral prednisone with methotrexate, azathioprine, or mycophenolate mofetil • Rixtuximab has been used in refractory cases
Systemic Sclerosis (scleroderma)	• Begin with methotrexate (or hydroxychloroquine) and corticosteroid injections • Later, vitamin D analogues (calcipotriene, calcitrol) and colchicine to halt fibrosis • Phototherapy can soften the skin
Brocq pseudopelade	• Topical triamcinolone acetonide, hydroxychloroquine oral prednisone and isotretinoin
Lichen planopilaris	• Scalp injections of triamcinolone acetonide with oral prednisone and retinoids • Hydroxychloroquine and mycophenolate mofetil have also been successfully used
Infectious alopecias	
Central centrifugal cicatricial	• Oral tetracycline and topical corticosteroids
Dissecting cellulitis	• First choice - Oral isotretinoid • Also useful - Oral antibiotics such as doxycycline, ciprofloxacin, rifampicin, and dapsone
Acne necrotica	• Oral tetracycline or oxacillin, cephalexin, cefuroxime, dicloxacillin, trimethoprim/sulfamethoxazole, antibacterial shampoos and oral retinoids
Folliculitis decalvans	• Minocycline, erythromycin, cephalosporins, sulfamethoxazole/ trimethoprim but these treatments tend to cause relapse infections • Rifampin, clindamycin, and fusidic acid show less relapse infections • Topical triamcinolone with topical antibiotics, such as mupirocin/fusidic acid/erythromycin are also effective
Tinea capitis	• First choice - Oral giseofulvin • Itraconazole, terbinafine and fluconazole are as effective and require shorter periods of treatment

Perspective and Prospects

The ancient Greek physician Hippocrates (460 BCE-379 BCE) originally called alopecia "Fox's disease." Centuries later in 30 CE, the great Roman scholar Cornelius Celsus described different types of alopecia. For many years no one had any idea what caused alopecia, but some proposed that parasite infestations caused it while others attributed hair loss to nervous conditions. Then in 1942, J. B. Hamilton demonstrated the link between the hormone testosterone and alopecia.

Hair transplantation procedures constitute the most permanent treatment for alopecia. Hair transplantation uses small patches of hair-bearing scalp and transplants them to a bald or thinning area. The number of grafts required to get proper coverage depends on the size of the grafts; minigrafts contain two to four hair follicles, micrografts, one to two hair follicles, slit graphs, which are inserted into slits created in the scalp, about four to ten hair follicles, and the long and thin strip graphs, about thirty to forty. Achieving satisfactory coverage usually requires several surgical sessions, and it usually takes about two years to see the final result.

—*Michael A. Buratovich, Ph.D.*

See also Dermatology; Dermopathology; Immunology; Immunopathology; Systemic Sclerosis

For Further Information:
Breitkopf, Trisia, Gigi Leung, Mei Yu, Eddy Wang, and Kevin J. McElwee. "The Basic Science of Hair Biology: What Are the Causal Mechanisms for the Disordered Hair Follicle." *Dermatologic Clinics* 31 (2013): 1-19.
Cohen, Nathan J. *Beat Alopecia*. Seattle, Wash.: Amazon Digital Services, Inc., 2012.
Smith, Gary. *Alopecia: The Complete Guide on Treatments and Remedies: Stop Hair Loss in Men*. Seattle, Wash.: Create Space Independent Publishing Platform, 2012.
Trüeb, Ralph M. *Female Alopecia: Guide to Successful Management*. Seattle, Wash.: Amazon Digital Services, 2013.

Alternative medicine

Specialty

Anatomy or system affected: All

Specialties and related fields: Osteopathic medicine, preventive medicine, and public health

Definition: A wide variety of medical practices and therapies which fall outside traditional (MD or DO), Western medical practice. The approaches emphasize the individual as a biopsychosocial whole, or, in some cases, as a biopsychosocial-spiritual whole. They deemphasize focusing treatment on specific diseases or symptoms.

Key terms:

physiological: characteristic of or appropriate to an organism's healthy or normal functioning

therapeutic: relating to the treatment of disease or disorders, but mostly pertaining to healing or curing and not merely the absence of disease or symptoms

toxin: a poisonous substance that is a product of the chemical processes of a living organism

Science and Profession

Alternative medicine—which can encompass modalities like natural healing, complementary medicine, integrative medicine, or holistic medicine—focuses on the relationship among the mind, body, and spirit. An underlying philosophy is that people can maintain health by preventing disease in the first place by keeping the body in "balance" and by utilizing the body's "natural" healing processes when people succumb to disease. Alternative medicine approaches contrast with Western medicine's traditional focus on treating symptoms and curing disease and its under emphasis of preventive medicine. Thought to be radical at one time, complementary medicines and therapies are gaining appeal as their anecdotal efficacy and reputation grow.

Alternative medicine practitioners treat a wide variety of disease processs, including cancer and acquired immuno-deficiency syndrome (AIDS) to chronic pain and fatigue, stress, insomnia, depression, high blood pressure, circulatory and digestive disorders, allergies, arthritis, diabetes mellitus, and drug and alcohol addictions.

Major risks associated with alternative medicine include costly delays in seeking appropriate treatment, misinformation, side effects from self-administered remedies, and psychological distress if patients believe that they are responsible for their illness or lack of recovery. Also, many alternative-medicine practitioners have little or no formal health training and may discourage traditional medical treatment or oppose proven health measures such as immunization and pasteurization.

Diagnostic and Treatment Techniques

Numerous alternative medicine treatments exist varying widely in the nature of their claims, their acceptability to conventional doctors, and the manner in which they can and cannot be tested. The treatments can be divided into three main types.

Treatments that deal with the mind/body connection or that have recognized benefits and accepted applications and are often used together with conventional medicine. These approaches include acupuncture and acupressure, biofeedback, chiropractic, hydrotherapy, light therapy, meditation, oxygen therapy, qi gong, sound therapy, Tai Chi Chuan, and yoga. The second type comprises treatments that can be tested by conventional methods and have some accepted applications. These treatments include aromatherapy, cell therapy, colon therapy, detoxification, energy medicine, enzyme therapy, homeopathy, kinesiology, magnetic field therapy, and neural therapy. Treatments of the third type are difficult to study because they seem to be at odds with Western medicine and cannot readily be tested through standard methods. An example of this type of treatment is herbal medicine.

Acupressureand acupuncture. These treatments are both based on the belief that the body has a vital energy that must be balanced in order to maintain good health. Acupressure uses pressure from the fingertips or knuckles to stimulate specific points on the body, while acupuncture uses needles inserted into the skin to restore the balance of energy. Both acupressure and acupuncture have been shown to stimulate the release of endorphins, the body's natural painkillers. Acupressure is useful for the relief of chronic pain and fatigue and increasing blood circulation. Acupuncture has been used successfully for relieving chronic pain and treat-

ing drug and alcohol withdrawal symptoms. Although hepatitis, transmission of infectious disease, and internal injuries have been reported in connection with acupuncture, such problems are uncommon.

Biofeedback. This technique involves learning to control automatic physiological responses such as blood pressure, heart rate, circulation, digestion, and perspiration to reduce anxiety, pain, and tension. The patient concentrates on consciously controlling the body's automatic responses while a machine monitors the results and displays them for the patient. Biofeedback may have some benefits in treating asthma, chronic pain, epilepsy, drug addiction, circulatory problems, and stress.

Chiropractic. Chiropractic treatment uses traditional medicine techniques such as x-rays, physical examinations, and various tests to diagnose a disorder. Muscle spasms or ligament strains are treated by manipulation or adjustment to the spine and joints, thus reducing pressure on the spinal nerves and providing relief from pain. Recent research suggests chiropractic should be considered in treating certain types of lower back pain, as it is often superior to conventional interventions. Practitioners should be state licensed, and caution should be taken with practitioners who often repeat full-spine x-rays or who ask patients to sign contracts at any time during treatment. Chiropractic is practiced either "straight," involving only spinal manipulation, or "mixed," involving other biomedical technologies such as electrical stimulation. Chiropractic treatment can be harmful if it is practiced in patients with fractures or undetected tumors or if it is practiced incorrectly.

Hydrotherapy. The use of water for healing or therapeutic purposes is termed hydrotherapy. It is used to treat chronic pain,and to relieve stress, mprove circulation, mobility, strength, and flexibility; to reduce swelling; and to treat injuries to the skin. Because the buoyancy of water offsets gravity, more intense exercise can be done when standing in water, while a lower heart rate is maintained and pain is decreased. The risks associated with hydrotherapy are minimal, such as overdoing exercise, or rare, such as slipping or drowning.

Light therapy. Phototherapy, or light therapy, is used to treat health disorders that are related to problems with the body's inner clock, or circadian rhythms. These rhythms govern the timing of sleep, hormone production, body temperature, and other biological functions. People need the full wavelength spectrum of light found in sunlight to maintain health. If the full wavelength is not received, the body may not be able to absorb some nutrients fully, resulting in fatigue, tooth decay, depression, hostility, hair loss, skin conditions, sleep disorders, or suppressed immune functions. Treatment involves spending more time outdoors, exercising, and using light boxes that mimic natural sunlight. Phototherapy is commonly used to treat seasonal affective disorder (SAD), a recognized subtype of depressive illness.

Meditation. Meditation is used to relax the mind and body, to reduce stress, and to develop a more positive attitude. By focusing on a single thought or repeating aa word

Chinese medicine may employ a technique called cupping, the application to the back of cups that create a vacuum, in order to restore proper circulation. (PhotoDisc)

or phrase, a person can release conscious thoughts and feelings and enter deep relaxation. Meditation can affect the pulse rate and muscle tension and so is effective in treating high blood pressure, migraines, insomnia, and some digestive disorders.

Oxygen therapy. Hyperbaric oxygenation therapy, or oxygen therapy, is used to treat disorders in which the oxygen supply to the body is deficient. This therapy can help with heart disease, circulatory problems, multiple sclerosis, gangrene, and strokes. Oxygen therapy is also used for traumas such as crash injuries, wounds, burns, bedsores, and carbon monoxide poisoning. Treatment consists of exposing the patient to 100 percent pure oxygen under greater-than-normal atmospheric pressure. The body tissues receive more than the usual supply of oxygen and so can compensate for conditions of reduced circulation. The increased oxygen helps keep tissues alive and promotes healing.

Qi gong. Qi gong (pronounced "chee-kung") translates from the Chinese as "breathing exercise." The Chinese believe that exercise balances and amplifies the vital energy force—Ch'i or qi—within the body. Qi gong is used to increase circulation; to reduce stress; to promote health, fitness, and longevity; and to cure illness. The most common exercises involve relaxation, strengthening, and inward training. Because the exercise involves movement done

with gentle circular and stretching movements, people with decreased flexibility or disabilities can participate.

Sound therapy. The use of certain sounds can reduce stress, lower blood pressure, relieve pain, improve movement and balance, promote endurance and strength, and overcome learning disabilities. The body has its own rhythm, and illness can arise when the rhythm is disturbed. Tests have shown that particular sounds can slow breathing and a racing heart, create a feeling of well-being, alter skin temperature, influence brain-wave frequencies, and reduce blood pressure and muscle tension.

Tai Chi Chuan. Originally designed as a form of self-defense, Tai Chi Chuan is now practiced as physical exercises based on rhythmic movement, equilibrium of body weight, and effortless breathing. The exercises involve slow and continuous movement without strain. Tai Chi Chuan is beneficial because it demands no physical strength initially. The exercises increase circulation, stimulate the nervous system and glandular activity, and increase joint movement and concentration.

Yoga. The ancient art of yoga seeks to achieve the balance of mind, body, and spirit. Practitioners believe that good health is created through proper breathing, relaxation, meditation, proper diet and nutrition, and exercise. The deep breathing and stretching exercises bring relaxation, release of tension and stress, improved concentration, and oxygenation of the blood. The exercises can also provide muscle toning and aerobic respiration, which are beneficial to the heart.

Aromatherapy. Used extensively in Europe and Japan, aromatherapy involves the use of the essential oils or essence from the flowers, stems, leaves, or roots of plants or trees. These essences can be absorbed through the skin, eaten, or inhaled in vapor form. There is evidence that inhaling some scents may help prevent secondary respiratory infections and reduce stress. Practitioners believe that aromatherapy can benefit people suffering from muscle aches, arthritis, digestive and circulatory problems, and emotional or stress-related problems. Absorption through the skin and inhalation are considered safe, but eating any essence could result in poisoning.

Cell therapy. Although not approved in the United States, cell therapy is widely used worldwide. It involves the injection of cells from the organs, fetuses, or embryos of animals and humans. These cells are used for revitalization purposes; that is, they promote the body's healing process for damaged or weak organs. Cell therapy seems to stimulate the immune system and is used to treat cancer, immunological problems, diseased or underdeveloped organs, arthritis, and circulatory problems.

Colontherapy. This technique involves the cleaning and detoxification of the colon by flushing with water, using enemas, or ingesting herbs or other substances. A healthy colon will absorb water and nutrients and eliminate wastes and toxins. Most modern diets, however, are low in fiber, a substance which helps clean out the colon. Further, most people are relatively sedentary and eat acidic foods. For adults, most digested food takes fifty to seventy hours after digestion to move through the bowels. (In contrast, evidence indicates that in the early twentieth century, fecal material was released within twelve to twenty hours after ingestion.) A baby's food is defecated within four to ten hours after ingestion. The theory is that the more time fecal material spends in the body, the more time there is for impacted feces, bacteria, viruses, fungi, parasites, and toxemia to develop. Although not a specific cure for any disease, colon therapy removes the source of toxins and allows the body's natural healing processes to function properly. Practitioners claim that symptoms related to colon dysfunction, such as backaches, headaches, bad breath, gas, indigestion and constipation, sinus or lung congestion, skin problems, and fatigue can be relieved when the toxins are removed from the colon.

A person trained in colonic therapy guides a speculum into the rectum and cleanses the area by gently guiding water, herbs, vitamins, or oxygen through the entire five feet of the colon. Enemas cleanse only the lower or sigmoid colon, which is only eight to twelve inches of the bowel.

Detoxification. This therapy focuses on ridding the body of the chemicals and pollutants present in water, food, air, and soil. The body naturally eliminates or neutralizes toxins through the liver, kidneys, urine, and feces, and through the processes of exhalation and perspiration. Detoxification therapy accelerates the body's own natural cleansing process through diet, fasting, colon therapy, and heat therapy. Symptoms of an overtaxed body system include respiratory problems, headaches, joint pain, allergy symptoms, mood changes, insomnia, arthritis, constipation, psoriasis, acne, and ulcers.

Energy medicine. Bioenergetic medicine, or energy medicine, uses an energy field to detect and treat health problems. A screening process to measure electromagnetic frequencies emitted by the body can detect imbalances that may cause illness or warn of possible chemical imbalances. One of several machines is then used to correct energy-level imbalances. Energy medicine claims to relieve conditions such as skin diseases, headaches, migraines, muscle pain, circulation problems, and chronic fatigue.

Enzymetherapy. This treatment uses plant and pancreatic enzymes to improve digestion and the absorption of nutrients. Since enzymes provide the stimuli for all chemical reactions in the body, improper eating habits may cause a lack of certain enzymes, resulting in general health problems.

Homeopathy. Based on the belief that "like cures like," homeopathy is thought to provide relief from most illnesses. During therapy, the patient receives small doses of prepared plants and minerals in order to stimulate the body's own healing processes and defense mechanisms. These substances mimic the symptoms of the illness. While studies on this approach remain inconclusive, homeopathic medicine has some appeal, possibly because some homeopathic practitioners are traditionally trained medical physicians.

Kinesiology. This therapy employs muscle testing and standard diagnosis to evaluate and treat the chemical, structural, and mental aspects of the patient. The principle behind kinesiology is that certain foods can cause biochemical reactions that weaken the muscles. Diet and exercise, as well as muscle and joint manipulation, are part of the treatment. There are risks of injury caused by an unqualified practitioner.

Magnetic field therapy. Also called biomagnetic therapy, magnetic field therapy uses specially designed magnets or magnetic fields applied to the body. Electrically charged particles are naturally present in the bloodstream, and when magnets are placed on the body, the charged particles are attracted to the magnets. As a result, currents and patterns are created that dilate the blood vessels, allowing more blood to reach the affected area. Magnetic field therapy is used to speed healing after surgery, to improve circulation, and to strengthen and mend bones. It is also used to improve the quality of healing in sprains, strains, cuts, and burns, as well as to reduce or reverse chronic conditions such as degenerative joint disease, some forms of arthritis, and diabetic ulcers.

Neural therapy. This therapy is used to treat chronic illness or trauma (injury) caused by changes in the natural electrical conductivity of the nerves and cells. Every cell has its own frequency range of electricity, and tissue remains healthy as long as the energy flow through the body is normal. Neural therapy uses anesthetics injected into the body to deliver energy to cells blocked by disease or injury. Conditions that respond to neural therapy are allergies; arthritis; asthma; kidney, liver, and heart disease; depression; head and back pain; and muscle injuries.

Herbal medicine. This field uses plants and flowers to treat most known symptoms of physical and emotional illnesses. Almost 75 percent of the world's population relies on herbal remedies as their primary source of health care, and much of traditional medicine is derived from plants. Herbal medicine mixtures can be complicated, however, and some, like any medications, are toxic if taken incorrectly.

Perspective and Prospects

While relatively new to Western society and medicine, many alternative or complementary therapies are ancient and derive from non technologically based understandings of how the human body and the world work. What specifically works for whom, when, and for what conditions remains a complex problem. Anecdote and hearsay, and the limits and failures of Western medicine, guide and motivate interest in these approaches.

Renewed interest in alternative therapies occurred in the 1970s and has grown since. By 2007, an estimated 38 percent of all Americans had used some form of complementary therapy. In 1992, with Americans spending more than fourteen billion dollars annually on alternative medicine, the US government established the Office of Alternative Medicine (which became the National Center for Complementary and Alternative Medicine, or NCCAM and is now named the National Center for Complementary and Integrative Health (NCCIH) as a part of the National Institutes of Health (NIH). This office evaluates complementary treatments on a scientific basis and provides public information. Health insurers maintain a key interest in alternative medicine, and an increasing number are paying for it. Some raditionally trained physicians are prescribing or recommending some form of alternative medicine as a complement to their own.

In 2007, NCCAM found that 38 percent of adults used some form of complementary or alternative medicine (CAM). A 2004 survey indicated that, if one included megavitamin therapy and prayer associated with health concerns, the number of adults who use CAM was 62 percent. The survey found that the main reasons that people used complementary and alternative medicine were beliefs that it would improve their health when combined with conventional medicine, that it would be interesting to try, or that conventional treatment either would not or did not work. People most likely to use CAM were women, those with a high level of education, those who had been hospitalized in the last year, and former smokers.

The American Holistic Medical Association had hundreds of members. Physicians can become board certified in holistic medicine, meaning that they are committed to treating the whole person, emphasize prevention rather than merely treating symptoms, believe in integrating other modes of treatment and not limiting themselves to only Western medicine, and believe in the importance of the healing relationship and in treating the patient as a unique individual. In 2005, the Association of the American Medical Colleges reported that 95 of 125 medical schools offer complementary and alternative coursework and training and the numbers are sure to increase.

—Virginia L. Salmon and Paul Moglia, PhD;
updated by LeAnna DeAngelo, PhD and
Richard P. Capriccioso, MD

For Further Information:
Abrams, D. I., and Weil, A. (editors). *Integrative Oncology*, second edition. Oxford University Press. Sep 3, 2014. https://global.oup.com/academic/product/integrative-oncology-9780199329724?cc=us&lang=en&#

Bauer, Brent A., Philip T. Hagen, and Martha Millman. *Mayo ClinicBook of Alternative Medicine and Book of Home Remedies.* New York: Time Home Entertainment, 2013.

Center for Applied Physiology. http://www.menninger.edu. Ditchek, Stuart, Andrew Weil, and Russell H. Greenfield. *Healthy Child, Whole Child: Integrating the Best of Conventional and Alternative Medicine to Keep Your Kids Healthy.* Rev. ed. New York: HarperCollins, 2009.

Complementary and alternative therapies for advanced cancer, http://www.cancer.org/treatment/understandingyourdiagnosis/advancedcancer/advanced-cancer-cam

Edens PhD, Patricia Stanfill, Integrative Oncology. *Salem Health: Cancer.* Ebsco Publishing, 2016

Freeman,Lyn. *Mosby's Complementary and Alternative Medicine: A Research-Based Approach.* 3d ed. St. Louis, Mo.: Mosby, 2009.

Jacobs, Jennifer, ed. *The Encyclopedia of Alternative Medicine: A Complete Family Guide to Complementary Therapies.* Rev. ed. Boston: Journey Editions, 1997.

Micozzi, Marc S. *Fundamentals of Complementary and Alternative Medicine.* 4th ed. St. Louis, Mo.: Saunders/Elsevier, 2011.

Minocha, Anil. *A Guide to Alternative Medicine and the Digestive System.* Thorofare, N.J.: Slack, 2013.

National Center for Complementary and Integrative Health, https://nccih.nih.gov.

Synovitz, Linda Baily, and Karl L. Larson. *Complementary and Alternative Medicine for Health Professionals: AHolisticApproach to Consumer Health.* Burlington, Mass.: Jones & Bartlett, 2013.

Trivieri, Larry, Jr., and JohnW. Anderson, eds. *Alternative Medicine: The Definitive Guide.* 2d ed. Berkeley, Calif.: Ten Speed Press, 2002.

Wang, Jianguo, and Hong Zhu. *Chinese Medicine: Acupuncture, Herbal Medicine, and Therapies.*NewYork: Nova Science, 2012.

Weil, Andrew. *Healthy Aging: ALifelong Guide to Your Physical and Spiritual Well-Being.* New York: Anchor Books, 2007.

Wu, Emily S. *Traditional Chinese Medicine in the United States: In Search of Spiritual Meaning and Ultimate Health.* Lanham, Md.: Lexington Books, 2013.

Altitude sickness

Disease/Disorder

Anatomy or system affected: Brain, ears, head, lungs, nervous system, respiratory system

Specialties and related fields: Emergency medicine, neurology, occupational health

Definition: A condition resulting from altitude-related hypoxia (low oxygen levels).

Causes and Symptoms

There are four types of altitude sickness: acute mountain sickness, high-altitude pulmonary edema (HAPE), high-altitude cerebral edema (HACE), and high-altitude

---

Information on Altitude Sickness

Causes: Rapid ascent to high altitudes, hypoxia (low oxygen levels)

Symptoms: Headache, decreased appetite, insomnia, fatigue, nausea, death in severe cases

Duration: A few days

Treatments: Descent to lower altitudes, corticosteroids, oxygen

---

retinopathy (HAR). Though most patients have mild symptoms, death is not uncommon in severe cases. Illness is associated with rapid ascent to mountain areas by tourists, skiers, and mountaineers. Residents of mountainous regions are less susceptible because their bodies have adapted to lower oxygen levels. It is estimated that up to one-quarter of tourists skiing in the mountains of the western United States have experienced some manifestations, although mild ones, of altitude sickness.

Acute mountain sickness is characterized by headache, decreased appetite, insomnia, fatigue, nausea, and onset at altitudes above 1,980 meters (6,500 feet). The risk of becoming affected increases with young age, quick ascent, and a past history of acute mountain sickness. Symptoms usually last for a few days. Between 5 and 10 percent of patients with acute mountain sickness progress to HAPE, which occurs when the small pulmonary blood vessels leak, allowing fluid accumulation in the lungs. Mortality from HAPE ranges from 11 to 44 percent. The related condition HACE occurs when fluid accumulation in the brain causes increased pressure within the skull. Neurologic signs such as confusion and coma may be noted.

Treatment and Therapy

Prevention is crucial to the reduction of morbidity and mortality from altitude sickness. Ascents should be slow, especially those involving physical exertion. Sedatives and salt should be avoided; alcohol should be avoided for the first forty-eight hours. Most people adapt to altitude changes within three days. Returning to lower altitudes at night is advised. Premedication with acetazolamide, a prescription drug, will hasten adaptation and reduce symptoms. In serious cases, descent to lower altitudes is vital. Corticosteroids, oxygen, and hyperbaric treatments may be used. Chronically ill persons should check with their doctors before attempting strenuous activity at high altitudes.

—*Louis B. Jacques, M.D.*

See also Asphyxiation; Brain; Brain disorders; Coma; Cyanosis; Edema; Hyperbaric oxygen therapy; Hyperventilation; Hypoxia; Lungs; Nervous system; Neurology; Neurology, pediatric; Oxygen therapy; Pulmonary diseases; Pulmonary edema; Pulmonary medicine; Pulmonary medicine, pediatric; Respiration.

For Further Information:

Auerbach, Paul S. *Medicine for the Outdoors*. Rev. ed. Boston: Little, Brown, 1999.
Hackett, Peter H. and David R. Shlim. "Altitude Illness." *CDC: Travelers' Health*, July 7, 2011.

Luks, A. M., et. al. "Wilderness Medical Society consensus guidelines for the prevention and treatment of acute altitude illness." In *Wilderness Eviron Med.* 21, 2. (June, 2010): 146-55.
Reeves, John T., and Robert F. Grover. *Attitudes on Altitude: Pioneers of Medical Research in Colorado's High Mountains*. Boulder: University of Colorado Press, 2001.
Rennie, D. "The Great Breathlessness Mountains." *Journal of the American Medical Association* 256 (July 4, 1986): 81-82.
Ward, Michael P., John B. West, and James S. Milledge. *High Altitude Medicine and Physiology*. 4th ed. New York: Oxford University Press, 2007.
Wilkerson, James A., ed. *Medicine for Mountaineering and Other Wilderness Activities*. 6th ed. Seattle: The Mountaineers Books, 2010.

Alzheimer's disease

Disease/Disorder

Anatomy or system affected: Brain, cells, nerves, nervous system, psychic-emotional system

Specialties and related fields: Geriatrics and gerontology, internal medicine, neurology, nursing, psychiatry

Definition: A relentlessly progressive disease resulting in the loss of higher cognitive function; the most common form of dementia.

Key terms:

Alzheimer's beta peptide (Aβ): the principal proteinaceous component of certain brain lesions in Alzheimer's disease

amyloid: extracellular proteinaceous deposits having distinctive tinctorial properties

neurofibrillary tangles: a hallmark lesion of Alzheimer's disease and several other disorders consisting of intracellular aggregates of the structural protein tau

presenilins: proteins linked to several forms of inherited Alzheimer's disease, which are believed to play a role in the production of Aβ

senile plaques: a hallmark lesion of Alzheimer's disease, composed of Aβ amyloid

Causes and Symptoms

In 1906, Alois Alzheimer described the pathological correlates of presenile dementia. Once considered rare, Alzheimer's disease is now recognized as the most common form of dementia, composing 60 to 80 percent of all dementias across different age groups. The disease affects one in every eight individuals age sixty-five and older and one in every seven age seventy-one and older. The cognitive impairments include agnosia, the loss of perceptual ability regarding the interpretation of sensory perceptions; apraxia, the inability to understand the meaning or appropriate use of things; and dysphasia, the failure to arrange words in a meaningful manner. It is a relentlessly progressive neurodegenerative disorder that leads ultimately to death. While neurological and psychiatric examination provide an assessment of impairment, definitive diagnosis is arrived at only through autopsy. On the level of observable behavior, in persons affected by Alzheimer's dementia the symptoms often develop gradually, usually after the age of sixty. However, the disease has also been known to develop in younger individuals and to have a more rapid onset. As such, when symptoms such as those noted develop at any age, they deserve attention.

On a more neurologic and cellular level, Alzheimer's disease is characterized by a triad of pathological changes in the brain including senile (or neuritic) plaques, which consist of extracellular proteinaceous deposits surrounded by dystrophic neurons; the presence of similar extracellular proteinaceous deposits in the brain vasculature, termed amyloid (or congophilic) angiopathy; and the presence within nerve cells of tangled fibrillary protein aggregates, called neurofibrillary tangles. These pathological hallmarks are accompanied by significant neuronal loss and brain atrophy, particularly in areas of the brain involved in memory and cognition, such as the hippocampus and temporal and prefrontal cortex. Neuronal loss disproportionately affects nerve cells that use the neurotransmitter acetylcholine (cholinergic neurons). It should be noted, however, that the tangles and plaques have also been found postmortem in the brains of individuals who did not have Alzheimer's disease, so the association of these hallmarks is not completely understood in all individuals.

The extracellular protein deposits in the plaques and brain vasculature have distinct optical and staining properties, suggesting that there is significant underlying organization of their constituent molecules. There are many distinct, typically rare, diseases in which proteins are deposited in this organized fashion in various parts of the body. In 1842, these deposits were called waxy degenerations or lardaceous diseases, and in 1854, they were termed amyloid ("starchlike"). The diseases are now termed amyloidoses. Examples of amyloidoses include the familial amyloidotic polyneuropathies and cardiomyopathies, senile systemic amyloidosis, lattice corneal dystrophy, the Dutch and Icelandic variants of hereditary cerebral hemorrhage with amyloid (HCHWA), and the spongiform encephalopathies, such as "mad cow disease" and kuru. In 1922, the most rigorous histological test for amyloid was devised, staining with congo red: amyloid deposits bind congo red (are congophilic) and rotate polarized light rays (are birefringent), resulting in a transition from red stain in bright-field microscopy to an apple green coloration under polarized light microscopy. Large segments of the proteins that form amyloid deposits have a particular molecular configuration called the beta pleated sheet. These proteins precipitate from solution and aggregate to form organized structures called amyloid fibrils. The parallel alignment of the congo red dye with the organized amyloid fibril results in the optical activity recognized as birefringence.

Because the beta pleated sheet was recognized as the principal configuration of the molecules in amyloid deposits, the primary component of the amyloid deposits in Alzheimer's disease was termed beta (for beta pleated sheet) amyloid protein (βAP), or, more recently, Alzheimer's beta peptide (Aβ).

The identity of the primary protein component of Alzheimer's amyloid was deduced in 1987. Aβ is derived from a much larger protein, the β-amyloid precursor protein (APP), and by two proteases, β-secretase and γ-secretase. When added to cultures of neurons, Aβ is toxic, and the de-

---

Information on Alzheimer's Disease

Causes: Unknown
Symptoms: Decreased ability to interpret sensory perceptions or to understand the meaning or appropriate use of things, dysphasia
Duration: Progressive, eventually fatal
Treatments: None for underlying cause; some second-generation drugs slow disease progression

---

gree of toxicity is correlated with the degree to which the Aβ has aggregated. APP is also a substrate for a third secretase, α-secretase, which cleaves in the middle of the Aβ sequence and thereby precludes formation of the neurotoxic Aβ peptide. In contrast to Aβ, the α-secretase-cleaved derivatives of APP are believed to be neurotrophic.

The identification of β- and γ-secretase has been a particularly vexing problem for biologists. A mutation in two amino acids of APP adjacent to the β-secretase site is known to increase β-secretase activity and thus to increase Aβ production. However, it is a matter of debate whether this mutation (lysine and methionine mutated to asparagine and leucine, or, in biochemical annotation, KM to NL) is due to the increased activity of β-secretase or to an unrelated "NLase" enzyme. Furthermore, although most Aβ is forty amino acids long, Aβ is heterogeneous in size, ranging from thirty-nine to forty-three amino acids in length, and the forty-two amino acid form appears to be particularly pathogenic. Most of this variation occurs at the γ-secretase site, and because of the variations in observed forms of Aβ, there are different hypotheses regarding the type of activity that would be expected of a γ-secretase. For example, Aβ 40 and 42 might be generated by two distinct secretases. Alternatively, both Aβ 40 and Aβ 42 might be generated from the same enzyme, but the particular cleavage site might be influenced by local factors: prior to γ-secretase cleavage the Aβ domain of APP resides in the membrane, and factors that influence membrane thickness, such as cholesterol content, may lead to preferential cleavage at one of the sites. Still a third possibility is that γ-secretase generates a peptide several amino acids longer than the mature Aβ 40/2 peptide and that a second enzyme chews back on this "pre-Aβ" to yield the mature Aβ 40/2. Here, too, factors such as membrane thickness might influence the relative abundance of the Aβ 40 and Aβ 42 forms.

Nevertheless, β-secretase has recently been identified by several groups as the beta-site APP cleaving enzyme (BACE), and animals whose expression of BACE has been "knocked out" produce virtually no Aβ. Although the identity of γ-secretase has long eluded researchers, γ-secretase activity is now closely associated and sometimes identified with expression of the presenilins (see below). However, since it has never been demonstrated that presenilins have γ-secretase-like catalytic activity, there is still debate regarding whether they are γ-secretase or a requisite component of a secretase complex. γ-secretase has been identified with tumor necrosis factor-alpha converting enzyme (TACE).

APP is a member of a family of proteins, including two

amyloid-precursor-like proteins (APLP1 and 2) for which several possible functions have been proposed, including the formation of specific brain structures, neurite outgrowth, and neurobehavioral development. Several mutations have been identified in APP in association with familial Alzheimer's disease, and these mutations are believed to influence the rate of secretase cleavage or to alter the solubility of the Aβ peptide. A further mutation in APP is associated with hereditary cerebral hemorrhage with amyloid-Dutch variant (HCHWA-Dutch), a rare disorder with Alzheimer's-like cerebrovascular pathology. APP has been localized to chromosome 21, and those afflicted with trisomy 21 (Down syndrome) suffer many of the same neurodegenerative hallmarks of Alzheimer's disease, perhaps through a gene dosage effect.

In addition to mutations in APP, mutations in other genes have been identified as causative factors in inherited forms of Alzheimer's disease that appear to affect APP processing. A tremendous amount of interest has recently focused upon presenilin 1, originally designated as S182, a gene associated with chromosome-14-linked Alzheimer's disease. Soon after the discovery of presenilin 1 in 1995, mutations in another gene, originally designated as STM2, were identified as causative in chromosome-1-linked Alzheimer's disease. The amino acid sequences of these proteins are remarkably similar, and STM2 is now called presenilin 2.

Mutations in either of these genes result in early-onset Alzheimer's disease, but presenilin 1 mutations result in a far more malignant disease. Presenilin 1 mutations often result in an extraordinarily early onset (third decade of life), and Alzheimer's plaques are abundant in regions of the brain, such as the cerebellum, which are unaffected in the sporadic disease. This results in motor signs, such as myoclonus and seizure, which are absent in the sporadic disease. Mutations in both presenilin 1 and presenilin 2 result in increased production of Aβ, especially of a slightly larger and more pathogenic peptide, Aβ 42. Because these mutations appear to primarily influence the length of Aβ, their activity has primarily been associated with γ-secretase activity.

Initially, the mechanisms by which the presenilin mutations might result in Alzheimer's disease were unclear. By coincidence, researchers in the field of programmed cell death, or apoptosis, found a gene they identified as ALG-3, which they believed rescued cells from programmed cell death. ALG-3 had significant identity with a portion of presenilin 2, and the researchers speculated that mutations in the presenilins might lead nerve cells to an aberrant entry into apoptosis, resulting in the neuronal cell atrophy and death observed in Alzheimer's disease. However, there is considerable debate about whether necrosis, as opposed to apoptosis, is the primary means of cell death in Alzheimer's disease, and the role of the presenilins in apoptosis remains controversial.

The presenilins had no similarity to any known mammalian proteins but had limited identity with two proteins found in the nematode worm *C. elegans*. One protein with very limited identity is spe-4, a protein involved in spermatogenesis in the worm. The other protein with more significant identity (43 percent) is sel-12, a protein involved in the signaling of Notch, a protein involved in many developmental processes. Attempts to knock out the expression of presenilin 1 result in severe defects that are lethal to the late-stage embryo and that closely resemble the defects obtained with knockout of Notch expression. Conversely, expression of the normal human presenilin in worm cells is defective for sel-12 expression and restores Notch signaling, suggesting that both γ-secretase activity and Notch expression converge in the activity of presenilin.

Notch signaling requires the proteolysis of a membrane-

Alzheimer's brain   Normal brain

Alzheimer's disease causes the volume of the brain to shrink substantially.

In the News:
Drugs to Slow the Progress of Alzheimer's Disease

Although there is no cure for Alzheimer's disease, certain drugs are shown to improve cognitive functioning. Pharmacological treatment of Alzheimer's disease consists of drugs that prevent the breakdown of acetylcholine in the synapses. Four cholinesterase inhibitors approved for mild to moderate forms of Alzheimer's disease are Cognex, Aricept, Reminyl, and Exelon. These agents inhibit an enzyme called acetylcholinesterase that degrades the neurotransmitter acetylcholine.

One of the most recent drugs to hit the market is called Namenda. It is the first approved medication to treat moderate to severe forms of Alzheimer's disease. Studies have shown that its use results in a slower decline in mental function. Namenda can be taken alone or in combination with donepezil (Aricept).

New drugs in clinical trial investigations include cholinesterase inhibitors such as epastigmine and physostigmine (Synapton)—a sustained release formation—and cholinergic agonist drugs such as milameline, AF 102B, and SB202026 (Memric). Clinical trials provide measurable means of hope for patients with Alzheimer's disease and their families. Two newer drugs in phase 2 of clinical trials include heptylphysostigmine (a cholinesterase inhibitor) and xanomeline (a cholinergic agonist).

In addition to approved Food and Drug Administration (FDA) medications, nonconventional treatment has been shown to improve the cognitive ability of some patients with Alzheimer's disease. Such treatments include vitamin E, ginkgo biloba, estrogen, coenzyme Q10, nonsteroidal anti-inflammatory drugs (NSAIDs) such as aspirin and ibuprofen, and cholesterol-lowering agents. More research is needed, for the effectiveness and safety of these remedies has not been evaluated by the FDA.

—Janet Mahoney, R.N., Ph.D., A.P.R.N.

bound precursor in a manner that is very similar to the γ-secretase cleavage of APP. While the presenilins do not resemble any known proteases, a certain class of proteases has an obligate amino acid residue which, when mutated in presenilin, eliminates both γ-secretase and Notch cleavage. Also, drugs that are believed to be γ-secretase inhibitors inhibit both γ-secretase cleavage and Notch cleavage. Thus, the presenilins appear to be intimately involved with the proteolysis of APP and Notch. Although Notch activity does not appear to be directly related to Alzheimer's pathology, there is a concern that drugs designed to reduce Aβ production by inhibiting γ-secretase activity might also have an impact on normal Notch signaling, thereby adversely influencing such things as blood cell maturation.

The presenilins are synthesized by all cells in the body, and they appear to be localized within the cell primarily if not exclusively in the endoplasmic reticulum/golgi apparatus. While Aβ was believed to be derived primarily from the cell-membrane-associated APP through a specific pathway (the endosomal/lysosomal pathway), the localization of the presenilins and their association with γ-secretase activity to the endoplasmic reticulum led to a reevaluation of the cellular site of Aβ generation. There is a consensus now that most Aβ, particularly the more pathogenic Aβ 42, is produced within the cells at the endoplasmic reticulum/golgi apparatus. These results are significant because they suggest that, rather than forming from extracellular circulating Aβ proteins, amyloid plaques may begin as aggregates of Aβ within the cell. Those aggregates may, in turn, lead to neuronal injury and death.

Although the presenilins are intimately associated with γ-secretase activity, there has not yet been any definitive proof that the presenilins are involved in proteolytic activity. One would expect, for example, that if the portion of human APP cleaved by γ-secretase and presenilin were coexpressed in a cell that has no endogenous γ-secretase activity (such as a yeast cell), that presenilin would cleave APP, yet this does not occur, and controversy remains over whether enzymatic activity resides with the presenilins or whether the presenilins are an obligate component of multiprotein complexes. Recently, a protein that forms a complex with presenilin and that binds APP was identified. This protein, Nicastrin, named for the Italian village of Nicastro, where key early studies on familial Alzheimer's disease took place, also appears to play an important role in γ-secretase activity and in Notch processing. It is possible that there are other key components to this γ-secretase complex that are yet to be elucidated. A number of additional proteins that interact with presenilin or with APP have been identified; their role in Alzheimer's disease pathogenesis is being investigated. These include calsenilin, Fe65, X11, and BBP-1 (β-amyloid binding protein-1).

Aβ is, therefore, a neurotoxic peptide and a component of two of the predominant features of Alzheimer's disease. Since senile plaques occur within specific regions of the brain, while sparing other regions (especially the cerebellum), investigators originally believed that this distribution of pathology was due to regional differences in the production of APP. However, it soon became apparent that APP was synthesized by virtually all cells and that Aβ is present in abundance throughout the brains and indeed in other tissues of normal nondemented individuals. How, then, does a normal biological molecule become a pathological agent in the aging brain to cause nonfamilial (sporadic) cases of Alzheimer's disease?

It has been proposed that multiple genetic and environmental factors may play a role in this transformation. Some investigators have proposed that one or more of the minor components of amyloid plaques may act as "pathological chaperone" molecules by binding Aβ and altering its solubility. The identification of such components might lead to new drug research strategies and to new insight into the mechanisms of amyloid formation. For example, heparin sulfated proteoglycans (HSPGs) have been identified as components of amyloid deposits, and some investigators have attempted to block amyloid formation by inhibiting the interaction of Aβ with HSPGs. Alpha-synuclein was identified as the nonamyloid component of Alzheimer's disease plaques (NAC peptide); interestingly, mutations in α-synuclein have been identified in familial forms of Parkinson's disease, and this protein is a major constituent of the inclusion bodies found in Parkinson's-disease-associated Lewy body dementia. Aluminum has been identified as a component of the senile plaques found in Alzheimer's disease, and aluminum toxicity results in the formation of neurofibrillary tangles. It has been proposed that aluminum exposure may be a predisposing factor, but this hypothesis is very controversial. Similarly, zinc has been implicated in the formation of Aβ plaques, and a drug that chelates (absorbs) zinc appears to reduce the abundance of plaques in transgenic animal models of Alzheimer's disease.

Soluble Aβ may circulate in the serum and cerebral spinal fluid bound to one of several chaperone proteins, including apolipoprotein E, apolipoprotein J, and transthyretin. Polymorphisms in these proteins might alter the affinity of these proteins for Aβ, thereby leaving more free Aβ available to aggregate into amyloid fibrils. A particular isoform of apolipoprotein E (ApoE4), for example, has an altered affinity for Aβ, and the inheritance of this isoform is associated with increased risk for Alzheimer's disease.

Genes that may play roles in the degradation of proteins may also be involved in the development of Alzheimer's disease pathology. For example, polymorphisms in the cystatin C gene may alter the susceptibility to late-onset Alzheimer's. Cystatin C is a protease inhibitor, and mutant cystatin C is an amyloid component in the Icelandic variant of hereditary cerebral hemorrhage with amyloid (HCHWA-I). Also, the normal process by which cells target proteins for disposal may be altered in Alzheimer's disease. Cells normally target proteins for degradation by conjugating them to the protein ubiquitin, and there are reports that the ubiquitination pathway is altered in the brain afflicted with Alzheimer's disease.

Neuritic plaques and less organized forms of plaques (diffuse plaques) are not unique to Alzheimer's disease but are also found in dementia pugilistica, as a sequelae to severe trauma, are found in Down syndrome, and are coexistent with other diseases, such as Parkinson's disease. Likewise, as already noted, the amyloid (congophilic) angiopathy is also found in other familial amyloidoses. It is the combination of these cardinal findings with the finding of neurofibrillary tangles that forms the triad of primary pathological signs of Alzheimer's disease.

Neurofibrillary tangles are intracellular aggregates of an unusually modified (hyperphosphorylated) form of the structural protein tau (t). Neurofibrillary tangles are not unique to Alzheimer's disease but occur in several other neurodegenerative diseases, such as amyotrophic lateral sclerosis (ALS)-Parkinson's dementia complex as a consequence of measles infections of the central nervous system (subacute sclerosing panencephalitis), in the rare spongiform encephalopathies (including Creutzfeldt-Jakob disease and kuru), and in frontotemporal dementia. The number of neurofibrillary tangles correlates well with the severity of behavioral impairment.

There has been a long-standing debate regarding the significance of the pathological findings in Alzheimer's disease. The debate has focused on whether Aβ-associated pathology or the tau-protein-associated pathology is the primary lesion in the disease, thus dividing investigators jocularly into βaptist and τaoist camps.

There has been a general consensus that Aβ plays a central causative role in the disease. According to this "amyloid hypothesis," the excessive production, rapid deposition, or aberrant metabolism of Aβ results in the formation of toxic aggregates of Aβ, which in turn result in injury to neurons, neuronal death, and behavioral impairment. The tau pathology manifested as neurofibrillary tangles is a consequence of Aβ effects. Consistent with this view is the fact that all genes that have thus far been associated with familial Alzheimer's disease play a role in Aβ processing or solubility.

However, others would argue that amyloid plaques in Alzheimer's disease are an epiphenomenon, that they are a result of the neurodegenerative process rather than its cause. According to this "tau hypothesis," neurofibrillary tangles are the central pathological finding in the disease, and Aβ plaques are a relatively inert consequence of normal aging or of neurofibrillary tangle-associated neuronal degeneration. Consistent with this viewpoint is the strong correlation between behavioral impairment and neurofibrillary tangle burden. In contrast, amyloid plaques may be found in the brains of normal nondemented individuals, and total plaque burden (the number of plaques found in a given brain section) does not correlate well with behavior. Indeed, it has been difficult to demonstrate significant behavioral impairment in transgenic animal models of Alzheimer's disease (animals that overproduce human APP in the brain), even in the presence of significant amyloid deposits in the brain. It is noteworthy that those animals fail to develop neurofibrillary tangles. However, there have been no direct links between the genetics of Alzheimer's disease and tau protein, although recently a mutation has been identified in tau associated with a non-Alzheimer's dementia (frontotemporal dementia).

Recently there has been a significant convergence of opinion that Aβ is central to Alzheimer's disease pathogenesis. This is due to recent reports that total brain amyloid protein burden (a measure of the total Aβ protein, including protein from plaques) and not plaque number correlates well with severity of dementia.

Treatment and Therapy

There are presently no therapies available for Alzheimer's disease that target the putative underlying mechanisms for the genesis and progression of the disease, although there are extraordinary efforts under way throughout the world to address these mechanisms. Treatment options at present are primarily palliative. This means that they address the symptoms, perhaps providing some temporary relief, but not providing any cure.

Since Alzheimer's disease neurodegeneration appears to affect primarily cholinergic neurons, cholinergic agents such as tacrine (Cognex), and other second-generation drugs that are better tolerated, such as donepezil (Aricept), rivastigmine (Exolon), and galantamine (Reminyl), have shown efficacy in terms of temporarily slowing progression of the disease. These agents all inhibit an enzyme (acetylcholinesterase) that degrades the neurotransmitter acetylcholine. Clinical trials using an agent that mimics the actions of acetylcholine (nicotine) ended abruptly due to side effects that included severe anxiety.

Because the amyloid lesions in Alzheimer's disease may elicit a limited inflammatory response in the brain, which in turn may be a major component of the neurotoxic effects of Aβ, nonsteroidal anti-inflammatory drugs (NSAIDs), such as aspirin and ibuprofen, have been proposed as agents having possible ameliorative effects.

Certain retrospective studies have shown a negative correlation between the use of estrogen replacement therapy (ERT) and both the age of onset and severity of Alzheimer's disease in postmenopausal women, suggesting that ERT may have a protective function in these subjects.

Cholesterol may influence the production of Aβ by altering the characteristics of cell membranes, and Aβ is transported by lipoproteins. Thus, lipid metabolism may have an impact on the development of Alzheimer's disease. It has recently been shown that the cholesterol-lowering agents lovastatin and pravastatin may significantly reduce the risk of Alzheimer's disease in older patients.

Perspective and Prospects

Alzheimer's disease is the sixth leading cause of death among Americans, costing $203 billion in annual costs. The disease is projected to affect between eleven million and sixteen million individuals in the United States by 2050.

The pharmaceutical manufacturer Lilly has patented the first orally active β-secretase inhibitor, and it is likely that there are many such drugs currently in development. It is possible that some of these drugs may suffer liabilities due to alterations of Notch signaling. Nevertheless, they will provide key information regarding the validity of the amyloid hypothesis. With the recent cloning of β-secretase, drug discovery efforts surrounding β-secretase will likely be greatly facilitated.

Another potential target for drug intervention in Alzheimer's disease is the inhibition of Aβ aggregation. Although a number of agents have been reported that inhibit aggregation, they are all characteristically large molecular weight peptides that have very limited access across the blood/brain barrier. Thus, although this approach may work in principle, the development of a useful drug from this approach may be severely limited by issues regarding access of the drug to the brain.

Neurofibrillary tangles are an additional feature of Alzheimer's disease that may serve as a target for drug development. Since neurofibrillary tangles are composed of hyperphosphorylated tau protein, inhibitors of tau phosphorylation might be developed as useful therapeutic entities.

It has recently been reported that experimental vaccination of transgenic animals, showing features of Alzhei-

mer's disease such as amyloid plaques with Aβ peptide, results in the reduction of amyloid burden. The exciting implications of these experiments are that Alzheimer's disease might one day be treated or even prevented by vaccination. This approach to the treatment of Alzheimer's disease has entered early clinical trials.

Other approaches to therapeutics for Alzheimer's disease include the development of neurotrophic factors that may enhance neuron survival. Research into stem cells has provided evidence for the presence of neuronal stem cells within the brain. Research into the mechanisms of stem cell migration and development might yield drugs that would enhance the recruitment of such primitive stem cells into dystrophic areas of the brain.

Because early detection of Alzheimer's disease increases the effectiveness of current drugs and treatments and helps keep some of the disease's more devastating symptoms at bay, research is focused on ways to detect the disease definitively. A Canadian study released in 2002 notes possible connections between scores of verbal memory tests and the likelihood of developing the disease. The study examined patients' performance on a variety of psychological tests to gauge the tests' reliability in detecting preclinical Alzheimer's disease. The researchers discovered that verbal memory tests-for example, recalling the categories of words or being able to remember terms for a short period of time-were highly accurate in determining which individuals went on to develop the disease. These findings seem to support what other researchers have found: the evident decline in verbal memory in elderly individuals in the one- to two-year period prior to the development of Alzheimer's disease symptoms.

The search for causes of Alzheimer's dementia remains a topic of interest in the effort to develop prevention strategies. For instance, recent research has demonstrated that isoflurane, a common anesthetic, can lead to the development of amyloid protein in cultured neuronal cells and to cell death. Research following this discovery may lead to recommendations to avoid the use of such anesthetics, in favor of others, as a way of preventing exposure of vulnerable persons to what may be a causative factor in Alzheimer's dementia.

In 2013, scientists at the National Institutes of Health discovered that blocking the activity of regulator protein CD33 may stem the disease process of Alzheimer's.

—Robert L. Martone;
updated by Nancy A. Piotrowski, Ph.D.

See also Aging; Aging: Extended care; Amnesia; Brain; Brain disorders; Dementias; Frontotemporal dementia (FTD); Geriatrics and gerontology; Hospice; Memory loss; Neurology; Pick's disease; Psychiatry, geriatric.

For Further Information:

Alzheimer's Association. http://www.alz.org.
Bellenir, Karen, ed. *Alzheimer's Disease Sourcebook: Basic Consumer Health Information About Alzheimer's Disease, Other Dementias, and Related Disorders.* 3d ed. Detroit, Mich.: Omnigraphics, 2003.

Brioni, Jorge D., and Michael W. Decker, eds. *Pharmacological Treatment of Alzheimer's Disease: Molecular and Neurobiological Foundations*. New York: Wiley-Liss, 1997.

Esiri, Margaret M., Virginia M.-Y. Lee, and John Q. Trojanowski, eds. *The Neuropathology of Dementia*. 2d ed. New York: Cambridge University Press, 2004.

Gauthier, Serge, ed. *Clinical Diagnosis and Management of Alzheimer's Disease*. 3d ed. Boca Raton, Fla.: Taylor & Francis, 2006.

Mace, Nancy L., and Peter V. Rabins. *The Thirty-Six-Hour Day: A Family Guide to Caring for Persons with Alzheimer Disease, Related Dementing Illnesses, and Memory Loss in Later Life*. 4th ed. Baltimore: Johns Hopkins University Press, 2006.

Rowland, Lewis P., ed. *Merritt's Textbook of Neurology*. 12th ed. Philadelphia: Lippincott Williams & Wilkins, 2010.

"Suppressing protein may stem Alzheimer's disease process." *nih.gov*. National Institutes of Health, 25 Apr. 2013. Web. 21 May 2013.

Wasco, Wilma, and Rudolph E. Tanzi, eds. *Molecular Mechanisms of Dementia*. Totowa, N.J.: Humana Press, 1997.

Whitehouse, Peter J., Konrad Maurer, and Jesse F. Ballenger, eds. *Concepts of Alzheimer Disease: Biological, Clinical, and Cultural Perspectives*. Baltimore: Johns Hopkins University Press, 2003.

Amebiasis

Disease/Disorder

Also known as: Entamebiasis, amebic dysentery, intestinal amebiasis, travelers' diarrhea

Anatomy or system affected: Abdomen, anus, gastrointestinal system, intestines, liver

Specialties and related fields: Bacteriology, epidemiology, gastroenterology, internal medicine, microbiology, public health

Definition: Infection of the colon or associated organs by the parasite *Entamoeba histolytica*.

Causes and Symptoms

Amebiasis entails infection of the colon by the single-cell parasite *Entamoeba histolytica*. The majority of people infected-about 80 to 90 percent-do not develop symptoms and may be chronic carriers, a fact that is difficult to detect. Most of those who are symptomatic experience loose stools, intermittent diarrhea, intensified flatulence, and stomach cramps. Severe cases involve bloody diarrhea (dysentery), abdominal tenderness, mucus in the stool, or fever.

The parasite spreads when a person swallows food or water containing infected feces. Infection occurs in two forms, the active parasite (trophozoite) or dormant parasite (cyst form, which may activate in the intestinal tract). The trophozoites attack the lining of the colon, feeding on bacteria and tissue, and may cause ulcers. Sometimes a lump (ameboma) forms that is large enough to obstruct the intestines.

Occasionally, the trophozoites penetrate the bowel wall and enter the abdominal cavity, causing peritonitis, or they may travel to other organs. The liver may be infected, with the parasite forming an abscess that can cause fever, chills, and weight loss. Much more rarely, the lungs, brain, or skin on the buttocks becomes infected.

Information on Amebiasis

Causes: Amoeba *Entamoeba histolytica*

Symptoms: Loose stools, diarrhea, nausea, fatigue, weight loss, abdominal cramping and tenderness, increased gas, fever

Duration: About ten days with treatment; relapses possible

Treatments: Antiparasitic medication

Treatment and Therapy

Physicians test for amebiasis by examining three to six stool samples for evidence of the parasite. A colonoscopy may be used to locate ulcers and take a tissue sample. Abscesses in the liver can be located by ultrasound or computed tomography (CT) scan but cannot directly confirm the presence of *Entamoeba histolytica*.

The standard treatment is to give the patient antibacterial drugs. For those who are not sick, one antibiotic is given; for those with symptoms, there are usually two. The most common combination is metronidazole and iodoquinol, administered orally for ten days. Paromomycin and diloxanide furoate are also used, and for liver abscess, tinidazole. Follow-up tests of stool samples after two to four weeks are used to check for the presence of the parasite, as relapses may occur. Antidiarrheal medications may be needed to help patients control their bowels.

Perspective and Prospects

The vast majority of amebiasis infections occur in countries with poor sanitation or that use human waste as a crop fertilizer. Therefore, amebiasis is a form of travelers' diarrhea for tourists in Mexico, Central America, parts of South America and Africa, and South Asia. Sexual transmission is possible. Mass outbreaks are rare, but one arose during the 1933 Chicago World's Fair when contaminated water led to about one thousand symptomatic cases and fifty-eight deaths.

—*Roger Smith, Ph.D.*

See also Abdomen; Abdominal disorders; Bacterial infections; Colon; Diarrhea and dysentery; Food poisoning; Gastroenterology; Gastroenterology, pediatric; Gastrointestinal system; Intestines; Liver; Liver disorders; Nausea and vomiting; Parasitic diseases; Protozoan diseases; Ulcers.

For Further Information:

"Amebiasis." *MedlinePlus*, Mar. 22, 2013.

Beers, Mark H. *The Merck Manual of Medical Information*. New York: Pocket Books, 2003.

Ericsson, Charles. *Travelers' Diarrhea*. 2nd ed. Hamilton, Ont.: B. C. Decker, 2008.

McCoy, Krisha, and Michael Woods. "Amoebic Dysentery." *Health Library*, Nov. 26, 2012.

"Parasites - Amebiasis." *Centers for Disease Control and Prevention*, Nov. 2, 2010.

Parker, James N. *The Official Patient's Sourcebook on Travelers' Diarrhea*. Urbana, Ohio: Icon Health, 2002.

Schwartz, Eli. *Tropical Diseases in Travelers*. Hoboken, N.J.: Blackwell, 2009.

Amenorrhea

Disease/Disorder

Anatomy or system affected: Endocrine system, reproductive system

Specialties and related fields: Endocrinology, family medicine, gynecology

Definition: The absence of menstrual cycles.

Key terms:

anorexia nervosa: a psychiatric disease characterized by a distorted body image in which the individual severely limits food intake because of fear of weight gain

estrogen: a hormone secreted from the ovaries that is crucial for the buildup of the uterine lining, ovulation, and bone density maintenance

premature ovarian failure: cessation of menses prior to the age of forty because of the early loss of ovarian follicles

prolactin: a hormone secreted from the posterior pituitary gland; at high levels (for example, resulting from tumors in the pituitary), prolactin can cause amenorrhea and increase breast secretions, a condition known as galactorrhea

secondary sexual characteristics: in females, the development of breast tissue and pubic hair

Causes and Symptoms

Amenorrhea, or the absence of menses, can be physiologic, such as during pregnancy, or pathologic. Amenorrhea can be primary or secondary in nature. Primary amenorrhea is defined as the absence of menses by age sixteen, even in the presence of normal growth and secondary sexual characteristics. In girls with abnormal growth, primary amenorrhea is defined as the absence of menses by age fourteen. Causes of primary amenorrhea include abnormalities of the reproductive outflow tract that prevent the flow of menstrual blood. Examples include imperforate hymen, transverse vaginal septum, and Asherman's syndrome, whereby scar tissue within the uterus prevents the outflow of menstrual fluid. Girls with these conditions may experience cyclic cramping and discomfort from the buildup of menstrual blood. Other causes of primary amenorrhea include genetic problems such as Turner syndrome, in which the individual has a single X chromosome, or androgen insensitivity syndrome, in which the individual appears female but is genetically male and lacks ovaries and a uterus. Turner syndrome and androgen insensitivity tend to be asymptomatic regarding their amenorrhea. Rare congenital causes of primary amenorrhea include Kallman syndrome and empty sella syndrome.

Secondary amenorrhea refers to the absence of menstrual periods after menstrual cycles have occurred previously. It is defined as the absence of menses for the duration of three regular menstrual cycles or six months. Physiological causes of secondary amenorrhea include pregnancy, the postpartum state, and the menopause. Pathologic causes of secondary amenorrhea include disorders of the central nervous system or hypothalamus, such as extreme stress or exercise and anorexia nervosa. Disorders of the pituitary gland, such as tumors, can cause secondary amenorrhea as well. These tumors may be accompanied by

---

Information on Amenorrhea

Causes: Stress, psychological disorders, hormone deficiency, extremely low body fat

Symptoms: Cessation of menstrual periods

Duration: Often chronic

Treatments: Hormone replacement, oral contraceptives, counseling

---

galactorrhea, from high levels of prolactin, or by visual impairment. Hormonal disturbances can also lead to secondary amenorrhea. One example is hypothyroidism, which is often accompanied by fatigue and cold intolerance. Polycystic ovary syndrome, an endocrinologic disorder characterized by insulin resistance and hirsutism, may also lead to amenorrhea. Another cause of secondary amenorrhea is premature ovarian failure, which may be attributable to radiation or chemotherapy. These individuals may experience the symptoms of early menopause, such as hot flashes and vaginal dryness.

Treatment and Therapy

The treatment for amenorrhea depends on the cause. If the disorder is the result of anatomic causes, then surgery may cure it. For instance, an imperforate hymen or transverse vaginal septum can be corrected surgically, allowing for normal outflow of menstrual fluid. If the disorder is the result of hormonal imbalances, then medications may be given, such as thyroid hormone for hypothyroidism or bromocriptine for hyperprolactinemia. In individuals with polycystic ovary syndrome, metoformin may be given to regulate the menstrual cycles. By correcting these hormonal imbalances, the resumption of regular menstrual cycles may occur, thus allowing for conception and pregnancy, if the individual so desires.

In cases of amenorrhea caused by extreme stress or exercise and anorexia nervosa, removal from the stressful conditions, a decrease in exercise levels, or an increase in caloric intake to maintain normal ideal body weight often remediates amenorrhea. Individuals who suffer from anorexia nervosa also require psychiatric treatment.

Individuals with genetic causes or premature ovarian failure leading to amenorrhea are unlikely to attain menstruation via medical therapy. For these individuals, therapy is aimed at preventing or treating the sequelae of estrogen deficiency that accompany amenorrhea. For instance, women with premature ovarian failure are at risk for the depletion of bone mineral density and osteoporosis. These individuals may benefit from hormone therapy in the form of estrogen and progesterone.

Perspective and Prospects

The cause for amenorrhea can often be found, since a vast array of diagnostic tests are available. Anatomic abnormalities may be detected on physical examination or via imaging of the reproductive structures such as ultrasound. Hormonal causes of amenorrhea can often be found through blood tests of hormones produced by the hypothalamus, pituitary gland, ovaries, thyroid gland, and adrenal glands. These tests can identify the hormone derangement and which organ is responsible. Genetic tests have allowed physicians to understand the basis of primary amenorrhea on a molecular level. While many cases of amenorrhea can be treated effectively once the cause has been identified, the future holds promise that better therapies with fewer side effects will be found.

—Anne Lynn S. Chang, M.D.

See also Anorexia nervosa; Dysmenorrhea; Eating disorders; Exercise physiology; Gynecology; Hormones; Menstruation; Puberty and adolescence; Reproductive system; Turner syndrome; Weight loss and gain; Women's health.

For Further Information:

Kasper, Dennis L., et al., eds. *Harrison's Principles of Internal Medicine*. 18th ed. New York: McGraw-Hill, 2012.

Kohnle, Diana, and Andrea Chisholm. "Absent Periods." *Health Library*, Sept. 27, 2012.

McPhee, Stephen J., and Maxine A. Papadakis, eds. *Current Medical Diagnosis and Treatment*. 50th ed. Los Altos: Lange Medical Pub, 2011.

Stenchever, Morton A., et al. *Comprehensive Gynecology*. 5th ed. St. Louis, Mo.: Mosby/Elsevier, 2007.

Vorvick, Linda J., and David Zieve. "Amenorrhea - Primary." *MedlinePlus*, May 31, 2012.

Vorvick, Linda J., and David Zieve. "Secondary Amenorrhea." *MedlinePlus*, May 31, 2012.

American Medical Association (AMA)

Organization

Definition: The largest voluntary association of physicians in the United States, with most of its members engaging directly in the practice of medicine.

Key terms:

Accreditation Council for Continuing Medical Education (ACCME): the organization that promotes and accredits continuing education for physicians, which the AMA sponsors

Accreditation Council for Graduate Medical Education (ACGME): the council that accredits physician residency programs in 1,500 U.S. medical schools; it is sponsored by the AMA and four other organizations

House of Delegates: the representative body that decides official policy and action on behalf of the AMA membership; state medical societies are allocated most of the delegate positions in the house, since 90 percent of all physicians affiliate with them, while medical specialty societies, military and other federal service groups, and five special sections also are given representation

Liaison Committee on Medical Education (LCME): an organization formed by the AMA and the Association of American Medical Colleges to set standards and accredit all U.S. and Canadian medical schools offering M.D. degrees

Role in the United States

Since its inception, the American Medical Association (AMA) has worked to improve the credibility of medicine as a profession in the United States. The AMA helped to shape and develop the physician licensing system used now in every state. Through the auspices of various accreditation bodies that it sponsors, such as the LCME, ACGME, and ACCME, the AMA monitors medical education programs to ensure that they continue to meet high standards. The AMA established a professional code of ethics for physicians and revises it periodically to guide physicians through the ever-changing health care environment. The AMA Council on Ethical and Judicial Affairs regularly issues interpretations of the principles of medical ethics; the council can censure, suspend, or expel a physician who violates the code of ethics. The *Journal of the American Medical Association* (or *JAMA*) was first published in July, 1883, and is now the world's most widely circulated medical journal. The AMA also publishes ten medical specialty journals and the weekly *American Medical News*. In addition, the AMA produces and distributes press releases, video news releases, and radio and television news programs.

The AMA advocates a "patient's bill of rights," which supports patient autonomy, dignity, confidentiality, and ongoing access to needed medical care. The AMA believes that the practice of medicine should be based on sound scientific principles, which are promulgated in *JAMA* and in the many specialty journals that it sponsors and publishes. The AMA also houses one of the nation's largest medical libraries, subscribes to more than 150 computer databases, and maintains comprehensive computer files on all physicians and medical students in the United States.

Guidelines for Health

The AMA acknowledged early in its development the role that it should play in promoting the improvement of public health. Among the public health initiatives that the AMA has sponsored are the clear labeling of poison containers, early childhood screening for hearing and vision problems, the inspection of milk to ensure its quality, the installation of seat belts in automobiles, low tolerance in state laws regarding drunk driving, and the banning of tobacco product advertisement. More recently, the AMA was among the first professional associations to advocate significant reform of the American health care delivery system, especially to respond to the needs of uninsured and underinsured people. The communications arm of the AMA produces services and products designed to increase public knowledge regarding significant health care issues and medical care advances.

Perspective and Prospects

Nathan Smith Davis, a medical doctor and a delegate of the New York State Medical Society, introduced resolutions that led to the holding of the first national medical convention in May, 1846. Davis's tireless leadership during the first convention enabled the establishment of the American Medical Association in May, 1847. Davis also served as an AMA president and the first editor-in-chief of the *Journal of the American Medical Association*.

The original AMA constitution set out several enduring principles for the organization. The AMA would be governed by representatives elected from the membership, and officers would serve only one year. The purposes of the AMA would be to advance medical knowledge, to work to improve medical education, to establish high ethical and practice standards, to encourage the formation and maintenance of state and local medical societies, and to work against medical quackery.

To ensure that the association speaks with a unified voice, the AMA has used, since its founding, the principle of representative democracy. State medical societies are entitled to a voting delegate and an alternate for each one thousand members; this represents the overwhelming majority of voting delegates. Other organizations, such as the Veterans Administration and medical schools sections, are also given one delegate and one alternate. The delegates form the AMA House of Delegates, which meets twice a year to evaluate and decide on policy issues. To prepare properly for a meeting of the House of Delegates, reference committees consider and hold open hearings on important medical issues, such as testing for acquired immunodeficiency syndrome (AIDS). The reference committees then make recommendations to the House of Delegates, which often decides hundreds of policies during each session.

The AMA is a powerful lobbyist in Washington, D.C., where it seeks to influence national legislation affecting the delivery of medical care. It also represents the interests of its members in important cases brought before various courts.

—*Russell Williams, M.S.W.*

See also Animal rights vs. research; Centers for Disease Control and Prevention (CDC); Education, medical; Ethics; Hippocratic oath; Law and medicine; Medical College Admission Test (MCAT); National Institutes of Health (NIH).

For Further Information:
American Medical Association. *Caring for the Country: A History and Celebration of the First 150 Years of the American Medical Association.* Chicago: Author, 1997. Written as a lively, thoughtful narrative, this book examines the role a great institution and its physician members have played in creating the world's finest system of medical care.

Baker, Robert B., ed. *The American Medical Ethics Revolution: How the AMA's Code of Ethics Has Transformed Physicians' Relationships to Patients, Professionals, and Society.* Baltimore: Johns Hopkins University Press, 1999. Twenty essays offer a detailed analysis of the political and philosophical maneuvering behind the preparation of the 1847 Code of Ethics and explore the resulting impact on modern health care.

Campion, Frank. *The AMA and U.S. Health Policy Since 1940.* Chicago: Chicago Review Press, 1984. A thorough study of the American Medical Association's medical policy since 1940. Includes bibliographical references and an index.

Fishbein, Morris. *A History of the American Medical Association, 1847 to 1947.* Philadelphia: W. B. Saunders, 1947. A historical look at the American Medical Association, including biographies of the organization's presidents and the histories of publications, councils, bureaus, and other official bodies.

Amnesia

Disease/Disorder

Anatomy or system affected: Brain, nervous system, psychic-emotional system

Specialties and related fields: Neurology, psychiatry, psychology

Definition: The loss of memory due to physical and/or psychological conditions.

Key terms:

anterograde: referring to amnesia in which events following a biological or psychological trauma are forgotten; new learning is impaired

episodic memory: the remembrance of personal information in one's life, such as the events of the previous day

procedural memory: the ability to reproduce learned skills, particularly perceptual-motor activities such as riding a bike

retrograde: referring to amnesia in which events preceding a biological or psychological trauma are forgotten; retrieving previously formed memories is impaired

semantic memory: the storage of factual information, such as the meaning of words

Causes and Symptoms

The primary attribute of amnesia is a loss of memory for a specific time period. The extent, duration, and type of that memory loss can vary greatly. In anterograde amnesia, the formation of new memories is impaired, while in retrograde amnesia, the retrieval of previously formed memories is impaired. In rare cases, anterograde amnesia is continuous, in which there is great impairment of memory formation for the remainder of a person's life. Retrograde amnesia in rare cases may be generalized, in which the totality of an individual's personal memory preceding the onset of amnesia is lost. More commonly, both anterograde and retrograde amnesias are localized, in which the memory of a period of time ranging from seconds to minutes (although occasionally days or longer) is lost. The memory loss may be selective, with only some aspects of a particular time period being absent. In all these forms of amnesia, the most common type of information lost is episodic; rarely are procedural memories destroyed.

Amnesia is typically caused by either psychological circumstances, in which case it is termed psychogenic, or by biological processes, in which it is referred to as biogenic or organic. Sometimes, however, the cause involves both psychological and biological factors. Psychogenic amnesias are usually caused by some sort of emotional trauma. Emotional trauma is the common thread that runs through the amnesia associated with the following disorders: dissociative amnesia (the inability to recall significant personal information); fugue (memory loss accompanied by sudden, unexpected travel from home); dissociative identity disorder (the presence of two or more distinct personalities, with the inability to recall extensive time periods); and post-traumatic stress disorder (significant distress and memory disturbances following an extreme traumatic event). Emotional trauma is typically absent in posthypnotic amnesia, which is induced by hypnotic suggestion, and childhood amnesia, in which adult memories of early childhood experiences before the age of five are typically vague and fragmentary. Psychogenic memories, while principally involving episodic information, may

---

Information on Amnesia

Causes: Head trauma, various diseases, psychological or emotional trauma
Symptoms: Loss of memory for a specific time period
Duration: Episodic, sometimes long term
Treatments: Psychological intervention, drugs affecting neurotransmitter levels

---

extend to semantic information, which is rarely seen in biogenic amnesia.

Biogenic amnesia is usually the result of trauma to the brain or disease processes. Anterograde and retrograde amnesia are common following a concussion or brain surgery, particularly involving the temporal lobe. Electroconvulsive treatments induced by a current passed through electrodes on the forehead (sometimes used to treat depression) tend to have a more anterograde effect. A diversity of toxic and infectious brain illnesses can lead to Korsakoff's syndrome, first described in chronic alcoholics. The primary feature is anterograde disturbance, with the ability to store new information limited to a few seconds. Dementia typically begins with the loss of recent memories and gradually spreads retrograde into the person's more distant past as the condition progresses. Hardening of the brain arteries, Alzheimer disease, and numerous infectious agents can lead to dementia. Transient global amnesia is an abrupt anterograde and retrograde loss leaving some degree of permanent memory loss; it is thought to be caused by temporary reductions in the blood supply to specific brain regions.

Treatment and Therapy

As time passes from the emotional and physiological traumas that precipitate amnesia, there is usually some degree of memory recovery. The less severe the trauma, the better the prognosis. Psychological interventions involving the use of careful interrogation, the use of emotionally significant stimuli, or hypnosis can help the amnesic fill in the gaps of memory deficits. Drugs that affect levels of neurotransmitters such as acetylcholine, aspartate, glutamate, norepinephrine, and serotonin can also have an impact on memory recovery. For example, John Krystal reported in 1993 that Vietnam War veterans given yohimbine, a drug that activates norepinephrine, experienced vivid flashbacks of combat trauma.

Some amnesias can be either prevented-using electrodes on only one side of the head in electroconvulsive treatment lessens the likelihood of amnesia-or significantly ameliorated by psychological and/or biological intervention. Severe amnesias, such as dementia, have no effective cure. However, drugs to may be prescribed to help manage symptoms, such as cholinesterase inhibitors and memantine, which help boost chemical messengers involved in memory. Major memory loss in the elderly has a particularly poor prognosis for recovery and is often indicative of imminent death. Where memory recovery is poor, optimizing the use of the remaining mental abilities and available environmental resources can help those with amnesia better adapt to their living environments.

Perspective and Prospects

The first scientific explanations of amnesia came in the late nineteenth century. Théodule-Armand Ribot (1839-1916) proposed a "law of regression," in which memory loss was thought to progress from the least stable to the most stable memories. Sergey Korsakoff (1853-1900) was one of the first to demonstrate that amnesia need not be associated with the loss of reasoning abilities found in dementia. While Ribot and Korsakoff focused on organic causes of amnesia, Pierre Janet (1859-1947) described amnesics who apparently had no underlying biological disease. He explained these cases in terms of mental fragmentation that he called dissociation.

Prevention, rather than treatment, of amnesia became the focus of attention as the twentieth century drew to a close. Two promising research areas in the twenty-first century are drugs to limit the effects of brain damage and the beneficial impact of a stimulating environment in staving off the effects of aging on the brain.

—Paul J. Chara, Jr., Ph.D., and Kathleen A. Chara, M.S.

For Further Information:
"Amnesia." *Mayo Clinic*, Oct. 11, 2011.
Baddeley, Alan, et al., eds. *Episodic Memory: New Directions in Research*. New York: Oxford University Press, 2002.
Berrios, German E., and John R. Hodges, eds. *Memory Disorders in Psychiatric Practice*. New York: Cambridge University Press, 2000.
Damasio, Antonio R. *Descartes' Error: Emotion, Reason, and the Human Brain*. New York: G. P. Putnam's Sons, 1994.
"Dissociative Disorders." *Mayo Clinic*, Mar. 3, 2011.
Herman, Judith. *Trauma and Recovery: The Aftermath of Violence-from Domestic Abuse to Political Terror*. Rev. ed. New York: Basic Books, 2003.
Jasmin, Luc, and David Zieve. "Memory Loss." *MedlinePlus*, Feb. 16, 2012.
Papanicolaou, Andrew C., et al. *The Amnesias: A Clinical Textbook of Memory Disorders*. New York: Oxford University Press, 2006.
Schacter, Daniel L. *Searching for Memory: The Brain, the Mind, and the Past*. New York: Basic Books, 1996.
Squire, Larry R., and Daniel L. Schacter, eds. *Neuropsychology of Memory*. 3d ed. New York: Guilford Press, 2002.

Amniocentesis

Procedure

Anatomy or system affected: Abdomen, reproductive system, uterus

Specialties and related fields: Embryology, genetics, obstetrics, perinatology

Definition: The removal of amniotic fluid from a pregnant woman for analysis; this fluid provides biochemical and genetic information about the fetus, enabling physicians to identify congenital problems in the second trimester as well as to determine the presence of fetal or intra-amniotic disease in the third trimester.

Key terms:

amniotic sac: a thin, tough, membranous sac that contains amniotic fluid and that encloses the embryo or fetus

chorionic villi: the fingerlike projections of the placenta that function in oxygen, nutrient, and waste transportation between a fetus and its mother

chromosomal defect: an abnormality in the chromosomes, the threadlike, darkly staining bodies found in all cells that carry genetic information in the form of deoxyribonucleic acid (DNA)

Down syndrome: a common genetic disorder characterized by mental retardation and a number of other abnormal findings, including heart malformations

gestational age: the age of a fetus, as determined from the first day of the last menstrual period, which is approximately two weeks before the date of conception; when the date of the last menstrual period is not known, the gestational age can be estimated via ultrasound

karyotype: the chromosomal makeup of an individual; also refers to the arrangement of chromosomes in standard paired fashion on a photomicrograph, which can facilitate analysis of the chromosomes

respiratory distress syndrome: a disease of lung immaturity that can be fatal and is found in children who are born prematurely

Rh isoimmunization: a condition in which a woman who is lacking a substance on red blood cells called Rh factor carries a fetus with the Rh factor on its red blood cells; in these cases, the woman may produce antibodies that attack the red blood cells of the fetus, leading to fetal anemia

trimester: any of the three consecutive three-month periods during pregnancy; the first trimester generally refers to weeks zero to twelve of gestation, the second trimester refers to weeks thirteen to twenty-four of gestation, and the third trimester refers to weeks twenty-five to forty-two of gestation

trisomy 18: a condition caused by extra pieces of chromosome 18 in the cells of the fetus; characterized by mental retardation and a number of other abnormalities, often including severe heart malformations

ultrasonography: the use of sound waves, directed at the body, to create visual images of the tissues being examined

Indications and Procedures

Human pregnancy begins after an egg cell and a sperm cell unite to become a fertilized egg. This process, called conception, occurs in one of the Fallopian tubes, and about a week later the fertilized egg enters the uterus. Cell division during the time period between fertilization and its entry into the uterus converts the fertilized egg into an organized cell cluster that attaches to the lining of the uterus. Following this attachment, the cluster penetrates the lining and becomes closely entwined with uterine tissues, developing three parts: the placenta, the embryo, and an amniotic sac (filled with the fluid within which the embryo is suspended). Two months after conception, the embryo-then an inch-long fetus-possesses all the anatomic features that will be present when it is born. During the remainder of the pregnancy, the fetus will grow much larger, and all its internal and external anatomic details will be elaborated.

Amniocentesis is used to provide diagnostic information before a fetus is born. It can be carried out anytime after

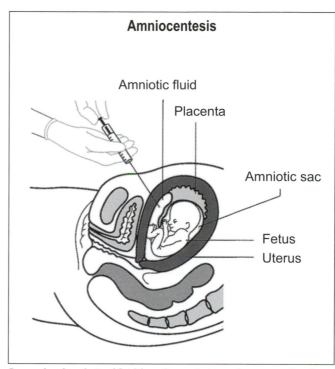

Amniocentesis

Amniotic fluid

Placenta

Amniotic sac

Fetus

Uterus

Removal and analysis of fluid from the amniotic sac that surrounds a fetus during gestation can be used to rule out or confirm the presence of serious birth defects or genetic diseases.

fourteen weeks gestational age. At this point, the amniotic fluid pockets are large enough to sample safely with minimal risk to the fetus, and an adequate volume of amniotic fluid may be obtained for genetic and biochemical analysis. In general, amniocentesis or other forms of prenatal diagnosis in early pregnancy (that is, before twenty-four weeks gestational age) are indicated when the risk that the fetus is abnormal is as least as great as the risk of miscarriage from the procedure.

Amniocentesis is indicated in cases where a fetal anomaly is suspected or found on ultrasound, and additional information can be gained through the amniotic fluid regarding the nature of the defect. It is also indicated in women over the age of thirty-five, as the risk for chromosomal defects increases with maternal age. At the age of thirty-five, the risk of Down syndrome outweighs the risk of performing amniocentesis, thereby making the procedure a reasonable one to perform routinely. Other indications for an amniocentesis include women with a previous pregnancy complicated by chromosomal abnormalities and in cases where either parent is a carrier for a chromosomal abnormality.

Another indication for amniocentesis is a known family history of a genetic defect. The types of disorders that can be ruled out via amniocentesis tend to be single-gene defects, and either parents have usually been diagnosed as having the disease or are known carriers of the disease. Examples of these diseases include cystic fibrosis, Duchenne or Becker muscular dystrophy, fragile X syndrome, hemophilia, Huntington's disease, neurofibromatosis type 1, sickle cell disease, Tay-Sachs disease, phenylketonuria (PKU), and thalassemias.

In the third trimester, amniocentesis is indicated if fetal developmental maturity and well-being need to be assessed. These factors help guide decision-making in treating a patient and her fetus. Commonly, amniocentesis is used to determine fetal lung maturity. This piece of information will help the obstetrician better weigh the risks of early delivery versus prolonging a pregnancy in cases where complications put the infant and/or mother at risk. Another indication for amniocentesis in the third trimester is to assess the level of fetal anemia, such as in cases of Rh isoimmunization. Amniocentesis can provide samples of amniotic fluid that can be analyzed to determine the degree of fetal red blood cell destruction and anemia. Futhermore, these samples also can be analyzed for fetal lung maturity. If the fetal lungs are mature and the fetal anemia is profound, then the obstetrician may opt for early delivery of the infant in order to minimize the risks posed to the fetus by remaining in utero.

Another indication for performing amniocentesis in the third trimester is to rule out an infection. When an intra-amniotic infection is suspected, an analysis of amniotic fluid via amniocentesis can determine the presence or absence of an infection and help the obstetrician determine a treatment plan, such as antibiotics or delivery of the infant.

Amniocentesis in the third trimester may also be indicated for therapeutic purposes. For instance, it may be performed in cases in which the amount of amniotic fluid is excessive, which is termed polyhydramnios. In this situation, the removal of amniotic fluid may relieve maternal symptoms of extreme discomfort and pressure. Another example of a therapeutic use for amniocentesis is in cases of twin gestation in which unequal sharing of the placenta is present. This can lead to a condition in which the amniotic sac of one twin contains dramatically more fluid than that of the other twin. In such cases, amniotic fluid may be aspirated from the twin with the excess amniotic fluid in order to relieve the uneven distribution of fluid between the two fetuses.

Amniocentesis can be an office procedure. The woman is usually supine or lying on her side. Ultrasound is performed to determine the location of the fetus, the location of the placenta, and the location of the largest and most accessible pockets of amniotic fluid. The optimal location for needle insertion is then determined, and the site of needle puncture on the abdomen is cleaned to prevent infection. Local anesthetic may be injected at the puncture site to minimize discomfort. Under ultrasound guidance, a needle attached to a syringe is inserted through the skin, subcutaneous fat, and uterine wall and finally into a pocket of amniotic fluid. Correct placement of the needle is confirmed by the aspiration of amniotic fluid. A sample of the fluid is then aspirated into the syringe. The syringe is disconnected from the needle, and the needle is removed. Obstetricians will almost always monitor the well-being of the fetus through fetal heart tones before and after the procedure in order to ensure that the fetus tolerated the procedure well.

Uses and Complications

In the second trimester, amniocentesis can be very helpful in identifying chromosomal abnormalities, particularly in women over the age of thirty-five. The amniotic fluid obtained from amniocentesis contains fetal cells that can be grown in tissue culture and examined for abnormalities in the chromosomes. Chromosomal problems can lead to a fetus with syndromes such as Down syndrome or trisomy 18. After a woman tests positive for a chromosomal abnormality, she should receive genetic counseling regarding the nature of the abnormality and known consequences of fetuses carrying it. Knowledge of the chromosomal abnormality can help the pregnant woman plan for the future and can help the obstetrician and pediatrician plan for the safest delivery possible for the baby. Some women who discover that they are carrying a fetus with a chromosomal abnormality may opt for termination of the pregnancy; others may wish to continue it. In cases in which the amniocentesis results are normal, the woman's anxiety and fears regarding having a baby with serious genetic defects may be greatly reduced.

Other uses of amniocentesis include analysis of the fetal cells to determine the presence of hereditary diseases such as cystic fibrosis. Amniocentesis can also identify the sex of the fetus. The amniotic fluid from amniocentesis may also be used to identify levels of biochemical markers such as acetyl cholinesterase, which may be indicative of structural abnormalities in the fetus.

In the third trimester, the most common use of amniocentesis is to determine fetal lung maturity in cases where the obstetrician anticipates an early delivery of the baby. The amniotic fluid can be analyzed for levels of substances secreted by the developing fetal lung (such as the ratio of lecithin and sphingomyelin). Because the respiratory system is one of the last organs to mature in the fetus, the level of these chemical markers that indicate fetal lung maturity enables physicians to assess whether the lungs are mature. Immature fetal lungs can lead to a serious condition called respiratory distress syndrome after the baby is born. In cases in which amniocentesis indicates that the fetal lungs are not yet mature, steroid injections may be given to the mother to induce fetal lung maturity prior to the delivery of the infant.

Another use of amniocentesis in the third trimester is to follow the severity of fetal anemia in Rh isoimmunization. In these cases, the mother produces an antibody, a type of protein, which attacks the fetus's red blood cells, leading to anemia. As the pregnancy progresses, fetal anemia can become very severe and can even lead to fetal death. Therefore, the ability to track the progression of fetal anemia is extremely important. This is possible through serial amniocenteses. The amniotic fluid obtained from amniocentesis is analyzed for its optical density. The result helps guide the physician in determining whether it is safer for the fetus to continue in the uterus or whether it should be delivered. In cases in which the fetus is very premature and early delivery is undesirable, drastic measures such as an intrauterine transfusion of blood to the fetus via the umbilical cord may be performed.

For most patients, amniocentesis is relatively painless and involves only an initial pinprick and/or a sensation of pressure. Amniocentesis is very safe for both mother and fetus, and it may be repeated more than once during a pregnancy if necessary. The chances of a complication from an amniocentesis are on average less than 0.5 percent. The risk is even lower in the hands of experienced practitioners. Potential complications include fetal loss when the amniocentesis is performed in early pregnancy. When performed in the third trimester of pregnancy, complications include precipitation of labor, placental trauma leading to bleeding, and injury to the fetus, for example, if the needle punctures delicate parts of the fetus. As with any invasive procedure, there is always a risk of bleeding or infection (in this case, to both the mother and the fetus). However, these risks are small when the proper procedures are followed.

Perspective and Prospects

The ability for physicians to diagnose fetal abnormalities essentially began with the development of amniocentesis in the 1950s. Its first application was in the diagnosis of Rh isoimmunization. In 1966, M. W. Steele and W. R. Breg Jr. demonstrated that the fetal cells from the amniotic fluid could be cultured and the chromosomal makeup of the fetus could be analyzed. This led to the development of the field of prenatal diagnosis.

Besides amniocentesis, a common technique used for prenatal diagnosis is chorionic villus sampling. In this procedure, placental tissue and amniotic fluid are sampled and sent for analysis. A catheter is inserted into the uterus through the vaginal opening and then guided by ultrasonography until its tip reaches the many chorionic villi that edge the placenta at its connection to the uterus. Gentle suction is applied, and a few of the villi are sucked out, first into the catheter and then into a sampling device. The cells that are obtained are tested in the same manner as with cells obtained through amniocentesis.

Chorionic villus sampling arose from the demonstration of the clear value of the information derived from fetal cells obtained from amniotic fluid. This useful procedure was devised to shorten the time period after amniocentesis, often several weeks long, that is needed to grow enough fetal cells in tissue culture to provide the amount of tissue required for successful karyotyping or DNA sequencing work. Another advantage of the chorionic villus sampling procedure is that it can be carried out with younger fetuses, as young as twelve weeks old, although the risk to such a fetus (fetal loss) is somewhat higher than that which is seen after amniocentesis. However, earlier diagnosis of a fetal abnormality allows for more time to obtain counseling and for decision-making. If termination of the pregnancy is desired, then the earlier it is performed, the safer it is for the mother.

Prenatal diagnosis has multiple purposes beyond the diagnosis of fetal abnormalities in utero. Traditionally, many couples have been discouraged from obtaining prenatal diagnosis if termination of the pregnancy is not an option for them. Nevertheless, prenatal diagnosis can be invaluable in helping parents make informed choices when their fetus is at risk for an abnormality. Often, couples find it difficult to make decisions regarding the pregnancy, and the more information available to them, the more likely the best decisions will be made in keeping with the couple's values. Another purpose of prenatal diagnosis is that normal results from prenatal testing can go a long way in reassuring women and their partners who are at high risk for an abnormal fetus. Finally, a third purpose of prenatal diagnosis is to allow couples who are afraid to have children because of a known familial or personal history of abnormalities to proceed with pregnancy, with the knowledge that abnormalities can be detected early in utero.

Unfortunately, most fetal abnormalities that are found are not easily repairable, reversible, or curable prior to birth. In recent years, a small number of research-oriented medical centers in the United States have started pioneering programs for fetal surgery. Fetal surgery involves surgical correction of anomalies while the fetus is in utero, with the hope that early correction will result in better results and fewer morbidities than waiting until after the baby is born. In fetal surgery, both the mother and the fetus must undergo surgery. The uterus is accessed through incisions on the mother's abdomen. The fetus may be temporarily removed from the uterus while the defect is being repaired. The fetus is then replaced in the uterus, and the woman's uterus and the abdominal incision are closed. Neural tube defects and congenital diaphragmatic hernias (in which a defect in the fetal diaphragm enables the fetal bowel to enter the thoracic cavity and prevent the fetal lungs from developing) are examples of fetal defects that can be repaired through fetal surgery. Fetal surgery carries considerable risks to the mother and fetus. There are the usual risks of major surgery to the mother, such as bleeding, infection, and risk of internal injury. The fetus is at increased risk of premature delivery and of persistent loss of amniotic fluid from leaks in the amniotic sac. Hence, fetal surgery is still considered experimental, and results from these procedures have been mixed at best.

Finally, amniocentesis has enabled physicians to minimize morbidity and mortality of infants in many situations in which an effective intervention exists, once the diagnosis of a disease state is established. This is especially true for maternal or fetal problems in the third trimester. Hence, the utility of amniocentesis not only involves potentially decreased stays in neonatal intensive care units but in many cases may be cost effective in the long run as well. However, the complexity of determining which specific parameters should be used to determine cost effectiveness (for example, relevant clinical options, variables, outcomes, and placement of values on the outcomes) makes this analysis extremely difficult.

—*Sanford S. Singer, Ph.D.;*
updated by Anne Lynn S. Chang, M.D.

See also Abortion; Birth defects; Chorionic villus sampling; Congenital disorders; Cystic fibrosis; Diagnosis; Down syndrome; Embryology; Fetal surgery; Genetic counseling; Genetic diseases; Genetics and inheritance; Gynecology; Intellectual disability;

Karyotyping; Laboratory tests; Obstetrics; Placenta; Pregnancy and gestation; Rh factor; Screening; Sickle cell disease; Spina bifida; Ultrasonography; Women's health.

For Further Information:

"Amniocentesis." *Health Library*, October 11, 2012.

Filkins, Karen, and Joseph F. Russo, eds. *Human Prenatal Diagnosis*. 2d ed. New York: Marcel Dekker, 1990.

Gabbe, Steven G., et al, eds. *Obstetrics: Normal and Problem Pregnancies*. 6th ed. Philadelphia: Saunders, 2012.

Heyman, Bob, and Mette Henriksen. *Risk, Age, and Pregnancy: A Case Study of Prenatal Genetic Screening and Testing*. New York: Palgrave, 2001.

Nussbaum, Robert L., Roderick R. McInnes, and Willard F. Huntington. *Thompson and Thompson Genetics in Medicine*. 7th ed. Philadelphia: Saunders/Elsevier, 2007.

Rapp, Rayna. *Testing Women, Testing the Fetus: The Social Impact of Amniocentesis in America*. New York: Routledge, 1999.

Sherwood, Lauralee. *Human Physiology: From Cells to Systems*. 8th ed. Pacific Grove, Calif.: Brooks/Cole/Cengage Learning, 2012.

Turnpenny, Peter, and Sian Ellard. *Emery's Elements of Medical Genetics*. 14th ed. New York: Churchill Livingstone/Elsevier, 2011.

Amniotic fluid

Biology

Anatomy or system affected: Embryo/Fetus

Specialties and related fields: Obstetrics, Maternal-fetal medicine, Neonatology

Definition: Protective fluid in the amniotic sac that surrounds the unborn baby.

Key terms:

AF: amniotic fluid

AFI: amniotic fluid index

AFV: amniotic fluid volume

amniotic sac: sac that contains the fetus and amniotic fluid during pregnancy and consists of the amnion and chorion membranes

anomaly: abnormality or deviation from the norm

embryo: from the 3rd through approximately the end of the 10th week of gestation

fetus: from approximately the beginning of the 11th week of gestation till birth

iIdiopathic: when the cause of a disease or condition is unknown

oligohydramnios: abnormally decreased amniotic fluid volume

polyhydramnios/hydramnios: abnormally increased amniotic fluid volume

Physiology/Structure

During pregnancy, the unborn baby, first as an embryo, then as the fetus, is surrounded by a covering, known as the amniotic sac. This sac contains a protective fluid, the amniotic fluid (AF), which starts to accumulate after the first few weeks of gestation.

AF consists of 98-99% water. The remaining 1-2% components of AF change as the pregnancy progresses.

Early in the pregnancy, the source of the AF is uncertain. It is likely derived from three sources. These are: 1) the fetal surface of the placenta,2) across the amniotic sac from the maternal blood flow of the uterus, and 3)secretions from the surface of the embryo. Presently it is unknown how much each contributes to the formation of AF.

Later in the pregnancy, production and excretion of fetal urine and fetal lung secretions become the major source of AF.

Between 8-11 weeks of gestation, the fetus begins to produce urine. This will become a major component of AF during the 2nd trimester, and by the 2nd half of the pregnancy, fetal urine will become the primary source of AF. The daily volume of urine produced by the fetus is approximately 30% of the fetal body weight.

Another source of AF is fetal lung secretions, which begins in the 2nd trimester. The fetal lungs secrete approximately 100x as much fluid as is needed for lung growth and development. Of the excess, approximately 50% is swallowed and the other approximately 50% enters the AF.

Secretions from the fetal oral-nasal cavity also contribute to AF, but as a minor source of AF production.

The production of AF is balanced by the clearance of the AF. The major source of clearance is through fetal swallowing and across the microscopic fetal vessels on the fetal surface of the placenta.

Fetal swallowing begins at 8-11 weeks, and is the major means of removal of AF from the amniotic cavity. The fetus swallows 20-25% of its body weight daily.

By late pregnancy, fetal urination contributes approximately 1000 ml and fetal lung secretions approximately 350 ml daily to the AF. Resorption by fetal swallowing is approximately 750 ml and flow across the fetal vessels on the placenta surface is approximately 400 ml daily.

The amniotic fluid volume (AFV) increases until approximately 34-36 weeks gestation, and then is stable till term. Post-term, the AF may decrease.

Function

AF is essential for normal growth and development of the fetus. It cushions and protects the fetus from trauma to the maternal abdomen. It also protects the umbilical cord from being compressed between the fetus and the uterus.

Not only does AF provide fluid and space, to permit fetal breathing, fetal movement, and fetal swallowing. It also contains important growth factors that are needed to promote normal development of the fetal lungs, musculoskeletal, and gastrointestinal systems.

The AF serves as a reservoir of fluid and nutrients for the fetus and aids in regulating temperature. It contributes to the stability of the pregnancy, by maintaining cervical length and consistency and averting contractions. In addition, the fetus receives some protection from infection through antibacterial properties of the AF.

Assessing and Monitoring

In clinical practice, assessment of AFV on prenatal sonography has become a standard component in fetal surveillance during the 2nd and 3rd trimester. This is especially important in the evaluation of high risk pregnancy. The most commonly used method is the amniotic fluid index (AFI). The deepest fluid pockets in each of the 4 quadrants of the gravid uterus are measured. The normal range of their sum is>5 and <25 cm. The average is 12-15 cm from 16 weeks until 40 weeks. Sonographic measurement of AFV is a semi-quantitative measurement. It is more accurate in assessing normal AFV. It has the potential to over or under estimate the extremes in AFV.

Volume extremes in AFV are of a concern, as they may be associated with increased risk for adverse pregnancy outcome. An evaluation for etiology is indicated when AFV abnormalities are identified.

We can asses more than just the AFV. Since AF contains fetal lung fluid, it can be tested to measure the level of AF surfactant and predict fetal lung maturity. In addition, the level of alpha-fetoprotein in AF can be used to predict open neural tube defects. AF also contains fetal cells, which can be used for prenatally genetic testing.

Polyhydramnios/Hydramnios

Polyhydramnios, also known as hydramnios, is an abnormally increased AFV and complicates 1-2% of pregnancies. It can be due to increased AF production and/or decreased AF removal. Polyhydramnios is clinically suspected if the size of the gravid uterus is larger than expected for the gestational age. The diagnosis is confirmed by sonographic examination. It can also be an incidental finding on a routine sonographic examination.

Mild polyhydramnios is an AFI of 25-29.9. It is the most common and accounts for approximately 2/3 of the incidences of polyhydramnios. Moderate is an AFI of 30-34.9, and accounts for approximately 20%, while severe is>/= to 35, and account for the remaining approximately 15%.

Mild polyhydramnios is frequently benign and idiopathic, and many cases will resolve spontaneously.

Severe polyhydramnios often has an underlying etiology and more likely to have consequences for the pregnancy. It is associated with preterm labor, preterm delivery, poor perinatal outcome, and a significant increase in congenital anomalies. The excess AF increases the possibility of fetal malpresentation, umbilical cord prolapsed, placental abruption, and postpartum hemorrhage.

Approximately 15% of pregnancies with polyhydramnios are found to be due to fetal congenital anomalies. These anomalies can prevent the resorption of AF, or increase production. Less common are congenital infections, such as cytomegalovirus, toxoplasmosis, syphilis and parvovirus.

Another 15-20% of pregnancies with polyhydramnios are due to maternal diabetes. Maternal hyperglycemia results in fetal hyperglycemia. The fetus responds to the increased glucose by increasing fetal urination, resulting in an increase in AFV

Polyhydramnios is often asymptomatic. When severe, or when it develops rapidly, the expectant mother may experience persistent shortness of breath, abdominal discomfort, edema of the lower extremities, uterine irritability and contractions.

Since etiologies are so varied, the treatments are also varied and tailored to the underlying cause in most cases. At present though, it is not clear that medical intervention for polyhydramnios improves the outcome.

Oligohydramnios

When the AFV is abnormally low, it is known as oligohydramnios. It also complicates about 1-2% of pregnancies. When there are no measurable pockets of AF on sonographic examination it is known as abhydramnios. It is clinically suspected when the size of the gravid uterus is smaller than expected for the gestational age. It is diagnosed on sonographic examination.

While polyhydramnios is often mild, with a benign prognosis, in the absence of an underlying etiology, this is not the case with oligohydramnios. More major malformations are noted with oligohydramnios than with normal AFV. Decreased production is the most common etiology, usually due to renal anomalies or impaired uteroplacental flow. It can also occur due to increased loss of AF, such as from premature rupture of membranes. It can be due to maternal dehydration, which is amenable to treatment. Medications, such as angiotensin-converting enzyme inhibitors (ACEI), angiotensin receptor blockers (ARB) and non-steroidal anti-inflammatory drugs (NSAIDS), can cause oligohydramnios by decreasing fetal urine production.

During the 1st trimester, oligohydramnios is an ominous finding. The etiology is often unclear. The pregnancy is usually not viable, and the pregnancy aborts.

With the 2nd trimester, prognosis depends on the cause and the severity of the oligohydramnios. Etiologies can include fetal anomaly, preterm premature rupture of membranes, placental abruption, and fetal growth restriction. Sometimes the cause is unknown.

When the AFV is borderline/low normal during the 2nd trimester, the prognosis is usually good. It is monitored by serial sonographic examination. When oligohydramnios is more severe, the pregnancy often ends in fetal or neonatal death. More than 50% are delivered preterm. The delivery may be spontaneous or medically indicated due to maternal or fetal complications.

When oligohydramnios develops in the 3rd trimester, etiologies include preterm premature rupture of membranes, uteroplacental insufficiency due to pre-eclampsia, maternal vascular disease, fetal anomalies, placental abruption, post-term decrease in AFV and idiopathic. There are also increased risks of poor outcome due to umbilical cord compression, uteroplacental insufficiency and meconium aspiration. In addition, there is an increased risk of cesarean deliveries, low Apgar scores, stillbirth and neonatal death.

The prognosis and treatment of oligohydramnios in the 3rd trimester depends on the cause, severity, gestational age of onset and duration of the oligohydramnios. If oligohydramnios is severe and longstanding, it is usually not amendable to intervention. No treatment has been proven to be effective long term.

The Future

AF contains fetal stem cells. These are easily collected from the AF of women undergoing amniocentesis. Amniocentesis is done as a prenatal diagnostic tool when genetic testing of the fetus is indicated. This is a potential source of stem cells for research of human genetics. This may become one of the main models for the research of human genetic diseases in the near future.

These stem cells are of interest, as they would avoid the ethic issue of using cells from human embryo tissue and animal experimentation. Also, results obtained from testing on animal models may not carry over to humans, as well as the excessive costs of animal models.

AF stem cells have shown, in vitro, the ability to differentiate into cells derived from all three germ layer. They are of interest as a model for cell therapy, due to this ability to differentiate into different cell types.

AF stem cells may have future use for tissue replacement, drug testing, study of diseases and their treatments, as well as further research on human genetics.

—*Linda Roethel, MD*

For Further Information:

Antonucci, Ivana, Martina Provenzano, Melissa Rodrigues, Andrea Pantalone, Vincenzo Salini, Patrizia Ballerini, Cesar V. Borlongan and Liborio Stuppia, "Amniotic Fluid Stem Cells: A Novel Source for Modeling of Human Genetic Disease, International Journal of Molecular Science, 2016, 17, 607. This article discusses the potential of fetal stem cells obtained from amniotic fluid. It notes the possible uses in disease research and treatment, while avoiding ethical issues of other sources of stem cells.

Beloosesky, Ron, MD, Michael G. Ross, MD, MPH, "Oligohydramnios," July 2017. An on-line reference source for health care professionals that is up dated on a regular schedule. It is concise and easy to read. The articles cross reference related topics in UpToDate, for the reader that desires further information.

Beloosesky, Ron, MD, Michael G. Ross, MD, MPH, "Polyhydramnios," July 2017. An on-line reference source for health care professionals that is up dated on a regular schedule. It is concise and easy to read. The articles cross reference related topics in UpToDate for the reader that desires further information.

Cunningham, F. Gary, Kenneth J. Leveno, Steven I. Bloom, Catherine Y. Spring, Jodi S. Dashe, Barbara L. Hoffman, Brian M. Casey, Jeanne S. Sheffield, eds, "Amniotic Fluid," Williams Obstetrics, 24th ed., McGraw-Hill Education 2014, 231-239. Well written, informative textbook on Obstetric for health care professionals.

Magann, Everett, MD, Michael G Ross., MD, MPH, "Assessment of amniotic fluid volume," July 2017. An on-line reference source for health care professionals that is up dated on a regular schedule. It is concise and easy to read. The articles cross reference related topics in UpToDate for the reader that desires further information.

Morris, RK, CH Meller, J Tamblyn, GM Malin, RD Riley, MD Kilby, SC Robson, KS Khan, "Assocoatopn amd prediction of amniotic fluid measurements for adverse pregnancy outcome: systematic riew and mets-analysis, BJOG 2014;121:686-699. Article designed for health care professionals. It reviews our present knowledge regarding the association of abnormal amniotic fluid volume with pregnancy outcome.

Nash, Patricia, NNP-BC, MSN, Amniotic Fluid Index, *NeonatalNetwork*, vol 32, no 1, January/February 2013, 46-49. An easy to read article regarding amniotic fluid index, what it measures and what an abnormal AFI may indicate.

Ross, Michael G., MD, MPH, Marie H. Beall, MD, "Physiology of amniotic fluid volume regulation," July 2017. An on-line reference source for health care professionals that is updated on a regular schedule. It is concise and easy to read.

Amphetamine

Treatment

Anatomy or system affected: Central nervous system

Specialties and related fields: Medicine, psychiatry, pediatrics, bariatrics, sleep disorders

Definition: Amphetamine is a potent central nervous system (CNS) stimulant that is used in the treatment of attention deficit hyperactivity disorder (ADHD), narcolepsy, and obesity.

Amphetamine is a stimulant drug that releases euphoric sensations and increases mental and physical performance, overcoming fatigue. The compound imitates natural stimuli, like food and water, that signal and allow the release of dopamine in the central nervous system. It has been previously prescribed to alleviate pain and ease attention-deficit hyperactivity disorder (ADHD)—especially in the 1960s, when American pharmaceutical companies distributed the drug widely and readily, eventually leading to substance abuse and a categorization of the compound as a Schedule II drug. Amphetamine misuse is still apparent, though now it is mostly evident and has a long history in three major groups: students, athletes, and the military forces.

Brief History

The use and production of stimulant compounds are as old as human records have been kept. More than 5,000 years ago, Chinese physicians would use the stimulant *ma huang* for weight loss and appetite suppression. In the 1880s, Japanese chemist Nagayoshi Nagai successfully synthesized methamphetamine from *ma huang* after discovering ephedrine, an amphetamine substitute, to be a primary and active agent in the compound. By 1887, Romanian chemist Lazar Edeleanu produced amphetamine, but the compound's effects on the central nervous system were not revealed until the 1930s, after which, reports of amphetamine abuse began to rise.

Amphetamine, like other fatigue-combatting drugs, increases the concentration of dopamine in the synaptic gap, or the space between the cell membrane of an axon terminal and the target cell, which allows a nerve cell (neuron) to pass electrical or chemical signals to other nerve cells. Dopamine increases the survival of an organism by aiding its attentiveness and learning to identify the natural threats against survival. Dopamine is a natural neuromediator that signals the brain to release sensations of pleasure following stimuli, such as food and water. Drug substances can either imitate, increase the secretion, or block natural neuromediators. Amphetamines have structures similar to that of dopamine and can use the dopamine transporters, or diffuse through the nerve cell membrane into the terminal button of the presynaptic region. Upon reaching the presynaptic region, amphetamines reverse the mechanism of the dopamine transporter to eject dopamine molecules out of their respective storage units and travel into the synaptic gap, ultimately increasing the dopamine concentrations in that gap.

The presence of amphetamine also reduces dopamine reuptake and constrains the production of monoamine oxydase A (MAO-A), an enzyme that eliminates dopamine and increases violent tendencies. Likewise, amphetamines use glutamate neurons to excite dopamine-connected neurons by removing any inhibitory effects, thus allowing the dopaminergic neurons to be easily available. The uptake of amphetamine increases the release of dopamine, simulating the presence of natural stimuli to increase the body's pleasure sensations.

Impact

Amphetamine abuse has been a widespread problem given its high toxicity levels and the resulting abnormalities in the brain's structure. Amphetamine and stimulant pills became readily available in the late 1960s in the United States and, consequently, stimulant abuse rose abruptly. Adult amphetamine abusers have lower gray-matter volume and higher striatal volumes, decreasing effective muscle control and sensory perceptions, while compensating for the excess dopamine. Children who were exposed to higher levels of amphetamine *in utero*, on the other hand, have lower striatal volumes and often develop white-matter abnormalities that affect the central nervous system.

Amphetamine affects the central nervous system, generally increasing the body's alertness, available energy, emotional stability, and presenting a sense of euphoria. Amphetamine abuse improves a person's performance, provides a feeling of euphoria and, in some cases, encourages anorexia. By the 1970s, amphetamine production was reduced by at least 80 percent and the U.S. Food and Drug Administration characterized it as a Schedule II drug, based on its stronger potential to addiction, in the hope of greatly minimizing the widespread addiction occurring across the country. As a Schedule II drug, doctors became more cautious when prescribing the drug for clinical use, given that amphetamine is often prescribed for those with attention-deficit hyperactivity disorder (ADHD).

Amphetamine abuse is prevalent in three main groups: the military, athletes, and students. Substance abuse is alluring given its effective increase in energy and improved performance that is essential in these particular fields of study and employment. Amphetamines were previously used during World War II to enhance soldier alertness during battle as well as fight mental and physical fatigue. However, as amphetamines were distributed by the members of the U.S. and British armies, the German and Japanese military followed suit, distributing methamphetamine to its brigades, thus spreading and starting the use of stimulant drugs by military forces.

Amphetamines restores performance skills that have been degraded by sleep deprivation or circadian rhythm-related deficiencies. However, the combination of sleep deprivation and stimulant drugs may have antagonistic effects, such as enhanced paranoia.

Amphetamine use in American athletes was first reported in the 1940s for American football and in the 1950s for other sports. Sleep deprivation and muscular pain is common in athletes. The use of amphetamines to combat these ailments and provide positive performances, especially the increased attention, focus, energy, self-confidence, and mood, outweigh the adverse health effects that follow, or so athletes reasoned. By the 1970s, deaths among athletes were associated to improper use of the amphetamines, causing high blood pressure from the mixture of amplified exercise performances and peripheral vasoconstriction that hinders the body from cooling down, thus leading to heat strokes and cardiac arrests. Augmented euphoria often masked the body's senses to the normal bodily warnings, deterring any possible signals of cardiac arrests.

Students and professionals use amphetamine for its effective increase in productivity and concentration. Students believe the drug increases one's alertness and ability to maintain information for longer periods of time, such that its usage enhances studying. Dependency upon amphetamines and other stimulant-related drugs has been shown to increase rates of binge alcohol-drinking, cannabis and cocaine use, as well as higher chances for heart attack and stroke for long-time users.

—*Pamela Rose V. Samonte and Rhea U. Vallente, PhD; updated by Geraldine Marrocco*

For Further Information:

Berman, Steven, et al. "Abuse of Amphetamines and Structural Abnormalities in Brain." *Annals of the New York Academy of Sciences* 1141 (2008): 195-220. PMC. Web. 5 Dec. 2015. http://www.ncbi.nlm.nih.gov/pmc/articles/PMC2769923/.

Cagniard, Barbara, et al. "The Dopamine Transporter Expression Level Differentially Affects Responses to Cocaine and Amphetamine." *Journal of Neurogenetics* 28.1-2 (2014): 112-21. Print.

Casey, Kevin F., et al. "Reduced Dopamine Response to Amphetamine in Subjects at Ultra-High Risk for Addiction." *Biological Psychiatry* 76.1 (2014): 23-30. Print.

Dubuc, Bruno. "How Drugs Affect Neurotransmitters." The Brain from Top to Bottom. Canadian Institutes of Health Research: Institute of Neurosciences, Mental Health and Addiction. Web. 5 Dec. 2015. http://thebrain.mcgill.ca/flash/i/i_03/i_03_m/i_03_m_par/i_03_m_par_amphetamine.html.

Ellinwood, E. H., G. King, and T. H. Lee. "Chronic Amphetamine Use and Abuse." Neuropsychopharmacology: The Fifth Generation of Progress. 2000. Web. 5 Dec. 2015. http://www.acnp. org/g4/gn401000166/ch162.htm.

Ruiz, P., E. C. Strain, and J. H. Lowinson. *Lowinson and Ruiz's Substance Abuse: A Comprehensive Textbook.* Wolters, 2011. Print.

Sandtner, Walter, et al. "A Quantitative Model of Amphetamine Action on the Serotonin Transporter." *Biophysical Journal* 106.2 (2014): 365a. Print.

Amputation

Procedure

Anatomy or system affected: Arms, bones, hands, joints, knees, legs, muscles, musculoskeletal system, nervous system, skin

Specialties and related fields: Critical care, emergency medicine, general surgery, oncology, orthopedics, physical therapy, plastic surgery, vascular medicine

Definition: The removal of a limb or other body part in order to prevent more serious harm to the patient.

Key terms:

disarticulation: the amputation of a limb through a joint, without cutting the bone

edema: the accumulation of an excessive amount of fluid in cells or tissues

fascia: a sheet of fibrous tissue which envelops the body beneath the skin and also encloses the muscles or groups of muscles, separating their many layers or groups

gangrene: necrosis (tissue death) caused by obstruction of the blood supply; it may be localized to a small area or involve an entire extremity

ischemia: a local anemia or area of diminished or insufficient blood supply caused by mechanical obstruction (commonly narrowing of an artery) of the blood supply

periosteum: the thick, fibrous membrane that covers the entire surface of a bone except for the cartilage within a joint

peripheral: referring to a part of the body away from the center

prosthesis: a fabricated, artificial substitute for a missing part of the body, such as a limb

prosthetist: an individual skilled in constructing and fitting prostheses

vascular: relating to or containing blood vessels

Indications and Procedures

Amputations are performed in order to preserve life or to avoid more extensive damage or destruction to an individual or a portion of the body. They are performed in response to pathological processes (bacterial or viral infections, ischemia, or cancer, for example) that do not respond to treatment or to address the aftereffects of violent trauma (accidents, crushing injuries, or bullet wounds) in which tissues have been injured so extensively that they cannot be repaired, restored, or otherwise salvaged or saved.

Extremities are the most common sites for amputations, and there are four principal reasons for removing all or part of an extremity. The first is trauma which is so severe that surgical or other repair is not possible. The second reason is the presence of a tumor in the bones, soft tissues, muscles, blood vessels, or nerves of the extremity. A third cause is extensive infection that does not respond to usual or conservative treatment or that may lead to septicemia, a generalized infection that spreads throughout the entire body through the bloodstream. The final indication for performing an amputation is the presence of peripheral vascular disease, a group of conditions that compromise or reduce the blood supply in an extremity.

Most amputations of the leg are performed because of impaired circulation, or ischemia. Several conditions may lead to ischemia, the most common of which is inadequately controlled diabetes mellitus. Others include atherosclerosis (a buildup of plaque in a blood vessel that restricts circulation), cellulitis, and vascular diseases. Bacterial infection can also lead to impaired circulation. When circulation continues to be inadequate, gangrene develops; infection can also contribute to or accelerate existing gangrene.

There are three general classes of amputation: provisional or open, conventional or standard, and osteomyoplastic. The techniques for each are briefly described.

The technique for a provisional amputation is often referred to as guillotine. In the past, this approach was commonly used in battle situations where speed was important to minimize both blood loss and subsequent infection. Cur-

rently, the technique is used mainly to remove a victim from a dangerous situation, typically one causing a crushing injury in which the alternative to amputation is death. All tissues are cut circularly. Skin is retained to the greatest degree possible, muscle and fascia are cut shorter, and the bone is cut shorter still. The hope is that the soft tissues (skin and muscles) will ultimately cover the bone, but the results are generally unsatisfactory. Large scars are common, and muscle frequently adheres to the bone. Long periods are required for healing, infections are common, and prostheses do not fit well. Another, more definitive amputation is usually required at a later date.

In a conventional amputation, skin, underlying tissues, muscle, and fascia are all cut in curved flaps that originate at the end of the remaining, unamputated bone. The muscles, fascia, bone, and major blood vessels are divided at the base of the remaining bone; nerves are cut at a slightly higher level, approximately 2.5 centimeters (1 inch) above the end of the bone. The nerves will retract somewhat into the muscle, minimizing postoperative pain. Muscles are tapered so that large masses of tissue are not present over the end of the stump; this will enhance the fit of a later prosthesis. At the cut end of the bone, the outer layer of bone is removed in order to reduce the possibility of bone spurs forming at some time in the future. The skin over the amputation site is closed loosely to avoid stretching as it heals.

The purpose of an osteomyoplastic amputation is to improve function after a prosthesis is fitted. The preparation of skin and fascia is the same as for a conventional amputation. Nerves and blood vessels are also divided. Muscles are separated for about 5 centimeters (2 inches) past the point where the bone will be cut. A portion of the outer surface (periosteum) from the bone to be amputated is sutured to the divided muscle. The bone is then cut. The prepared flap of periosteum and muscle is sutured to the periosteum of the stump. This procedure covers the marrow cavity of the stump, helps to preserve the remaining bone, and reduces postoperative infections. The remaining muscles are then sutured across the end of the stump. The skin is closed as in a conventional amputation. In an alternative procedure, holes are drilled in the bone of the stump. Muscles are inserted in the holes and sutured in place. The net effect of these osteomyoplastic procedures is to strengthen the musculature of the stump and to improve mobility for a prosthesis.

There are several common sites or levels for amputations of the leg. Syme's amputation is performed when most of the foot has been destroyed by trauma or compromised by poor circulation. In this type of amputation, the bones of the foot are removed, and the end of the tibia becomes the weight-bearing surface for the prosthesis.

A below-the-knee (BK) amputation is used to provide additional mobility for a prosthesis. It also leads to more complete rehabilitation because the knee is still available for movement. It is also associated with a reduction in phantom limb pain.

An above-the-knee (AK) amputation is frequently selected when gangrene extends into the muscles or skin of the calf. When the muscles of the leg are contracted, a prosthesis is not likely to be fitted or used; thus there is no advantage to a BK amputation in this situation. The AK amputation is associated with the highest healing rate for amputations among patients with peripheral vascular disease. The rate of a repeat amputation performed at a higher level on the leg is also low. Prostheses that permit walking, however, are less efficient with amputations at this level.

Both amputations have about the same rate of healing, but a higher percentage of individuals with BK amputations walk on prostheses than do those with AK amputations. The choice between BK and AK amputation is determined by the general health of the patient and the potential for rehabilitation. The most important determinant of level of amputation, however, is the vascular status of the patient.

The leg can also be amputated at either the knee or the hip; such a procedure is a disarticulation, an amputation through a joint. A knee disarticulation is most commonly used with children to preserve the growing portion (epiphysis) of the remaining thigh bone. A hip disarticulation is used with tumors or extensive soft tissue injuries in the thigh. Special prostheses that permit walking after such procedures are available but are relatively uncommon; however, as technology improves, such prostheses are becoming more widely available and increasingly comfortable and functional.

Portions of the upper extremity are usually amputated after extensive trauma. Malignant disease of the bone or muscle is a less common reason for amputation at these sites. The considerations described for the lower extremity are applicable for the upper extremity, namely, preserving as much tissue as possible for later rehabilitation and recovery of function. The sites for amputation are also analogous. Individual fingers can be amputated, or the entire hand can be amputated at the wrist (a location similar to the Syme's amputation of the foot). Similarly, the forearm can be amputated either below the elbow or above the elbow. Portions of the arm can be disarticulated at the elbow or at the shoulder. Restoration of function is far more difficult, however, in an upper extremity amputation than for a lower extremity amputation. It is easier to restore the ability to walk than it is to restore hand function.

Uses and Complications

The level or site of an amputation is critical to recovery and rehabilitation. When an amputation is performed because of cancer or some other malignant disease, the principal concern is a wide excision of any apparent tumor. When amputation is performed after the patient has sustained significant trauma or to treat peripheral vascular disease, the major factor determining the best site is usually the extent of healthy tissue. Other important factors include preserving sufficient length in the remaining bone or stump so that a prosthesis may be used. Furthermore, the prosthesis must be functional, must have adequate space for attachment, and must be cosmetically acceptable. The scar must be placed so that it will not break down from mechanical traction or interfere with the fit of the prosthesis.

In general, the more bone that can be left in place, the more functional a prosthetic limb will be; patients will also have better control of their prostheses. Frequently, special procedures will have to be used to save skin or to graft skin to the site of an amputation so as to preserve the length of

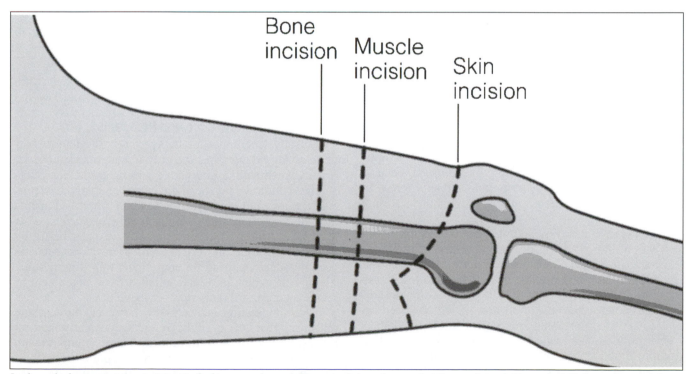

In above-the-knee amputation, incisions in the bone, muscles, and skin are made in such a way that the muscles and skin can be folded over the remaining bone, thus creating a stump to which a prosthesis may later be molded and attached.

the bone. The issue of bone length is especially critical in amputations of the upper extremities, as arms, hands, and fingers are so important in daily functions. The prospects for rehabilitation are also considered when an amputation is contemplated. For example, there is less need to preserve bone for a prosthesis if an individual is not inclined-because of temperament, age, or physical condition-to rehabilitate a lost body part.

There are different regional considerations for patients requiring an amputation for peripheral vascular disease. The ability of the skin and other tissues to heal is directly dependent on an adequate supply of blood. Injections of dye into local small arteries, a procedure called arteriography, are used to determine if the vessels can deliver sufficient blood to a proposed amputation site or around joints such as the knee.

Amputations for extensive trauma should be performed soon after the injury is sustained in order to reduce the chances for contamination or infection. This practice will also assist in subsequent psychological adjustment to the loss of the body part.

Bedridden patients frequently suffer from ulcers of the skin, or bedsores, lesions that do not heal well if at all. In combination with impaired circulation (ischemia), these ulcers can lead to the need for amputations. This group of patients must be carefully prepared for surgery by conditioning muscles that will remain after the amputation. Before an amputation is attempted, extensive efforts must be made to heal all skin ulcers. Physical therapy is frequently used before the surgery to strengthen and improve the tone of muscles. Antibiotics and frequently changed dressings are employed to fight infection. Patients should be moved frequently to avoid the formation of new skin ulcers. Special beds are often used to avoid concentrating pressure on body parts; this can be accomplished with pillows and lambskin mats. In some cases, ice packs are used in the days immediately prior to amputation to limit the spread of infection and to reduce pain.

Conventional postoperative care for amputation focuses on providing optimal tissue care: movement and specific exercises to prevent contractures (the loss of use for muscles), the compression of tissue to prevent edema, and the initiation of physical therapy to regain or retain the optimum use of the remaining body part. The ultimate goal is to provide a prosthesis wherever possible and appropriate in order to improve the patient's quality of life and vocational opportunities.

Edema is minimized by applying tight dressings to the amputation site. After sutures are removed, elastic bandages are used for the next several weeks. Exercises and movement of the stump will prevent contractures. These exercises should be started as soon as possible after the amputation. When a portion of an arm or leg has been removed, it is important to move and stretch the entire limb.

One problem associated with amputations is called phantom limb pain: the perception of pain in a body part that is no longer attached to the body. Typically, a patient who has lost a limb will experience pain or other sensation as if the limb were still intact. This phenomenon occurs because of stimulation in the nerve endings of the remaining stump. Such sensations are amplified in the posterior horn, a portion of the spinal cord. The nervous impulses are processed by the brain and interpreted as pain; it is this subjective feeling that the patient experiences. Phantom limb pain can usually be prevented by surgical techniques employed at the time of amputation.

Traumatically amputated body parts can sometimes be reattached. Portions of fingers, hands, and entire upper extremities have been successfully reattached; lower extremity reattachments are less common. The regeneration of nerves, however, is not uniformly accomplished. The myelin sheaths of nerves-the cells that surround many nerves to provide insulation and to increase the velocity of nerve impulse conduction-must be approximated for successful regeneration. The lack of nerve regeneration can affect either motor or sensory aspects of the body part. Lack of motor nerve regeneration leads to disuse atrophy and loss of functional use of the body part. Cosmetically, the body usually appears normal. Loss of sensory innervation requires adaptation, but the ability to move the body part is not affected. If the sensory loss is from skin only, the deficit is usually not significant. Sensory loss in fingers and toes is more serious; other senses such as sight and position receptors in joints must be relied upon to compensate for the lack of direct input from fingers or toes. These deficits can be overcome with rehabilitation.

Amputations performed by surgeons skilled in techniques appropriate for ischemic or necrotic tissue have the lowest incidence of postoperative complications and the highest degree of success for subsequent rehabilitation. The death rate for amputations required for isolated trauma, infection, or tumors is less than 3 percent. In contrast, amputations related to vascular diseases result in death for approximately one patient in four. Mortality rates rise with the removal of increasing amounts of a body part: The removal of a toe or foot is less likely to end in death than the removal of an entire leg.

Perspective and Prospects

Historically, techniques for amputation evolved on the battlefield. Amputation was the only treatment available for battle casualties; the alternative was death. Military surgeons were known for speed. In the early part of the twentieth century, antibiotics were discovered. Improved instrumentation and operative techniques were first developed in the 1950s. Microscopic procedures have been perfected more recently. The net effect of these developments has been to reduce the need for amputation following trauma. These same techniques have enabled the reattachment or reimplantation of fingers or other extremities.

When amputation is necessary, however, the surgeon must weigh the desires of the patient against his or her best interests. It is natural for patients to want to retain as much original tissue as possible, but surgeons prefer to perform an amputation only once. Impaired circulation compromises tissues. When individuals with conditions such as diabetes require amputation and insufficient tissue is removed, the result is frequently another amputation. Individuals with poorly controlled diabetes may lose their entire legs in a series of amputations.

After an amputation, physical therapy begins the rehabilitation process. As soon as the patient can tolerate movement, exercises are undertaken. The goal of these activities is to return the person to as normal a level of function as possible. The services of an occupational therapist are used to regain old motor skills or to learn new ones. An artificial body part is fitted by a prosthetist. The sooner a prosthesis is fitted, the greater is the probability that the patient will adapt successfully to it. Temporary prostheses initially fitted within the first twenty-four hours following surgery have had high degrees of acceptance.

Prostheses typically are of two varieties: functional and cosmetically appealing. Prostheses with wires attached to movable hooks allow limited motor function of hands. Muscles of the forearm are retrained to provide movement of the hook. Lower limb prostheses are usually more anatomically correct and cosmetically appealing. They allow walking and other movements but do not usually allow fine motor control of toes. This does not preclude the adaptation and eventual recovery of fairly complex motor skills, including those required for participation in sports activities. Research is ongoing to test the viability of implantable brain-computer interfaces that would enable patients to control their prosthetic limbs with thoughts; however, at present, these devices pose a high risk of infection and remain in the experimental stage.

One predictor of eventual success with the prosthesis is the age at which it is fitted. Young children adapt rapidly, but the older the patient is, the more difficult adaptation to a prosthesis becomes. Older persons often merely tolerate an artificial limb while younger persons accept the prosthesis and continue with the activities of their lives. Much of the rehabilitation after an amputation is psychological. With appropriate support and therapy, the potential for a nearly normal life exists for most persons experiencing an amputation.

—*L. Fleming Fallon, Jr., M.D., Ph.D., M.P.H.*

See also Arteriosclerosis; Bacterial infections; Blood vessels; Bone cancer; Bone disorders; Bone grafting; Bones and the skeleton; Cancer; Circulation; Critical care; Critical care, pediatric; Diabetes mellitus; Emergency medicine; Fracture and dislocation; Fracture repair; Frostbite; Gangrene; Grafts and grafting; Ischemia; Lower extremities; Muscles; Necrosis; Oncology; Orthopedic surgery; Orthopedics; Orthopedics, pediatric; Osteonecrosis; Physical rehabilitation; Plastic surgery; Prostheses; Skin; Tumor removal; Tumors; Upper extremities; Vascular medicine; Vascular system; Wounds.

For Further Information:

Barnes, Robert W. *Amputations: An Illustrated Manual.* Philadelphia: Hanley & Belfus, 2000.
Brunicardi, F. Charles, et al., eds. *Schwartz's Principles of Surgery.* 9th ed. New York: McGraw-Hill, 2010.
Kellicker, Patricia Griffin. "Amputation-General Overview." *Health Library*, December 30, 2012.
May, Bella J. *Amputations and Prosthetics: A Case Study Approach.* 2d ed. Philadelphia: F. A. Davis, 2002.
Smith, Douglas G. "General Principles of Amputation Surgery." In *Atlas of Amputations and Limb Deficiencies: Surgical, Prosthetic, and Rehabilitation Principles*, edited by Smith, John W. Michael, and John H. Bowker. 3d ed. Rosemont, Ill.: American Academy of Orthopaedic Surgeons, 2004.
Townsend, Courtney M., Jr., et al., eds. *Sabiston Textbook of Surgery.* 19th ed. Philadelphia: Saunders/Elsevier, 2012.

Amylase

Biology

Also known as: Ptyalin

Anatomy or system affected: Digestive

Specialties and related fields: Gasteroenterology

Definition: An enzyme from the salivary glands and pancreas that breaks down (digests) starch and glycogen to maltose, a disaccharide, trisaccharides and some glucose.

Key terms:

amylaseblockers: drugs that inhibit the action of amylase

hyperamylasemia: elevated levels of amylase in the blood and digestive system

hypoamylasemia: elevated levels of amylase in the blood and digestive system

pancreatic enzymereplacement therapy: a technique that introduces amylase into the digestive system via capsules.

Structure and Functions

Amylase refers to a class of specialized digestive enzymes synthesized by the salivary glands and pancreas. This enzyme breaks down complex carbohydrates (polysaccharides) such as starch found in rice, potatoes, breads, and grains to maltose, a disaccharide, trisaccharides and some glucose which is the primary energy source used by cells. Maltose and trisaccharides are digested by other enzymes to glucose. Amylase is produced by the salivary glands and the pancreas.

In humans, the conversion of complex carbohydrates, primarily starch, which account for a substantial percentage of the average person's diet, is essential to providing the body with glucose. Amylase begins to digest starch almost immediately as the salivary glands that line the inside of the mouth and along the throat release amylase, also known as ptyalin. Additional amylase is produced by the pancreas; that enables the body to continue to digest starch.

Disorders and Diseases

Hyperamylasemia refers to elevated levels of blood amylase. The condition can be caused by a variety of conditions including primarily perforated stomach, pancreatitis, pancreatic cancer, inflammation of the gall bladder, kidney disease and certain medications.

Hypomylasemia refers to low levels of blood amylase. It may be caused by conditions such as obesity, diabetes mellitus and metabolic syndrome. These conditions seem to be related to insufficient insulin. Amylase can be administered to patients with pancreatic amylase insufficiency via capsules in a process known as Pancreatic Enzyme Replacement Therapy. Several amylase preparations are commercially available.

The measurement of amylase in the blood and urine can help detect the onset of several diseases. Amylase measurement can also be used to detect pancreatic failure, pancreatic cancer and kidney failure. Tests that measure the level of amylase have been used to diagnose long term alcohol abuse (the enzyme works overtime to try to convert all the fermented liquid into usable sugars) and side-effects of prescription birth control pills.

Amylase inhibitors, known as starch blockers, prevent amylase from breaking down starch and other complex carbohydrates to glucose thereby preventing the absorption of glucose that would be derived from amylase action. Potentially, amylase inhibitors could be used as a weight loss treatment and as a treatment for diabetes.

Perspective and Prospects

Amylase was the first enzyme to be discovered, isolated and named. Anselm Payen (1795-1871), a French industrial biochemist, was the first to classify natural enzymes as part of a wider research project centered on refining and purifying sugar in sugar beets. Payen was specifically interested in removing the signature reddish coloration from the sugar. In that research, he isolated the enzyme and named it diastase, from a Greek word meaning to separate or set apart. In 1833, while working with Jean Françoise Persoz (1805-1868) to define the principal processes in large-scale beer and wine production, Payen further isolated amylase as a naturally occurring catalyst in the concentrated barley or grain mixture that stimulated the production of sugar from the grains, an elemental step in the fermentation process.

The diet of modern humans contains a substantially more complex carbohydrate than did the diet of our paleolithic ancestors. Our paleolithic ancestors did not produce salivary amylase. With the changing of the diet to one that is composed of more complex carbohydrates, it became an advantage for the salivary glands to produce amylase. The gene coding for pancreatic amylase (*AMY1*) duplicated and evolved into one active in the salivary glands. Research has demonstrated that cultures that consume higher amounts of complex carbohydrates in their diets have more copies of the *AMY1* gene than cultures that consume diets lower in complex carbohydrates.

Amylase can be used commercially in the production of beer and some liquors. Yeast produces amylase which can digest the starch in grain to glucose which the yeast further metabolizes into alcohol.

—*Joseph Dewey, PhD;*
updated by Charles L. Vigue, PhD

For Further Information:
"Amylase." *United States National Library of Medicine.* Web. 10 June 2015.
"Amylase: The Importance of Carbhydrates." *EnzymeEssentials.* Web. 10 June 2015.

Filaire, Edith, et al. "Dietary Intake, Eating Behaviors, and Diurnal Patterns of Salivary Cortisol and Alpha-Amylase Secretion among Professional Young Adult Female Tennis Players." *International Journal of Sport Nutrition& ExerciseMetabolism* 25.3 (2015): 233-242. *Academic Search Complete.* Web. 2 Aug. 2015.
Lark, Susan M. *Enzymes: The Missing Link to Health.* Washington's Crossing: Women's Wellness, 2013. Print.
Sandor, Ellix Katz. *The Art of Fermentation: An In-Depth Exploration of Essential Concepts and Processes from around the World.* White River Junction: Chelsea Green, 2012. Print.
Shelton, C. D. *Carbohydrates: The Facts about Starches and Sugars.* Harrisonburg: *Choice,* 2013. Print.
Shinga, Hiromi. *The EnzymeFactor.* Graham: Millichap, 2011. Print.
Silverman, Richard B. *The OrganicChemistryof EnzymeCatalyzed Reactions.* London: Academic P, 2002. Print.
Xian, Liang, et al. "Purification and Characterization of a Highly Efficient Calcium-Independent α-Amylase from Talaromyces Pinophilus 1-95." *Plos ONE* 10.3 (2015): 1-18. *Academic Search Complete.* Web. 2 Aug. 2015.

Amyotrophic lateral sclerosis (ALS)
Disease/Disorder
Also known as: Lou Gehrig's disease
Anatomy or system affected: Musculoskeletal system, nervous system, respiratory system
Specialties and related fields: Alternative medicine, biochemistry, family medicine, gastroenterology, internal medicine, neurology, physical therapy, psychiatry, psychology, pulmonary medicine, speech pathology
Definition: A progressive, degenerative neurological disorder that affects neurons in the brain and spinal cord.
Key terms:
electromyography(EMG): a technique used to diagnose various nerve and muscle disorders, entailing continuous recording of the electrical activity in a muscle with electrodes
motorneuron: one of several units that make up the nerve pathway between the brain and the specific organ connected to it
fasciculation: a brief, spontaneous contraction of muscle fibers associated with disorders of the lower motor neurons
lower motorneuron: a type of nerve with its cell body in the spinal cord and an axon that extends from the spinal cord into a peripheral or cranial nerve that eventually connects with and directs the activity of a skeletal muscle. Lower motor neurons that connect (synapse) with upper motor neurons in the brain stem or spinal cord.
spasticity: a rigidity or resistance to passive limb movement, usually occurring in limbs that are weak, respond in an impaired way to voluntary control, and whose weakness is thought to be due to observed lesions in the upper motor neurons
upper motorneuron: a type of nerve with a cell body in the brain and an axon that extends down the brain stem and/or spinal column and connects (synapses) with a lower motor neuron.

Causes and Symptoms

Amyotrophic lateral sclerosis (ALS) refers to a group of progressive diseases involving neurons that control voluntary muscle contraction. Both upper neurons originating in the brain and lower neurons originating in the spinal cord are affected. These neurons progressively deteriorate and eventually die, leaving atrophied muscles in their wake. Between fourteen and fifteen thousand Americans are affected with ALS, with five thousand new cases diagnosed each year. Although the disease affects people of all races and ethnicities, Caucasians and non-Hispanics are affected more commonly. Males are affected slightly more often than females. ALS tends to affect individuals between the ages of fifty-five to seventy-five, although it can affect people of all ages.

Despite extensive epidemiological, controlled, and clinical research, the cause or causes of ALS are unknown. The disease is random and sporadic in 90 percent of the cases. It does not run in families. There are no known risk factors, and it does not seem to develop following exposure to toxins, radiation, or any particular environmental sources. Diet appears to have no effect. Five to ten percent of all ALS cases are inherited in what is referred to as the familial form. Familial cases usually only require one parent to be a carrier for the disease gene. Several ALS causative genes have been discovered. In familial cases and in some sporadic cases, twenty-five to forty percent have a mutation in chromosome 9 open reading frame 72, or *C9ORF72*, which is also involved with certain forms of dementia. *C9ORF72* codes for a protein that localizes in neurons, although the mechanism of its involvement with ALS is unknown. Twelve to twenty percent of familial cases have a mutation in the gene that encodes the copper-zinc superoxide dismutase 1 (*SOD1*). It is not known how a mutation in *SOD1* can lead to the symptoms associated with ALS, but the SOD1 protein detoxifies superoxide radicals (O_2^-) and an inability to clear these reactive oxygen species may cause increased cell damage and cell death. The causes of most other cases are unknown but may involve defects in RNA and/or protein processing and/or metabolism. Research has not identified any specific and consistent association between any environmental factor and ALS.

ALS researchers have also noted the presence of increased glutamate in the spinal cord and serum in some familial and nonfamilial cases. It is theorized that glutamate may play a key role in the mechanism of nerve damage. Other theories about what causes ALS assign important roles to the body's own immune system, suggesting that ALS may be an autoimmune disease, similar in mechanism (if not effect) to systemic lupus erythematosus.

The early symptoms of ALS are almost always gradual and subtle in its early stages and often include muscle weakness. People may slur speech or experience weakening grip. Fasciculations, cramps and spasticity are common. They become clumsy and unsteady, penmanship worsens, and their limbs weaken. Although the rate of progression of the disease varies widely from individual to individual, the course or stages of deterioration remain fairly universal. As the disease progresses and attacks voluntary motor functions, patients develop increasing difficulty with walking, swallowing, talking, and dressing. Further progression may require more aggressive support with

---

Information on Amyotrophic Lateral Sclerosis

Causes: Unknown
Symptoms: Slurred speech, weakening grip, clumsiness and unsteadiness, weakened limbs
Duration: Progressive and fatal
Treatments: None; symptomatic relief and comfort measures

---

feeding tubes and mechanical ventilators. In the later stages of ALS, patients become very susceptible to pneumonia. Most ALS patients die of respiratory failure within three to five years after diagnosis.

Perhaps the most insidious aspect of ALS is that while voluntary muscles deteriorate, thinking and emotions remain completely unaffected. Individuals are aware of the entire disease process, loss of independence, and decreasing ability to express themselves. Perhaps even more important than the medical management of the disease is the attention to the existential, psychological, and family challenges that ensue.

There is no single definitive diagnostic test for ALS. Diagnosis usually involves an analysis of symptoms. For the neurological specialist, the key to diagnosing and differentiating ALS is ruling out other motor neuron disorders that mimic ALS. The presence of simultaneous upper neuron and lower motor neuron damage is often indicative of ALS. The diagnosis of ALS is made because other, more common and more treatable, motor neuron diseases have been excluded.

There are several diagnostic procedures helpful in determining the patient's diagnosis. Electromyography (EMG) is a diagnostic technique that detects electrical activity in the muscles. Specific EMG patterns and findings can be diagnostic of ALS, though not all patterns are clear, distinct, and unambiguous. Nerve conduction studies that measure the nerve's ability to transmit signals are also used to help differentiate ALS from peripheral neuropathy or myopathies. Magnetic resonance imaging (MRI) provides visual images of the brain and spinal cord. While MRI readings are usually normal in ALS patients, an MRI is often ordered to help the physician determine that the symptoms are not from another disorder, evident in an abnormal or significant MRI reading. Laboratory tests for various infections can rule out the cause of symptoms as an infectious disease.

Treatment and Therapy

There is no specific treatment or cure for ALS. The mainstays of therapy rely on supportive assistance with mobility and communication, symptomatic relief, and comfort measures. Medications such as riluzole (*Rilutek*) can decrease the release of glutamate, and a few studies have shown that riluzole may prolong survival and slow the rate of deterioration. Unfortunately, it does not halt or reverse neuron damage. Pain is usually not a symptom of ALS. Edaravone (*Radicava*) seems to slow "the decline in clinical assessment of daily functioning". More problematic are feelings of stiffness, soreness, and discomfort. Both pharmacologic and non-pharmacologic treatments can bring symptomatic relief of spasticity, fatigue, and fasciculations, significantly improving patients comfort and quality of life. Allied health care providers such as nutritionists, physical, occupational, respiratory and speech therapists play an important role in helping to keep patients, and often their families, functional, maintaining independence and mobility as much as possible. As muscle weakness progresses, assistive devices such as communication and sign boards, leg splints, and wheelchairs may be needed. Mental and behavioral health specialists, as well as hospice programs, provide much needed support and relief for both patients and family members who are typically the caregivers of the ALS patient.

Perspective and Prospects

The National Institute of Neurological Diseases and Stroke (NINDS) continues to search for genetic, biochemical, molecular, cellular and environmental causes of ALS and its subsequent neuronal degeneration and progression. Research continues on possible genetic and epigenetic causes of ALS by studying several genes in various animal models. Skin cells from ALS patients have been induced to form stem cells which can differentiate into neurons. Scientists are searching for a biological marker for ALS. Such a discovery may yield a method of early detection and possible prevention. The NINDS is also searching for new treatments for ALS such as gene, biochemical, cellular, immunological and drug therapies.

Updated by Charles L. Vigue, PhD

For Further Information:
Dunsky, Eliot H. *ALS: An Orientation*. Self-published. North Charleston, South Carolina: CreateSpace, 2016.
Feigenbaum, David, ed. *Journeys with ALS*. Virginia Beach, Va.: DLRC Press, 1998.
Hoffmann, Michael. *The Origin of Amyotrophic LateralSclerosis*. Amazon Kindle, 2015.
Kimura, Jun, and Ryuji Kaji, eds. *Physiologyof ALS and Related Diseases*. New York: Elsevier Science, 1997.
McFarlane, Rodger, and Philip Bashe. *The Complete Bedside Companion: No-Nonsense Advice on Caring for the Seriously Ill*. New York: Simon & Schuster, 1998.
Mitsumoto, Hiroshi, and Theodore L. Munsat, eds. *Amyotrophic LateralSclerosis: A Guide for Patients and Families*. 3d ed. New York: Demos Health, 2009.
National Institute of Neurological Disorders and Stroke. "Amyotrophic lateral sclerosis (ALS) Fact Sheet." https://www.ninds.nih.gov/Disorders/Patient-Caregiver-Education/Fact-Sheets/Amyotrophic-Lateral-Sclerosis-ALS- Fact-Sheet.
Oliver, David, Gian Domenico Borasio, and DeclanWalsh, eds. *PalliativeCare in Amyotrophic LateralSclerosis*. 2d ed. New York: Oxford University Press, 2006.
Parker, James N., and Philip M. Parker, eds. *Official Patient's Sourcebook on Amyotrophic LateralSclerosis*. San Diego, Calif.: Icon Health, 2003.

Anal cancer
Disease/Disorder
Also known as: Cancer of the anal canal, anorectal cancer, rectal cancer, anal neoplasia, Bowen's disease, Paget's disease, HPV-related anal dysplasia, anal intraepithelial neoplasm

Anatomy or system affected: Anus, gastrointestinal system
Specialties and related fields: Gastroenterology, oncology, proctology
Definition: Cancer affecting the lower alimentary tract, including the interior anal canal from the anorectal ring to the anal verge with 5 centimeters of skin extending beyond, including the perianal skin.
Key terms:
anal intraepithelial neoplasia (AIN): precursor lesions to the development of anal cancer
anoscopy: examination of the anal canal via a small tubal instrument inserted a few inches into the anus
human papillomavirus (HPV): a virus with numerous serotypes, including types 16 and 18, implicated in cervical and anal cancer

Causes and Symptoms

The human papillomavirus (HPV), especially serotypes 16 and 18, is believed to be a major risk factor for anal cancer. Receptive anal intercourse is a risk (but not a necessary factor) in acquisition of the virus. A history of sexually transmitted infection and/or multiple sexual partners and immunosuppression, including from HIV-AIDS, are also associated with an increased risk. Women with cervical or vulvar cancer are at an increased risk for developing anal cancer.

The symptoms depend on the area affected and the cell types. Some cell types, such as squamous cell carcinoma and basaloid squamous carcinoma, are most likely to cause bleeding. A mass may be present upon examination, but it will not be noticed by most patients, and constipation or obstruction is not a significant symptom in most cases. Perianal carcinoma is more likely to cause itching.

Treatment and Therapy

Physical examination may include any of the following: a digital rectal exam, cytology (anal Pap), high-resolution anoscopy with 3 percent acetic acid, proctoscopy, and palpation of the inguinal lymph nodes. Biopsy must be done to confirm the diagnosis of abnormalities, with examination of the inguinal lymph nodes for metastatic disease. Additional studies for metastasis include lung films, liver enzyme serum studies, computed tomography (CT) scans, endoscopic ultrasound, and examination of any additional presenting symptoms related to other body systems.

Anal cancer is staged from 0 to IV, with stage 0 having the best prognosis. Outcomes for anal cancer depend on the following: the size of the lesions (smaller lesions correlate with improved prognosis over larger lesions); the location of the lesions (those in the perianal skin have a better prognosis than those deeper in the anal canal); differentiation of the tumors (well-differentiated tumors correlate with a better prognosis than tumors that are poorly differentiated); and lymph node involvement or other extension of the tumor (lack of nodal involvement or other tumor extension improves prognosis). About 50 percent of anal cancer is di-

Information on Anal Cancer

Causes: Human papillomavirus (HPV) serotypes 16 and 18, high-risk sexual activity, immunosuppression

Symptoms: Bleeding, itching, pain; may be asymptomatic

Duration: Chronic

Treatments: Surgery, radiation, chemotherapy

agnosed through localized lesions. General mortality rates are estimated at 14 percent, meaning that most patients have a good prognosis.

Because of the rare nature of this cancer, studies on preferred treatments have been limited, and treatment is guided by individual factors such as site of involvement, size of lesion, cell type and differentiation, and extension beyond the primary lesion. Treatment may involve surgical removal of the lesion, chemotherapy, and radiation. Most management is now done with radiation therapy and chemotherapy with 5-fluorouracil (5-FU) and mitomycin. Radiation accounts for most of the treatment-related toxicities; however, new developments such as intensity-modulated radiation therapy (IMRT) may decrease adverse effects, and there are ongoing investigations into less toxic and more efficacious chemotherapeutic regimens, especially the substitution of cisplatin for mitomycin or combination of the two agents. Recommendations call for close medical follow-up after treatment.

Perspective and Prospects

Anal cancer is relatively uncommon, making up only about 4 percent of cancers of the alimentary tract. However, rates are increasing, especially among men and, in particular, HIV-positive men. Approximately 4,700 cases are diagnosed yearly in the United States. It is estimated that about 7,000 cases will be diagnosed and 900 will die of the disease in 2013.

Prevention may be conferred by the expanded availability of vaccines against HPV and by lifestyle modifications to reduce sexual risk. Screening guidelines for the performance of anal Paps are in flux, but these tests have become more widely available with liquid-based cytology. Discussion of the use of anal Pap tests is ongoing, particularly for HIV-positive individuals at an increased risk for anal cancer. Anal Pap screening may diagnose anal intraepithelial neoplasia (AIN), the development of precursor lesions similar to cervical intraepithelial neoplasia (CIN), the development of precursor lesions to cervical cancer. Detection of precursor lesions by Pap testing can then be followed by high-resolution anoscopy, similar to cervical colposcopy. Early diagnosis of AIN may lead to effective treatment, similar to diagnosis of CIN; however, the lack of standard screening recommendations and limited resources for the referral of patients with positive anal Pap findings limit many clinicians from screening.

For Further Information:

Chiao E. Y., et al. "Screening HIV-infected Individuals for Anal Cancer Precursor Lesions: A Systematic Review." *Clinical Infectious Diseases* 43 (2006): 223-33.

Czito B. G., and C. G. Willett. "Current Management of Anal Canal Cancer." *Current Oncology Reports* 11 (2009): 186-92.

Das, P., C. H. Crane, and J. A. Ajani. "Current Treatment for Localized Anal Carcinoma." *Current Opinion in Oncology* 19 (2007): 396-400.

Fox, P. "Anal Cancer Screening in Men Who Have Sex with Men." *Current Opinion in HIV/AIDS* 4 (2009): 64-67.

Franceschi, S., and H. De Vuyst. "Human Papillomavirus Vaccines and Anal Carcinoma." *Current Opinion in HIV/AIDS* 4 (2009): 57-63.

Gervaz, P., N. Buchs, and P. Morel. "Diagnosis and Management of Anal Cancer." *Current Gastroenterology Reports* 10 (2008): 502-6.

Jemal, A., et al. "Cancer Statistics, 2006." *CA: A Cancer Journal for Clinicians* 56 (2006): 106-30.

MedlinePlus. "Anal Cancer." *MedlinePlus*, Apr. 10, 2013 (updated Aug. 28, 2012).

National Cancer Institute. "Anal Cancer." *National Cancer Institute*, n. d..

National Cancer Institute. "SEER Stat Fact Sheets: Anal Cancer." *National Cancer Institute: Surveillance Epidemiology and End Results*, n. d.

Raper, J. L. "Anal Pap Screening in Men with HIV." *ADVANCE for Nurse Practitioners* 14 (2006): 30-35.

Seaman, Andrew M. "Anal Cancer May Be on the Rise in the U.S." *Reuters Health Information*, Mar. 22, 2013.

Analgesic

Treatment

Anatomy or system affected: Peripheral or central nervous system

Specialties and related fields: Pain management, oncology, medicine, nursing

Definition: An analgesic or painkiller is any member of the group of drugs used to achieve analgesia, relief from pain.

An analgesic is a medication taken to alleviate pain. "Painkiller" is the common term for an analgesic. The outcome of taking an analgesic is analgesia, being without pain. Analgesia is not associated with loss of consciousness as in anesthesia. Most analgesics provide pain relief rather than reducing inflammation, although some varieties have an anti-inflammatory quality. Certain analgesics are available without a prescription and can be purchased over the counter at a pharmacy or local store. Others can only be obtained with a prescription provided by a doctor. The long-term use of an analgesic may result in a detrimental effect on body organs. While an analgesic may be safe under certain circumstances, in other instances it may not be.

Background

There are different types of analgesics, available either as over-the-counter or opioid analgesics. Over-the-counter analgesics do not require a prescription; these include brand names such as Tylenol (generic name acetaminophen). They may also be termed simple analgesics. Aspirin or paracetamol provide the generic makeup. An opioid analgesic can only be obtained through a licensed professional's prescription (MD, DO, APRN). When pain is severe, certain medications are available as a combination of acetaminophen and opioid analgesic. An analgesic is generally recommended to any person suffering from pain, with opioids often prescribed only for severe or acute pain. Often, chronic pain may also be treated by an opioid analgesic.

An opioid is also called a narcotic analgesic. Opioids contain opium or morphine derivatives. There is an increased risk of side effects when talking a narcotic. Moreover, the potential toward addiction of an opioid needs to be taken into account, particularly if the patient shows a propensity to addiction. Often when pain is severe and warrants an opioid, the practitioner has an assessment instrument to evaluate the diagnosis, intractability, risk and efficacy (DIRE). By means of a score system including what caused the pain, as well as the physical and psychological health of the patient, the adverse effects versus the benefits can be determined.

A non-steroidal anti-inflammatory drug (NSAID) is another type of analgesic. These medicines are generically known as ibuprofen, diclofenac sodium, or naproxen sodium. An NSAID is an analgesic drug that also acts as an anti-inflammatory. Aspirin, while primarily an analgesic, functions to reduce inflammation as well.

It is essential to follow the dosage and instructions for usage when taking an analgesic. The maximum amount for adults should not exceed 3,000 mg per day. This equals six 500 mg tablets or two tablets up to three times in a day. At times up to four times a day (4,000 mg) is permitted. The number of days one can continue taking the analgesic is clearly stated or will be advised by the doctor. Some stronger versions contain more than 500 mg, and this needs to be checked accordingly. In some instances, an analgesic is taken as needed, or at regular intervals as prescribed to control pain relief. With opioid analgesics, there is an added warning not to stop taking the medication abruptly to prevent withdrawal effects.

Overview

An analgesic creates pain relief by the medication blocking the pain signal on route to the brain. The inhibition of an enzyme, or diverting an interpretive message to the brain, may also be factors contributing to the modulation or alleviation of pain.

Simple analgesics and NSAIDS do not usually result in a dependency on the drug. Taking an opioid might. Over a period of time when taking an opioid, the body becomes tolerant to the drug. What transpires as a result is that the medication becomes less effective, and the person experiencing pain feels that he or she requires more medication. There is a cycle that occurs whereby the level of tolerance leads to a breakthrough withdrawal sensation. In this case, there is an increased degree of pain, often greater than when the analgesic was first taken. More medication is then consumed, and combined with the feeling that additional and more frequent use is required, a system of addiction sets in. Opioids create a physical dependency when used on a long-term basis. Checking that the dosage is not raised indiscriminately is crucial to avoid consumption overload. The problem with chronic pain is the requirement of regular analgesic use and the tolerance that comes about.

Side effects when taking analgesics may be mild or extremely severe. These effects depend largely on how much and how often the drug is taken. For instance, paracetamol may be considered a harmless drug, even when taken on a regular long-term basis. However, if too much paracetamol is taken, damage can occur to the liver and kidneys. Aspirin can likewise have an adverse effect on the renal system. This type of analgesic is not indicated for children or during pregnancy. Anyone with asthma cannot take aspirin, nor should a person with stomach issues such as ulcers. NSAIDS can cause potentially serious or life-threatening side effects when taken in large doses or for a prolonged time. Circulatory or heart problems can occur, with the threat of a cardiac attack or stroke. The gastrointestinal system may be severely compromised. Bleeding or perforation may happen. Conditions such as these may result in fatalities. The elderly are at a higher risk. Damage to the kidneys is particularly pertinent regarding the use of analgesics. Over-the-counter analgesics, especially when medicines are mixed, can result in analgesic nephropathy (kidney damage). Acetaminophen and NSAIDS like aspirin or ibuprofen taken over a long duration can be responsible for this type of damage to the inner structures of the organ. When self-medicating and without following doctor's guidance, this is more likely to occur. An opioid analgesic may cause drowsiness or dizziness; other effects can include constipation, vomiting, blood pressure changes, or confusion, and even hallucinations. Driving when taking an opioid is not advised. Serious side effects are equivalent to other analgesics, in addition to the increased risk of tolerance and addiction.

Severe side effects often come about because of the mixture of medicines or taking more than the recommended daily dosage for a few years. A medical doctor will take into account the patient's history and other prescriptions in order to best ascertain the appropriate medicinal combination, where relevant. The reaction to incorrect usage or interactions with other medicines may be experienced immediately, or the damage may set in on an incremental basis. Interactions with other drugs or alcohol can be detrimental or fatal.

—*Leah Jacob, MA*

For Further Information:
"Analgesics." *ArthritisFoundation.* Arthritis Foundation National Office, n.d. Web. 7 June 2016.
"Analgesics (Pain Relievers)." *Reconnexion.* Reconnexion, 2013. Web. 7 June 2016.
"Analgesic Nephropathy." *US National Library of Medicine.* US National Library of Medicine, 3 May 2016. Web. 7 June 2016.
"Analgesics Overview." *ArthritisFoundation.* Arthritis Foundation National Office, n.d. Web. 7 June 2016.
Campbell, John Dr. "Pain 5, Analgesic Pathways." Online video clip. *YouTube.* YouTube, 29 Nov. 2013. Web. 7 June 2016.
Eustice, Carol. "Analgesic Medication: What You Should Know." *Verywell.* Verywell, 29 Apr. 2016. Web. 7 June 2016.

"Over-the-counter Pain Relievers." *US National Library of Medicine.* US National Library of Medicine, 3 May 2016. Web. 7 June 2016.

"Painkillers (Analgesics)." *ArthritisResearch UK.* Arthritis Research UK, Sept. 2011. Web. 7 June 2016.

Anatomy

Anatomy or system affected: All
Specialties and related fields: All
Definition: The structure of the human body-its parts, systems, and organs.
Key terms:

abdomen: the rib-free part of the trunk, below the diaphragm

head: the part of the body containing the major sense organs (such as the eyes and ears) and the brain

lower extremities: the thigh, lower leg, and foot

thorax: the part of the trunk above the diaphragm, containing the ribs; the chest

trunk: the central part of the body, to which the extremities are attached

upper extremities: the arm, forearm, and hand

Structure and Functions

The body's parts can be categorized either regionally or functionally. Regionally, the body consists of a trunk to which are attached two upper extremities, two lower extremities, and a head that is attached by means of a neck. Functionally, the body consists of a digestive system, a circulatory system, an excretory system, a respiratory system, a reproductive system, a nervous system, an endocrine system, an integument (skin), a skeleton, and a series of muscles.

Regionally, the trunk can be divided into an upper portion called the chest (or thorax), containing ribs, and a lower, rib-free portion called the abdomen. Internally, the thorax and abdomen are separated by a muscular sheet called the diaphragm. The upper extremities of the trunk include the arms, forearms, and hands; the lower extremities include the thighs, lower legs, and feet. The head includes the brain and the major sense organs such as the eyes and ears; the neck is the narrower, flexible part that connects the head to the trunk. The ventral (front) surface of the abdomen is often divided around the umbilicus into upper-left, upper-right, lower-left, and lower-right quadrants.

Functionally, the body consists of a number of organ systems. The digestive system breaks down foods into simpler substances and absorbs them. The circulatory system transports oxygen and other materials around the body. The excretory system rids the body of many waste products, while the respiratory system rids the body of carbon dioxide and adds oxygen to the blood. The reproductive system produces sex cells and, in females, provides an environment for the development of an embryo. The nervous system sends signals in the form of nerve impulses from one part of the body to another, and the endocrine organs send chemical messengers (hormones) through the bloodstream. The integument, or skin, protects the outer surface of the body from infection, from injury, and from drying out (desicca-

Directional Terms for the Body
Superior: upward; toward the top of the head
Inferior: downward; toward the ground or the feet
Cranial: toward the head; the same as superior in humans
Caudal: toward the tail
Dorsal: toward the back
Ventral: toward the belly surface
Medial: toward the midline
Lateral: away from the midline
Radial: on the medial side (or thumb side) of the arm, forearm, and hand
Ulnar: on the lateral side (or little finger side) of the arm, forearm, and hand; the same side that contains the ulna
Anterior: forward, in the customary direction of motion; equivalent to ventral in humans, but the same as cranial in other animals
Posterior: toward the rear, opposite to the customary direction of motion; equivalent to dorsal in humans, but the same as caudal in other animals

tion); it also maintains the body's internal temperature by providing insulation and preventing the body from overheating during exercise through sweating. The skeleton serves as the body's framework and consists of 206 separate bones; these bones support the body's other organs and also protect the heart, the lungs, and especially the central nervous system (including the brain and the spinal cord). The muscles contract and produce movements.

Each major organ system is constructed of several major organs. The major organs contained within the thorax, for example, are the heart, lungs, and thymus body. The major organs contained within the abdomen include the stomach, spleen, liver, pancreas, small intestine (consisting of the duodenum, ileum, and jejunum), large intestine (consisting of the cecum, colon, and rectum, with the colon further divided into an ascending colon, transverse colon, descending colon, and sigmoid colon), and bladder. The kidneys and urinary ducts lie along the dorsal body wall of the abdomen. Also contained within the lower abdomen are the uterus, ovaries, and Fallopian tubes in the female and the vas deferens and prostate gland in the male. In males, two downward extensions of the abdominal cavity form the scrotal sacs that surround the testes.

The thoracic and abdominal cavities (and the scrotal cavities in males) are all considered part of the general body cavity, or coelom. Each part of the coelom is lined on all sides with a thin, single layer of flat (squamous) cells known as the peritoneum. The peritoneum forming the outer wall of these cavities is called the parietal peritoneum; the peritoneum on the outer surface of the internal organs, or viscera, is called the visceral peritoneum.

Each type of organ is made of a number of different tissues. The four major types of tissues are epithelial tissues, connective tissue, muscle tissue, and nervous tissue. Epithelial tissues (or epithelium) include those tissues that originate in broad, flat surfaces; their functions include protection, absorption, and secretion. Epithelia can be one-layered (simple) or many-layered (stratified). Their cells can be flat (squamous), tall and skinny (columnar), or equal in height and width (cuboidal). Some simple epithelia have nuclei at two different levels, giving the false appearance of different layers; these tissues are called pseudostratified. Some simple squamous epithelia have special names: The inner lining of most blood vessels is called the endothelium, while the lining of the body cavities (including all parts of the coelom) is called the mesothelium. Kidney tubules and most small ducts are also lined with simple squamous epithelia. The pigmented layer of the eye's retina and the front surface of the lens are examples of simple cuboidal epithelia. Simple columnar epithelia form the inner lining of most digestive organs and the linings of the small bronchi and the gallbladder. The epithelia lining the Fallopian tubes, nasal cavities, and bronchi are ciliated, meaning that the cells have small, hairlike extensions called cilia.

The outer layer of skin is a stratified squamous epithelium; other stratified squamous epithelia line the inside of the mouth, esophagus, and vagina. Sweat glands and other glands in the skin are lined with stratified cuboidal epithelia. Most of the urinary tract is lined with a special kind of stratified cuboidal epithelium, called a transitional epithelium, that allows a large amount of stretching. Parts of the pharynx, the larynx, the urethra, and the ducts of the mammary glands are lined with stratified columnar epithelium.

Glands are composed of epithelial tissues that are highly modified for secretion. They may be either exocrine glands (in which the secretions exit by ducts to targets nearby) or endocrine glands (in which the secretions are carried by the bloodstream to targets some distance away). The salivary glands in the mouth, the glandular lining of the stomach, and the sebaceous glands of the skin are examples of exocrine glands. The thyroid gland, adrenal gland, and pituitary gland are examples of endocrine glands. The pancreas has both exocrine and endocrine portions: The exocrine parts secrete digestive enzymes, while the endocrine parts, called the islets of Langerhans, secrete the hormones insulin and glucagon.

Connective tissues are tissues containing large amounts of material called extracellular matrix, located outside the cells. The matrix may be a liquid (such as blood plasma), a solid containing fibers of collagen and related proteins, or an inorganic solid containing calcium salts (as in bone). Blood and lymph are connective tissues with a liquid matrix (plasma) that can solidify when the blood clots. In addition to plasma, blood contains red cells (erythrocytes), white cells (leukocytes), and the tiny platelets that help form clots. The many kinds of leukocytes include granular types (basophils, neutrophils, and eosinophils, all named according to the staining properties of their granules), the monocytes, and the several types of lymphocytes. Lymph contains lymphocytes and plasma only.

Most connective tissues have a solid matrix, which includes fibrous proteins such as collagen and elastic fibers in some cases. If all the fibers are arranged in the same direction, as in ligaments and tendons, the tissue is called regular connective tissue. The dermis of the skin is an example of an irregular connective tissue in which the fibers are arranged in all directions. Loose connective tissue and adipose (fat) tissue both have very few fibers. The simplest type of loose connective tissue with the fewest fibers is sometimes called areolar connective tissue. Adipose tissue is a connective tissue in which the cells are filled with fat deposits.

Hemopoietic (blood-forming) tissue occurs in bone marrow and in the thymus, and it contains the immature cell types that develop into most connective tissue cells, including blood cells. Cartilage tissue matrix contains a shock-resistant complex of protein and sugar-like (polysaccharide) molecules. Cartilage cells usually become trapped in this matrix and eventually die, except for those closest to the surface. Bone tissue gains its supporting ability and strength from a matrix containing calcium salts. Its typical cells, called osteocytes, contain many long strands by which these cells exchange nutrients and waste products with other osteocytes and ultimately with the bloodstream. Bone also contains osteoclasts, large cells responsible for bone resorption and the release of calcium into the bloodstream.

Mesenchyme is an embryonic connective tissue made of wandering, amoeba-like cells. During embryological development, the mesenchyme cells develop into many different cell types, including hemocytoblasts, which give rise to most blood cells, and fibroblasts, which secrete protein fibers and then usually differentiate into other cell types.

Muscle tissues are specially modified for contraction. When a nerve impulse is received, overlapping fibers of the proteins actin and myosin slide against one another to produce the contraction. The three types of muscle tissue are smooth muscle, cardiac muscle, and skeletal muscle. The term *striated muscle* is sometimes used to refer to cardiac and skeletal muscle, both of which have cylindrical fibers marked by cross-bands, which are also called cross-striations. The striations are caused by the lining up of the contractile proteins actin and myosin. Smooth muscle contains cells with tapering ends and centrally located nuclei. Muscular contractions are smooth, rhythmic, and involuntary, usually not subject to fatigue. The cells are not cross-banded. Smooth muscle occurs in many digestive organs, reproductive organs, and skin, as well as in many other organs. Cardiac muscle occurs only in the heart. Its cross-striated fibers branch and come together repeatedly. Contractions of these fibers are involuntary, rhythmic, and without fatigue. Nuclei are located in the center of each cell; cell boundaries are marked by dark-staining structures called intercalated disks. Skeletal muscle occurs in the voluntary muscles of the body. Their cylindrical, cross-striated fibers contain many nuclei but no internal cell boundaries; a multinucleated fiber of this type is called a syncytium. Skeletal muscle is capable of rapid, forceful contractions, but it fatigues easily. Skeletal muscle tissue always attaches to connective tissue structures.

Nervous tissues contain specialized nerve cells (neurons) that respond rapidly to stimulation by conducting nerve impulses. All neurons contain RNA-rich granules, called Nissl granules, in the cytoplasm. Neurons with a single long extension of the cell body are called unipolar. Those with two long extensions are called bipolar, and neurons with more than two long extensions are called multipolar. There are two types of extensions: Dendrites conduct impulses toward the cell body, while axons generally conduct impulses away from the cell body. Many axons are surrounded by a multilayered fatty substance called the myelin sheath, which is composed of many layers of cell membrane wrapped around the axon.

Nervous tissues also contain several types of neuroglia, cells that hold nervous tissue together. Many neuroglia cells have projections that wrap around the neurons and help nourish them. The many types of neuroglia include the tiny microglia and the larger protoplasmic astrocytes, fibrous astrocytes, and oligodendroglia.

Two major tissue types make up most of the brain and spinal cord, or central nervous system. The first type, gray matter, contains the cell bodies of many neurons, along with smaller amounts of axons, dendrites, and neuroglia cells. The second type, white matter, contains mostly the axons (and sometimes also the dendrites) of neurons whose cell bodies lie elsewhere along with the myelin sheaths that surround many of the axons. Clumps of cell bodies are called *nuclei* when they are found within the brain and *ganglia* when they occur elsewhere. Bundles of axons are called *tracts* within the central nervous system and *nerves* when they appear peripherally.

The body can be described by the use of directional terms, which are defined in a relative manner according to the location of a given body part or segment. Some important directional terms are *superior, inferior, cranial, caudal, dorsal, ventral, medial, lateral, radial, ulnar, anterior,* and *posterior.*

Disorders and Diseases

Diseases or disorders that affect the entire body are called systemic or multisystem diseases. For example, fevers or febrile diseases raise the body's temperature. Many fevers are caused by infectious diseases such as influenza (actually a series of different viral infections). Influenzas cause fever, sore throat, muscle aches, coughs, headache, fatigue, and a general feeling of malaise.

Edema, or tissue swelling, is marked by an increase in the amount of extracellular fluid in several parts of the body at once. In the case of pulmonary edema, the fluid stains pink and fills the usually empty lung spaces (alveoli).

Most cancers are recognized by abnormalities of the cells in which they occur. The most dangerous cancers are marked by large tumors with ill-defined, irregular margins. If the cancer tumor is well defined, is small, and has a smooth, circular margin, then it is much less of a threat. Cancers are especially dangerous when they undergo metastasis, a process by which they produce wandering cells that spread throughout the body.

Juvenile diabetes mellitus (also called diabetes mellitus, type 1, and insulin-dependent diabetes mellitus, or IDDM), like most endocrine disorders, has systemic consequences throughout the body, including damage to nearly all the blood vessels. The primary defect in this disorder is a lack of insulin, which impairs the body's ability to use glucose. Another endocrine disorder with systemic consequences is Addison's disease, which is caused by a deficiency of the hormone adrenocorticotropic hormone (ACTH) that normally stimulates the cortex of the adrenal gland. Symptoms include weakness, loss of appetite, fatigue, weight loss, and reduced tolerance to cold. These symptoms result from imbalances in the levels of glucose and mineral salts throughout the body.

Systemic lupus erythematosus, a connective tissue disease, often produces red skin lesions marked by degeneration and flattening of the lower layers of the epidermis, drying and flaking of the outermost layer, dilation of the blood vessels under the skin, and the leakage of red blood cells out of these vessels, adding to the red color. (The word "erythematosus" means "red.")

Muscular dystrophy has several forms; the most common is marked in its advanced stages by enlarged muscles in which the muscle tissue is replaced by a fatty substance. Another muscular disease, myasthenia gravis, is often marked by overall enlargement of the thymus and an increase in the number of thymus cells. Myocardial infarction, a form of heart disease marked by damage to the heart muscle, is noticed in histological section by dead, fibrous scar tissue replacing the muscle tissue in the heart wall. In patients with arteriosclerosis, the usually elastic walls of the arteries become thicker and more fibrous and rigid; many of the same patients also suffer from atherosclerosis, a buildup of deposits on the inside of the blood vessel, partially or completely blocking blood flow.

In nervous tissue, damage to peripheral nerves often results in a process called chromatolysis in the cell bodies of the neurons from which these axons arise. The nuclei of these cells enlarge and become displaced to one side, while the Nissl granules disperse and the cell body as a whole undergoes swelling. Increased deposits of fibrous tissue characterize multiple sclerosis and certain other disorders of the nervous system. Some of these diseases are also marked by a degeneration of the myelin sheath around nerve fibers. In the case of a cerebrovascular stroke, impaired blood supply to the brain causes degeneration of the neuroglia and is followed by general tissue death and the replacement of the neuroglia by fibrous tissue. Cranial hematoma (abnormal bleeding) results in the presence of blood clots (complete with blood cells and connective tissue fibers) in abnormal locations. Alzheimer's disease is marked by granules of a protein-like substance called amyloid, often containing aluminum, surrounded by additional concentric layers of similar composition.

Perspective and Prospects

The Latin names that are used today for most body parts are derived in large measure from the writings of Galen, or

Claudius Galenus, the physician to the Roman army in the second century. The study of anatomy was furthered in the Renaissance by artists such as Leonardo da Vinci (1452-1519) and Michelangelo (1475-1564), both of whom dissected human corpses illegally in order to gain further knowledge of the anatomical structures visible on the body's surface. Such studies were followed by the well-illustrated anatomical texts of Andreas Vesalius (1514-64), who corrected many of Galen's errors regarding the structure of the human body.

A medical understanding of the circulatory system began with the studies of the Renaissance physician William Harvey (1578-1657), who examined the veins in the arms of many patients. It was Harvey who first described the presence of valves in the veins and who proved that the blood circulates outward from the heart, throughout the body, and then back again to the heart.

Microscopes were first developed around 1700 by Antoni van Leeuwenhoek (1632-1723) and others. Electron microscopes first became commercially available in the 1950s. Microscopy using instruments of these two types was widely used for distinguishing between healthy and diseased tissue taken either from bodies at autopsy or from biopsies of living patients. Modern diagnostic radiology began with the discovery of x-rays by Wilhelm Conrad Röntgen (1845-1923). Computed tomography (CT) scanning, which was developed in the 1960s and 1970s, allows for the creation of a three-dimensional x-ray picture.

—*Eli C. Minkoff, Ph.D.*

See also Genomics; Physiology; Systems and organs; *specific parts or systems.*

For Further Information:

Abrahams, Peter H., Johannes M. Boon, and Jonathan D. Spratt. *McMinn's Color Atlas of Human Anatomy.* 6th ed. St. Louis, Mo.: Mosby/Elsevier, 2008.

Agur, Anne M. R., and Arthur F. Dalley. *Grant's Atlas of Anatomy.* 13th ed. Philadelphia: Wolters Kluwer Health/Lippincott Williams & Wilkins, 2013.

Crouch, James E. *Functional Human Anatomy.* 4th ed. Philadelphia: Lea & Febiger, 1985.

Marieb, Elaine N. *Essentials of Human Anatomy and Physiology.* 10th ed. Harlow, England: Pearson Education, 2012.

Moore, Keith L., and Anne M. R. Agur. *Essential Clinical Anatomy.* 4th ed. Philadelphia: Lippincott Williams & Wilkins, 2011.

Netter, Frank H. *The CIBA Collection of Medical Illustrations.* West Caldwell, N.J.: CIBA Pharmaceutical, 1995.

Poewe, Werner, and Joseph Jankovic, eds. *Movement Disorders in Neurologic and Systemic Disease.* New York: Oxford University Press, 2014.

Preston, David C., and Barbara Ellen Shapiro. *Electromyography and Neuromuscular Disorders: Clinical-electrophysiologic Correlations.* 3d ed. Philadelphia: Elsevier/Saunders, 2013.

Rohen, Johannes W., Chihiro Yokochi, and Elke Lütjen-Drecoll. *Color Atlas of Anatomy: A Photographic Study of the Human Body.* 7th ed. Baltimore, Md.: Lippincott Williams & Wilkins, 2006.

Rosse, Cornelius, and Penelope Gaddum-Rosse. *Hollinshead's Textbook of Anatomy.* 5th ed. Philadelphia: Lippincott-Raven, 1997.

Standring, Susan, et al., eds. *Gray's Anatomy.* 40th ed. Edinburgh: Churchill Livingstone/Elsevier, 2008.

Wright, Thomas. *William Harvey: A Life in Circulation.* New York: Oxford University Press, 2013.

Anemia

Disease/Disorder

Anatomy or system affected: Blood, heart, kidneys

Specialties and related fields: Cardiology, family medicine, geriatric medicine, hematology, internal medicine, nephrology, oncology, preventive medicine

Definition: Anemia is defined as a decrease in the oxygen-carrying capacity of blood with a reduction in the red blood cell count and/or hemoglobin.

Key terms:

erythrocytes: red blood cells of the circulatory system that contain hemoglobin and are responsible for delivering oxygen to the tissues

erythropoietin: the hormone protein that is produced in the kidneys and acts on the bone marrow helping in red blood cell synthesis

hematopoiesis: the process of production of red blood cells by bone marrow

hemoglobin: the pigmented protein that imparts red color to the blood and carries oxygen from the lungs to the rest of the body

hemolyticanemia: anemia attributable to increased destruction of red blood cells

macrocytic anemia: anemia with red blood cells of increased size

microcytic anemia: anemia with red blood cells of decreased size

normocytic anemia: anemia with red blood cells of normal size

Causes and Symptoms

Red blood cells or erythrocytes are continuously produced in the bone marrow by a process known as hematopoiesis. This complex process requires adequate amounts of iron, vitamins such as B12 and folic acid, and hormones such as erythropoietin. Iron is required to form hemoglobin, which is the oxygen carrying protein contained in red blood cells. Deficiency of any of the above can cause a decrease in hemoglobin or red blood cell counts, resulting clinically in anemia. Certain medications, environmental toxins, and cancers that affect the bone marrow can also cause anemia. As erythropoietin is produced in the kidneys, anemia is seen with chronic kidney disease as well.

The normal life span of a red blood cell, from its production in the bone marrow to its destruction in the liver and spleen, is about 120 days. If the life span is decreased in any way, either by increased destruction due to various reasons or through blood loss (during trauma, vaginal bleeding, gastrointestinal bleeding, or surgery), anemia can result. Increased destruction can also occur if the red blood cells are abnormal or if the liver or spleen are enlarged. Anemia is recognized by laboratory tests when the hemoglobin falls below the normal values expected for the age and sex of the patient. The normal range of hemoglobin is 13.5 to 17.5 milligrams per deciliter in males and 12 to 16 milligrams per deciliter in females. Anemia is generally classified into three broad categories: microcytic, macrocytic, and normocytic, based on red blood cell size measured as the mean corpuscular volume (MCV) of red blood cells in blood tests. Microcytic anemia refers to decreased red blood cell size, usually with decreased hemoglobin as well. The most common cause of microcytic anemia is iron deficiency. Other causes include lead poisoning, thalassemia, sideroblastic anemia, and anemia of chronic disease.

Iron-deficiency anemia is a type of microcytic anemia with low serum iron caused by decreased intake, malabsorption, or increased loss of iron. The most common cause of iron deficiency in the United States is chronic blood loss, usually seen in women of reproductive age (menstrual loss) and the elderly (gastrointestinal blood loss due to tumors, cancers, or side effect of medication that irritates the stomach). Pregnant women may have iron deficiency as a result of inadequate intake that does not meet the requirements of the growing fetus; they require iron supplementation. Iron is absorbed in the small intestine, and any disease or procedure that causes problems with absorption, such as celiac sprue, inflammatory bowel disease (IBD), or intestinal surgery, can lead to iron-deficiency anemia. Iron-deficiency anemia is also prevalent in developing nations due to parasitic infestations such as hookworm. Iron deficiency is usually diagnosed by blood tests, but occasionally a bone marrow biopsy may be required in which absent iron stores are noted.

Chronic lead poisoning can also cause anemia by a direct toxic effect on the bone marrow. Lead is found in old house paints, pipes, bullets, batteries, and other items. Children living or playing in old houses are usually affected and may develop learning and behavioral problems in addition to anemia. The characteristic feature of lead poisoning in anemia is basophilic stippling of red blood cells.

Thalassemias are inherited disorders of the hemoglobin involving alpha or beta chains. These defective hemoglobin chains result in very small red blood cells that are fragile and destroyed in the spleen, causing hemolytic anemia. Patients with thalassemia may be revealed to suffer from anemia early in their childhood. Hydrops fetalis is a very severe form of thalassemia that results in fetal death. Thalassemia is most commonly seen in people of Mediterranean and Southeast Asian origin. Cooley's anemia or beta thalassemia major occurs early in childhood and causes growth retardation. Sideroblastic anemia is also caused by defective hemoglobin in red blood cells, resulting in hemolytic anemia. Certain toxins such as lead, alcohol, drugs such as chloramphenicol, and hypothermia can cause acquired sideroblastic anemia. Occasionally, sideroblastic anemia may be normocytic. A diagnosis is made when blood tests reveal an excess of iron and a characteristic bone marrow study shows ringed sideroblasts.

Macrocytic anemia is characterized by an increase in red blood cell size. Common causes of macrocytic anemia are vitamin B12 and folic acid deficiencies, alcoholism, hypothyroidism, myelodysplastic syndromes (MDS), and hemolytic anemias. Vitamin B12 and folate deficiency cause megaloblastic or macrocytic anemia. Vitamin B12 or cobalamin is essential for DNA synthesis. Cobalamin that is ingested in food is bound to the intrinsic factor that is es-

Information on Anemia

Causes: A deficiency in the oxygen-carrying material of the blood and/or vitamin B_{12}

Symptoms: Pallor, shortness of breath, heart palpitations, lethargy and fatigue, low blood pressure

Duration: Acute or chronic

Treatment: Replacement of deficient iron, vitamin B_{12}, or folate; blood transfusions

sential for absorption of the vitamin in the small intestine. Most cobalamin deficiency is the result of chronic dietary deficiency or pernicious anemia, which is a deficiency in the intrinsic factor. Folate (folic acid) is present in green leafy vegetables and fruits such as bananas. Folate deficiency is generally attributable to dietary deficiency, increased need as in pregnancy, or decreased absorption in the small intestine. Dietary deficiency is especially common in alcoholics. Pregnant women and patients on certain medications such as metformin, methotrexate, proton pump inhibitors, sulfazalazine have increased folic acid needs and require folic acid supplements. Hemolytic anemias are characterized by increased fragility of the red blood cells and hence their increased destruction in the spleen and liver. The types of hemolytic anemias are sickle cell anemia, hereditary spherocytosis, thalassemia, and autoimmune hemolytic anemias.

Sickle cell anemia is common in those with African ancestry. It is characterized by an abnormal "sickle" shape to the red blood cell that occurs when it is exposed to certain triggers. These abnormal red blood cells are unable to carry adequate oxygen to the tissues. As these fragile cells pass through the capillaries of the spleen, they rupture easily, resulting in anemia. In hereditary spherocytosis, red blood cells are spherical and rigid instead of being biconcave flexible discs. These cells are trapped in the spleen and are destroyed before completing their normal life span of 120 days. In autoimmune hemolytic anemia, antibodies are produced against the red blood cells, which enable them to be targets of destruction by the white blood cells of the immune system. This type of anemia is seen with unmatched blood transfusion or with the ingestion of certain drugs.

Normocytic anemia is characterized by a normal red blood cell size and is seen in anemia of chronic disease, acute blood loss, and anemia of chronic kidney disease. Chronic inflammatory diseases such as rheumatoid arthritis or lupus result in the production of certain toxins that act directly on the bone marrow and decrease red blood cell production. Normocytic anemia ensues, in which there is simply an overall decrease in red blood cell production without a maturation defect. The anemia usually improves when the chronic inflammation subsides. In chronic kidney disease, a decrease in erythropoietin production results in decreased red blood cell production. Aplastic anemia is another condition characterized by a marked decrease in red blood cell production because of the effect of toxins, medications, or infections such as parvovirus B19 (fifth disease). Other blood cell types may also be affected in

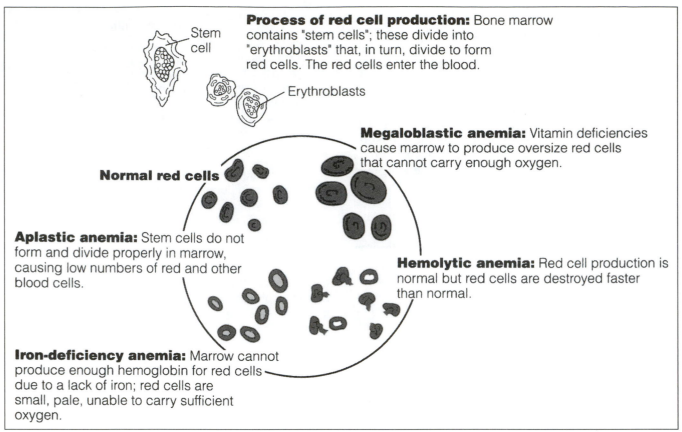

Anemia may take several different forms.

aplastic anemia, resulting in severe infections and bleeding problems.

The symptoms of anemia are generally the same irrespective of the cause. Patients are generally pale and fatigue easily and can experience dizziness, weakness, and palpitations or rapid heartbeat. Most of the symptoms are attributable to compensatory mechanisms of the body trying to overcome decreased oxygenation. These compensatory mechanisms result in an increased circulating fluid volume that can eventually cause heart failure. Patients may have symptoms of heart failure such as foot swelling, shortness of breath, palpitations, chest pain, lightheadedness, or episodes of passing out. Patients whose anemia is caused by blood loss may have these symptoms if the loss is chronic and the body has adequate time to compensate. In cases of acute blood loss or when hemoglobin falls below 5 milligrams per deciliter, however, patients may experience shock, low blood pressure, heart attack, stroke, and confusion, sometimes leading to death. On the other hand, chronic mild anemia may be asymptomatic and is detected as an incidental finding on a routine laboratory test.

Other symptoms may be specific to the cause of the anemia. Iron deficiency may sometimes manifest itself as pica (a craving for materials such as clay or ice) and flattened or spoon-shaped nails. Severe thalassemia in children is usually displayed in multiple fractures, a characteristic chipmunk face, an enlarged liver and spleen, heart failure, and gallstones. Patients with anemia caused by vitamin B_{12} deficiency may have neurological and psychiatric problems. There may be an associated thick red tongue and cracking at the angles of the mouth due to other associated vitamin deficiencies. Patients with hemolytic anemia can suffer from jaundice, dark urine, and gallstones because of the bilirubin released from the hemolysed red blood cells and enlarged spleen. Patients with sickle cell anemia may have acute pain crises and multiple infections. As a result of decreased oxygenation in peripheral tissues, stroke, angina, or lung clots may be the primary presentation in sickle cell disease. Patients with anemia of chronic disease usually have an obvious source of inflammation. Patients with bone marrow failure may also display symptoms of infection and bleeding.

Treatment and Therapy

The most important step in the management of anemia is an evaluation of the patient's condition and the cause of anemia by a physician or a nurse practitioner. A detailed history is usually elicited and should include dietary habits, occupation, associated symptoms, family history, medication history, and other medical problems. A complete physical examination is performed looking specifically for jaundice, pallor, signs of heart failure, and enlarged liver and spleen. The most helpful tool in the diagnosis of anemia is the blood test. The physician may order further tests when the diagnosis is difficult, which may include invasive tests such as a bone marrow biopsy. The treatment of anemia is directed toward the cause and acuteness of the problem. The use of blood transfusion is based on a person's signs and symptoms. In those without symptoms, they are not recommended unless hemoglobin levels are less than 6 to 8 milligrams per deciliter. These recommendations may also apply to some people with acute bleeding. Acute blood loss is an emergency and requires close monitoring in a hospital. It is treated with blood transfusions and fluid resuscitation. Some patients displaying signs of shock may need to be monitored in an intensive care setting. Patients with chronic anemia may be managed on an outpatient basis.blood

Iron deficiency is usually treated with oral iron sulfate tablets. Antacids and calcium supplements interfere with iron absorption and hence should not be taken simultaneously. Patients who cannot tolerate oral iron may be given iron intravenously. Lead poisoning is treated with chelating agents to remove the lead from the body. Thalassemia requires multiple blood transfusions and, if severe enough, bone marrow transplantation. Iron overload may become a problem with multiple blood transfusions, and chelating treatment with desferrioxamine may be needed to remove the excess iron. Hereditary spherocytosis may be treated with pyridoxine, and acquired spherocytosis caused by alcohol and medications is treated with discontinuation of the offending agent. Megaloblastic anemia due to vitamin B_{12} and folic acid deficiency is treated with oral supplements of these vitamins. Vitamin B_{12} may also be given intramuscularly. The neurological abnormalities are reversible if treated early. Autoimmune hemolytic anemias are treated by removal of the offending agent and with steroids. Some patients may require splenectomy (surgical removal of the spleen). Sickle cell crises are treated in the hospital with intravenous fluids, oxygen, and blood transfusion. Supportive care is generally required, and patients may need antibiotics for infections and high doses of painkillers. The number of attacks may be reduced by oral hydroxyurea therapy as an outpatient. The treatment of anemia caused by chronic kidney disease due to low erythropoietin will require supplementation with weekly subcutaneous erythropoietin and iron. In patients undergoing dialysis, hemoglobin must be maintained above 10 milligrams per deciliter. Patients with aplastic anemia will require multiple blood transfusions and immunosuppressive therapy and may benefit from bone marrow transplantation.

Perspective and Prospects

The earliest mention of iron therapy is in Greek mythology in the story of Iphiclus being cured of impotence by drinking a tea made from the rust of an iron blade. The use of iron for the treatment of anemia, however, occurred much later, after the discovery of blood and blood transfusion. Jan Swammerdam first described red blood cells in 1658, and the first blood transfusion was dog-to-dog in 1665 by Oxford physician Richard Lower. The first human-to-human blood transfusion was performed successfully in 1818 by British obstetrician James Blundell for the treatment of postpartum hemorrhage. Death from hemolytic anemias caused by mismatched blood transfusions, however, was a problem until Karl Landsteiner identified the ABO blood groups in 1901, for which he received the Nobel Prize in Medicine in 1930. He subsequently discovered Rh groups in blood that further reduced the incidence of hemolytic anemias resulting from blood transfusions. The first case of sickle cell anemia was described by James Herrick in 1910, but it was Linus Pauling who postulated that the disease was the result of the presence of mutant hemoglobin HbS. The mortality rate of anemia has improved significantly over the past century thanks to advances in blood transfusion and bone marrow transplantation. Current research is focusing on the therapeutic potential of anemia correction in cancer, rheumatoid arthritis, human immunodeficiency virus (HIV) infection, heart failure, and kidney disease. It is being shown that the correction of anemia improves quality of life significantly. Synthetic blood may become the treatment of anemia in the future.

—*Venkat Raghavan Tirumala, MD, MHA; updated by Ophelia Empleo-Frazier, MSN, GNP-BC, WCC, DCP and Geraldine Marrocco*

See also: Blood and blood disorders; Blood testing; Hematology; Hematology, pediatric; Phlebotomy; Serology; Sickle cell disease; Thalassemia; Vitamins*and minerals.*

For Further Information:
Greer, John, et al., eds. *Wintrobe's Clinical Hematology*. 13th ed. Philadelphia: Wolters Kluwer/Lippincott Williams & Wilkins Health, 2013.
"Iron and Iron Deficiency." *Centers for Disease Control and Prevention*, Feb. 23, 2011.
Kasper, Dennis L., et al., eds. *Harrison's Principles of Internal Medicine*. 19th ed. New York: McGraw-Hill, 2015.
McCoy, Krisha, and Kari Kassir. "Anemia." *Health Library*, Mar. 28, 2013.
National Anemia Action Council. http://www.anemia.org.
Oral Iron for Anemia: A Review of the Clinical Effectiveness, Cost-effectiveness and Guidelines Rapid Response Report: Summary with Critical Appraisal Ottawa (ON): Canadian Agency for Drugs and Technologies in Health; 2016 Jan 6.

Anesthesia
Procedure
Anatomy or system affected: Brain, muscles, musculoskeletal system, nerves, nervous system, psychic-emotional system, skin, spine
Specialties and related fields: Anesthesiology, critical care, dentistry, emergency medicine, general surgery, neurology, ophthalmology
Definition: The administration of drugs to block the transmission of nerve impulses to prevent pain, especially during surgery or childbirth; anesthesia may be general (causing total unconsciousness) or regional and local (deadening sensation and decreasing awareness without causing loss of consciousness).
Key terms:
epiduralanesthesia: anesthesia caused by injecting a local anesthetic between the vertebra and beneath the ligamentum flavum into the extradural space; also known as extradural anesthesia
local anesthesia: anesthesia produced by injecting a local

anesthetic solution directly into the tissues; also known as local block

local anesthetics: drugs that produce a reversible blockade of nerve impulse conduction

regional anesthesia: insensibility caused by the interruption of nerve conduction in a region of the body

spinal anesthesia: anesthesia produced by injecting a local anesthetic around the spinal cord; also known as subarachnoid block

Indications and Procedures

Anesthetics are primarily used to prevent pain during surgical operations, though they are also used to reduce fear, relax tissues, and prevent a sympathetic nervous system response to surgery. Some believe, erroneously, that being "put to sleep" with a general anesthetic is the only way an operation can be performed pain-free.

General anesthesia is a type of anesthesia that causes total unconsciousness and affects the entire body. Regional anesthesia, on the other hand, does not cause unconsciousness but allows surgery to be performed without pain by producing loss of sensation in a region of the body through the interruption of nerve-impulse transmission from the area to be incised.

General anesthetics produce a neurophysiological state characterized by five primary effects: (1) unconsciousness, (2) amnesia, (3) analgesia, (4) inhibition of autonomic reflexes, and (5) skeletal muscle relaxation. No general anesthetic can achieve all five of these primary effects by itself. Thus, patients receive a cocktail of general anesthetics drugs that are delivered both intravenously and by inhalation.

The goal is to induce rapid, smooth loss of consciousness that can be rapidly reversed and is safe. The composition of the anesthetic cocktail is determined by the type of procedure to be performed. For example, for minor superficial surgeries or invasive diagnostic procedures, oral or IV sedatives are administered in combination with local anesthetics (monitored anesthesia care). This technique retains the patient's ability to breathe on his/her own and respond to verbal commands. For more invasive surgical procedures, anesthesia can begin with oral or parenteral benzodiazepines prior to surgery, followed by intravenous anesthetics, such as thiopental or propofol to induce unconsciousness, which can be maintained during surgery with a combination of inhaled or intravenous drugs.

General anesthetics target neurons in the central nervous system. These drugs usually affect the connection between neurons known as the synapse. When neurons connect, one neuron is downstream of the synapse (presynaptic) and the other is upstream of the synapse (postsynaptic). In some cases, the presynaptic neuron generates stimulatory signals that activate the postsynaptic neurons. In other cases, the presynaptic neuron provides inhibitory signals that disable the postsynaptic neuron. General anesthetics seem to increase the inhibitory signals from presynaptic neurons to postsynaptic neurons or diminish the excitatory signals. The primary components of inhibitory signals include chloride ion channels (bound by the neurotransmitters

gamma-aminobutyric acid or GABA and glycine) and potassium ion channels. The primary excitatory ion channels include those activated by acetylcholine, excitatory amino acids, and serotonin. All these ion channels are potential targets of general anesthetics. Benzodiazepines, for example, bind to GABA channels and potentiate their activity, inhibiting postsynaptic neurons. See the table below for examples of general anesthetics.

General Anesthetics		
Anesthetic	Inhaled or intravenous (IV)	Comments
Nitrous oxide	Inhaled	Gaseous anesthetic, incomplete anesthetic, rapid onset and recovery
Desflurane	Inhaled	Volatile anesthetic, low volatility; pungent, rapid recovery
Sevoflurane	Inhaled	Volatile anesthetic, rapid onset and recovery
Isoflurane	Inhaled	Volatile anesthetic, medium rate of onset and recovery
Enflurane	Inhaled	Volatile anesthetic, medium rate of onset and recovery
Halothane	Inhaled	Volatile anesthetic, medium rate of onset and recovery
Dexmedetomidine	IV	Used for short-term sedation
Diazepam	IV	Barbiturate, intermediate-acting, has muscle-relaxation effects
Etomidate	IV	Minimal effects on heart rate and blood pressure, rapid recovery
Ketamine	IV	Analgesic activity, multiple modes of administration are possible
Lorazepam	IV	Barbiturate, slow onset and prolonged duration
Methohexital	IV	Barbiturate, short-acting and rapid onset of action
Midazolam	IV	Barbiturate, rapid onset but slow recovery
Propofol	IV	Rapidly turned over, fast recovery, well tolerated
Fospropofol	IV	Prodrug, converted to propofol in body, tends to cause paresthesias (including burning, tingling, stinging) and/or pruritus in the perineal region
Thiopental	IV	Rapid-onset, short-acting barbiturate

In regional anesthesia, the anesthetic agents are deposited either on the surface of the area to be anesthetized or near a specific nerve or pathway that lies between the area and receptors for painful stimuli that are part of the central nervous system. Thus, transmission of noxious stimuli to the brain is effectively blocked, allowing a surgical procedure to be performed without the patient feeling pain. Regional anesthesia is frequently referred to as regional nerve blockade.

Local anesthetics operate in several ways. Those injected near the nerves diffuse into the nerves and bind to receptors on their membranes. Once in the nerve sheath, local anesthetic agents prevent sodium from moving into the nerve interior by physically occluding sodium channels. Impulses traveling from the surgical area to the central nervous system are blocked so that nerves transmitting touch, temperature, and pain sensation are temporarily interrupted. Nerve impulses traveling from the central nervous system to the surgical area are also blocked, leading to an interruption of motor power to the surgical area. The number of nerves blocked depends on where the local anesthetic is deposited.

The duration of the nerve blockade depends on the type and dosage of local anesthetic injected as well as on the technique utilized. Diffusion of the local anesthetic out of the nerve and its absorption into the vascular bed causes the effect of the local anesthetic to be terminated. The blood flowing around the nerve removes the drug from the area. Decreasing the flow of blood to the area by adding vasoconstricting agents such as epinephrine to the local anesthetic to be injected is a common method used to prolong the duration of the nerve block.

Local anesthetics are weak bases whose structure consists of an aromatic moiety connected to a substituted amine through an ester or amide linkage. The two major families of local anesthetics are the amino amides and the amino esters. The clinical differences between the ester and amide local anesthetics involve their potential for producing adverse side effects and the mechanisms by which they are metabolized. Local anesthetics are also classified based on their potency and duration of action: a short duration of action (thirty to forty-five minutes), an intermediate duration of action (one to two hours), or a long duration of action (four to eight hours). The range in duration of nerve blockade is attributable primarily to two factors: the concentration of the drug used and the addition of vasoconstricting agents, such as epinephrine. Local anesthetics are listed in the table below.

Local Anesthetics		
Drug	Potency relative to procaine	Duration
Procaine (Novocain)	1	Short
Prilocaine	2	Short
Chloroprocaine	2	Short
Tetracaine (Pontocaine)	8	Long
Benzocaine	Surface use only	
Lidocaine (Xylocaine)	4	Medium
Mepivacaine (Carbocaine, isocaine)	2	Medium
Bupivacaine (Marcaine) & Levobupivacaine (Charaxine)	8	Long
Ropivacaine (Naropin)	8	Long

Local and regional anesthetics are excellent ways of supplying surgical and postoperative analgesia (pain control). Local anesthetics are now being given in combination with narcotic analgesics (painkillers). Narcotics are almost always given in combination with local anesthetics and bind to narcotic receptors in the area and provide analgesia (pain relief) without interrupting nerve transmission. The combination of local anesthetic agents with narcotics is gaining popularity in postoperative pain control; the patient can experience longer durations of pain relief while avoiding the systemic side effects of intravenously administered narcotics.

There are six categories of regional anesthesia: topical anesthesia, local block and field block, nerve block, intravenous (IV) neural blockade, subarachnoid block (spinal anesthesia), and epidural anesthesia, including caudal block. These are primarily differentiated based on the size of the region that is anesthetized and the duration of the neural blockade.

Topical anesthesia. In this technique, also known as surface anesthesia, an anesthetic drug is sprayed or spread onto the area to be desensitized. This short-acting form of anesthesia blocks nerve endings in the skin as well as mucous membranes, such as those of the nasopharynx (nose and throat), mouth, rectum, and vagina. Topical anesthesia is employed in minor procedures such as eye or rectal examinations. The advantages of topical anesthesia include quick onset of action, ease of administration, and general nontoxicity. Disadvantages include lack of deeper-tissue anesthesia and lack of tissue relaxation. A frequently used topical anesthetic is the drug benzocaine, often utilized for the treatment of traumatic tissue pain secondary to sunburn.

Local blocks and field blocks. In local blocks, the local anesthetic is injected with a needle and syringe into the skin and tissues of an area to be incised. As a result, the nerves around the incision are blocked. Local blocks are used in short, minor operations and prior to the insertion of intravenous or spinal needles. A field block is another type of local block. In a field block, the area surrounding the incision is also injected with local anesthetics, preventing impulses transmitted from a larger area from reaching the central nervous system.

Nerve blocks. Nerve blocks interrupt the transmission of nerve impulses by nerves or by bundles of nerves that are further removed from the surgical site. Nerve blocks may be used to anesthetize a single finger or toe (digital nerve block), a foot (ankle block) or hand, or an entire arm (axillary, supraclavicular, and interscalene blocks) or leg (leg block). In each type of neural blockade, the physician or nurse anesthetist injects local anesthetic agents around the major nerves that supply the area to be incised. The number of injections depends on the location of the nerves to be blocked.

may be blocked individually. An arm block can be accomplished by a single injection of a larger volume of local anesthetic into the axillary sheath or between the middle and anterior scalene muscles in the neck. Upper extremity blocks can be performed with a single injection because the brachial plexus (the nerves innervating the arm) is collectively encased in a sheath. Distal to the axillary area, the nerves innervating the arm are no longer encased in a sheath. Consequently, separate injections of the radial, median, and ulnar nerves are required to block the arm at the elbow or wrist.

Intercostal nerveblocks. Intercostal nerves innervate the outer and inner surfaces of the abdominal wall. Intercostal nerve blockade is utilized for postoperative pain control following thoracic or upper abdominal surgeries. A sterile needle is inserted into the skin over the lower margin of the rib along the posterior axillary line. The needle is then directed toward the intercostal groove located inferior to the rib. A local anesthetic is injected into the intercostal space containing the intercostal nerve, vein, and artery. The anesthetic lasts from six to twelve hours and may be prolonged by the addition of epinephrine to the solution.

Intravenous neural blockade. Intravenous (IV) neural blockade was discovered by August Bier in 1908; he was also the first to routinely utilize spinal anesthesia. Today, IV regional neural blockade is also referred to as Bier blockade. With Bier blockade, the local anesthetic agent is injected into a leg or arm vein just below a tourniquet. Inflation of the tourniquet prevents the local anesthetic from being released into general circulation. This local anesthetic, thus contained in the extremity, travels to the major nerves in the limb and blocks neural transmission. The duration of the neural blockade is governed by the length of time that the tourniquet is inflated. Once the tourniquet is deflated, the local anesthetic enters the systemic circulation, the neural blockade recedes, and normal sensation and power to the extremity are rapidly returned. Intravenous regional blockade of the extremities has many advantages: ease of performance, rapid onset, controllable duration of action, and rapid recovery. The disadvantages include possible tourniquet discomfort, possible reaction to the local anesthetic when it is released into general circulation, and rapid return of sensation, including pain, upon removal of the tourniquet.

Spinal anesthesia. Spinal anesthesia, also called subarachnoid block, is a commonly utilized form of anesthesia. Spinal anesthesia can be used for almost any type of surgical procedure below the umbilicus, such as surgical procedures performed on the legs and hips, hysterectomies, appendectomies, and cesarean sections.

A lumbar puncture (spinal tap) is performed in the lower back, usually between the second and third lumbar vertebrae, the third and fourth lumbar vertebrae, or the fifth lumbar and first sacral vertebrae. The patient is placed on his or her side in a flexed position (or sometimes in a sitting position). The physician or nurse anesthetist, wearing sterile gloves, prepares the skin in the area to be punctured with a skin antiseptic, such as betadine, and drapes the area with a sterile towel. The anesthetist then infiltrates the area of the puncture with lidocaine, producing a local block. Once the skin is anesthetized, a needle is inserted through the intraspinous space into the subarachnoid space. The needle passes through the supraspinous ligament, intraspinous ligament, and ligamentum flavum. Proper placement of the needle is identified through an observation of freely flowing spinal fluid. A local anesthetic agent is then injected into the spinal fluid. Cerebrospinal fluid (CSF) is a clear, colorless ultrafiltrate of the blood that fills the subarachnoid space. The total volume of CSF is 100 to 150 milliliters; the volume contained in the subarachnoid space is 25 to 35 milliliters.

Once injected into the subarachnoid CSF, the local anesthetic agent spreads in both a cephalad (toward the head and anterior) and caudad (toward the feet and posterior) direction. Factors influencing this spread include the dose and volume of the agent used, patient position, and the specific gravity (weight) of the anesthetic solution relative to the CSF. One of three types of solutions—isobaric, hypobaric, or hyperbaric—can be used. Hyperbaric solutions are heavier than CSF; thus, placing the patient in Trendelenburg's position (with the head tilted downward) will increase the cephalad spread of the anesthetic. With the patient in Trendelenburg's position, hypobaric solutions (with a specific gravity less than that of CSF) of local anesthetic agents spread caudally. Spread of the local anesthetic in the subarachnoid space usually stops (fixation) within five to thirty-five minutes after injection. After fixation has occurred, patient position changes will not influence the spread of local anesthetic or the subsequent level of anesthesia. Within minutes after a subarachnoid injection of a local anesthetic, patients experience a warm sensation in their lower extremities, followed by a loss of sensation and inability to move the legs. The duration of the neural blockade is dependent on the type of local anesthetic utilized, as well as the addition of any vasoconstrictor.

Epiduralanesthesiaand caudal block. Like spinal anesthesia, epidural blockade can be used for the prevention of pain during surgery. It can also be used to relieve pain after surgery, chronic pain, or labor pains; to supplement a light general anesthetic; and to diagnose and treat autonomic nervous system dysfunction. The technique is excellent for operations performed on the lower abdomen, pelvis, and perineum; for laminectomies; and in obstetrics for the relief of labor pains.

As with spinal anesthesia, the patient is placed on his or her side in a flexed position (or sometimes in a sitting position). The physician or nurse anesthetist, wearing sterile gloves, prepares the skin around the puncture with an antiseptic such as betadine and drapes the area with a sterile towel. The anesthetist infiltrates the area of the puncture with lidocaine, producing a local block. Once the skin is anesthetized, an epidural needle is inserted between the appropriate lumbar vertebrae (occasionally between thoracic vertebrae). With epidural blockade, however, the needle is not advanced into the subarachnoid space. Instead, needle advancement is terminated when the needle tip is in the epidural space. Thus, the dura is not penetrated as in spinal anesthesia, and postdural puncture headache does not occur with a properly placed epidural needle. Once the epidural space has been identified, local anesthetic agents (in larger volumes than utilized with subarachnoid anesthesia) are injected through the needle or through a small catheter threaded through the needle. Placement of a catheter through the needle allows reinjection to take place without subsequent needle punctures. This is particularly desirable for long surgeries, postoperative pain control, and the control of labor pains. Local anesthetic agents injected through a catheter for postoperative or labor pain control are usually given at lesser concentrations so that nerve motor fibers are not interrupted.

Caudal block is another type of epidural anesthesia. In this case, the needle (with or without a catheter) is placed through the sacrococcygeal ligament just superior to the coccyx. The technique is gaining popularity as an adjunct to general anesthesia in children for postoperative pain control.

Uses and Complications

Regional anesthesia has several advantages over general anesthesia. The first is ease of administration. The agents used are injectable, the equipment required is minimal, and the costs are reasonable. Second is the relative safety of the technique. A localized area of the body can be operated upon without the patient experiencing most of the undesirable and potentially harmful side effects of general anesthesia, such as loss of consciousness and the depression of the cardiovascular and respiratory systems. In addition, advantages include excellent muscle relaxation, which is often required to facilitate surgical procedures; improved peripheral blood flow; an antithrombotic effect; a decreased loss of blood in some cases; and postoperative pain relief. Regional anesthesia is also utilized in combination with general anesthesia to increase the benefits of both while decreasing adverse side effects.

Yet regional anesthesia has some disadvantages. First, some operations, such as major surgical procedures involving the brain, heart, and lungs, cannot be performed under regional anesthesia. Second, some patients may be allergic to the local anesthetics. Local anesthetics of the amino ester type may result in allergic reactions because of the metabolite p-aminobenzoic acid. Local anesthetics of the amino amide class are essentially devoid of allergic potential. Many anesthetic solutions, however, contain methylparaben as a preservative, and this compound can produce an allergic reaction in persons sensitive to p-aminobenzoic acid. Third, some patients desire to be unaware of the operation and may be anxious at the thought of being "awake." They erroneously believe that the total unconsciousness produced by general anesthesia is the only method to produce unawareness. In most cases, patients who receive a regional anesthetic also receive intravenous sedation to decrease their level of awareness. Subsequently, many patients report having no recollection whatsoever of the surgical procedure. In addition, the advantages of spinal anesthesia, one of the most popular types of regional anesthesia, far outweigh the disadvantages, which include hypotension, a high required dosage of anesthesia, and postdural puncture headache. Hypotension is treated with intravenous fluids and, if necessary, the administration of vasoconstricting drugs. Postdural puncture headache (spinal headache) is thought to be caused from a loss of spinal fluid (which cushions the brain) through the dural hole produced by the spinal needle. Advances in the technique of spinal anesthesia administration, including the use of very small needles introduced in a manner that separates the dural fibers, have significantly decreased the incidence of postdural puncture headache. Should this complication arise, however, it is treated with analgesics, intravenous fluids, and, if necessary, an injection of saline (or a sample of the patient's own blood) around the site of the dural puncture, effectively "patching" the dural hole created by the spinal needle.

Perspective and Prospects

The first successful demonstration of anesthesia (diethyl ether) by William T. G. Morton occurred in 1846 at the Massachusetts General Hospital. The discovery of anesthesia occurred prior to the discovery of germ theory and aseptic techniques. Therefore, although anesthesia made surgery painless in the early nineteenth century, there was still a high rate of surgical morbidity and mortality because of infection. In the late 1860s, germ theory had evolved from the work of Robert Koch and Louis Pasteur, and Joseph Lister's subsequent work on principles of asepsis contributed significantly to a decline in surgical mortality from infection by the late 1880s. There remained, however, a high surgical mortality rate caused by anesthesia. At that time, general anesthetic agents were commonly utilized, and few, if any, practitioners specialized in the administration of anesthesia.

Regional anesthesia was first utilized in 1884 when a German physician named Carl Koller performed an operation to correct glaucoma using a local anesthetic. In this case, cocaine, an alkaloid obtained from the coca plant, was instilled into the eye. This successful operation brought significant acceptance to the principle of local anesthesia. The great advantage of local anesthesia was that it anesthetized only the part of the body on which the operation was to be performed. Patients could be spared the depressive effects of general anesthesia, especially on the cardiovascular and respiratory systems. By the 1930s, various regional anesthesia techniques had been developed, including subarachnoid block (spinal anesthesia), lumbar epidural, caudal epidural, intravenous, and brachial plexus anesthesia. The occurrence of these regional anesthetic techniques, along with the evolution of local anesthetic agents, allowed anesthetists to tailor the type and duration of regional anesthesia to the requirements of each patient. Thus, regional anesthesia has become a popular choice among surgeons, anesthetists, and patients.

—*Maura S. McAuliffe;*
updated by Michael A. Buratovich PhD

See also: Acupuncture; Anesthesiology; Catheterization; Hypnosis; Local anesthesia; Lumbar puncture; Narcotics; Nervous system; Neurology; Neurology, pediatric; Pain; Pain management; Pharmacology; Surgery, general; Surgical procedures.

For Further Information:

Cousins, Michael J., P. O. Bridenbaugh, et al., eds. *Neural Blockade in Clinical Anesthesiaand Management of Pain*. 4th ed. Philadelphia: J. B. Lippincott, 2008.

"General Anesthesia—Interactive Tutorial." *Medline Plus*, 2013.

Katz, Jordan. *Atlas of Regional Anesthesia*. 4th ed. Norwalk, Conn.: Appleton & Lange, 2010.

Hines, Roberta L., and Katherine Marschall. *Stoelting's Anesthesiaand Co-Existing Disease*, 7th ed. Philadephia, PA: Elsevier, 2017.

Kellicker, Patricia. "General Anesthesia." *Health Library*, September 10, 2012.

Miller, Scott, and David Zieve. "Spinal and Epidural Anesthesia." *Medline Plus*, March 28, 2011.

Sweeney, Frank. *The AnesthesiaFact Book: Everything You Need to Know Before Surgery*. Cambridge, Mass.: Perseus, 2003.

Winnie, A. P. *Plexus Anesthesia: Perivascular Techniques of Brachial Plexus Block*. Reprint. Philadelphia: W. B. Saunders, 1993.

Anesthesiology

Specialty

Anatomy or system affected: Brain, muscles, musculoskeletal system, nerves, nervous system, psychic-emotional system, skin, spine

Specialties and related fields: Anesthesiology, critical care, dentistry, emergency medicine, general surgery, neurology, ophthalmology

Definition: The science of administering anesthesia during a surgical procedure.

Key terms:

anesthesia: a new word coined in the 1840s, derived from a Greek word meaning "not feeling"

electric anesthesia: the use of pulses of electricity to deaden nerve cells or cause unconsciousness

endotracheal tube: a flexible tube inserted through the mouth or nose into the trachea (windpipe) to carry anesthetic gas and oxygen directly to the lungs

ether: a volatile liquid that causes unconsciousness when inhaled; first demonstrated during surgery in 1846

nitrous oxide: called "laughing gas" because people appeared to become intoxicated from inhaling it; first used in 1844 to pull a tooth painlessly

novocaine: a local anesthetic, commonly used in dentistry, whose chemical structure is similar to that of cocaine

sodium pentothal: a fast-acting anesthetic that is injected into the vein; first developed for military hospitals during World War II

spinal anesthesia: the injection of an anesthetic at the base of the spine to produce loss of feeling in the lower part of the body and legs

The History of Anesthesiology

In a modern hospital, the surgical operating room normally is a very quiet place. The anesthesiologist, surgeon, assisting doctors, and nurses perform their duties with little conversation while the patient sleeps. Family members sit quietly in a nearby waiting room until the operation is over. Before the advent of anesthesiology in the 1840s, however, surgery was a thoroughly gruesome experience. Patients might drink some whiskey to numb their senses, and several strong men were recruited to hold them down. Surgeons cut the flesh with a sharp knife and sawed quickly through the bone while patients screamed in agony. The operating room in the hospital was located as far as possible from other patients awaiting surgery so that they would not hear the cries so plainly.

Many kinds of operations were performed before anesthetics were discovered. Among these were the removal of tumors, the opening of abscesses, amputations, the treatment of head wounds, the removal of kidney stones, and cesarean sections and other surgeries during childbirth. The frightful ordeal of "going under the knife," however, often caused patients to delay surgery until it was almost too late. Also, for the surgeon it was nerve-racking to work without anesthetics, trying to operate while the patient screamed and struggled.

Sir Humphry Davy (1778-1829) was a distinguished British chemist who studied the intoxicating effect of a gas called nitrous oxide. While suffering from the pain of an erupting wisdom tooth, he sought relief by inhaling some of the gas. In 1800, he published a paper suggesting the use of nitrous oxide to relieve pain during surgery. There was no follow-up on his idea, however, and it was forgotten until after anesthesia had been discovered independently in the United States.

The next episode in the history of anesthesiology was the work of Crawford W. Long (1815-78), a small-town doctor in Georgia. In the early nineteenth century, "ether frolics" had become popular, in which young people at a party would inhale ether vapor to give them a "high" such as from drinking alcohol. One young man was to have surgery on his neck for a tumor. Long was the town druggist as well as the doctor, so he knew that this fellow had purchased ether and enjoyed its effects. Long suggested that he inhale some ether to ready himself for surgery. On March 30, 1842, the tumor was removed with little pain for the patient. It was the first successful surgery under anesthesia.

Unfortunately, Long did not recognize the great significance of what he had done. He did not report the etherization experiment to his colleagues, and it remained relatively unknown. He used ether a few more times in his own surgical practice, one time while amputating the toe of a young slave. Long finally wrote an article for a medical journal in 1849 telling about his pioneering work, three years after anesthesia had been publicly demonstrated and widely adopted by others.

The story of anesthesiology then moved to Hartford, Connecticut, where a young dentist named Horace Wells (1815-48) played a major role. P. T. Barnum, of show business and circus fame, was advertising an entertaining "GRAND EXHIBITION of the effects produced by inhaling NITROUS OXIDE or LAUGHING GAS!" Wells decided to attend. He was one of the volunteers from the audience and "made a spectacle of himself," according to his wife.

Another volunteer who had inhaled the gas began to shout and stagger around; finally he ran into a bench, banging his shins against it. The audience laughed, but the observant Wells noticed that the man showed no pain, even

Gas mask

Gas cylinder
pressure meters

Hoses carrying
anesthetic
gas supply

The anesthesiologist, as a crucial team member in every major surgery, must constantly monitor the vital signs and level of consciousness of the anesthetized patient.

though his leg was bleeding. This demonstration gave Wells a sudden insight that a person might have a tooth pulled or even a leg amputated and feel no pain while under the influence of the gas.

Wells became so excited by the idea of eliminating pain that he arranged to have some nitrous oxide gas brought to his office on the next day. Then he had a long talk with a young dentist colleague, John Riggs, about the potential risks of trying it out on a patient. Finally, Wells decided to make himself the first test case, if Riggs would be willing to extract one of his wisdom teeth.

On the morning of December 11, 1844, a bag of nitrous oxide gas was delivered by the man who had been in charge of the previous evening's exhibition. Wells sat in the dental chair and breathed deeply from the gas bag until he seemed to be asleep. Riggs went to work with his long-handled forceps to loosen and finally pull out the tooth, with no outcry from the patient. After a short time, Wells regained consciousness, spit out some blood, and said that he had felt "no more pain than the prick of a pin."

After this success, Wells immediately set to work on further experiments. He acquired the apparatus and chemicals to make his own nitrous oxide. Within the next month, he used the gas on more than a dozen patients. Other dentists in Hartford heard about the procedure and started using it. By the middle of January 1845, Wells was confident enough to propose a demonstration to a wider audience.

Wells was able to arrange for a demonstration at Massachusetts General Hospital in Boston. While the audience watched, he anesthetized a volunteer patient with gas and extracted his tooth. Unfortunately, the patient groaned at that moment, causing laughter and scornful comments from the onlookers. Wells was viewed as another quack making grandiose claims without evidence. His demonstration had failed, and he returned to Hartford in discouragement. He later commented that he had probably removed the gas bag too soon, before the patient was fully asleep.

It was another dentist, William T. G. Morton (1819-68), who finally provided a convincing demonstration of anesthesia. Morton tried to obtain some nitrous oxide from a druggist, who did not have any on hand and suggested that ether fumes could be substituted. Morton then used ether on several dental patients, with excellent results. In 1846, he obtained permission for a demonstration at the same hospital where Wells had failed two years earlier. Famous

Boston surgeon John Warren and a skeptical audience watched as Morton instructed a patient to breathe the ether. When the patient was fully asleep, Warren removed a tumor from his neck. To everyone's amazement, there was no outcry of pain during the surgery. After the patient awoke, he said that he felt only a slight scratch on his neck. Warren's words have been recorded for posterity: "Gentlemen, this is no humbug!" Another doctor said, "What we have seen here today will go around the world."

The result of this dramatic demonstration of October 16, 1846, spread quickly to other hospitals in the United States and Europe. Several hundred surgeries were performed under anesthesia in the next year. In England, John Snow experimented with a different anesthetic, chloroform, and began to use it for women in childbirth. In 1853, Queen Victoria took chloroform from Snow during the delivery of her eighth child. Acceptance of anesthesia, and the science of anesthesiology, by the medical profession and the general public grew rapidly.

Science and Profession

Nitrous oxide, ether, and chloroform were the big three anesthetics for general surgery and dentistry for nearly a hundred years after their discovery. All three were administered by inhalation, but there were differences in safety, reliability, and side effects for the patient.

Wells, the dentist who had unsuccessfully tried to demonstrate nitrous oxide anesthesia in 1844, came to a tragic end in 1848 because of chloroform. He was testing the gas on himself to find out what an appropriate dosage should be. Unfortunately, he became addicted to the feeling of intoxication that it gave him. While under the influence of a chloroform binge, he accosted a woman on the street and was arrested. He committed suicide while in prison.

Nitrous oxide is a nearly odorless gas that must be mixed with oxygen to prevent asphyxiation. Storing the gases in large, leakproof bags was awkward. By comparison, ether and chloroform were much more convenient to use because they are liquids that can be stored in small bottles. The liquid was dripped onto a cloth and held over the patient's nose. Ether is hazardous, however, because it is flammable, and it also has a disagreeable odor. Chloroform is not flammable but is more difficult to administer because of the danger of heart stoppage.

Anesthesiology was practiced primarily by dentists, eye doctors, chemists, and all types of surgeons for many years. The Mayo Clinic in Rochester, Minnesota, was one of the first hospitals to recognize the need for specialists to administer anesthesia. In 1904, a nurse from Mayo named Alice Magaw gave a talk on what she had learned from eleven thousand procedures performed under anesthesia. Her concluding comment was that "ether kills slowly, giving plenty of warning, but with chloroform there is not even time to say good-by." Ether takes more time to induce anesthesia, but Magaw asserted that the patient's life was in less danger than from chloroform.

A Scottish physician, James Y. Simpson, was one of the early advocates of using chloroform for partial anesthesia during childbirth. The woman could breathe the vapor intermittently for several hours as needed without the disagreeable odor of ether. She would remain conscious, but the anesthetic apparently produced a kind of amnesia so that the pain was not fully remembered. Simpson received much public acclaim for his help to women in labor, including a title of nobility. (One humorist of the day suggested a coat-of-arms for Sir Simpson, showing a newborn baby with the inscription, "Does your mother know you're out?")

In the 1920s, several new anesthetic gases were created by chemists working closely with medical doctors. The advantages and drawbacks of each new synthesized compound were tested first on animals, then on human volunteers, and finally during surgery. One of the most successful ones was cyclopropane: it was quick acting and nontoxic and could be mixed with oxygen for prolonged operations. Like other organic gases, however, it was explosive under certain conditions and had to be used with appropriate caution.

A major development in 1928 was the invention of the endotracheal tube by Arthur Guedel. A rubber tube was inserted into the mouth and down the trachea (windpipe) to carry the anesthetic gas and oxygen mixture directly to the lungs. The space around the rubber tube had to be sealed in some way in order to prevent blood or other fluid from going down the windpipe. Guedel's ingenious idea was to surround the tube with a small balloon. When inflated, it effectively closed off the gap between the tube and the trachea wall. He gave a memorable demonstration at a medical meeting using an anesthetized dog with a breathing tube in its throat. After inflating the seal, the dog was submerged under water for several hours and then revived, showing that no water had entered its lungs.

The first local anesthetic was discovered in 1884 by Carl Koller, a young eye doctor in Vienna. He was a colleague of the famous psychoanalyst Sigmund Freud, and together they had investigated the psychic effects of cocaine. Koller noticed that his tongue became numb from the drug. He had the sudden insight that a drop of cocaine solution might be usable as an anesthetic for eye surgery. He tried it on a frog's eye, with much success. Following the tradition of other medical pioneers, he then tried it on himself. The cocaine made his eye numb. Koller published a short article, and the news spread quickly. Within three months, other doctors reported successful local anesthesia, using cocaine for dentistry, obstetrics, and many kinds of general surgery.

Chemists investigated the molecular structure of cocaine and were able to develop synthetic substitutes such as novocaine, which was faster and less toxic. Another improvement was to inject local anesthetic under the skin with a hypodermic needle. With this technique, it was possible to block off pain from a whole region of the body by deadening the nerve fibers. A spinal or epidural block is often used to relieve the pain of childbirth or for various abdominal surgeries.

There is another class of anesthetic drugs called barbiturates, which were originally developed for sleeping pills.

Any medication that induces sleep automatically becomes a candidate for use as an anesthetic. The most successful barbiturate anesthetic has been sodium pentothal. It is normally administered by injection into a vein in the arm and puts the patient to sleep in a matter of seconds. When the surgery is over, the needle is withdrawn and consciousness returns, with few aftereffects for most people. The anesthesiologist may use sodium pentothal in combination with an inhaled anesthetic if the surgery is expected to be lengthy.

Diagnostic and Treatment Techniques

Suppose that a man is scheduled to have some kind of abdominal surgery, such as the repair of a hernia or hemorrhoids or the removal of the appendix, an intestinal blockage, or a cancerous growth. The anesthesiologist would select a sequence of anesthetics that depends primarily on the expected length of the operation and the physical condition of the patient.

About an hour before surgery, the patient receives a shot of morphine to produce relaxation and drowsiness. After he is wheeled into the operating room, the anesthesiologist inserts a needle into a vein in the patient's arm and injects a barbiturate such as sodium pentothal. This drug puts him to sleep very quickly because it is rapidly distributed through the body, but it is not suitable for maintaining anesthesia.

A muscle-paralyzing agent such as curare is now injected, which allows the anesthesiologist to insert an endotracheal tube into the lungs. The tube delivers a mixture of nitrous oxide and oxygen, supplemented with a small amount of other organic additives or of a more potent gas such as ether. The seal around the tube must be inflated to prevent fluids from entering the windpipe. The patient is now in a state of surgical anesthesia.

For a difficult surgery, additional curare may be injected to paralyze the abdominal muscles completely. In this case, the breathing muscles would also become paralyzed, which means that a mechanical respirator would be needed to inflate and deflate the lungs.

The anesthesiologist monitors the patient's condition with various instruments, such as a stethoscope, blood pressure and temperature sensors, and an electrocardiograph (EKG or ECG) with a continuous display. A catheter may be inserted into a vein to inject drugs or to give a blood transfusion if necessary. When the surgery is completed, the anesthesiologist is responsible for overseeing procedures undertaken in the recovery room as the patient slowly regains consciousness.

Perspective and Prospects

Many modern surgeries would be impossible without anesthesia. Kidney or other organ transplants, skin grafts for a burn victim, or microsurgery for a severed finger all require that the patient remain still for an extended period of time. Anesthesiologists choose from a variety of local and general anesthetics as the individual situations require.

In the emergency room of a hospital, patients are brought in with injuries from industrial, farm, or car accidents. Gunshot and knife wounds, the ingestion of toxic chemicals, or sports injuries often require immediate action to reduce pain and preserve life. Soldiers who are wounded or burned in battle can be given relief from pain because of the available anesthetics. Beyond operating room patients, another category of people who benefit greatly from anesthesia are those who suffer from chronic pain, including that from arthritis, back pain, asthma, brain damage, cancer, and other serious ailments.

A more recent innovation is electric anesthesia, which employs an electric current. It is widely used for animals and is gaining acceptance for humans. A marine biologist can submerge two electrodes into water and cause nearby fish to become rigid and unable to swim. After being netted and tagged, the fish are released with no harmful aftereffects. Veterinarians can use a commercially available device with two electrodes that attach to the nose and tail of a farm animal. Pulses of electricity are applied, causing the animal to remain immobilized until surgery is completed.

The most common human application of electric anesthesia is in dentistry. The metal drill itself can act as an electrode, sending pulses of electric current into the nerve to deaden the sensation of pain. The discomfort of novocaine injections and the possible aftereffects of the drug are avoided. Another application is to provide relief for people with chronic back pain, using a small, battery-powered unit attached to the person's waist.

Experiments have been done using electricity for total anesthesia, both on animals and on human volunteers. Electrodes are strapped to the front and back of the head. When an appropriate voltage is applied, the subject falls into deep sleep in a short time. When the electricity is turned off, consciousness is regained almost immediately. In one experiment, two dogs underwent "electrosleep" for thirty days with no apparent ill effects. Long-term studies with more subjects are needed to establish this new technology.

—*Hans G. Graetzer, Ph.D.*

See also Acupuncture; Anesthesia; Hypnosis; Local anesthesia; Narcotics; Neurology; Neurology, pediatric; Nursing; Pain management; Pharmacology; Physician assistants; Surgery, general; Surgical procedures.

For Further Information:

Gregory, George A., ed. *Pediatric Anesthesia*. 4th ed. New York: Churchill Livingstone, 2002.

Gross, Amy, and Dee Ito. "All About Anesthesia: What Are the Choices When It Comes to Childbirth and Surgery?" *Parents Magazine* 65 (April, 1990): 213-21.

Longnecker, David E., and Frank L. Murphy. *Dripps, Eckenhoff, Vandam Introduction to Anesthesia*. 9th ed. Philadelphia: W. B. Saunders, 1997.

Matthes, Kai, et al., eds. *Anesthesiology*. New York: Oxford University Press, 2013.

Mayo Clinic. "General Anesthesia." *Mayo Foundation for Medical Education and Research*, January 19, 2013.

MedlinePlus. "Anesthesia." *MedlinePlus*, August 6, 2013.

Miller, Ronald D., ed. *Miller's Anesthesia*. 7th ed. Philadelphia: Churchill Livingstone/Elsevier, 2010.

Palmer, C. M., M. Paech, and R. D'Angelo, eds. *Handbook of Obstetric Anesthesia*. 6th ed. Oxford, England: Bios Scientific, 2002.

Rushman, G. B., N. J. H. Davies, and R. S. Atkinson. *A Short History of Anaesthesia*. Oxford, England: Butterworth-Heinemann, 1996.

Sweeney, Frank. *The Anesthesia Fact Book: Everything You Need to Know Before Surgery.* Cambridge, Mass.: Perseus, 2003.

Wolfe, Richard J. *Tarnished Idol: William Thomas Green Morton and the Introduction of Surgical Anesthesia-A Chronicle of the Ether Controversy.* San Francisco: Norman, 2000.

Aneurysmectomy

Procedure

Anatomy or system affected: Abdomen, brain, chest, heart

Specialties and related fields: Anesthesiology, critical care, emergency medicine, preventive medicine

Definition: A surgical procedure to repair an aneurysm, which occurs when an arterial or venous wall balloons.

Indications and Procedures

An aneurysm occurs when an artery or vein swells as pressure builds within it. Although aneurysms can occur wherever there are arteries or veins, typical occurrences are cranial (called cerebral aneurysms), thoracic, or abdominal. A major cause of aneurysms is a narrowing or blockage of clogged arteries or veins.

People who experience acute aneurysms are sometimes mistaken for stroke victims. Typical indications are a cessation of eye movement accompanied by a drooping of the eyelids and dilation of the pupil, rigidity in the neck, intense headache, and loss of consciousness.

Many aneurysms are repaired through bypass surgery, in which the affected area is clamped shut and excised. The area is then replaced by a section of artery or vein from the patient's leg, which is sutured into place. Controlling blood loss during such surgery is essential. If an aneurysm has ruptured, then numerous blood transfusions are likely to be required during the surgery, and preoperative blood typing is indicated. Patients are anesthetized when the surgeon is ready to make the first incision. A sterile surgical field is of the utmost importance for this procedure. As they are exposed, blood vessels are sealed immediately with hemostats (forceps) to control bleeding.

Uses and Complications

Aneurysmectomies are used to remove weakened tissue in arteries and veins at the site where ballooning has occurred or is imminent. The immediate danger posed by aneurysms is rupture, which can lead quickly to fatal blood loss. It is, therefore, imperative that medical assistance be rendered immediately. Treatment usually involves surgery to remove the aneurysm. In cases requiring emergency surgery, the prognosis is poor.

Aneurysms are sometimes diagnosed through x-rays and angiograms before they become symptomatic. Cerebral aneurysms are best detected through computed tomography (CT) scans or magnetic resonance imaging (MRI). When an early diagnosis is made, surgery can be performed under more controlled conditions than those that accompany emergency surgery. For aortic aneurysms, surgery before a rupture occurs usually has a recovery rate of 80 to 90 percent, whereas the recovery rate for surgery performed after an aneurysm has ruptured is less than 5 percent.

An aneurysm that occurs in the aorta is particularly dangerous because it creates a buildup in pressure around the heart so intense that it can cause the heart to stop beating. Although blood loss presents the greatest immediate risk in aneurysmectomy, seizures, cerebral edema, hydrocephalus, and infection may also present significant risks for patients.

—R. Baird Shuman, Ph.D.

See also Aneurysms; Angiography; Blood vessels; Brain; Brain disorders; Cardiology; Circulation; Computed tomography (CT) scanning; Craniotomy; Heart; Hematomas; Neurosurgery; Subdural hematoma; Vascular medicine; Vascular system.

For Further Information:

"Aneurysm Repair." *Texas Heart Institute*, August 2012.

"Aortic Aneurysm Repair-Endovascular." *Medline Plus*, December 10, 2012.

"Brain Aneurysm Repair." *Medline Plus*, July 19, 2012.

"How Is an Aneurysm Treated?" *National Heart, Lung, and Blood Institute*, April 1, 2011.

Melander, Sheila Drake, ed. *Case Studies in Critical Care Nursing: A Guide for Application and Review.* 3d ed. Philadelphia: W. B. Saunders, 2004.

Phillips, Nancymarie Fortunato. *Berry and Kohn's Operating Room Technique.* 12th ed. St. Louis, Mo.: Mosby/Elsevier, 2012.

Phippen, Mark L., and Maryanne Papanier Wells. *Patient Care during Operative and Invasive Procedures.* Philadelphia: W. B. Saunders, 2000.

Aneurysms

Disease/Disorder

Anatomy or system affected: Blood vessels, brain, circulatory system, head, heart, nervous system

Specialties and related fields: Cardiology, emergency medicine, general surgery, neurology, vascular medicine

Definition: A localized dilatation of a blood vessel, particularly an artery, that results from a focal weakness and distension of the arterial wall.

Causes and Symptoms

The arterial distension associated with aneurysms will take one of several forms. For example, fusiform aneurysms create a uniform bulge around an artery, while those of the saccular variety distend on one side of the blood vessel. Some saccular aneurysms found in the brain are called berry aneurysms for their protruding shapes.

Hypertension and arteriosclerosis commonly produce dilatation of the thoracic aorta. Very large aneurysms of the abdominal aorta (possibly the most common type) are usually caused by advanced atherosclerosis. The pathologic processes associated with the production of aortic aneurysms are varied, but certain factors are common to all.

Information on Aneurysms

Causes: Dilatation of a blood vessel (particularly an artery) from hypertension, arteriosclerosis, blunt trauma, bacterial endocarditis

Symptoms: Often none; sometimes sudden and severe pain, lump, or pulsing sensation near blood vessels

Duration: Acute

Treatments: Surgery

Types of Aneurysm

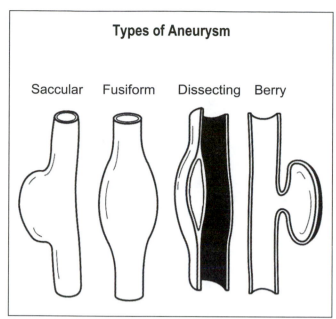

Saccular   Fusiform   Dissecting   Berry

Aneurysms may cause a variety of different shapes of distension of the affected blood vessel.

The media (middle arterial layer) of the normal aorta must remain intact in order for the aorta to withstand the systolic blood pressure. When the media is damaged, there is progressive dilation of the weakened area and an aneurysm develops. An aortic aneurysm is a serious disease with poor prognosis. Many such aneurysms rupture and cause death before surgical intervention can take place.

There are several types of aneurysms. Dissecting aortic aneurysms are those in which blood enters the wall of the blood vessel and splits the media of the vessel. The dissection of the media usually begins as a transverse tear in the region above the aortic valve and works downward between the layers of the aortic wall. Some believe that hypertension promotes the tear by increasing the tension on the aorta. Traumatic aneurysm is usually caused by penetrating wounds or by blunt trauma; the most common cause of such injuries is automobile accidents. Mycotic aneurysms of the aorta may be associated with bacterial endocarditis and sometimes with organisms such as salmonella. Aneurysms of the sinuses of Valsalva may be attributable to syphilitic aortitis, bacterial endocarditis, or congenital defect.

Treatment and Therapy

Surgical therapy for thoracic aortic aneurysms varies with the type and location of the lesion. Aneurysms involving the aortic arch are often surgically corrected by employing a bypass technique. One method sutures a large prosthetic graft between the ascending and descending aortas, thus bypassing the diseased area. Surgical techniques sometimes offer the only hope for the survival of a patient with aneurysm. A 2013 study identified that small aneurysms grow more slowly than larger aneurysms. It suggested that diagnostic imaging of patients with small aneurysms can occur with less frequency, increasing the cost effectiveness of treatment.

—*Jane A. Slezak, Ph.D.*

See also Aneurysmectomy; Arteriosclerosis; Blood vessels; Brain; Brain disorders; Bypass surgery; Cardiology; Cardiology, pediatric; Circulation; Heart; Hematomas; Hypertension; Neurology; Neurology, pediatric; Neurosurgery; Subdural hematoma.

For Further Information:
Adelman, Mark. "News release." *Journal of the American Medical Association.* (2013): Web. 22 May. 2013.
Goldman, Lee, and Dennis Ausiello, eds. *Cecil Textbook of Medicine.* 23d ed. Philadelphia: Saunders/Elsevier, 2007.
Keen, Richard R., and Philip B. Dobrin, eds. *Development of Aneurysms.* Georgetown, Tex.: Landes Bioscience, 2000.
Parker, James N., and Philip M. Parker, eds. *The Official Patient's Sourcebook on Cerebral Aneurysm.* San Diego, Calif.: Icon Health, 2002.
Yao, James S. T., and William H. Pearce, eds. *Aneurysms: New Findings and Treatments.* Norwalk, Conn.: Appleton & Lange, 1994.

Angelman syndrome

Disease/Disorder

Also known as: Happy Puppet Syndrome

Anatomy or system affected: Brain, eyes, gastrointestinal system, hair, head, joints, knees, mouth, nerves, nervous system, psychic-emotional system, skin, teeth

Specialties and related fields: Dermatology, family practice, genetics, neonatology, neurology, occupational health, pediatrics, physical therapy, psychiatry, psychology, speech pathology

Definition: A complex genetic disorder that causes developmental disabilities and neurological problems.

Key terms:

ataxia: lack of coordination during voluntary muscle movement

neuron: cells in the nervous system that are electrically excitable and generate, propagate, and transmit electrochemical signals called nerve impulses

ubiquitin: a small regulatory protein found in almost all nucleated cells that, when attached to other proteins, directs the cell to degrade them or use them for some other function

Causes and Symptoms

Angelman syndrome, an inherited neurological condition, provides a prime example of genetic imprinting. Genetic imprinting consists of the expression of particular genes in a parent-of-origin-specific manner. To illustrate genetic imprinting, Angelman syndrome (AS) results from mutations in the UBE3A gene that are inherited from the mother and not the father. AS shows this unusual inheritance pattern because in particular parts of the brain, the maternal copy of the UBE3A gene is expressed, but the paternal copy is inactive. This parent-of-origin-specific mode of expression of UBE3A characterizes those genes regulated by genetic imprinting.

The UBE3A gene is on chromosome 15, and encodes an enzyme called the E6 associated protein or E6-AP. E6-AP is a member of the E3 ubiquitin ligase family of enzymes. Ubiquitin is a small protein that is attached to other proteins to either mark them for destruction, or activate them to perform a specific function. In the brain, E6-AP attaches ubiquitin to proteins involved in neuron function and marks them for degradation. By recycling these proteins, E6-AP tightly regulates the levels of those proteins inside neurons. In the absence of E6-AP, the proteins in neurons lose their tight regulation, causing neuronal malfunction.

Children with AS show profoundly delayed development, severe speech impediment, intellectual disability, movement and balance problems (ataxia), trembling movement of the arms and legs, an excitable personality, and a happy demeanor with frequent smiling, laughing and hand-flapping movements. Hyperactivity and a short attention span are also common. By age 2, over 80 percent of AS children have a smaller than average head, and by age 3, most suffer from seizures. Other symptoms shown by some but not all AS children include crossing of the eyes (strabismus), a flatness at the back of the head (microbrachycephaly), a fascination with water (particularly running water), light pigmentation of the eyes, skin and hair, tongue thrusting accompanied by swallowing and sucking disorders, walking with the arms up in the air, sleep disturbances, stiff, jerky movements (hyperactive tendon reflexes), and an increased sensitivity to heat.

One in 12,000 to one in 20,000 people have AS.

Treatment and Therapy

No cure exists for AS. Treatments focus on managing the medical and developmental problems of AS children.

Antiepileptic medicines can help control the seizures. These include sodium valproate (Epilim), clonazepam, (Rivotril), lamotrigine (Lamictal), carbamazepine (Tegretol), and levetiracetam (Keppra). Another medication called piracetam (Nootropil) may help control the jerky movements seen in AS children.

Physical therapy can help AS children learn to walk better and overcome some of their other movement problems. Communication therapy can help AS children communicate better. AS children have severe speech disabilities, but some can learn to communicate with sign language. However, even though sign language is simply beyond the abilities of many AS patients, most AS children learn to communicate through nonverbal cues. Communication therapy can help AS children develop these skills. Behavior therapy can help AS children address their hyperactivity and short attention span. Most AS children are extroverted and can build strong relationships with family and friends.

Many AS children have circadian rhythm sleep disorder, and tend to sleep irregularly and for short periods of time. Such irregular sleep patterns can unduly stress their parents. Small studies have established that AS children have lower than normal levels of the hormone melatonin, which regulates sleep and wake cycles, in their bloodstream. Therefore, giving AS children oral melatonin can normalize their sleep patterns. AS children also may have poor bowel motility, which may cause constipation; however, laxatives can alleviate such problems.

Perspective and Prospects

An English pediatrician named Harry Angelman from Warrington (then in the county of Lancashire, but now in

---

Information on Angelman Syndrome

Causes: The inheritance of a mutant copy of the UBE3A gene from the mother

Symptoms: Developmental delay, speech impairment, trembling movement of arms and legs, seizures, happy disposition with frequent laughter, and excitable personality

Duration: Symptoms present at birth and remain for the remainder of life

Treatment: No cure available, anticonvulsant medicines for seizures, physical therapy for movement

---

the county of Cheshire) first described the syndrome that bears his name in 1965. Angelman's initial case report came from his observation of three handicapped children who all showed severe mental retardation and speech disability, a "marionette-like" gait, similar facial appearances, and unusual happiness. Angelman called it the "Happy Puppet Syndrome," which, in 1982, was changed to AS.

In 1987, researchers at Children's Hospital in Boston, Massachusetts identified a small piece of chromosome 15 that was missing in an AS patient. Two years later, Charles Williams at the University of Florida discovered that twelve different AS patients possessed a deletion on the long arm of chromosome 15 that removed the same segment (15q12). The following year Williams and his group identified that these deletions all originated in the patient's maternal chromosome. In 1997, Wagstaff and Beaudet identified maternal mutations in the UBE3A gene as the cause of AS.

In 2011, Benjamin Philpot's laboratory at the University of North Carolina School of Medicine showed that drugs called topoisomerase inhibitors (e.g., topotecan, irinotecan, etoposide and dexrazoxane) unsilenced the UBE3A gene in the brains of laboratory mice with a form of AS. This suggests that pharmacological agents might activate the UBE3A gene in the brains of AS patients, and may provide a much more potent treatment for AS in the future.

—*Michael A. Buratovich Ph.D.*

See also Genetic counseling; Genetic imprinting; Neurology

For Further Information:

Hewitt, John. *Angelman Syndrome: Causes, Tests, and Treatments.* Seattle, Wash.: CreateSpace Independent Publishing Platform, 2011.

Lyman, Pamela Jean. *In the Company of Angels.* Mustang, Okla.: Tate Publishing, 2013.

Williams, Charles A., Daniel J. Driscoll, and Aditi I. Dagli. "Clinical and Genetic Aspects of Angelman Syndrome." *Genetics in Medicine* 12 (2010): 385-395.

Angina

Disease/Disorder

Anatomy or system affected: Circulatory system, heart

Specialties and related fields: Cardiology, family medicine, internal medicine

Definition: Chest pain ranging from mild indigestion to a severe crushing, squeezing, or choking sensation.

Causes and Symptoms

Usually located below the sternum, angina may radiate down the left arm and/or left jaw, or down both arms and jaws. It is ischemic in nature, meaning that the pain is produced by a variety of conditions that result in insufficient supply of oxygen-rich blood to the heart. Some examples include arteriosclerosis (hardening of the arteries), atherosclerosis (arteries clogged with deposits of fat, cholesterol, and other substances), coronary artery spasms, low blood pressure, low blood volume, vasoconstriction (a narrowing of the arteries), anemia, and chronic lung disease.

Precipitating factors for angina include physical exertion, strong emotions, consumption of a heavy meal, temperature extremes, cigarette smoking, and sexual activity. These factors can cause angina because they may increase heart rate, cause vasoconstriction, or divert blood from the heart to other areas, such as the gastrointestinal system. Angina usually lasts from three to five minutes and commonly subsides when the precipitating factors are relieved. Typically, it should not last more than twenty minutes after rest or treatment.

Diagnosis consists of a physical examination which includes a chest X ray to determine any obvious lung or structural cardiac abnormalities; blood tests to screen risk factors such as lipids or to detect enzymes that can indicate if a heart attack has occurred; electrocardiography (ECG or EKG) to look at the electrical activity of the heart for evidence of damage or insufficient blood flow; nuclear studies such as thallium stress tests, which measure myocardial perfusion; and cardiac catheterization and coronary angiography to evaluate the anatomy of the coronary arteries, the location and nature of artery narrowing or constriction, and to assess the muscular function of the heart, including cardiac output.

Treatment depends on the specific cause of the angina. Three types of drugs are the most common form of treatment: nitrates, to increase the supply of oxygen to the heart by dilating the coronary arteries; beta-blockers, to lower oxygen demand during exercise and improve oxygen supply and demand; and calcium blockers, to decrease the work of the heart by decreasing cardiac contractility. A study published in March 2013 found that the drug Ranexa (ranolazine) might reduce symptoms of angina in patients with type 2 diabetes.

—*John A. Bavaro, Ed.D., R.N.*

See also Arteriosclerosis; Cardiology; Cardiology, pediatric; Chest; Echocardiography; Heart; Heart attack; Heart disease; Hyperlipidemia; Hypertension; Ischemia; Pain; Thrombosis and thrombus.

For Further Information:

Dranov, Paula. *Random House Personal Medical Handbook: For People with Heart Disease*. New York: Random House, 1991.

McGoon, M. *The Mayo Clinic Heart Book*. 2d ed. New York: William Morrow, 2000.

Pantano, James. *Living with Angina: A Practical Guide to Dealing with Coronary Artery Disease and Your Doctor*. New York: First Books, 2000.

Parker, James M., and Philip M. Parker, eds. *The 2002 Official Patient's Sourcebook on Angina*. San Diego, Calif.: Icon Health, 2002.

Zaret, Barry L., Marvin Moser, and Lawrence S. Cohen, eds. *Yale University School of Medicine Heart Book*. New York: William Morrow, 1992.

Angiography

Procedure

Anatomy or system affected: Blood, blood vessels, brain, circulatory system, head, heart

Specialties and related fields: Cardiology, emergency medicine, radiology, vascular medicine

Definition: The X-ray analysis of the cardiovascular system following the injection of a radiopaque contrast dye into an artery.

Indications and Procedures

Angiography (also called arteriography) is a procedure utilized for the detection of abnormalities in arteries of the heart, brain, or other organs. The procedure is carried out when symptoms suggest the narrowing or blockage of an artery, most frequently in the heart or brain. Such

An angiogram showing the path of the carotid artery through the head and neck. (Digital Stock)

symptoms include chest pain or similarly associated discomfort in the region of the stomach or left side of the body. Even if pain is absent, shortness of breath may indicate a cardiac or pulmonary problem. Slurred speech or vision may likewise suggest narrowing of an artery in the brain. Angiography can therefore indicate the likelihood of a heart attack or stroke, as well as other problems which may produce similar symptoms, such as blood clots or cancer.

The patient must avoid food or drink for approximately eight hours prior to the procedure. A catheter is inserted through the skin, usually in the groin area, and placed into the artery to be examined. A sedative is not necessary, although it may be given to the patient to aid in relaxation.

Once the catheter is in place, a radiopaque dye is injected, and x-ray photographs of the area in question are taken. The procedure generally takes about three hours.

Uses and Complications

Since any blockage or narrowing of an artery will result in accumulation of the radiopaque dye, the radiologist can pinpoint the site of the block. Based on the symptoms, the physician can discuss the diagnosis and recommend further procedures.

The most common complication associated with angiography is the mild discomfort resulting from insertion of the catheter. The dye itself may cause a slight burning sensation, and on rare occasions it may trigger an allergic response. In 1 to 2 percent of cases, more serious complications develop. If the blockage results from an atherosclerotic plaque or from a blood clot, in rare circumstances a piece of this material may break off and lodge elsewhere in the arterial system. The result can be a stroke or heart attack.

—Richard Adler, Ph.D.

See also Angioplasty; Arteriosclerosis; Blood vessels; Bypass surgery; Cardiology; Catheterization; Circulation; Echocardiography; Heart; Heart attack; Heart disease; Imaging and radiology; Plaque, arterial; Radiopharmaceuticals; Strokes; Vascular medicine; Vascular system.

For Further Information:
"Coronary Angiography." *Medline Plus*, June 22, 2012.
"CT Angiography (CTA)." *Radiological Society of North America*, July 2, 2012.
Dranov, Paula. *Heart Disease*. New York: Random House, 1990.
"Extremity Angiography." *Medline Plus*, December 10, 2012.
Higgins, Charles B., and Albert de Roos. *Cardiovascular MRI and MRA*. Philadelphia: Lippincott Williams & Wilkins, 2002.
Karch, Amy Morrison. *Cardiac Care: A Guide for Patient Education*. New York: Appleton-Century-Crofts, 1981.
Ludinghausen, Michael. *Clinical Anatomy of Coronary Arteries*. New York: Springer, 2003.
Prince, Martin R., et al. *3-D Contrast MR Angiography*. New York: Springer, 2003.
Rosenblum, Laurie. "Angiography." *Health Library*, May 20, 2013.
Rutherford, Robert B., ed. *Vascular Surgery*. 7th ed. Philadelphia: Saunders/Elsevier, 2010.

Angioplasty

Procedure

Anatomy or system affected: Blood vessels, circulatory system, heart

Specialties and related fields: Cardiology, vascular medicine

Definition: The insertion of a long, flexible tube into a narrowed or blocked blood vessel in order to repair it; in balloon angioplasty, a small balloon at the end of the tube is inflated to compress a fatty blockage in the blood vessel and thus increase blood flow.

Indications and Procedures

Angioplasty, particularly balloon angioplasty, may be performed on any blocked or narrowed blood vessel, such as in the legs, but it is most commonly used to open heart vessels blocked by coronary artery disease.

Worldwide, an estimated seventeen million people die each year from cardiovascular disease, a condition often signaled by chest pain known as angina pectoris. Other symptoms include shortness of breath, heart palpitations, or an actual heart attack. Probable causes of heart disease can be diagnosed by stress tests and angiography. If the cause is blockage of the coronary arteries, the cardiologist may order angioplasty to open the blocked vessels and restore a better blood flow to the heart.

The patient cannot eat or drink anything after midnight the day before the procedure is to be performed. A mild sedative may be given. The site for insertion of the catheter, often the inside of the elbow or the groin, is shaved and is cleaned with an antiseptic solution. A local anesthetic is injected at the insertion site, but the patient remains awake during the procedure. The surgeon makes a small opening in the skin at the insertion site, inserts the catheter into an artery, watches the progress of the catheter on an x-ray monitor, and guides the tip into the blocked arteries.

In balloon angioplasty, the most common type, the tube is equipped with a balloon. Once the tip is in place in the blocked area, the balloon is inflated and deflated several times in order to compress the fatty material (plaque) and increase blood flow through the artery. The catheter then is slowly withdrawn.

If the arm site was used, the small incision is stitched closed. If the groin site was used, the puncture opening is closed with pressure. A dressing is applied to the insertion site. Barring any complications, the patient may return home later the same day or the next day.

Uses and Complications

The cardiac catheters used in angioplasty can also remove plaque with special cutting or laser tips. The balloon tip may be used to place a stent, a metal mesh tube that is placed permanently in the coronary artery to keep it open. Blood thinning medication may be prescribed to keep blood from clotting on the stent and closing it.

About 80 percent of the angioplasty treatments are successful, with the patient being able to resume a reasonably normal lifestyle and enjoy a good quality of life. Complications of coronary artery angioplasty seldom occur, but they may include bleeding or clotting, an abnormal heartbeat, perforation of the heart muscle or artery, and, rarely, a heart

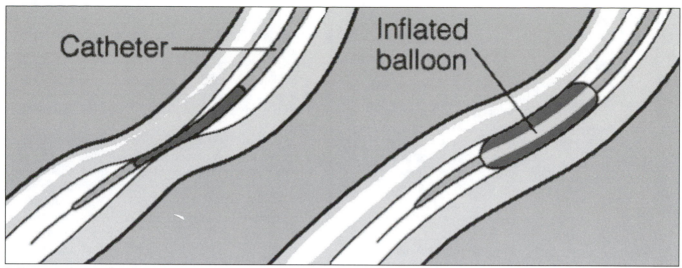

Balloon angioplasty involves the insertion of a catheter into an artery that has narrowed and the inflation of a small balloon in order to expand the vessel; this procedure is usually performed to counteract the effects of atherosclerotic disease, in which plaque deposits accumulate in the arteries.

attack, stroke, or even death.

—*Albert C. Jensen, M.S.*

See also Angina; Angiography; Arteriosclerosis; Blood vessels; Bypass surgery; Cardiology; Catheterization; Heart; Heart attack; Heart disease; Heart valve replacement; Palpitations; Plaque, arterial; Stents; Thrombolytic therapy and TPA; Vascular medicine; Vascular system.

For Further Information:
American Heart Association. *AHA Focus Series: Arteriosclerosis.* Washington, D.C.: American Heart Association, 1988.
"Angioplasty and Stent Placement-Heart." *Medline Plus*, August 24, 2012.
"Coronary Angioplasty." *Health Library*, February 7, 2013.
McGoon, M. *The Mayo Clinic Heart Book.* 2d ed. New York: William Morrow, 2000.
Ohman, Magnus, Gail Folger Cox, and Victoria K. Folger. *So You're Having a Heart Cath and Angioplasty.* Hoboken, N.J.: John Wiley & Sons, 2003.
Rutherford, Robert B., ed. *Vascular Surgery.* 7th ed. Philadelphia: Saunders/Elsevier, 2010.
Tcheng, James E. *Primary Angioplasty in Acute Myocardial Infarction.* Totowa, N.J.: Humana Press, 2002.
"What Is Coronary Angioplasty?" *National Heart, Lung, and Blood Institute*, February 1, 2012.

Animal rights vs. research
Ethics
Definition: The debate concerning medical research techniques using animals as test specimens in order to obtain information regarding procedures, drugs, or products to be used on humans.
Key terms:
amyloidosis: a condition characterized by the deposit of waxy substances in animal organs
Aneurysm: dilatation of a blood vessel
atherosclerosis: thickening of the artery wall due to accumulation of fatty materials such as cholesterol and triglycerides.
biomedical research: investigation or experimentation relating to biological, medical, and physical science
biomedicine: the branch of medical science concerned with the capacity of human beings to survive and function in abnormally stressful environments and with the protective modification of such environments
cardiomyopathy: a typically chronic disorder of heart muscle that may involve obstructive damage to the heart
commissurectomy: the removal of a connecting band of tissue in the brain or spinal cord
endocarditis: inflammation of the lining of the heart and its valves
hemophilia: a hereditary blood defect (occurring almost exclusively in males) characterized by delayed clotting of the blood and consequent difficulty in controlling hemorrhage after even minor injuries
neuritis: an inflammatory or degenerative lesion of a nerve, marked by pain and the loss of normal reflexes
toxoplasmosis: an infection caused by parasitic microorganisms that invade tissues and that may cause damage to the central nervous system, especially in infants
tumor: abnormal mass of tissue as a result of abnormal growth or division of cells
uveitis: inflammation of the uvea of the eye
vivisection: surgery conducted for experimental purposes on a living organism

Controversy Surrounding Animal Experimentation
The practice of utilizing animals as test subjects in research has resulted in the informal formation of two basic factions: those who support its role as providing information regarding the contagion and transmission of diseases, their treatment, and their potential cure; and those who deplore the use of animals, citing miserable living conditions for captive animals, which are subjected to painful and debilitating experiments that sometimes result in disfigurement, permanent injury, or death.

Those in the first party include doctors, medical researchers, sick patients and their families who have benefited from the information gained. They believe that the performance of experiments on animals has been invaluable, leading to the discovery of many medical treatments and cures for humans afflicted with disease, as well as information related to the risks and benefits of drugs or other products. The second party, often referred to as animal rights activists, is made up of people dedicated to halting the testing and killing of animals in experiments. These groups include People for the Ethical Treatment of Animals (PETA), the Animal Liberation Front (ALF, and the American Anti-Vivisection Society (AAVS), to name a few. Some animal rights activists groups have picketed laboratories, incensed critics, and, in extreme cases, destroyed testing facilities and released the animals kept in them in order to prevent or impede further testing. These groups believe that animals have a right to live in their normal habitats without human intrusion.

Since second century Rome, doctors and scientists have conducted experiments on animals, including dissections. The discoveries have yielded immeasurable amounts of information which can be assimilated to human medical conditions. On the other hand, animal experiments have become so commonplace, that animals are sometimes regarded as mere tools in the laboratory. "To me, a monkey was as expendable as a screwdriver or a pair of pliers," indicates Donald Barnes, a former experimental psychologist who has become an animal activist.

Animal rights activists seek an end to animal experimentation, claiming that much of it is unnecessary. According to PETA, the major infectious diseases, such as poliomyelitis, tuberculosis, cholera, and typhoid fever, are dying out in developing countries mostly because of improved living conditions and sanitation, rather than because of vaccines. Furthermore, the ALF reminds scientists that insulin, a treatment for diabetes mellitus that was created using animal research, is not a cure for the disease. Some test procedures, such as scalding or electrocution, are pointless, as the outcome of the experiment is already known. Barnes explains why he was fired from a research position: "One day I refused to carry out a particular military experiment on four perfectly healthy primates, but only because we already knew the answer to the question. It was an invalid experiment, and as the principal investigator I knew that its only purpose was to ensure further funding for the lab."

Animal rights activists can take different approaches to the issue. The more conventional and more peaceful method is the pursuit of stricter regulations for animal research. In announcements and letters to researchers, activists may state that they are seeking the enactment of laws and regulations that ban all research using animals. Bills to prevent or limit animal research have been introduced in several American states. Other efforts include an attempt to win legal standing to act on behalf of animals and endeavors to divert federal funds earmarked for biomedical research into the development of alternatives for experimentation.

The more conservative approach to promoting animal rights is through advocacy and educational organizations. For example, the American Anti-Vivisection Society (AAVS), founded in 1883, works with schools, the media, government officials, and community members to develop alternative methods to animal use. The AAVS uses two types of educational activities. The first is Animalearn, an education program which focuses on ending vivisection in the classroom setting. The second is the Science Bank, which provides alternatives to using animals in basic dissections. The Science Bank provides over 500 CD-ROMS, models, videos, and mannikins?all offered for free for students ranging from Pre-K all the way through medical school.

Other activists have taken extreme measures to display their disgust through demonstrations, break-ins, and vandalism to research laboratories across the United States. Such acts cost research firms more than $17 million annually. Damage to the laboratories and equipment and the releasing or stealing of animals impede the research process and call attention to the activists' concerns. The efforts of some of these activists have become increasingly violent, including the use of bombs and other explosives at or near testing facilities. PETA, an organization of more than 325,000 members, says that it disavows violence, but the ALF has actually claimed credit for some of the attacks. In 2006, US President George W. Bush signed the Animal Enterprise Terrorism Act, which made it a crime to deliberately cause economic damage to an institution engaged in animal research. However, activists are still continuing to display vandalism. In direct contrast to the activists' perceptions of animal research are doctors, scientists, beneficiaries, and others who argue in favor of animal biomedical testing. According to David Chernof, the former president of the Los Angeles County Medical Association, "Animal research has been the basis for every medical advance which has benefitted humanity in the past 100 years-from insulin to heart surgery to polio and a cure for childhood leukemia." The American Medical Association (AMA) and other medical organizations support the use of animal testing for its importance in advancing the treatment and cure of human diseases. Animals are considered indispensable in biomedical research because of structural similarities between animals and humans, who often react to illnesses in the same way and suffer from many of the same diseases. The AMA actively opposes all laws, regulations, and social protesting that seek to limit such research. The medical field believes that it is only through continued support of the research process, including funding and experimentation, that the United States can continue to be a leader in medical discoveries.

Consumers of a variety of health, hygiene, and beauty products also benefit from animal testing. Such testing has protected consumers from pain, discomfort, and allergic reactions to such products as shampoo, lipstick, and dyes. While testing that does not involve the use of animals often can achieve these goals, sometimes animal testing is the only way to establish the safety of a product for use by humans.

Scientists point out that the information gained from the research often benefits the animals as well. For example, research has shown that feeding monkeys a low-cholesterol diet helps to relieve arteriosclerosis in that particular animal. Other experiments have resulted in the discovery of vaccines to treat infected cattle, poultry, horses, cats, and dogs. In addition, the researchers indicate that the federal government's rules and regulations regarding the housing conditions and care of test animals are so strict that the medical centers probably provide better care for these animals than that received by human patients.

Another group that supports animal biomedical research is the patients who have survived an illness or catastrophe because research had allowed the development of proper treatments, or patients currently receiving treatment. The Incurably Ill for Animal Research (IIFAR), a US organization made up of people suffering from chronic diseases (and their families), supports the humane use of animals for research. In 1990, the group presented the US Congress with a petition signed by 70,000 members requesting that such research be allowed to continue. While the members of IIFAR express regret that animals have been sacrificed, they argue that the technology and information gained have helped many of them cope with illness and receive treatment and have sometimes cured diseases that otherwise would have proven fatal to humans.

Caught in the middle of the controversy are veterinarians, who by trade seek to alleviate pain and illness of animals. Veterinarians are the caretakers of research animals and at the same time are the targets of the campaigns of animal rights activists. The American Veterinary Medical Association basically agrees with the AMA on this issue, but it has not taken such a high-profile role in proclaiming this position. Some veterinarians believe that they are fighting a war of facts versus emotions and that education is the only answer, that the public should be informed that animal welfare is not necessarily equated with animal rights.

Many recent guidelines have been established that may help to assuage the fears of animal rights activists, while still promoting humane methods of experimentation with animals. Major guiding documents have been published to enforce humane care in the use of animals in research. For example, the American Psychological Association developed guidelines for the acquisition, housing, use, and disposition of nonhuman animals in research. These guidelines are all in compliance with federal, state, and local laws and regulations.

The Benefits of Animal Research

Whether the use of animals in experiments is ethical is a matter of debate. Not all animal experimentation is equal. The goals of animal experimentation for product safety, such as for cosmetics versus a drug for heart disease, may need to be weighed separately. The merit and the pros and cons may differ substantially in the eyes of both animal testing advocates and animal rights advocates.

Nevertheless, such research has had many successes. Breakthroughs using animal research have resulted in the development of a vaccine for polio, treatments for cancer, safer heart surgery, and even the artificial heart. Some other medical discoveries made through animal research, listed in the Journal of the American Medical Association, are in aging, anesthesia, behavioral studies, cardiovascular medi-

cine, the study of hearing (audiology), ophthalmology, organ transplantation, pulmonary medicine, radiology, reproductive biology, virology, the treatment and study of AIDS, immunology, cancer, hemophilia, hepatitis, malaria, rabies, and toxoplasmosis.

Aging. Direct relationships between infections and immunologic disease have made dogs an excellent example to study in cases of amyloidosis. Dogs also serve as models for the study of Alzheimer's disease because of similar pathological changes-an increase in neuritic plaques-seen with Alzheimer's disease in humans. Primates also exhibit this abundance of neuritic plaques. Rodents have been used extensively in aging studies because their functional ability declines with age in a fashion similar to that of humans. Researchers have now been able to create genetically engineered mice to make them vulnerable to DNA damage and damage their mitochondria. As a result, scientists are able to gather information regarding the ways in which DNA or mitochondrial damage contributes to the disease of aging. In addition, targeted genetic manipulated mice are providing novel insights into the aging process.

Anesthesia. The development of equipment and use of positive-pressure ventilation in performing chest surgery on dogs led to an adapted use for humans. A classic success story in the development of anesthetic techniques was when the first lung cancer patient to have a lung removed survived another forty years.

Behavioral studies. Research involving dogs, rats, and mice provides feedback on environmental adaptation, hereditary characteristics, and learned behaviors. Relationships between behaviors such as fear and stress and between physiological changes such as cardiac rate changes and anorexia nervosa can provide assimilations for humans. Research on depression in primates provides information about sleep disturbances, which can resemble depression and disordered physiology in humans. The study of the communicative abilities of primates helps in the development of teaching practices for mentally retarded children. Animals who suffered from intractable epilepsy have undergone commissurectomy, which has led to the understanding of left-right brain hemisphere cognitive differences in humans. Experiments with rats have shown that obesity shortens the life span. Mice have been utilized as principal research subjects because of the availability of inbred strains and mutants with differing neuroanatomy and biochemistry. The generally short life span of a mouse allows researchers to observe the animal and its changes in its normal lifetime, yielding information within a short time frame. Lastly, a study using birds has recently shown, for the first time, the gene involvement in speech and language impairments that are associated with autistic disorders.

Cardiovascular medicine. Endocarditis develops naturally in dogs-no inducement or intervention is necessary-and provides scientists with information on bacterial endocarditis in humans. Many inherited cardiovascular problems occur in dogs, and the surgical techniques to correct such defects have also proven effective in humans. Rats develop hypertension spontaneously, increasing with age and occurring more frequently in male rats. As a result, they can be used as tests of blood pressure controls in the study of antihypertensive agents. Mouse models have also been proven to be useful to study the development and progression of atherosclerotic lesions, which leads to heart disease. Recent insights into the pathophysiology of abdominal aortic aneurysms have be a result of mouse models. Cats are used as models to evaluate therapeutic approaches to cardiomyopathy, as well as the role of the liver and how the gastrointestinal tract functions.

Audiology. Hearing loss patterns in mice closely resemble those in humans. The mouse has become an excellent source of information about age-induced hearing loss as well as about the effects of noise exposure.

Ophthalmology. Common retinal diseases such as glaucoma, cataracts, and uveitis occur in dogs; these animals have been used to find effective strategies for alleviating these eye conditions in humans. Cat research involving cataracts has provided information on postsurgical corneal healing. Primates have also been used in the study of vision disorders and visual maturation in children.

Organ transplantation. The first successful kidney transplants were performed on dogs in the late 1950s, which led to correct procedures for human organ transplantation. Studies of tissue rejection in rats can be assimilated to the same affliction in humans.

Pulmonary medicine. Rats have proven valuable in the study of decompression sickness as well as of the effects of air emboli in the lungs. Dogs have been used to study emphysema, pulmonary edema, and thermal burns of the lung associated with fire or the ingestion of chemicals. Lung surgery on dogs led to the development of the pulmonary pump oxygenator.

Radiology. Research in radiology shows that some animals are more sensitive to radiation than others and that survival is dependent on the age when the first dosages of radiation were received.

Reproductive biology. Primates, rats, and mice are excellent subjects for reproductive research, including studies on endocrinology and menstruation. This research has led to advances in fertility control methods for humans. Pregnancy, fetal development, and birth are studied in primates because of their similarities to the human condition of pregnancy. The identification of the Rh factor was an immunological breakthrough resulting from tests on primates. The discovery of human papilloma viruses causing cervical cancer was made using hamsters, mice, and cows. The development of in vitro fertilization was made from rabbits.

Virology. Understanding of viral transmissions and diseases has been furnished by research done on mice; these findings have led to the formulation of vaccines for influenza, polio, encephalomyelitis, and rabies.

Acquired immunodeficiency syndrome (AIDS). Simians provide an excellent study population for AIDS because their immunodeficiency symptoms, syndromes, and viruses are almost identical to those of humans. In addition, the AIDS virus itself was isolated in captive rhesus monkeys.

Immunology. Discoveries concerning the activation of innate immunity and adaptive immunity were made using mice. This may lead to newer drugs that treat various illnesses more efficiently.

Cancer. One of the first studies of chemotherapy was performed on dogs, which resulted in the knowledge that some cancers may be caused by infectious agents. Cats are used as subjects in breast cancer studies because of similarities in structure to humans. In addition, rats and mice are used extensively in cancer research, especially in the study of tumors. For example, mice were used as animal models to evaluate the response of targeted treatment of Gastrointestinal Stromal Tumors (GISTs). This approach of cancer research on GISTs can be essential for innovative treatments for other types of cancers.

Hemophilia. Hemophilia in dogs is nearly identical to that in humans, so the dog has served as a model for this research. The first successful bone marrow transplant occurred in laboratory mice and served as the example for such transplants in humans.

Hepatitis. The dog is used as a research subject because viral hepatitis occurs naturally in dogs. The dog also is used for comparative studies of cirrhosis of the liver. Research involving chimpanzees led to the discovery of the hepatitis B vaccine.

Malaria. Potential therapies for malaria, which affects 200 million people worldwide, can be discovered through tests on primates.

Rabies. The original vaccine produced for the treatment of rabies resulted from experimentation on rabbits.

Toxoplasmosis. The study of cats infected with toxoplasmosis has led to treatments for the 4,500 human babies born annually in the United States with this infection.

Perspective and Prospects

Through the use of animals as test subjects, benefits have been gained for both humans and animals. Many therapies and cures have been discovered through careful experimentation with animals in which a particular animal is found to be suited to a particular test. Animal research has been performed for centuries, and the information gleaned from the procedures has provided modern medicine with many vaccines and treatments that probably would not have been possible without such research.

Animal rights activists have struck a nerve in the field of research and have increased awareness among animal researchers about ensuring the use of humane methods of experimentation. Continued dialogue between these groups will be necessary to avoid the halting of important medical research and to discourage the unnecessary use of animals when other methods are available.

—Carol A. Holloway; updated by Krystal Jenkins, OMS-IV, and Maisah Shaikh, OMS-IV

See also American Medical Association (AMA); Ethics; Laboratory tests; National Institutes of Health (NIH); Veterinary medicine

For Further Information:

Breo, Dennis L. "Animal Rights vs. Research? A Question of the Nation's Scientific Literacy." *Journal of the American Medical Association* 264 (November 21, 1990): 2564. An excellent source of information regarding all aspects of animal biomedical research.

"Bruce A. Beutler-Interview." Nobelprize.org. *Nobel Media* AB 2013. Web. 25 Oct 2013. http://www.nobelprize.org/nobel_prizes/medicine/laureates/2011/beutler-interview.html. A great source for current awards given in medical research.

Cohen, Carl, and Tom Regan. *The Animal Rights Debate.* Lanham, Md.: Rowman & Littlefield, 2001. An exploration of the philosophical debate with the authors representing the opposite poles.

Cooke, Patrick. "A Rat Is a Pig Is a Dog Is a Boy: The Debate over Animal Rights Is Full of Equations That Don't Add Up." *Health* 5 (July/August, 1991): 58-64. An excellent article examining the highly emotional issue of animal experimentation in medical research.

Fox, James G., et al., eds. *Laboratory Animal Medicine.* 2nd ed. New York: Academic Press, 2002. A text that covers the biological and disease aspects of laboratory animal medicine. Also explores the biohazards associated with the use of animal experimentation and factors complicating the bioethics of animal research.

Groves, Julian McAllister. *Hearts and Minds: The Controversy over Laboratory Animals.* Philadelphia, Pa.: Temple University Press, 1997. This book describes the controversies involved in the use of laboratory animals for different types of testing.

"Harald zur Hause-Nobel Lecture: The Search for Infectious Causes of Human Cancers: Where and Why. " Nobelprize.org. *Nobel Media* AB 2013. Web. 25 Oct 2013. http://www.nobelprize.org/nobel_prizes/medicine/laureates/2008/hausen-lecture.html. A great source for current awards given in medical research.

Horner, J., and F.D. Minifie (2011). "Research Ethics I: Responsible Conduct of Research (RCR)-Historical and Contemporary Issues Pertaining to Human and Animal Experimentation." *Journal of Speech, Language and Hearing Research* (Online), 54(1), S303-S329A. Retrieved from http://search.proquest.com/ docview/858020215?accountid=12917. A publication that demonstrates the rule and regulations involved in using animals in research experiments.

Jackson, Christine. "Dissection: Science or Violence?" *Mothering* 9 (Spring, 1991): 91. A list of sources for further information is provided at the end of the article, as well as a directory of sources offering alternatives to the dissection of animals.

Kistler, John M., and Marc Bekoff. *Animal Rights: A Subject Guide, Bibliography, and Internet Companion.* Westport, Conn.: Greenwood Press, 2000. A comprehensive bibliography of 916 annotated entries that cover a range of topics surrounding animal rights, from vegetarianism to vivisection to feminist perspectives. Topic discussions are balanced and accompanied by web page information that lists reviews, related articles, and books available online.

Louisiana State University Health Sciences Center. "Bird Study Finds Key Info about Human Speech-Language Development." *ScienceDaily,* 17 Oct. 2013. Web. 25 Oct. 2013. A publication which studies behavioral science in birds.

Pantaleo, M.A., L. Landuzzi, G. Nicoletti, C. Nanni, S. Boschi, G. Piazzi, and G. Biasco. "Advances in Preclinical Therapeutics Development Using Small Animal Imaging and Molecular Analyses: The Gastrointestinal Stromal Tumors Model." *Clinical and Experimental Medicine* 9, no. 3 (2009): 199-205. doi:http://dx.doi.org/10.1007/s10238-009-0033-5. A journal article that explains the use of small animals in the development of novel cancer treatments.

"Robert G. Edwards-Nobel Lecture: Robert Edwards: Nobel Laureate in Physiology or Medicine." Nobelprize.org. *Nobel Media* AB 2013. Web. 25 Oct 2013. http://www.nobelprize.org/nobel_prizes/medicine/laureates/2010/edwards-lecture.html. A great source for current awards given in medical research.

Rudacille, Deborah. *The Scalpel and the Butterfly: The War Between Animal Research and Animal Protection.* New York: Farrar, Straus & Giroux, 2000. In this useful survey, Rudacille takes a middle ground between biomedical researchers who defend animal experimentation and animal rights activists who would abolish such research.

Sterna, James P. *Earth Ethics: Introductory Readings on Animal Rights, and Environmental Ethics.* 2d ed. Upper Saddle River, N.J.: Prentice Hall, 2000. An anthology of writings that explore the opposing debates of a range of ethical issues, including the use of animals for scientific research.

Wise, Stephen M. *Drawing the Line: Science and the Case for Animal Rights.* Cambridge, Mass.: Perseus, 2002. The former president of the Animal Legal Defense Fund explores the intelligence and abilities of myriad animals in an effort to demonstrate how animals often meet the criteria for legal personhood.

"Working to End the Use of Animals in Science-The American Anti-Vivisection Society (AAVS)." N.p., n.d. Web. 28 Oct. 2013. The American Anti-Vivisection webpage, which provides access to further information.

Zaragoza, Carlos, Carmen Gomez-Guerrero, Jose Luis Martin-Ventura, Luis Blanco-Colio, Begoña Lavin, Beñat Mallavia, Carlos Tarin, Sebastian Mas, Alberto Ortiz, Jesus Egido. "Animals in Cardiovascular Disease." *Journal of Biomedical Biotechnology.* 2011; 2011: 497841. Published online 2011 February 16. doi: 10.1155/2011/497841. A good source of information for how the use of animal models have led to advancements in cardiovascular disease.

Ankylosing spondylitis

Disease/Disorder

Anatomy or system affected: Back, bones, eyes, gastrointestinal system, hips, immune system, joints, ligaments, musculoskeletal system, spine, tendons

Specialties and related fields: Immunology, rheumatology

Definition: A chronic, progressive, inflammatory disease of the spine and other joints

Key terms:

allele: an alternative form of a gene

ankylosis: a condition of joint rigidity or fusion

autoimmune disorder: a condition in which the immune system damages the body's tissues

chronic: a disease or disorder of long duration, from weeks to months or a lifetime

kyphosis: abnormal forward curvature of the upper spine

risk factor: aspects of genetics, environment, or behavior that increase the chance for developing a disease or disorder

Causes and Symptoms

Ankylosing spondylitis is an inflammatory disease of the spine and other joints. The disease is thought to be an autoimmune disorder in which the immune system attacks joint tissues. Although its cause remains unknown, risk factors have been identified. Risk factors are aspects of a person's genes, environment, or behavior that increase the chance of developing a disease. The main risk factor for ankylosing spondylitis is an allele of the HLA-B gene, HLA-B27. This allele is found in about ninety-five percent of people with ankylosing spondylitis. Ankylosing spondylitis affects men more than women and usually begins in adolescence and young adulthood. Frequent gastrointestinal infections raise the risk for having ankylosing spondylitis.

Symptoms begin gradually and include dull pain and stiffness in the lower back or hips, especially in the morning and after periods of inactivity. Moderate physical activity or hot showers relieve pain and stiffness. Sites affected include joints of the spine, hips, shoulders, the joints between ribs and the sternum, and small joints in the hands and feet. Tendons and ligaments become painful where they attach to bones. Other symptoms include fatigue, loss of appetite, low fever, and malaise, which is a vague sense of ill health. Some people develop eye pain, redness, inflammation, and blurred vision. The disease is progressive, which means that symptoms become severe over time. Symptoms often "flare," growing severe and then subsiding.

Inflammation damages joint tissue and stimulates bone deposition at the joint. Over time, some joints stiffen and fuse, a condition called ankylosis. Fusion is most evident in the lower spine and hips. Spinal fusion causes a characteristic forward-bending spine, a deformity called kyphosis. In some cases, fusion causes the head and neck to bend down to the chest, making it difficult to raise and turn the head and neck. Hip damage can impair mobility.

Complications of ankylosing spondylitis vary in severity. About one-third of people with ankylosing spondylitis have uveitis, inflammation of the eye. Symptoms include sensitivity to light, eye pain, and blurred vision. Bones and joints of the spine become brittle and susceptible to fracture. The rib cage grows stiff, making breathing difficult. Some people experience inflammation of the aorta, the large artery that carries blood from the heart to the body. An inflamed aortic valve impairs blood flow from the heart.

Treatment and Therapy

Diagnosis includes assessment of the ability to bend and twist in different directions. Measurement of chest circumference allows changes to be tracked should the rib cage become affected. Diagnosis also considers the person's symptoms and history. The hallmark diagnostic sign is telltale damage to the sacroiliac joint, the joint between the sacrum and the hip. This damage can be visualized using X-ray or computed tomography (CT), a form of X-ray imaging that uses a computer to construct detailed three-dimensional pictures. Magnetic resonance imaging is used if CT or X-ray results are unclear. A blood test detects the presence of HLA-B27, which occurs in nearly all people with ankylosing spondylitis. Other blood tests measure signs of inflammation. These tests include the erythrocyte sedimentation rate, which is elevated in this disease.

No cure exists for ankylosing spondylitis. Treatments relieve symptoms, reduce the risk for complications, and maintain mobility. Ankylosing spondylitis is usually treated with nonsteroidal anti-inflammatory medications to reduce inflammation, pain, and stiffness. Although effective, these medications entail a risk for stomach bleeding, especially after prolonged use. Disease-modifying anti-rheumatic medications control the autoimmune reactions. Tumor necrosis factor blockers interfere with cell signals responsible for autoimmunity. Tumor necrosis factor

Information on Ankylosing Spondylitis

Causes: Inherited inflammatory, autoimmune disorder
Symptoms: Gradual onset of chronic lower back pain, stiff, painful joints, difficulty expanding chest to breathe, eye inflammation
Duration: Chronic
Treatments: Anti-inflammatory medication, alleviation of symptoms, physical therapy

blockers are given intravenously in the hospital.

Physical therapy assists breathing, develops good posture, and maintains muscle strength, joint flexibility, and range of motion. Usually surgery is unnecessary. Severe hip damage can be corrected with hip replacement surgery. To cope with the effects of the disease, people should stop smoking, get adequate sleep, eat a healthful diet, and get regular, low impact exercise.

Perspective and Prospects

Five-thousand-year-old mummified remains from Egypt suggest that ankylosing spondylitis has been affecting humans for millennia. Signs and symptoms consistent with ankylosing spondylitis have been reported by several physicians and anatomists, from the second century Greek physician Galen to the sixteenth century Italian anatomist Realdo Colombo. In 1691, the Irish physician Bernard Connor first described the hallmark skeletal abnormalities of this disease. Connor described a skeleton with fused, brittle vertebrae, the sacrum fused to the ilium, and ribs fused to the sternum. In the nineteenth century, several physicians recorded spinal deformities consistent with ankylosing spondylitis. The first case in the United States was described in 1858. The defining features and diagnosis of ankylosing spondylitis were spelled out in the late nineteenth century by Vladimir Bekhterev, Adolph Strümpell, and Pierre Marie. In recognition of their work, ankylosing spondylitis was once called Bekhterev Disease and Marie-Strümpell Disease.

Ankylosing spondylitis affects one percent of adults in the United States. It is one of a group of inflammatory spine diseases called spondylarthropathies or spondyloarthritis. These in turn are examples of a larger group of autoimmune disorders that include rheumatoid arthritis, Reiter's Syndrome, and many others. The mechanism underlying these diseases remains only partly understood. In ankylosing spondylitis, most people with the HLA-B27 allele do not develop the disease, and research suggests that five to six other genes are involved. Research suggests that intestinal immunity is defective, leading to bacterial infections of the intestine. When these bacteria enter the blood, they trigger the autoimmune response and tissue damage of ankylosing spondylitis. In 2013 scientists found an association between intestinal infection with the bacterium Klebsiella pneumoniae and the autoimmune damage seen in ankylosing spondylitis.

—*Mark Zelman, Ph..D.*

See also Cardiology; Immunology; Immunopathology; Occupational health; Orthopedics; Physical rehabilitation; Pulmonology; Rheumatology; Surgery, general

For Further Information:

Professional Guide to Diseases. 10th ed. Springhouse, Pa.: Lippincott Williams & Wilkins, 2013.

Rashid, Taha, Clyde Wilson, and Alan Ebringer. "The Link between Ankylosing Spondylitis, Crohn's Disease, Klebsiella, and Starch Consumption." *Clinical and Developmental Immunology* no. 5 (May 27, 2013): 1-9.

Reveille, John D., Anne-Marie Sims, et al. "Genome-wide Association Study of Ankylosing Spondylitis Identifies Non-MHC Susceptibility Loci." *Nature Genetics* 42, no. 2 (February, 2010): 123-127

Weisman, Michael H. *Ankylosing Spondylitis.* New York: Oxford University Press, 2011.

Anorexia nervosa

Disease/Disorder

Anatomy or system affected: Brain, endocrine system, gastrointestinal system, hair, heart, immune system, kidneys, musculoskeletal system, nails, nervous system, psychic-emotional system, reproductive system, skin

Specialties and related fields: Family medicine, neurology, nutrition, psychiatry, psychology

Definition: Self-induced malnutrition resulting in a body weight 15 percent or more below normal for age and height, and, in women, characterized by the absence of three or more consecutive menstrual periods.

Key terms:

eating disorder: weight gain or loss resulting from compulsive overeating, anorexia nervosa, or bulimia

obsessive-compulsive: having a preoccupation with a specific idea (such as body image) and showing uncontrollable related behavior (such as dieting)

refeeding: the reintroduction of nutritional substances into the diet of a patient suffering from malnutrition

Causes and Symptoms

Anorexia nervosa is an obsessive-compulsive disorder characterized by a body weight at or below 85 percent of normal and an intense fear of weight gain. Anorexia nervosa is typically a physical manifestation of underlying emotional conflicts such as guilt, anger, and poor self-image. Eating disorders such as anorexia nervosa are the third most common chronic condition among girls ages fifteen to nineteen. Approximately 90 percent of people with anorexia are female.

Anorexia nervosa often occurs following a successful dieting experience, and frequent dieting may contribute to the development of the disorder. Dieters may experience positive feedback regarding weight loss and feel compelled to continue losing weight.

Although the term "anorexia" means "loss of appetite," most anorectics continue to experience hunger but ignore the body's normal craving for food. Anorectics frequently identify specific areas of the body that they believe are "fat," despite their emaciated condition. Secrecy and ritual eating habits may be signs of anorexia nervosa. Sufferers often lie to family and friends to avoid eating meals and may eat only a set diet at a specific time of day.

Information on Anorexia Nervosa

Causes: Emotional and psychological disorders pertaining to body image

Symptoms: Extreme weight loss, amenorrhea, malnutrition, forgetfulness, attention deficits, confusion, fatigue, apathy, irritability, brittle nails, hair loss, dry skin, cold hands and feet

Duration: Chronic

Treatments: Medical refeeding, individual and/or family counseling, antidepressants

---

Many people with anorexia are high achievers, exhibiting perfectionist or "people-pleasing" personalities. In addition, a strong correlation exists between anorexia nervosa and athletic activities that emphasize the physique, such as track, tennis, gymnastics, cheerleading, and dance. People with anorexia may demonstrate additional obsessive-compulsive behaviors such as weighing themselves and/or examining themselves in the mirror several times per day, being overly concerned with calorie or fat content, exercising compulsively, maintaining unusually consistent eating patterns, and kleptomania (compulsive stealing).

Anorexia nervosa is frequently a symptom of depression, and the accompanying weight loss can be seen as a cry for help. Eating disorders tend to run in families, particularly those that equate thinness with success and happiness. The condition may also occur as a result of a traumatic situation such as death, divorce, pregnancy, or sexual abuse.

Symptoms and resulting physical conditions include amenorrhea, the abnormal interruption or absence of menstrual discharge, which can occur when body fat drops below 23 percent. Anorexia nervosa may also be characterized by a distended abdomen as a result of a buildup of abdominal fluids and the slowing of the digestive system.

Resulting malnutrition can impair the immune system and cause anemia or decreased white blood cell counts. Brain and central nervous system functions may also be affected, resulting in forgetfulness, attention deficits, and confusion. Anorectics frequently experience fatigue, apathy, irritability, and extreme emotions.

Additional symptoms can include thyroid abnormalities, fainting spells, irregular heartbeat, brittle nails, hair loss, dry skin, cold hands and feet, hypotension (low blood pressure), infertility, broken blood vessels in the face, and the growth of downy body hair called lanugo as the body attempts to insulate itself because of the loss of natural fat.

The occurrence of eating disorders in adolescents is especially dangerous because the condition can retard growth and delay or interrupt puberty. Anorexia nervosa can also result in the erosion of heart muscle, which lowers the heart's capacity and can lead to congestive heart failure. Anorectics may experience musculoskeletal problems such as muscle spasms, atrophy, and osteoporosis as a result of potassium and calcium deficiencies. In extreme cases, patients may also experience kidney failure.

Brittany Bethel, a college student battling anorexia nervosa, who was expelled from school in 2007 after suffering a heart attack while running on campus. (AP/Wide World Photos)

Treatment and Therapy

Treatment of anorexia nervosa generally consists of medical treatment, including electrolyte balance, and diagnosing and addressing any related health problems, such as heart problems, depression, and osteoporosis; psychotherapy, either group, family, individual, or some combination; and nutrition counseling, as most people with anorexia need to focus away from weight loss and toward nutritional gain.

Research indicates that eating disorders are one of the psychological problems least likely to be treated, and anorexia nervosa has the highest mortality rate of all psychosocial problems. The National Institute of Mental Health estimates that one in ten anorexia cases ends in death from starvation, suicide, or medical complications such as heart attacks or kidney failure.

Psychologists play a vital role in the successful treatment of eating disorders and are integral members of the multidisciplinary team that may be required to provide patient care. As part of this treatment, a physician may be called on to rule out medical illnesses and determine that the patient is not in immediate physical danger. A nutritionist may be asked to help assess and improve nutritional intake.

It is frequently necessary first to treat the acute physical symptoms associated with anorexia nervosa. Most patients-especially those with severe cases-benefit from treatment in a controlled environment that allows medically supervised "refeeding" to achieve a target rate of weight gain. Less severe cases may be treated on an outpatient basis.

During the initial phase of refeeding, the patient may receive a low-calorie diet to avoid overwhelming low-functioning organs. Patients who do not comply with the recommended diet may receive caloric supplements and, in serious cases, intravenous feeding.

Successful treatment also involves resolution of underlying emotional conflicts through individual and/or family counseling and may also include use of antidepressants such as fluoxetine (Prozac).

Anorexia nervosa is extremely difficult to treat, with a fatality rate of 5 percent to 10 percent within ten years. Nearly half of all sufferers never recover fully from the condition.

Perspective and Prospects

Anorexia is a multifaceted problem that has physical, emotional, and cultural components. More than three-quarters of adolescent girls in the United States report being unhappy with their bodies and, on average, 25 percent of women are on a diet at any given time.

Most eating disorders were not recognized as illnesses until the late nineteenth century. Conditions such as anorexia nervosa gained the attention of medical professionals during the 1960s and beyond as a result of the media's obsession with thinness.

The media are prime contributors to this trend. Television and magazines send confusing messages to young consumers, such as depicting painfully thin models promoting high-fat snacks. Most models weigh about 23 percent less than the average American woman, and up to 60 percent of models suffer from eating disorders. In addition, the media frequently portray overweight people as having a lower socioeconomic status than people who are thin. Obese people are generally portrayed as comical, while thin people are often depicted as more intelligent, sophisticated, and successful, and as happier with their lives.

In March 2013, the medical journal The Lancet published a study on the use of deep brain stimulation (DBS). The small study invovling six female patients reported improvements in mood and increases in body-mass index in those who recieved what is referred to as a brain pacemaker. The surgery is reversable and minimally invasive.

It appears likely that the incidence of eating disorders will continue to escalate as the media persist in depicting an idealized female body image significantly below normal body weight.

—Cheryl Pawlowski, Ph.D.;
updated by LeAnna DeAngelo, Ph.D.

See also Addiction; Amenorrhea; Anxiety; Appetite loss; Bulimia; Depression; Eating disorders; Hyperadiposis; Malnutrition; Menstruation; Nutrition; Obesity; Obesity, childhood; Obsessive-compulsive disorder; Psychiatric disorders; Psychiatry, child and adolescent; Puberty and adolescence; Sports medicine; Stress; Vitamins and minerals; Weight loss and gain; Weight loss medications; Women's health.

For Further Information:

Broccolo-Philbin, Anne. "An Obsession with Being Painfully Thin." *Current Health 2* 22, no. 5 (January, 1996): 23.

Brumburg, Joan Jacobs. *Fasting Girls: The History of Anorexia Nervosa*. Rev. ed. New York: Vintage Books, 2000.

Costin, Carolyn. *The Eating Disorder Sourcebook*. 3d ed. New York: McGraw-Hill, 2007.

Dallas, Mary Elizabeth. "Brain 'Pacemaker' May Help Ease Tough-to-Treat Anorexia." *Health Day*. 7 Mar 2013: Web. 22 May. 2013.

Gordon, Richard A. *Eating Disorders: Anatomy of a Social Epidemic*. 2d ed. Malden, Mass.: Blackwell Scientific, 2000.

Lucas, Alexander R. *Demystifying Anorexia Nervosa: An Optimistic Guide to Understanding Healing*. Updated ed. New York: Oxford University Press, 2008.

Parker, James N., and Philip M. Parker, eds. *The 2002 Official Patient's Sourcebook on Binge Eating Disorder*. San Diego, Calif.: Icon Health, 2002.

Anosmia
Disease/Disorder

Anatomy or system affected: Brain, nervous system, nose
Specialties and related fields: Family medicine, neurology, otorhinolaryngology
Definition: A complete loss in the ability to detect odors.

Causes and Symptoms

One of the causes of anosmia is a blockage in the nasal cavity such that odorant molecules cannot reach the olfactory receptors. This blockage can be the result of conditions such as nasal polyps, foreign bodies, or the temporary swelling that accompanies colds or allergies.

If the person was born without a sense of smell and the air passageways are open, then the cause of the loss is likely congenital. If there was once a sense of smell, then causes of the loss may include head trauma, an upper respiratory infection, drug toxicity, and a brain tumor. With head trauma-such as from a fall or an automobile accident-or degenerative brain diseases, there is a disruption in the ability of the olfactory nerves to send signals to the brain. When the cause is a viral infection, the person usually reports a cold or flu during which loss of the sense of smell occurred but did not return as the cold resolved. The reasons for permanent loss are not clear but likely involve a disruption in the neural pathways.

Treatment

Removing the blockage is the treatment in the case of a blocked air passageway. In the case of allergies, flu, or the common cold, as the swelling resolves the sense of smell usually returns. Nasal polyps can be reduced by steroids or surgically removed.

If the cause of the loss is head trauma, then a systemic and/or topical course of steroids may help, although the prognosis is not good. For anosmia following a viral infection, the sense of smell sometimes returns gradually over a year or so. Steroids taken during or soon after the infection

Information on Anosmia
Causes: Blockage, viral infection, head trauma
Symptoms: Inability to detect odors
Duration: Several days to lifelong
Treatments: Surgery to remove blockage, oral or systemic steroids

may be helpful. If the loss is from drug toxicity, then changes in medications may help.

Perspective and Prospects

Anosmia can present serious problems in the detection of smoke, spoiled food, body odors, or natural gas. People with anosmia should consider the use of smoke detectors (including one in the car) and natural gas detectors in the house. Because it is difficult to detect spoiled food, items in the refrigerator should be labeled with the date of purchase and care should be taken not to consume green or slimy foods. Concerns about body or breath odors can be addressed by practicing reasonable hygiene.

Because of the relationship between the sense of smell and the perception of flavor, most common foods do not "taste" right to those with anosmia. In this case, the perception of the flavor of food can be enhanced somewhat by adding texture or more salt or sugar. If the patient is preparing food for others, however, then these enhancements will not be well received by people with a functioning sense of smell.

—*David Hornung, Ph.D.*

See also Common cold; Influenza; Nasal polyp removal; Nasopharyngeal disorders; Nervous system; Neurology; Sense organs; Smell; Taste; Viral infections.

For Further Information:
Engen, Trygg. *The Perception of Odors*. New York: Academic Press, 1982.

Finger, Thomas E., Wayne L. Silver, and Diego Restrepo, eds. *Neurobiology of Taste and Smell*. 2d ed. New York: Wiley-Liss, 2000.

Gilbert, Avery. *What the Nose Knows: The Science of Scent in Everyday Life*. New York: Crown, 2008.

Wolfe, Jeremy M., et al. *Sensation and Perception*. 2d ed. Sunderland, Mass.: Sinauer, 2009.

Anthrax
Disease/Disorder

Also known as: Woolsorter's disease
Anatomy or system affected: Gastrointestinal system, immune system, nervous system, respiratory system, skin
Specialties and related fields: Bacteriology, critical care, dermatology, emergency medicine, internal medicine, microbiology, pathology
Definition: A bacterial infection of humans and other animals, especially herbivores, which occurs following entrance into the body of *Bacillus anthracis* spores through abrasions in the skin or by ingestion or inhalation.
Key terms:
eschar: a thick, crusty, blackish skin lesion that follows a burn, other injury, or some unusual types of infection;

derived from the Greek *eschara*, meaning "fireplace"
spores: highly resistant structures produced by certain gram-positive bacteria under environmental pressure to allow survival until more favorable conditions exist
virulence: the degree of pathogenicity, or ability to cause disease; derived from the Latin *virulentus*, meaning "full of poison"

Causes and Symptoms

The bacterium that causes anthrax is a large, encapsulated, gram-positive rod which produces exotoxins and spores. The capsule and exotoxins are important virulence factors, and both are necessary for disease to occur. Spores are ellipsoidal or oval and are located within the bacilli. The endospores have no reproductive significance, as only one spore is formed by each bacillus and a germinated spore yields a single bacillus. Spores form in soil or dead tissue and with no measurable metabolism may remain dormant for years. They are resistant to drying, heat, and many disinfectants.

Anthrax is primarily a disease of herbivorous animals that has spread to humans through association with domesticated animals and their products. Herbivorous animals grazing in pastures with soil contaminated with endospores become infected when the spores gain entry through abrasions around the mouth and germinate in the surrounding tissues. Omnivores and carnivores can become infected by ingesting contaminated meat. Human infection is often a result of a close association with herbivores, particularly goats, sheep, or cattle (including their products of hair, wool, and hides). Anthrax has been an uncommon infection in the United States, and only 233 human cases were reported from 1955 to 1987.

The most common clinical illness in humans is skin in-

> ### Information on Anthrax
> **Causes:** Infection with bacterial spores through skin or by ingestion or inhalation
> **Symptoms:** After skin exposure, vesicle that ruptures to leave an ulcer; after inhalation, flulike symptoms a few days later (cough, fever, chills, respiratory distress); systemic spread causes fever, headache, malaise, and sometimes meningitis
> **Duration:** Two weeks, with long-term effects; inhalation type often fatal
> **Treatments:** Prolonged antibiotic therapy and intensive supportive measures

fection acquired when spores penetrate through cuts or abrasions. After an incubation period of three to five days, a papule develops and evolves into a vesicle, which ruptures to leave an ulcer that dries to form a characteristic black eschar. Inhaled spores reach the alveoli of the lung, where they are engulfed by macrophages and germinate into bacilli. Bacilli are carried to lymph nodes, where release and multiplication are followed by bloodstream invasion and spread to other parts of the body, including the brain, causing meningitis. The illness begins with flulike symptoms a few days after the inhalation of anthrax spores and may be associated with substernal (under the breastbone) discomfort. Cough, fever, chills, and respiratory distress with dyspnea (abnormal or uncomfortable breathing) and stridor (noisy breathing) ensue. The least common type of infection is that of the gastrointestinal tract.

The laboratory criteria for the diagnosis of anthrax are cultural growth of *Bacillus anthracis* from a clinical specimen collected from an affected tissue or site or other supportive laboratory data, such as polymerase chain reaction (PCR), immunohistochemical staining, or serology that shows evidence of anthrax infection.

Treatment and Therapy

Antibiotic treatment of cutaneous anthrax does not change the course of the evolving skin lesion, but it reduces edema (swelling) and systemic symptoms such as fever, headache, and malaise which may be part of the illness. Antibiotic therapy is also initiated to prevent complications from spreading infection and, most important, bloodstream invasion. The mortality rate of cutaneous infection with appropriate antibiotic treatment is less than 1 percent. Virtually all patients with inhalation anthrax will die if untreated. Antibiotic therapy, especially if administered during the early part of this biphasic illness, combined with other intensive supportive measures, may save up to 50 percent of patients, although long-term effects

In October, 2001, a firefighter decontaminates an FBI agent after they emerge from the American Media building where anthrax sent through the mail caused the death of a photo editor. (AP/Wide World Photos)

may be noted. The paucity of gastrointestinal anthrax cases has resulted in limited mortality data, but mortality has been estimated to be as high as 50 percent, with disease limited to the mouth and throat having a better prognosis. If recovery ensues, the disease subsides within two weeks. Antibiotic therapy is indicated for all cases.

Initial antibiotic therapy is with either ciprofloxacin or doxycline, plus one or two additional antibiotics for more severe cases until the patient is stable. Prolonged antibiotic therapy (one hundred days) is indicated for more serious illness. Antibiotics may also be used to prevent illness in the case of possible exposure, and an anthrax vaccine is available for persons at high risk of exposure.

Perspective and Prospects

A disease killing cattle in 1491 BCE, likely to have been anthrax, is recounted in the Book of Genesis. In Exodus 9, the Lord instructs Moses to take "handfuls of ashes of the furnace" and "sprinkle it toward the heaven in the sight of the Pharaoh." Moses performed the deed, and "it became a boil breaking forth with blains upon man and upon beast." This may represent the first use of anthrax as a biological agent. Greek peasants tending goats suffered from anthrax. *Anthrax* in Greek means "coal," which refers to the coal-black center of the skin lesion.

Anthrax was the first pathogenic bacillus to be seen microscopically when it was described in infected animal tissue by Aloys-Antoine Pollender in 1849. Studies by Robert Koch in 1876 resulted in the four postulates which form the basis for the study of infectious disease causation. In 1881, Louis Pasteur demonstrated the protective efficacy of a vaccine for sheep made with his attenuated vaccine strain.

Anthrax spores can be easily packaged to act as aerosolized agents of war, and the genome may be bioengineered to alter the virulence of anthrax or the ability of current vaccines to protect against it. In 1979, anthrax spores were accidentally released from a Soviet biowarfare facility in the city of Sverdlovsk, resulting in at least seventy-seven human cases, with sixty-six deaths. In the United States, a bioterrorism attack with anthrax spores placed in letters and sent through the mail caused twenty-two infections and five deaths in 2001.

In the future, more rapid molecular based diagnostic methods promise to identify cases earlier so that appropriate antibiotic therapy can be initiated, ensuring a maximum opportunity for recovery. A need also exists for safer and more effective vaccines that would offer protection even against bioengineered strains.

—*H. Bradford Hawley, M.D.*

See also Bacterial infections; Bacteriology; Biological and chemical weapons; Epidemiology; Immunization and vaccination; Microbiology; Toxicology; Zoonoses.

For Further Information:

Bartlett, John G., Thomas V. Inglesby, Jr., and Luciana Borio. "Management of Anthrax." *Clinical Infectious Diseases* 35 (October 1, 2002): 851-858.

Centers for Disease Control and Prevention. "Bioterrorism-Related Anthrax." *Emerging Infectious Diseases* 8 (October, 2002): 1013-1183.

Dixon, Terry C., et al. "Anthrax." *New England Journal of Medicine* 341 (September 9, 1999): 815-826.

Kyrincou, Demetrios N., Alys Adamski, and Nanci Khardori. "Anthrax: From Antiquity and Obscurity to a Front-runner in Bioterrorism." *Infectious Disease Clinics of North America* 20 (2006): 227-251.

Antianxiety drugs

Treatment

Anatomy or system affected: Brain, psychic-emotional system

Specialties and related fields: Family medicine, forensic medicine, internal medicine, pharmacology, psychiatry

Definition: Medications used to treat anxiety that is causing impairment.

Indications and Procedures

Anxiety disorders are the most common mental health disorders. The fifth edition of the American Psychiatric Association's *Diagnostic and Statistical Manual of Mental Disorders* (2013)-the most widely used reference manual for research, clinical assessment, and insurance purposes in the field of psychiatry-lists several anxiety disorders, including generalized anxiety disorder, panic disorder, social anxiety disorder, separation anxiety disorder, agoraphobia, selective mutism, and specific phobias. Anxiety is also a pronounced symptom of other mental illnesses, such as depression, schizophrenia, avoidant personality disorder, dependent personality disorder, post-traumatic stress disorder, and obsessive-compulsive disorder.

Although the physiological responses (sympathetic nervous system activation) and behavioral tendencies (fight-or-flight reaction) are similar, fear and anxiety differ fundamentally in their causes. Anxiety is triggered by the anticipation of a future, life-altering, or adverse event (real or imagined) or the recollection of a past adverse event. Fear is triggered by an encounter with immediate danger. Worrying about an upcoming dentist's appointment is experienced as anxiety, while facing an armed robber in the hallway is experienced as fear. In both instances, people's hearts race, their pupils dilate, and their breathing accelerates. The former involves a future orientation, whereas the latter involves a present orientation. Anxiety can be elicited by an excessive concern with "worst-case-scenarios" or irrational thoughts or beliefs about performance or social acceptance. When symptoms of anxiety become distressful and cause impairment in functioning (for example, the inability to work or attend school), then diagnosis of an anxiety disorder and the use of antianxiety medications and other therapeutic interventions are indicated.

Uses and Complications

The first line of treatment for anxiety disorders is cognitive behavioral therapy, which has been shown to be as effective as medications in the treatment of anxiety. In cases where psychotherapy alone is insufficient to treat the anxiety, antianxiety medications may be prescribed to help control symptoms. Three major categories of antianxiety medications, also known as anxiolytics, are used to treat anxiety disorders, and each of these act on similar neural transmitters and pathways: benzodiazepines, selective serotonin reuptake inhibitors (SSRIs), and selective norepinephrine reuptake inhibitors (SNRIs). Tricyclic antidepressants are also used in the treatment of anxiety disorders, although SSRIs are preferred due to their greater safety and tolerability. Barbituates, which act as central nervous system depressants, were once the first line of treatment for anxiety disorders, but their clinical use in the treatment of anxiety has been phased out due to the high risk of overdose and dependence.

Selective serotonin reuptake inhibitors. Selective serotonin reuptake inhibitors (SSRIs) are the most widely prescribed medications for the treatment of anxiety. As their name suggests, SSRIs act by increasing the levels of serotonin (5-hydroxytryptamine) in the brain by preventing its reuptake by neurons. When first approved for use, SSRIs were widely acclaimed as breakthrough medications in the treatment of depression, and clinical practice soon demonstrated their effectiveness in alleviating the symptoms of anxiety as well. Medications in this class include fluoxetine (Prozac), sertraline (Zoloft), fluvoxamine (Luvox), paroxetine (Paxil), citalopram (Celexa), and escitalopram (Lexapro).

SSRIs require four to six weeks to reach maximum efficacy and can cause withdrawal symptoms if their use is stopped abruptly. The ingestion of large doses of SSRIs can result in severe toxicity, but fatal overdoses are rare. Hence, the risk of lethality from excessive SSRI use is minimal, especially when compared to other anxiolytics. In addition, SSRIs are nonaddictive and do not cause memory impairment. However, the list of potential side effects associated with SSRI use is lengthy: anhedonia, photosensitivity, drowsiness, headache, bruxism, vivid and bizarre dreams, dizziness, fatigue, urinary retention, changes in appetite, weight gain, suicidal ideation, tremors, orthostatic hypotension, and increased sweating. In addition, the sexual side effects that stem from SSRI use include reduced libido, erectile dysfunction, anorgasmia, genital anesthesia, and premature ejaculation.

Serotonin norepinephrine reuptake inhibitors. Serotonin norepinephrine reuptake inhibitors (SNRIs) work by blocking the reuptake of serotonin and norepinephrine in the brain. Various SNRIs block the reuptake of these neurotransmitters with differing affinity ratios, so that an SNRI that causes uncomfortable side effects in a patient may be replaced with another that does not have the same negative effects. The most common side effect of SNRIs is nausea, followed by dry mouth, sweating, constipation, and heart palpitations. Medications in this class include venlafaxine (Effexor), duloxetine (Cymbalta), and desvenlafaxine (Pristiq).

Benzodiazepines. The first benzodiazepine, chlordiazepoxide (Librium), was discovered in 1955. Benzodiazepines enhance the effects of gamma-aminobutyric acid (GABA), which is the chief inhibitory neurotransmitter in the central nervous system, making them useful in the treatment of anxiety. Benzodiazepines are fast-acting and typically relieve symptoms within thirty to sixty minutes of ingestion. Although cognitive impairment and paradoxical effects such as aggression, agitation, mania, or suicidality can occasionally occur with benzodiazepine use, these drugs are generally safe and effective in the short term. Benzodiazepines possess sedative and hypnotic properties that are useful in treating agitation and insomnia. Most benzodiazepines are administered orally; however, they can also be given intravenously, intramuscularly, or rectally. Other benzodiazepines are alprazolam (Xanax), clonazepam (Klonopin), diazepam (Valium), lorazepam (Ativan), and oxazepam (Serax).

Benzodiazepines can cause many side effects, including blurred or double vision, slowed reflexes, impaired thinking and judgment, dizziness, slurred speech, and depression. These effects are especially evident with prolonged use and at higher dosages, which can lead to abuse and dependence. The fastest-acting benzodiazepines (for example, Xanax) have the greatest potential for addiction and are listed as Schedule IV controlled substances. A sudden decrease in the dosage or abrupt cessation of benzodiazepine use can result in symptoms of rebound, which is a return of anxiety but at intensities that are higher than initial levels, and of withdrawal, which causes insomnia, sweating, shaking, confusion, and tachycardia (elevated heart rate). Hence, a gradual reduction in the dosage and administration of these medications is recommended.

Tricyclic antidepressants. Antidepressants are also used in the treatment of anxiety. The first class of antidepressants prescribed as anxiolytics are known as tricyclic antidepressants (TCAs), which are named for the chemical structure of the drugs in the class-three rings. The first TCA, imipramine (Tofranil), was discovered in the late 1950s. Other examples of tricyclic antidepressants are amitriptyline (Elavil), amoxapine (Asendin), clomipramine (Anafranil), desipramine (Norpramin), doxepin (Sinequan), nortriptyline (Pamelor), protriptyline (Vivactil), and trimipramine (Surmontil). The side effects of TCAs include hypotension (low blood pressure), blurry vision, dizziness, constipation, dry mouth, drowsiness, increased appetite, and weight gain. In addition, an overdose of TCAs can often be fatal. The severe morbidity and mortality associated with these drugs is well documented because of their cardiovascular and neurological toxicity. Due to their greater safety and tolerability, SSRIs are the preferred treatment for anxiety.

Perspective and Prospects

Anxiety disorders are among the most common types of psychiatric illnesses worldwide, with a lifetime prevalence of 15 percent and a twelve-month prevalence of more than 10 percent. Research into safer and more effective treatments for these disorders is ongoing.

—*Arthur J. Lurigio, Ph.D.*

See also Antidepressants; Anxiety; Appetite loss; Depression; Emotions: Biomedical causes and effects; Grief and guilt; Hyperhidrosis; Hyperventilation; Hypochondriasis; Midlife crisis; Neurosis; Obsessive-compulsive disorder; Palpitations; Panic attacks; Paranoia; Phobias; Postpartum depression; Post-traumatic stress disorder; Psychiatric disorders; Psychiatry; Psychiatry, child and adolescent; Psychiatry, geriatric; Psychoanalysis; Psychosomatic disorders; Sexual dysfunction; Stress; Stress reduction; Suicide; Sweating.

For Further Information:

American Psychiatric Association. *Diagnostic and Statistical Manual of Mental Disorders*. 5th ed. Washington, D.C.: American Psychiatric Association, 2013.

Bourne, Edmund J. *The Anxiety and Phobia Workbook*. 5th ed. Oakland, Calif.: New Harbinger Press, 2011.

Gorman, Jack M. *The Essential Guide to Psychiatric Drugs*. New York: St. Martin's Press, 1998.

Griez, Eric J. L., Carlo Faravelli, and David Nutt. *Anxiety Disorders: An Introduction to Clinical Management and Research*. Hoboken, N.J.: John Wiley & Sons, 2001.

Sadock, Benjamin J., and Virginia A. Sadock. *Kaplan & Sadock's Synopsis of Psychiatry: Behavioral Sciences/Clincal Psychiatry*. 10th ed. Philadelphia, Pa.: Lippincott, Williams & Wilkins, 2007.

Schiffman, Jason E. "Anti-Anxiety Medications Explained." *Psychology Today*, November 25, 2011.

Toufexis, Donna, Sayamwong E. Hammack, and David J. Triggle. *Anti-Anxiety Drugs*. New York: Chelsea House, 2006.

"What Is Anxiety Disorder?" *National Institute of Mental Health*, 2013.

Antibiotic resistance

Disease/Disorder

Anatomy or system affected: All

Specialties and related fields: Bacteriology, genetics, microbiology, pharmacology, public health.

Definition: The ability of micro-organisms to survive and reproduce in the presence of a drug that formerly killed or inhibited it.

Key terms:

antibiotic: a substance that kills or prevents the growth of a pathogen

bacteria: microscopic, single-celled organisms that do not have an organized nucleus

bacterial chromosome: a circular deoxyribonucleic acid (DNA) molecule cell in bacteria that stores the entire organism's genetic information

bacteriophage: a virus that infects bacteria

conjugation: the direct exchange of genetic material between bacteria by cell-to-cell contact

microbiome: the ecological community of micro-organism that share our body space

nosocomial infection: an infection that is acquired in a hospital

pathogen: organism that causes disease

plasmids: circular pieces of DNA within bacteria that are much smaller than bacterial chromosomes

transduction: the indirect transfer of genetic material between bacteria by bacteriophage

transformation: the exchange of genetic material between strains of bacteria by the uptake of naked DNA

transposons: segments of DNA that can jump or transpose from one DNA molecule to another or can change their location on the same DNA molecule

Causes and Symptoms

Antibiotics inhibit crucial life-sustaining processes in bacteria. They inhibit such processes as cell wall synthesis, protein synthesis, membrane function, and DNA and RNA synthesis. Additionally, some antibiotics act as "antimetabolites" that interfere with normal metabolic processes within cells. Antibiotics are classified according to the biochemical processes they inhibit and their structure.

Inhibitors of cell wall synthesis include the beta-lactams, which consist of the penicillins, cephalosporins, monobactams, and carbapenems, the glycopeptides (vancomycin), and fosfomycin. Protein synthesis inhibitors include the aminoglycosides, MLSK (macrolides, lincosamides, streptogramins, ketolides) group, tetracyclines, glycylcyclines, phenicols, oxazolidionones, and the ansamycins. A group of antibiotics called the lipopeptides disrupt cell membrane function and contains polymyxin B, colistin, and daptomycin. The antibiotic combination trimethoprim/sulfamethoxazole is an antimetabolite that inhibits the synthesis of the vitamin folic acid. Folic acid is essential for the synthesis of components used in the replication of DNA. Since humans do not synthesize folic acid but acquire from their diets, this biosynthetic pathway represents an excellent selective target. Finally inhibitors of DNA and RNA synthesis include the quinolones and the furanes (Table 1).

Antibiotic resistance occurs when bacteria develop the ability to resist an agent that has been designed to destroy it. Bacteria resist antibiotics by employing several different strategies. First, they can use enzymes that degrade or modify the antibiotic so that it no longer inhibits its target. For example, bacteria become resistant to beta-lactam antibiotics by acquiring the genes that encode enzymes called beta-lactamases. Beta-lactamases degrade beta lactam antibiotics and prevent them from inhibiting cell wall synthesis. Drug modification also mediates resistance to chloramphenicol, aminoglycosides, and fosfomycin.

The second mechanism of antibiotic resistance is modification of the target that the antibiotic usually inhibits. Streptococcus pneumoniae, which causes pneumonia and meningitis, has become resistant to several beta-lactam antibiotics by altering its cell wall synthesizing proteins. Vancomycin resistance also results in changes in the way bacteria make their cell walls. Resistance to most of the protein synthesis inhibitors and quinolones is caused by changes in their targets.

The third resistance strategy involves preventing the antibiotic from achieving a high enough concentration in the cell to accomplish its task. Efflux proteins that pump the drug from the cell, drive tetracycline and erythromycin resistance in several bacterial cells. Alternatively, some bacteria prevent the antibiotic from entering the cell. For example, the so-called "gram-negative" bacteria, whose cell wall consists of an outer membrane that surrounds a thin cell wall, have a natural resistance to certain antibiotics (e.g., the glycopeptides and members of the MKLS group), since these drugs cannot pass through the outer membrane.

Bacteria can develop resistance to an antibiotic either through a random mutation or the acquisition of new genes. Once antibiotic resistance has been acquired, the process of natural selection spreads this advantageous new trait throughout the population. Natural selection "weeds out" those bacteria unable to tolerate the antibiotic and leaves a smaller population better adapted to withstand it. Those antibiotic-resistant bacteria will reproduce and pass their genes onto the next generations.

Table 1	
Antibiotic class	**Mode of Action**
Beta-lactams	Inhibitor of cell wall synthesis
Penicillins Penicillin G Penicillin M Extended-spectrum penicillins Aminopenicillins Ampicillin Amoxicillin Bacampicillin Carboxypenicillins Carbenicillin Ticarcillin Ureidopenicillins Azlocillin Piperacillin Mezlocillin Amidinopenicillins Mecillinam Pivmecillinam	Inhibitor of cell wall synthesis
Cephalosporins 1st generation cephalosporins Cephalothin Cefazolin 2nd generation cephalosporins Cefuroxime Cefamandole Cephamycin Cefoxitin 3rd generation cephalosporins Cefotaxime Ceftazidime Ceftriaxone 4th generation cephalosporins Cefepime Oral 3rd generation cephalosporins Cefixime Cefpodoxime Next Generation Cephalosporins Ceftobiprole Ceftaroline	Inhibitor of cell wall synthesis
Monobactams Aztreonam	Inhibitor of cell wall synthesis
Carbapenems Imipenem Meropenem Ertapenem Doripenem Penems Faropenem	Inhibitor of cell wall synthesis
Glycopeptides Vancomycin Dalbavancin Oritavancin Telavancin Teicoplanin	Inhibitor of cell wall synthesis
Fosfomycins Fosfomycin	Inhibitor of cell wall synthesis
Aminoglycosides Streptomycin Kanamycin Gentamicin Tobramycin Amikacin	Protein synthesis inhibitors
MLSK Macrolides Erythromycin Clarithromycin Azithromycin Lincosamines Lincomycin Clindamycin Streptogramins Quinupristin/Dalfopristin Pristinamycin Ketolides Telithromycin	Protein synthesis inhibitors
Tetracyclines Tetracycline Minocycline Doxycycline	Protein synthesis inhibitors
Glycylcyclines Tigecycline	Protein synthesis inhibitors
Phenicols Chloramphenicol	Protein synthesis inhibitors
Oxazolidinones Linezolid	Protein synthesis inhibitors
Ansamycins Rifampin	Protein synthesis inhibitors
Lipopeptides Polymyxin B Colistin Daptomycin	Disruptors of cell membranes
Trimethoprim/Sulfamethoxazole	Antimetabolites
Fluoroquinolones Garenoxacin Ciprofloxacin Levofloxacin Norfloxacin, Ofloxacin Sparfloxacin Gatifloxacin Moxifloxacin	Inhibitors of DNA and RNA synthesis

Antibiotic resistance is genetically encoded in deoxyribonucleic acid (DNA) molecules. Bacterial DNA is a circular bacterial chromosome in the bacterial cell. Additionally, bacteria may contain small, circular fragments of DNA called plasmids, which are separate from the bacterial chromosome. Some plasmids also harbor genes for conjugation, a process by which plasmids are transferred from one bacterial cell to another by means of direct contact. When plasmids that carry genes that make a bacterium resistant to a particular antibiotic also contain conjugation genes, they can transfer antibiotic resistance between bacteria. Not all plasmids contain conjugation genes and can be exchanged in this way.

In addition to conjugation, antibiotic resistant genes can be transferred to different DNA molecules by means of transposons, which are small segments of DNA that have the ability to actively jump from one DNA molecule to another. A transposon may jump from a bacterial chromosome and insert itself elsewhere on the chromosome or onto a plasmid. Some transposons contain antibiotic resistant genes and when they move they can transfer antibiotic resistance to bacterial chromosomes or plasmids that formerly did not possess capabilities. Transposons can also be inserted on either side of an island of genes that encode antibiotic resistance or other useful functions and elicit transfer of groups of genes.

Viruses that infect bacteria can also mistakenly transfer antibiotic resistant genes between bacteria in a process called transduction. Bacteriophages are viruses that attach to bacterial cells, inject their own DNA, and co-opt the bacterial cellular machinery to replicate the viral DNA and bacteriophage components. Sometimes, the virus mistakenly incorporates DNA from the host bacterial cell into its own DNA. The virus may then transfer this DNA to the next bacterial host to which it attaches. In this way, it can transfer drug resistant genes between bacteria that are unable to undergo conjugation.

Some bacterial species can acquire traits such as antibiotic resistance by taking up whole DNA molecules and incorporating its genes into their own chromosomes. This process is called transformation. Bacteria cells that have the ability to take up DNA are called "competent." In many bacterial species, competence is inducible and some species of bacteria (e.g., members of the genera Neisseria and Hemophilus) possess cellular machinery dedicated to scrounging their environment for new genes.

Given the multiple ways that bacteria can procure antibiotic resistant genes, and the constant selection for antibiotic resistance, many pathogenic and nonpathogenic bacteria have become resistant to many different types of commonly used antibiotics. The increasing levels of antibiotic resistance have generated tremendous anxiety among public health professionals, and have also generated several public health concerns.

At one time, Mycobacterium tuberculosis, the causative agent of tuberculosis, was susceptible to one of two drugs: isoniazid or rifampin. However, by 1991, in New York City, 33 percent of all tuberculosis infections were resistant to at least one drug, and 19 percent were resistant to both rifampin and isoniazid. The disease caused by these M. tuberculosis strains that are resistant to isoniazid and rifampin is called multidrug resistant tuberculosis (MDR-TB). Globally, 3.7 percent of new cases and 20 percent of previously treated cases are estimated to consist of MDR-TB. MDR-TB patients require treatment with four drugs for several months. Also, the treatment of those MDR-TB patients who are at risk for noncompliance (e.g., indigent, prisoners, mentally-challenged, elderly) must be directly supervised by health care workers to ensure compliance because antibiotic noncompliance places patients at risk for treatment failure and increases the risk of the emergence of antibiotic resistance. Such measures increase the cost of treating MDR-TB. In 2011 there were an estimated 630,000 cases of MDR-TB among the world's 12 million cases of TB. In 2006, a report jointly published by the US Centers for Disease Control and Prevention and the World Health Organization (WHO) described a more severe form of tuberculosis known as extremely drug resistant tuberculosis (XDR-TB). XDR-TB is resistant to rifampin and isoniazid, plus three of the injectable second-line drugs (kanamycin, capreomycin, and amikacin), and all the fluoroquinolones (gatifloxacin, levofloxacin, oflaxacin, and moxifloxacin). Treatment of XDR-TB requires up to five drugs at a time, or experimental drugs, all of which show high toxicities and are more expensive. XDR-TB has been identified in 84 countries globally.

Another health care challenge involves the common skin organism Staphylococcus aureus, a gram-positive bacterium that has a thick cell wall and no outer membrane. This microorganism has, through the acquisition of several antibiotic resistant genes, become resistant to a variety of antibiotics, including particular macrolides, penicillins, cephalosporins, several quinolones, and tetracycline. These antibiotic resistant Staphylococcus aureus strains, or methicillin-resistant Staphylococcus aureus (MRSA), cause severe skin and soft tissue infections, sepsis (bacterial colonization of the bloodstream), pneumonia, abscesses, infection of catheters and orthopedic implants and ventilator-associated pneumonia. MRSA infect patients with defective or weakened immune systems and cause diseases that are very difficult to treat. There are two main types of MRSA: community-acquired MRSA (CA-MRSA) and hospital-acquired MRSA (HA-MRSA). CA-MRSA tends to produce a large number of toxins and have a predilection for the skin. HA-MRSA are comparatively more drug resistant. The drug of choice for MRSA infections is vancomycin, but in 1997, vancomycin-resistant Staphylococcus aureus (VRSA) emerged (possibly acquired from vancomycin-resistant Enterococcus), which threatened to eliminate the only treatment for MRSA and produce a new major public health crisis. Fortunately, in part owing to strict practices of isolation, disinfection, identifying MRSA carriers, and judicious use of vancomycin, VRSA has not yet become a frequent cause of infection.

Places with routinely high antibiotic use such as hospitals and nursing homes or densely-populated cities in developing countries with inadequate drug regulations and chronic antibiotic overuse or misuse are breeding grounds for high-level antibiotic resistance. Several gram-negative bacterial species have acquired antibiotic resistance and frequently cause nosocomial (hospital-acquired) pneumonia, urinary tract infections, surgical wound infections, and other complications. Two examples should suffice. First, in 2008 micro-organisms isolated from an Indian patient being treated in a Swedish hospital were resistant to all beta-lactam antibiotics, including carbapenems. These bacteria were resistant to these antibiotics because they harbored the New Delhi metal-containing beta-lactamase (NDM-1), which was encoded on a plasmid that could be transferred by conjugation. Presently, NDM-1 is one of the most widespread beta-lactamases throughout northern Europe and the Asia Pacific region. Typically NDM-1 appears in bacteria that already show resistance to multiple antibiotics, making its eradication nigh impossible. Second between 1977 and 2000 outbreaks of respiratory disease in hospital intensive care units (ICUs), typically among mechanically ventilated patients, yielded an organism called Acinetobacter baumannii, which normally does not cause disease. Other outbreaks in military field hospitals also in Afghanistan and Iraq were also caused by this organism. Acinetobacter lives in some people without causing disease, but in these clinical cases it contained a host of genetic elements that made it resistant to a broad range of antibiotics, including carbapenem. Carbapenem resistance in Acinetobacter results from the presence of type D beta-lactamases that are distinct from NDM-1 and this organism remains a growing threat in hospitals. This shows how the acquisition of antibiotic resistance can turn a member of the normal human microbiome into an opportunistic pathogen.

Treatment and Therapy

From an evolutionary perspective, antibiotic resistance is inevitable, but this does not mean that we cannot benefit from better stewardship of antibiotics. Frequent antibiotic exposure intensifies the selective pressure in bacterial populations and increases the likelihood that resistance emerges. Overprescription of antibiotics and improper usage has contributed to the present antibiotic resistance problem. Several studies have shown that antibiotics are prescribed for a host of cases that are almost certainly caused by viruses. Antibiotics in this case do no good and simply give the bacteria in our bodies further opportunities to develop resistance to them. Also poor patient compliance with medical directions such as the failure to take the full course of antibiotics may encourage the development of drug resistance. Bacteria that survive the partial course may be more likely to be resistant to that drug, making future administrations less effective.

Agricultural use of antibiotics also contributes to the present increase in the rates of antibiotic resistance. In the United States, millions of pounds of antibiotics are administered to farm animals to keep them healthy and help them to grow larger. The role such widespread agricultural use of antibiotics plays in the spread of antibiotic resistance is illustrated by the actions of the Danish government, who ended the administration of antibiotics as growth-promoters in the late 1990s. At the behest of the Danish government, WHO established an international review panel to determine if this ban affected the health of Danish farm ani-

> ### Information on Antibiotic Resistance
> **Cause:** Mutations in genes that encode antibiotics targets, the acquisition of antibiotic resistant genes, and natural selection for antibiotic resistance
> **Symptoms:** Infectious diseases that do not respond to the usual drugs and require newer, more powerful, and sometimes more expensive drugs
> **Duration:** As along as selection for antibiotic resistance exists
> **Treatment:** Newer drugs and more judicious use of the present antibiotics we have

mals. However, the WHO panel concluded that livestock and poultry production increased following the ban and levels of antibiotic resistance on farms and in meat decreased. On the strength of the Danish model, the 27 countries of the European Union (EU) banned the use of antibiotics as growth promoters in livestock in 2006.

Additionally, the overuse of antibiotics in the developing contributes where over-the-counter sales of antibiotics without a physician's prescription encourage overuse and misuse of antibiotics and increased levels of antibiotic resistance. In such circumstances, regulatory authorities can make a difference as in the case of Chile, for example, where the mandatory prescription of antibiotics and the ban of over-the-counter sales have decreased the rates of antibiotic resistance. Also the presence of substandard antibiotics in developing countries substantially contributes to the problem of antibiotic resistance, since the exposure of micro-organisms to low concentrations of antibiotics selects for resistant strains. Presently, of the 191 WHO member states, 30 percent have no or limited drug regulation in place. This encourages the unregulated importation, manufacture, and distribution of drugs, which leads to the proliferation of counterfeit drugs. Clearly better and more consistent drug regulation is needed.

With respect to drug development, several new antimicrobial agents have entered large clinical trials (phase 3 trials). New quinolones include nemonoxacin, and delafloxicin, two drugs that kill a broad spectrum of pathogenic bacteria and are well tolerated: finafloxacin, a drug that is acid-activated, works particularly well in the stomach, wounds, abscesses, and urine; zabofloxacin, a drug that shows excellent activity against pneumonias, and ozenaxacin, works well as a topical agent. A new tetracycline, omadacycline, evades many of the resistance mechanisms that confer resistance to tetracycline and has been designated by the Food and Drug Administration (FDA) as a qualified infectious disease product for community-acquired bacterial pneumonia and acute bacterial skin and skin-acquired infections. A new ketolide called solithromycin shows less toxicity than other ketolides and a low minimal inhibitory concentration (MIC) against several bacterial species. It has recently entered phase 3 clinical trials. An exciting new oxazolidinone, tedizolid, has the efficacy of linezolid but fewer side effects, and has entered phase 3 clinical trials.

To combat beta-lactamases, pharmaceutical companies designed "beta lactamase inhibitors" that are given in combination with beta-lactam antibiotics. For example, the drug Augmentin consists of the beta-lactam antibiotic amoxicillin and clavulanic acid, which inhibits beta-lactamases. The problem with these ingenious combinations is that bacteria have evolved inhibitor-resistant TEM beta-lactamases (IRTs). To overcome this problem, several new beta-lactam-inhibitor combinations have been developed. Combination of the new beta-lactamase inhibitor avibactam with several beta-lactam antibiotics forms several potent new antimicrobial combinations.

Perspective and Prospects

To tackle the problem of antibiotic resistance we must address the supply side (developing new drugs to replace ineffective old ones) and the demand side (changing the way we use antibiotics) of this issue. In both cases incentives are essential. Without a doubt new antibiotic development has diminished. A 2004 study showed that of 506 drugs in development by 15 large pharmaceutical companies and seven major biotechnology companies, only six of these were antibiotics. Between 1998 and 2002, the approval of new antibacterial agents by the FDA decreased by 56 percent, and a 2008 study revealed that only 15 of 167 antibiotics under development had a new mechanism of action. The reason for this decrease is that pharmaceutical companies receive little financial compensation for developing new antibiotics. The remuneration for antibiotics remains miniscule compared to cancer drugs, heart medicines, or antihypertensive drugs that patients take for the rest of their lives rather than temporarily. Consequently, pharmaceutical companies have stopped developing antibiotics and put their resources in more financially fruitful ventures. To restore incentives to the supply side of the issue, governments should provide new patent protections for new antibiotics and even develop tradeable intellectual rights for the development of new antibiotics that companies can use for financial benefit. Such incentives would reignite antibiotic research and development.

To address the demand side, physicians feel a duty to serve those patients presently at their door and not those they will see in ten years. However, studies have shown that incentives to improve patient follow-up in order to improve compliance with physician instructions increases compliance. Second, government regulators must do a better job of policing substandard or counterfeit drugs, since the use of these cultivates resistance. Finally, health care providers must learn to educate patients and learn to be assertive with patients as to why certain infections do not merit antibiotic prescriptions. Patients also must learn to trust their primary health care provider and not demand antibiotics when the diagnosis does not merit it.

—*Michael A. Buratovich Ph.D.*

See also Bacteriology; Dermatology; Dermopathology; Epidemiology; Hospitals; Intensive care units (ICU); Microbiology; Pathology; Pharmacology; Pharmacy; Pulmonary medicine; Urology

For Further Information:
Gallagher, Jason, C., and Conan MacDougall. *Antibiotics Simplified*. Burlington, Mass.: Jones and Bartlett Learning, 2013. A nicely written and easily understood introduction to the different types of antimicrobials and their pharmacology and clinical use.
Gualerazi, Claudio, O., Letzia Brandi, Attilio Fabbretti, and Cynthia Pon, eds. *Antibiotics: Targets, Mechanisms, and Resistance*. Weinheim, Germany: Wiley-VCH, 2013. A broad but detailed treatment of current and future antibiotic development.
Pucci, Michael J., and Karen Bush. "Investigational Antimicrobial Agents of 2013." *Clinical Microbiology Reviews* 26, no. 4 (2013): 792-821. A detailed summary of the new antimicrobials in the drug pipeline.
Walsh, Christopher. *Antibiotics: Actions, Origins, Resistance*. Washington, DC: ASM Press, 2013. A magisterial treatment of the biochemistry, mechanisms and synthesis of antibiotics and antibiotic resistance.
World Health Organization: http://www.who.int/en/.

Antibiotics

Treatment
Anatomy or system affected: All
Specialties and related fields: Bacteriology, immunology, microbiology, pharmacology
Definition: The use of drugs that are selectively toxic to microorganisms.
Key terms:

chemotherapeutic index: for antibiotics, the ratio of the maximum dose that can be administered without causing serious damage to a person to the minimum dose that will cause serious damage to the infecting microorganism; a measure of selective toxicity

minimal inhibitory concentration: the amount of an antibiotic needed to inhibit the growth of a microorganism in the laboratory; may be correlated to the dose of the antibiotic needed to control an infection

normal microbiota: the collection of microorganisms that inhabit tissues of healthy persons and that to some degree establish environments hostile to pathogens (the causative agents of disease)

resistance determinants: genes found in some bacteria that permit them to resist the action of particular antibiotics; these genes can be transferred between cells, allowing rapid spread of antibiotic resistance among bacteria

semisynthetic: used to refer to natural products, such as antibiotics, that have been chemically modified to be more useful for a particular application

spectrum of activity: the range of microbial species that can be inhibited by an antibiotic; broad-spectrum antibiotics can control more than one kind of infection, but narrow-spectrum antibiotics avoid unintentional damage to the normal microbiota

superinfection: an infection caused by destruction of the normal microbiota by antibiotic therapy, which allows for proliferation of a pathogen other than the one targeted by the antibiotic

Indications and Procedures

Humans live in the midst of a microbial world of bacteria, fungi, and protozoa. Microorganisms were the first inhabitants of the earth. When multicellular animals arose, some microbes adapted to use them as a source of nutrients. Most of these microorganisms did no harm to their hosts. In fact, humans carry around bacteria numbering in the trillions. Some were not harmless and possessed the means to penetrate tissues and invade internal organs. As a result, animals evolved a variety of defensive strategies, referred to as immune responses, to resist such invasion. Infections develop when these responses fail to repel the invading bacteria. To combat such infections, humans can turn to antibiotics for help.

Antibiotics are drugs that kill, or inhibit the reproduction of, bacteria. In the strict use of the term as defined by Selman Waksman, the discoverer of streptomycin, an antibiotic is "a chemical substance produced by microorganisms which has the capacity to inhibit the growth of bacteria and even destroy bacteria and other microorganisms in dilute solution."

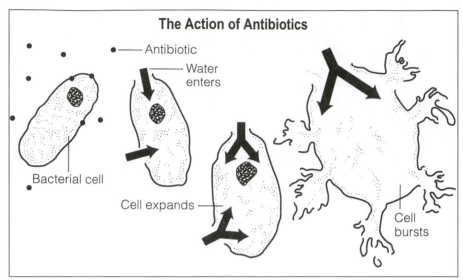

The Action of Antibiotics

An antibiotic destroys a bacterium by causing its cell walls to deteriorate; water will then enter the bacterium unchecked until it bursts.

The effectiveness of antibiotics arises from their selective toxicity, which relies on differences between the fundamental biology of pathogenic bacteria and that of an infected person. The sulfonamides, or sulfa drugs, the first class of antibiotic compounds to achieve widespread use, are chemically similar to molecules used by bacteria for the synthesis of folic acid, an essential vitamin. When sulfonamides are present, they interfere with folic acid synthesis, preventing growth of the bacteria. Because humans lack the ability to synthesize folic acid (which is obtained from food), their cells are unaffected by sulfonamides. The beta-lactams, a class of antimicrobial chemicals that includes the penicillins and cephalosporins, interfere with the synthesis of peptidoglycan, an essential component of bacterial cell walls that is totally lacking in human cells. Other antibiotics target unique aspects of microbial protein synthesis and nucleic acid metabolism. Antibiotics are sometimes used in combination; for example, beta-lactams may be used to weaken bacterial cell walls, promoting access of a second antibiotic directed against an internal target.

The clinical microbiology laboratory can assist physicians in determining appropriate antibiotic therapy by identifying infectious agents and determining the susceptibility or resistance of the agent to a range of potential antibiotics. In the early days of antimicrobial chemotherapy, it was often sufficient to diagnose an infection from its symptoms, from which one could infer the type of microorganism causing the infection (for example, gram-positive or gram-negative bacteria) and prescribe one of a limited number of broad-spectrum agents with confidence that it would be effective. Today, while immediate application of broad-spectrum antibiotics may be called for to contain a serious infection, concern over creating resistant pathogens leads more physicians to request the identification and testing of microorganisms. Furthermore, the extensive resistance encountered among pathogens suggests that a broad-spectrum agent may be ineffective.

Advances in clinical microbiology are directed toward increasing the speed and accuracy of the identification of infectious agents, with a primary goal of providing information useful in prescribing antimicrobial chemotherapy. Clinical samples (infected fluids, biopsy samples, or tissue swabs) are used to inoculate selective and differential media that favor the growth of a suspected pathogen. Material from isolated colonies is then subjected to a variety of tests designed to characterize aspects of the microorganism's physiology and metabolic biochemistry, which provide criteria for the taxonomic identification of the organism. While some smaller laboratories rely on the manual inoculation of test media and reference to printed diagnostic tables for identification, the trend is toward greater automation to allow more rapid processing of multiple samples. Panels of test media prepared in multiwell plates can be simultaneously inoculated, and because many of the tests are evaluated by color changes, test results can be read with spectrophotometers designed to scan the individual tests. Test data are entered into computer programs that match the test results with probability matrices to provide a probable identification of the organism used to inoculate the tests. In the largest laboratories, efficiency can be enhanced by using robotics to conduct many of the steps, from inoculation to the reporting of test results and probable identification.

While automation can help to speed up the rate at which test information is obtained, classic identification tests are limited by the need for the incubation and growth of the test organism; this limitation can be particularly burdensome in the case of microorganisms that are especially slow-growing, among which are the mycobacteria that cause tuberculosis. In response, laboratories increasingly rely on identification methods that allow direct examination of the microorganism. Serological tests, which use antibodies directed against antigens specific to a particular microbe, and DNA probes, targeted to species-specific genes, are being applied to an increasing range of pathogenic microorganisms. Some of these tests have advanced to the point that infectious agents can be identified directly in clinical samples, circumventing the need for isolation in the laboratory. In 2013, a research team from the University of Toronto announced the creation of an electronic chip that can analyze blood for pathogens in a matter of minutes, far more quickly than previous methods. The chip can simultaneously test for multiple viruses and bacteria, which will facilitate rapid detection and more targeted treatment of the infectious agent.

In evaluating the susceptibility of a microorganism to an antibiotic, microbiologists seek to determine the minimal inhibitory concentration (MIC) at which an antibiotic will inhibit the growth of the microbe in a standard growth medium; the MIC can be correlated with an effective dose of the antibiotic. In broth dilution tests, a defined number of microbial cells is inoculated into a series of broth tubes containing different concentrations of an antibiotic; the MIC is reported as the lowest concentration of the antibiotic that prevents growth of the organism in the broth. The same technologies used to automate identification can be used to allow a large number of broth dilution tests to be carried out in multiwell plates, so that susceptibility to a range of antibiotics can be determined simultaneously.

Where automation is unavailable, broth dilution testing is impractical because of the labor involved, and laboratories may rely on an indirect method called a disk diffusion test, or Kirby-Bauer assay. In this method, disks of filter paper impregnated with a defined amount of antibiotic are placed on a plate of solid growth medium that has been seeded with cells of the microorganism being tested. During incubation, the antibiotic diffuses from the disk, leading to a gradient of antibiotic concentration extending in all directions from the disk. If the microbe is susceptible to the antibiotic, its growth will be inhibited in a circular zone surrounding the disk; the diameter of the zone of inhibition varies directly with the MIC for that antibiotic. As with traditional identification methods, tests for antibiotic susceptibility are limited by the requirement that the test organism be allowed time to grow in the laboratory. It is likely that commercial DNA probes will be developed to allow the direct detection of genes that encode resistance to individual antibiotics.

Uses and Complications

Given the importance of differences between the biology of infectious microorganisms and the biology of the infected host to the effectiveness of antibiotics, it is not surprising that antibiotics have been used most successfully to control infections caused by bacteria, whose molecular and cellular biology differs vastly from that of humans. Consequently, most antibiotics directed against bacteria show a favorable chemotherapeutic index, which is the ratio of the maximum dose that can be administered without causing serious harm to the recipient of the drug to the minimum dose that will be effective in controlling the infection.

Infections caused by eukaryotic fungi and protozoa are particularly difficult to treat because of the similarities between the cell structure and function of these organisms and those of human cells. While the topical application of antifungal agents such as miconazole is very effective in the treatment of fungal skin infections and vaginal candidiasis, the treatment of systemic fungal infections (usually with amphotericin B) is much more difficult to perform and is more likely to cause serious side effects. Amphotericin B, the mainstay of antifungal therapy for decades, was particularly toxic. Newer antifungal agents, such as the azoles and echinocandins, are better tolerated and sometimes more effective, but antifungal therapy remains a challenge. Similar complications accompany efforts to treat protozoal infections with antimicrobial agents; this situation is especially frustrating, since parasitic infections such as malaria and schistosomiasis pose a major worldwide health problem. The number of methods available for the chemical treatment of viral infections is extremely limited, in view of the fact that viruses rely on the molecular machinery of the infected host for their reproduction. One antiviral strategy that has met with limited success is to design nucleotide analogues that interfere with viral nucleic acid synthesis; both acyclovir, used for infections caused by the herpes simplex virus, and azidothymidine, the first agent shown to affect the course of human immunodeficiency virus (HIV) infection, belong to this class of drugs.

In addition to potential toxicity, other factors need to be considered when choosing an antibiotic for treatment of a particular infection. Attention must be given to the course of treatment when an antibiotic is administered, so that a sufficient concentration is maintained at the site of infection. If an antibiotic is administered orally, then it must be able to survive the environment of the gastrointestinal tract in order to reach the targeted tissues. Only certain antibiotics are able to cross the blood-brain barrier for effective treatment of infections of the central nervous system.

Antibiotics can be classified according to their spectrum of activity (the range of pathogenic organisms that they effectively kill or inhibit); broad-spectrum antibiotics are effective against many species, while narrow-spectrum antibiotics target a specific group. A broad-spectrum antibiotic can be prescribed upon diagnosis of an infection, without identification of the particular pathogen responsible; this trait can be important when immediate containment of the infection is essential to the health of the patient. Yet the indiscriminate use of broad-spectrum antibiotics can harm microorganisms other than those causing an infection. External surfaces, including the skin, gastrointestinal tract, upper respiratory tract, and vagina, are inhabited by large numbers of microorganisms, collectively referred to as the normal microbiota. While this relationship is hardly a symbiotic one, such organisms do help to maintain environments that inhibit the growth of pathogenic microbes. Administration of broad-spectrum antibiotics can cause the depletion of normal microbiota organisms, leading to conditions favoring superinfection by a pathogen other than the one targeted by the antibiotic. For example, vaginal candidiasis (often called a yeast infection) can develop with the administration of antibacterial drugs. The bacteria that normally inhabit the vagina maintain an acidic environment that inhibits the growth of the pathogenic fungus *Candida albicans*, which may nevertheless persist in low numbers. If these bacteria are adversely affected by antibiotic treatment, then the vagina may become less acidic, allowing *C. albicans* to grow and cause tissue damage. Other superinfections can lead to serious damage to the gastrointestinal tract. There is also concern that the use of broad-spectrum antibiotics may encourage the growth of antibiotic-resistant strains among the microorganisms that constitute the normal microbiota. Because antibiotic resistance can be transferred from one bacterial species to another, conditions that favor the growth of any antibiotic-resistant microbes can contribute to the development of antibiotic-resistant pathogens.

Specific resistance to the action of antibiotics is a matter of great concern to medical personnel who deal with infectious diseases. In the early 1940s, when the first antibiotics came into widespread use, virtually all strains of *Staphylococcus aureus* (a bacterium that causes a variety of infections) were susceptible to penicillin G, a beta-lactam that can be administered orally. By the 1990s, it was rare to isolate a strain of *S. aureus* from an infection that was not resistant to multiple beta-lactams. Similar situations prevail with other pathogenic microorganisms, seriously impairing the ability to control many infections. Antibiotic resistance usually develops when a pathogen possesses specific genes encoding proteins that allow the organism to avoid the action of the antibiotic. Such proteins may inactivate the antibiotic molecule, interfere with the uptake of the antibiotic, or modify the target of the antibiotic so that it is no longer affected by the antibiotic. In bacteria, the genes encoding antibiotic resistance (called resistance determinants, or R-factors) are usually found on plasmids, small circular deoxyribonucleic acid (DNA) molecules that are separate from the bacterial chromosome. A single plasmid may contain genes for resistance to several antibiotics. Many plasmids also contain genes that allow them to be transferred from one cell to another, even if the cells are of different species. These genes can cause antibiotic resistance to spread rapidly among microorganisms.

Because the presence of an antibiotic in an animal's tissues favors the survival of bacteria carrying resistance determinants for that antibiotic, continued application of an antibiotic tends to increase the incidence of resistance to that antibiotic. Overcoming this dilemma is difficult. Narrow-spectrum antibiotics should be used whenever practical, since they limit the range of species subject to selection for antibiotic resistance. Some microbiologists have urged that the nontherapeutic application of antibiotics, such as the use of tetracycline as a growth-promoting factor in animal feeds, be discontinued because it can contribute to the spread of resistance determinants. The identification of new natural and synthetic compounds for which resistance has not yet been encountered can help to defeat pathogens that have developed resistance to the current repertoire of antibiotics, but experience teaches one to expect that such victories will be temporary; the implementation of each new antibiotic will lead to the discovery of new resistance determinants.

Perspective and Prospects

The latter decades of the nineteenth century are often referred to as the golden age of microbiology, because it was during this time that microbiologists identified many of the pathogenic microorganisms responsible for infectious diseases. Although such knowledge was useful in helping to control the transmission of infectious diseases in populations through public health measures and vaccination programs, it did little to alleviate the suffering of the individual already infected with now-identifiable pathogens. Actual treatment of infections required the identification of chemical compounds that would be selectively toxic to the microorganisms, and such compounds were unknown at that time. Nevertheless, the potential value of such compounds motivated many scientists to devote their research to the search for chemicals that would destroy microorganisms without damaging an infected person.

The few compounds used at this time (mostly heavy metal salts) tended to exhibit a very low chemotherapeutic index, and some scientists despaired of finding poisons that were poisonous for only some forms of life. Then, in 1910, Paul Ehrlich demonstrated that Salvarsan (arsphenamine), an arsenical compound, was selectively toxic to the bacterial agent of syphilis. Although Salvarsan was useless for other infections, it provided evidence that selective toxicity was possible and encouraged the medical community to find other selective toxins. Extensive chemical screening programs led, in 1935, to the commercial production of the sulfanilamides, which are active against multiple species of bacteria.

The greatest conceptual advance in the development of antimicrobial drugs was made by those bacteriologists who concentrated on the phenomenon of antagonism, whereby certain microorganisms produce compounds that inhibit others. Study of these compounds eventually led to the practical application of gramicidin (described by René Dubos in 1939), penicillin (described by Alexander Fleming in 1928), and streptomycin (described by Selman Waksman in 1943). Penicillin receives special attention in the history of antibiotics because the industrial processes developed to allow production of massive quantities of the drug proved valuable in the commercial exploitation of other antibiotics. With the goal of increasing the yield of penicillin, motivated in part by a desire to have an alternative to the sulfonamides for the treatment of infections attending World War II, industrial microbiologists optimized the composition and aeration of the growth media and selected mutant strains of the penicillin-producing fungus that secreted the drug in amounts far greater than those seen by Fleming. In doing so, they established some of the engineering principles that allowed for the growth of biotechnology.

Eventually, major pharmaceutical companies committed

themselves to extensive screening programs to identify additional natural antibiotics. Microorganisms isolated from soil were tested for their ability to inhibit the growth of pathogens. Eventually it was realized that although a diverse range of organic molecules possess antibiotic properties, such compounds are produced by a limited range of microorganisms. More than half of the natural antibiotics currently in use are produced by mycelial bacteria called actinomycetes. One approach that has complemented the identification of new natural antibiotics is the chemical modification of such drugs through the addition or removal of groups of atoms. Compared to natural antibiotics, such semisynthetic derivatives may have properties that promote accumulation at high levels in the target tissue or prevent recognition of the antibiotic molecule by products of resistance determinants. All the beta-lactams in common use today are semisynthetic molecules.

While microbiologists have been discovering further natural antibiotics and synthesizing others, they have also been learning more about the molecular biology of infectious pathogens. Research is also progressing on ways to decrease the unnecessary use of antibiotics. Rapid flu tests can now be used by doctors to determine whether patients need antibiotics at all. New uses for antibiotics are also being discovered every day. For instance, researchers have begun to explore ways to attach powerful implants to medical devices in order to decrease infection postoperatively. Together, all these types of knowledge will allow antibiotic development to become increasingly useful.

—Kenneth A. Pidcock, Ph.D.;
updated by Nancy A. Piotrowski, Ph.D.

See also Bacterial infections; Bacteriology; Candidiasis; Chemotherapy; Cytology; Cytopathology; Drug resistance; Fungal infections; Genetic engineering; Gram staining; Herbal medicine; Immune system; Immunology; Immunopathology; Infection; Laboratory tests; Microbiology; Parasitic diseases; Pharmacology; Pharmacy; Protozoan diseases; Viral infections.

For Further Information:
"Antibiotics: Misuse Puts You and Others at Risk." *Mayo Clinic*, February 4, 2012.
"Antibiotics: When They Can and Can't Help." *American Academy of Family Physicians*, November 2010.
Black, Jacquelyn G. *Microbiology: Principles and Explorations*. 8th ed. Hoboken, N.J.: John Wiley & Sons, 2012.
Brock, Thomas, ed. *Milestones in Microbiology*. Englewood Cliffs, N.J.: Prentice Hall, 1961.
Conte, John E. *Manual of Antibiotics and Infectious Diseases: Treatment and Prevention*. 9th ed. Philadelphia: Lippincott Williams & Wilkins, 2002.
Gale, E. F., et al. *The Molecular Basis of Antibiotic Action*. London: John Wiley & Sons, 1981.
Levinson, Warren. *Review of Medical Microbiology and Immunology*. 12th ed. New York: McGraw-Hill Medical, 2012.
Levy, Stuart B. *The Antibiotic Paradox: How the Misuse of Antibiotics Destroys Their Curative Powers*. Cambridge, Mass.: Perseus, 2001.
Moberg, Carol L., and Zanvil A. Cohn, eds. *Launching the Antibiotic Era*. New York: Rockefeller Press, 1990.
Neu, H. C. "The Crisis in Antibiotic Resistance." *Science* 249 (August 21, 1992): 1064-1073.
Walsh, Christopher. *Antibiotics: Actions, Origins, Resistance*. Washington, D.C.: ASM Press, 2003.

Antibodies
Biology
Also known as: Gamma globulin proteins, immunoglobulin (Ig)
Anatomy or system affected: Blood, cells, circulatory system, immune system, lymphatic system
Specialties and related fields: Bacteriology, biochemistry, biotechnology, immunology, internal medicine, microbiology, oncology, pathology, pharmacology, preventive medicine, public health
Definition: An antibody is a protein that is produced by the body to recognize and eliminate specific foreign antigens, such as bacteria, viruses, or other microorganisms, by way of triggering the immune system. It is produced by white blood cells, also called B lymphocytes.
Key terms:
constant region: The C-terminal portion of the antibody that is highly conserved across species
Fc-fusion proteins: specific proteins of interest fused to the Fc region of the antibody at its C-terminal end
heavy chain: the bigger subunits of an antibody
isotypes: the different classes of antibodies
light chain: the smaller subunits of an antibody
monoclonal antibodies: antibodies derived from a single parent clonal cell
variable region: the N-terminal portion of the antibody, which possesses antigen-binding sites and has variable amino acid sequences

Structure and Functions
An antibody is a Y-shaped protein unit, or tetramer, made of four individual subunits: two identical smaller subunits called light chains and two identical bigger subunits called heavy chains. There are two families of light chain, called kappa and lambda. Each immunoglobulin (Ig) class consists of either one of these two families of light chains and does not change through its life. There are approximately ten different types of heavy chain, and they contribute to the different classes of antibodies or immunoglobulins. The five major types of heavy chains are a, d, e, g, and m types. Each possesses a distinct number of amino acids. Depending on the type of heavy chain present, the antibodies are classified into five major classes or isotypes: IgA, IgD, IgE, IgG, and IgM. Each isotype has a specific function, and more than one Ig isotype is required for complete elimination of a certain antigen. The presence of specialized proteins called cytokines can trigger switching of one type of isotype to another.

Each light or heavy chain possesses a constant region, which is conserved in its amino acid composition across different Ig types, and a variable region, which differs between different B cells. The constant region is present in the C-terminal portion of the protein, and the variable region is present at the N-terminal portion. The variable region contains the antigen-binding sites and is thus responsible for binding to the specific antigen. The antibody displays maximum versatility in this region in possessing hundreds of binding sites and as a result is able to recognize and bind hundreds of different antigens. The tips of the variable region are called fragment antigen-binding (Fab) regions. The constant region remains identical in all heavy or light chains of the antibodies. It is responsible for activating the complement system and can also initiate phagocytosis. The constant region is also identical between different isotypes. The base of this region consists of the fragment crystallizable (Fc) region. Once the antigen is bound to the antibody surface, the constant region of the antibody elicits an appropriate immune response.

When there is an exposure to the antigen, the B cells in the blood transform into specific cells called plasma cells and begin producing antibodies, utilizing the aid of helper T cells of the immune system. Antibodies, through their antigen-binding sites, bind with the antigen and form antigen-antibody complexes. Each antigen presents a surface that can be recognized and bound by the specific antibody. The antigen-antibody complex is a signal for destruction. The complex can be engulfed by other specialized cells called macrophages or can be lysed by triggering a proteolytic pathway called a complement pathway. This whole response is called the humoral response of the immune system.

Disorders and Diseases

The most important function of an antibody is to distinguish between "self" and "nonself" proteins. An antibody should bind only to nonself proteins. When this recognition capability is compromised, the result is the development of autoimmune diseases or disorders. An autoimmune disease can occur in specific organs, such as the thyroid gland, or in the entire body, as with lupus or rheumatoid arthritis. Scleroderma, multiple sclerosis, vitiligo, psoriasis, and alopecia are other examples of autoimmune diseases that can develop because of an attack on the body's own proteins by antibodies.

Perspective and Prospects

The study of antibodies began in the late nineteenth century when scientists discovered a "factor" or antitoxin that could react with antigens or the toxin. The term "antibody" was introduced by Emil von Behring and Shibasaburo Kitasato in 1890. In the early twentieth century, the specificity of antibodies was demonstrated and the methodology for studying antigen-antibody complexes was deduced. The structure of the antibody was realized in 1960. Since then, the field of antibody research has grown and important discoveries have been made about the structure, functions, and utility of antibodies. Different types of antibodies have been discovered and their genetic basis inferred.

In addition to affording immunity against pathogens, antibodies are used as important agents in clinical diagnostics and the treatment of a variety of human diseases, including cancer and a number of infectious diseases. Antibody engineering involves the development of monoclonal antibodies directed against specific antigens involved in diseases. Some of these antibodies can be modified to carry drugs or radioactive substances to be delivered specifically to tumor cells in the case of cancer. A number of monoclonal anti-

bodies such as Herceptin (trastuzumab), Rituxan (rituximab), and Remicade (infliximab) have been approved by the Food and Drug Administration (FDA) to treat various diseases. Fc-fusion proteins such as Enbrel (etanercept) have also been developed in the last decade for treatment of various diseases. Many monoclonal antibodies and Fc-fusion proteins are being tested in clinical trials. In addition, diagnostic tests may involve the detection of antibodies. Polyclonal antibodies were initially used to prevent viral illnesses and later in the treatment of antibody deficiencies.

Another major application of antibodies is in scientific research. A number of extremely useful scientific techniques involve the use of antibodies, such as Enzyme-Linked Immuno-Sorbent Assay (ELISA), Western blotting, flow cytometry, immunohistochemistry, immunohistochemistry, and immunocytochemistry. These techniques are regularly employed in scientific experiments to understand the structure and function of proteins involved in a variety of diseases.

—*Geetha Yadav, Ph.D.; updated by Samar Aslam, M.D.*

See also Autoimmune disorders; Blood and blood disorders; Cancer; Cells; Cytology; Cytopathology; Hair loss and baldness; Hematology, Hematology, pediatric; Host-defense mechanisms; Immune system; Immunology; Multiple sclerosis; Psoriasis; Rheumatoid arthritis; Scleroderma; Systemic lupus erythematosus (SLE); Vitiligo

For Further Information:

An, Zhiqiang, ed. *Therapeutic Monoclonal Antibodies: From Bench to Clinic.* Hoboken, N.J.: John Wiley & Sons, 2009.
Lewin, Benjamin. *Genes IX.* 9th rev. ed. Sudbury, Mass.: Jones & Bartlett, 2008.
McCullough, Kenneth, and Raymond Spier. *Monoclonal Antibodies in Biotechnology: Theoretical and Practical Aspects.* New York: Cambridge University Press, 1990.

Anticoagulants

Biology

Anatomy or system affected: Blood vessels, heart, brain, lower limbs, site of implantation of embryo or placental blood vessels

Specialties and related fields: Hematology, coagulation, cardiovascular disease, stroke, obstetrics and gynecology

Definition: Drugs that delay or halt blood clotting by acting on clotting factors or platelets

Key terms:

thrombosis: the occurrence of blood clots (thrombus) in blood vessels

venous thromboembolism: blood clots that originate in veins; includes deep vein thrombosis (clots that form mostly in the deep veins of the legs) and pulmonary embolism (deep vein thrombosis clots that detach from the walls of veins and travel to the lungs, where they block blood flow)

platelet: blood cells that cluster together to form a blood clot with the help of clotting factors

clotting factors: proteins in the blood that are involved in the formation of blood clots, such as prothrombin and Factor VIII; produced primarily by platelets, the liver, and the lining of blood vessels, but many other tissues are now thought to be sources

therapeutic index(therapeutic range): range of drug dosages within which the drug is effective and safe (i.e., does not cause significant adverse events)

Structure and Functions

In the body, the tendency towards clotting (fibrosis) and the opposing tendency towards clot disruption and bleeding (fibrinolysis) are in a dynamic balance. Tipping the balance in one direction can lead to too much clotting (thrombosis) while too high a shift in the other direction causes excessive bleeding.

Platelets are involved in the normal process of clot formation. When a blood vessel is injured, platelets attach to the walls of the injured blood vessels and emit chemical signals that attract and activate other platelets, resulting in aggregation of the platelets to form a platelet plug that staunches bleeding from the damaged blood vessel. This platelet plug alone, however, is not strong enough to curtail blood loss from the injured blood vessel; the platelet plug must be reinforced by a cable-like protein called fibrin. This fibrin-formation process involves two pathways: 1) the contact activation pathway and 2) the tissue factor pathway. Together, the two pathways result in the conversion of the clotting factor, factor X to an active form called factor Xa. Factor Xa and other cofactors convert prothrombin to thrombin. Thrombin processes a blood-based protein called fibrinogen into a smaller protein called fibrin. Fibrin self-assembles into long, rigid, fibers that reinforce platelet plugs.

Anticoagulants are drugs used in the treatment of thrombosis or the prevention of thrombosis in people who have certain conditions or are undergoing procedures that increase risk of blood clots. Anticoagulants delay the clotting of blood or prevent clots from expanding in blood vessels by blocking the action of clotting factors. Examples of anticoagulants include warfarin, heparin, direct thrombin inhibitors, and factor Xa inhibitors. Another group of drugs, the thrombolytic agents, dissolve clots that have already formed.

Warfarin, one of the oldest anticoagulants, is still in use today. It works by inhibiting a liver-based enzyme called vitamin K epoxide reductase (VKORC1). VKORC1 modifies clotting factors II, VII, IX, and X and proteins C and S so that they bind calcium ions more tightly. Inhibition of VKOR1 by warfarin reduces the vitamin K-dependent modification of these clotting factors, rendering them non-functional and slowing the clotting process. However, warfarin treatment requires constant monitoring because of its narrow therapeutic index (the dosage range within which a drug is effective and safe). Heparin, a complex polysaccharide, inhibits clotting by acting on antithrombin III, thrombin II, and factor Xa during the clotting process. Previously, only unfractionated heparin was used, but now low-molecular-weight heparins (LMWHs) such as enoxaparin, dalteparin, and tinzaparin are also available. LMWHs have become the preferred type of anticoagulant for treating pulmonary embolism and unstable angina because their kinetics are more predictable than unfractionated heparin, but LMWHs are associated with safety concerns in people with kidney disease. Factor Xa inhibitors include idraparinux (indirect inhibitor), fondaparinux, rivaroxaban, apixaban, edoxaban, and betrixaban (direct inhibitors). Direct thrombin inhibitors (e.g., dabigatran) and factor Xa inhibitors bind to thrombin and factor Xa, respectively, and prevent them from participating in the clotting process. Thrombolytic agents (or fibrinolytic agents) activate plasmin, which degrades the fibrin cross-links in blood clots and causes the clots to break up. Examples of thrombolytic agents are alteplase (tissue plasminogen activator), reteplase, tenecteplase, and urokinase.

Although antiplatelet drugs are a separate class of drugs from anticoagulants, they are used for similar indications. Antiplatelet medications disrupt platelet activation and aggregation, thus reducing clot formation. The most well-known antiplatelet is aspirin, which inhibits the cyclooxygenase (COX)-1 and COX-2 enzymes, thus preventing the release of thromboxane A2, which is involved in platelet aggregation. More recently, antiplatelets with a different mechanism of action became available and are now widely used. These drugs, which include clopidogrel, prasugrel, ticagrelor, and cangrelor, inhibit a protein called P2Y12 that is crucial for platelet function and aggregation.

Indications and Procedures

Anticoagulants are used to treat or prevent prevalent conditions such as venous thromboembolism (including deep venous thrombosis and pulmonary embolism) and ischemic stroke. Depending on the acuteness and nature of the thrombotic incident, different anticoagulants may be appropriate. For example, warfarin is a very effective treatment for acute thrombotic episodes. However, warfarin is a somewhat difficult drug to use because of its varied effectiveness from person to person and narrow therapeutic index, which necessitates continuous monitoring. On the other hand, heparin is a popular option for preventing blood clots during surgery, kidney dialysis, and blood transfusions.

Individuals with thrombophilia or hypercoagulability, a condition characterized by an increased risk of thrombosis, often need anticoagulants to prevent clots in their arteries and veins. The type of anticoagulant, dosage, and duration of treatment depends on the underlying cause. The condition may be caused by inherited disorders (e.g., deficiencies in clotting factors), acquired conditions (e.g., antiphospholipid syndrome or pregnancy), or a combination of both. Other individuals who frequently need anticoagulants are those undergoing surgery, especially orthopedic surgery, and those with acute coronary syndromes. Short-term anticoagulant therapy is typically used in these patients. On the other hand, patients with mechanical heart valves and those who have had repeated thrombotic incidents could be prescribed anticoagulants for life.

For antiplatelets, the American Diabetes Association and the American Heart Association jointly recommend aspirin for the prevention of heart disease in people over 40 who have diabetes or those who have additional risk factors for heart disease but do not have elevated risk for gastrointestinal hemorrhage (an adverse effect of aspirin). Clopidogrel, prasugrel, and ticagrelor are given to patients with atherosclerosis who are getting a stent implanted via catheter, a process known as percutaneous coronary intervention. In these patients, the antiplatelet drugs can prevent heart attacks, stroke, and stent thrombosis, which refers to common and often fatal clots that form in stents.

Administration

Warfarin may be administered either orally or by injection. Foods that contain vitamin K such as kale, Swiss chard, broccoli, and spinach, can interfere with the drug's function. For this reason, clinicians may recommend diet changes for patients prescribed warfarin. Heparin is always administered by injection, most commonly intravenously or subcutaneously (just under the skin). Direct thrombin inhibitors are currently administered only by injection, although an orally administered drug is in development. For factor Xa inhibitors, the indirect inhibitors must be given by injection, while the direct inhibitors can be given either orally or by injection. Thrombolytic agents are often used to treat emergency conditions arising from a sudden clot. The therapy is administered either intravenously through a vein in the arm or through a catheter for durations ranging from 1 hour (for a heart attack) to 48 hours (for deep vein thrombosis). Antiplatelet therapies are mainly orally administered.

Monitoring

Among the anticoagulants, warfarin requires the most stringent monitoring because of its narrow therapeutic index-the range of doses within which warfarin is effective yet safe (bleeding risk is not excessive). This index needs to be monitored throughout the course of therapy, using the prothrombin time/international normalized ratio (PT/INR) test, which gives a number (the INR) that indicates whether or not the level of warfarin in the blood is within the therapeutic window (usually 2-3). Besides PT/INR monitoring, patients being considered for warfarin therapy should also be tested for mutations in the *VKORC1* and *CYP2C9* genes. The *VKORC1* gene test detects a mutation in the *VKORC1* gene (a change of guanine to adenosine). This mutation causes the VKORC1 enzyme, warfarin' target, to be more susceptible to the effects of warfarin. Patients with this mutation will likely require a lower dose of warfarin. CYP2C9 metabolizes warfarin, helping to clear it from the body after it has fulfilled its function. Changes in the *CYP2C9* gene called *CYP2C9*2* and *CYP2C9*3* are linked to poorer metabolism of warfarin, meaning that more of the drug stays in the body for a longer time, which could have toxic effects. Thus, clinicians should consider lowering the warfarin dosage in patients with these gene changes.

The efficacy of the antiplatelet agent clopidogrel is also dependent on the form of the *CYP2C19* gene present. CYP2C19*2 and *3 forms are associated with poor re-

sponses to clopidogrel, while a healthier response is associated with the *17 form. Prasugrel and ticagrelor are less affected and unaffected, respectively, by *CYP2C19* genotype.

Another anticoagulant that may require monitoring is unfractionated heparin. The activated partial thromboplastin time (aPTT) test is most frequently used to monitor the anticoagulant effect of the drug, although heparin anti-Xa tests are sometimes used instead. Based on the aPTT or heparin anti-Xa test results, clinicians may make changes to the dosage of unfractionated heparin to maintain the anticoagulant effect/bleeding risk balance. LMWH use is generally not monitored, unless the patient has a kidney disorder or is pregnant or obese, since such individuals may have problems clearing LMWHs from the body.

Since thrombolytic agents are frequently used in emergency settings to treat suddenly arising blood clots, patients treated with these agents require close monitoring. Besides monitoring for excessive bleeding and the anticoagulant effect of the drugs in the affected organ, clinicians will also closely monitor the blood pressure of the patient, and their heart and lung function. However, the situation could potentially be complicated if, during dissolution of the blood clots by the thrombolytic agent, pieces of the clots travel deeper into the affected organ, obstruct other, smaller blood vessels, and aggravate the situation.

Uses and Complications

The main complication that can occur with all anticoagulants (and antiplatelets) is excessive bleeding or hemorrhage. Thus, patients on anticoagulants need to be monitored for excessive bleeding and if bleeding becomes a problem, the medication should be reduced in dosage or discontinued. Patients who are treated with two anticoagulants simultaneously are at even greater risk than those receiving a single anticoagulant and need to be very carefully monitored for excessive bleeding. Treatment for bleeding includes prothrombin complex concentrate (PCC) and recombinant factor VIIa. If a patient receives too large a dose of an anticoagulant, or if an emergency necessitates quenching anticoagulant activity in the patient, antidotes to these drugs do exist. For example, the antidote for warfarin is vitamin K, the antidote for heparin is a salt called protamine sulfate, and the antidote for dabigatran is an antibody against it called idarucizumab, which must be given intravenously. A genetically-engineered form of Factor Xa called andexanet is being researched as an antidote for apixaban, rivaroxaban, edoxaban, and betrixaban. The administration of thrombolytic agents may cause premature dissolution of clots and excessive bleeding. In such cases, a drug called aminocaproic acid, which acts as an antidote for thrombolytic agents, may be given either orally or intravenously.

Other adverse effects are often specific to the particular therapies. For example, heparin can cause heparin-induced thrombocytopenia and thrombosis (HITT), which is an immune disorder that causes severe thrombosis. HITT typically appears 4 to 10 days after heparin exposure and is characterized by a drastic drop in platelet count (half of baseline levels). Paradoxically, although the number of platelets drop, the hallmark of the condition is venous thromboembolism. In the longer term, unfractionated heparin treatment carries a risk of osteoporosis.

Perspective and Prospects

Anticoagulant therapy has progressed considerably in the past several decades. Many alternatives to the traditional anticoagulants, warfarin and unfractionated heparin, are now available. These therapies have wider therapeutic indices than warfarin does, and some have more favorable adverse effect profiles, less interaction with food, or more predictable pharmacokinetics (behavior of the drug in the body that relates to its activity) than warfarin or heparin. Many of these newer therapies do not require monitoring in most situations. However, they tend to be more expensive and some cause safety concerns in specific groups of patients. For example, fondaparinux could be dangerous to patients with kidney disease. The risk of bleeding continues to be the major serious adverse effect of anticoagulants and antiplatelets and necessitates much of the monitoring and testing in patients taking the drugs. As new anticoagulant drugs continue to be developed, we can envision drugs that combine excellent anticoagulant effects with a lower risk of excessive bleeding, as well as better antidotes to bleeding.

—*Ing Wei Khor*

For Further Information:

American Association for Family Practitioners. 2016 FP Comprehensive: Anticoagulation. http://www.aafp.org/test/fpcomp/FP-E_422/pt1.html. Accessed September 7, 2017.

American Heart Association. What Are Anticoagulants and Antiplatelet Agents. https://www.heart.org/idc/groups/heart-public/@wcm/@hcm/documents/downloadable/ucm_300338.pdf. Updated 2017. Accessed September 7, 2017.

Mayo Clinic. Heparin: Intravenous Route or Subcutaneous Route. Available at: http://www.mayoclinic.org/drugs-supplements/heparin-intravenous-route-subcutaneous-route/description/drg-20068726. Updated March 01, 2017. Accessed September 7, 2017.

Society for Vascular Biology. https://vascular.org/patient-resources/vascular-treatments/thrombolytic-therapy. Accessed September 7, 2017.

Antidepressants

Treatment

Anatomy or system affected: Brain, nervous system, psychic-emotional system

Specialties and related fields: Biochemistry, family medicine, neurology, psychiatry, psychology

Definition: A group of drugs used for the treatment of clinical depression.

Key terms:

bipolar disorders: mood disorders characterized by significant swings in mood from depression to persistent feelings of elation; also known as manic-depressive illness

depression: a mood disorder characterized by loss of energy, depressed mood, diminished interest in pleasurable activities, feelings of worthlessness, and difficulty in concentrating

fluoxetine: the generic name for the antidepressant commonly called Prozac

monoamine oxidase inhibitors (MAOIs): a class of drugs that relieve the symptoms of depression by inhibiting the enzyme that deactivates the brain chemical monoamine oxidase

neurotransmitters: chemicals produced by the brain that allow for cells to transmit electrical signals

obsessive-compulsive disorder: a psychiatric disorder that causes a person to ruminate on a particular thought and then act out a ritualistic behavior

selective serotonin reuptake inhibitors (SSRIs): a class of antidepressant drugs, first introduced in 1987, that work by inhibiting the reuptake of the neurotransmitter serotonin, thus making more of it available to brain cells

tricyclics: antidepressant drugs that interfere with several neurotransmitters, making more of them available to the brain

Indications and Procedures

Antidepressants are prescribed most often to individuals suffering from symptoms of clinical depression, a severe form of depression that interferes with the person's ability to function (for example, to hold down a job or to handle the responsibilities of being a student). The symptoms of depression must be present for at least two weeks before a diagnosis is made and treatment is recommended. Depression may be treated with antidepressant medications, brief psychotherapy, or a combination of both. Antidepressants are also used in the treatment of anxiety disorders.

Several classes of antidepressants can be considered as treatment options for depression. Each class of drugs acts on the nervous system in its own unique way, and each class produces different kinds of side effects. Monoamine oxidase inhibitors (MAOIs) and tricyclic antidepressants are regarded as two different classes of first-generation drugs. These two classes and the new-generation selective serotonin reuptake inhibitors (SSRIs), including fluoxetine (Prozac), all affect the nervous system by increasing the availability of neurotransmitters such as norepinephrine or serotonin.

Although physicians have several classes of drugs at their disposal to combat the effects of depression, no single drug or class of drugs has been found to be significantly more effective in treating symptoms. In fact, no reliable test exists to discover which antidepressant will be most effective for a particular patient. However, it is clearly the case that most patients will respond favorably to one class of drugs over the others. The effectiveness of antidepressants can be evaluated on two fronts: the degree to which symptoms of clinical depression are reduced and the pervasiveness of any adverse side effects that may result from a particular medication.

Uses and Complications

Because all antidepressant medications cause some adverse side effects, physicians attempt to determine the minimum clinically effective dose. For some patients, antidepressants may cause suicidal ideation in the first few weeks of their use. Anyone taking antidepressants should be closely monitored by a physician, especially when the medication is first prescribed. Patients should discuss how they are feeling with their doctor after a new antidepressant medication is prescribed so that the physician can evaluate the effectiveness of the antidepressant and identify any adverse side effects. Because there are several different types of antidepressants available, some experimentation may be necessary to determine which medication works best for a given patient.

In terms of specific side effects of drugs, MAOIs may produce a serious adverse side effect known as a hypertensive crisis, which results in a rapid elevation of blood pressure. This condition is caused by an interaction of the drug with foods containing tyramine, such as aged cheeses, aged meats, and red wines; thus, these foods must be avoided while MAOIs are in use. Less serious side effects produced by MAOIs include constipation, diarrhea, and difficulty falling asleep.

Tricyclic antidepressants may produce dry mouth, blurred vision, or weight gain. However, the most serious aspect of tricyclics is the danger if an overdose is taken, as fatal cardiac rhythm disturbances can occur. Given that patients suffering from depression may have thoughts of suicide, the amount of prescription given at one time must be carefully monitored and should be limited. SSRIs have fewer and more easily tolerated side effects than the first-generation antidepressants, although some patients will experience weight gain and sexual dysfunction resulting in the loss of the sexual drive.

Abruptly stopping an antidepressant prescription will lead to a range of withdrawal symptoms, from feeling more depressed to becoming irritable to developing flulike symptoms. Although the withdrawal symptoms are not dangerous, it is recommended that antidepressants be reduced in dosage over a period of several days.

Perspective and Prospects

Since the late 1980s, individuals suffering from depression have had access to medications that produce fewer adverse side effects than first-generation antidepressants. Investigators are also learning that antidepressants can help patients with other psychological conditions, such as bipolar disorders, anxiety disorders, panic attacks, and obsessive-compulsive disorder.

Despite the successes that have come with the availability of several classes of antidepressants, there still remains a group of patients suffering from depression who do not benefit from them. Investigators are continuing to look for more effective treatments, particularly ones that can alleviate the symptoms of depression more quickly. Group therapy and cognitive behavioral therapy are also effective in the treatment of depression and should be used in combination with antidepressants to improve treatment outcome.

—*Bryan C. Auday, Ph.D.*

See also Anxiety; Bipolar disorders; Depression; Emotions: Biochemical causes and effects; Grief and guilt; Neurology; Neurology, pediatric; Obsessive-compulsive disorder; Panic attacks; Pharmacology; Postpartum depression; Psychiatric disorders; Psychiatry; Psychiatry, child and adolescent; Psychiatry, geriatric; Stress; Stress reduction; Suicide.

For Further Information:

American Psychiatric Association. *Diagnostic and Statistical Manual of Mental Disorders.* 5th ed. Arlington, Va.: American Psychiatric Association, 2013.
"Antidepressants: Selecting One That's Right for You." *Mayo Clinic,* November 8, 2011.
"Depression." *National Institute of Mental Health,* 2013.
Diamond, Ronald J. *Instant Psychopharmacology: Up-to-Date Information About the Most Commonly Prescribed Drugs for Emotional Health.* 3d ed. New York: W. W. Norton, 2009.
Feldman, Robert S., Jerrold S. Meyer, and Linda F. Quenzer. *Principles of Neuropsychopharmacology.* Sunderland, Mass.: Sinauer, 1997.
Hart, Carl, and Charles Ksir. *Drugs, Society, and Human Behavior.* 15th ed. New York: McGraw-Hill, 2012.
Lickey, Marvin E., and Barbara Gordon. *Medicine and Mental Illness: The Use of Drugs in Psychiatry.* New York: W. H. Freeman, 1991.

Antihistamines

Treatment

Anatomy or system affected: Chest, circulatory system, ears, eyes, head, immune system, lungs, nose, psychic-emotional system, respiratory system, throat, skin

Specialties and related fields: Family medicine, immunology, otorhinolaryngology, pharmacology, preventive medicine, pulmonary medicine

Definition: Over-the-counter and prescription-type drugs that are commonly prescribed for allergy symptoms to reduce the effects of histamines.

Key terms:

allergic rhinitis: an uncomfortable condition of the nose resulting from the sensitivity of the nasal passageway to pollen or other substances

arrhythmias: problems with the rhythm of the heart, such as irregular heartbeat

decongestants: drugs that are taken to reduce swelling of the nasal passages and decrease production of mucus, the fluids commonly found in the sinuses during allergic reactions and colds

drug synergy: a process by which drugs taken in combination with each other interact and can have a greater effect than the drugs taken separately

histamines: proteins released by the immune system as part of allergic reactions

mucous membranes: the lining covering the parts of the body in the major air passageways and in the alimentary tract

Indications and Procedures

Antihistamines provide a rapid form of treatment for controlling histamine-based physical reactions, including cold and allergy symptoms, rashes and hives, and insect bites and stings. They are also especially helpful for the allergic condition known as hay fever, which is related to seasonal allergies and allergic rhinitis. Antihistamines serve largely to decrease the discomfort and symptoms caused by histamine reactions. Symptoms of histamine reactions may include sneezing, itchy skin, rashes, a swollen throat, watery or itchy eyes, and a runny nose. In reducing these effects, antihistamines may also be useful in helping to decrease the risk of additional infections caused by the swelling of sensitive mucous membranes in the body, particularly in the sinuses, nose, and throat. Typically, if such membranes remain swollen, the passageways of the body, such as the sinuses, can become congested, making it easier for infections to develop.

Antihistamines are typically administered orally, in pill form, one or more times per day, but they are also available in the form of eye drops, nose sprays, and liquids. They are also combined frequently with other drugs such as decongestants to ameliorate further any uncomfortable cold symptoms and to prevent consequent problems such as sinus infections. Antihistamines alone are generally considered to be ineffective at reducing nasal congestion.

Uses and Complications

In addition to reducing histamine reactions, antihistamines have several side effects, including dry mouth, drowsiness, dizziness, nausea and vomiting, blurred vision, restlessness in some children, confusion, and difficulty urinating. Newer, or second-generation antihistamines (e.g., loratadine, desloratidine, fexofenadine, cetirizine), cause significantly less drowsiness.

Furthermore, any drug, including antihistamines, can be abused if used in larger quantities than prescribed or recommended. For instance, some individuals may use high quantities of antihistamines to experience a more pronounced sedating effect or other psychoactive effects. This is dangerous, as use of any substance outside its recommended use, particularly in situations requiring safety (for instance, driving, operating machinery, being around strangers, being in strange places) may lead to unexpected negative consequences. Of the side effects mentioned, drowsiness persists in being the most problematic, as people needing to take the drugs more than once a day may have their daytime activities interrupted by feeling sleepy. Additionally, if antihistamines are combined with other substances, both prescription drugs or others such as alcohol, then drug synergies can occur. With sedating drugs such as alcohol, for instance, the onset of drowsiness can hasten and its strength can be greater than might be expected with either the antihistamine or the alcohol alone. As such, the use of antihistamines, particularly in combination with other sedating drugs (opioids, barbiturates, anesthetics, benzodiazepines, sedating pain medications), or even sedating alternative medicines, is not advised in situations requiring attention and alertness, such as driving or operating machinery.

Because of issues such as drug interactions and how the drug may affect the body, antihistamines should be taken cautiously. They also should not be used by women who are pregnant or breast feeding, people with liver or kidney problems, acute glaucoma, or enlarged prostate unless directed by a provider. Other contraindications may exist as well. The advice of a physician or pharmacist is best followed when taking any drug.

Perspective and Prospects

Antihistamines have been paired with substances such as decongestants so that they may relieve more symptoms. In the past, however, some additions have come with both advantages and disadvantages. The addition of pseudoephedrine to antihistamine medications, for example, increased their ability to address symptoms and decreased some of the drowsiness. Pseudoephedrine, however, has stimulating properties that have been identified as problematic and has had to be removed from many types of medications.

Antihistamine development is also driven by a desire to make them more specific. For instance, one person may need an antihistamine to reduce nasal irritation while another may need one to alleviate itchy eyes. As such, it is expected that antihistamines will be developed to have much more specific effects on the body and to have little to no sedating or other side effects while still being effective at reducing allergy and cold symptoms. Nevertheless, some of the familiar antihistamines known today are likely to remain available, as they are generally useful. Also, mildly sedating medicines, such as antihistamines taken at a normally recommended dose, may continue to have a place in medicine, as they serve as a good substitute for individuals needing non-addictive sleep medication and who are unlikely to abuse these substances.

—*Nancy Banasiak, MSN, APRN*

See also: Allergies; Anti-inflammatory drugs; Bites and stings; Common cold; Decongestants; Hay fever; Hives; Host-defense mechanisms; Immune system; Immunology; Itching; Multiple chemical sensitivity syndrome; Nasopharyngeal disorders; Over-the-counter medications; Otorhinolaryngology; Pharmacology; Pharmacy; Rashes; Sinusitis; Skin; Skin disorders; Sleep disorders; Smell; Sneezing.

For Further Information:
"Antihistamines: Understanding Your OTC Options." *American Academy of Family Physicians*, February 2012.
Bozek, A. *"Pharmacological Management of Allergic Rhinitis in the Elderly." Drugs & Aging,* January 2017.
Sur, DK, & Plesa, ML "Treatment of Allergic Rhinitis." *American Family Physician*, December 2015.
Web MD, Accessed September 20, 2017 http://www.webmd.com/allergies/antihistamines-for-allergies

Antihypertensives

Treatment

Also known as: Blood pressure medicines

Anatomy or system affected: All

Specialties and related fields: Cardiology, family practice, pharmacology, preventative medicine, vascular medicine

Definition: Medicines that lower blood pressure.

Key terms:

diastole: period of time during which the heart relaxes and fills with blood

hyperkalemia: excessively high blood levels of potassium

hypokalemia: abnormally low blood levels of potassium

orthostatic hypotension: a sudden fall in blood pressure

when a person stands up

systole: the contraction of the heart and the forcible expulsion of blood into large blood vessels

vasoconstriction: narrowing of blood vessels as a result of the contraction of the smooth muscles that surround the walls of blood vessels

vasodilation: expansion of blood vessels as a consequence of the relaxation of the smooth muscles that surround the walls of blood vessels

Indications and Procedures

Blood pressure (BP) refers to the force exerted by the circulating blood against the walls of blood vessels. BP consists of the product of two physiological parameters: the pumping of the heart that propels blood through blood vessels and the resistance provided by those vessels against which the heart must work. These two parameters are referred to as cardiac output (CO) and peripheral vascular resistance (PVR). Mathematically, BP = CO x PVR. Consequently, if either CO or PVR increase, BP increases, and, conversely, if either of these decreases, BP decreases.

The heart undergoes a cycle of contracting and relaxing. When the heart contracts and ejects blood from its chambers, it undergoes systole. After systole, the heart relaxes and allows its chambers to fill; a period known as diastole. At systole, the BP has its highest reading and at diastole, its lowest reading. BP is measured units called torr or 1/760 of standard atmospheric pressure. BP measurements always record a higher number (the systolic pressure) and a lower number (the diastolic pressure). Normal BP is defined as a systolic pressure of 120 torr and a diastolic pressure of 80, which is reported as 120 / 80 or "120 over 80."

Even though the BP rises and falls during the day, if someone's BP remains above normal over time that person has high BP or hypertension. A systolic BP between 120 and 139 torr or a diastolic BP between 80 and 90 torr constitutes a condition known as prehypertension. People with prehypertension have a greater risk of developing hypertension. If an individual has a systolic BP between 140 and 159 torr or a diastolic BP between 90 and 99 torr, they have stage 1 hypertension. If they have a systolic BP above 160 or greater or a diastolic BP above 100 torr or greater they have stage 2 hypertension. Hypertension increases the risk of heart disease, congestive heart failure, kidney disease, blindness, and stroke. Also, hypertension tends to have no symptoms until the patient suffers a cardiovascular catastrophe. For this reason, hypertension has been called "the silent killer." Controlling hypertension remains one of the most important goals of preventative medicine.

In many cases, a patient's hypertension does not have an obvious direct cause. In such cases the patient has essential or idiopathic hypertension. In other cases, the patient's hypertension results from an underlying condition. In such cases the patient has secondary hypertension, and kidney disease, tumors, and adrenal gland abnormalities constitute some of the most common causes of secondary hypertension.

Not all strategies for controlling hypertension include medications. Particular lifestyle choices increase some-

one's risk for hypertension: cigarette smoking, obesity, diabetes, physical inactivity, chronic alcohol consumption, a family history of hypertension or heart disease, excessive consumption of sodium, and age or sex (women older than 55 and men older than 45). Therefore, nondrug strategies to manage hypertension include weight loss, stress reduction, regular aerobic exercise, smoking cessation, moderation of alcohol consumption, and dietary changes. Some people have a physiological sensitivity to salt and must decrease their consumption of sodium in order to control their BP. These people can usually reduce their BP by adhering to the Dietary Approaches to Stop Hypertension or DASH diet. Those who use the DASH diet eat fruits, vegetables, low-fat dairy foods, poultry, nuts, and fish that are low in sodium, saturated fat, and cholesterol, and avoid sweets, sugared drinks, red meats, and fats.

If nondrug strategies fail to properly low the BP to normal levels, then the next step requires the administration of an antihypertensive agent. One of the first agents used to lower BP are diuretics. Diuretics drugs work in the kidney to increase the amount of water filtered from the blood by the kidney and increase urine output. Because PVR depends on blood volume, the reduction of blood volume lowers BP. A second class of antihypertensive agents is the beta blockers. Beta blockers bind to receptors on the surfaces of heart muscle cells called beta receptors and prevent them from receiving signals from sympathetic nerves. The sympathetic nervous system mediates the "fight or flight" response, and sympathetic nerve inputs increase the heart rate. An increase in heart rate increases CO and therefore increases BP. By blocking sympathetic nerve inputs to the heart, beta blockers decrease CO and BP.

If BP remains high after administration of a diuretic or a beta blocker, then the physician either increases the dosages of these drugs or prescribes an additional antihypertensive agent. Such drugs include calcium channel blockers, angiotensin-Converting Enzyme (ACE) inhibitors, or angiotensin II Receptor Blockers (ARBs). Calcium channel blockers (CCBs) inhibit L-type calcium channels that reside in the membranes of the smooth muscles that surround blood vessels and heart cells. Since they prevent the entry of calcium ions into these cells, CCBs dilate blood vessels, reduce the force of contraction of heart muscles, and slow the conduction of electrical activity within the heart. In doing so, CCBs decrease PVR and CO and lower BP.

ACE inhibitors irreversibly inactivate the enzyme angiotensin-converting enzyme (ACE). Present mainly in the capillary beds of the lungs, ACE converts the polypeptide angiotensin I to angiotensin II, a molecule that causes blood vessels to narrow (vasoconstriction), thus increasing PVR. The liver produces a blood protein called angiotensinogen and an enzyme called renin converts angiotensinogen to angiotensin I. The kidney secretes renin in response to lower arterial BP, decreased salt in the urine, or sympathetic nerve activity. Angiotensin II also signals to the adrenal glands to release the hormone aldosterone, which directs the kidney to retain more salt.

Table 1			
Generic Name	**Trade Name**	**Use**	**Side Effects**
Thiazides diuretics			
bendroflumethiazide	Naturetin	Hypertension, edema associated with congestive heart failure (CHF)	Dizziness, vertigo, lightheadedness, headache (transient) weakness, loss of appetite, upset stomach, diarrhea, constipation, blood problems (rarely), high blood sugar (hyperglycermia), hypokalemia, electrolyte disturbances, allergies
hydrochlorothiazide	HydroDiuril, Esidrix, Microzide, Oretic	Hypertension, edema due to CHF, liver disease, and steroid treatment	
chlorothiazide	Diuril		
chlorothalidone	Thalitone		
hydroflumethiazide	Saluron		
indapamide	Lozol		
metolazone	Zaroxolyn		
methyclothiazide	Enduron		
polythiazide	Renese		
Loop diuretics			
bumetanide	Bumex	Edema due to CHF, liver kidney, and lung disease	Electrolyte and blood imbalances, loss of appetite, upset stomach, dizziness, sugar in urine, lightheadedness when getting up (orthostatic hypotension), sun sensitivity, ringing in the ears (tinnitus)
ethacrynic acid	Edecrin	Same as bumetanide and fluid retention in the stomach (ascites) due to malignancy, unexplained edema and fluid retention in the lymph system	Same as bumetanide plus diarrhea
furosemide	Lasix	Same as bumetanide plus hypertension	Same as bumetanide
torosemide	Demadex		Same as bumetanide plus headache
Potassium-sparing diuretics			
amiloride HCl	Midamor	CHF, hypertension, preventing hypokalemia, prevents the constant urination in those who take lithium	Headache, dizziness, nausea, loss of appetite, diarrhea, vomiting, weakness, fatigue, rash, low blood pressure (hypotension)
spironolactone	Aldactone	Hypertension, edema due to CHF, liver and kidney disease, prevents hypokalemia in at-risk patients (i.e. hyperaldosteronism)	Headache, diarrhea, drowsiness, lethargy, hyperkalemia, erectile dysfunction, gynecomastia
triamterene	Dyrenium	Prevention of hypokalemia, edema due to CHF, liver and kidney disease and hyperaldosteronism	Diarrhea, nausea, vomiting, hyperkalemia, sun sensitivity
Osmotic diuretics			
Glycerol	–	Glaucoma, before and after surgery	Headache, nausea, vomiting
Isosorbide	–		
mannitol	Osmitrol	Promote urine formation in acute kidney disease, reduce internal eye pressure (interocular pressure or IOP), brain swelling (cerebral edema), irrigation solution in prostate surgical techniques	Edema, electrolyte and fluid imbalance, blurred vision, nausea, vomiting, diarrhea, urinary retention
urea	Ureaphil	Reduction of IOP and pressure inside the head	Headache, nausea, vomiting, fluid, and electrolyte imbalance, fainting
Carbonic anhydrase inhibitors			
acetazolamide	Diamox	Glaucoma, edema due to CHF, liver and kidney disease and drugs, epilepsy	Weakness, fatigue, loss of appetite, nausea, vomiting, rash, sun sensitivity, tingling feeling in skin
methazolamide	Neptazane	Glaucoma	

This signaling pathway, the renin-angiotensin-aldosterone system, raises BP. By blocking the production of angiotensin II, ACE inhibitors prevent vasoconstriction and sodium retention, which leads to wider blood vessels, reduced PVR and BP. ARBs prevent angiotensin II from binding to its receptor on the surfaces of the smooth muscles that surround blood vessels and adrenal gland cells. Thus, even though ARBs do not prevent the synthesis of angiotensin II, they prevent angiotensin II from causing vasoconstriction and sodium retention, and consequently lower PVR and BP.

If, after adding these additional antihypertensive agents, the patient's BP still remains abnormally high, then the physician prescribes a combination of two or three antihypertensive agents and may consider other drugs such as alpha blockers, direct-acting blood vessel dilators, or the centrally or peripherally acting antiadrenergics. Alpha blockers bind alpha1 receptors on the surfaces of the smooth muscles that surround blood vessels and prevent them from receiving signals that tell them to contract. Thus, alpha blockers cause blood vessels to dilate, reducing PVR and BP. Direct-acting blood vessels dilators (or vasodilators) work through a variety of different mechanisms to cause blood vessel dilation or vasodilation and reduce PVR and, therefore, BP. Antiadrenergics inhibit the sympathetic nervous system. Some work in the brain and spinal cord (central nervous system), and others work at the level of the peripheral nervous system. Typically some combination of these drugs reduces the blood pressure into the normal range.

Uses and Complications

The first-line drugs for treating hypertension tend to be diuretics and beta blockers. These drugs tend to work quite well, are usually rather inexpensive and, for the most part, well tolerated.

Several different types of diuretics exist: thiazides, loop diuretics, potassium-sparing diuretics, osmotic diuretics, and carbonic anhydrase inhibitors. All diuretics prevent the reabsorption of salts and water by the kidney, increase water loss and urine output, and, consequently, reduce PVR and BP. Diuretics are used to reduce BP, but also to treat the swelling (edema) that results from congestive heart failure, liver and kidney disease, glaucoma, and swelling in the brain (cerebral edema). After beginning any antihypertensive agent, many patients feel lightheaded when they change from a sitting to a standing position (orthostatic hypotension). These symptoms typically fade after taking the drug for some time. Most antihypertensives also cause sexual dysfunction. The most common side effects of diuretics are dehydration and low potassium levels (hypokalemia), but other rarer side effects occur as well (Table 1). These represent the side effects patients have experienced while taking these drugs; no one has experienced all these side effects. Potassium-sparing diuretics can cause excessively high blood potassium levels (hyperkalemia).

Beta blockers can treat hypertension or the chest pain that results when the heart receives too little oxygen to perform its work (angina pectoris). Beta blockers may cause diarrhea, stomach pain, nausea, vomiting, rash, blurred vision, muscle cramps, fatigue, headache, depression, confusion, dizziness, nightmares, and hallucinations (Table 2). They may cause heart failure in heart patients and interfere with blood sugar readings in diabetics. If withdrawn suddenly they can cause heart attacks or sudden death. Beta blockers can also aggravate asthma attacks in asthmatics because of the presence of a different type of beta receptor in the lungs. This, however, can be alleviated by using cardioselective beta blockers that have a higher affinity for the heart-specific beta receptor (ß1) than the lung-specific beta receptor (ß2).

Table 2. Beta Blockers	
Generic name	**Trade name**
acebutolol*	Sectral
atenolol*	Tenormin
betaxolol*	Kerlone
bisprolol*	Zebeta
carteolol	Cartrol
metoprolol*	Lopressor, Toprol-XL
nadolol	Corgard
penbutolol	Levatol
pindolol	Visken
propranolol	Inderal
timolol	Biocadren
carvedilol	Coreg
labetalol	Normodyne, Trandate
*Note: * cardioselective beta blocker*	

ACE inhibitors and ARBs can treat hypertension, congestive heart failure, or diabetics suffering kidney problems. The side effects of ARBs and ACE inhibitors are a dry cough (ACE inhibitors usually), hyperkalemia, diarrhea (ARBs mainly), orthostatic hypotension, headache, drowsiness, weakness, a salty or metallic taste in one's mouth, and a rash (Table 3). Rarely, ARBs and ACE inhibitors cause a massive shift of fluid to areas under the skin (angioedema), allergies, a decrease in white blood cells, and kidney failure. Neither ARBs nor ACE inhibitors should be taken during pregnancy because they can cause birth defects.

CCBs are used to treat angina and hypertension. CCB side effects include dizziness, lightheadedness, nervousness, loss of muscle strength (asthenia), fatigue, nausea, constipation and upset stomach, edema, low blood pressure (hypotension), irregular heart rate, rash, flushing, nasal congestion and cough. CCBs also interact with several other drugs (Table 4).

CCBs interact with cimetidine (for ulcers, increases effects of CCBs), theophylline (for asthma, CCBs increase toxic effects of theophylline), St. John's Wort (herb, for depression, reduces blood concentrations of CCBs), digoxin (heart medicine, CCBs increase toxicity of digoxin), and rifampin (antituberculosis drug, decreases effects of CCBs).

Table 3. ACE Inhibitors and ARBs

Generic name	Trade name
ACE Inhibitors	
benzapril	Lotensin
captopril	Capoten
enalapril	Vasotec
fosinopril	Monopril
lisonipril	Prinivil, Zestril
moexipril	Univasc
perinopril	Aceon
quinapril	Accupril
ramapril	Altace
trandolapril	Mavik
ARBs	
candesartan	Atacand
eprosartan	Teveten
irbesartan	Avapro
losartan	Cozaar
olmesartan	Benicar
telmisartan	Micardis
valsartan	Diovan

Table 4. Calcium-Channel Blockers

Generic name	Trade name
amlodipine	Norvasc
bepridil	Vascor
diltiazem	Cardizem, Dilacor
felodipine	Plendil
nicardipine	Cardene
nifedipine	Adalat, Procardia
nisoldipine	Sular
verapamil	Calan, Isoptin, Verelan

Alpha blockers might be useful for treating hypertension in older men because these drugs have a tendency to shrink the prostate. Doxazosin (Cardura), prazosin (Minipress), and terazosin (Hytrin) may cause these side effects: dizziness, weakness, fatigue, upset stomach and loss of appetite, drowsiness, edema, and nasal congestion.

The antiadrenergic drugs include peripherally acting drugs, such as guanadrel (Hylorel) and guanethidine (Ismelin), and the centrally acting drugs, such as clonidine (Catapres), guanabenz (Wytensin), guanfacine (Tenex), and methydopa (Aldomet). The side effects of guanadrel and guanethidine include blurred vision, orthostatic hypotension, sexual dysfunction, diarrhea, and swelling of feet or lower legs. Drugs that work within the central nervous system cause more severe side effects and typically are only used as a last resort or for emergencies. Heavy sedation, fainting, dry mouth, constipation, impotence, dizziness and drowsiness are some of the most common side effects. Psychological side effects that range from depression, nightmares, mood changes, and psychosis also occur. Despite these side effects, methydopa is the drug of choice to treat high blood pressure during pregnancy (gestational hypertension).

The peripheral vasodilators include hydralazine (Apresoline), minoxidil (Loniten), diazoxide (Hyperstat) and nitroprusside (Nitropress). These drugs cause many serious side effects and are only used in emergencies.

Perspective and Prospects

In 2600 BC, the ancient Chinese diagnosed hypertension by the quality of one's pulse and treated it with bleeding and leeches. Revolutionary work in 1733 by the English Reverend Stephen Hales, Riva-Rocci in 1896, and Nikolai Korotkoff in 1905 culminated in the invention of the blood pressure cuff, which gave clinicians a way to easily measure blood pressure.

Hypertension remained an untreated disease over the initial part of the twentieth century. Even President Franklin Delano Roosevelt's hypertension was treated with phenobarbital, a low-sodium diet, and rest. Then in 1957-58, thiazide diuretics were shown by the US Veterans Administration (VA) to significantly reduce cardiovascular morbidity and mortality. These successes led to the establishment of the Joint National Committee on the Detection, Evaluation, and Treatment of High Blood Pressure (JNC), which established national clinical guidelines for hypertension management and treatment.

For recalcitrant cases of hypertension, composite drugs that combine two or more antihypertensives in one dose have been developed and these have revolutionized hypertension treatment. For example, Zestoretic combines hydrochlorothiazide and lisinopril. Because ACE inhibitors can cause hyperkalemia and decrease urine output, hydrochlorothiazide nullifies those side effects by increasing potassium and water loss and increasing the reduction in BP. Timolide combines hydrochlorothiazide with the beta blocker timolol. Since beta blockers sometimes can cause edema in some people, the thiazide diuretic gets rid of all that extra swelling and further reduces blood pressure. Such combinations have made treating the harder hypertension cases much easier to treat and much more convenient for patients.

—*Michael A. Buratovich, Ph.D.*

See also Cardiology; Hypertension; Hypotension; Kidneys; Pharmacology; Vascular medicine

For Further Information:

Appel, Lawrence J. "The Verdict from ALLHAT-Thiazide Diuretics Are the Preferred Initial Therapy for Hypertension." *Journal of the American Medical Association* 288, no. 23 (2002): 3039-3042. A sound, informed, and digestible summary of the ALLHAT study, the largest and most comprehensive clinical study of antihypertensives.

Ellerbeck, Susan. *DASH Diet for Beginners-Lose Weight, Lower Blood Pressure, and Improve Health.* Seattle, Wash.: Amazon Digital Services, 2013. An introduction to the DASH diet and the benefits that it can provide.

Mann, Samuel J. *Hypertension and You: Old Drugs, New Drugs, and the Right Drugs for Your High Blood Pressure.* Lanham, Md.: Rowman and Littlefield, 2012. A hypertension specialist provides sound medical advice on how to think about hypertension and how to treat it.

Manning, Loretta, and Sylvia Rayfield. *Pharmacology Made Insanely Easy.* Duluth, Ga.: I Can Publishing Inc., 2013. Two veteran medical educators team up to produce an easily read, enjoyable, and slightly off-beat presentation of pharmacology.

McArthur, John. "Hypertension-High Blood Pressure: How to Lower Blood Pressure Permanently in 8 Weeks or Less, the Hypertension Treatment, Diet, and Solution." Carrara, Queensland, Australia: *Natural Health Magazine,* 2012. A compilation of nondrug strategies for treating high blood pressure accompanied by corroborating clinical data.

Anti-inflammatory drugs

Treatment

Anatomy or system affected: All

Specialties and related fields: Dermatology, endocrinology, family medicine, internal medicine, ophthalmology, orthopedics, otorhinolaryngology, rheumatology, vascular medicine.

Definition: Medicines used to relieve inflammation, pain, redness, and swelling; generally grouped into two categories: nonsteroidal anti-inflammatory drugs (NSAIDs) and corticosteroids (steroid hormones that have an anti-inflammatory effects).

Key terms:

arthritis: a painful condition that involves inflammation of one or more joints.

bursitis: inflammation of the sac of lubricating fluid located between joints.

hormone: a substance made by the body that travels through the bloodstream to reach its target organ and have its effect.

inflammation: the body's response to injury that may include redness, pain, swelling, and warmth in the affected area.

salicylates: a group of drugs (including aspirin) derived from salicylic acid, used to relieve pain, reduce inflammation, and lower fever.

steroids: a class of hormones produced by the adrenal glands; can also be made synthetically.

tendinitis: inflammation of a tendon, a tough band of tissue that connects muscle to bone.

Indications

Nonsteroidal anti-inflammatory drugs (NSAIDs), often referred to as aspirin, are utilized to relieve painful conditions such as arthritis, bursitis, gout, menstrual cramps, tendinitis, sprains, and strains. Additionally, aspirin is commonly prescribed to patients who have had one myocardial infarction (heart attack) to decrease the risk of a second. While some NSAIDs require a prescription, many are sold over the counter. Some common NSAIDs, with brand names in parentheses, are diclofenac (Voltaren), etodolac (Lodine), flurbiprofen (Ansaid), ibuprofen (Motrin, Advil, Rufen, Nuprin), nabumetone (Relafen), naproxen (Naprosyn or Aleve), and oxaprozin (Daypro). These drugs can come in the form of capsules, caplets, tablets, liquids, and suppositories.

Corticosteroids make up the second group of anti-inflammatory drugs used to ameliorate the symptoms associated with conditions such as asthma, lupus, arthritis, and allergic reactions. Like NSAIDs, corticosteroids are available in various forms including inhalants, creams, ointments, and oral (systemic) medications. Common corticosteroids are beclomethasone (Beconase, Vancensase, Vanceril), betamethosone (Diprolene, Lotrisone), hydrocortisone, mometasone (Elocon), prednisone (Deltasone, Orasone), and triamcinolone (Azmacort, Nasacort).

Complications

Although used across many medical specialties and for a plethora of reasons, NSAIDs are not without their dangers. Common side effects are mild and can include stomach pains or cramps, nausea, vomiting, indigestion, headache, and dizziness. Despite these relatively mild side effects, individuals currently taking other medications, women who are pregnant or who plan to become pregnant, women who are breast-feeding, and persons with stomach or intestinal problems, liver disease, heart disease, high blood pressure, bleeding diseases, diabetes, Parkinson's disease, or epilepsy should consult their physicians prior to taking NSAIDs. While side effects are rare, some can be life-threatening. In fact, research has shown that some NSAIDs can increase the risk of strokes and heart attacks. Any feelings of tightness in the chest, irregular heartbeat, swelling, or fainting are reasons to discontinue the use of NSAIDs and consult a physician. It is important to note that children should not be given aspirin if they are recovering from a viral infection as it can lead to Reye's syndrome -a potentially fatal condition that results in swelling of the liver and brain.

That said, there is research underway for new, anti-inflammatory painkillers that elicit fewer side effects. One example is licofelone, an NSAID that can inhibit both cyclooxygenase 1 and 2 (COX-1 and COX-2) as well as lipoxygenase (LOX), three of the enzymes involved in inflammation pathways. Licofelone is being tested on its ability to help in osteoarthritis management and is reported to be gentler on the stomach.

Corticosteroid therapy produces dramatic, immediate relief from pain, swelling, and inflammation due to arthritis. Small amounts of steroid may be injected directly into the inflamed joint or they can be taken by mouth. However, the beneficial effects tend to be temporary and long-term use can lead to the development of cataracts, increased blood sugar which can worsen a person's diabetes, reduced resistance to infections, as well as gastrointestinal ulcers and bleeding. It follows that the advent of other highly effective alternatives has led to less frequent use of steroids in the setting of arthritis.

Additionally, corticosteroids are a common treatment for persons suffering from more serious asthmatic conditions or when treatment with bronchodilators has not proven effective. Corticosteroids, which are not bronchodilators and do not open the airways, instead work to reduce inflamma-

In the News: Dangers of COX-2 Inhibitors

In a 2001 issue of the *Journal of the American Medical Association*, Debabrata Mukherjee and coauthors summarized the results of two major randomized trails of COX-2 inhibitors: the Vioxx Gastrointestinal Outcomes Research Study (VIGOR), with 8,076 patients, and the Celecoxib Long-Term Arthritis Safety Study (CLASS), with 8,059 patients, as well as several smaller trials of these drugs. The VIGOR study found that treatment with rofecoxib (trade name Vioxx), a popular pain reliever for arthritis, increased the risk of developing a thrombotic cardiovascular event (myocardial infarction, unstable angina, cardiac thrombus, resuscitated cardiac arrest, sudden or unexplained death, ischemic stroke, and transient ischemic attacks) by twofold over naproxen treatment. Myocardial infarction rates for COX-2 inhibitors were found to be significantly higher than for the placebo group in both large studies. Other smaller-scale studies are consistent with the findings from the VIGOR and CLASS trials.

Some of these adverse effects of Vioxx could be mitigated by simultaneous treatment with aspirin; however, such an approach significantly detracts from the utility of nonsteroidal anti-inflammatory drugs (NSAIDs) such as Vioxx, since one would experience the same degree of stomach irritation from the aspirin that NSAIDs are prescribed to avoid. In September, 2004, the pharmaceutical company Merck pulled Vioxx off the market because of the preponderance of evidence suggesting that it poses serious risks of heart attack and stroke. It has been estimated that as many as 30,000 to 100,000 patients have had heart attacks or strokes as a result of taking Vioxx.

—*Michael R. King, Ph.D.*

tion to allow the lungs to function properly. They should be used regularly and for the complete course as prescribed to achieve full benefits. Corticosteroids may be sprayed into the nose for relief of stuffy nose, irritation, hay fever, or other allergies, while oral corticosteroids are used primarily for the prevention of asthma attacks.

Ophthalmic anti-inflammatory medicines can be used to reduce problems that occur during or following eye surgery. by alleviating eye inflammation. These can be obtained only with a doctor's prescription. Corticosteroids also serve to relieve inflammation of the temporal arteries, the blood vessels that run along the temples. Inflammation here can disrupt the blood supply and result in blindness, partial loss of vision, strokes, and even heart attacks.

Individuals who have medical conditions such as allergies, diabetes, pregnancy, osteoporosis, glaucoma, infections, thyroid problems, liver disease, kidney disease, heart disease, or high blood pressure should discuss these conditions with their physician before taking corticosteroids. If corticosteroids are used for a short time, development of side effects is rare. However, breathing problems or tightness in the chest, pain, rash, swelling, extreme exhaustion, irregular heartbeat, or wounds that do not heal should be reported to a physician. Steroids should not be stopped abruptly without consulting a physician, especially if the steroids have been taken for a long time, as the body requires a weaning process to adapt.

Perspective and Prospects

The bark of the willow tree, which contains salicylates, was known in 18th Century England to reduce fever and aches. In 1876, the first successful treatment of acute arthritis with sodium salicylate (aspirin) was reported. In the 1970s, pharmacologist John Vane amassed evidence of the effectiveness of NSAIDs.

The earliest demonstration of the importance of corticosteroids as anti-inflammatory agents occurred in the 1940s regarding rheumatoid arthritis. The challenge of corticosteroid therapy lies in achieving the desired results with a minimum of side effects.

—*Mary Hurd;*
updated by Lillian Dominguez, MD

See also: Allergies; Antihistamines; Arthritis; Asthma; Back pain; Bursitis; Dermatitis; Dermatology; Dermatology, pediatric; Eye surgery; Fever; Gout; Hay fever; Inflammation; Itching; Narcotics; Over-the counter medications; Pain; Pain management; Pharmacology; Poisonous plants; Rashes; Rheumatoid arthritis; Rheumatology; Skin disorders; Steroids; Tendinitis; Tendon disorders.

For Further Information:

American Medical Association. *American Medical AssociationFamily Medical Guide*. 4th ed. Hoboken, N.J.: John Wiley & Sons, 2004.
"Anti-Inflammatories and Corticosteroids." *American Association for Respiratory Care*, 2013.
Liska, Ken. *Drugs and the Human Body, with Implications for Society*. 8th ed. Upper Saddle River, N.J.: Pearson/Prentice Hall, 2009.
"NSAIDs: Nonsteroidal Anti-Inflammatory Drugs." *American College of Rheumatology*, August 2012.
Subak-Sharpe, Genell J., and Thomas O. Morris, eds. "Drug Therapy." In *The Columbia University College of Physicians and Surgeons Complete Home Medical Guide*. 3d ed. New York: Crown, 1995.
"What is an inflammation?" *PubMed Health*, January 2015.

Antioxidants

Treatment
Anatomy or system affected: All
Specialties and related fields: Alternative medicine, family medicine, internal medicine, nutrition, oncology
Definition: A group of vitamins, minerals, and enzymes that help protect the body from damage-causing free radicals.

Free Radicals and Cell Damage

The role of antioxidants in preventing cell damage by free radicals has received considerable interest in recent years. Antioxidants are substances that may neutralize the harmful effects of free radicals in the body. Free radicals are highly reactive chemicals that form in normal metabolism or are produced by radiation and environmental stress. These volatile chemicals react with cell components, causing mutations in deoxyribonucleic acid (DNA) and destroying cell proteins and lipids. The aging process and various degenerative diseases are believed to be caused in part by the lifetime accumulation of cell damage caused by free radicals. Both antioxidants and free radicals are produced naturally by the body to help the body stay in a balanced state of health. Aging, stress, and pollution all damage

DNA in the cells. Antioxidants may provide protection and reduce the risk of stroke, heart disease, cancer, and other health problems associated with aging.

Antioxidant defenses occur naturally in the body to inactivate free radicals and repair damaged tissues. The body's natural supply of antioxidants is limited, however, and a small amount of destruction occurs to cells daily. Dietary antioxidants-in the form of fruits and vegetables or vitamin supplements-are believed to improve health and to prevent cell damage by boosting the body's natural supply of antioxidants.

Extensive research, including many large-scale studies, has demonstrated the beneficial role of dietary antioxidants in preventing such age-related disorders as cardiovascular disease, cancer, immune dysfunction, brain and neurological disorders, and cataracts. Fruits and vegetables, long recognized for their protective and healthful effects, are particularly rich sources of antioxidants.

Important Antioxidants

Vitamin E, vitamin C, and beta carotene are the main dietary antioxidants. Vitamin E (tocopherol) is a fat-soluble antioxidant found in oil, nuts, seeds, and whole grains. This antioxidant appears to protect arteries against damage. In addition, the results of Women's Health Study suggest that taking natural-source vitamin E may help to reduce the risk of cardiovascular mortality. Vitamin C (ascorbate) works in the water-soluble part of tissues. Citrus fruits, strawberries, sweet peppers, and broccoli are good sources of vitamin C. This antioxidant boosts the immune system, strengthens blood vessel walls, and increases levels of a natural antioxidant, glutathione. Vitamin C also helps restore levels of active vitamin E in the body. Beta carotene, a precursor of vitamin A, is found in carrot juice, sweet potatoes, and apricots. The Physicians' Health Study has found that taking beta carotene slowed cognitive decline..

Other antioxidants include lycopene, lutein, coenzyme Q_{10}, gingko, lipoic acid, grapeseed, and various substances found in green and black teas. The micronutrients zinc and selenium also have antioxidant properties; they aid the immune system and boost the levels of natural antioxidant enzymes in the body. Antioxidants appear to work together, as a combination of antioxidants is more potent than each substance alone.

Perspective and Prospects

Evidence for the beneficial role of antioxidants in human health is limited. Clinical studies have not definitively confirmed whether consuming large amounts of antioxidants offers increased protection against aging or age-related diseases. It is not clear what the optimal levels of antioxidants are to prevent the damaging effects of free radicals. Adequate levels of vitamins may vary greatly for each person, depending on levels of environmental stress, smoking, how well supplements are absorbed, and other factors. In addition, it is unclear whether vitamin supplements are superior to fruits and vegetables, since other factors in these foods (fiber, micronutrients) may be responsible for their healthful effects.

In general, people who eat five to eight servings of fruits and vegetables per day are thought to be getting an adequate amount of antioxidants. Taking antioxidant supplements is controversial, as some researchers believe that they may interfere with the body's natural production of antioxidants.

—*Linda Hart, M.S., M.A.;*
updated by LeAnna DeAngelo, Ph.D.

See also Aging; Alternative medicine; Cancer; Food biochemistry; Herbal medicine; Immune system; Melatonin; Nutrition; Phytochemicals; Self-medication; Supplements; Vitamins and minerals.

For Further Information:

"Antioxidants." *Academy of Nutrition and Dietetics*, 2013.

"Antioxidants: Beyond the Hype." *Harvard School of Public Health*, 2008.

Balch, Phyllis A. *Prescription for Nutritional Healing: A Practical A-to-Z Reference to Drug-Free Remedies Using Vitamins, Minerals, Herbs, and Food Supplements.* 5th rev. ed. Garden City Park, N.Y.: Avery, 2010.

Bourassa, Martial G., and Jean-Claude Tardif, eds. *Antioxidants and Cardiovascular Disease.* New York: Springer, 2006.

Busch, Felicia. *The New Nutrition: From Antioxidants to Zucchini.* New York: Wiley, 2000.

Cadenas, Enrique, and Lester Packer, eds. *Handbook of Antioxidants.* 2d ed. New York: Marcel Dekker, 2002.

Knight, Joseph A. *Free Radicals, Antioxidants, Aging and Disease.* Washington, D.C.: AACC Press, 1999.

Morello, Michael J., et al., eds. *Free Radicals in Food: Chemistry, Nutrition, and Health Effects.* Washington, D.C.: American Chemical Society, 2002.

Weil, Andrew. *Healthy Aging: A Lifelong Guide to Your Physical and Spiritual Well-Being.* New York: Anchor Books, 2007.

Antipsychotic drugs

Anatomy or system affected: Brain, Central Nervous System (CNS), Thyroid, Pituitary, Hypothalamus

Specialties and related fields: Neuroscience, Neurology, Psychiatry, Psychology, Schizophrenia, Bipolar Disorder

Definition: a group of drugs, also known as neuroleptics, used primarily to treat psychotic disorders

Key terms:

central nervous system: comprised of the brain and spinal cord. It controls thoughts, emotions and actions by electrical signals traveling though neural pathways.

neurotransmitter: a chemical messenger that transmits a neural signal across a synapse

neurons: highly specialized cell found in the nervous system, which produces an electrical signal to transmit information

dopamine: a neurotransmitter that helps send electrical signals for emotion, movement, and other processes.

positive symptoms: symptoms of schizophrenia that involve the production of an abnormal behavior

psychosis: a mental disorder in which one's emotions and thoughts are impaired, causing a person to lose touch with reality. Primarily characterized by experience of delusions, personality shifts, discontinuous thought patterns and speech, and unrefined social behavior.

schizophrenia: a type of psychotic disorder involving a detachment among one's thoughts, emotions and behaviors.

How are Antipsychotic Drugs Used in Medicine?

Antipsychotic drugs are most commonly used to treat schizophrenia; however, they are also used to treat other psychiatric illnesses such as bipolar disorder and depression. Additionally, recent studies indicate antipsychotic drugs can improve symptoms associated with obsessive-compulsive disorder (OCD), aggressive behavior, and cancer induced bone pain (CIPB). In extension, first-generation antipsychotics are also used to treat nausea and vomiting, to sedate patients before anesthesia, relieve sever itching, and can manage psychosis caused by drugs and alcohol.

Types of Antipsychotic Drugs

In the 1950's, researchers began using a class of drugs known as phenothiazines after recognizing its calming effects in psychiatric patients. Phenothiazines became what is commonly known today as conventional antipsychotics. Antipsychotics primarily reduce the positive symptoms of schizophrenia, a psychiatric illness that is characterized by delusions (irrational beliefs), hallucinations, and disorganized speech (incoherent speech with frequent changes of topic). Some frequently prescribed examples of first-conventional antipsychotics (these used to be called first-generation antipsychotics) include chlorpromazine, haloperidol, both in generic formulations and the brand name drugs Loxitane, Moban, Serentil, and Navane.

Beginning in the 1960's, a new class of antipsychotics was introduced as an alternative to patients who might not respond well to conventional drugs. This new class, known as atypical antipsychotics, is characterized by having fewer deleterious side effects. Some frequently prescribed examples include the brand name drugs Abilify, Clozaril, Zyprexa, and Risperdal. Both conventional and atypical antipsychotics do not produce drug dependence and it is extremely rare for patients to commit suicide using them. However, many patients may experience several unpleasant side effects. The most common side effects involve a range of movement disorders such as facial tics, hand tremors, and muscular rigidity. One of the more serious complications from using antipsychotics is tardive dyskinesia. This condition results in rhythmic, repetitive sucking and smacking movements of the lips and tongue. Usually, tardive dyskinesia appears only after using these drugs for many years, sometimes decades. Typically, this condition can be treated by early identification of the symptoms and lowering the amount of medication. Additional symptoms of these drugs can include weight gain, photosensitivity, and dry mouth. While conventional and atypical antipsychotics have been shown to be equally effective, the advantage of atypical medicines is that they have fewer incidents of adverse side effects, which allow patients to experience an overall higher quality of life.

The vast majority of antipsychotics are taken orally; however, some can be administered by intermuscular injection. Long lasting injectable antipsychotic medication have relatively fewer side effects than oral antipsychotic medications in that it is associated with less relapses and lower hospitalization. In extension, those who use long lasting injectable antipsychotic drugs are more likely to continue treatment because of the reduced undesirable side effects and patients do not have to be reminded each day to take their medication.

How do Antipsychotic Drugs Work?

Psychosis often results from an excess of the chemical dopamine. Antipsychotics primarily work by inhibiting D2 receptors in the brain to block dopamine, which in turn reduces the positive symptoms of psychosis. While blocking dopamine receptors reduces psychosis symptomology, it can lead to manifestation of abnormal motor functions common in Parkinson's disease such involuntary tremor. Both conventional and atypical antipsychotics impact additional neurotransmitters such as serotonin and noradeline. However, the mechanism of action between the conventional and atypical antipsychotics differ in that conventional drugs primarily act by inhibiting dopaminergic receptors in four distinct dopaminergic pathways. In contrast, atypical antipsychotics block D2 receptors and a subtype serotonin receptor known as 5HT2A.

Psychedelic drugs, such as LSD, produce hallucinations comparable to those that schizophrenics experience as a result of excess serotonin secretion. Therefore, researchers reasoned that inhibiting serotonin along with dopamine would mitigate positive symptoms. Antipsychotics have an indirect effect on glutamate input and output because dopamine receptors regulate glutamine neurotransmission. Researchers further explored the relationship between glutamate delusional episodes after examining the psychedelic drug PCP that causes delusions and hallucinations by interfering with the NMDA glutamate receptor in the brain. Studying drugs that cause schizophrenia-like symptoms can shed light on the mechanism in the CNS that brings on psychosis.

Antipsychotics do not cure psychosis; rather they treat the symptoms. Therefore, a large percentage of patients will remain on medication for their entire lives. Women are more prone to adverse side effects from a lower dose of antipsychotics than men. Researchers found that in general, women are more sensitive to the total dose of antipsychotics. Therefore, lower doses should be used in women.

—*Bryan C. Auday, PhD and Michelle Satava, BA*

For Further Information:

Hart, C. L., and C.K. Ksir. Drugs, Society, & Human Behavior. 16th ed. New York, NY: McGraw-Hill Publishers, 2015.

Bartolomeis, A. D., Fiore, G., & Iasevoli, F. (2005). Dopamine-Glutamate Interaction and Antipsychotics Mechanism of Action: Implication for New Pharmacological Strategies in Psychosis. *Current PharmaceuticalDesign, 11*(27), 3561-3594. doi:10.2174/138161205774414538

Sørup, F. K., Hallas, J., Brunak, S., & Andersen, S. E. (2017). Adverse Drug Events with Antipsychotics—A Sex Difference. Adverse Drug Events with Antipsychotics—A Sex Difference, 39(8), 56.

The Antivaccine Movement

Anatomy or system affected: Immune system
Specialties and related fields: Infectious Disease, Immunology, Pediatrics, Vaccinology
Definition: Organized conspiracy theorist movement mostly led by people with no medical or scientific qualifications opposed to the use of vaccines that blames the medical practice of vaccinations for a wide range of health problems.

Key terms:

antigen: A foreign substance that evokes an immune response when introduced into the body by any means.

CDC: The Centers for Disease Control and Protection, which serves as the main public health and epidemiology institute in the United States.

epidemiology: A branch of medicine that examines the patterns, causes and long- and short-term effects of disease and health in specific populations.

herd immunity: (also known as herd effect, community immunity, or population immunity) is a form of indirect protection from infectious disease that occurs when a large percentage of a population has become immune to an infection, through vaccination or natural infection, thereby providing a measure of protection for individuals who are not immune.

inoculation: the introduction of a pathogen or antigen into a living organism to stimulate the production of antibodies.

MMR: measles-mumps-rubella combination vaccination that contains live, attenuated measles, mumps, and rubella viruses that grow inside young patients but do not cause the disease and sensitize the immune system against these viruses, conferring life-long immunity in most cases. The CDC recommends two doses of MMR vaccine; a first dose at 12-15 months of age and a second dose at 4 through 6 years of age.

vaccination: treating someone with a vaccine against a specific disease or diseases to make them immune to that disease or group of diseases.

vaccine: material derived from disease-causing agents that do not cause the disease but are given to individuals by any means to sensitize the immune system against those agents and confer long-term immunity against the diseases caused by those agents.

variolation: the first technique used to immunize an individual against smallpox (Variola. The process involved collecting dried smallpox scabs taken from an infected patient and then giving them to a healthy person via inhalation or by inserting them into scratches in the skin resulting in a milder but protective infection that would confer immunity against smallpox.

Historical Perspective

Opposition to vaccines has been around since the conception of the very first "vaccine" or variolation against smallpox. Smallpox, for instance, was a feared disease due to its high mortality rate and severe sequela for survivors. However, as early as 430 B.C., people recognized that those who fell ill with smallpox and survived would not contract the disease again. This observation led early civilizations to practice the act of "variolation," the precursor to modern-day vaccination, in which material from an infected person was introduced to an uninfected patient to provide protection against smallpox. This practice, however, was not always successful. Between 1 and 20 out of every 1,000 persons who were variolated died from the inoculation.

Various fears regarding variolation have been described since the 17th century. Religious fears included the idea that vaccine-preventable diseases were sent by God to punish the sinful. Variolation was perceived as a "diabolical operation" because it interfered with God's will. Public health concerns rose with the discovery that those variolated could infect others if they themselves did not remain in quarantine. Significant epidemics of smallpox, such as one in Paris in 1762, provided proof. As a result of these epidemics, laws against inoculation became common in cities across Europe in an effort to control the spread of smallpox. People fearing smallpox and lacking scientific knowledge were left forced to choose between unregulated inoculation or taking a chance on natural infection, with its well-known and devastating consequences.

Edward Jenner replaced inoculation with vaccination in 1796, using fluid from a cowpox pustule instead of from a smallpox lesion to prevent smallpox. Because vaccination with cowpox was noted to be safer than variolation, laws were passed in Europe, notably in London, that mandated vaccination to prevent smallpox outbreaks. These laws were not well received by all, leading to establishment of the Anti-Vaccination League and the Anti-Compulsory Vaccination League. Arguments then by critics of variolation and vaccination bear similarities to those of modern day "anti-vaxxers." Some people cite "religious beliefs" as a reason not to vaccinate. Others claim compulsory vaccination is a violation of their "personal liberties." Many question the safety of vaccine components and scrutinize the current recommended vaccination schedule. In spite of the controversies and fears, the benefits of vaccinations cannot be denied. Furthermore, smallpox was the first vaccine-preventable disease to be eradicated from the earth, in 1980.

The Primary Current Issues

Over the past couple of decades, certain individuals have emerged as the modern-day leaders of the antivaccine movement. *Andrew Wakefield* may be the most prominent antivaccine activist of today, continuing to perpetuate a mythical link between autism and the measles, mumps, and rubella (MMR) vaccine. Wakefield became widely known with the publication of a fraudulent paper in 1998 in the journal *The Lancet*, in which he proposed a causal association between the MMR vaccine and autism. His original theory was that autism was a result of a chronic enterocolitis (inflammation of the digestive tract) that developed following administration of the MMR vaccine, which caused a leaky intestine that led to absorption of substances damaging to the brain of children. More importantly, he concluded that the damage was "reversible" once the trigger was removed. Wakefield's association of the

Don't mix your ethyls with your methyls.

ETHYLS	METHYLS
Ethyl alcohol is a type of alcohol found in alcoholic beverages and some medicines.	**Methyl alcohol** is found in antifreeze, and may cause blindness or death. No amount of methyl alcohol is safe for consumption.
Ethyl mercury (a metabolite of thimerosal) is found in some multi-dose vaccines to prevent contamination of the vaccine vial. It is quickly metabolized and does not accumulate in the body.	**Methyl mercury** is found in deep sea fish, and is a known and potent toxin. It is slowly metabolized and can accumulate in the body.

MMR vaccine with autism captured public attention, but failed to consider errors in the study design or the numerous ethical issues that eventually emerged. It was revealed that Wakefield had been receiving payments from attorneys attempting to prove that the MMR vaccine had injured their clients' children. Some of the patients in his study were enrolled through anti-MMR campaigns. Aside from the many undisclosed conflicts of interest, Wakefield was also found to have manipulated the data to his benefit. All 12 children in the study were reported as having had normal development, when in fact almost half had documented developmental concerns prior to receiving the MMR vaccine. Soon after the paper's publication and resulting media coverage, the public's confidence in MMR vaccine plummeted. Although Wakefield's paper was later retracted and his license to practice medicine was revoked, the damage was done. In some areas, vaccination rates dropped to 80%, and doubts caused by Wakefield's theory persist today. No one seems to have noticed that autism is not reversible as he originally proposed. Even now, as recently as 2017, a measles outbreak in the Somali community in Minnesota was directly associated with Wakefield's message linking MMR vaccine to autism.

It is easy to understand why vaccines have become a favorite in the autism blame game. Most childhood vaccines are administered before the age of two. National guidelines recommend autism screening within this same time frame, at 18 and 24 months, since a cardinal feature of autism spectrum disorder is language delay—and significant expressive speech development does not occur before 15-18 months. Numerous scientific studies have repeatedly shown there is no causal relationship between vaccination and the development of autism. If the MMR vaccine causes autism, one would expect that unvaccinated children would have lower rates of autism. However, well-designed studies have shown the risk of autism is no different in MMR-vaccinated children compared to unvaccinated children. Rates of autism are rising despite an increasing number of unvaccinated children.

In part because of the influence of antivaccine activist and former *Playboy* cover girl *Jenny McCarthy*, many people fear that ingredients in vaccines are not safe. Public concern has focused particularly on mercury as an ingredient in vaccines. In 1999, the Food and Drug Administration (FDA) was tasked with assessing the amount of mercury in all the products regulated by the agency. To assuage the public, the U.S. Public Health Service recommended removing thimerosal, a mercury-containing preservative, from vaccines, despite evidence showing that the very low amounts of thimerosal in vaccines were safe. This move caused an uproar among those who saw this move by public health officials as affirming their views that thimerosal itself was the "trigger" for autism. But several reputable studies have demonstrated no association between thimerosal and autism. In fact, the incidence of autism has not declined since thimerosal-containing vaccines were removed, and actually has continued to rise.

Finally, it is worth noting that thimerosal was never an ingredient in the MMR vaccine. To clarify, there are two different types of mercury: methylmercury and ethylmercury. Methylmercury is part of the earth's crust and thus found ubiquitously in the environment in sources such as water and in our bodies, even in breast milk. When ingested, typically by consuming fish and shellfish, it can accumulate and becomes toxic to the nervous system. Ethylmercury, on the other hand, is formed when the body breaks down thimerosal, and is cleared from the body within days. Unlike methylmercury, ethylmercury does not accumulate in the body. Thus, ethyl and methyl are not the same type of mercury. Similarly, ethyl and methylalcohol are two different chemicals. Ethyl alcohol is found in beer, wine, and liquor, commonly consumed safely, while methyl alcohol is a toxic chemical found in antifreeze, extremely toxic when consumed, leading to blindness or death.

A less obvious advocate of the antivaccine movement is *Dr. Robert Sears*, who in 2007 published *The VaccineBook*, promoting a "safer" delayed immunization schedule. He reasoned that vaccines contain aluminum and too much aluminum is harmful. Aluminum has been a component in vaccines for over 50 years. It serves as an adjuvant—a material that improves the immune response of a vaccine. Sears argues that immunizations given at 2 months of age can contain up to 1,225 micrograms (μg) of aluminum. However, he fails to mention that infants ingest far more aluminum in their diet alone. By 6 months of age babies have consumed 6,700 μg if breastfed; 37,800 μg if formula fed; and 116,600 μg if fed a soy-based formula. Sears further suggests that a baby's immune system cannot handle multiple simultaneous immunizations. However, a normal newborn's immune system is actually prepared. The moment a baby is born, she becomes saturated with microorganisms, since the birth canal is anything but sterile. Furthermore, infants and young children encounter exponentially more antigens in their daily lives than they do from all vaccines combined. A delayed or spaced-out immunization schedule can be dangerous, because it leaves infants susceptible to vaccine-preventable diseases that can result in permanent disability or even death. The current Centers for Disease Control and Prevention (CDC) deliberately schedules childhood immunizations to protect children from disease when they are most at risk.

Religious or moral concerns also continue to be cited as a reason some parents choose not to vaccinate their children in this era. One current concern is about the liceity of vaccinating children with specific vaccines made from cells obtained from aborted fetuses. Developing vaccines can be challenging. For example, to develop the lifesaving poliovirus vaccine, scientists first had to successfully grow the virus. For instance, by infecting monkey kidney cells, scientists were able to use these cells as a "laboratory" to continue growing the poliovirus that was used to produce the vaccine. However, not all viruses are able to grow in animal cells. Some cells die too quickly, while others do not grow at all. In addition, after developing the polio vaccine, researchers found that monkey cells could contain a virus that caused cancer in monkeys. Afraid of giving cancer to humans instead of preventing diseases, researchers needed to try other kinds of cells. Fetal cells appeared to be a good possibility because fetal cells can replicate indefinitely and they knew that a fetus could become infected with rubella and survive inside of the mother only to be born with the devastating rubella syndrome. That meant the virus, then, could replicate in those cells and survive. Scientists tested their assumption and were able to successfully grow the virus inside fetal cells obtained from a therapeutic abortion, and then produce the rubella virus that continues to be used for vaccines today. A common misconception is that ongoing abortions are required to continue to produce these vaccines. The fetal cells that were used originally are the same cell lines that are used now to produce the rubella vaccine, varicella-containing vaccines, hepatitis A vaccine, and one type of rabies vaccine. It is important to note that religious leaders and the Vatican have weighted in saying this shouldn't deter parents from vaccinating their children, and that the greater good is to use vaccines to protect children.

Perspective and Prospects

The current vaccine schedule approved by the CDC, American Academy of Pediatrics, and American Academy of Family Physicians is continuously being examined and improved. Though the number of recommended immunizations has grown in the past few decades, the overall number of antigens has decreased from over 3,000 proteins to fewer than 150. Additionally, the FDA and CDC collect ongoing data regarding vaccine safety and efficacy to make policy decisions. For example, RotaShield, the first vaccine developed against rotavirus, was removed from the market less than a year after its introduction due to concerns that infants might be at increased risk of developing an intestinal disorder called *intussusception*. This recommendation came despite rotavirus being the leading cause of profound dehydration due to diarrhea, accounting for more than 50,000 hospitalizations each year in the U.S. In 2016, the CDC recommended against the use of FluMist, an intranasal version of the influenza vaccine that was a popular choice among the needle wary. Compared to its intramuscular counterpart, FluMist was far inferior in its protection against the flu. When the CDC put forth their recommendations, AstraZeneca, the manufacturer of FluMist, lost tens of millions of dollars in revenue. Another example of a policy change following continued vaccine research is the recent CDC recommendation of only 2 doses of the HPV vaccine rather than the previously recommended 3-dose series for children ages 9-14 years. Two doses separated by 6 months was found to be just as efficacious in preventing cancers caused by the human papillomavirus.

Vaccine refusal is not a choice that affects only individuals; it is a choice that affects public health. If an outbreak of a disease occurs due to decreasing vaccination rates, even immunized children are at risk of contracting disease. In recent years, herd immunity protection has been fading due to under-vaccination. Herd immunity is especially important for those most vulnerable—infants, individuals with congenital or acquired immune problems, and the elderly. In order to protect the vulnerable through herd immunity, a certain percentage of the population needs to be vaccinated against the disease. Unfortunately, diseases once considered all but eradicated or incredibly rare are now making a comeback in the U.S. due to under vaccination. Meanwhile, some of these diseases remain prevalent in other nations. With global commerce and travel, the threat of biological warfare, and dwindling herd immunity, these diseases can quickly be re-introduced in the U.S. An unprotected population—either by choice or because they are too young or have medical conditions that preclude them from vaccination—faces the risk of illness and the associated morbidity and mortality from infection. Outbreaks happen when immunization rates decline. Recent outbreaks of whooping cough and measles in the U.S. have been more common in communities with a rising number unvaccinated individuals.

Paradoxically, the very success of vaccines poses a particular challenge in countering the modern-day antivaccine movement. The incidence of vaccine-preventable diseases has declined so dramatically that most young parents (and physicians) have no experience with these life-altering and potentially fatal diseases. The fear of polio, measles, and smallpox has largely disappeared. Because these diseases occur so infrequently, many parents fear the rare potential side effects of a vaccine or the pain of the injection more than the disease itself. We must remember, though, that these diseases are now rare thanks to widespread vaccination.

—*Kayleigh McBride, DO and Barbara Pahud, MD*

For Further Information:

Mnookin, S. (2011). *The panicvirus: A true story of medicine, science, and fear*. New York: Simon & Schuster.

Rothstein, A. "Vaccines and Their Critics, Then and Now." *The New Atlantis*, Number 44, Winter 2015, pp. 3-27.

Wolfe RM, Sharp LK. "Anti-vaccinationists past and present." *British Medical Journal*. 2002;325(7361):430- 432.

Deer B. "How the case against the MMR vaccine was fixed". *British Medical Journal*. 342: c5347. PMID 21209059. DOI: 10.1136/bmj.c5347.

Porter D, Porter R. "The politics of prevention: anti-vaccinationism and public health in nineteenth-century England." *Medical History*. 1988;32(3):231-252.

Nelson, MC, Rogers J. "The Right to Die? Anti-vaccination Activity and the 1874 Smallpox Epidemic in Stockholm." *Social History of Medicine*, Volume 5, Issue 3, 1 December 1992, Pages 369-388, https://doi.org/10.1093/ shm/5.3.369.

Jain A, Marshall J, Buikema A, Bancroft T, Kelly JP, et al. "Autism occurrence by MMR vaccine status among US children with older siblings with and without autism." *JAMA* 313: 1534-1540.

Riedel S. *Edward Jenner and the history of smallpox and vaccination*. Proceedings (Baylor University Medical Center). 2005;18(1):21-25.

Institute of Medicine. *ImmunizationSafety Review. Vaccinesand AutismBoard of Health Promotionand Disease Prevention, Institute of Medicine* (National Academy Press, Washington, DC, 2004).

Paul A. Offit, Charlotte A. Moser. "The Problem with Dr Bob's Alternative Vaccine Schedule." *Pediatrics* Jan 2009, 123 (1) e164-e169; DOI: 10.1542/peds.2008-2189.

Anus

Anatomy

Anatomy or system affected: Gastrointestinal system, intestines

Specialties and related fields: Gastroenterology, internal medicine, oncology, proctology

Definition: The anus ends the gastrointestinal tract, the point most distant from the mouth. It controls defecation.

Structure and Functions

The anus terminates the long tube through the body where digestion takes place and that begins with the mouth. It consists of the anal canal, located immediately below the rectum, and the anal sphincter. The sphincter itself has a double ring of strong muscles, the interior and external sphincters. In the anus, the tissue type changes from that of the intestinal tract to external skin.

The anus controls defecation: the expulsion of the semisolid waste matter of digestion (feces) from the body. The anal sphincter is controlled by the autonomic nervous system, which keeps it shut. As feces fill the rectum, pressure on its walls creates the urge to defecate. The muscles of the anal sphincter then relax. Most adults and children, but not infants, can force the lower sphincter to remain tight until they are ready to defecate and then aid the process by consciously relaxing the muscles involved. During defecation, a muscular contraction pulls the anus back over the feces until the sphincter shuts.

Disorders and Diseases

The anus is subject to several common mechanical injuries and infections. Most common of all are hemorrhoids, which are varicose (swollen) veins. They can protrude from the anus (external hemorrhoids) or lie inside the anal canal (interior hemorrhoids). Pregnancy, exertion while lifting heavy objects, and straining during defecation are the typical causes. Sometimes a hard or large bowel movement or anal sex causes a tear in the anus, called an anal fissure. Both fissures and hemorrhoids can cause pain and light bleeding during defecation.

An anal abscess is a pocket of bacteria that has filled a mucus-secreting gland in the anal wall. It can cause severe pain and damage to surrounding tissue. An anal fistula is a tube that opens between one part of the anal wall to another or to a separate organ, such as the vagina. All these defects can be repaired surgically. Additionally, pruritus (itching) can occur from a variety of causes, such as bacteria, poor hygiene, allergic reactions, parasites, and the anxiety-itch-anxiety cycle.

Injury to the anus or infection may impair or prevent control of the anus, which leads to fecal incontinence (uncontrollable bowel movements). Primary cancer in the anus is rare, occurring in about 0.0001 percent of the population. It usually involves squamous cell carcinoma in the skin near the anus or in the transition between the anus and the rectum.

—*Roger Smith, Ph.D.*

See also Anal cancer; Colon; Colonoscopy and sigmoidoscopy; Colorectal cancer; Colorectal polyp removal; Colorectal surgery; Digestion; Gastroenterology; Gastroenterology, pediatric; Gastrointestinal system; Hemorrhoids; Incontinence; Intestinal disorders; Intestines; Rectum; Stomach, intestinal, and pancreatic cancers.

For Further Information:

"Anal Cancer Treatment." *National Cancer Institute*. March 25, 2013.

Beers, Mark H., ed. *The Merck Manual of Medical Information: Second Home Edition*. New York: Pocket Books, 2004.

Ehrenpreis, Eli, Shmuel Avital, and Marc Singer. *Anal and Rectal Diseases: A Concise Manual*. New York: Springer, 2012.

Kaneshiro, Neil K. "Imperforate Anus." *MedlinePlus*, May 1, 2011.

Keshav, Satish. *The Gastrointestinal System at a Glance*. 2d edition. Oxford: Wiley-Blackwell, 2013.

Maimonides, Moses, Gerrit Bos, and M. R. McVaugh. *On Hemorrhoids*. Provo, Utah: Brigham Young University Press, 2012.

Parker, Steve. *The Human Body Book*. 2d ed. New York: Dorling Kindersley, 2013.

Thibodeau, Gary A., Kevin T. Patton, and Catherine Parker Anthony. *Structure and Function of the Human Body*. 14th ed. St. Louis: Mosby Elsevier, 2012.

Anxiety

Disease/Disorder

Anatomy or system affected: Heart, nervous system, psychic-emotional system, skin

Specialties and related fields: Cardiology, internal medicine, psychiatry, psychology

Definition: Heightened fear or tension that causes psychological and physical distress; the American Psychiatric Association recognizes six types of anxiety disorders, which can be treated with medications or through counseling.

Key terms:

anxiety: abnormal fear or tension, which may occur without any obvious trigger

brain imaging: any of several techniques used to visualize anatomic regions of the brain, including X rays, magnetic resonance imaging, and positron emission tomography

compulsion: a repetitive, stereotyped behavior performed to ward off anxious feelings

GABA/benzodiazepine receptor: an area on a nerve cell to which gamma aminobutyric acid (GABA) attaches and that causes inhibition (quieting) of the nerve; benzodiazepine drugs enhance the attachment of GABA to the receptor

obsession: a recurrent, unwelcome, and intrusive thought

panic: a sudden episode of intense fearfulness

Causes and Symptoms

Anxiety is a subjective state of fear, apprehension, or tension. In the face of a naturally fearful situation, anxiety is a normal and understandable condition. When anxiety occurs without obvious provocation or is excessive, however, anxiety may be said to be abnormal or pathological (existing in a disease state). Normal anxiety is useful because it provides an alerting signal and improves physical and mental performance. Excessive anxiety results in a deterioration in performance and in emotional and physical discomfort.

There are several forms of pathological anxiety, known collectively as the anxiety disorders. According to the Anxiety and Depression Association of America (ADAA), as a group, anxiety disorders constitute the most common mental illness in the United States, where 14.6 percent of the population will experience anxiety at some point in their lives. More women suffer from anxiety disorders than do men, by a 2:1 ratio.

The anxiety disorders are distinguished from one another by characteristic clusters of symptoms. These disorders include generalized anxiety disorder, panic disorder, obsessive-compulsive disorder, phobias, adjustment disorder with anxious mood, and post-traumatic stress disorder.

The first three disorders are characterized by anxious feelings that may occur without any obvious precipitant, while the latter three are closely associated with anxiety-producing events in a person's life.

Generalized anxiety disorder is thought to be a biological form of anxiety disorder in which the individual inherits a habitually high level of tension or anxiety that may occur even when no threatening circumstances are present. Generally, these periods of anxiety occur in cycles that may last weeks to years. The prevalence is unknown, but this disorder is not uncommon. The male-to-female ratio is nearly equal.

Evidence suggests that generalized anxiety disorder is related to an abnormality in a common neurotransmitter receptor complex found in many brain neurons. These complexes, the GABA/benzodiazepine receptors, decrease the likelihood that a neuron will transmit an electrochemical signal, resulting in a calming effect on the portion of the brain in which they are found. These receptors exist in large numbers in the cerebral cortex (the outer layer of the brain), the hippocampus (a structure inside the temporal lobe shaped like a sea horse), and the amygdala (the almond-shaped gray matter inside the temporal lobe). The hippocampus and amygdala are important parts of the limbic system, which is significantly involved in emotions. Benzodiazepine drugs enhance the efficiency of these receptors and have a calming effect. In contrast, if these receptors are inhibited, feelings of impending doom result.

According to the ADAA, panic disorder is found in 2.7 percent of the United States population, and the female-to-male ratio is 2:1. This disorder usually begins during the young adult years. Panic disorder is characterized by recurrent and unexpected attacks of intense fear or panic. Each discrete episode lasts about five to twenty minutes. These episodes are intensely frightening to the individual, who is usually convinced he or she is dying. Because people who suffer from panic attacks are often anxious about having another one (so-called secondary anxiety), they may avoid situations in which they fear an attack may occur, in which help would be unavailable, or in which they would be embarrassed if an attack occurred. This avoidance behavior may cause restricted activity and can lead to agoraphobia, the fear of leaving a safe zone in or around the home. Thus, agoraphobia (literally, "fear of the marketplace") is often secondary to panic disorder.

Panic disorder appears to have a biological basis. In those people with panic disorder, panic attacks can often be induced by sodium lactate infusions, hyperventilation, exercise, or hypocalcemia (low blood calcium). Highly sophisticated scans show abnormal metabolic activity in the right parahippocampal region of the brain of individuals with panic disorder. The parahippocampal region, the area surrounding the hippocampus, is involved in emotions and is connected by fiber tracts to the locus ceruleus, a blue spot in the pons portion of the brain stem that is involved in arousal.

In addition to known biological triggers for panic attacks, emotional or psychological events may also cause an attack. To be diagnosed as having panic disorder, however, a person must experience attacks that arise without any apparent cause. The secondary anxiety and avoidance behavior often seen in these individuals result in difficulties in normal functioning. There is an increased incidence of suicide attempts in people with panic disorder; up to one in five have reported a suicide attempt at some time. The childhoods of people with panic disorder are characterized by an increased incidence of pathological separation anxiety and/or school phobia.

Obsessive-compulsive disorder (OCD) is an uncommon anxiety disorder with an equal male-to-female ratio. It is characterized by obsessions (intrusive, unwelcome thoughts) and compulsions (repetitive, often stereotyped behaviors that are performed to ward off anxiety). The obsessions in OCD are often horrifying to the afflicted person. Common themes concern sex, food, aggression, suicide, bathroom functions, and religion. Compulsive behavior may include checking (such as repeatedly checking to see if the stove is off or the door is locked), cleaning (such as repetitive hand washing or the wearing of gloves to turn a doorknob), or stereotyped behavior (such as dressing by using an exact series of steps that cannot be altered). Frequently, the compulsive behaviors must be repeated many times. Sometimes, there is an exact, almost magical number of times the behavior must be done to ward off anxiety. Although people with OCD have some conscious control over their compulsions, they are driven to perform them because intense anxiety results if they fail to do so.

The most common psychological theory for OCD was proposed by Sigmund Freud, who believed that OCD symptoms were a defense against unacceptable unconscious wishes. Genetic and brain imaging studies, however, suggest a biological basis for this disorder. Special brain scans have shown increased metabolism in the front portion of the brain in these patients, and it has been theorized that OCD results from an abnormality in a circuit within the brain (the cortical-striatal-thalamic-cortical circuit). Moreover, OCD is associated with a variety of known neurological diseases, including epilepsy, brain trauma, and certain movement disorders.

Phobias are the most common anxiety disorders. A phobia is an abnormal fear of a particular object or situation. Simple phobias are fears of specific, identifiable triggers such as heights, snakes, flying in an airplane, elevators, or the number thirteen. Social phobia is an exaggerated fear of being in social settings where the phobic person fears he or she will be open to scrutiny by others. This fear may result in phobic avoidance of eating in public, attending church, joining a social club, or participating in other social events. Phobias are more common in men than in women, and they often begin in late childhood or early adolescence.

In classic psychoanalytic theory, phobias were thought to be fears displaced from one object or situation to another. For example, fear of snakes may be a displaced fear of sex because the snake is a phallic symbol. It was thought that this process of displacement took place unconsciously. Many psychologists now believe that phobias are either ex-

Information on Anxiety
Causes: Abnormality in common neurotransmitter receptor complex, genetics, emotional or psychological events
Symptoms: Motor tension (muscle tension, trembling, fatigue) and autonomic hyperactivity (shortness of breath, palpitations, cold hands, dizziness, gastrointestinal upset, chills, frequent urination)
Duration: Often chronic, with discrete episodes lasting five to twenty minutes
Treatments: Sedatives, psychotherapy

aggerations of normal fears or that they develop accidentally, without any symbolic meaning. For example, fear of elephants may arise if a young boy at a zoo is accidentally separated from his parents. At the same time that he realizes he is alone, he notices the elephants. He may then associate elephants with separation from his parents and fear elephants thereafter.

Adjustment disorder with anxious mood is an excessive or maladaptive response to a life event in which the individual experiences anxiety. For example, an individual may become so anxious after losing a job that he or she is unable to eat, sleep, or function and begins to entertain the prospect of suicide. While anxiety is to be expected, this person has excessive anxiety (the inability to eat, sleep, or function) and a maladaptive response (the thought of suicide). The exaggerated response may be attributable to the personality traits of the individual. In this example, a dependent person will be more likely to experience an adjustment disorder than a less dependent person.

Adjustment disorders are very common. In addition to adjustment disorders with anxious mood, people may experience adjustment disorders with depressed mood, mixed emotional features, disturbance of conduct, physical complaints, withdrawal, or inhibition in school or at work. These disorders are considered to be primarily psychological.

Post-traumatic stress disorder (PTSD) is similar to adjustment disorder because it represents a psychological reaction to a significant life event. PTSD only occurs, however, when the precipitating event would be seriously emotionally traumatic to a normal person, such as war, rape, natural disasters such as major earthquakes, or airplane crashes. In PTSD, the individual suffers from flashbacks to the precipitating event and "relives" the experience. These episodes are not simply vivid remembrances of what happened but a transient sensation of actually being in that circumstance. For example, a Vietnam War veteran may literally jump behind bushes when a car backfires.

People who suffer from PTSD usually are anxious and startle easily. They may be depressed and have disturbed sleeping and eating patterns. They often lose normal interest in sex, and nightmares are common. These individuals usually try to avoid situations that remind them of their trauma. Relationships with others are often strained, and the patient is generally pessimistic about the future.

In addition to the anxiety disorders described, abnormal anxiety may be caused by a variety of drugs and medical illnesses. Common drug offenders include caffeine, alcohol, stimulants in cold preparations, nicotine, and many illicit drugs, including cocaine and amphetamines. Medical illnesses that may cause anxiety include thyroid disease, heart failure, cardiac arrhythmias, and schizophrenia.

Treatment and Therapy

When an individual has difficulty with anxiety and seeks professional help, the cause of the anxiety must be determined. Before the etiology can be determined, however, the professional must first realize that the patient has an anxiety disorder. People with anxiety disorders often complain primarily of physical symptoms that result from the anxiety. These symptoms may include motor tension (muscle tension, trembling, and fatigue) and autonomic hyperactivity (shortness of breath, palpitations, cold hands, dizziness, gastrointestinal upset, chills, and frequent urination).

When an anxiety disorder is suspected, effective treatment often depends on an accurate diagnosis of the type of anxiety disorder present. Accurate diagnosis requires both physical and psychological evaluations, as it is very important to rule out nonpsychiatric medical conditions causing anxiety. A variety of medications can be prescribed for the anxiety disorder. In addition, several types of psychotherapy can be used. For example, patients with panic disorder can be educated about the nature of their illness, reassured that they will not die from it, and taught to ride out a panic attack. This process avoids the development of secondary anxiety, which complicates the panic attack. Phobic patients can be treated with systematic desensitization, in which they are taught relaxation techniques and are given graded exposure to the feared situation so that their fear lessens or disappears.

The origin, diagnosis, and treatment of anxiety disorders can best be portrayed through case examples. Three fictional cases are described below to illustrate typical anxiety disorder patients.

Mrs. Smith is a twenty-four-year-old married mother of two young children. She works part time as a bookkeeper for a construction company. Her health had been good until a month ago, when she began to experience spells of intense fearfulness, a racing heart, tremors of her hands, a dry mouth, and dizziness. The spells would come on suddenly and would last between ten and fifteen minutes. She was convinced that heart disease was causing these episodes and was worried about having a heart attack. As a result, she consulted her family physician.

Physical examination, electrocardiogram, and laboratory studies were all normal. Her physician had initially considered cardiac arrhythmia (abnormal rhythm of the heartbeat) as a cause but diagnosed panic disorder on the basis of Mrs. Smith's history and the outcome of the tests. Treatment consisted of medication and comforting explanations of the nonfatal nature of the disorder. Within three weeks, the panic attacks stopped altogether.

This case illustrates many common features of panic disorder. The patient is a young adult female with classic panic attacks striking "out of the blue." Most patients fear that they are having a heart attack or a stroke or that they are going insane. Typically, they present their symptoms to general medical physicians rather than to psychiatrists. Treatment with medication and simple counseling techniques is usually successful.

Mr. Jones is a thirty-five-year-old single man who works as an accountant. He has always been shy and has adopted leisure activities that he can do alone, such as reading, gardening, and coin collecting. As a child, he was bright but withdrawn. His mother described him as "high-strung," "a worrier," and "easily moved to tears." Recently, he has been bothered by muscle achiness, frequent urination, and diarrhea alternating with constipation. He thinks constantly about his health and worries that he has cancer.

Mr. Jones makes frequent visits to his doctor, but no illness is found. His doctor tells him that he worries too much. The patient admits to himself that he is a worrier and has been his whole life. He ruminates about the details of his job, his health, his lack of friends, the state of the economy, and a host of other concerns. His worries make it hard for him to fall asleep at night. Once asleep, however, he sleeps soundly. Finally, Mr. Jones is given a tranquilizer by his physician. He finds that he feels calm, no longer broods over everything, falls asleep easily, and has relief from his physical symptoms. To improve his social functioning, he sees a psychiatrist, who diagnoses a generalized anxiety disorder and an avoidant (shy) personality disorder.

This case illustrates many features of patients with generalized anxiety disorder. These individuals have near-continuous anxiety for weeks or months that is not clearly related to a single life event. In this case, some of the physical manifestations of anxiety are prominent (muscle tension, frequent urination, and diarrhea). Difficulty falling asleep is also common with anxiety. In contrast, patients who are depressed will often have early morning wakening. In this case example, the patient also has a concomitant shy personality that aggravates his condition. Such a patient usually benefits from treatment. Medication may be required for many years, although it may be needed only during active cycles of anxiety. Because some patients attempt to medicate themselves with alcohol, secondary alcoholism is a potential complication.

Mrs. Johnson is a forty-two-year-old married homemaker and mother of four children. She works part time in a fabric store as a salesclerk. She is friendly and outgoing. She has also been very close with her family, especially her mother. She comes to her family physician because her mother has just had a stroke. Because her mother lives on the other side of the country, Mrs. Johnson needs to take an airplane if she is to get to her mother's bedside quickly. Unfortunately, she has a long-standing fear of flying; even the thought of getting into an airplane terrifies her. She has not personally had a bad experience with flying but remembers reading about a plane crash when she was a teenager. She denies any other unusual fears and otherwise functions well.

Her family physician refers her to a psychologist for systematic desensitization to relieve her phobia for future situations. As a stopgap measure for the present, however, she is taught a deep-muscle relaxation technique, is shown videotapes designed to reduce fear of flying, and is prescribed a tranquilizer and another drug to reduce the physical manifestations of anxiety (a beta-blocker). This combination of treatments allows her to visit her mother immediately and, eventually, to be able to fly without needing medication.

This case illustrates a typical patient with an isolated phobia. Phobias are probably the most common anxiety disorders. Treatments such as those described above are usually quite helpful.

Perspective and Prospects

Anxiety has been recognized since antiquity and was often attributed to magical or spiritual causes, such as demoniac possession. Ancient myths provided explanations for fearful events in people's lives. Pan, a mythological god of mischief, was thought to cause frightening noises in forests, especially at night; the term "panic" is derived from his name. An understanding of the causes of panic and other anxiety disorders has evolved over the years.

Sigmund Freud (1856-1939) distinguished anxiety from fear. He considered fear to be an expected response to a specific, identifiable trigger, whereas anxiety was a similar emotional state without an identifiable trigger. He postulated that anxiety resulted from unconscious, forbidden wishes that conflicted with what the person believed was acceptable. The anxiety that resulted from this mental conflict was called an "anxiety neurosis" and was thought to result in a variety of psychological and physical symptoms. Psychoanalysis was developed to uncover these hidden conflicts and to allow the anxiety to be released.

Freud's theories about anxiety are no longer universally accepted. Many psychiatrists now believe that several anxiety disorders have a biological cause and that they are more neurological diseases than psychological ones. This is primarily true of generalized anxiety disorder, panic disorder, and obsessive-compulsive disorder. It is recognized that anxiety can also be triggered by drugs (legal and illicit) and a variety of medical illnesses.

Psychological causes of anxiety are also recognized. Adjustment disorder with anxious mood, phobias, and PTSD are all thought to be primarily psychological disorders. Unlike with Freud's conflict theory of anxiety, most modern psychiatrists consider personality factors, life experiences, and views of the world to be the relevant psychological factors in such anxiety disorders. Nonpharmacological therapies are no longer designed to uncover hidden mental conflicts; they provide instead support. Specific therapies include flooding (massive exposure to the feared situation), systematic desensitization (graded exposure), and relaxation techniques.

—*Peter M. Hartmann, M.D.*

See also Antianxiety drugs; Antidepressants; Appetite loss; Arrhythmias; Bipolar disorders; Death and dying; Depression; Emotions: Biomedical causes and effects; Grief and guilt; Gulf War syndrome; Hyperhidrosis; Hyperventilation; Hypochondriasis; Midlife crisis; Neurosis; Obsessive-compulsive disorder; Palpitations; Panic attacks; Paranoia; Phobias; Postpartum depression; Post-traumatic stress disorder; Psychiatric disorders; Psychiatry; Psychiatry, child and adolescent; Psychiatry, geriatric; Psychoanalysis; Psychosomatic disorders; Sexual dysfunction; Stress; Stress reduction; Suicide; Sweating.

For Further Information:

American Psychiatric Association. *Diagnostic and Statistical Manual of Mental Disorders: DSM-IV-TR*. 4th rev. ed. Arlington, Va.: Author, 2010.

Barlow, David H. *Anxiety and Its Disorders*. 2d ed. New York: Guilford Press, 2004.

Bourne, Edmund J. *The Anxiety and Phobia Workbook*. 5th ed. Oakland, Calif.: New Harbinger, 2011.

Davidson, Jonathan, and Henry Dreher. *The Anxiety Book*. New York: Penguin, 2003.

Ghinassi, Cheryl Winning. *Anxiety*. Santa Barbara, Calif.: Greenwood/ABC-CLIO, 2010.

Kahn, Jeffrey P. *Angst: Origins of Anxiety and Depression*. New York: Oxford University Press, 2013.

Kleinknecht, Ronald A. *Mastering Anxiety: The Nature and Treatment of Anxious Conditions*. New York: Plenum Press, 1991.

Leaman, Thomas L. *Healing the Anxiety Diseases*. New York: Plenum Press, 1992.

Muskin, Philip R., Patricia L. Gerbarg, and Richard P. Brown. *Complementary and Integrative Therapies for Psychiatric Disorders*. Philadelphia: Elsevier, 2013.

Saul, Helen. *Phobias: Fighting the Fear*. New York: Arcade, 2001.

Sheehan, David V. *The Anxiety Disease*. New York: Bantam Books, 1983.

Stahl, S. M., and Bret A. Moore. *Anxiety Disorders: A Guide for Integrating Psychopharmacology and Psychotherapy*. London: Routledge, 2013.

Tompkins, Michael A. *Anxiety and Avoidance: A Universal Treatment for Anxiety, Panic, and Fear*. Oakland, Calif.: New Harbinger, 2013.

Aortic aneurysm

Disease/Disorder

Anatomy or system affected: The aorta

Specialties and related fields: Cardiology, vascular and endovascular specialists

Definition: A dilation or ballooning of the arterial vessel wall to twice its original size, creating an area of weakness.

Key terms:

adventitia: the outer most collagen layer of the aortic vessel

aorta: largest artery in the body carrying freshly oxygenated blood to the peripheral vascular system

computed tomography (CT): a scan that uses x-rays to visualize cross-sections of the body

false aneurysms: a weakening and dilation of an arterial vessel caused by trauma

true aneurysms: dilation of an arterial vessel caused by a congenital or acquired problem

fusiform aneurysm: dilation of the circumference of the arterial vessel

saccular aneurysm: arterial wall dilation confined to one area causing a ballooning effect

abdominal aortic aneurysms (AAA): a dilation of the aorta in the abdominal cavity

thoracic aortic aneurysms (TAA): a dilation of the aorta in the thoracic cavity

intima: the innermost layer of endothelial cells in the aortic *vessel*

media: the middle layer of the aortic vessel made up of thick elastic tissue

ultrasound: a method of diagnostic imaging using high-frequency sound

Overview

Aortic aneurysms can be described in terms of their location, type, and if they are true or false. While it is possible for an aneurysm to develop in the ascending, transverse, or descending portions of the aorta, it is most commonly seen in the abdominal aorta area between the renal arteries and the aortic bifurcation. Aortic aneurysms can be thoracic (above the diaphragm) or abdominal (below the diaphragm). A fusiform aneurysm describes dilation of the circumference of the aorta compared to saccular, which describes a dilation confined to one area of the vessel wall. Aneurysms may also be described as true, caused by a congenital or acquired problem, or false, caused by trauma to the layers of the arterial wall.

Three tissue layers construct the vessel walls of the aorta: the intima is the inner most layer of endothelial cells; the media, the middle layer, is thick elastic tissue; and the adventitia is the outer most collagen layer. When the media layer is weakened by either true or false causes, stretching of the intima and adventitia ensues, allowing for widening and increased tension within the arterial wall. A history of smoking, elevated blood pressure, and other factors can accelerated the rate of aneurysm enlargement and thus risk for rupture. While the normal abdominal aorta has diameter less than 3 cm, an aneurysm diameter of greater than 5.5 cm is the most indicative clinical feature of an impeding rupture. A rupture causes an abrupt and massive hemorrhage resulting in shock that is life threatening. Approximately 90 percent of all ruptured abdominal aortic aneurysms (AAA) result in death.

Diameter of AAA	Risk of Rupture
> 5 cm	20%
> 6 cm	40%
> 7 cm	50%

Causes and Symptoms

Thoracic aneurysms tend to be asymptomatic until they rupture. Depending on where the dilation of the aorta pushes on surrounding structures, such as the esophagus, left vagus, laryngeal nerve, or phrenic nerve, a person may experience dyspnea, wheezing, dysphagia, or cough, as well as pain in their neck, substernal area, or back, worsened by supine positioning. If the aneurysm develops in the ascending region or the aortic root, heart failure or a myocardial infarction may be the initial presenting symptoms.

Similarly, an AAA can also be asymptomatic. Usually an AAA is discovered during a physical examination or through imaging. The most common complaint related to an AAA is lower back or flank pain. Other associated symptoms may include: a pulsating abdominal mass, the sensation of a "heartbeat" in the abdomen with supine posturing, cool or cyanotic extremities, and pain or tiredness in the legs with walking.

Diagnosis

Thoracic aortic aneurysms (TAA) are not usually identified on physical exam, as they are obscured by the rib cage and sternum. AAAs can often be identified during a physical exam, but it can be difficult to accurately determine the size. In obese individuals, palpation of a large AAA may not be possible.

If a clinician suspects an AAA in an asymptomatic patient, the definitive diagnosis is made by a fasting abdominal ultrasound. However, if an AAA is suspected, the patient presents with symptoms (back or flank pain) and is hypotensive (systolic Z mmHg), a computed tomography (CT) scan is used to locate or rule out a hemorrhage walking. A CT scan is a highly accurate tool for assessing aneurysm size, and is often used to monitor aneurysm growth. A CT scan is also used to definitively diagnose a TAA.

Treatment

While there are no recommended medical management guidelines, the mainstay of treatment is reducing the risk of expansion and rupture. This includes smoking cessation and modification of other risk factors. Blood pressure reducing agents such as angiotensin-converting enzyme inhibitors, and cholesterol reducing agents such as statins can be helpful in the reducing the aneurysm rate of growth. Surgical repair of the aneurysm is the most effective means of preventing rupture. For those with an AAA less than 5.5cm, the recommendation is close monitoring through serial CT scans; and for an AAA greater than 5.5cm in otherwise healthy patients, surgical repair is recommended.

Risk Factors and Screening

Several compounding risk factors predispose an individual for abdominal aortic aneurysms including: male gender, advancing age (over 65), history of smoking, family history of AAA, history of peripheral artery aneurysm, atherosclerosis, and Caucasian race. Atherosclerosis coupled with hypertension, hyperlipidemia, and smoking is the most common cause of aneurysms. Ehlers-Danlos syndrome, Marfan syndrome, Syphilis, chronic inflammation, and blunt trauma are other less common causes of AAA. The U.S. Preventive Services Task Force (USPSTF) defines the screening criteria for an AAA, recommending a one-time abdominal ultrasound for men ages 65-75 years that have ever smoked. The USPSTF also recommends screening men over the age of 60 years with a family history of AAA.

—*Marisela Fermin-Schon, RN*

See also Atherosclerosis, Hypertension, Hyperlipidemia, Ehlers-Danlos Syndrome, Marfan Syndrome, Syphilis

For Further Information:

"Abdominal Aortic Aneurysm Screening." Medicare.gov: Your Medicare Coverage. Retrieved November 9, 2013. http://www.medicare.gov/coverage/ab-aortic-aneurysm-screening.html

Chaikof, E.L., D.C. Brewster, R. L. Dalman, et al. "The Care of Patients with an Abdominal Aortic Aneurysm: The Society for Vascular Surgery Practice Guidelines." Journal of Vascular Surgery 50, no. 4 (2009): S2-S49.

Clouse, W.D., J.W. Hallett, H.V. Schaff, M.M. Gayari, D.M. Ilstrup, and L.J. Melton. "Improved Prognosis of Thoracic Aortic Aneurysms: A Population-Based Study." Journal of the American Medical Association 280, no. 22 (1998): 1926-1929.

Collins, K.A. (2013). "Overview of abdominal aortic aneurysm." In UpToDate, edited by J.F. Eidt, J.L. Mills, and J.L. Duda. Retrieved from http://www.uptodate.com/contents/overview-of-abdominal-aortic-aneurysm?detectedLanguage=en&source=search_result&search=Overview+of+abdominal+aortic+aneurysm&selectedTitle=1%7E150&provider=noProvider

Dalman, R.L., and M. Mell, M. "Management of Asymptomatic Abdominal Aortic Aneurysm." In UpToDate, edited by J.L. Mills, J.F. Eidt, E.R. Mohler, and D.L. Clement. Retrieved from http://www.uptodate.com/contents/management-of-asymptomatic-abdominal-aortic-aneurysm?detectedLanguage =en&source= search_result&search=abdominal+aortic+aneurysm&selected Title=1~126&provider=noProvider# H909597049

Forsdahl, S. H., K. Singh, S. Solberg, and B.K. Jacobsen. "Risk Factors for Abdominal Aortic Aneurysms: A 7-Year Prospective Study: The Tromsø Study, 1994-2001." Circulation, 119, no. 16 (2009): 2202-2208.

Hiratzka, L.F., G.L. Bakris, J.A. Beckman, et al. "Guidelines for the Diagnosis and Management of Patients with Thoracic Aortic Disease." Journal of the American College of Cardiology 55, no. 14 (2010):e27-e129.

Isselbacher, Eric Michael. "Diseases of the Aorta." In Goldman's Cecil Medicine, 24th ed., edited by Lee Goldman and Andrew I. Schafer, 482-486. Philadelphia: Elsevier Saunders, 2011.

Jim, J., and R.W. Thompson. "Clinical Features and Diagnosis of Abdominal Aortic Aneurysm." In UpToDate, edited by J.L. Mills, J.F. Eidt, E.R. Mohler, and K.A. Collins. Retrieved from http://www.uptodate.com/contents/clinical-features-and-diagnosis-of-abdominal-aortic-aneurysm?detectedLanguage=en&source=search_result&search=aortic+aneurysm&selected Title=4%7E150&provider=noProvider

Little, Tami. "Care of Patients with Vascular Problems." In Medical-Surgical Nursing: Patient-Centered Collaborative Care, 7th ed., edited by Donna D. Ignatavicius and M. Linda Workman, 792-796. St. Louis: Elsevier, 2013.

Mohler, E.R. "Epidemiology, Risk Factors, Pathogenesis and Natural History of Abdominal Aortic Aneurysm." In UpToDate, edited by J.L. Mills, J.F. Eidt, and K.A. Collins. Retrieved from http://www.uptodate.com/contents/epidemiology-risk-factors-pathogenesis-and-natural-history-of-abdominal-aortic-aneurysm?detectedLanguage=en&source=search_result&search=Epidemiology%2C+risk+factors%2C+pathogenesis+and+natural+history+of+abdominal+aortic+aneurysm&selectedTitle=1~126&provider=noProvider

"Screening for Abdominal Aortic Aneurysm." U.S. Preventive Services Task Force, 2005. Retrieved November 9, 2013 from http://www.uspreventiveservicestaskforce.org/uspstf/uspsaneu.htm

Woo, Y.J., and E.R. Mohler. "Clinical Features and Diagnosis of Thoracic Aortic Aneurysm." In UpToDate, edited by C.M. Otto, J. Hoekstra, J.F. Eidt, J.L. Mills, and K.A. Collins. Retrieved from http://www.uptodate.com/contents/clinical-features-and-diagnosis-of-thoracic-aortic-aneurysm?detectedLanguage=en&source=search_result&search=aortic+aneurysm&selected Title=3%7E150&provider=noProvider

Aortic stenosis

Disease/Disorder

Anatomy or system affected: Cardiovascular system, heart, brain

Specialties and related fields: Cardiology, internal medicine

Definition: Narrowing of the bicuspid or tricuspid valve, preventing blood flow from the left ventricle to the aorta.

Key terms:

angina: pain in the chest caused by insufficient blood flow to the heart muscle

calcification: the deposit of lime salts in organic tissue, leading to the buildup of calcium in the arterial wall

heart failure: a condition in which the heart cannot pump enough blood to meet the body's needs

hypertrophic left ventricle: enlargement of the muscle tissue of the heart's main pumping chamber

murmur: the sound made by blood flowing backward through a heart valve

syncope: fainting, passing out, temporary loss of consciousness

Epidemiology

Aortic stenosis can be a result of a congenital malformation, calcification, or rheumatic disease. Congenital malformations are sometimes missed early in childhood and need correction during adolescence. Aortic stenosis due to calcification is more typical, generally affects the tricuspid valves, and usually manifests in men in their 60s to 80s. Aortic stenosis resulting from rheumatic disease primarily affects the mitral valve and is rare in developed countries.

Pathobiology

With aortic stenosis, the blood must work harder to get through the calcified or malformed leaflets. In order for this to occur, the muscles of the left ventricle (LV) become thickened and hypertrophic. This increase in muscle thickness preserves the heart's ejection fraction and the cardiac output, allowing the body to receive the necessary blood. Although LV hypertrophy serves as a preserving mechanism, it also leads to some of the pathological symptoms associated with aortic stenosis.

Symptoms

Angina. Chest pain, shortness of breath, and fatigue during

Pathologic specimen of severely stenotic trileaflet aortic valve. Gross nodular atherocalcific changes on the aortic sides of the leaflet can be seen. (Cleveland Clinic)

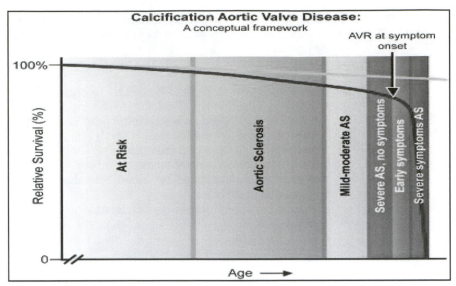

Calcific aortic valve disease: outflow obstruction is the end stage of a systemic disease process. (European Heart Journal)

which ultimately leads to heart failure.

Signs

During the physical exam, a systolic ejection murmur is typically heard in the aortic area with a delayed pulse in the carotid artery. The hypertrophic LV is not displaced but is enlarged and demonstrates a bounding pulse. A co-occurring bounding pulse in the apex with a delayed and weak pulse in the carotid is characteristic of aortic stenosis.

Diagnosis

Echocardiography is most diagnostic due to its ability to identify a LV hypertrophy, systolic ejection performance, and any aortic valve deformities. When echocardiography shows severe aortic stenosis and the patient is exhibiting the signs and symptoms mentioned, no further testing is necessary.

exercise can be signs of angina. In order for the hypertrophic LV to maintain its adequate ejection fraction, it must use up the blood supply coming into the heart. Reduced blood flow to the rest of the heart causes angina.

Syncope. Syncope is due to poor blood flow to the brain during exertion. The brain's increased blood demand and the heart's decreased cardiac output due to the narrowing of the tricuspid valves results in inadequate cerebral perfusion, culminating in syncope.

Heart Failure. Heart failure in aortic stenosis is a result of both systolic and diastolic failure. Systolic failure occurs due to the heart's inability to contract properly. Diastolic failure is due to the inability of the hypertrophic LV to relax completely. As aortic stenosis progresses, deposition of collagen on the heart further stiffens the heart muscles,

Treatment

No medicinal interventions are efficacious in treating aortic stenosis. Avoiding strenuous exercise, careful follow-ups, and periodic echocardiograms are suggested for asymptomatic patients. For symptomatic patients, aortic valve replacement is the only proven treatment. All patients, regardless of age, benefit from valve replacement. Antibiotics are needed in those with mechanical valves undergoing surgical or dental procedures.

Illustration of aortic valve stenosis and thickened ventricular wall. (Mayo Clinic, 2013)

Prognosis

In asymptomatic patients, survival is age-matched. With symptomatic patients, survival declines dramatically, averaging at three-year mortality without aortic valve replacement.

—Roushig Grace Kalebjian, MA, RN

See also Aortic insufficiency, Stenosis, Mitrial Stenosis, Heart valve disease

For Further Information:

Armstrong, Guy P. "Aortic Stenosis." *The Merck Manual: Home Health Handbook for Patients and Caregivers.* Retrieved from http://www.merckmanuals.com/home/heart_ and_blood_ves-sel_disorders/heart_valve_disorders/aortic_ steno-sis.html?qt=aortic%20stenosis&alt=sh

Carabello, A.B. "Valvular Heart Disease." *Goldman's Cecil Medicine,* edited by Lee Goldman and Andrew I. Schafer, 453-457. Philadelphia: Elsevier Saunders, 2008.

Otto, C.M. "Clinical Features and Evaluation of Aortic Stenosis in Adults." *UpToDate,* edited by D.S. Basow. Retrieved from http://www.uptodate.com/contents/clinical-features-and- evaluation-of-aortic-stenosis-in-adults

Otto, C. "Calcific Aortic Valve Disease: Outflow Obstruction Is the End Stage of a Systemic Disease Process." *European Heart Journal,* 30 (2009):1940-1942. Retrieved from http://eurheartj.oxfordjournals.org/content/30/16/1940.full.

Apgar score

Procedure

Anatomy or system affected: Circulatory system, heart, lungs, muscles, nervous system, respiratory system

Specialties and related fields: Critical care, neonatology, obstetrics

Definition: Virginia Apgar, an obstetrical anesthesiologist, developed the Apgar score in 1952 to assess the clinical status of newborns and the effectiveness of resuscitation.

Indications and Procedures

The five categories evaluated by the Apgar score-heart rate, respiratory effort, muscle tone, response to stimulus (reflex response), and color-reflect functions necessary to sustain life. The accompanying table lists the components in descending order of importance. The Apgar score is the sum of scoring (0, 1, or 2) each of the five parameters.

The first Apgar score is traditionally assigned at one minute after birth. It reflects the baby's condition in the womb and indicates the degree of resuscitation that may be required. A low one-minute score is not predictive of adverse neurologic outcome.

A second Apgar score is assigned at five minutes after birth. A score of 7 to 10 is considered normal, while a score of 4 to 6 is considered borderline. A five-minute Apgar score of 3 or less has been associated with cerebral palsy in full-term infants; however, only approximately 4 to 5 percent of infants with low five-minute Apgar scores have long-term neurologic abnormalities. A stronger relationship exists between low Apgar scores and future neurologic disability when the assessment is taken at times greater than ten minutes after birth.

Perspective and Prospects

Approximately 1.4 percent of all babies have Apgar scores of less than 7 at five minutes after birth. The highest proportions of infants with low Apgar scores at five minutes are among infants born to mothers under sixteen years of age or over forty years of age and to those who did not receive adequate prenatal care.

Current research using the Apgar score focuses increasingly on the neonatal heart rate and respiratory effort, looking for long-term subtle behavioral disabilities that may be associated with low and borderline Apgar scores.

—David A. Clark, M.D.

See also Birth defects; Blue baby syndrome; Cardiovascular system; Childbirth; Childbirth complications; Jaundice; Multiple births; Neonatology; Physical examination; Pregnancy and gestation; Premature birth; Reflexes, primitive; Respiration; Respiratory distress syndrome; Screening; Well-baby examinations.

For Further Information:

"APGAR." *Medline Plus,* December 2, 2011.

"Apgar Scores." *American Academy of Pediatrics,* May 31, 2013.

Apgar, Virginia, and Joan Beck. *Is My Baby All Right?* New York: Pocket Books, 1974.

Barness, Lewis A. *Manual of Pediatric Physical Diagnosis.* 6th ed. St. Louis, Mo.: Mosby Medical, 1991.

Schwartz, M. William, et al., eds. *Schwartz's Clinical Handbook of Pediatrics.* 5th ed. Philadelphia: Wolters Kluwer/Lippincott Williams & Wilkins, 2012.

Zitelli, Basil J., and Holly W. Davis, eds. *Atlas of Pediatric Physical Diagnosis.* 6th ed. St. Louis, Mo.: Mosby/Elsevier, 2012.

Aphasia and dysphasia

Disease/Disorder

Anatomy or system affected: Brain, nervous system

Specialties and related fields: Neurology, speech pathology

Definition: Aphasia is loss of the comprehension or production of language, while dysphasia is impairment of comprehension or production of language.

Key terms:

angiography: a series of X-ray films taken in a fixed sequence using contrast dye so that pictures of the arteries, smaller vessels, and veins can be obtained

ataxia: lack of coordination and irregularity of voluntary,

The Apgar Score			
Sign	**0**	**1**	**2**
Heart rate (beats per minute)	Absent	Below 100	Above 100
Respiratory effort	Absent	Slow, irregular	Good crying
Muscle tone	Limp	Some	Active motion
Response to nasal catheter	None	Grimace	Cough, sneeze
Color	Blue or pale	Body pink, extremities blue	Pink

purposeful movements

computed tomography (CT) scan: a noninvasive diagnostic study consisting of a series of X-ray films scanning different levels of the brain and resulting in pictures that show hemorrhages, tumors, cysts, edema, infarction, atrophy, and hydrocephalus

electroencephalography (EEG): recording of the electrical activity of the brain by using eight to sixteen electrodes placed on specific areas of the scalp; used to evaluate cerebral disease, as well as metabolic and systemic disorders, and to diagnose brain death

hemiparesis: weakness on one side of the body

myoclonus: a series of shocklike contractions that cause throwing movements of a limb

nystagmus: involuntary oscillations of one or both eyes

paresthesia: numbness and tingling sensations in the extremities

ptosis: sagging or drooping; often refers to ptosis of the eyelids, usually as a result of muscle weakness

---

Information on Aphasia and Dysphasia

Causes: Dysfunction in the left cerebral hemisphere, primarily from stroke but also from various vascular, neoplastic, traumatic, degenerative, metabolic, or infectious diseases or injuries

Symptoms: Various language dysfunctions (fluency, volume, or quantity of speech)

Duration: Acute, chronic, or progressive, depending on cause

Treatments: Speech therapy, treatment of underlying cause

Causes and Symptoms

Dysphasias are usually associated with cerebrovascular accident (CVA), or stroke, involving the middle cerebral artery or one of its many branches. Language disorders may arise, however, from a variety of injuries and diseases: vascular, neoplastic, traumatic, degenerative, metabolic, or infectious.

Dysphasia results from dysfunction in the left cerebral hemisphere, most commonly in the frontotemporal region of the brain and particularly around the insula. Most language disorders are attributable to acute processes that either resolve or cause a chronic residual deficit, while others result from degenerative disorders that cause the dysfunction to be progressive.

Dysphasias have been classified both anatomically and functionally. Other classifications are linguistic and describe the fluency, volume, or quantity of speech. Pure forms of any language dysfunction, however, are very rare. Expressive dysphasias are primarily characterized by expressive deficits, but a verbal comprehension deficit may be present. Receptive dysphasias have expressive deficits. Transcortical dysphasias involve the ability to repeat and to recite. Speech is fluent but with striking paraphrases. The individual is unable to read and write, and comprehension is impaired.

Transcortical dysphasias are caused by hypoxia (oxygen deficiency) from prolonged hypotension (low blood pressure), carbon monoxide poisoning, or other mechanisms that destroy the border zone between the anterior, middle, and posterior cerebral arteries. Blood supply is marginal in this region. Hypoxia in this area may occasionally isolate the posterior speech areas or all the speech areas from the remainder of the cortex, although both areas remain intact. The sensory and motor speech areas are, therefore, functional, but connections with other sensory or motor areas are impaired. Information from the remaining areas of the cortex cannot be transmitted to be transformed into language.

Aphasias can be classified into Broca's, Wernicke's, anomic, or global aphasias. Aphasia reflects damage to one or more of the brain's primary language centers, which, in most persons, are located in the left hemisphere. Broca's area lies next to the region of the motor cortex that controls the muscles necessary for speech, and presumably coordinates their movement. Wernicke's area, which helps control the content of speech and affects its auditory and visual comprehension, lies between Heschl's gyrus, the primary receiver of auditory stimuli, and the angular gyrus, a "way station" between the auditory and visual regions. Connecting Wernicke's and Broca's areas is a large nerve bundle, the arcuate fasciculus, which also helps control the content of speech and enables repetition.

The left hemisphere is dominant for language in all right-handed people and in the majority of left-handed people. When a stroke occurs in the dominant hemisphere, the patient may experience dysphasia or aphasia. Language disorders involve the expression and comprehension of written or spoken words. When the lesion involves Wernicke's area of the brain, the patient experiences receptive aphasia; neither the sounds of speech nor its meaning can be distinguished, and comprehension of both written and spoken language is impaired. The lesion causing expressive aphasia affects Broca's area, the motor area for speech. The patient has difficulty speaking and writing. Aphasias may be classified as either nonfluent or fluent. In nonfluent aphasia, the patient speaks very little and produces speech slowly and with obvious effort. In fluent aphasia, the patient may speak, but the phrases have little meaning because of impaired comprehension. Conduction aphasia is a type of fluent aphasia in which the lesion is in the pathway between Broca's and Wernicke's areas. Most aphasias are mixed, with some impairment of both expression and understanding. A massive lesion may result in global aphasia, in which virtually all language function is lost.

Stroke is the most common cause of aphasia. Associated findings usually include decreased level of consciousness, right-sided hemiparesis, and paresthesia. Another communication problem experienced by many stroke patients is dysarthria, or slurred speech. Dysarthria results from a disturbance in muscular control and produces impairment of pronunciation, articulation, and phonation. Dysarthria does not result in any disturbance of language function itself. However, an occasional stroke patient may be unfortunate enough to have both aphasia and dysarthria.

A transient ischemic attack (TIA) can produce any type of aphasia. Usually, the aphasia occurs suddenly and resolves within twenty-four hours of the TIA. Brain abscess may result in any type of aphasia. Usually, the aphasia develops insidiously and may be accompanied by hemiparesis, ataxia, facial weakness, and signs of increased intracranial pressure. A brain tumor may cause anomic aphasia, which may be an early sign of the condition. Encephalitis (brain inflammation) usually produces transient aphasia. Its earlier signs include fever, headache, and vomiting. Accompanying the aphasia may be convulsions, confusion, stupor or coma, hemiparesis, asymmetrical deep tendon reflexes, positive Babinski's reflex, ataxia, myoclonus, nystagmus, ocular palsies, and facial weakness. Head trauma may cause any type of aphasia. Typically, aphasia resulting from severe trauma occurs suddenly and may be transient or permanent, depending on the extent of brain damage. Anomic aphasia may begin insidiously and then progress; associated signs include behavioral changes, memory loss, poor judgment, restlessness, myoclonus, and muscle rigidity. Alzheimer's disease, a degenerative dementia, may also cause aphasia. Drug abuse, particularly heroin overdose, can cause any type of aphasia.

Depending on its severity, aphasia may impede communication slightly or may make it impossible. Anomic aphasia eventually resolves in more than 50 percent of patients, but global aphasia is irreversible.

In the pediatric population, aphasia is sometimes mistakenly attributed to children who fail to develop normal language skills but who are not considered mentally retarded or developmentally delayed. Aphasia refers solely to loss of previously developed communication skills, however, and should not be used in this context. Brain damage associated with aphasia in children most commonly follows anoxia (oxygen deprivation), the result of near-drowning or airway obstruction.

Treatment and Therapy

If a person suddenly develops aphasia, a physician should be notified immediately. The patient is assessed quickly for signs of increased intracranial pressure, such as papillary changes, decreased level of consciousness, vomiting, seizures, bradycardia (slow heart rate), widening pulse pressure, and irregular respirations. If signs are detected related to increased intracranial pressure, appropriate medications are administered to decrease cerebral edema. Emergency resuscitation equipment may be used to support respiratory and cardiac function, if necessary. Emergency surgery may be indicated.

If the patient does not display signs of increased intracranial pressure, or if the aphasia has developed gradually, then a thorough neurologic assessment is performed, starting with the patient history. Information may be obtained from the patient's family or companion because of the patient's impairment. The staff member assigned to the patient's care will ask about a history of headaches, hypertension, or seizure disorders, as well as about any drug use.

The patient's ability to communicate and to perform routine activities before the aphasia began is assessed. The patient is checked for obvious signs of neurologic deficit, such as ptosis or fluid leakage from the nose and ears. The patient's vital signs are taken and level of consciousness assessed. Assessing the level of consciousness is often difficult, however, because the patient's verbal responses may be unreliable. In addition, dysarthria or speech apraxia (the inability to control voluntarily the muscles of speech) may accompany aphasia. The patient should be allowed ample time to respond and should be spoken to slowly. Assessment of pupil response, eye movements, and motor function, especially mouth and tongue movement and swallowing, is conducted. To best assess motor function, the care provider will first demonstrate and then have the patient imitate responses, rather than merely providing verbal directions.

Immediately after aphasia develops, the patient may become confused or disoriented. The care provider can help restore a sense of reality by frequently telling the patient what has happened, where he or she is and why, and the date. The patient needs careful explanation of diagnostic tests, such as computed tomography (CT) scans, angiography, and electroencephalography (EEG). Later, periods of depression are expected as the patient recognizes the handicap. The patient can be aided in attempts at communication through a relaxed, accepting environment with a minimum of distracting stimuli. When speaking to the patient, the staff assigned to care cannot assume that he or she understands. The patient may simply be interpreting subtle clues to meaning, such as social context, facial expressions, and gestures. To help avoid misunderstanding, care providers should speak in simple phrases and use demonstration to clarify verbal directions. Because aphasia is a language disorder, not an emotional or auditory one, a normal tone of voice should be used when speaking to the patient. Necessary aids, such as eyeglasses or dentures, should be provided to facilitate communication. Referrals to speech pathologists early in the development of the problem will help the patient cope with aphasia.

—*Jane C. Norman, Ph.D., R.N., C.N.E.*

See also Brain; Brain disorders; Neurology; Neurology, pediatric; Speech disorders; Strokes; Transient ischemic attacks (TIAs).

For Further Information:
Aminoff, Michael J., David A. Greenberg, and Roger P. Simon. *Clinical Neurology.* 7th ed. New York: McGraw-Hill Medical, 2009.
Rowland, Lewis P., ed. *Merritt's Textbook of Neurology.* 12th ed. Philadelphia: Lippincott Williams & Wilkins, 2010.
Samuels, Martin A., ed. *Manual of Neurologic Therapeutics.* 7th ed. New York: Lippincott Williams & Wilkins, 2004.
Victor, Maurice, and Allan H. Ropper. *Adams and Victor's Principles of Neurology.* 9th ed. New York: McGraw-Hill, 2009.

Aphrodisiacs
Treatment
Also known as: Love potions
Anatomy or system affected: Genitals (theoretically), psychic-emotional system
Specialties and related fields: Alternative medicine

Definition: Substances capable of inducing sexual desire or lust or enhancing sexual performance.

Indications and Procedures

The word "aphrodisiac," derived from Aphrodite, the mythical Greek goddess of love, describes a number of animal and plant products reputedly capable of promoting sexual desire. Aphrodisiacs are thought to function in one of three ways: promote a desire for sexual stimulation or sexual appetite, increase the ability to indulge in sexual activity, or increase the capability and prolong the ability to maintain successful sexual activity.

The concept of natural substances being used to promote sexual activity has been a feature of art and literature throughout history, but modern medical and scientific opinions have been dismissive, concluding that no such substances that can be quantitatively measured exist in natural products. Despite this knowledge, the market for aphrodisiacs flourishes, in many cases to the detriment of rare or endangered plants and animals whose natural characteristics are falsely considered to harbor the means of enhancing sexual pleasure.

At the same time, a number of modern drugs are being manufactured, prescribed, and used in clinical medicine to restore the sexual capability of patients who suffer either physical or pathological disorders resulting in organic impotence (lack of the physical capability for sexual performance). Modern pharmaceutical manufacturers aggressively market numerous proprietary hormone and testosterone replacement therapies and priapitic drugs. A clinical drug prescribed for penile dysfunction, such as Viagra (sildenafil), by strict definition could be considered an aphrodisiac.

Uses and Complications

One major motive for the use of aphrodisiacs is a feeling of sexual inadequacy. For individuals who consider themselves sexually adequate yet still use aphrodisiacs, mere physical performance and sexual stamina are less important. These people tend to use aphrodisiacs in the hope of increasing their sexual pleasure. However, there is little evidence to support the efficacy of substances commonly thought to be natural aphrodisiacs. Individuals interested in increasing their sexual desire should talk to their doctor. Limiting stress, treating any underlying medical conditions that may affect sexual performance, or consulting a therapist who specializes in sexuality and intimate relationships may help to improve sexual function and satisfaction.

—*Randall L. Milstein, Ph.D.*

See also Hormones; Masturbation; Reproductive system; Sexual dysfunction; Sexuality.

For Further Information:

Stanley, Autumn. *Mothers and Daughters of Invention*. Metuchen, N.J.: Scarecrow Press, 1993.
Stark, Raymond. *The Book of Aphrodisiacs*. New York: Stein and Day, 1981.
Swanson, Janice B. "Do Natural Aphrodisiacs Actually Work?" *Mayo Clinic*, July 14, 2012.
Taberner, P. V. *Aphrodisiacs: The Science and the Myth*. Philadelphia: University of Pennsylvania Press, 1985.

Apnea

Disease/Disorder

Anatomy or system affected: Brain, lungs, nervous system, respiratory system

Specialties and related fields: Internal medicine, neonatology, neurology, pulmonary medicine

Definition: Cessation of breathing, from the Greek meaning "without wind."

Causes and Symptoms

People normally experience brief pauses in breathing. When these pauses last more than twenty seconds or are accompanied by bradycardia (slow heart rate) or cyanosis (bluish skin from poor blood oxygenation), however, they can be life threatening. This condition is referred to as apnea.

Apnea can be categorized into three types based on whether inspiratory muscle activity is present. In central apnea, which has a neurological cause, there is no activity of inspiratory muscles following expiration. Central apnea is uncommon except in cases of prematurity in infants. Obstructive apnea, the most common type, occurs when the person is making an effort to breathe, so inspiratory muscles are moving. As a result of a blockage, however, air cannot flow into or out of the person's nose or mouth. This condition typically occurs while the patient is asleep and is characterized by snoring, gasping for air, or stridor (noisy breathing). It is seen in people who have a physical obstruction in the airway, who experience gastroesophageal reflux, or who are overweight. The third type of apnea is mixed apnea, which is a combination of central and obstructive apnea. It is usually seen in young children and can occur while asleep or awake.

Individuals with apnea will often show decreases in heart rate, oxygen saturation, peripheral blood flow, and muscle tone. Adults suffering from sleep apnea may exhibit depression, irritability, learning difficulty, and sleepiness during the day. With sleep apnea, there can be up to sixty apneic episodes per hour, with snoring or choking in between.

All forms of apnea can be diagnosed by electrophysiological testing. Pneumograms are often done on premature babies to record their pattern of breathing over a twelve-hour period. Polysomnography is used for older children and adults to record electrical activity of the brain, muscle activity, heart rate, airflow, oxygen levels in the body, and eye movement.

Treatment and Therapy

The treatment of apnea can be based on medication, mechanical treatment, or surgery. The category of drugs used to treat apnea is xanthines. Mechanical treatment involves the use of continuous positive airway pressure (CPAP), a mask worn over the nose during sleep that forces air through the nasal passages. Another potential treatment

Information on Apnea

Causes: Inspiratory muscle inactivity, airway obstruction

Symptoms: Choking, snoring, gasping, stridor, bradycardia, cyanosis, depression, irritability, learning difficulty, daytime sleepiness

Duration: Chronic, with multiple episodes during sleep

Treatments: Medication (xanthines), mechanical treatment (continuous positive airway pressure mask), surgery

involves the use of a mandibular advancement device (MAD), a specially designed and fitted oral appliance that prevents obstruction of the throat during sleep. Surgery may be performed to remove an obstruction or to increase the size of the airway. Overweight patients are often encouraged to exercise and improve their diet.

Perspective and Prospects

Studies have indicated that people with obstructive sleep apnea have less gray matter in their brains. Research is being done to determine if the lack of gray matter leads to the apnea or the lack of oxygen caused by apnea causes deterioration in the brain.

—*Robin Kamienny Montvilo, R.N., Ph.D.*

See also Asphyxiation; Cyanosis; Hypoxia; Lungs; Pulmonary diseases; Pulmonary medicine; Pulmonary medicine, pediatric; Respiration; Resuscitation; Sleep; Sleep apnea; Sleep disorders; Wheezing.

For Further Information:

George, Ronald B. *Current Pulmonology and Critical Care Medicine*. Vol. 17. Philadelphia: Mosby, 1996.

Klaus, Marshall H., and Avroy A. Fanaroff, eds. *Care of the High-Risk Neonate*. 5th ed. Philadelphia: W. B. Saunders, 2001.

Pack, Allan, ed. *Sleep Apnea: Pathogenesis, Diagnosis, and Treatment*. 2d ed. New York: Marcel Dekker, 2008.

"Sleep Apnea." *MedlinePlus*, Apr. 19, 2013.

White, Emily, Thomas Workman, Amir Sharafkhaneh, and Michael Fordis. "Treating Sleep Apnea: A Review of the Research for Adults." *Agency for Healthcare Research and Quality*, Aug. 8, 2011.

Appendectomy

Procedure

Anatomy or system affected: Abdomen, gastrointestinal system, intestines

Specialties and related fields: Emergency medicine, general surgery

Definition: Corrective surgery to remove the appendix, which is required when acute appendicitis produces severe abdominal pain and the probability of peritonitis or health complications, which may be fatal if untreated.

Key terms:

cecum: a pouchlike portion of the large intestine

fecalith: a hardened piece of fecal matter which often begins events leading to appendectomy by blocking the appendix

peritonitis: infection of the abdominal (peritoneal) cavity in which the visceral organs are found

septic pyelophlebitis: inflammation of the veins which carry blood away from the kidneys; it results from neglecting symptoms of acute appendicitis and can be fatal

Indications and Procedures

The appendix, more correctly named the vermiform appendix, is a hollow tube of muscle attached to the pouchlike beginning of the large intestine (the cecum) and closed at the end farthest from this point of attachment. It does not serve a known purpose and is thought to be a disappearing vestige of an organ that once had a purpose. Hence the appendix is called a vestigial organ.

A vermiform appendix exists only in humans and other primates. In humans, it is approximately 7.6 to 10.2 centimeters (3 to 4 inches) long and 1.3 centimeters (0.5 inches) in diameter. The cavity of the appendix (its lumen) is narrowest at the point of attachment to the cecum, and the muscular walls of the organ normally contract periodically to expel into the cecum both mucus made by the appendix and intestinal contents that may have accidentally entered the lumen.

When the narrow opening of the appendix into the cecum is blocked so as to prevent expulsion of mucus or fecal material, the organ becomes infected, a condition called appendicitis. The most frequent obstructions found in appendix openings are fecaliths. These objects are hardened pieces of fecal matter that entered the appendix from the large intestine. Swelling of the inner walls of the appendix as a result of other causes (such as bacterial infection) can also begin such a blockage.

Following blockage, the events leading to appendicitis usually occur in the following order. First, fluids and mucus secreted by the cells lining the walls of the appendix collect in the blocked organ. This makes the appendix swell, causing the blood vessels that feed the organ's tissues gradually to close off. In the absence of an adequate blood supply, the tissue begins to die. At the same time, bacteria originating in the cecum grow vigorously in the affected appendix, increasing the inflammation and swelling of the dying organ.

Quick and appropriate treatment by surgical removal of the infected appendix-appendectomy-is required at this time. Otherwise, the walls of such an appendix, one weakened by tissue death and subjected to increasing pressure by both bacterial growth and the buildup of mucus, may burst. When this happens, the contents spill into the abdominal cavity and infect the membranes that line it. Such infection, peritonitis, is very serious and painful. In most cases, however, the use of antibiotics will keep peritonitis from becoming fatal.

Where open-surgery appendectomy is required, the patient is usually given a general anesthetic and a 5.1- to 7.6-centimeter(2- to 3-inch) incision is made directly over the site of the appendix. Where laparoscopic surgery is performed, three small incisions (1.2 centimeters or 0.5 inches long) will be made in the abdomen; a small camera called a laparoscope is then passed through one incision and surgical tools are inserted into the other incisions. In both procedures, the surgeon then ties off and cuts the blood vessels

The Removal of the Appendix

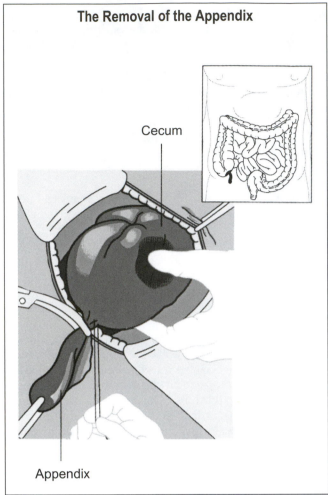

Cecum

Appendix

Inflammation of the appendix, a vestigial organ attached to the colon, usually requires an emergency appendectomy to avoid rupture and more extensive, life-threatening infection; the inset shows the location of the appendix.

that feed the organ. Next, the appendix is tied off near its connection to the cecum and carefully cut free without allowing its contents to enter the abdominal cavity. The operation usually takes under an hour and produces minor postoperative discomfort for a few days. The surgical risks of this procedure are very slight. Some of the benefits of laparoscopic surgery include less scar tissue and a shorter duration of postoperative discomfort.

Uses and Complications

Acute infection of the appendix, requiring its surgical removal, is the most frequent cause for abdominal surgery. It is most likely to occur between the ages of eight and thirty, but no age group is exempt. Acute appendicitis is often symptomized by initial generalized abdominal pain that rapidly becomes localized. The pain, which can be quite severe and which is felt whenever the patient moves or coughs, frequently occurs in the lower-right quadrant of the abdomen (an area between the navel and the front edge of the right hipbone). This location is common because many appendixes are located in the underlying abdominal cavity. The appendix may be found, however, in any of several

other positions. Hence, the pain can occur elsewhere in the abdomen, and acute appendicitis may be mistaken for other abdominal disorders.

Other symptoms useful in diagnosing acute appendicitis are nausea and vomiting, increased pulse rate, and mild fever. In addition, the patient's white blood count will often increase from the normal range of 7,000 to 10,000 per cubic millimeter to 25,000. Doctors can also use computed tomography (CT) scanning for diagnostic purposes. When symptoms of acute appendicitis occur, medications should not be given unless quick access to surgical facilities is available. For example, cathartics are a poor treatment choice because they stimulate intestinal contractions that may accelerate intestinal rupture. Similarly, the use of hot water bottles to relieve pain is inappropriate because it may also speed rupture. In cases of acute pain, the patient should be taken to a hospital emergency room as quickly as possible.

The dangers associated with appendicitis arise from its neglect. Peritonitis is rarely fatal because of the timely use of antibiotics. Much more serious are localized abscesses of the abdominal wall and the inflammation of the veins that carry blood away from the kidneys (septic pyelophlebitis). Both of these problems can be fatal, even when extensive and aggressive antibiotic therapy is carried out.

—*Sanford S. Singer, Ph.D.*

See also Abdomen; Abdominal disorders; Appendicitis; Emergency medicine; Gastroenterology; Gastroenterology, pediatric; Gastrointestinal system; Infection; Inflammation; Intestinal disorders; Intestines; Laparoscopy; Pediatrics; Peritonitis.

For Further Information:

"Appendectomy-Laparoscopic Surgery." *Health Library*, November 30, 2012.

"Appendectomy-Open Surgery." *Health Library*, November 7, 2012.

"Appendectomy: Surgical Removal of the Appendix." *American College of Surgeons*, 2012.

Krahenbuhl, L. *Acute Appendicitis: Standard Treatment or Laparoscopic Surgery?* New York: Karger, 1998.

Papadakis, Maxine, et al., eds. *Current Medical Diagnosis and Treatment 2013*. New York: McGraw-Hill Medical, 2012.

Porter, Robert S., et al., eds. *The Merck Manual of Diagnosis and Therapy*. 19th ed. Whitehouse Station, N.J.: Merck Research Laboratories, 2011.

Zinner, Michael J., et al., eds. *Maingot's Abdominal Operations*. 12th ed. New York: McGraw-Hill, 2012.

Appendicitis
Disease/Disorder

Anatomy or system affected: Abdomen, gastrointestinal system, intestines

Specialties and related fields: Emergency medicine, gastroenterology, pediatrics

Definition: Inflammation of the human vermiform appendix.

Causes and Symptoms

Appendicitis may be acute or chronic. The inflammation characteristic of the condition may be associated with infection, or the causes may be various or even unknown.

Information on Appendicitis

Causes: Infection or unknown
Symptoms: Abdominal pain, nausea, fever, elevated white blood cell count
Duration: Acute or chronic
Treatments: Surgical removal of appendix

In the human digestive system, the small intestine empties into the large intestine, or colon, in the lower right abdomen. Movement of waste from that point is generally upward through the ascending colon, but the colon begins with a downward-projecting blind end called the cecum, to which is attached the vermiform ("wormlike") appendix. The appendix has no known function. Occasionally, its opening into the cecum becomes obstructed, and inflammation, swelling, and pain follow. Sometimes the cause of the obstruction is identifiable, such as parasitic pinworms or hardened fecal material; more often, it is not. Symptoms, including pain that is general at the outset but localizes in the lower right abdomen, can include nausea, fever, and an elevated white blood cell count. If the swollen appendix bursts, peritonitis-infection and poisoning of the abdominal cavity-can result. Peritonitis is usually signaled to the patient by an abrupt cessation of pain, when the swelling is relieved, but is followed by serious and life-threatening complications.

Treatment and Therapy

The treatment of choice is almost invariably surgical removal of the inflamed appendix, an operation that is no longer considered major surgery. The patient is usually out of bed in a day or two and fully recovered in a few weeks. Peritonitis, however, calls for emergency surgery to remove the toxic material released by the ruptured appendix, as well as the appendix itself. Because a greater or lesser portion of the abdominal cavity must be cleansed with saline solution and treated with antibiotics, this surgery can become a major procedure.

—*Robert M. Hawthorne, Jr., Ph.D.*

See also Abdomen; Abdominal disorders; Appendectomy; Gastroenterology; Gastroenterology, pediatric; Gastrointestinal disorders; Gastrointestinal system; Infection; Intestinal disorders; Intestines; Obstruction; Pediatrics; Peritonitis.

For Further Information:

A.D.A.M. Medical Encyclopedia. "Appendicitis." *MedlinePlus,* July 22, 2011.
Brodsky, Jason A., ed. "Appendicitis." *National Digestive Diseases Information Clearinghouse,* February 16, 2012.
Clayman, Charles B., ed. *The American Medical Association Encyclopedia of Medicine.* New York: Random House, 1994.
Krahenbuhl, L. *Acute Appendicitis: Standard Treatment or Laparoscopic Surgery?* New York: Karger, 1998.
Litin, Scott C., ed. *Mayo Clinic Family Health Book.* 4th ed. New York: HarperResource, 2009.
Wagman, Richard J., ed. *The New Complete Medical and Health Encyclopedia.* 4 vols. Chicago: J. G. Ferguson, 2002.
Wood, Debra, and Marcin Chwistek. "Appendicitis." *Health Library,* November 8, 2012.

Aromatherapy

Treatment

Anatomy or system affected: Brain, nervous system, nose, psychic-emotional system
Specialties and related fields: Alternative medicine, otorhinolaryngology, preventive medicine, psychology
Definition: The use of scents to facilitate physical, mental, and emotional well-being.

Indications and Procedures

Aromatherapy is best thought of as a complement to other procedures or treatments. Essential oils and aromatic plants are used to stimulate memories, bring about feelings of calm, aid meditation, and enhance visualization exercises. Aromatherapy helps create to conditions that enhance the ability to concentrate, to mentally or physically relax, or to discuss or recall personal information or memories. As such, aromatherapy may be an appropriate adjunctive treatment for stress-related disorders and other disorders treated with psychotherapies. Some practitioners suggest that specific scents have extraordinary properties (such as memory enhancers or aphrodisiacs), but little scientific evidence exists for such claims.

Methods of aromatherapy are

The vermiform appendix, located in the lower-right abdomen at one end of the large colon, may become inflamed as a result of obstruction; surgery is nearly always required to avoid bursting and the release of deadly toxins into the body.

Appendix

varied but chiefly involve scent inhalation alone or in combination with massage. With massage, essential oils (oils from aromatic plants) are applied directly to the body and massaged into the skin. Otherwise, essential oils are inhaled briefly, as one might use "smelling salts," or in a more diffuse manner, as with incense or perfume. Oils may be dabbed on pulse points, dispersed by fragrance diffusers, simmered in potpourri vessels, added to boiling water to be diffused by steam, or added to baths.

Uses and Complications

Allergic reactions to the aromatic oils are the greatest complication of aromatherapy. The substances typically used are highly concentrated and not safe for internal use. In the hands of an unskilled user, the oils may create unpleasant odors or allergic reactions. In addition, the long-term effects of such inhalants on lung functioning are not well documented; caution must be advised.

Perspective and Prospects

Historically, perfumes were offered to the gods by the Greeks, were essential for burial rites among the Egyptians, and were said to attract good spirits among American Indians. Today, scents are used widely by therapists and individuals alike to facilitate well-being. Future work will likely include greater research on aromatherapy's safety and the role of olfaction on memory functioning.

—*Nancy A. Piotrowski, Ph.D.*

See also Allergies; Alternative medicine; Anxiety; Herbal medicine; Smell; Stress; Stress reduction.

For Further Information:

"Aromatherapy." *American Cancer Society*, April 2012.

Bauer, Brent A. "What Are the Benefits of Aromatherapy?" *Mayo Clinic*, May 27, 2011.

Lawless, Julia. *The Complete Illustrated Guide to Aromatherapy: A Practical Approach to the Use of Essential Oils for Health and Well-Being.* New York: HarperCollins, 2002.

Ryman, Daniele. *Aromatherapy: The Complete Guide to Plant and Flower Essences for Health and Beauty.* New York: Bantam, 1993.

Arrhythmias

Disease/Disorder

Also known as: Dysrhythmias, conduction disturbances

Anatomy or system affected: Heart

Specialties and related fields: Cardiology

Definition: A disturbance of electrical conduction activity in the heart. Potential causes range from medications to diseases or conditions that delay or block an impulse in the conduction system.

Key terms:

atria: the two upper chambers of the heart, which receive blood from the body and lungs and send it to the ventricles; the sinoatrial node is located in the upper right atrium

conduction pathway: a system of nodes and tracts through the heart that conduct electrical impulses to its muscle cells, creating coordinated contraction

electrocardiogram (ECG or EKG): a recording of the electrical activity of the heart

sinoatrial (S-A) node: the pacemaker of the heart; also called the sinus node

ventricles: the two lower chambers of the heart, which receive blood from the atria and send it to the body and lungs

Causes and Symptoms

The heart is a unique muscle with characteristics of each of the other two types of muscle, skeletal and smooth. Like skeletal muscle cells, myocardial cells are striated and contract following the all-or-none principle, but individual cells can contract independently. Like smooth muscle, the heart is controlled by the autonomic nervous system but able to contract independently because it has its own unique conduction system, composed of the sinoatrial (S-A) node; the interatrial and internodal conduction tracts; the atrioventricular (A-V) junction, including the A-V node and bundle of His; the right and left bundle branches; and the Purkinje fibers.

The heart delivers blood to all tissues needing nutrients and oxygen. The ability to contract effectively twenty-four hours a day, seven days a week for years requires a system with good internal control and many backup systems. Blood flow through the heart needs to move progressively through the right atrium and ventricle to the lungs in order to oxygenate the blood and through the left atrium and ventricle and out to the body to deliver the nutrients and oxygen. Control of heart rate and rhythm by the autonomic nervous system and conduction tissues creates effective pumping.

When something goes awry with the electrical impulses controlling this pumping, the condition is called an "arrhythmia" and is defined by where the problem originates. Arrhythmias range from benign to life threatening, depending on which portion of the heart is involved. The description of arrhythmias follows the conduction system, from S-A node or sinus arrhythmias to independent ventricular myocardial cells producing ectopic (extra) beats, called "premature ventricular contractions (PVCs)." These may be occasional single irregular beats of little consequence or a series of irregular beats that compromise regular blood flow. The determination of what type of arrhythmia is present is made by interpreting the results of one or more tests, which may include an electrocardiogram (ECG or EKG), exercise stress test, or electrophysiological test.

Two types of arrhythmias may occur: impulse propagation, in which an area of the heart or conduction tissue blocks the passage of an impulse, or impulse initiation, in which an area of the heart or conduction tissue becomes excited and creates one or more extra beats. They may occur because of something acute and reversible, such as inadequate oxygenation (myocardial infarction, or heart attack), or a chronic condition, possibly from damage to the myocardial tissue or the conduction system.

Treatment and Therapy

Depending on the diagnosis, treatments range from nothing

Information on Arrhythmias

Causes: Inadequate oxygenation (as from heart attack), medications, various conditions
Symptoms: Often none; blood clots possible
Duration: Acute or chronic
Treatments: None, medications, or surgery (pacemaker implantation, heart transplantation), depending on severity

to hospitalization. An example of a benign arrhythmia is sinus bradycardia, a normal rhythm but a very slow rate, less than sixty beats per minute. Athletes often have well-conditioned cardiovascular systems that pump more blood each beat than do those of nonathletes; thus, their heart rates are slower when the same amount of blood needs to be delivered.

The other extreme, ventricular fibrillation, is characterized by ventricular cells contracting wildly. Blood flow is totally disrupted, and if the arrhythmia is not controlled by defibrillation (the application of electricity), then sudden death will occur. In between these extremes would be someone who reacts to caffeine. Premature atrial contractions (PACs), isolated early beats coming from irritated cells in the atrium, may occur when a person is under stress or has taken stimulants. The obvious treatment is to remove the stress or the stimulant in order to return the heart to normal.

The treatment of arrhythmia may depend on whether it has an impact on blood flow. It is important to keep blood moving smoothly and progressively through the heart to maintain blood flow and oxygenation of body tissues. Additionally, when blood flow is turbulent, the cells suspended in the blood bump into one another, and some are damaged. When this happens, blood clots can form. If an abnormal number of clots occur, a greater chance exists that they could also block a blood vessel in the brain, heart, or lungs, which can be life threatening.

The decision to treat the arrhythmia or to try to prevent complications, such as blood clots, is a question for patients and physicians. Medications can be used to reduce clotting, but this requires long-term treatment with possible side effects. Surgical procedures-such as radiofrequency ablation, which destroys an abnormal electrical pathway causing an arrhythmia, or the Maze procedure, which forms new pathways using scar tissue-may result in permanent cure, avoiding the need for lifelong medication. Knowing the risks and benefits of each treatment helps the patient decide.

If damaged myocardium is the cause of the arrhythmia, then the physician will determine the extent of the damage and offer treatment options, ranging from medications to surgery. The medication may interrupt or keep the arrhythmia from occurring, or it may help the weakened muscle pump blood, which will increase the flow of oxygen and help reduce the chance for further arrhythmias.

If the conduction system is not functioning, then a pacemaker may be inserted and attached to the heart to create a regular rhythm. If the problem is ventricular fibrillation that cannot be controlled with medication, an internal defibrillator may be placed to shock the heart back to a normal rhythm. At the extreme, a heart transplant has the ability to correct an arrhythmia, but this is not usually the reason that a transplant occurs. A transplanted heart has its internal conduction system intact and so should be able to beat on its own.

Perspective and Prospects

The longer one lives, the greater the chance that the heart muscle or conduction system will be damaged. Therefore, it is essential that pharmaceutical companies continue to search for effective drugs and that surgeons continue to refine the techniques required to best treat arrhythmias. Pacemakers have advanced dramatically since the early 1980s, from bulky instruments with nonrechargeable batteries to sophisticated, miniature combination machines that can adjust the heart rate depending on need and, in the extreme, defibrillate with a shock to convert a problem arrhythmia. A concerted effort by emergency medical personnel and technicians has created automatic external defibrillators (AEDs) that anyone can use to allow those people suffering from fibrillation to be saved. Such devices are necessary because cardiopulmonary resuscitation (CPR) is effective in only about 20 percent of cases, often because fibrillation persists during CPR and continues to interrupt blood flow.

—*Wendy E. S. Repovich, Ph.D.*

See also Arteriosclerosis; Atrial fibrillation; Cardiology; Cardiology, pediatric; Cardiopulmonary resuscitation (CPR); Defibrillation; Echocardiography; Heart; Heart attack; Heart disease; Hypertension; Ischemia; Mitral valve prolapse; Pacemaker implantation; Palpitations; Panic attacks.

For Further Information:

A.D.A.M. Medical Encyclopedia. "Arrhythmias." *MedlinePlus*, June 22, 2012.
Angelopoulos, Theodore J. "Electrocardiography." In *ACSM's Clinical Certification Review*, edited by Michael S. Wegner, Jeanne E. Ruff, and Walter R. Thompson. Philadelphia: Lippincott Williams & Wilkins, 2001.
Carson-DeWitt, Rosalyn, and Michael J. Fucci. "Arrhythmias." *Health Library*, November 8, 2012.
"Heart Arrhythmias." *Mayo Foundation for Medical Education and Research*, February 27, 2013.
Pappano, Achilles J., Withrow Gil Wier, and Matthew N. Levy. *Cardiovascular Physiology*. 9th ed. St. Louis, Mo.: Mosby, 2006.
Boyer, Mary Jo. *Lippincott's Need-to-Know ECG Facts*. Philadelphia: Lippincott Williams & Wilkins, 1997.

Arteriosclerosis

Disease/Disorder

Anatomy or system affected: Blood vessels, circulatory system, heart

Specialties and related fields: Cardiology, internal medicine, vascular medicine

Definition: Also called atherosclerotic disease or "hardening of the arteries," a generalized disease that causes narrowing of the arteries because of deposits on the arterial walls and leads to a multitude of serious medical conditions, notably stroke and heart attack.

Key terms:

angina: chest, jaw, or shoulder pain with exercise or stress- a symptom of atherosclerotic heart disease

embolus: a small piece of atherosclerotic plaque, thrombus, or other debris that breaks off and lodges in a blood vessel

infarct: tissue death resulting from lack of blood flow

intermittent claudication: a symptom of lower extremity arteriosclerosis manifested by pain or cramping in the leg while walking, relieved by rest; from the Latin word *claudicatio*, "to limp"

ischemia: lack of blood in a particular tissue

rest pain: pain noted in the most distal portion of the extremity at rest, relieved by analgesics

revascularization: procedures to reestablish the circulation to a diseased portion of the body

thrombosis: aggregation of platelets and other blood cells to form a clot

Causes and Symptoms

The human body's arterial system is designed to carry oxygen, hormones, various types of blood cells (such as red and white blood cells), and other nutrients in the blood from the heart to the periphery and all organ structures of the body. The arteries are composed of three separate layers: adventia (the outer layer), media (the middle layer), and intima (the inner layer). Atherosclerosis or arteriosclerosis, derived from the Greek words that mean "hardening of the arteries," refers to the different diseases that compromise one or more of the layers of the large or medium-sized arteries or smaller arterioles. Most commonly, fat, cholesterol, and calcium deposits are laid down along the intima and inner portion of the media. These components build up, forming plaques, which then may produce stenosis (narrowing) or occlusion (closure) of the arterial lumen. Accumulation of platelets and other blood cells can form a thrombus along with plaque buildup, which also obstructs the arteries. Pieces of plaque or thrombotic material can break off, causing emboli to lodge in the vessels acutely. Atherosclerosis begins with some form of damage to the delicate lining of the intima (the endothelium), by infections, inflammation, hypertension, or even natural toxins. That damage induces platelet adherence and other repair mechanisms, creating an opportunity for the accumulation of fat and calcium deposits in plaques.

Depending on the arterial segment in the body that is affected, various diseases and symptoms may occur. As the blood vessels become diseased with plaque buildup, the body will try to compensate by the development of collaterals, small vessels that bypass the diseased artery. Collateral vessels are smaller than the native arteries and cannot accommodate the same amount of blood. Normally, during exercise, there is an increased demand for additional blood flow to the muscles; flow will increase and the arteries will dilate. With atherosclerosis, since the arteries are blocked and collaterals cannot accommodate the additional blood volume, waste products in the muscles build up, causing pain. In the heart, this process affects the flow in the coronary arteries, and angina (chest pain) may occur.

Information on Arteriosclerosis

Causes: Increased levels of fat, cholesterol, and/or calcium deposits that form plaques in arteries

Symptoms: Angina, cramping in extremities, pallor, parathesias

Duration: Chronic

Treatments: Drugs, bypass surgery, lifestyle changes

In lower extremity arteriosclerosis, stenosis or occlusions of the aorta, iliac, femoral, popliteal, or tibial arteries may occur, producing intermittent claudication.

As the disease progresses, more blood vessels become stenosed or occluded and collateral formation will maximize, but the circulation is severely limited and ischemia may result. In atherosclerotic heart disease, significant ischemia may then result in a myocardial infarct, or heart attack. In the lower extremities, patients may develop rest pain. The most severe symptoms of lower extremity arteriosclerosis are the development of nonhealing ulcers and gangrene (tissue death) in the lower portion of the foot, similar to a heart attack. When the disease process has become this severe, there are multisegmental areas of arterial occlusions and no further compensatory mechanisms. Monckeberg's sclerosis, not usually thought of as a true form of atherosclerosis, refers to the disease in which calcification of the tibial arteries is noted, often in diabetic patients.

Acute arterial ischemia is a sudden onset of ischemia as opposed to the more common chronic processes described above. The usual cause of acute arterial ischemia is an embolus (portion of a clot) that lodges in thearteries. The most common source of embolization is the heart; embolization from the heart occurs in patients who have recently had a heart attack, who have mitral valvular disease, or who have atrial fibrillation (irregular heartbeats). Another cause of acute arterial ischemia is thrombosis of, or embolization from, an aneurysm. An aneurysm, another disease process, produces a weakening of the adventia and a "ballooning" of the arteries with a thrombus (clot). Rupture or thrombosis (clotting off) may be a consequence of aneurysmal disease. In such cases, because no significant collaterals have developed in the area of the acute blockage, immediate revascularization is mandatory to prevent significant tissue death.

In cerebrovascular disease, atherosclerosis affects the arteries supplying the circulation to the brain (the carotid and vertebral-basilar system). The most common symptoms noted are transient ischemic attacks (TIAs), also referred to as ministrokes. TIAs usually last less than twenty-four hours. Most TIAs are produced by embolization, in which pieces of plaque in the major arteries break off and temporarily block the blood flow to certain areas of the brain. Once the symptoms last more than twenty-four hours, a cerebrovascular accident (CVA), cerebral infarct, or stroke has occurred. Atherosclerosis in the cerebrovascular system will behave in a manner similar to that previously described, with increasing stenosis and eventual occlusion.

Collateral development seems to be especially prominent in the cerebrovascular system, since the brain is a greedy organ needing blood at all times. The majority of CVAs are caused by occlusion or thrombosis of a major vessel, producing significant ischemia in a portion of the brain.

Cerebral aneurysms due to atherosclerosis can rupture (sometimes as the result of uncontrolled hypertension) and bleed, causing tissue destruction from both the presence of blood and the compensatory vasospasm and ischemia. The result is a CVA or even death.

Contributing or significant risk factors in the development of atherosclerosis include hypertension (high blood pressure), hyperlipidemia (high amounts of fats or lipids in the blood), smoking, diabetes mellitus, and family history. Inflammation, especially from infections, is a significant risk factor as well. Also, depending on the significance and the location of atherosclerosis, a variety of symptoms and conditions can result. In atherosclerotic heart disease, the first symptom is angina. As in intermittent claudication, chest, shoulder, or upper back pain may occur during exercise or stress as a result of the decreased blood supply to the tissues of the end organ, the myocardium (heart muscle). As the disease progresses, the angina will become more unstable and patients will become progressively limited in minor activities. Symptoms of a heart attack may include severe, crushing chest pain, shortness of breath, pain in the left arm, and tingling of the fingers. Cessation of breathing and cardiac arrest indicate a significant heart attack. Immediate medical attention during the severe symptomatic phase or with cardiac arrest will aid in reducing further damage to the heart muscle and may prevent death. Many heart attacks are "silent" in that, although portions of the cardiac muscle are "dead," symptoms will have been negligible or minor, because of sufficient collateralization.

In lower extremity atherosclerosis, patients with intermittent claudication will complain of pain or cramping in their calves, thighs, or buttocks while walking or exercising; symptoms will be relieved by rest. Claudication is usually described by distances, such as "one block" claudication or "half a mile" claudication. Rest pain occurs mostly at night at the most distal portion of the extremity, usually the toes and forefoot. Often patients will sleep in chairs or with their legs hanging off the bed to relieve the pain. On physical examination, the foot is usually cool to the touch, with a slightly bluish discoloration. There is hardening of the nails, dryness of the skin, and loss of hair in the lower portion of the leg. Pulses are absent or diminished. Often, when the leg is in a dependent position, dependent rubor, a purplish discoloration of the leg, is seen, produced by dilation of the small blood vessels in the skin to provide the maximum amount of blood. Elevating the leg will produce a cadaverous white pallor. Because of the limited blood supply, ulcers will not heal and gangrene can develop. Patients with symptoms of severe claudication, rest pain, or neuropathic diabetes should be evaluated prior to undergoing any podiatry procedures because their compromised circulation will result in poor healing. Patients with acute arterial ischemia of the lower extremity will

Arteriosclerosis leads to the buildup of fatty plaques on the walls of arteries, which inhibits blood flow and may lead to obstructions resulting in stroke, heart attack, and other life-threatening events.

complain of the "five P's": pain, pallor, pulselessness, paresthesia (decrease of feeling), and paralysis. As previously described, emergent revascularization of the acutely ischemic limb is necessary to prevent limb loss or amputation.

Although aneurysmal disease is a separate entity, it may be associated with atherosclerotic disease in certain cases. Most aneurysms produce no symptoms. Detection of aneurysms is usually incidental; during a physical examination, for example, a physician may note a pulsatile mass in the abdomen (aorta, iliac), in the groin (femoral), or behind the knee (popliteal). Incidental diagnosis of aneurysms may also occur during routine chest X rays; the X ray may reveal a calcium rim around the body of the aneurysm. As aneurysms increase in size, the probability of rupture increases; therefore, elective surgery is usually recommended once certain sizes are achieved: more than six centimeters for an abdominal aneurysm and more than two centimeters for femoral and popliteal aneurysms. Symptoms of a rupturing abdominal aneurysm include severe lower back pain and a decrease in blood pressure, whereas thrombosis of a popliteal or femoral aneurysm will cause an acutely ischemic leg. Symptomatic aneurysms are considered medical emergencies, since ruptures may result in death and thrombosis in limb loss.

Symptoms of TIAs due to thrombosis in the carotid arteries, which supply the front of the brain, include hemiparesis (weakness) or paresthesia, aphasia (speech disorder) when the left carotid is affected, and amaurosis fugax (loss of vision likened to seeing a window shade being pulled down) resulting from blockage of the ophthalmic artery (which branches off the carotid) on the side of the blindness. Other symptoms include dizziness, vertigo, imbalance, and other visual disturbances. These more generalized symptoms are referable to the vertebral-basilar circulation, which supplies the back portions of the brain, or are a result of multisegmental cerebrovascular disease in which a low-flow state can affect multiple areas of the brain and produce diverse symptoms. A stroke is an event whose symptoms will last more than twenty-four hours. Often these are permanent deficits, affecting the patient for the rest of his or her life.

Many patients will be asymptomatic (have no symptoms) and not develop TIAs but will have a stroke, which may result from eventual occlusion or thrombosis of the cerebral vessels and infarcts in a particular section of the brain. Asymptomatic cerebrovascular disease is often detected by the presence of a bruit (French for "noise"). Stenosis in arteries resembles rapids in a river: Flow will go very fast through the blockage and then be turbulent. The turbulence will produce a bruit which can be detected with a stethoscope. Turbulence from stenoses ranging from 20 to 80 percent can cause a bruit. The absence of a bruit does not mean that the arteries are disease-free. Once the stenosis reaches critical proportions, the flow is diminished and turbulence may be negligible. An occluded artery will also have no bruit, since there is no flow. Once the narrowing has reached 60 to 80 percent, many doctors will recommend elective surgery to reestablish flow and prevent eventual occlusion and possible stroke. About 75 percent of strokes are ischemic, resulting from this process. Bruits may be appreciable in other parts of the body and can also indicate the presence of atherosclerosis in those areas.

Atherosclerosis of the renal arteries, which supply the kidneys, may cause a condition known as renovascular hypertension. This type of high blood pressure is often difficult to control with medication, and continued high blood pressure will contribute to progression of the atherosclerotic process elsewhere in the body.

Another condition that results from atherosclerosis is chronic mesenteric ischemia. Here the blood vessels supplying the intestines, the stomach, and many of the organs associated with the digestive process are affected. Patients may experience pain with eating and significant weight loss. This condition is often missed until an extensive workup for cancer or other chronic diseases yields negative results. In acute mesenteric ischemia, by contrast, thrombosis of the superior mesenteric artery occurs. As with other acute arterial conditions, emergent revascularization is necessary to prevent gangrene of the intestines.

Treatment and Therapy

A complete history and physical examination are usually the first methods of diagnosing atherosclerosis. Eliciting symptoms, noting significant risk factors and physical findings, will aid the physician in determining areas at risk.

In lower extremity atherosclerosis, a common noninvasive method utilizes Doppler ultrasound. A series of blood pressure cuffs are attached to the extremity, and segmental blood pressure and plethysmographic wave-

forms are measured. A drop of more than twenty millimeters of mercury (mm Hg) of pressure between segments or extremities is indicative of a significant stenosis at that level, or a ratio of less than 0.5 when the ankle pressure is compared to the brachial pressure (a normal ratio is 1.0). Exercise testing will demonstrate whether there are significant drops in pressure, confirming the diagnosis and severity of claudication.

Duplex ultrasound machines utilize B-mode (brightness-mode) ultrasound to visualize the vessels and type of plaque, while Doppler ultrasound can audibly evaluate the blood flow in the vessels. Using real-time spectrum analyzers, the Doppler signals are then analyzed in terms of velocities and waveform characteristics. The greater the velocities, the greater the amount of stenosis. Absence of blood flow will denote occlusions. The use of color duplex ultrasound, in which the Doppler signals are color-coded in terms of flow direction and speed to denote the various flow patterns in normal and diseased vessels, has enhanced the diagnostic accuracies in the examinations. The use of color Doppler in many of the ultrasound machines is aiding in more rapid detection of arterial lesions in cardiac, cerebrovascular, and lower extremity arterial circulation.

Arteriography or angiography is an invasive procedure. The delineation of the blockages and collateral pathways detected through this method-in which the patient is hospitalized and a catheter is used to inject dye containing iodine into the arteries-is then used to plan a revascularization procedure.

Ultrasound is the primary diagnostic tool for detecting and measuring the size of aneurysms. Computed tomography (CT) scanning is an alternative radiological modality to visualize aneurysms.

The majority of patients with mild to moderate intermittent claudication can be treated conservatively. Cessation of smoking, alterations to diet, and a carefully controlled exercise plan will alleviate or decrease the progression of symptoms. Less than 5 percent of patients with intermittent claudication will develop gangrene sufficient to warrant a major amputation within a five-year period.

Some medications available work by decreasing the stickiness of the platelets in the blood; these are often prescribed for patients with claudication. Aspirin is often prescribed to alleviate symptoms of TIAs and to protect patients from strokes or heart attacks. Although it is a powerful drug in decreasing the incidence of embolization, a national study has demonstrated that patients with TIAs and severe stenosis of the carotid arteries should undergo surgical revascularization to protect against major strokes. It has become clear that aspirin may also be helpful because of its anti-inflammatory properties, particularly now that the role of damage to the endothelium from inflammation and infections is understood.

Severe disabling claudication, rest pain, ulceration or gangrene of the lower extremity, and unstable angina and heart attacks require some sort of surgical intervention. Usually bypass surgery is planned to revascularize the ischemic portion of the extremity or myocardial tissue to prevent limb loss or further cardiac events. The arteriogram will illustrate the areas of blockage, and, depending on the results of this test, various types of bypasses can be performed. Inflow procedures refer to bypasses performed above the groin. Aorto-iliac or aorto-femoral are the most common types performed, usually utilizing a prosthetic (plastic) material. Outflow procedures are those performed below the groin; these include femoral-popliteal or femoral-tibial bypasses. Prosthetics are sometimes used, but the best bypass material in terms of durability is the patient's own vein, either removed and reversed, or in situ (in place). Depending on the type of bypass procedure performed, the five-year patency rates (number of bypasses open at five years) exceed 85 percent for aorto-iliac/aorto-femoral bypasses and 75 percent for lower extremity reconstructions. Coronary artery bypass grafts (CABGs) typically employ the saphenous veins of the legs or the mammary artery of the chest wall to bypass the diseased segments in the heart vessels.

Endarterectomy, a surgical technique in which the intima and part of the media are excised, effectively "scrapes out" atherosclerotic plaques. Although used in other arterial segments, endarterectomy is the most common surgical procedure used to revascularize the carotid arteries.

Other interventional modalities have been developed. Percutaneous balloon angioplasty involves placing a balloon catheter in the diseased segment during an angiogram and opening up the area of stenosis or small segmental occlusion. This method has been employed in the coronary arteries as well as in the vessels of the aorta, iliacs, and lower extremities.

New lytic drugs, which "dissolve" clots, are sometimes employed alone, or in combination with balloon angioplasties or surgery, especially in the more acute cases of lower extremity arterial ischemia and myocardial infarctions.

Perspective and Prospects

Atherosclerosis of the coronary and cerebrovascular system is a major cause of death. Heart attacks are the primary cause of death in the United States, with approximately 650,000 people dying annually. Half of those deaths are sudden, with no prior significant symptoms. Stroke is the third leading cause of death in the United States, with approximately 155,000 deaths annually. There are 400,000 strokes annually, and about one-fourth of all nursing home patients are permanently impaired from strokes. These statistics have a great impact on the amounts of health care moneys spent annually to care for victims of heart disease and strokes.

Since the 1960s, the rates of death from both heart attacks and strokes in the United States have decreased significantly. Control of blood pressure and diet, the development of new drugs and diagnostic techniques, and the advent of cardiovascular surgery in the early 1950s have aided in this decrement. Unfortunately, atherosclerotic diseases are still prevalent. Autopsies of Korean War and Vietnam War American soldiers demonstrated that atherosclerotic plaque was evident even at an early age. This was attributed to the high-fat diet of most Americans. It is recognized that this disease is more prevalent in young males and that females are more protected until the onset of menopause; then the death rates tend to equalize. High-salt diets, which may increase the incidence of hypertension, also contribute to the development and progression of atherosclerosis. Since the 1960s, extensive education of the American public regarding dietary control has had a favorable impact. More recently, the benefits of exercise have helped to stem the atherosclerotic process.

The 1950s saw the development of cardiovascular surgery. The first bypass (arterial autograft) probably occurred during the Korean War. Coronary artery bypass surgery and carotid endarterectomies are among the most common surgical procedures performed today. Recognition of and prompt treatment of cardiac and cerebrovascular symptoms remain the key to better survival rates. With development of newer bypass materials for lower extremity bypass surgery in the 1970s, as well as better surgical techniques for utilization of the saphenous veins, the amputation rate has significantly decreased. Research into graft materials that better mimic the native arteries and veins continues.

Since the 1950s, a number of noninvasive and invasive procedures have been developed to diagnose atherosclerotic disease. The development of ultrasound devices in the 1950s initiated the research into using these noninvasive devices to diagnose atherosclerotic disease. The duplex devices, introduced commercially in the late 1970s and early 1980s, opened a new diagnostic field for detection of atherosclerotic disease. These devices allow for visualization of plaque morphology (composition of the plaque such as thrombus, calcium, and hemorrhage) and the blood-flow characteristics for a better understanding of the atherosclerotic process. Future developments in the field of ultrasound include holographic imaging for three-dimensional visualization of plaques. These noninvasive technologies will also allow physicians to monitor the effects of new drugs and techniques in the treatment of atherosclerosis. Advances in digital subtraction and computer enhancement of angiographic techniques, along with new contrast media, are making arteriograms safer and more accurate.

Current diagnostic technologies include magnetic resonance imaging (MRI), a nonradiological modality for visualizing structures in the brain and other portions of the body. MRI is used with the aid of computerization to do MR angiography. Magnetic resonance is also utilized to measure, noninvasively, actual flow in individual arterial segments of the body in terms of cubic centimeters per minute. Positron emission tomography (PET) scanning, a non-X-ray method, gives brilliant, color-enhanced visualization of blood flow to tissues.

—*Silvia M. Berry, M.Sc., R.V.T.;*
updated by Connie Rizzo, M.D., Ph.D.

See also Angina; Angiography; Angioplasty; Bypass surgery; Cardiac arrest; Cardiology; Cholesterol; Circulation; Claudication; Edema; Embolism; Endarterectomy; Echocardiography; Heart; Heart attack; Heart disease; Heart failure; Hypercholesterolemia;

Hyperlipidemia; Hypertension; Ischemia; Metabolic syndrome; Phlebitis; Plaque, arterial; Stents; Strokes; Thrombolytic therapy and TPA; Thrombosis and thrombus; Transient ischemic attacks (TIAs); Vascular medicine; Vascular system; Venous insufficiency.

For Further Information:

Crawford, Michael, ed. *Diagnosis and Treatment in Cardiology.* New York: McGraw, 2002.

Eagle, Kim A., and Ragavendra R. Baliga, eds. *Practical Cardiology: Evaluation and Treatment of Common Cardiovascular Disorders.* 2d ed. Philadelphia: Lippincott, 2008.

Goldman, Lee, and Dennis Ausiello, eds. *Cecil Textbook of Medicine.* 23d ed. Philadelphia: Saunders, 2007.

Hoffman, Gary S., and Cornelia M. Weyand. *Inflammatory Diseases of Blood Vessels.* New York: Dekker, 2002.

MedlinePlus. "Atherosclerosis." *MedlinePlus*, Apr. 24, 2013.

The New Good Housekeeping Family Health and Medical Guide. New York: Hearst, 1989.

Rosenblum, Laurie. "Atherosclerosis." *Health Library*, Nov. 11, 2012.

Rutherford, Robert B., ed. *Vascular Surgery.* 6th ed. Philadelphia: Saunders, 2005.

Tierney, Lawrence M., Stephen J. McPhee, and Maxine A. Papadakis, eds. *Current Medical Diagnosis and Treatment 2007.* New York: McGraw, 2006.

Arthritis

Disease/Disorder

Anatomy or system affected: Bones, hands, hips, immune system, joints, knees, legs, musculoskeletal system

Specialties and related fields: Internal medicine, orthopedics, physical therapy, rheumatology

Definition: A group of more than one hundred inflammatory diseases that damage joints and their surrounding structures, resulting in symptomatic pain, disability, and systemwide inflammation.

Key terms:

anti-inflammatory drugs: drugs to counter the effects of inflammation locally or throughout the body; these drugs can be applied locally or introduced by electric currents (in a process called ionthophoresis), by injections into the joint or into the muscles, or by mouth; the three classes of these drugs are steroidal, immunosuppressant, and nonsteroidal

cartilage: material covering the ends of bones; it does not have a blood supply or nerve supply but may swell or break down

inflammation: the body's defensive and protective responses to trauma or foreign substances by dilution, cellular efforts at destruction, and the walling-off of irritants; characterized by pain, heat, redness, swelling, and loss of function mediated through a chemical breakdown

physical modalities: the physical means of addressing a disease, which include heat, cold, electricity, exercises, braces, assistive devices, and biofeedback

rehabilitation: a physician-led program to evaluate, treat, and educate patients and their families about the sequelae of birth defects, trauma, disease, and degenerative conditions, with the goals of alleviating pain, preventing complications, correcting deformities, improving function, and reintegrating individuals into the family and society

synovium: the cellular lining of a joint, having a blood supply and a nerve supply; the synovium secretes fluid for lubrication and protects against injury and injurious agents

Causes and Symptoms

Approximately one in six people (more than 15 percent) suffers from one of approximately one hundred varieties of arthritis, and 2.6 percent of the population suffers from arthritis that limits their activities. Although many people over seventy-five years of age experience arthritis, the disease can occur in the young as a result of infections, rheumatic conditions, or birth defects. Young and middle-aged adults experience the disease as a result of trauma, infections, and rheumatic or immune reactions. Arthritis may be located in joints, joint capsules, the surrounding muscles, or diffusely throughout the body. Inflammation of the joint lining (synovium) can similarly afflict the linings of other organs: the skin, colon, eyes, heart, and urinary passage. Those suffering from the disease may therefore suffer from psoriasis and rashes, spastic colitis and diarrhea, dryness of the eyes, inflammations of the conjunctiva or iris, frequent urination, discharge and burning upon urination, and other symptoms.

The collagen-type arthritic diseases involve the binding materials in the body or connective tissues and may be rheumatologic, generally more diffuse and in the distal joints (as in juvenile rheumatoid arthritis and rheumatic fever), or located in the skin and muscles (dermatomyositis). Psoriatic arthritis causes severe punched-out defects in the joints. Reiter's and Sjögren's syndromes involve the eyes and the joints. Genetic conditions, such as Gaucher's disease, frequently run in families. Metabolic disturbances, such as gout, can leave uric acid deposits in the skin and in the joints. Gout sufferers experience very painful, hot, tender, and swollen joints-often in the large toe. Immunologically mediated arthritides may be associated with infections, liver diseases, bowel disturbances, and immune deficiencies. Localized infections may be bacterial, viral, or fungal. "Miscellaneous disorders," a basket category, include conditions that do not fit into any of the aforementioned categories: Psychogenic disorders and arthritis associated with cystic disorders are examples. Arthritis may also be associated with tumors that grow from cartilage cells, blood vessels, synovial tissue, and nerve tissue. Blood abnormalities may give rise to hemorrhages into joints (a side effect of sickle cell disease and hemophilia) and can be disabling and very painful, sometimes requiring surgery. Traumatic and mechanical derangements-sports and occupational injuries, leg-length disparity, and obesity-may elicit acute synovial inflammation with subsequent degenerative arthritis. Finally, wear-and-tear degeneration can occur in joints after years of trauma, repetitive use, and (especially in the obese) weight-bearing. The most common arthritic entities are rheumatoid arthritis (also called atrophic or proliferative arthritis), osteoarthritis, hypertrophic arthritis, and degenerative arthritis.

The inflammatory reactions in response to injury or disease consist of fluid changes-the dilation of blood vessels accompanied by an increase in the permeability of the blood vessel walls and consequent outflow of fluids and proteins. Injurious substances are immobilized with immune reactions and removed by the cellular responses of phagocytosis and digestion of foreign materials, resulting in the proliferation of fibrous cells to wall off the injurious substances and in turn leading to scar formation and deformities. The chemical reactions to injury commence with a degradation of phospholipids when enzymes are released by injured tissue. Phospholipids-fatty material that is normally present-break down into arachidonic acid, which is further broken down by other enzymes, lipoxygenase and cycloxygenase, resulting in prostaglandins and eicosanoid acids. Most anti-inflammatory medications attempt to interfere with the enzymatic degradation process of phospholipids and could be damaging to the liver and kidneys and to the body's blood-clotting ability.

The physician bases the diagnosis of arthritic disease on the patient's medical history and a physical examination. Specific procedures such as joint aspiration, laboratory studies, and X-ray or magnetic resonance imaging (MRI) may help to establish the diagnosis and the treatment. The history will elicit the onset of pain and its relation to time of day and difficulties performing the activities of daily living. A functional classification has evolved that is similar to the cardiac functional classification: Class 1 patients perform all usual activities without a handicap; class 2 patients perform normal activities adequately with occasional symptoms and signs in one or more joints but still do not need to limit their activities; class 3 patients find that they must limit some activities and may require assistive devices; and class 4 patients are unable to perform activities, are largely or wholly incapacitated, and are bedridden or confined to a wheelchair, requiring assistance in self-care.

A person's medical history or surgical conditions and the medications that he or she is taking can influence the physician's diagnosis and prescription for treatment. Patients may present a gross picture of the body to the physician showing the joints involved in their symmetry (whether distal or proximal, and whether weight-bearing or post-traumatic in distribution). Physicians may ask (verbally or by questionnaire) for a history of other system complaints, which can then be checked more thoroughly. During a physical examination, the physician will check the joints, skin, eyes, abdomen, heart, and urinary tract. The neuromuscular evaluation may reveal localized tenderness of the joints or muscles, swelling, wasting, weakness, and abnormal motions. Joints may have weakened ligamentous, muscle, and tendon supports that could give rise to instability or grinding of joints, with subsequent roughening of cartilage surfaces. The arthritides are frequently associated with muscular pains, called fibrositis and myofascial pain syndromes.

Fibrositis is a diffuse muscular pain syndrome with tenderness in the muscles, no muscle spasm, and no limitations in motion; all laboratory tests are within normal limits. It is frequent in postmenopausal women who have a history of migraines, cold extremities, spastic colitis, softening of the bone matrix accompanied by loss of minerals,

---

Information on Arthritis

Causes: Infection, rheumatic conditions, birth defects, trauma, immune reactions, wear-and-tear degeneration

Symptoms: Joint pain, psoriasis and rashes, spastic colitis and diarrhea, dryness of the eyes, frequent urination

Duration: Chronic

Treatments: Anti-inflammatory drugs; application of heat, cold, or electricity; exercise; biofeedback; assistive devices

---

and irritability. Myofascial trigger points can be found in both men and women, at all ages, with acutely tender nodules or cords felt in muscles. The pain of these trigger points is referred to more distal areas of the muscles that may not be tender to touch. Physicians may frequently miss the acutely tender trigger points. Tests will show whether pain is elicited when muscles are contracted with motion, when muscles are contracted without motion, or when motion is carried out passively by the examiner without muscular effort by the patient.

Joint pathology is generally associated with some limitation in the range of motion. Sensation testing, muscle strength, and reflex changes may also indicate nerve tissue damage. Nerves occasionally pass close to joints and may be pinched when the joint swelling encroaches upon the passage opening. This condition may result in carpal tunnel syndrome, in which the median nerve at the wrist becomes pinched, causing pain, numbness, and weakness in the hand. Pinched nerves may also be associated with tarsal tunnel syndrome, in which the nerve at the inner side of the ankle joint may be compressed and cause similar complaints in the feet. Other nerves may be constricted in exiting from the spine and when passing through muscles in spasm.

The medications used to treat arthritis can involve the nervous system. An evaluation and estimation of the severity of the disease can be obtained by electrical testing, as in electroneuromyography. The nerves are stimulated, and their rate of transmitting the stimulus is measured. The normal transmission rate for nerves is forty-five meters per second. Delays at areas of impingement can be determined by measuring the transmission rate of a stimulus from different points along the nerve paths. Abnormal or damaged muscles will cause muscle fibers to contract spontaneously, or fibrillate. Chest expansion during inspiration and after expiration may be limited because of arthritis at the spine or because of lung pathology. Involvement of the spine can also be measured by the posture, the ability to move the neck, and the ability to move the lower back.

Arthritis of the spine leads to progressive loss in motion. The amount lost can be measured by comparing the normal motion with the restricted motion of the patient. The neck may be limited in all directions, rotation of the head to the sides can restrict the driving view, and the head may gradually tilt forward. The lower back may also exhibit restriction in all directions; for example, it may be limited in forward bending because of spasms in the muscles in the back. Tilting backward of the trunk may be limited and painful when the vertebral body overgrowth of osteoarthritis or degenerative arthritis restricts the space for the spinal cord. The nerves pinched in their passage from the vertebrae may thus cause radiculitis, irritation of the nerves as they exit from the spine that leads to pain and muscle involvement. Circumferential measurements of the involved joints and the structures above and below can confirm swelling, atrophy from disuse or inaction, or atrophy from a damaged nerve supply. When measurements are repeated, they can indicate improvement or deterioration. One type of arthritis that most often affects the spine, ankylosing spondylitis, occurs predominantly in males in their late teenage and early adult years.

Testing of blood for cells, chemicals, or enzymes is helpful. The simplest test-the sedimentation (or "sed") test-measures the rate at which blood cells settle out of the plasma. Normally, women have a more rapid rate of sedimentation than men. When this rate exceeds the normal range, active inflammation in the body is indicated. Comparisons of sed tests performed at different stages can reveal the disease's rate of progression or improvement. The chemicals tested may include uric acid for gout and sugar for diabetes. Blood tests for immune substances and antibodies are also possible, although the American College of Rheumatology recommends avoiding broad testing of antibodies. The joint fluid can be aspirated and analyzed, particularly for appearance, density, number of blood cells, and levels of sugar. Cloudy fluid, the tendency to form clots, a high cell count, and lower-than-normal levels of sugar in the joint fluid (compared to the overall blood sugar level) indicate abnormalities. With inflammatory arthritides, the X-rays will show the results of synovial fluid and cellular overabundance. Clumps of pannus break off and may destroy the cartilage and bone. Bones about these joints, because of increased vascularity and blood flow, have less minerals and will appear less dense, a condition known as osteoporosis.

Deformities in inflammatory arthritis may be the result of unequal muscle pulls or the destruction or scarring of tissues; such deformities can occasionally be prevented by the use of resting splints, which is most important for the hands.

Degenerative and post-traumatic arthritis show joint narrowing, thinning of the cartilage layer, hardening of the underlying bone (called eburnation), and marginal overgrowth of the underlying bone (called osteophytes),

---

In the News: Glucosamine and Chondroitin

Medical, surgical, and rehabilitative techniques have been used in the treatment of arthritis. Recently more people have turned to complementary and alternative medicine for treatment of medical disorders, including arthritis. Two nutritional supplements that have been widely used to treat osteoarthritis are glucosamine (a substance involved in cartilage formation and repair) and chondroitin sulfate (which provides cartilage with elasticity). While these substances are produced naturally by the human body, when marketed as dietary supplements glucosamine is usually derived from shellfish, while chondroitin comes from either cow or shark cartilage. Because dietary supplements are not regulated by any federal agency, consumers must be sure to deal with a reputable manufacturer to assure product quality.

A large-scale study of glucosamine and chondroitin in treating osteoarthritis of the knee was undertaken at sixteen rheumatology centers in the United States with funding from the National Institutes of Health. The first phase of the Glucosamine/Chondroitin Arthritis Intervention Trial (GAIT) compared five groups taking 1,500 milligrams of glucosamine, 1,200 milligrams of chondroitin sulfate, 1,500 milligrams of glucosamine with 1,200 milligrams chondroitin sulfate, 200 milligrams of a COX-2 inhibitor (a nonsteroidal anti-inflammatory drug, or NSAID, available by prescription to treat osteoarthritis), and a placebo. All substances used in this study were assessed to ensure their purity and quality. For patients who suffered moderate to severe pain (but not those suffering mild pain), the combination of glucosamine and chondroitin sulfate provided greater pain relief than did the placebo or the COX-2 inhibitor. Phase two of GAIT found that glucosamine and chondroitin were no more effective than a placebo at preventing joint damage caused by arthritis; the supplements did not slow the destruction of cartilage that leads to narrowing in knee joints.

Based on this study, the Arthritis Foundation suggests that these nutritional supplements should be used in conjunction with prescription medications and with exercise, weight control, and possibly surgery. Individuals considering glucosamine/chondroitin therapy should be aware that glucosamine is contraindicated for people with shellfish allergies and that it may affect blood sugar levels in diabetics. Chondroitin may affect blood-clotting ability in individuals taking anticoagulants. Research into the usefulness of glucosamine and chondroitin sulfate continues.

—*Robin Kamienny Montvilo, R.N., Ph.D.*

---

resulting in osteoarthritis. Osteophytes, or marginal lipping in the back, may enhance symptoms of lower back pain. The cushions between the vertebrae, called discs, are more than 80 percent water, a figure which diminishes with aging, bringing the joints in the back (the facets) closer together and compressing the facet joints between the vertebrae. Irritation and arthritis of these joints are the result. Other organ structures may be involved as well.

A diagnosis of rheumatoid arthritis should include two to four of the following criteria: morning stiffness, three or more joints involved symmetrically (especially the hands), six weeks or longer in duration, rheumatoid nodules that can be felt under the skin, blood tests showing a serum rheumatoid factor, and the radiographic evidence described above.

Treatment and Therapy

Treatment of arthritis may vary from home treatment to outpatient treatment to hospitalization for acute, surgical, and/or rehabilitative care. Educating patients as to their condition, the prognosis, the treatment goals, and the methods of treatment is necessary. Patients must be made aware of warning signs of progression, drug effects, local and systemic side effects of drug therapy, and diet associated with relieving pain, stiffness, and inflammation. If surgery is contemplated for joint replacement or other reasons, patients should be fully informed as to expectations and rate of functional activities. Postoperative restrictions in the range of motion must be given; in hip replacement, for example, hip bending should not exceed ninety degrees. The rotation and overlapping of legs must be limited initially after surgery.

Some physicians provide a questionnaire that outlines the activities of daily living and recommends how a patient should perform such activities and how much time should be spent at rest. The goals generally are to maintain function, to alleviate pain, to limit the progression of deformities, to prevent complications, and to treat associated and secondary disease states. In patients with degenerative arthritis-most often the elderly, who are at risk for other organ failures-arthritides associated with systemic diseases and other organ involvements may require care. Patients with rheumatoid arthritis, for example, frequently are anemic. Anti-inflammatory drugs, normally used to treat the arthritis, may cause blood loss through the gastrointestinal tract and even ulcerations. The physician may therefore prescribe alternative therapies.

Other therapies can include assistive devices, counseling patients and their families regarding home management, medicinal regimen and compliance, behavior modification, sexual advice, and biofeedback. The aim is to reduce the need for and frequency of medical care, through a balance between rest and activity and between effective drug dose, toxicity, and physical modalities. To protect joints and allow function, various braces and assistive devices may be needed. Scarring of a wrist joint can be alleviated by avoiding positions that inhibit function. Shoulders should not be left with arms close to the body, since frozen shoulders aggravate neck and arm problems.

Physicians may offer physical therapy, occupational therapy, assistive devices for self-care, ambulation, or home and automobile modifications. Assistive devices may include reachers, an elongated shoehorn handle, thickened handles for utensils, walkers, canes, crutches, and wheelchairs. Homes may require ramps for easier access, widened doors to allow wheelchair passage, grab bars in bathtubs, or raised toilet seats for easier transference from a wheelchair.

Heat therapy may reduce the pain, loosening and liquefying tightened tissues. Somewhat like gelatin, tissue liquefies when heated and solidifies when cooled. Patients frequently will be stiffer after protracted rest periods (for example, on waking) and feel better after some activity and exercise. Heated pools offer an excellent heating and exercise modality. The type of heat modality used will depend upon the depth of heating desired. Hot packs and infrared lamps will heat predominantly the skin surface areas and some underlying muscles. Diathermy units heat the muscular layers, and ultrasound treatments heat the deepest bony

layers. Ultrasound (but not diathermy) can even be used in patients who have metallic implants such as joint replacements.

Transcutaneous electrical nerve stimulation can be used to alleviate pain. The units can regulate the frequency of electrical impulses. The usual starting rate is 100 cycles, which can alleviate pain in a few minutes; this rate is later changed to 4 cycles, which will give hours of relief even when discontinued. The intensity can also be varied. The sensation desired is a slight tingle. The effect described induces an increase in the release of beta endorphin, a substance naturally produced by the body with effects similar to those of morphine. Endorphin is produced by other physical therapy procedures as well: hypnosis, acupuncture, suggestion, and stress, among others.

Patients in chronic pain may show a reduced level of the beta endorphin and an increase in a substance P, and they may find no relief of pain with physical therapy. The P chemical increases the nerves' sensitivity to stimuli, producing greater pain. Patients with chronic pain may show depression, hysteria, and hypochondriasis on the Minnesota Multiphasic Personality Inventory and may require antidepressants. Exercise programs can help to increase endorphin levels. These exercises may range from simple movements performed by a therapist (the patient remaining passive) to active exertion against loads for strength. Stretching or gentle, intermittent traction may gradually decrease contractures, but neck traction should not be used in patients with rheumatoid arthritis of the neck.

Surgery may occasionally be necessary to alleviate pain, to replace joints, or to alleviate contractures. Isometric or static exercises can mobilize muscles without joint movement and maintain muscle viability during joint pain. Individuals can, however, be trained to perform activities more efficiently and effectively, thus saving energy. Posture training may alleviate postural muscle fatigue. In acute stages of inflammation, the treatment choices are rest, ice, compression, and proper positioning and medicinals for pain and inflammation. The stepped-up medicinal approach utilizes nonsteroidal anti-inflammatory drugs (NSAIDS)-such as aspirin, indomethacin, ibuprofen, naproxen, piroxicam, and nabumetone-and adds other drugs as necessary, including antimalarials and gold, immune suppressants, and systemic corticosteroids. Irradiation of lymphoid tissues may also be used at the acute stages. Heat modalities should not be used in acute cases, since the speed of chemical reactions increases on heating; the chemical enzyme activity of collagenase that destroys cartilage could increase the rate and extent of damage. The simplest way to prepare cold applications is to fill a plastic container with water and refrigerate it. Physicians may also use fluoromethane or other refrigerant sprays. The hot packs sold in pharmacies can similarly be soaked in water and placed in the refrigerator to create an ice pack.

In 2002, researchers announced a new type of anti-inflammatory painkiller that showed promise in initial studies on people with arthritis in their knees. Licofelone works just as well as NSAIDs but seems to be gentler on the stomach. Medical experts believe that it will prove a better alternative to NSAID arthritis drugs such as Vioxx, Bextra, and Celebrex. Vioxx was removed from the market in September, 2004, and Bextra in April, 2005. All three are COX-2 selective inhibitors. These drugs selectively block the enzyme COX-2, the enzyme controlling the production of prostaglandins, natural chemicals that contribute to body inflammation and cause the pain and swelling of arthritis. They do not affect COX-1, however, so the selective aspect offers the benefit of diminishing inflammation without accelerating the risk of stomach ulceration and bleeding.

Perspective and Prospects

Historically, arthritis was treated with electric eels (as the source of electric shocks) and warm baths or sands. Some experimental treatments presently being tried include electric current to joints to bring about reductions in intra-articular pressures and in the fluid and cellular content in joints. Acupuncture has been shown to bring an increase in the beta endorphin levels and consequent relief of pain. Topical use of capsaicin, an extract from peppers, is reported to counteract substance P. One group is attempting the experimental procedure of washing out inflamed joints with a saline-type solution. Exercises continue to maintain and improve strength, dexterity, the range of motion, and endurance. Good health habits-including adequate rest, good nutrition, and nutritional supplements-can be beneficial.

—*Eugene J. Rogers, M.D.;*
updated by Victoria Price, Ph.D.

See also Anti-inflammatory drugs; Bone disorders; Bones and the skeleton; Bursitis; Fracture and dislocation; Gout; Hip fracture repair; Hip replacement; Inflammation; Joints; Juvenile rheumatoid arthritis; Massage; Muscle sprains, spasms, and disorders; Orthopedic surgery; Orthopedics; Orthopedics, pediatric; Osteoarthritis; Over-the-counter medications; Pain management; Physical rehabilitation; Reiter's syndrome; Rheumatoid arthritis; Rheumatology; Spinal cord disorders; Spine, vertebrae, and disks; Tendon disorders; Tendon repair.

For Further Information:

Aesoph, Lauri M. *How to Eat Away Arthritis*. Englewood Cliffs, N.J.: Prentice, 1996.
Arthritis Foundation. *The Arthritis Foundation's Guide to Good Living with Fibromyalgia*. Atlanta: Author, 2001.
Flynn, John A., and Lora Brown Wilder, eds. *Recipes for Arthritis Health*. New York: Rebus, 2003.
Fries, James F. *Arthritis: A Take-Care-of-Yourself Health Guide to Understanding Your Arthritis*. 5th ed. Reading, Mass.: Addison, 1999.
Hunder, Gene G. *Mayo Clinic on Arthritis*. Rev. ed. Rochester, Minn.: Mayo Clinic, 2002.
Lahita, Robert G. *Rheumatoid Arthritis: Everything You Need to Know*. Rev. ed. New York: Avery, 2004.
Lane, Nancy E., and Daniel J. Wallace. *All About Osteoarthritis: The Definitive Resource for Arthritis Patients and Their Families*. New York: Oxford UP, 2002.
Lorig, Kate, and James F. Fries, eds. *The Arthritis Helpbook: A Tested Self-Management Program for Coping with Arthritis and Fibromyalgia*. Updated ed. Cambridge, Mass.: Da Capo, 2007.
MedlinePlus. "Arthritis." *MedlinePlus*, Apr. 24, 2013.
Nelson, Miriam E., et al. *Strong Women and Men Beat Arthritis*. New York: Putnam, 2003.
Preidt, Robert. "HealthDay: 5 Rheumatology Procedures You Might Not Need." *MedlinePlus*, Mar. 5, 2013.
Sands, Judith K., and Judith H. Matthews. "Medications: Arthritis Drugs Hit Their Mark." *Harvard Health Letter* 24, no. 4 (February, 1999): 4-5.
Shlotzhauer, Tammi L., and James L. McGuire. *Living with Rheumatoid Arthritis*. 2d ed. Baltimore: Johns Hopkins UP, 2003.
Weinblatt, Michael E. *The Arthritis Action Program: An Integrated Plan of Traditional and Complementary Therapies*. New York: Fireside, 2001.

Arthroplasty

Procedure

Anatomy or system affected: Musculoskeletal system; joints of shoulder, elbow, wrist, hands, hips, knees, ankles.

Specialties and related fields: Anesthesiology, general surgery, geriatrics and gerontology, orthopedics, rheumatology, sports medicine, occupational and physical therapy.

Definition: A surgical procedure also referred to as joint replacement surgery in which parts of a degenerated and/or damaged joint are removed and replaced with a metal, plastic, or ceramic device called a prosthesis. The prosthesis is designed to replicate the movement of a normal, healthy joint.

Key terms:

acetabulum: the portion of the pelvic bone joining the femoral head to create the hip joint

cartilage: flexible connective tissue between bones

epidural: the injection of an anesthetic into the fluid around the spine or into the epidural space in the back

femur: the leg bone extending from the knee to the hip

orthopedics: a medical specialty emphasizing the prevention and correction of skeletal deformities

patella: the flat, triangular bone in the front of the knee; also called the kneecap

tibia: the shin bone

rheumatoid arthritis: a long-term autoimmune disorder that primarily affects joints resulting in warm, swollen, and painful joints

viscosupplementationinjections: injections to add lubrication into the joint to make joint movement less painful

Indications and Procedures

Cartilage within a joint covers the ends of the bones, preventing bone from pressing on bone and allowing smooth, pain-free movement. Joints can become painful when cartilage on the end of each adjoining bone deteriorates, a process called osteoarthritis. A fracture, trauma, or another medical condition such as rheumatoid arthritis can also cause joint pain and disability, any of which may lead an individual to consider arthroplasty. Should initial nonsurgical treatments such as medications, physical therapy, and joint injections prove to be unsuccessful, arthroplasty, a surgery undertaken to replace deteriorating joints, becomes an option, particularly among the elderly.

Arthroplasty may be performed on the fingers, wrists, shoulders, elbows, and ankles but the most common sites of the surgery are the hips and knees. Most patients requiring hip or knee replacements are over the age of fifty, but arthroplasty may be indicated for younger people who have suffered advanced joint deterioration or trauma. Specialists in sports medicine who are typically orthopedic surgeons also frequently prescribe arthroplasty.

The hip is a ball-and-socket joint comprising the top of the femur (ball) inserted into the acetabulum (socket). During walking, the top of the femur slides within the acetabulum. Cartilage of the hip joint normally covers both bones where they join permitting smooth, painless contact between the surfaces. When the cartilage deteriorates, bones rub against each other, causing pain and restriction in movement that is eventually best relieved by hip replacement surgery.

In hip surgery, an incision, varying in length from 2 to 12 inches, is made over the back of the hip (and more recently, the front of the hip, referred to as an anterior approach). Tissue and muscles are cut or pushed aside to expose the hip joint. The femur and acetabulum are separated. A cavity made in the acetabulum accommodates the replacement cup and allows for the insertion of a plastic-lined metal shell. The ball on the femur end of the joint is removed and replaced with a metal ball attached to a metal stem, usually made of titanium that is inserted into the femoral canal. The two parts are then cemented into place, making them adhere to the bone. Damaged muscles and tendons are repaired before the incision is closed with staples or sutures.

A similar situation can afflict the knee. In some instances, an orthopedist makes a small incision in the knee using a surgical instrument called an arthroscope or endoscope. The device inserts a narrow, illuminated tube with a camera attached into the affected site for a visual examination viewed on a monitor. If this examination, as well as previous x-rays, reveal worn bone and cartilage, a knee replacement is potentially indicated.

Knee arthroplasty consists of the worn knee joint being replaced with metal and plastic components. In knee arthroplasty, a long incision is made in the front of the knee and the patella is removed to make the joint accessible. Holes are drilled into the lower femur to affix the metal replacement. Holes are also drilled in the upper tibia to anchor a plastic plate. The back part of the patella is excised to create a flat surface into which holes are drilled to receive a plastic button. In most cases, the prosthesis is secured with cement, and the incision closed, usually with sutures or staples. Because polymethylmethacrylate cement is usually used in both the hip and knee procedures, the individual, under the guidance of a physical therapist, can gradually place weight on the surgical limb and progress as tolerated. Knee and hip arthroplasties are performed without cement and use implants with a textured or coated surface that the new bone actually grows into. Such implants may also use screws or pegs to stabilize the implant until the completion of bone ingrowth. Since cementless implants depend on new bone growth for stability, they require a longer healing time than cemented replacements. Typically, hip and knee replacements are performed on patients under general anesthesia, although a local anesthetic, either spinal or epidural, is sometimes used. In most cases, general anes-

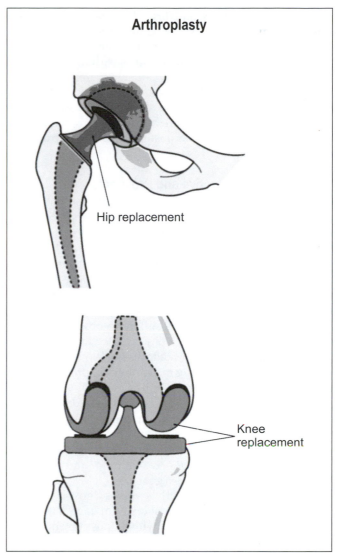

Arthroplasty

Hip replacement

Knee replacement

The hip and knee joints can be replaced by metal or plastic ball-and-socket prostheses when disease or injury is too extensive to repair the existing joints.

thesia is preferred because patients must remain completely still during this surgery and general anesthesia causes temporary paralysis.

Uses and Complications

Arthroplasty is used to relieve pain and restore mobility in patients who have been disabled by their conditions and are reasonable surgical risks. Because many such patients are elderly, extensive preoperative evaluation is necessary. Arthroplasty may be used when medical treatments no longer effectively relieve joint pain and disability. Some medical treatments for osteoarthritis tried before arthroplasty include physical therapy, cortisone joint injections, anti-inflammatory medicines, viscosupplementation injections, and pain medicines.

Conditions such as diabetes mellitus, hypertension, heart or lung disease, and anemia increase the surgical risk. Open lesions increase the risk of infection. Nerve damage can result from cutting muscles and tendons during surgery. Blood clots can form in the lungs or legs of patients undergoing arthroplasty, and this risk may continue for two months following surgery. Blood thinners are usually administered postoperatively. Infection and loosening of prosthetic parts are additional surgical risks and complications.

Physical therapy, essential following arthroplasty of any joint, usually begins two or three days after the surgery and continues for eight weeks. Most patients are completely ambulatory within six weeks postoperatively of hip or knee arthroplasty.

Perspective and Prospects

Joint replacement is becoming more common and more than 1 million Americans have a hip or knee replaced each year. Research has shown that despite increases in age, joint replacement can help overall mobility and general wellbeing. As life expectancy increases, incidence of joint problems is increasing exponentially. In the early twentieth century, many people who lived beyond their sixties were immobilized by chronic arthritis, osteoporosis, and painful joints. When an elderly person suffered a broken hip, it often marked the beginning of a physical decline with a fatal outcome. Medical advances made during World War II had a profound effect on treating many physical problems that, although experienced in combat by relatively young people, required treatment that was soon used in dealing with the joint problems of the elderly. Hip and knee surgery were once more disabling than they currently are. Hip surgery now requires incisions as small as one inch long, although four-inch incisions are more common and ten-inch incisions are used by some surgeons.

Although arthroplasty usually involves a hospital stay of two days depending on the complexity of each individual case, some low-risk individuals without post-op complications become outpatient procedures. The use of titanium in prostheses has extended the effectiveness of such surgery, with these devices currently expected to last for over two decades. People who have arthroplasty generally have substantial improvement in their joint pain, ability to perform activities, and quality of life.

—*R. Baird Shuman, PhD*

See also: Arthritis; Arthroscopy; Bones and the skeleton; Fracture and dislocation; Fracture repair; Hip fracture repair; Joints; Kneecap removal; Orthopedic surgery; Orthopedics; Osteoarthritis; Rheumatoid arthritis; Rheumatology; Rotator cuff surgery; Sports medicine.

For Further Information:

"Arthroscopy". Department of Research & Scientific Affairs, American Academy of Orthopaedic Surgeons. Rosemont, IL; AAOS; May 2014. Based on data from the HCUP Nationwide Inpatient Sample, 2011; Agency for Healthcare Research and Quality. Accessed 9-15-2017.

"What is arthroplasty?" *John Hopkins Medicine. Health Library.* The Johns Hopkins University, The Johns Hopkins Hospital, and Johns Hopkins Health System. August 2016. Accessed 9-15-2017. http://www.hopkinsmedicine.org/healthlibrary/test _procedures/orthopaedic/arthroplasty_92,P07677

"What Is Joint Replacement Surgery?" *National Institutes of Health. Joint Replacement Surgery*: Health Information Basics for You and Your Family. National Institute of Arthritis and Musculoskeletal and Skin Diseases (NIAMS) Information Clearinghouse. National Institutes of Health. 2016. Accessed 9-14-2017. https://www.niams.nih.gov/health_info/Joint_Replacement/default.asp

Lewis, Sarah, PharmD. Arthroplasty. *Healthgrades Operating Company, Inc.* 2017. Accessed 9-16-2017. https://www.healthgrades.com/procedures/arthroplasty.

Arthroplasty. *American Academy of Orthopedic Surgeons.* http://orthoinfo.aaos.org/glossary.cfm

Arthroplasty. *Yale School of Medicine Patient Care.* http://www.yalemedicalgroup.org/stw/Page.asp?PageID=STW028955

Joint Replacement Surgery. *Arthroplasty Association of North America.* http://www.aana.org/EducationLibrary/Articles/JointReplacementSurgery/tabid/128/Default.aspx

Kellicker, Patricia Griffin. "Hip Replacement." *Health Library*, May 6, 2013.

"Knee Replacement." *Health Library*, May 3, 2013.

Rothrock, Jane C., ed. *Alexander's Care of the Patient in Surgery.* 14th ed. St. Louis, Mo.: Mosby/Elsevier, 2010.

"Total Knee Replacement." *American Academy of Orthopaedic Surgeons*, December 2011.

Arthroscopy

Procedure

Anatomy or system affected: Hips, joints, knees, legs
Specialties and related fields: Orthopedics, rheumatology
Definition: A technique for examining joints through a thin scope inserted into the joint; it may be used to visualize and perform surgical procedures.

Indications and Procedures

The arthroscope is a rigid tube enclosing a series of lenses around which are wrapped glass fibers for transmitting light. The arthroscope is placed inside a larger metal sheath, which allows fluid to flow between the components. After disinfecting the skin, the surgeon inserts a cannula (tube) into the desired cavity using an obturator, a prosthetic device which is removed and replaced by the arthroscope.

Instruments passed through the cannula include probes, forceps, knives, scissors, and a variety of clamps. Cutting may be done manually or with a motor-driven tool. The surgeon uses a small light and lens on the instrument to see the operative field. The eyepiece of an arthroscope may be replaced by a video camera to allow viewing on a television monitor.

After the skin is prepared and the instruments are inserted, diagnostic or operative procedures are begun. The joint or tissue is thoroughly explored before any further steps are taken. An assistant positions the body part, freeing the surgeon to operate. The most common site for an arthroscopic procedure is the knee; other sites include the elbow, shoulder, and ankle.

After the procedure is completed, the joint is flushed to remove all debris. The instruments are withdrawn, and the skin punctures are closed with a single suture or bandage closure. The patient returns in a week for a postarthroscopic examination and removal of sutures. Rehabilitation is important; it should begin on the day follow-

Arthroscopy is a diagnostic procedure in which a fiber-optic instrument is inserted into a joint for direct examination without the complications that accompany a larger incision; sometimes surgical instruments are also passed through the arthroscope.

ing arthroscopy and can require up to several months, depending on the site and procedure.

Uses and Complications

Arthroscopy is a technique originally developed for diagnosis in joints; it is now used for surgical procedures as well. Typically, arthroscopy is used for knee and shoulder joint injuries, but it can also be used in the ankle, hip, or elbow. The technique has also been applied in innovative ways by podiatric foot and ankle surgeons to relieve different ankle problems, including ligament damage, bone chips, and recurrent pain from end-stage arthritis.

Many simple procedures can be done using local anesthesia, although regional or general anesthesia is preferred. Arthroscopy can be carried out in either a fluid or a gas environment within the joint. A saline solution is often used; it disperses light more evenly but requires a system to pump the fluid in and out. A gas environment is more useful for visualizing surface irregularities of cartilage.

Such techniques have significantly changed orthopedic surgery. The use of arthroscopy for diagnosis and treatment reduces postoperative infections, the time needed for rehabilitation, and costs. Most arthroscopic procedures are now done on an outpatient basis.

—*L. Fleming Fallon, Jr., M.D., Ph.D., M.P.H.*

See also Arthritis; Arthroplasty; Bones and the skeleton; Endoscopy; Fracture and dislocation; Fracture repair; Hip fracture repair; Joints; Kneecap removal; Laparoscopy; Orthopedic surgery; Orthopedics; Osteoarthritis; Rheumatoid arthritis; Rheumatology; Sports medicine.

For Further Information:

Chow, James C. Y., ed. *Advanced Arthroscopy*. New York: Springer, 2001.

Clark, Glenn T., Bruce Sanders, and Charles N. Bertolami, eds. *Advances in Diagnostic and Surgical Arthroscopy of the Temporomandibular Joint*. Philadelphia: W. B. Saunders, 1993.

Geissler, William. *Wrist and Elbow Arthroscopy: A Practical Surgical Guide to Techniques*. London: Springer, 2013.

Johnson, Donald H. *Operative Arthroscopy*. Philadelphia: Kluwer, 2013.

Miller, Mark D., Daniel E. Cooper, and Jon J. P. Warner. *Review of Sports Medicine and Arthroscopy*. 2d ed. Philadelphia: W. B. Saunders, 2002.

Saxena, Amol. *Sports Medicine and Arthroscopic Surgery of the Foot and Ankle*. New York: Springer, 2013.

Sherman, Orrin Howard, and Jeffrey Minkoff, eds. *Arthroscopic Surgery*. Baltimore: Williams & Wilkins, 1990.

Tibone, James E., Felix H. Savoie III, and Benjamin S. Shaffer, eds. *Shoulder Arthroscopy*. New York: Springer, 2003.

Zarins, Bertram, and Richard A. Marder, eds. *Revision of Failed Arthroscopic and Ligament Surgery*. Malden, Mass.: Blackwell Science, 1998.

Asbestos exposure

Disease/Disorder

Anatomy or system affected: Gastrointestinal system, lungs, respiratory system

Specialties and related fields: Environmental health, occupational health, oncology

Definition: Asbestos is a naturally occurring fire-resistant mineral fiber historically used in a variety of applications ranging from lamp wicks to roofing shingles. Asbestos fibers consist of silica compounds that can irritate human tissue, resulting in disorders such as asbestosis as well as cancers of the lung, larynx, and gastrointestinal system.

Key terms:

asbestos: a naturally occurring mineral fiber composed of silica compounds

mesothelioma: a specific type of cancer occurring when asbestos fibers irritate the pleural lining of the lungs

metastasis: the migration of cancer from its original location in the body to other organs

pleura: the thin membrane that lines the interior of the chest walls and covers the lungs

silicon dioxide: a compound formed when silica is exposed to air

Causes and Symptoms

Asbestos is a naturally occurring mineral fiber whose fire-resistant properties have been known since antiquity. Although there are a variety of forms of asbestos, with some being more associated with occupational illness and disease than others, all asbestos shares a common characteristic: Because asbestos consists of silica crystals, the fibers are inherently irritating to human tissue. On the surface of the skin, they can become embedded and lead to the formation of calluslike growths, termed "asbestos warts," as the body attempts to encapsulate the irritating fibers.

Asbestosis

Asbestosis-the progressive destruction of respiratory tissues via inhalation of dust-sized asbestos fibers that attach

Information on Asbestos Exposure

Causes: Irritation of tissue of skin or lungs by silica fibers

Symptoms: For skin, calluslike growths; for lungs, scarring resulting in asbestosis and mesothelioma (cancer)

Duration: Chronic and progressive

Treatments: None; support for symptoms

to the walls of the lung and then spread outward-is often the result of prolonged exposure to asbestos-containing materials in such environments as shipyards, office buildings, and manufacturing plants. It is one of a wide variety of environmental diseases.

Asbestosis, a lung disorder caused by fiber-related scarring of lung tissue, was one of the first disorders recognized as being associated with asbestos exposure. It is now known that the fibers do not scar the lungs directly; rather, they trigger the production of acid by the lung tissue as the body attempts to break down the silica crystals. Asbestosis is similar to disorders such as silicosis, "black lung," and "brown lung" in that lung capacity is reduced as cumulative damage reduces victims' ability to breathe.

Mesothelioma, a particularly invidious cancer, is also associated with asbestos exposure. With this form of cancer, the cells between the walls of the pleura (the outer covering of the lungs that separates the lungs from the chest wall) or the peritoneum (the sac containing the abdominal organs) form malignant growths.

Both asbestosis and mesothelioma may take many years to develop, with some victims not developing mesothelioma until as many as forty years after the initial exposure. On the other hand, there have been cases of adolescents developing mesothelioma within only a few months of initial asbestos exposure.

Treatment and Therapy

Localized "asbestos warts" on the skin may be unattractive, but they are generally benign. The lung diseases associated with asbestos exposure, however, are progressive and ultimately fatal. In asbestosis, the scarred lung tissue becomes increasingly stiff, and the person becomes unable to take in sufficient oxygen.

Mesothelioma has a high mortality rate, as it is rarely detected in its early stages. Symptoms such as shortness of breath are attributed to more common diseases such as asthma. As the cancer spreads, lung capacity is diminished, and the victim eventually dies from the inability to take in sufficient oxygen, if he or she has not already succumbed to other organs failing after the cancer metastasizes.

Perspective and Prospects

The ancient Romans mined asbestos for use in manufacturing fireproof mats and garments, as did various other cultures throughout recorded history. During the nineteenth century, asbestos became a popular material for lamp wicks, as it could convey the lamp oil without being consumed by the flame itself. As industrialization progressed, asbestos became widely used in such applications as brake shoes for automobiles, oven linings in electric stoves, and building materials. Asbestos was impregnated into siding and shingles for exterior walls and roofs, insulation for attics and walls, and ceiling and floor tiles. By the mid-twentieth century, asbestos had become ubiquitous in society, from the materials on which people walked to the roofs over their heads. The Romans recognized that mining asbestos was effectively a death sentence, as slaves working

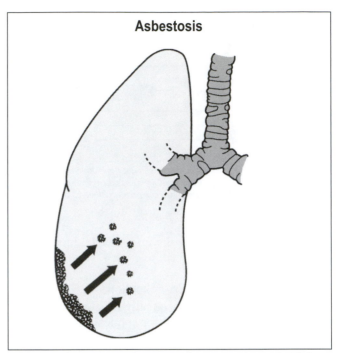

Asbestosis

Asbestosis—the progressive destruction of respiratory tissues via inhalation of dust-sized asbestos fibers that attach to the walls of the lung and then spread outward—is often the result of prolonged exposure to asbestos-containing materials (in shipyards, office buildings, manufacturing plants); it is one of a wide variety of environmental diseases.

in asbestos production quickly developed coughs and wasted away from lung diseases. As mining was generally a dusty and dangerous occupation, however, the special risks that asbestos presented were not well recognized. For centuries, many physicians assumed that all miners' lung ailments were forms of consumption (tuberculosis), when in fact tuberculosis was an opportunistic infection that followed after a miner became weakened by disorders such as silicosis and asbestosis.

By the 1930s, researchers had established that asbestos presented especially high risks of causing lung diseases in miners, shipyard workers, and others who either manufactured or worked with materials incorporating asbestos, such as insulation. By the mid-twentieth century, it had become evident that extremely small amounts of asbestos exposure could lead to asbestos-related disorders. Miners' spouses developed mesothelioma after being exposed to asbestos through doing laundry, for example, while children became victims through exposure to their parents' work clothes in the home.

The widespread use of asbestos fibers in multiple applications means that exposure remains a concern in the twenty-first century. Although asbestos is no longer as widely used in industry, reducing the prevalence of workplace exposures, people can still risk asbestos exposure when engaging in home improvement projects as they rip out old flooring or replace ceiling tile.

—*Nancy Farm Mannikko, Ph.D.*

See also Cancer; Chronic obstructive pulmonary disease (COPD); Environmental diseases; Environmental health; Interstitial pulmonary fibrosis (IPF); Lung cancer; Lungs; Mesothelioma; Occupational health; Pulmonary diseases; Pulmonary medicine; Pulmonary medicine, pediatric; Skin disorders.

For Further Information:
"Asbestos." *American Cancer Society*, May 10, 2013.
"Asbestos." *MedlinePlus*, June 17, 2013.
Bowker, Michael. *Fatal Deception: The Terrifying True Story of How Asbestos Is Killing America*. New York: Touchstone, 2003..
Frank, A. L. "Global Problems from Exposure to Asbestos." *Environmental Health Perspectives Supplements* 101, no. 3 (1993): 165-68.
National Heart, Lung, and Blood Institute. "What Are Asbestos-Related Lung Diseases?" *National Institutes of Health*, May 1, 2011.
Roggli, Victor L., et al. *Pathology of Asbestos-Associated Diseases*. 2d ed. New York: Springer, 2004.

Asperger syndrome

Disease/Disorder

Also known as: Asperger's syndrome, Aspergers syndrome, Asperger's disorder

Anatomy or system affected: Psychic-emotional system

Specialties and related fields: Psychiatry, psychology, neurology, physical therapy, psychiatry, speech therapy

Definition: A pervasive developmental disorder involving clinically significant impairment in social interactions and repetitive or stereotyped patterns of behavior, but no particular problem with cognitive functioning.

Key terms:

autism: a disorder characterized by disturbed language development, a lack of interpersonal responsiveness, odd and repetitive behaviors, and resistance to changes in the environment

autismspectrum disorder(ASD): a neurological and developmental disorder that begins early in childhood and continues throughout adulthood.

pervasive developmental disorders: disorders characterized by delayed and severely impaired social interaction or communication skills, or stereotyped behavior, interests, and activities

Causes and Symptoms

Asperger syndrome was first described in 1944 by the Austrian pediatrician, Hans Asperger (1906—1980). There is controversy as to whether Asperger syndrome should be classified as an autism spectrum disorder or as a separate syndrome. Originally, the syndrome was classified separately from autism, but now most experts consider the syndrome to be a mild form of autism spectrum disorder (ASD).

Asperger syndrome is characterized by normal intelligence and normal but often precocious language skills with unusual language usage. Symptoms usually develop around the age of two years and may improve as the child ages, but symptoms persist for life. Since the classification of the syndrome has varied over the years, the number of people with the disease is difficult to determine, but it is estimated that over 37 million people world-wide are affected. Boys are affected three to four times more often than girls.

Asperger syndrome has social and behavioral compo-nents. The person is socially awkward and significantly impaired in the ability to engage in meaningful social interaction. Behaviorally, the person has restricted, repetitive patterns of behaviors, interests (often obsessive), and activities. Unlike autism, however, Asperger syndrome does not involve severe delays in language or other cognitive skills, although subtle aspects of social communication, such as give-and-take conversation, may be impaired. Affected children express normal curiosity and age-appropriate learning skills and adaptive behavior and have no clinically significant delays in cognitive development.

The impairment in social interaction is gross and sustained. The child may be unable to maintain normal eye-to-eye contact or may show unusual facial expressions, body posture, or gestures. The child may fail to develop age-appropriate peer relationships. A younger child may show little or no interest in establishing friendships. An older person may have an interest in friendship but lack understanding of the conventions of social interaction. The individual may not share enjoyment, interests, or achievements. The individual may lack social or emotional reciprocity, preferring solitary activities, involving others in activities only as tools or mechanical aids, or not participating actively in simple social play or games. The social impairment typically is manifested as an eccentric and one sided approach to others, such as pursuing a conversational topic regardless of others' reactions, rather than as social and emotional indifference.

The behavioral impairment takes the form of stereotypical behavior. Persons with Asperger syndrome may pursue specific and narrow areas of interest such as preoccupations about a specific topic about which they can amass a great deal of information and pursue with great intensity, often to the exclusion of other activities. In contrast to autism, however, language development is normal, with the exception that these individuals are preoccupied with talking about their own arcane interests. They can be verbose, and they fail to self-monitor. Physical development is often delayed leading to clumsiness and poor coordination. The course of Asperger syndrome is continuous and lifelong.

The patient's verbal abilities may, to some extent, mask the severity of the social dysfunction and may prove misleading for parents and teachers, who are blinded by the child's vocabulary. Despite these problems, however, follow-up studies suggest that, as adults, many individuals with Asperger syndrome are capable of gainful employment and personal self-sufficiency.

Asperger syndrome is diagnosed by a pattern of symptoms rather from a single symptom. Not all people diagnosed with Asperger syndrome will exhibit the same symptoms, and there is considerable overlap between the symptoms of Asperger syndrome and other ASDs. Since the classification of the syndrome has changed over the years and controversies exist concerning the precise definitions of these autistic spectrum disorders and the boundaries between the milder manifestations of these disorders and non-autistic conditions, clinicians may have difficulty diagnosing Asperger syndrome.

Information on Asperger Syndrome

Causes: Unknown, possibly genetic
Symptoms: Gross and sustained social impairment; restricted and repetitive patterns of behaviors, interests, and activities
Duration: Lifelong
Treatments: Primarily drug, physical, social, cognitive, behavioral and speech therapy

Although the *Diagnostic and Statistical Manual of Mental Disorders*, 5th. Edition (DSM-V), published by the American Psychiatric Association in 2013 includes Asperger syndrome in the category of ASD, The *Diagnostic and Statistical Manual of Mental Disorders*, 4th. Edition (DSM-IV), included Asperger syndrome separately from other ASDs and described the diagnostic criteria of Asperger syndrome as "severe and sustained impairment in social interaction, and the development of restricted, repetitive patterns of behavior, interests and activities that must cause clinically significant impairment in social, occupational or other important areas of functioning." Intelligence and verbal skills are normal although language usage may be unusual including speaking loudly with unusual intonation and pitch. There is often a delay in the development of coordination, motor dexterity and motor skills.

Because language development is normal, parents or caregivers are not usually concerned about the child's development until the child begins to attend a preschool or is exposed to peers, and since the child's verbal abilities may, to some extent, mask the severity of the social dysfunction, diagnosis can be significantly delayed.

Diagnosis often involves interviews with the parents and child and is usually made between the ages of four and eleven, but since some diagnosticians are relatively unfamiliar with Asperger syndrome and several screening instruments are in use, some experts believe that many individuals go undiagnosed or misdiagnosed for many years even into adulthood. Often Asperger syndrome is misdiagnosed as attention deficit hyperactivity disorder (ADHD). Asperger is often over-diagnosed. Under-diagnosis, over-diagnosis and misdiagnosis can often be devastating for both patient and families.

The cause(s) of Asperger syndrome is/are unknown, but genetics and the environment may play a role. The evidence for a genetic cause is that Asperger syndrome has a tendency to run in families and family members of Asperger syndrome people often have ASD symptoms. No specific gene(s) associated with Asperger syndrome has/ have been conclusively identified although some scientists have reported the discovery of Asperger syndrome susceptibility genes indicating that the syndrome may be polygenic. Research has not identified any environmental factor associated with Asperger syndrome.

Treatment and Therapy

As with the other pervasive developmental disorders, no completely effective treatment exists for Asperger syndrome. Most treatment efforts focus on enhancing communication skills and reducing repetitive and obsessive behaviors and clumsiness. Although there is not agreement among professionals on a single treatment protocol, treatment has generally focused on physical, social, cognitive, behavioral and speech therapy either individually or in groups. Research has yet to confirm the effectiveness of social therapy. Medication such selective serotonin reuptake inhibitors (SSRIs) (fluoxetine, fluvoxamine, and sertraline), antipsychotics (risperidone and olanzapine) and stimulants have typically been used to focus on treating mood and/or anxiety. Risperidone often helps to reduce repetitive behaviors and impulsivity. SSRIs have been shown to reduce repetitive behaviors. The earlier the intervention the better the results. Up to 20% of children diagnosed with Asperger syndrome may not meet the diagnostic criteria for Asperger syndrome as adults. Persons with Asperger syndrome may be quite successful as adults, especially in professions in which their attention to routine, concentration on detail, and relative indifference to sentiment are an asset.

Perspective and Prospects

Since its first description in 1944 by Hans Asperger, there has been considerable progress in describing, defining, diagnosing and treating the syndrome. Although the cause(s) is/are unknown, studies of the genetics of the syndrome are ongoing. Many books and online resources are available for people of all academic levels. Many people with Asperger syndrome and other ASDs suggest that society should look at ASDs as complex syndromes rather than as diseases that need to be cured. Some scientists have argued that Asperger syndrome should be viewed as an alternative cognitive style rather than a disorder.

—Lillian M. Range, PhD;
updated by Nancy A. Piotrowski, PhD
and Charles L. Vigue, PhD

See also: Autism; Bonding; Cognitive development; Developmental disorders; Developmental stages; Learning disabilities; Psychiatric disorders; Psychiatry; Psychiatry, child and adolescent.

For Further Information:
American Psychiatric Association. *Diagnostic and Statistical Manual of Mental Disorders: DSM-5*. 5th ed. Arlington, Va.: Author, 2013.
Ariel, Cindy N., and Robert A. Naseef, eds. *Voices from the Spectrum: Parents, Grandparents, Siblings, People with Autism, and Professionals Share Their Wisdom*. Philadelphia: Jessica Kingsley, 2006.
Aspergers 101. https://aspergers101.com/changes-to-aspergers-syndrome-in-the-dsm-v/
Autism Society. http://www.autism-society.org/what-is/ aspergers-syndrome/
Grossberg, Blythe, Psy. D. *Aspergers and Adulthood: A Guide to Working, Loving, and Living With Aspergers Syndrome*. Berkeley: Althea Press. 2015.
Roberson, Kenneth E. *Adult Asperger's Syndrome: The Essential Guide: Adult Aspergers, Aspergers in Adults, Adults with Aspergers*. Self published with CreateSpace, 2016.
Wood, Debra. "Asperger Syndrome." *Health Library*, Mar. 15, 2013.

Aspergillosis
Disease/Disorder

Anatomy or system affected: Blood, bones, brain, ears, eyes, heart, kidneys, liver, lungs, spleen

Specialties and related fields: Cardiology, family medicine, immunology, internal medicine, microbiology, nephrology, ophthalmology, otorhinolaryngology, pulmonary medicine, radiology

Definition: Infection with fungi from the genus *Aspergillus*, which initially produces pulmonary hypersensitivity reactions or colonizes the lung, and then either grows within a pulmonary cavity, or disseminates through the blood to other organs.

Causes and Symptoms

Members of the fungal genus *Aspergillus* are widely distributed in soil and decaying plant material. Inhalation of fungal spores can cause allergic reactions in people with asthma, a condition called allergic bronchopulmonary aspergillosis. In someone with a preexisting lung cavity caused by tuberculosis or cystic fibrosis, the fungus can grow within this cavity and form a fungus ball (aspergilloma) that moves within the cavity but does not invade the cavity wall. However, if the immune system works poorly because of chronic steroid treatment, alcoholism, or underlying lung disease, then the fungus ball can invade the surrounding lung tissue, a condition called chronic necrotizing pulmonary aspergillosis. If the immune system is profoundly weakened because of a recent organ transplant, advanced acquired immunodeficiency syndrome (AIDS), or genetic diseases that cripple the immune system, then initial colonization of the lung with *Aspergillus* leads to dissemination of the organism through the bloodstream to other organs (invasive aspergillosis). This results in a rapidly progressing and often fatal systemic infection. Allergic reactions to *Aspergillus* or fungus balls usually cause fever, coughing that sometimes produces blood or brownish mucus, wheezing, recurrent episodes of lung obstruction, and sometimes sinus infections. The symptoms of invasive aspergillosis may additionally include chills, headaches, shortness of breath, chest pain, coughs that produce blood-filled material, bone pain, blood in the urine, decreased urine output, and symptoms involving specific organs, such as meningitis (brain), blindness or visual impairment (eye), sinusitis, and endocarditis (heart).

Information on Aspergillosis

Causes: Infection with *Aspergillus* fungal spores

Symptoms: Fever, coughing, wheezing, lung obstruction, sinus infections; sometimes also chills, headaches, shortness of breath, chest pain, bone pain, blood in the urine, decreased urine output

Duration: Acute

Treatments: Oral corticosteroids, antifungal agents, surgical resection if needed

---

Treatment and Therapy

For allergies to *Aspergillus*, oral corticosteroids are used, since inhaled steroids are typically ineffective. Addition of the antifungal drug itraconazole to steroids might be necessary for patients whose allergies fail to resolve. Fungus balls are usually not treated unless they cause symptoms. Surgical resection of the affected part of the lung can cure fungus balls permanently, but only in people who have enough lung capacity to survive such a procedure. Invasive aspergillosis requires immediate therapy, and voriconazole is the usual first treatment choice. Lipid amphotericin B formulations are a viable option, but its toxicity makes voriconazole the better choice. Isuvaconazole, itraconazole, caspofungin, micafungin or posaconazole are also effective in those patients who do not tolerate or respond to other drugs. Fungus balls that invade the lung require prolonged treatment with voriconazole, itraconazole, or lipid amphotericin B formulations to cure the patient completely, but surgical resection of the affected portion of the lung might be necessary.

—Michael A. Buratovich, PhD;
updated by Steffan Kim

See also: Acquired immunodeficiency syndrome (AIDS); Alcoholism; Allergies; Asthma; Corticosteroids; Cystic fibrosis; Fungal infections; Immune system; Immunodeficiency disorders; Immunology; Lungs; Pulmonary diseases; Pulmonary medicine; Respiration; Steroids; Transplantation; Tuberculosis.

For Further Information:
Badii, Chitra and Marijane Leonard. "Aspergillosis." *Healthline*, Jan. 5, 2016.

Centers for Disease Control and Prevention, "Aspergillosis." *Fungal Diseases*, Jan. 21, 2016.

Kumar, V., Abbas, A. K., Aster, J. C. eds. *PathologicBasis of Disease*. 9th ed. Philadelphia, PA: Elsevier, 2015.

Murray, Patrick R, Rosenthal, Ken S., Pfaller Michael A. *Medical Microbiology*. Philadelphia, PA: Elsevier, 2016.

Polsdorfer, Ricker, MD. "Aspergillosis." *Health Library*, Dec. 30, 2011.

Asphyxiation
Disease/Disorder

Anatomy or system affected: Lungs, respiratory system

Specialties and related fields: Emergency medicine, occupational health

Definition: The state of unconsciousness or death resulting from oxygen deprivation

The phenomenon whereby the body experiences a decrease in oxygen below normal levels is called hypoxia; extreme cases of hypoxia lead to anoxia, a complete lack of oxygen. The difference between anoxia and asphyxia is that in asphyxia an accumulation of excess carbon dioxide (hypercapnia) takes place, as the normal exchange of oxygen and carbon dioxide in the lungs is obstructed.

Respiration is regulated in the medulla, while chemoreceptors present in the aortic arch and the carotid sinus respond to levels of oxygen, carbon dioxide, and the pH in blood and the cerebrospinal fluid. The concentration of carbon dioxide pressure in the plasma is proportional to the oxygen pressure. Generally, oxygen deprivation may be the consequence of one or more of several conditions. In all cases, damage results that leads first to hypoxia and eventually to death.

Types of oxygen deprivation. In the first condition, respiration may be slowed or stopped by injury or foreign material blocking the air passage. The most common example of this case is asphyxia that results from the inhalation of water by exhausted swimmers or persons who cannot swim. Large quantities of water fill the lungs and cut off the oxygen supply. Other examples include the entrapment of food or liquid in the respiratory tract, strangulation, and residence in high altitude. In these cases, the carbon dioxide pressure is drastically increased. Artificial respiration may save the victim's life; it should be performed as soon as possible and after the removal of the inhaled foreign substance via vomiting. Strangulation provides the more serious problem of capillary rupturing and internal bleeding.

A second condition, hypoxic anoxia, is caused by an inadequate concentration of oxygen in the atmosphere, which occurs in poorly ventilated enclosed spaces such as mine tunnels, sewers, or industrial areas. Odorless gases such as methane (which is produced in decomposing sewage) or nitrogen may be dangerous because they generally go undetected. A former way of detecting such gases involved taking along a bird in a cage and monitoring its well-being during the exploration of unknown caves or ancient tombs.

In anemic anoxia, respiration may not be effective because of the reduced capacity of the blood to become oxygenated; as a result, less oxygen is transferred to the tissues. Carbon monoxide behaves differently from methane or nitrogen, since it binds much more strongly to hemoglobin than oxygen does. Thus the hemoglobin, which is the oxygen-carrying component of blood, does not transfer oxygen to the tissues, which are starved of it. The passage of oxygen from the lung alveoli to the adjacent blood capillaries may also be affected, such as with chronic lung disease, infections, or developmental effects.

A fourth category is stagnant anoxia, whereby a reduced flow of blood through the blood tissues takes place. This may be a generalized condition, attributable to heart disease, or localized, which may take place in a pilot during aerial maneuvers, for example. A blackout of an aviator is a result of the heart's inability to pump enough blood to these regions against the high centrifugal force. In some cases, the carbon dioxide pressure cannot be removed in the usual manner by the lung. Any lung disease will decrease the effective removal of carbon dioxide and therefore result in elevated levels of it in the blood. Thus in emphysema, a disease in which the alveoli increase in size and which leads to a reduction of the surface area available for gas exchange, carbon dioxide will be retained in the blood. In bronchopneumonia, the alveoli contain secretions, white cells, bacteria, and fibrin, which prevent an efficient gas exchange.

In histotoxic anoxia, the failure of cellular respiration is observed. The body's cells are unable to utilize oxygen as a result of poisoning, as from cyanide. The supply of oxygen

---

Information on Asphyxiation

Causes: Injury, airway obstruction, strangulation, high altitude, poor ventilation, anemia, trauma, hemorrhage, circulatory disease

Symptoms: Increased heart and pulse rate, vision and hearing impairment

Duration: A few minutes

Treatments: Resuscitation with oxygen

---

is normal, but the cells are unable to metabolize the oxygen that is delivered to them.

Symptoms. All cases of anoxia may lead to oxygen deprivation in the brain, which may be fatal if it lasts more than a few minutes. Nerve cell degeneration may start and continue, despite the fact that the original cause of anoxia is removed and normal breathing is resumed. Many health conditions may interfere with the blood transport of oxygen, which is accomplished via the red blood cells. Such diseases include cases of anemia, trauma, hemorrhage, and circulatory disease.

The body responds to oxygen deprivation with an increase in the rate or depth of breathing. The normal, sea-level oxygen pressure of the air is approximately 160 millimeters (6.2 inches) of mercury. When the oxygen pressure is reduced to 110 millimeters (4.2 inches) of mercury at an altitude of about three thousand meters (ten thousand feet), the pulse rate increases and the volume of blood pumped from the heart also increases. Although prolonged exposure to low oxygen pressure may bring the pulse rate back to normal, the output of the heart remains elevated. Despite the lack of oxygen, both the heart and the brain function because of the dilation of their blood cells and the increased oxygen extraction from the blood. Anoxia leads to vision problems first, while hearing is generally the last sense to go. It is not unusual for a person who is suffering from anoxia to be incapable of moving but able to hear.

—*Soraya Ghayourmanesh, Ph.D.*

See also Altitude sickness; Amyotrophic lateral sclerosis; Apnea; Asthma; Choking; Cyanosis; Drowning; Emphysema; Heimlich maneuver; Hyperbaric oxygen therapy; Hyperventilation; Hypoxia; Lungs; Pulmonary medicine; Pulmonary medicine, pediatric; Respiration; Resuscitation; Unconsciousness.

For Further Information:

Heartsaver Manual: A Student Handbook for Cardiopulmonary Resuscitation and First Aid for Choking. Dallas, Tex.: American Heart Association, 1987.

Hendrick, David J. *Occupational Disorders of the Lung: Recognition, Management, and Prevention.* New York: W. B. Saunders, 2002.

Kittredge, Mary. *The Respiratory System.* Edited by Dale C. Garell. Philadelphia: Chelsea House, 2000.

Krementz, Jill. *How It Feels to Fight for Your Life.* Boston: Little, Brown, 1989.

Lutz, Peter L., and Goran E. Nilsson. *The Brain without Oxygen: Causes of Failure-Physiological and Molecular Mechanisms for Survival.* 3d ed. Boston: Kluwer Academic, 2003.

West, John B. *Pulmonary Pathophysiology: The Essentials.* 8th ed. Philadelphia: Wolters Kluwer/Lippincott Williams & Wilkins, 2013.

West, John B. *Respiratory Physiology: The Essentials*. 9th ed. Philadelphia: Wolters Kluwer/Lippincott Williams & Wilkins, 2012.

Aspirin
Biology
Also known as: *acetylsalicylic acid*

Anatomy or system affected: nervous system, immunological system

Definition: a drug that has analgesic, anti-inflammatory, antipyretic and antiplatelet properties

Key terms:

antipyretic: a substance that reduces body temperature

analgesic: a substance that reduces pain

cyclooxygenase: an enzyme in the synthesis of prostaglandins and thromboxanes

non-steroidal anti-inflammatory drug(NSAID): drugs that do have the steroid structure and reduces inflammation

prostaglandin: hormones synthesized by many tissues that are vasodilators and inhibitors of platelet aggregation

Reye's syndrome: an encephalopathy of unknown cause but is most commonly associated with aspirin use in children

thromboxane: hormones synthesized by many tissues that are vasoconstrictors and stimulators of platelet aggregation

Structure and Functions

Aspirin is the commercial name of a drug developed by Bayer in the Nineteenth Century using an extract of the bark of the willow tree. Its active ingredient is acetylsalicylic acid. There is evidence in the archaeological record showing that willow tree bark has been used for medicinal purposes as far back as 2000 BCE.

Aspirin is a non-steroidal anti-inflammatory drug (NSAID) used to treat pain, inflammation, swelling and fever. It is commonly used to treat mild to moderate aches and pain such as what one would experience in a headache or muscle cramps, to reduce fever during mild infection, to reduce inflammation such as experienced in arthritis and to reduce blood clotting. Aspirin also seems to be able to prevent the development of colorectal cancer. The most common side effects are upset stomach and stomach ulcers in adults and Reye's syndrome in children. Occasionally, more severe side effects can occur.

In 1971, John Vane determined that aspirin functions by interfering with the synthesis of prostaglandins and thromboxanes by inhibiting cyclooxygenase (COX) enzymes which are also known as prostaglandin-endoperoxide synthase. Prostaglandins and thromboxanes are synthesized by COX-1 and COX-2 enzymes. Prostaglandins and thromboxanes are produced by many cells and tissues and have many functions such as raising body temperature (pyretic), stimulating local muscle contraction (pain and cramps) and stimulating platelet aggregation (blood clotting), inhibiting platelet aggregation, constricting blood vessels and dilating blood vessels.

Aspirin can potentially prevent platelet aggregation and prevent heart attack and reduce pain and fever by inhibiting thromboxane and prostaglandin synthesis through its irreversible inhibition of COX-1. While the exact scope of its benefits as a preventative of heart attacks is still subject to debate, there is general agreement that aspirin does help reduce the risk of heart attacks.

Aspirin alters COX-2 so that it synthesizes lipoxins which have anti-inflammatory properties thus alleviating the symptoms of conditions such as rheumatoid arthritis.

Perspective and Prospects

Medical texts that date back to the ancient civilization of Sumer contain the oldest references to the beneficial effects of tea made from willow bark. The Egyptians were also aware of its beneficial properties, and the Greek and Roman civilizations were likewise familiar with it. During Europe's Middle Ages, physicians and folk healers remained aware of willow bark's uses. Finally, in the eighteenth century, scientific research was begun to determine the substance and the mechanism responsible for willow bark's effects. Several researchers were able to isolate the active ingredient and identify it as salicin by the early nineteenth century, and Charles Frederic Gerhardt synthesized a more stomach friendly "buffered" compound, acetylsalicylic acid, in 1853.

In 1899, drug manufacturer Bayer began selling its product, named Aspirin, for the treatment of fever and for pain relief. The drug quickly grew in popularity around the world, helped in part by the Spanish flu epidemic after World War I, which provided a venue for the drug to showcase its potency. Aspirin generated huge profits for drug companies all over the world, most of them producing the drug independently, without the authorization of Bayer. The trademarked name Aspirin soon came into the lexicon as the generic "aspirin," which is commonly listed as an ingredient in non-Bayer products.

Aspirin's popularity slowed in the 1950s and 1960s when alternatives to aspirin—acetaminophen and ibuprofen, most notably—entered the marketplace. These alternative drugs appealed primarily to the small portion of the population who experienced an allergic reaction or stomach irritation attributable to aspirin. In 1981, aspirin was also linked to Reye Syndrome in children, a potentially fatal complication following viral infections such as influenza or chickenpox. Aspirin came back into wide use not long after, however, as researchers noticed its ability to prevent blood clots that can block the flow of blood to various parts of the body, reducing the risk of stroke and heart attack. It is now common for doctors to prescribe one aspirin per day (often at 81mg strength, commonly called a 'baby aspirin.') for their patients who may be at risk for strokes and/or heart disease, since aspirin is unlikely to cause negative side effects and has been shown to reduce the incidence of heart attacks.

—Scott Zimmer, MLS, MS, JD;
updated by Charles L. Vigue, PhD

For Further Information:
"Answers About Aspirin." *Harvard Heart Letter* 24.5 (2014): 1-7. *Health Source—Consumer Edition*. Web. 1 June 2015.

"Aspirin: Heart Healthy but Know the Risks." *Harvard Men's Health Watch* 19.3 (2014): 1-7. *Health Source—Consumer Edition*. Web. 1 June 2015.

"Is Aspirin a Dangerous Drug?" *Jama* 312.23 (2014): 2577. *MEDLINEwith Full Text*. Web. 1 June 2015.

Largent, Mark A. *Keep Out of Reach of Children: Reye's Syndrome, Aspirin, and the Politics of Public Health*. New York: Bellevue, 2015. Print.

Russell, Jesse, and Ronald Cohn. *History of Aspirin*. Edinburgh: Pubmix, 2013. Print.

Smith, Tom, et al. "The Aspirin Foundation Scientific Conference: The History, the Present State and the Future of Aspirin Prophylaxis." *Ecancermedicalscience* 8.(2014): 388. *MEDLINEwith Full Text*. Web. 1 June 2015.

Souter, Keith. *An Aspirina Day: The Wonder Drug That Could Save Your Life*. London: O'Mara, 2011. Kindle file.

Williams, Craig D., *et al.* "Aspirin Use Among Adults in the U.S.: Results of a National Survey." *American Journal of Preventive Medicine* 48.5 (2015): 501-508.*MEDLINEwith Full Text*. Web. 1 June 2015.

Assisted living facilities

Health care system

Specialties and related fields: Geriatrics and gerontology, organizations and programs, preventive medicine, public health

Definition: Long-term care alternatives to nursing homes where routine daily tasks, such as housekeeping and meal preparation, are provided for the residents. Generally, residents are retired seniors who can live independently with general assistance from the in-house staff.

Key terms:

activities of daily living: general personal care activities such as eating, dressing, and bathing

independence, autonomy, and dignity: the philosophical principles of assisted living facilities

long-term care: health care or personal care performed for those who are unable to do so themselves; the cornerstone of assisted living

Background

Assisted living care is a form of long-term care. Although assisted living facilities (ALFs) cater to populations other than senior citizens (for example, individuals with disabilities), most facilities provide services for retired senior citizens. Those individuals who require assistance with general activities of daily living such as housekeeping and cooking but do not need significant medical care can often avoid an unnecessarily early entry into a nursing home by first living in an assisted living facility. Therefore, these facilities provide varying degrees of daily assistance for otherwise healthy and independent seniors.

Although assisted living as a practice is regulated throughout the United States, not all states use the same terminology, making comparisons difficult. States use various terminology-senior housing, board and care, adult foster care-that may or may not espouse the principles of ALFs. Accordingly, state regulation of a particular facility may be minimal to nonexistent. For example, some states regulate the type of services while others regulate the building itself. Many of the states with a high percentage of seniors, such as Florida, have adopted an inclusive umbrella model that regulates the entire ALF. However, this lack of consistent federal oversight throughout all states proves confusing for many individuals-especially those searching for long-term care. However, "assisted living facility" is the most common term for longterm care that provides some, but not all, assistance in activities of daily living for its residents.

The ongoing cost of long-term care often consumes the retirement savings of many seniors. The combined expenses of medications, visits to the primary care provider and personal assistance often outweigh simple housing costs, and elderly individuals are often at risk for injury when performing household chores at home. However, seniors now have the option of an ALF, which often provides individual treatment plans that maintain privacy and dignity by permitting broad independence at a fraction of what nursing homes charge. To contain costs, assisted living facilities have replaced comprehensive in-house medical services, such as those available at traditional nursing homes, with individual treatment plans that provide their residents with the optimal amount of help for their particular situations.

Assisted living facilities are fundamentally different from other senior-oriented care options. Similar to childcare facilities, adult day-care facilities provide daytime care for seniors who live with their children. Often, adult day-care facilities cater to individuals who have cognitive dysfunction (for example, memory loss or Alzheimer's disease). Adult daycare facilities typically operate during the weekday work hours, providing caregivers respite either during the day or during their work commitments. In contrast to ALFs, residents leave the facility at the end of the day. Another senior-oriented care option is a nursing home. Nursing homes are similar to ALFs in that the resident lives full time at the facility; however, nursing homes manage

Elderly residents of an assisted living facility. (© Rabbitsfoot/Dreamstime.com)

medical routines, provide intensive medical and nursing care, and all of daily care-often including dressing, bathing, and additional self-care activities.

Types of Assisted Living Facilities

Although differences abound in ALFs, there are basic similarities. Assisted living facilities typically require residents to be generally in control of the majority of their activities of daily living. Residents are expected to perform their own bathing, dressing, and personal care, including medication routines. Although some residents might have minor memory impairments, most are generally in good physical and psychological health, and ALFs strive to create an environment to foster the continued good health of their residents. Strong social connections can often form between residents at cohesive ALFs, an important element of the aging process. Research suggests maintaining strong social interactions is key to maintaining health and well-being as one ages.

There are as many living arrangements as there are ALFs. Some ALFs resemble hostels with eight or more beds in one room, several rooms to a floor, and a separate communal bathroom. Because of the high volume of residents, these ALFs often do not offer individualized treatment plans and, in a situation reminiscent of nursing homes, independence and autonomy are often replaced by resident infantilization. Although these ALFs lack privacy and the staff-to-resident ratio, by necessity, is high, these are generally the least expensive among all the ALFs. General health and well-being often decline rapidly after admittance, forcing relocation to a more care-intensive facility. Accordingly, these ALFs have the quickest resident turnover of all the long-term care facilities.

On the opposite end of the ALF spectrum is the assisted living retirement community. These facilities mimic in-home care as precisely as possible. Whereas retirement communities are generally populated by completely healthy and independent older adults, assisted living retirement communities offer all the amenities and privacy of retirement communities as well as daily in-home care. Often these communities have extensive amenities, including recreation facilities, swimming pools, and other outside sport facilities. In addition, they frequently have numerous staff members dedicated to organizing and maintaining these amenities. Accordingly, these facilities are generally the most expensive but offer the greatest privacy and most closely resemble the aging-athome experience.

Between crowded communal living and luxurious retirement- style living is the most common form of ALFs, the apartment-style assisted living facility. Constructed as typical apartments, these facilities provide each resident with a complete and separate living facility. Each unit generally has a complete bathroom, bedroom, and living room-full kitchens are often not included. Each resident lives independently but eats in a communal dining room with other residents. Communal social rooms and twenty-four-hour security and staff presence are standard amenities. High-end facilities may provide shuttle services, hairdressers, comprehensive exercise facilities-often with a full-time activity director- and monthly visits from nurse practitioners or medical doctors. Regardless of their size, most ALFs often look and feel like home for the residents and their visitors.

Safety Concerns

The expansion of assisted living facilities benefits the long term care industry writ large. Prior to the large numbers of ALFs, nursing homes bore the brunt of aging seniors. Seniors experiencing even the smallest impediment in independence were forced into nursing homes. Because nursing homes are designed to cater to the most dependent seniors, even the most functional seniors often experience precipitous drops in functioning from early entry. The same health impediments that nursing homes cater to are, conversely, also a struggle for ALFs.

The line between whether someone should remain in his or her home versus residing in an ALF can be difficult to determine for a spouse and other family members. Often safety concerns become the final determinant. An inability to cook for themselves or minor memory concerns (for example, forgetfulness with the stove) are often used to rationalize a difficult decision. This decision may be easier in the future, however, as research suggests that ALFs prolong independence compared to remaining in one's residential setting. Often removing one's responsibility for a few activities of daily living relieves stress and mental reserves, allowing the senior to focus on other personal care routines. The independent orientation of ALFs stands in contrast to nursing homes, which often contribute to dependency rather than facilitate independence. Just as safety concerns may lead to the move to an ALF, the decision to discharge a resident from an ALF is also often driven by safety concerns. Because ALFs do not provide twenty-four-hour intensive service, residents are free to come and go from the facility and use the bathroom or other accident-prone areas. Residents who are either cognitively impaired or whose health has declined dramatically are often asked to leave the ALF, and for many seniors the next move is into a nursing home.

Regardless of the size, philosophical orientation, or services provided, ALFs provide a much-needed option in longterm care. Seniors with minor impairments can extend their functional independence for many years, and seniors in ALFs actually experience prolonged independence over remaining in home. In tandem with the rapidly aging population, ALFs are evolving even as they struggle with their own identity nationally and within each state.

Perspective and Prospects

Assisted living facilities burgeoned as the aging baby boomers approached retirement. Baby boomers, the generation born between 1946 and 1964, are healthier and more independent than retirees of the past, and the long-term care industry responded to this demographic shift with the expansion ofALFs. Prior to the broad expansion of ALFs, seniors in need of even the smallest amount of assistance were forced into nursing homes unless they could afford costly in-home care. More recent developments in long-term care involve graduated levels of care in one facility to accommodate residents' needs as they age. In contrast to assisted living-only facilities, where residents must move out after they become unable to bathe, dress, or manage their general health successfully, facilities that offer an increased level of care as needed permit residents to move through their retirement years in a single location. Providing flexible services is especially important to a senior's quality of life, as familiarity and daily routines often can mask advancing stages of mental confusion. These facilities, sometimes referred to as continuing-care retirement communities, have residence fees that are typically higher-most facilities require an entrance fee of more than $60,000-thus limiting this option to the most wealthy of seniors. Nevertheless, these facilities are an important part of the ongoing redefinition of independent living. Where pure ALFs provide a designated set of services, continuing care communities can adapt to the particular needs of each resident throughout the aging process.

This revolution in long-term care has also carried over to nursing homes and has led to the creation of green nursing homes. These nursing homes house approximately ten residents in a large house like structure and provide a full range of personal care and medical services. As in ALFs, the focus in these green homes is on independent thriving. Whereas nursing homes were historically viewed as the last option for seniors, these new green nursing homes are often abundant with plants, domestic animals, homelike furnishings, and daily visitors and volunteers who try to keep the residents and staff cheerful and healthy.

Irrespective of any particular facility or philosophy of care, assisted living facilities are the favored choice of aging seniors. No spouse or family member wants to watch a loved one lose control of daily functioning. Overworked and economically strapped children of aging parents often find themselves faced with a difficult decision. By focusing on dignity, independence, and freedom, assisted living facilities make these choices easier for many.

—*Dana K. Bagwell;*
updated by Ophelia Empleo-Frazier,
MSN, GNP-BC, WCC, DCP

See also: Aging; Aging: Extended care; Alzheimer's disease; Dementias; Geriatrics*and gerontology; Home care; Psychiatry, geriatric.*

For Further Information:
Allen, James E. *Assisted Living Administration: The Knowledge Base*. New York: Springer, 2004.
Connell, Linda H. *NursingHomes and Assisted Living Facilities: Your Practical Guide for Making the Right Decision*. Naperville, Ill.: Sphinx, 2004.
Eldercare Locator. "Assisted Living." *US Department of Health and Human Services*, December 8,2017. https://www.usa.gov/federal-agencies/eldercare-locator
Health in Aging. "Assisted Living." *American GeriatricsSociety Foundation for Health in Aging*, December 8, 2017.
Levin, Mora Jean. How to Care for Your Parents: A Practical Guide to Eldercare. New York: W. W. Norton, 1997.
Mollica, R.Assisted Living and Residential Care in the States in 2010-AARP Public Policy Institute. https://www.aarp.org/.../residential-care-insight-on-the-issues-july-2012-AARP
Mollica, Robert, et al. Residential Care and Assisted Living Compendium: 2007.Washington, D.C.: Department of Health and Human Services, 2007.
Namazi, Kevan H., and Paul K. Chaftez, eds. *Assisted Living: Current Issues in Facility Management and Resident Care*.Westport, Conn.: Auburn House, 2000.
NIH Senior Health. "Long-Term Care." *National Institutes of Health*, 2012.
Polzer, Karl. *Assisted Living State Regulatory Review*. Washington, D.C.: National Center for Assisted Living, 2012.
Weisstub, David N. *Aging: Caring for Our Elders*. Boston: Kluwer Academic, 2001.

Assisted reproductive technologies
Procedure
Anatomy or system affected: Endocrine system, genitals, glands, reproductive system, uterus

Specialties and related fields: Biotechnology, embryology, endocrinology, ethics, genetics, gynecology, obstetrics, perinatology

Definition: A range of medical procedures that are used to assist couples in conception and prenatal care, with special focus on infertility and its cure. Assisted reproductive technologies currently include techniques such as in vitro fertilization, artificial insemination, and surgical procedures to repair or diagnose reproductive problems and in the future may include cloning or gene therapy.

Key terms:

endometriosis: excessive growth of the endometrium, which can result in large clumps of tissue called fibroids that can interfere with ovulation and menses and in some cases can fill the uterus

endometrium: the lining of the uterus, which thickens around the time of ovulation in preparation for an embryo to implant, should conception occur

ovulation: release of an egg from an ovary into a Fallopian tube

tubal ligation: a surgical procedure to prevent the possibility of pregnancy permanently by blocking the Fallopian tubes, thus preventing eggs from passing into the uterus

vasectomy: a surgical procedure for preventing sperm from being released during ejaculation; involves the removal of a portion of the vas deferens

Indications and Procedures
Although most couples experience little or no difficulty conceiving and carrying a child to term, about 15 percent experience infertility. Infertility is defined as an inability to conceive after a year of having regular, unprotected intercourse. Not all couples can be helped, but an increasing number of reproductive technologies are available, from in vitro fertilization (IVF) and artificial insemination to drug therapies and surgical repair.

Typically, the first step is to determine whether the man's sperm is fertile by performing a simple sperm count. If sperm counts are low or the sperm are abnormal, then the primary treatment is artificial insemination, also called intrauterine insemination (IUI). Cryopreserved sperm are obtained from a sperm bank, which collects ejaculate from healthy, fertile men. The donors of the sperm remain anonymous, and the samples are usually a mixture of sperm from two or more men. This method maintains even greater anonymity and increases the amount of sperm available, thus increasing the chances of conception.

To ensure the highest probability of success, IUI should be performed when the woman is ovulating and is most fertile. Most women experience a slight rise in their basal body temperature when they ovulate, and monitoring daily body temperature upon waking can be used in some cases. A more reliable method is detection of a surge in luteinizing hormone (LH) in the urine. LH usually stimulates ovulation within thirty-six to forty hours after the surge. A home urine LH analysis kit can be used, and when the LH surge is detected, insemination can be scheduled for the following day. Self-observation of cervical mucus changes can also be used to detect ovulation. Insemination is a simple office procedure in which the physician uses a special catheter to transfer the semen sample into the uterus.

If adequate numbers of sperm are present, and they appear normal and active, then the diagnostic focus shifts to the woman. Because the female reproductive system is primarily internal, diagnosis is often more complicated and expensive and in some cases can pose risks to the woman. The primary cause of infertility in women is inability to ovulate. Factors that may prevent ovulation include lifestyle factors (drug abuse, obesity, weight loss, prolonged acute stress), hormone imbalance, ovarian tumors or cysts, previous infection, an unusually short menstrual cycle, previous surgery, or birth defects. Sorting out the specific cause or causes can be a daunting task, and the causes remain unknown in some cases.

The initial diagnosis involves extensive consultation on health status and lifestyle, a complete physical examination, urine and blood tests to check for infection or hormone imbalance, and often tests on samples of cervical mucus and a portion of the endometrium (lining of the uterus). The primary goal of these initial tests is to determine whether ovulation is occurring. If ovulation is occurring, the problem likely involves an abnormal uterine condition or an endocrine imbalance that is interfering with implantation. Other problems might include some fault with the eggs that are released or with the ability of sperm to penetrate or fuse with the nucleus of the egg.

If the ova (eggs) are abnormal, then donor ova can be collected from another woman, followed by IVF with the male partner's sperm. Often the fault with abnormal ova is with the cytoplasm, so another possible treatment is to remove the nucleus from an abnormal ovum and place it into a donor ovum from which the nucleus has been removed. The resulting ovum would then have a nucleus derived from the mother and a cytoplasm derived from the donor. Although this approach is technically feasible, it has ignited ethical concerns similar to those raised about cloning.

If ovulation is not occurring, which is true in the majority of cases, then additional tests are required. Continued monitoring of hormone levels may identify an imbalance or timing problem that can be corrected with hormone treatments. Sometimes hormone treatments alone are able to normalize ovulation and restore fertility. In other cases, the problem involves a blockage or abnormal shape of the Fallopian tubes or uterus. Diagnostic procedures at this stage typically involve some form of imaging technology so that the condition of the reproductive organs can be assessed.

Hysteroscopy is a procedure for viewing the interior of the uterus; it can be done either in a doctor's office or in an outpatient setting at a hospital. In preparation for the procedure, the woman is usually given a mild analgesic such as acetaminophen or ibuprofen, as some minor cramping is common. The doctor then washes the vagina and cervix. A local anesthetic is administered to the cervix. The cervix is carefully dilated, and the hysteroscope is inserted through the cervix into the uterus. The hysteroscope contains a small light for illuminating the interior of the uterus and a small camera for viewing. Some conditions that can be detected using hysteroscopy include a septum that divides the uterus, fibroid growths or polyps, and cancerous or precancerous lesions. Often, the location where the Fallopian tubes enter the uterus can also be viewed. Many of these conditions can be asymptomatic. Surgical removal of a septum or other growths may restore fertility. If a woman is able to produce an egg to fertilize but is unable to carry the child herself, another option is surrogacy, which then involves legal procedures to establish parentage.

Hysterosalpingography can be used to view both the uterus and the Fallopian tubes. This x-ray procedure uses a contrast dye to visualize internal structures. Placing the dye into the uterus involves insertion of a special flexible catheter through the cervix. A balloon at the end of the catheter is inflated to hold the catheter in place as the contrast dye is pumped into the uterus. X rays are taken every few seconds as the dye travels through the uterus. Eventually, the dye travels the length of the Fallopian tubes. The images obtained can be used to identify many of the anomalies also detectable using hysteroscopy and can also identify problems with the Fallopian tubes. If the Fallopian tubes are blocked, then the dye will not travel their length, which will be visible in the x-ray photographs.

In some cases, none of these minimally invasive diagnostic procedures identifies a problem. In such cases, diagnostic laparoscopy can be used. Using a laparoscope, a flexible tube with a light and special lens at the end, a doctor can view internal organs directly. After administering regional or general anesthesia, an incision is made near the region of the peritoneal cavity to be imaged. Carbon dioxide is used to fill the peritoneal cavity to improve viewing conditions. The laparoscope is then inserted through the incision. If an abnormality is detected, then the doctor may insert another instrument to collect tissue for a biopsy. After laparoscopic examination is completed, the incision is closed. Laparoscopy is usually done in a hospital as an outpatient procedure, and the patient can go home the same day. Even after diagnostic laparoscopy, the cause of infertility may remain unknown.

Uses and Complications

Assisted reproductive technologies are best suited to couples in which one or the other is infertile but otherwise in good health. Age may also be an important factor for the woman, as fertility, implantation, and normal development of the fetus are all affected as a woman ages, especially beyond thirty-five. Although these technologies can be successful in older women, the risks involved need to be assessed carefully with a doctor. They can also be more costly in older women, because more attempts using IUI and IVF are often required.

Hysteroscopy and hysterosalpingography are the most commonly used procedures for diagnosing infertility, once the more obvious causes have been ruled out. Although both can cause mild to moderate discomfort, they have very few associated risks and can be performed in most obstetrics/gynecology (OB/GYN) offices. If a clear diagnosis is obtained, then a number of problems may require surgery. Blockage, abnormalities of the Fallopian tubes or other reproductive organs, ectopic pregnancies, and abnormal growths (cysts or tumors) can be treated or repaired surgically. In most cases, laparoscopic surgery is used, as it is less invasive than traditional abdominal surgery. Laparoscopic surgery is performed in the same way as diagnostic laparoscopy and may be done at the same time if a problem is discovered in the process.

Diagnostic laparoscopy is typically the method of last resort, as some potentially life-threatening risks are involved, such as damage to abdominal organs, inflammation or infection of the peritoneum or other organs, hemorrhaging, and formation of embolisms that may block an important artery. The procedure can also be more painful in cases where anesthesia is only partially effective. Current research suggests that the benefits may outweigh the risks, but some women choose not to have diagnostic laparoscopy, and not all doctors consider the risks appropriate.

When surgical intervention is unable to restore fertility, the most common option is in vitro fertilization (IVF). As long as the woman's uterus is anatomically and physiologically normal, IVF can be an effective, although expensive, option. It is the method of choice for women who have blocked Fallopian tubes or an abnormal pelvic anatomy or who have had tubal ligation and are considering reversal. It also tends to increase the chances of pregnancy in older women and women with endometriosis. Low sperm count or vasectomy reversal in the male partner may also require IVF, as the sperm may require concentration for effective fertilization. IVF can also be an effective solution for women who cannot ovulate or who have very few or faulty eggs, in which case donated eggs can be used. Gamete intrafallopian transfer (GIFT) collects multiple eggs and places them into a catheter along with sperm. Ovum and sperm are then together injected surgically into the Fallopian tubes, where conception may take place. In zygote intrafallopian transfer (ZIFT), ovum are mixed with sperm in the laboratory, and the resulting zygotes are surgically placed into the Fallopian tubes.

IVF is not without its risks and potential failings. Carefully designed hormone injection protocols are used to stimulate multiple follicle formation and to prevent premature ovulation. Progress is typically monitored using ultrasound. If the number of follicles is too small, then the cycle may be canceled, as the cost of retrieval, given the number of eggs that could be available, is too high. Overstimulation can also occur, which can lead to abnormal levels of estrogen that may pose a health threat. If an appropriate number of follicles are produced, then eggs are retrieved using a needle inserted through the top of the vagina. The placement of the needle is guided using ultrasound, and once the ovaries are reached, the eggs are aspirated into it.

A final concern with IVF is the increased incidence of multiple pregnancies. To increase the chance of a pregnancy, multiple fertilized eggs are placed in the uterus. When only a single embryo is transferred, live births occur less than 10 percent of the time. In recent years, as IVF procedures have steadily improved, the incidence of multiple pregnancies has increased. A study published in 2003 showed that when two embryos were transferred and a live birth resulted, approximately 16 percent of the time twins resulted. This percentage rose to almost 30 percent when three embryos were transferred. When more than three embryos were transferred, triplets and higher numbers occurred with increasing frequency as well. Due to the number of premature births resulting from in vitro fertilization, most reproductive endocrinologists limit the number of embryos transferred in order to limit the number of multiple births.

IVF is a solution only when sperm quantity is adequate or donor sperm is acceptable to the couple. In some cases the sperm count for the male may be so low that even concentrating the sperm would be insufficient to achieve fertilization. Sperm can still be obtained from the male in some cases. If no sperm are found in the ejaculate, there may be an obstruction, and sperm may still be obtained by using a needle inserted near the obstruction. In some cases, the male's sperm may lack the ability to penetrate the egg. If a couple insists that they do not want to use donor sperm, then the last option available is typically intracytoplasmic sperm injection (ICSI), in which a single sperm is injected directly into the cytoplasm of an egg. This technique has been so successful that even males with only a few sperm have been able to father a child. If sperm count is low or motility is poor, sperm from the male may be mixed with donor sperm, so that if pregnancy occurs, the identity of the father can remain uncertain if so desired by the parents.

Perspective and Prospects

Assisted reproductive technologies arose during the latter half of the twentieth century. Prior to this period, infertility was poorly understood and treatments were essentially nonexistent. The first attempt at treating infertility involved artificial insemination in 1785 by the Scottish surgeon John Hunter. A child was born that same year, apparently as a result of his attempts. The next documented attempt at IUI was by Robert Dickinson in 1890. His attempts were highly secretive because the Anglican Church condemned such procedures. The first comprehensive guidelines for determining male infertility based on sperm count and quality were published in 1934.

In 1945, a report of early IUI experiments was published in the *British Medical Journal*. As a result, in 1948 the archbishop of Canterbury proposed making IUI a criminal offense. Although the British government did not follow his advice, it did discourage the use of IUI. During the 1950s, the public demand for solutions to infertility far exceeded medical solutions. By 1955, there had been four successful pregnancies using frozen donor sperm. In spite of these successes, IUI was not to become an acceptable and widely used procedure until the 1970s.

The first fertility drug was developed in 1949, but it took until 1962 for this discovery to be applied successfully, resulting in ovulation and a successful birth. Throughout the 1960s and beyond, the use of fertility hormones was further refined, allowing more infertile women to ovulate and bear children. Use of fertility hormones has become a key part of IVF as well, allowing the harvesting of viable eggs.

The first step toward IVF occurred in 1944, when the first in vitro fertilization took place. It took another thirty-one years for the first IVF pregnancy, and unfortunately it was an ectopic pregnancy. Three years later, in 1978, Louise Brown became the first "test tube" baby born as a result of IVF. In 1981, Elizabeth Jordan Carr became the first IVF baby in the United States. Use of IVF is now routine, and success rates continue to rise.

The 1980s and 1990s saw even greater improvements. Surgical procedures using laparoscopy continued to improve, and diagnostic procedures became ever more sensitive. In the 1980s, donor eggs became widely available. One of the difficulties in using donor eggs had always been preserving them until use, because they seemed much more sensitive than sperm. The first baby derived from a frozen egg occurred in 1983, and methods of preservation are now even better. In 1986, the first baby derived from a frozen donor egg was born in Australia.

In 1992, researchers in Belgium reported the first pregnancies resulting from ICSI, and a year later the first successful birth from ICSI was reported in the United States. IVF was so routine by this time that in 1994 a sixty-two-year-old woman gave birth, and a year later a sixty-three-year-old woman who lied to her doctor about her age also gave birth.

To work around the use of defective eggs, in 1997 the first cytoplasmic transfer birth occurred and ignited controversy over the continued use of the technique. Some ethicists saw it as being too much like human cloning and germline genetic manipulation, and they advocated banning the technique. In the United States, the Food and Drug Administration (FDA) quickly stepped in and claimed jurisdiction over use of the technique. It remains an experimental technique, and its implications are still being addressed.

The cloning of the first mammal from adult cells, Dolly the sheep, brought the possibility of reproductive cloning in humans to the forefront. In response to the many concerns about the potential for cloning humans, President Bill Clinton issued a moratorium on funding to those performing research on human cloning. Human cloning remains a very controversial issue and has been banned by most countries.

The future of assisted reproductive technologies will probably include ever more improved techniques and may also include germline gene modification. Embryos can currently be screened for a number of genetic defects, so that parents can be given the opportunity to use only healthy embryos. The potential for screening for a variety of genetic defects or traits means that parents in the future could choose embryos that meet certain criteria such as sex, intelligence, or personality. It may even be possible to engineer improvements in embryos. The ethics of using these kinds of techniques are still being debated and are considered questionable by many. Regardless of the outcome of these discussions, the future certainly will hold the prospect for almost all couples to have a baby derived from their own genetic material, a dream that was once unattainable for many infertile couples.

—*Bryan Ness, Ph.D.;*
updated by Robin Kamienny Montvilo, R.N., Ph.D.

See also Cloning; Conception; Embryology; Ethics; Gamete intrafallopian transfer (GIFT); Genetic engineering; Gynecology; In vitro fertilization; Infertility, female; Infertility, male; Multiple births; Obstetrics; Pregnancy and gestation; Reproductive system; Uterus.

For Further Information:

American Society for Reproductive Medicine. *Guidelines on Number of Embryos Transferred: A Practice Committee Report-A Committee Opinion*. Birmingham, Ala.: Author, 1999.

Blackley, Michelle. "'Eggs for Sale': The Latest Controversy in Reproductive Technology." *USA Today* 132, no. 2698 (July, 2003): 56-58.

De Jonge, Christopher J., and Christopher L. R. Barratt, eds. *Assisted Reproductive Technology: Current Accomplishments and New Horizons*. New York: Cambridge University Press, 2002.

Gardner, David K, Botros Rizk, and Tomasso Falcone, eds. *Human Assisted Reproductive Technology: Future Trends in Laboratory and Clinical Practice*. New York: Cambridge University Press, 2011.

Henig, Robin Marantz. "Pandora's Baby." *Scientific American* 288, no. 6 (June, 2003): 62-67.

Khamsi, F., et al. "Recent Advances in Assisted Reproductive Technologies." *Endocrine* 9, no. 1 (August, 1998): 15-25.

Parekattil, Sijo J., and Ashok Agarwal, eds. *Male Infertility: Contemporary Clinical Approaches, Andrology, ART, and Antioxidants*. New York: Springer, 2012.

Powledge, Tabitha M. "Looking at ART." *Scientific American* 286, no. 4 (April, 2002): 20-21.

Rizk, Botros, and Eric Jauniaux, eds. *Pregnancy After Assisted Reproductive Technology*. New York: Cambridge University Press 2012.

Schultz, Richard M., and Carmen J. Williams. "The Science of ART." *Science* 296, no. 5576 (June, 2002): 2188-90.

Shanley, Mary Lyndon. *Making Babies, Making Families*. Boston: Beacon Press, 2001.

Steiger, Samantha P., ed. *In Vitro Fertilization*. New York: Nova Science, 2011.

Tan, Seang Lin, and Togas Tulandi, eds. *Reproductive Endocrinology and Infertility: Current Trends and Developments*. Basel, Switzerland: Marcel Dekker, 2003.

Wilcox, Melynda Dovel, and Josephine Rossi. "What Price a Miracle?" *Kiplinger's Personal Finance* 56, no. 9 (September, 2002): 116-19.

Yoshida, T. M. "Infertility Update: Use of Assisted Reproductive Technology." *Journal of the American Pharmaceutical Association* 39, no. 1 (January/February, 1999): 65-72.

Assisted suicide

Ethics

Specialties and related fields: Oncology, palliative care, hospice, pharmacology

Definition: Suicide involving the indirect or direct assistance of a second party.

Assisted suicide is a broad term referring to the involvement of a second party in the termination of a consenting person's life. The legal and ethical debate surrounding assisted suicide has stratified the polarizing topic into several different categories, but the most medically relevant version in the United States is known as physician-assisted suicide (PAS). PAS is legal in three U.S. states and is defined as suicide resulting from the self-administration of a lethal dose of a medication prescribed by a physician explicitly intended for the self-termination of life. This is not to be confused with euthanasia, where the physician or a second party actively administers the life-ending medication, as opposed to the patient.

PAS is currently legal in Oregon, Washington, and Vermont via legislation, and in Montana via a court ruling. However, the restrictions vary from state to state. PAS is only legal in cases of terminally ill patients with a prognosis of less than six months. Currently, there is active legislation for PAS in Montana. In Hawaii, while there is no law restricting or sanctioning PAS, aid-in-dying is a widely accepted practice in the medical community. In contrast, euthanasia is illegal in all states, and physicians could face criminal charges if they directly administer life-terminating medication to a patient, even with an explicit request and informed consent.

Several European countries have less restrictive laws regarding physician involvement in suicide. In the Netherlands, Belgium, and Switzerland, it is legal to directly administer medication that ends another person's life with an explicit request and their full informed consent, a set of conditions known as "voluntary active euthanasia." In the Northern Territory of Australia, euthanasia was legal for a short time in the 1990s, but the law was rescinded. Several other countries are currently debating the legal and ethical implications of assisted suicide.

Proponents of assisted suicide argue that patients with terminal illnesses should be afforded the right to die "with dignity" in a comfortable, nonviolent manner, and with the aid and expertise of a medical professional, if they so choose. Opponents of PAS argue that more widespread adoption of physician-assisted suicide could be a "slippery slope." That is, if physician-assisted suicide becomes widely adopted and accepted practice with terminally ill patients, it may be utilized in the disabled community, people with normal life expectancy, and those who are unable to consent to death, such as comatose patients. Other arguments against PAS are based upon on moral, legal, and religious beliefs.

—Sarah Acker and Nicole Mitchell

For Further Information:

Dees, Marianne, Myrra Vernooij-Dassen, Wim Dekkers, and Chris van Weel. "Unbearable Suffering of Patients with a Request for Euthanasia or Physician-Assisted Suicide: An Integrated Review." *Psycho-Oncology* 19, no. 4 (2010): 339-352.

Hendry, Maggie, et. al. "Why Do We Want the Right to Die? A Systematic Review of the International Literature on the Views of Patients, Carers and the Public on Assisted Dying." *Palliative Medicine* 27, no. 1 (2013): 13-26.

Rosenfeld, Barry. *Assisted Suicide and the Right to Die: The Interface of Social Science, Public Policy, and Medical Ethics.* Arlington, Va.: American Psychological Association, 2004.

Asthma

Disease/Disorder

Anatomy or system affected: Chest, immune system, lungs, respiratory system

Specialties and related fields: Environmental health, immunology, pulmonary medicine

Definition: A chronic inflammatory obstructive pulmonary disease that obstructs the airways to the lungs and makes it difficult or, in severe attacks, nearly impossible to breathe.

Key terms:

allergen: any substance that causes an overreaction of the immune system; also called an antigen

allergic reaction: the presence of adverse symptoms that are part of the body's overreaction to an antigen

allergy: an overreaction of the immune system to a substance that does not affect the general population; the tendency to be allergic is inherited

beta-agonists: chemicals that attach to the beta-receptors on cells; often used in inhalers, they cause the bronchioles to dilate, or open

bronchioles: small air tubes leading to the air sacs of the lungs; the functional units of the airway that are involved in asthma

mast cells: cells in connective tissue capable of releasing chemicals that cause allergic reactions

trigger: the substance or event that sets off an asthma attack; triggers may be allergens or some other type of stimulus

Causes and Symptoms

Asthma is a Greek word meaning "gasping" or "panting." It is a chronic obstructive pulmonary (lung) disease that

---

Information on Asthma

Causes: Environmental factors, allergens, viral infections, stress, exercise

Symptoms: Tightening of the chest, sudden breathlessness, wheezing, coughing

Duration: Chronic, with acute episodes

Treatments: Medications (bronchodilators, anti-inflammatory drugs, trigger-sensitivity reducers); lifestyle modification to avoid triggers

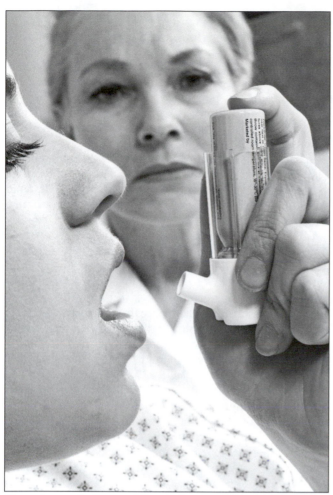

Many asthma medications are delivered using an inhaler. (PhotoDisc)

become smaller and continue to divide. The air finally moves into the smallest tubes, called "bronchioles," and then flows into the millions of small, thin-walled sacs called "alveoli." Vital gas exchange occurs in the alveoli.

This gas exchange involves two gases in particular, oxygen and carbon dioxide. Oxygen must cross the membrane of the alveoli into the blood and then travel to all the cells of the body. Within the cells, it is used in chemical reactions that produce energy. These same reactions produce carbon dioxide as a by-product that is returned by the blood to the alveoli. This gas is removed from the body through the same pathway that brings oxygen into the lungs.

The parts of this airway that are involved in asthma are the bronchioles. These tubes are wrapped with smooth, involuntary muscles that adjust the amount of air that enters. The lining of the bronchioles also contains many cells that secrete a substance called "mucus." Mucus is a thick, clear, slimy fluid produced in many parts of the body. Normal production of mucus in the lungs catches foreign material and lubricates the pathway to allow smooth airflow. People suffering from asthma have very sensitive bronchioles.

Three pathological processes in the bronchioles contribute to an asthma attack. One is an abnormal sensitivity and constriction of the involuntary muscles surrounding the airway, which narrows the diameter of the airway. Another is an inflammation and swelling of the tissues that make up the bronchioles themselves. The third is an increased production of mucus, which then blocks the airways. These three mechanisms may work in combination and are largely caused by the activation of mast cells in the airways. The result can be extreme difficulty in taking air into the lungs until the attack subsides. The characteristic "wheeze" of asthma is caused by efforts to exhale, which is more difficult than inhaling. In the most serious attacks, the airways may close down to the point of suffocating the patient if medical help is not given.

Attacks can vary in severity at different times because of variations in tension within the bronchiole muscles. Although there is still debate about the general function of these muscles, they probably help to distribute the air entering the alveoli evenly. Control of the tension in these smooth muscles is involuntary and follows a circadian (twenty-four-hour) rhythm influenced by neurohormonal control. Accordingly, for most people, this cycle causes maximum constriction to occur at about 6 a.m. and maximum relaxation to occur at about 6 p.m. Hence, asthma attacks tend to be more severe in the late night and early morning.

Following a given asthma attack, patients are sometimes susceptible to additional, more severe attacks. This period of high risk, called a "late-phase response," occurs five or six hours after the initial symptoms pass and may last as long as several days. Some researchers believe that the increase in deaths from asthma in the United States may be tied to this danger, which often goes unrecognized.

The initial cause and mechanism of an asthma attack can vary from person to person. Accordingly, asthma is usually divided into two types. One type is extrinsic-that is, caused

involves repeated attacks in which the airways in the lungs are suddenly blocked. The disease is not completely understood, but asthma attacks cause the person to experience tightening of the chest, sudden breathlessness, wheezing, and coughing. Death by asphyxiation is rare but possible. Fortunately, the effects can be reversed with proper medication. The severity of symptoms and attacks varies greatly among individuals, and sufferers can be located on a continuum running from mild to severe. Mild asthmatics have fewer than six minimal attacks per year, with no symptoms between attacks, and they require no hospitalizations and little or no medication between attacks. Severe asthmatics have more than six serious attacks each year, have symptoms between attacks, lose more than ten school days or workdays, and require two or more hospitalizations per year. Attacks are typically spaced with symptom-free intervals but may also occur continuously. Rather than focusing only on the specific attacks, one should view and treat asthma as a chronic disease, a nagging, continuing condition that persists over a long period of time.

A review of the path of air into the body during normal breathing helps in understanding asthma. During inhalation, air travels into the nose and mouth and then into the trachea (windpipe); it then divides into the two tubes called "bronchi" and enters the lungs. Inside each lung, the tubes by external triggers that bring about an allergic response. Allergic reactions involve the immune system. Normal functioning of the immune system guards the body against harmful substances. With an allergy, the body incorrectly identifies a harmless substance as harmful and reacts against it. This substance is then called an "allergen." If the symptoms of this reaction occur in the lungs, the person has extrinsic or allergic asthma.

Researchers have discovered that many people with asthma have elevated levels of immunoglobulin E (IgE), a substance that indicates an allergic reaction within the body. Allergic triggers for asthma include dust, pollens, animal dander, cockroaches, and other substances. Infants may have an IgE response to respiratory syncytial virus. Improved asthma treatments may lie in substances that interfere with interleukin-4 (IL-4), which promotes IgE production in the body.

When allergens enter the body, the white blood cells make specific IgE antibodies that can bond with the invaders. Next, the IgE antibodies attach to the surfaces of mast cells; these cells are found all over the body and are numerous in the lungs. The allergens attach to the IgE antibodies located on the mast cells, and the mast cells are stimulated to produce and release chemicals called "mediators," such as histamine, prostaglandin D2, and leukotrienes. These mediators cause sneezing, tighten the muscles in the bronchioles, swell the surrounding tissues, and increase mucus production.

The second type of asthma is intrinsic and does not involve allergies. People who suffer from intrinsic asthma have hyperactive or twitchy airways that overreact to irritating factors. The mechanism for this form is not always understood, but no IgE antibodies for the irritant are placed on the mast cells. Examples of such nonallergic stimuli are cigarette smoke, house dust, artificial coloring, aspirin,

ozone, or cold air. Odors from insecticides, cleaning fluids, cooking foods, and perfume can also trigger attacks. Also included in this category are attacks that are caused by viral infections (including colds and flu), stress, and exercise. Asthma can be triggered by many different substances and events in different people. While the symptoms are the same whether the asthma is intrinsic or extrinsic, asthmatics need to identify what substances or events trigger their attacks in order to gain control of the disease.

In addition to tightening of the chest, sudden breathlessness, wheezing, coughing, and chest pain common to an asthma attack, symptoms of a severe attack include rapid pulse, blue lips or skin, perspiration, anxiety, or extreme fatigue.

Why people develop asthma is not well understood. Asthma can begin at any age, but it is more likely to arise in childhood. While it is known that heredity predisposes an individual to asthma, the pattern of inheritance is not a simple one. Most geneticists now regard allergies as polygenic, which means that more than one pair of genes is involved. Height, skin color, and intelligence are other examples of polygenic traits. Exposure to particular external conditions may also be important. The children who develop asthma are more likely to be boys, while girls are more likely to show signs of the disease at puberty (about age twelve). Childhood asthma is also most likely to disappear or to be "outgrown" at puberty; about half of the cases of childhood asthma eventually disappear.

Early exposures to some triggers may be a key in the development of asthma. Increasingly, studies indicate that air pollution is an important risk factor for developing asthma, especially in children. Smoking by mothers can cause children who have a genetic disposition to develop asthma, as early exposure to secondhand smoke can cause an allergy to develop. Early studies in this area were confusing until the data were sorted by level of education. Lung specialist Fernando Martinez of the University of Arizona believes that less-educated women who smoke are more likely to cause this effect because their homes tend to be smaller and therefore expose the children to more concentrated levels of smoke. A British study indicated that more frequent and thorough housecleaning might keep children from developing asthma. Early exposure by genetically susceptible children to dust and the mites that thrive in dust may also cause some to develop asthma.

While attacks can cause complications, there is no permanent damage to the lungs themselves, as there is in emphysema. Complications include possible lung collapse, infections, chronic dilation, rib fracture, a permanently enlarged chest cavity, and respiratory failure. However, millions of days of work and school are lost as victims recuperate; asthma is the leading cause of missed school days. Even though attacks can be controlled by medication, occasionally fatalities do occur.

Treatment and Therapy

The key to gaining control of asthma is discovering the particular factors that act as triggers for an attack in a given

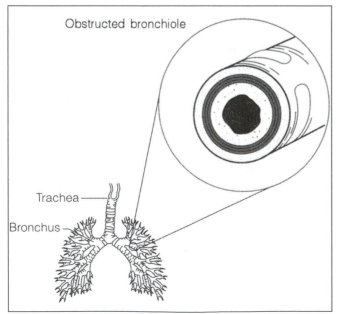

During an asthma attack, obstructed bronchioles limit or halt airflow, resulting in severely restricted breathing.

In the News: Increased Asthma Rates in the United States

Asthma rates in the United States are increasing, especially in children, but the cause has yet to be determined. The American Lung Association reported a rise in prevalence of the disease from 34 cases per 1,000 people in 1982 to 56 cases per 1,000 in 1994. The Environmental Protection Agency reported that in the last two decades of the twentieth century, cases of childhood asthma more than doubled.

A study covered in the August, 2002, issue of *Pediatrics* reported that the prevalence of asthma in children increased on average 4.3 percent per year between 1980 and 1996. From 1997 to 2000, asthma attacks leveled off and may have reached a plateau. Another study—by the Air Pollution and Respiratory Health branch of the National Center for Environmental Health—showed that the prevalence of asthma in adults increased each year between 2000 and 2008.

Office visits for children with asthma increased 3.8 percent from 1980 to 1999 (and continued to increase each year through 2004). Hospitalization of children with asthma grew 1.4 percent each year during this period, and child deaths from asthma increased 3.4 percent per year from 1980 to 1998. Statistics also show that children four years of age and younger had the greatest increase in prevalence and use of health care, but the highest mortality was in adolescents. There was a highly disproportionate number of cases in African American children.

Causes for the increase are unknown, but theories include factors in the environment, such as increasing air pollutants and allergens. The hygiene hypothesis suggests that more sterile living environments, the use of antibiotics and antibacterial products, and vaccinations may be contributing factors. Another possibility, according to Lara J. Akinbami of the Centers for Disease Control and Prevention's National Center for Health Statistics, is diagnostic transfer, which refers to a change in the labeling of other respiratory diagnoses of children to asthma. Diagnostic transfer may be the result of greater awareness of the disease but alone would not account for the rise in rates. Adding to the complexity of this issue is that, in 1997, the National Health Interview Survey was redesigned and began using a different childhood asthma measure.

Public health efforts may have contributed to the recent plateau by providing greater access to care for children through the State Children's Health Insurance Program. Other public health interventions have promoted prevention and a decline in mortality from the disease. Although it is not completely clear that rates have reached a true plateau, or what the exact causes of increased rates may be, most researchers and physicians agree that more research and data are needed.

—*Martha Loustaunau, Ph.D.*

individual. These factors vary and at times can be surprising; for example, one person found that a mint flavoring in a particular toothpaste was a trigger for his asthma. Nevertheless, most common triggers fall in the following groups: allergies; irritants, including dust, fumes, odors, vapors, molds, mildew, and red tide; air pollution, temperature, and dryness; colds and flu; and stress. Even types of food may be important. Diets low in vitamin C, fish, or a zinc-to-copper ratio, as well as diets with a high sodium-to-potassium ratio, seem to increase the risk of asthma attacks and bronchitis. There have also been correlations between low niacin levels in the diet and tight airways and wheezing. Food allergies and sulfites, chemical preservatives found in wine and dried fruits, may also act as triggers.

Some doctors have improved their diagnosis of asthma with a tool called the "peak flow meter." The meter can also be used by patients at home to predict impending attacks. This inexpensive device measures how quickly air can be moved out of the lungs. Therefore, it can be discovered that airways are beginning to tighten before other symptoms occur. The early warning allows time to adjust medications to head off attacks. This tool can help asthmatics take charge of their disease.

Various medications are available to keep the airways open and to lower their sensitivity. In an emergency, drugs may be injected, but medications are usually either inhaled or taken orally as pills. Because inhalation transports the medication directly to the lungs, lower doses can be used. Many asthmatics carry inhalers, which allow them to breathe in the medication during an attack. Because this action requires a person to coordinate inhaling with the release of the spray, young children are sometimes better off with a device that requires them to wear a mask. The choice and dosage of medicine vary with the patient, and physicians need to determine what is safest and most effective for each individual. Self-treatment with nonprescription drugs should be avoided.

Some of the most commonly prescribed drugs are bronchodilators, inflammation reducers, and trigger-sensitivity reducers. The bronchodilators include albuterol, metaproterenol, and terbutaline. They are beta-agonists that mimic the way in which the body's nervous system relaxes or dilates the airways. (Any drug that functions as a beta-blocker should be avoided by asthmatics because of its opposite effects.) Another bronchodilator is adrenaline (or epinephrine), but it is a less specific drug that also affects the heart and increases the pulse rate. Theophylline, a stimulant chemically related to caffeine, relaxes the airways and also helps clear mucus. Cromolyn sodium decreases sensitivity to triggers and is sometimes inhaled on a daily basis as a long-term treatment to prevent attacks. Injections of omalizumab (Xolair) may be prescribed in combination with other medications to control difficult-to-treat cases.

The use of inflammation reducers known as "corticosteroids" plays an important role in the treatment of asthma. Whether administered orally or via an inhaler, these powerful medications can both prevent and treat the airway inflammation that leads to asthma attacks. Their anti-inflammatory effects mean fewer symptoms and attacks, better airflow, and airways that are less likely to react to triggers in an exaggerated or hyperresponsive manner. Inhaled steroids are preferred for long-term treatment of asthma. Inhalation delivers the medication directly to the site of inflammation and is associated with fewer side effects, which can include osteoporosis, thinning and easily bruised skin, cataracts, and suppression of the adrenal glands. However, oral steroids play an important role in the treatment of asthma, especially during periods of sudden, life-threatening symptoms or for patients with severe and ongoing disease. To minimize possible side effects, oral steroids are given every other day or in decreasing dosage over a limited period of time. Initially, corticosteroids were used if other drugs were ineffective, but since 1991 they have been strongly recommended for long-term preventive use. Calcium and vitamin D supplements are used to prevent bone loss in these patients.

Concerns about safety with these medications increase when asthmatics use high doses (more than two hundred inhalations monthly) of beta-agonist inhalers or take combined beta-agonist/anti-inflammatory drugs for a long period of time. According to a 2006 study, higher risks of fatal or near-fatal attacks and of hospitalization may be associated with high, long-term usage of the beta-agonists fenoterol, which is not used in the United States, and salmeterol, an ingredient in the popular inhaler Advair. Because beta-agonists can cause a worsening of symptoms, inhalers containing this combination are not recommended as the first line of treatment for asthmatics. The risks and benefits of long-term use of long-acting beta-agonists should be discussed with a physician.

Individuals should not exceed their prescribed dosage when using an inhaler. An individual who feels the need to use an inhaler more often to obtain adequate relief should see a doctor. The increased need is a sign of worsening asthma, and a doctor needs to investigate and perhaps change the treatment.

Drugs that interfere with the chemical moderators such as leukotriene have also been approved for treatment. Zileuton (Zyflo) interferes with leukotriene production in the mast cells. Montelukast sodium (Singulair) blocks the actions of leukotrienes as they attach to receptors on the outside of airway cells and turn on the cellular responses that lead to the asthma reaction: contraction of the airway muscles, swelling of the airway lining, and flooding of the remaining airway space with sticky mucus.

Over-the-counter drugs are often used by asthmatics to treat their symptoms. These drugs often use ephedrine, metaraminol, phenyl- ephrine, methoxamine, or similar chemicals. All these drugs are structurally related to amphetamine or adrenaline. Unfortunately, some people may be getting relief without discovering the cause of their asthma. Self-treatment without a doctor's guidance is risky.

That asthmatics should generally avoid exercise is a myth. With a doctor's approval, regular sports and exercise may be pursued. Furthermore, exercise may be helpful in reducing the frequency and severity of attacks. Many athletes compete at high levels in spite of their asthma. Sports that do not require continuous activity or exposure to cold, dry air are preferred. Swimming is considered ideal. Doctors can help the athlete with a pre-exercise medication plan and a backup plan if symptoms occur during or after the exercise.

Another damaging belief about asthma needs comment.

Early Freudian psychology held that asthma could be caused by a mother who failed to answer her baby's crying. Accordingly, the onset of asthma, with its gasping for air, was seen as a continuation of that crying. This sad hypothesis is false: asthma is not connected to any abnormal relationships between mother and child, and it is not caused by early or deep psychological problems.

Asthmatics are advised to avoid allergens and other asthma triggers and to consider installing air conditioning and HEPA air filtering units. Anti-allergy shots and breathing techniques may also offer relief.

Perspective and Prospects

Asthma was recognized in ancient times in both the East and the West. The Chinese people have a rich collection of traditional remedies going back more than two thousand years that includes the use of *ma huang*, an Asiatic species of the genus *Ephedra*, for asthma and other lung conditions. *Ma huang* is a shrubby, almost leafless gymnosperm. In 1887, the alkaloid ephedrine was isolated from *Ephedra* as the active ingredient in the plant; the drug is similar in effect to adrenaline. Alkaloids are bitter in taste and often affect the nervous system. Scientists used the ending -*ine* to identify alkaloids, many of which have strong physiological effects on humans (such as caffeine, morphine, nicotine, and cocaine). *Ma huang* was used in both ancient China and India.

Pliny the Elder (23-79 CE) believed that everything had been created for the sake of humans and therefore that nature was a complete storehouse of natural remedies. His encyclopedia *Historia Naturalis* recommended ephedron, a source of ephedrine, for asthma, coughing, and hemorrhages. Some believe that Pliny may have suffered from asthma. He died from the fumes of Mount Vesuvius while investigating the volcano and trying to help refugees.

In the eighteenth century, the discovery of oxygen, nitrous oxide, and other gases led to serious efforts to determine medical uses for these gases. Inhalation allowed a gaseous medication to be removed as soon as the effect was achieved; precise dosage did not have to be calculated. There were legitimate efforts to find painkillers for surgery and dentistry. Soon, charlatans falsely claimed, however, to be able to use the new gases to cure asthma and other diseases. Anesthetics such as ether, nitrous oxide, and chloroform were used by doctors in the 1850s to treat asthma and other conditions.

As early as 1190, Maimonides, the physician to the court of Saladin, the sultan of Egypt, noted that asthma tended to run in families. Unfortunately, Maimonides's thoughts about heredity were forgotten until much later. Early in the twentieth century, researchers did find that 48 percent of the asthmatics surveyed had an immediate family history of allergies.

In 1991, the NAEP, a panel of experts brought together by the US National Heart, Lung, and Blood Institute, issued guidelines for the diagnosis and treatment of asthma urging a focus on long-term prevention, increasing the use of inhaled steroids (especially with severe and moderate asthmatics) and use of the peak flow meter to predict attacks.

—*Paul R. Boehlke, Ph.D.; Shih-Wen Huang, M.D.;*
updated by Caroline M. Small

See also Allergies; Asphyxiation; Bronchi; Environmental diseases; Lungs; Multiple chemical sensitivity syndrome; Pulmonary diseases; Pulmonary medicine; Pulmonary medicine, pediatric; Respiration; Wheezing.

For Further Information:

A.D.A.M. Medical Encyclopedia. "Asthma." *MedlinePlus*, July 9, 2012.

Adams, Francis V. *The Asthma Sourcebook*. 3d ed. New York: McGraw-Hill, 2007.

American Lung Association. http://www.lung.org.

American Medical Association. *Essential Guide to Asthma*. New York: Pocket Books, 2000.

Barnes, Peter J., and Simon Godfrey. *Asthma*. 2d ed. London: Martin Dunitz, 2000.

Berger, William E. *Asthma for Dummies*. New York: John Wiley & Sons, 2004.

Carson-DeWitt, Rosalyn, and Brian Randall. "Asthma-Adult." *Health Library*, September 30, 2012.

Clark, T. J. H., et al., eds. *Asthma*. 4th ed. New York: Oxford University Press, 2001.

Haas, François, and Sheila Sperber Haas. "Living with Asthma." In *The World Book Medical Encyclopedia*. Chicago: World Book, 1988.

Kellickerm, Patricia Griffin, and Michael Woods. "Asthma-Child." *Health Library*, September 30, 2012.

Krementz, Jill. *How It Feels to Fight for Your Life*. Boston: Little, Brown, 1989.

National Center for Environmental Health. "Asthma." *Centers for Disease Control and Prevention*, May 6, 2013.

Ostrow, William, and Vivian Ostrow. *All About Asthma*. Morton Grove, Ill.: Albert Whitmany, 1989.

Parker, James M., and Philip M. Parker, eds. *The Official Patient's Sourcebook on Asthma*. Rev. ed. San Diego, Calif.: Icon Health, 2005.

Welch, Michael J., and the American Academy of Pediatrics. *American Academy of Pediatrics Guide to Your Child's Asthma and Allergies: Breathing Easy and Bringing up Healthy, Active Children*. New York: Random House, 2000.

Astigmatism

Disease/Disorder

Anatomy or system affected: Eyes

Specialties and related fields: Ophthalmology, optometry

Definition: A slight deformation of the eyeball that makes it impossible for a person to form a sharp image of two perpendicular lines simultaneously.

Causes and Symptoms

The problem of astigmatism is caused by a difference in the focal length of the eye for two perpendicular directions, which can occur if the eyeball becomes slightly deformed, like a grape being squeezed between two fingers. The curvature of the cornea (outer eye surface) would be flattened in one plane but remain more rounded in the other one. A deformed eye lens can also cause astigmatism.

During an eye examination, the optometrist tests for astigmatism by showing the patient a diagram of straight lines radiating outward from the center of the picture. A person with normal eyes will see all the lines in focus, but someone with astigmatism will see only one line sharply focused while the other ones are fuzzy. For example, if the horizontal line is perceived to be in focus, then the vertical line will be blurred while the lines in between will be partially out of focus. Each eye must be tested individually because the amount of astigmatism can differ.

Treatment and Therapy

To correct for astigmatism, the optometrist can add a cylindrical correction to the eyeglass prescription, which changes the focal length of the eye in only one plane. A cylindrical lens can be pictured to be thick in the middle and thin at the edges, like a slice cut off from the outside edge of a cylindrical object.

Normal eye

Irregular cornea

Irregular lens

Astigmatism results when either the cornea or the lens is irregular, distorting the image that reaches the retina.

A typical prescription for a person who is farsighted and also has astigmatism might be "+2.0D + 0.5 cyl axis 90." The "+2.0D" is the strength of a typical converging lens for a farsighted person, expressed in diopters. Diopters are equal to the inverse of the focal length, so 2.0 diopters equals a focal length of 0.5 meter, or 50 centimeters. The correction for astigmatism here specifies a cylindrical lens of +0.5 diopters situated at an angle of 90 degrees to the horizontal axis.

Astigmatism can be corrected with hard contact lenses because the lens makes contact with the cornea over a layer of tears. The tears fill the space between the lens and the misshapen eyeball, providing the extra focusing that is required.

Laser surgery has become a highly successful procedure to correct for vision problems, including astigmatism. The most common forms of refractive surgery for astigmatism are laser in situ keratomileusis (LASIK), photorefractive keratectomy (PRK), and laser epithelial keratomileusis (LASEK). In laser surgery, a computer-controlled laser beam is used to reshape the inner cornea to restore horizontal and vertical symmetry for the eyeball.

—Hans G. Graetzer, Ph.D.

See also Blurred vision; Eye infections and disorders; Eye surgery; Eyes; Laser use in surgery; Myopia; Ophthalmology; Optometry; Refractive eye surgery; Sense organs; Vision; Vision disorders.

For Further Information:

A.D.A.M. Medical Encyclopedia. "Astigmatism." *MedlinePlus*, September 3, 2012.

American Medical Association. *American Medical Association Family Medical Guide*. 4th rev. ed. Hoboken, N.J.: John Wiley & Sons, 2004.

Cameron, John R., James G. Skofronick, and Roderick M. Grant. *Medical Physics: Physics of the Body*. Madison, Wis.: Medical Physics, 1992.

Haughton, Alison N., and Eric L. Berman. "Astigmatism." *Health Library*, September 1, 2011.

"ISRS Refractive Surgery: Procedures." *International Society of Refractive Surgery*, 2013.

McCall, Richard P. "Optics of the Eye." In *Physics of the Human Body*. Baltimore: Johns Hopkins University Press, 2010.

Slade, Stephen G., Richard Baker, and Dorothy Brockman. *The Complete Book of Laser Eye Surgery*. Naperville, Ill.: Sourcebooks, 2002.

Astym® therapy

Procedure

Anatomy or system affected: Soft tissues of the body; muscles; tendons; ligaments; musculoskeletal systems and neural pathways

Specialties and related fields: Rehabilitation, Physical Therapy, Occupational Therapy, Athletic Training, Athletic Enhancement

Definition: Astym® treatment is regenerative soft tissue therapy that rebuilds and heals the soft tissues of the body, non-invasively and without pharmaceuticals. Astym® treatment safely and effectively stimulates internal scar tissue to be resorbed by the body and regenerates damaged soft tissues. This non-invasive therapeutic approach utilizes handheld instrumentation, applied topically, to locate underlying dysfunctional soft tissue and then transfer specific pressures and shear forces via that instrumentation to the dysfunctional tissue through specific protocols and application patterns developed from scientific and clinical study. The particular pressures and shear forces are aimed at inducing a cellular response, whereby cellular mediators and growth factors assist in activating scar tissue resorption, stimulating tissue turnover and regenerating soft tissues.

Indications and Procedures

Astym® therapy is typically provided in a physical or occupational therapy setting. However, elite athletes are frequently treated as part of their team care to optimize performance and treatment may occur at the site of competitions. In addition, large employers and the military routinely have Astym® therapy provided in their facilities or in the field in order to minimize interruption by resolving injuries effectively and efficiently.

Developed methodically from theory through basic science investigation to clinical study and practice, Astym® therapy engages the regenerative mechanisms of the body. It has been shown to be consistently safe and effective in the treatment of internal scar tissue that is causing pain or movement restriction, chronic tendonitis, traumatic soft tissue injury, post-surgical pain/restrictions and other soft tissue dysfunctions.

Tendinopathies and tendonitis are a widespread problem and often present a challenge to healthcare professionals, in many cases remaining unresolved. Astym® treatment is highly effective in the treatment of tendinopathy and clinical trials have demonstrated Astym® therapy to reduce pain, and increase motion and functional ability in this population. Effective both as a first-line treatment, and as a last resort when other treatments have failed, Astym® therapy is an attractive treatment option. It has a relatively short treatment course of four to six weeks (8-10 visits), and during treatment, there are usually no restrictions on activity, which is a welcome change from other more restrictive treatment options. Randomized clinical trials have shown Astym® therapy to be more effective than the standard-of-care treatments for lateral elbow tendinopathy (tennis elbow), patellar (knee) tendinopathy and Achilles tendinopathy.

Astym® therapy has also been found to reduce pain and increase function in cases where internal scar tissue is interfering with movement or causing pain. Internal scar tissue may result from a number of factors, including overuse, problematic biomechanics, trauma or surgery. Although Astym® therapy routinely demonstrates considerable success in the treatment of conditions where scar tissue is present, extraordinary improvement has been shown when Astym® therapy is used post-surgically.

There is also evidence that Astym® therapy can improve the brain-to-body connection by stimulating neuroplastic changes in damaged nervous systems. This is critically important, since Astym® therapy may alter the natural progression or prognosis for such disorders as cerebral palsy and brain injury, which has not yet been possible. The positive neural effects of Astym® therapy were demonstrated in a large, three-arm randomized controlled trial, which revealed that Astym® therapy immediately and significantly improves muscle performance after injury. These results are supported by other clinical studies indicating improvement in neural conditions such as carpal tunnel syndrome, restricted movement due to cerebral palsy and brain injury.

Uses and Complications

Some of the diagnoses that show strong clinical results from Astym® therapy		
General Conditions	Specific Conditions	
Chronic tendinopathy	Achilles Tendinopathy	Trochanteric Bursitis
Joint and muscle stiffness	Anterior and Posterior Tibialis Tendinopathy	Lateral Epicondylopathy
Sprains and strains	Arthrofibrosis	Low Back Pain (nonradicular)
Conditions resulting from dysfunctional scar tissue or fibrosis (e.g. post-traumatic, post-surgical	Carpal Tunnel Syndrome	Medial Epicondylopathy
	Chronic Ankle Pain and Stiffness	Patellar Tendinopathy
	Chronic Wrist Pain and Stiffness	Plantar Fasciopathy
	DeQuervain's Tenosynovitis	Post-Mastectomy Scarring
	Golfer's Elbow	Post-Surgical Scarring/Fibrosis
	Hamstring Strain	Rotator Cuff Tendinopathy
	IT Band Syndrome	Scar Tissue/Fibrosis
	Jumper's Knee	Tennis Elbow

Astym® therapy is generally well-tolerated by patients. The treating therapist/clinician should adjust the topical pressures and forces to be within the tolerance of each patient. General contraindications include: compromised skin integrity; open wound(s); active infection; skin ulcerations; acute deep venous thrombosis (DVT); treatment involving the area of a pacemaker or internal defibrillator; active primary or metastatic tumor site; clotting disorders; and any medical condition or disorder that may be exacerbated by the application of topical pressures on the skin or underlying structures.

In order to receive proper treatment, it is important to confirm that the clinician is officially certified in Astym® therapy. Certification training educates clinicians in the scientifically developed protocols and specific treatment parameters that have been studied in the randomized controlled trials. Astym® therapy has consistently demonstrated safety and effectiveness in clinical study and is also well tolerated by patients. Astym® therapy is distinctly different from instrument-assisted soft tissue mobilization (IASTM) interventions, and it is important to recognize that IASTM interventions show neither the effectiveness nor the safety of Astym® therapy. Although the IASTM methods use tools to treat tissue, the methods and results are quite different from those of Astym® therapy, and IASTM methods are often not well tolerated by patients. IASTM methods use tooled cross-friction massage to, it is argued, break apart the tissue, whereas Astym® therapy engages the regenerative mechanisms of the body aiming to repair damaged tissue and stimulate the resorption of scar tissue. A recent systematic review evaluated the research on IASTM and concluded the research does not support the efficacy of IASTM for treating musculoskeletal pathologies.

Perspective and Prospects

Historically, treatment for soft tissue disorders centered upon treating inflammation. However, with the discovery that tendinopathies and some other soft tissue conditions are primarily degenerative in nature, scholars emphasize that treatment should now be focused on regeneration and restoration. Astym® therapy was the first conservative treatment scientifically developed to engage the regenerative mechanisms of the body and has been proven to be effective in treating a variety of soft tissue disorders. Although many available treatments today still focus on reducing inflammation, they often have little to no scientific evidence supporting their effectiveness.

—*Thomas L. Sevier, MD*

For Further Information:

Cheatham SW, Lee M, Cain M, Baker R. "The Efficacy of Instrument Assisted Soft Tissue Mobilization: A Systematic Review." *Journal of the Canadian Chiropractic Association* 60, no. 3 (September 2016): 200-211. Research does not support the efficacy of IASTM for treating musculoskeletal pathologies.

Chughtai M, Mont MA, Cherian C, Cherian JJ, Elmallah RD, Naziri Q, Harwin SF, Bhave A. "A Novel, Nonoperative Treatment Demonstrates Success for Stiff Total Knee Arthroplasty after Failure of Conventional Therapy ." *Journal of Knee Surgery* 29, no. 3 (April 2016): 188-193. In a large study of post-surgical patients suffering from persistent knee stiffness, patients who underwent Astym® treatment reported significant improvements in their ability to move and function. These dramatic improvements were achieved despite the fact that the subject patients had already failed standard rehabilitation intervention.

Davies CC, Brockopp D, Moe K. "Astym® Therapy Improves Function and Range of Motion Following Mastectomy." *Breastcancer: Targets and Therapy* 8, (March 2016): 39-45. Following a course of treatment with Astym® therapy, which included treatment application to the thickened scar tissue and hypersensitive soft tissue adhesions in the affected area, patients experienced less pain, increased function and reduced hypersensitivity.

Kivlan BR, Carcia CR, Clemente FR, Phelps AL, Martin RL. "The Effect of Astym® Therapy on Muscle Strength: A Blinded, Randomized, Clinically Controlled Trial." *BMC Musculoskeletal Disorders* 16, (October 2015): 325. Subjects that received Astym® therapy increased maximal force output of the lower extremity immediately following treatment by an average of 15% from pretreatment values. This was significantly greater than the average 1% and 6% decrease in maximal force output demonstrated in the control and placebo treatment groups, respectively.

Ryan SL, Wallace P. "Use of Astym® Treatment to Improve Contractures and Dyskinesia in an Individual with Anoxic Encephalopathy." Combined Sections Meeting, APTA, (February 2009) Las Vegas, Nevada. In a patient with a traumatic brain injury, Astym® therapy improved movement and range of motion; prior to Astym® therapy, patient was bed-bound in need of total care. After Astym® therapy, patient had dramatic improvement in range of motion, could perform functions on his own, and self-propel a wheel chair.

Sevier, TL, Stegink-Jansen CW. "Astym® Treatment vs. Eccentric Exercise for Lateral Elbow Tendinopathy: A Randomized Controlled Clinical Trial." *PeerJ* 3, (May 2015): e967; DOI 10.7717/peerj.96. This large randomized, controlled trial showed Astym® therapy to be highly effective in resolving chronic tendinopathy, and also showed Astym® therapy to be highly effective on tendinopathy that failed to resolve with other treatment.

Scheer NA, Alstat LR, Van Zant RS. "Astym® Therapy Improves Bilateral Hamstring Flexibility and Achilles Tendinopathy in a Child with Cerebral Palsy: A Retrospective Case Report." *Clinical Medicine Insights: Case Reports* 9, (October 2016): 95-98 doi: 10.4137/CCRep.S40623. After being treated with Astym® therapy, a child with cerebral palsy improved flexibility and strength and could discontinue wearing braces.

Wilson JK, Sevier TL, Helfst RH, Honing EW, Thomann AL. "Comparison of Rehabilitation Methods in the Treatment of Patellar Tendinitis." *Journal of Sport Rehabilitation* 9, no. 4 (November 2000): 304-314. Astym® therapy resolved tendinopathy better than other treatments, and was also effective in treating patients whose tendinopathy would not resolve with other treatments.

Ataxia

Disease/Disorder

Anatomy or system affected: Brain, musculoskeletal system, nervous system

Specialties and related fields: Exercise physiology, family medicine, geriatrics and gerontology, internal medicine, neurology, nursing, occupational health, orthopedics, pediatrics, physical therapy, speech pathology

Definition: A lack of coordination while performing voluntary movements that may appear as clumsiness, inaccuracy, or instability.

Causes and Symptoms

Ataxia most often results from disorders of the cerebellum (a large structure at the lower back of the brain, just above where the spinal cord enters the skull at the bottom) or its connections. Disorders resembling ataxia can also be seen following parietal or frontal lobe lesions of the brain. Ataxia is a symptom, not a diagnosis. Ataxia may affect any part of the body.

Some medical conditions can cause ataxia to appear suddenly, such as head trauma, stroke, brain hemorrhage, brain tumor, congenital abnormality, postviral infections, exposure to certain drugs or toxins (for example, alcohol or seizure medications), and cardiac or respiratory arrest. Other conditions may cause ataxia to appear gradually, such as

---

Information on Ataxia

Causes: Head trauma, stroke, brain hemorrhage, brain tumor, congenital abnormality, postviral infections, exposure to certain drugs or toxins, cardiac or respiratory arrest, hypothyroidism, some vitamin deficiencies, certain cancers, multiple sclerosis, syphilis

Symptoms: Lack of coordination while performing voluntary movements (clumsiness, inaccuracy, instability)

Duration: Acute, chronic, or progressive, depending on cause

Treatments: Medications or surgery, depending on underlying condition; physical and occupational therapy

---

hypothyroidism, some vitamin deficiencies (vitamins E or B_{12}), exposure to certain drugs or toxins (heavy metals, chronic alcohol use, and some cancer drugs), certain kinds of cancer (ovarian and lung cancer), congenital abnormality, heredity disorders, multiple sclerosis, syphilis, and unknown causes of cerebellar degeneration disorders.

Treatment and Therapy

A careful neurologic and general physical examination, including blood tests and X-rays, can determine whether other parts of the nervous system are impaired and whether a medical illness may be causing ataxia. No medicine specifically treats the symptom of ataxia. If ataxia is the result of a stroke, a low vitamin level, or exposure to a toxic drug or chemical, then treatment would involve minimizing the effects of the current stroke and preventing further ones, instituting vitamin therapy, or avoiding the toxic drug or chemical, respectively. In some cases, the metabolic disorders that cause ataxia may be treated with controlled diet and medication. If ataxia is the result of a tumor, then surgery may be necessary. Many people with hereditary or idiopathic forms of ataxia have additional symptoms. Medications or other therapies might be appropriate for some of these symptoms, such as tremor, stiffness, spasticity, depression, and sleep disorders.

The mainstay of treatment for ataxia is the provision of physical and occupational therapy directed at maintaining function for as long as possible. Gait training and assistive devices such as canes, crutches, or a walker are useful to prevent falls and enhance mobility. Other adapted utensils and tools may be helpful to assist with writing, feeding, and self-care if hand or arm coordination is impaired, as may be speech therapy and communication devices for those with impaired speech.

Extremity ataxia that interferes with activities of daily living, such as feeding or dressing, may be treated with proximal splinting. Distal weights may dampen intention tremor. If the ataxia is exacerbated by weakness, strengthening exercises can be beneficial. Specific coordinated exercises are often helpful in treating static causes of ataxia (stroke or head injury) but not as useful in treating progressive disorders such as hereditary ataxias. Ataxia of eye movements rarely requires treatment, but it may be disabling if the patient has difficulty reading.

—*Linda L. Pierce, Ph.D., R.N.*

See also Alcoholism; Brain; Brain damage; Brain disorders; Brain tumors; Head and neck disorders; Multiple sclerosis; Muscle sprains, spasms, and disorders; Muscles; Nervous system; Neuroimaging; Neurology; Occupational health; Speech disorders; Strokes; Vitamins and minerals.

For Further Information:

Braddom, Randall L., ed. *Physical Medicine and Rehabilitation*. 3d ed. Philadelphia: Saunders, 2007.

Gillen, G. "Improving Activities of Daily Living Performance in an Adult with Ataxia." *American Journal of Occupational Therapy* 54, no. 1 (January/February, 2000): 89-96.

Gillen, G. "Improving Mobility and Community Access in an Adult with Ataxia." *American Journal of Occupational Therapy* 56, no. 4 (July/August, 2002): 462-66.

MedlinePlus. "Cerebellar Disorders." *MedlinePlus*, Apr. 19, 2013.

Athlete's foot

Disease/Disorder

Also known as: Tinea pedis

Anatomy or system affected: Feet, nails, skin

Specialties and related fields: Dermatology, podiatry

Definition: A microscopic fungal infection that lives on the outer layers of skin, nails, or hair on the feet.

Causes and Symptoms

Several different dermatophytes (microscopic fungi) can cause tinea pedis through contact with the skin on the bottom of the foot. Once contact is made, the dermatophytes grow if the environmental conditions are right. These fungi thrive in warm, moist surroundings such as wet shoes and socks or swimming pools, showers, and locker rooms. Since sweat is a common source of moisture for fungal growth, this disorder is often associated with athletes-thus the term "athlete's foot." It is commonly believed that athlete's foot is highly contagious. However, the presence of the fungus on the healthy foot does not necessarily result in the disorder; a warm, moist environment is also required.

The most common symptom of athlete's foot is constant itching or burning of the skin between the toes, particularly the outside, smaller toes. The skin turns white and begins to peel. A scaly, red dry rash develops and frequently progresses to cracks or fissures. A clear fluid may be released. If untreated, the infection may spread to the toenails and other areas of the foot. Also, the person becomes more susceptible to secondary bacterial infections.

Another form of athlete's foot results in a red, scaly rash that spreads across the bottom and sides of the foot. Because the rash pattern resembles a moccasin, this form is often called "moccasin foot."

Treatment and Therapy

With good hygiene and the removal of moist, warm environmental conditions, the fungus may die off on its own. If these conditions are not treated, however, the fungus can persevere for years. The best results occur with the use of antifungal drugs. Many types are available over the counter

---

Information on Athlete's Foot

Causes: Presence of fungi and warm, moist surroundings

Symptoms: Constant itching or burning between toes; peeling skin; dry, scaly rash; skin cracks or fissures

Duration: Acute or chronic

Treatments: Good hygiene; removal of moist, warm environment; antifungal drugs (creams, powders, sprays, liquids)

---

in creams, powders, sprays, or liquids. Imidazole drugs attack the cell walls of the fungus and keep the cells from growing and reproducing. Eventually, the infection will die off. More severe infections are treated with allylamine drugs. These drugs, which must be obtained with a prescription, cause a buildup of toxins that kill the fungi. If the nail is involved, systemic antifungal medication maybe needed.

The best treatment for athlete's foot is to prevent it by using good foot hygiene. Feet should be washed daily with soap and water. Wet feet should always be dried thoroughly, especially between the toes. Shoes and socks should be kept dry by regular changing and the use of foot powder to absorb moisture, if needed. Wearing light, airy shoes to reduce perspiration of the feet is also beneficial. Proper footwear is needed for public showers, gyms and bathrooms.

—*Bradley R. A. Wilson, PhD;*
updated by Nancy Banasiak

See also: Dermatology; Feet; Foot disorders; Fungal infections; Itching; Lower extremities; Over-the-counter medications; Podiatry; Rashes; Skin; Skin disorders.

For Further Information:

Donowitz, Leigh G., ed. *Infection Control in the Child Care Center and Preschool*. 8th ed. Philadelphia: Lippincott Williams & Wilkins, 2012.

Fink, Brett Ryan, and Mark S. Mizel. *The Whole Foot: A Complete Program for Taking Care of Your Feet*. New York: Demos Health, 2012.

Flint, Wesley and Cain, Jarrett. (2014). "Nail and Skin Disorders of the Foot." *Medical Clinics of North America, 98*, 213-225.

Goroll, Allen and Mullery, Albert. (2014). *Primary Care Medicine: Office Evaluation and Management of the Adult Patient*. Phili: Lippincott Williams & Wilkens.

Richardson, Malcolm D., and Elizabeth M. Johnson. *The Pocket Guide to Fungal Infection*. 3d ed. Malden, Mass.: Blackwell, 2012.

Walkins, Leon. *Walkins' Manual of Foot and Ankle Medicine and Surgery*. 4th Ed. Philadelphia: Wolters Kluwer, 2017

Atrial fibrillation

Disease/Disorder

Anatomy or system affected: Cardiovascular system, heart

Specialties and related fields: Cardiology, emergency medicine, intensive care, gerontology

Definition: Abnormal heart rhythms or muscle contractions in the atria resulting from disorganized electrical impulses.

Key terms:

anticoagulant: chemical substances that prevent or reduce

the coagulation of blood; also known as blood thinners

arrhythmia: improper beating of the heart; can be too fast, too slow, or irregular

electrocardiogram: device that records the electrical activity of the heart over a period of time using electrodes placed on the skin

embolus: unattached mass that travels through the bloodstream and is capable of clogging a blood vessel

fibrillation: rapid, irregular, and unsynchronized contraction of muscle fibers

Causes and Symptoms

In the normal heart, the sinoatrial node (SA node) generates regular, organized electrical impulses in the right atrium. In atrial fibrillation, also called A-Fib or AF, the sinoatrial node is overwhelmed by disorganized electrical impulses generated throughout both the left and right atria. These irregular electrical impulses may or may not be conducted to the ventricles, resulting in irregular ventricular contractions. An electrocardiogram (ECG or EKG), which analyzes the heart's electrical rhythm, can reveal electrical conduction abnormalities with atrial fibrillation. The electrical impulses seen on an ECG with atrial fibrillation are often described as "irregularly irregular".

Atrial fibrillation can present with a variety of symptoms, but often patients will present without any symptoms. Patients might describe feeling either a slow heartbeat (for example, heart "pauses") or palpitations (fast heartbeat). Other symptoms that can occur during an episode of atrial fibrillation are shortness of breath, lightheadedness or dizziness, fatigue, and chest discomfort. One of the biggest risks for patients with atrial fibrillation is the development of blood clots. Atrial fibrillation prevents the atria from contracting regularly, which causes blood to pool in the atria between skipped atrial contractions. This increases the risk of blood clotting in the atria and then embolizing to the brain, resulting in a stroke.

Atrial fibrillation may occur with or without other heart abnormalities. Commonly, atrial fibrillation occurs with an underlying heart condition. Patients who develop atrial fibrillation often also have a stiffening of the arteries, aortic stenosis, or enlargement of the left ventricle. Hypertension (high blood pressure) is another predisposing factor for this conduction irregularity. Other risk factors linked to atrial fibrillation include aging, obesity, sleep apnea, diabetes, and myocardial infarction (heart attack). It is important to consider the interdependence between genetics, the heart's response to risk factors, and aging when thinking about a patient's risk for developing atrial fibrillation.

Treatment and Therapy

The primary goal of therapy, when possible, is restoring the heart to a sinus rhythm. Additionally, treatments focus on preventing thromboembolic (blood clot) complications of atrial fibrillation. If the patient is experiencing acute atrial fibrillation, then the causative factors should be addressed. Electrical cardioversion, which maintains normal heart rhythms using coordinated electrical shocks, is the

---

Information on Atrial Fibrillation

Causes: Hypertension, acute myocardial infarction, coronary artery disease, valvular heart disease, heart surgery, thyroid disorders, pulmonary clots, acute alcohol ingestion, cocaine use, pneumonia, congenital or other heart defects, surges in vagal tone, idiopathic

Symptoms: Often asymptomatic; sometimes heart palpitations or fluttering, angina (chest tightness), shortness of breath, lightheadedness

Duration: Acute or chronic

Treatments: Electrical cardioversion, antiarrhythmics, anticoagulants, catheter ablation

---

treatment of choice. Heart rates can also be controlled effectively with antiarrhythmic medications such as beta-blockers, calcium channel blockers, or digoxin. Rare complications, such as embolic stroke, may arise due to lack of proper blood flow within the atria as a result of abnormal contractions (fibrillation). Anticoagulants (blood thinners) such as aspirin or warfarin can be prescribed to prevent stroke. Ablation therapy to destroy heart tissue producing the irregular electrical impulses or the Maze procedure, which creates new electrical pathways through the heart using scar tissue, can also be used if antiarrhythmics or cardioversion do not work. Lifestyle changes such as trigger avoidance and regular exercise may help patients avoid recurrences of acute atrial fibrillation.

Perspective and Prospects

It is projected that atrial fibrillation will continue to increase in incidence worldwide over the next few decades. Therefore, improvements in both the classification and the characterization of the disease are imperative. Refining the understanding of genetics, such as chromosome 4 variants, offer prospects for intervention. Stroke prevention, comprehensive treatment including both rate and rhythm control, and management of underlying conditions may also help mitigate atrial fibrillation.

—*Jesse Fishman, Pharm.D.;*
updated by Steffan Kim

See also: Arrhythmias; Cardiology; Cardiology, pediatric; Cardiopulmonary resuscitation*(CPR); Defibrillation; Echocardiography; Heart; Heart attack; Heart disease; Hypertension; Ischemia; Mitral valveprolapse; Pacemaker implantation; Palpitations.*

For Further Information:

A.D.A.M. Medical Encyclopedia. "Atrial Fibrillation or Flutter." *MedlinePlus*, June 22, 2012.

Camm,A. John, Thomas F. Lüscher, and PatrickW. Serruys, eds. *The ESC Textbook of Cardiovascular Medicine*. 2d ed. NewYork: Oxford University Press, 2009.

Fauci, Anthony S., et al. *Harrison's Principles of Internal Medicine*. 18th ed. New York: McGraw-Hill Medical, 2012.

Fox, C.S., et al. "Parental Atrial Fibrillation as a Risk Factor for Atrial Fibrillation in Offspring." *JAMA: Journal of the American Medical Association* 291, no. 23 (2004): 2851-2855.

Mosby's Medical Dictionary. 8th ed. St Louis: Mosby, 2009.

Wood, Debra, and Michael J. Fucci. "Atrial Fibrillation." *Health Library*, November 9, 2012.

Atrophy

Disease/Disorder

Also known as: Muscle wasting

Anatomy or system affected: Musculoskeletal system, nervous system, spine

Specialties and related fields: Family medicine, geriatrics and gerontology, neurology, nursing, orthopedics, osteopathic medicine, pathology, physical therapy, radiology, rheumatology, sports medicine

Definition: A wasting away or decrease in size and/or activity of a body part because of disease or other influences such as inactivity. Skeletal muscle can undergo atrophy because of disuse or neurological and musculoskeletal disease.

Key terms:

isokinetic: referring to the resistance training that provides muscular overload

neuromuscular electrical stimulation (NMES): the application of electrical and current to elicit a muscle contraction

Causes and Symptoms

Atrophy of any body organ can result from inadequate nutrition and lack of activity. However, other pathological conditions resulting in poor circulation, an interruption of nerve supply to the affected organ, and disease of the organ tissue itself can also cause atrophy. Muscle atrophy is a common form of atrophy that can result from various diseases of the nervous and musculoskeletal system. The body's metabolism of protein is also directly related to the condition of muscle atrophy, as muscle and liver protein can be used for energy. This research supports the finding that muscles atrophy during periods of inactivity. Muscle weakness can also be an early manifestation of thyroid or parathyroid disease.

The symptoms of atrophy are dependent upon the organ affected. Muscle atrophy is most evident with loss of function and general mobility. When muscles of the lower extremities become atrophied, the individual becomes easily fatigued with activity and may be at risk for falls.

Treatment and Therapy

The organ that is affected by atrophy dictates the treatment and therapy to be provided. Once any loss of circulation, nerve, or hormone support is regained, the atrophy normally diminishes and is replaced by growth to allow the return of normal function. As a general rule, muscles worked close to full capacity will increase in strength. The overload can be applied with standard weights, pulleys, springs, or a variety of isokinetic devices. Muscle growth in response to overload training occurs primarily from an enlargement of the individual muscle fibers.

Neuromuscular electrical stimulation (NMES) is the application of electrical current to elicit a muscle contraction. The use of NMES in orthopedic and neuromuscular rehabilitation has increased significantly over the years. A nerve action potential may be elicited either by a command originating in the motor cortex of the brain or by an electrically induced stimulus at the periphery. In either case, the

---

Information on Atrophy

Causes: For organs, inadequate nutrition, lack of activity, poor circulation, nerve supply interruption, organ disease; for muscles, nervous and musculoskeletal system disease, thyroid or parathyroid disease, protein metabolism, inactivity

Symptoms: For organs, dependent upon organ affected; for muscles, loss of function and general mobility, fatigue

Duration: Chronic, may be temporary

Treatments: Depends on causes; diminishes with recovery of circulation, nerve, or hormone support; strength exercises (weights, pulleys, springs, isokinetic devices); rehabilitation with neuromuscular electrical stimulation

---

action potential and release of transmission substances are the same.

Perspective and Prospects

Advances in medicine and rehabilitation have helped individuals afflicted with atrophy. The development of functional electrical stimulation allows individuals to carry out tasks by artificially stimulating muscles that have become too weak to carry out normal activity. Research in the area of spinal cord injuries is ongoing and advancing, addressing the causes and result of muscle atrophy from an interruption in nerve input.

—*Jeffrey P. Larson, P.T., A.T.C.*

See also Exercise physiology; Hypertrophy; Muscle sprains, spasms, and disorders; Muscles; Neurology; Neurology, pediatric; Overtraining syndrome; Physical rehabilitation.

For Further Information:

A.D.A.M. Health Encyclopedia. "Muscle Atrophy." *MedlinePlus*, March 22, 2013.

Genetics Home Reference. "Multiple System Atrophy." *National Institutes of Health*, August 20, 2013.

Gersh, Meryl R. *Electrotherapy in Rehabilitation*. Philadelphia: F. A. Davis, 1992.

Magee, D. G. *Orthopedic Assessment*. Philadelphia: W. B. Saunders, 1992.

McArdle, William, et al. *Exercise Physiology*. Philadelphia: Lea & Febiger, 1991.

National Human Genome Research Institute. "Learning About Spinal Muscular Atrophy." *National Institutes of Health*, February 19, 2012.

Noback, Charles R. *The Human Nervous System Introduction and Review*. 4th ed. Malvern, Pa.: Lea & Febiger, 1991.

Attention-deficit disorder (ADD)

Disease/Disorder

Also known as: Attention-deficit hyperactivity disorder (ADHD)

Anatomy or system affected: Brain, nervous system, psychic-emotional system

Specialties and related fields: Family medicine, genetics, neurology, pediatrics, psychiatry, psychology

Definition: A condition characterized by an inability to focus attention or to inhibit impulsive, hyperactive behavior; it is associated with poor academic performance and behavioral problems in children but also may be diagnosed in adults under certain conditions.

Key terms:

antianxiety medication: a medication that acts in the brain to decrease negative reactions to stress and anxiety and to decrease avoidance behavior

antidepressant: a medication that acts in the brain to decrease a sad or depressed mood and other behaviors associated with depression

nervous system: the system in the body, including the brain, that receives and interprets stimuli and transmits impulses to other organs; the brain is the center of thinking and behavior

neurotransmitter: a chemical in the brain that sends a signal from one brain cell to another

Causes and Symptoms

Most experts think that 3 to 7 percent of children may have attention-deficit disorder (ADD), which is more formally known as attention-deficit hyperactivity disorder (ADHD). The cause of ADD is unknown, although the fact that it often occurs in families suggests some degree of genetic inheritance. The condition is more common in boys, but it does occur in girls. ADD is usually diagnosed when a child enters school, but it may be discovered earlier. Adolescents and even adults who were not diagnosed earlier in life may be diagnosed later in life when their symptoms cause particularly severe problems. Some causes of ADD that have been suggested, but never proved, include low blood sugar, food additives, the sweetener aspartame, allergies, and vitamin deficiencies. Other causes being explored include head injury, exposure to emotionally traumatic situations such as abuse or violence, and exposure to environmental contaminants such as lead or substances of abuse such as nicotine in utero.

Children who do not have ADD may, at times, have some of the symptoms of this disorder, but children who can be diagnosed with ADD must have most of the symptoms most of the time-in school, at home, or during other activities. The symptoms are usually grouped into three main categories: inattention, hyperactivity, and impulsiveness.

Children who have symptoms of inattention often make careless mistakes at school or do not pay close attention to details in play or work. They may have problems sustaining attention over time and frequently do not seem to listen when spoken to, especially in groups. Children with ADD have difficulty following instructions and often fail to finish chores or schoolwork. They do not organize well and may have messy rooms and desks at school. They also frequently lose things necessary for play or school. Because they have trouble sustaining attention, children with ADD dislike tasks that require this skill and will try to avoid them. One of the key symptoms is distractibility, which means that children with ADD are often paying attention to extraneous sights, sounds, smells, and thoughts rather than focusing on the task that they should be doing. Particularly frustrating to parents is the symptom of forgetfulness in

---

Information on Attention-Deficit Disorder (ADD)

Causes: Unknown, possibly genetic
Symptoms: Inattention, hyperactivity, impulsiveness
Duration: Chronic
Treatments: Medication, counseling

---

daily activities, in spite of numerous reminders from parents about such common, everyday activities as dressing, hygiene, manners, and other behaviors. Children with ADD have a poor sense of time; they are frequently late or think that they have more time to do a task than they really do.

Not all children with ADD have symptoms of hyperactivity, but many have problems with fidgeting, or squirming. It is common for these children to be constant talkers, often interrupting others. Other symptoms of hyperactivity include leaving their seat in school, church, or similar settings and running around excessively in situations where they should be still. Children with ADD have difficulty playing quietly, although they may watch television or play video games for long periods of time. Some of these children seem to be driven by a motor, or are continuously on the go.

All children with ADD will have some symptoms of impulsiveness, such as blurting out answers before questions are completed. Another example of impulsiveness would be or intruding upon others in conversation or in some activity. They may also have difficulty standing in lines or waiting for their turn in games.

It is important to recognize that children with ADD are not bad children who are hyperactive, impulsive, and inattentive on purpose. Rather, they are usually bright children who would like to behave better and to be more successful in school, in social life with peers, and in family affairs, but they simply cannot. One way to think about ADD is to consider it a disorder of the ability to inhibit impulsive, off-task, or undesirable attention. Consequently, the child with ADD cannot separate important from unimportant stimuli and cannot sort appropriate from inappropriate responses to those stimuli. It is easy to understand how someone whose brain is trying to respond to a multitude of stimuli, rather than sorting stimuli into priorities for response, will have difficulty focusing and maintaining attention to the main task.

It is also important to remember that it is not only the presence of symptoms that categorizes a child as having ADD but also the intensity and prevalence of the symptoms in more than one setting. For example, a child may not seem to pay attention in school and often may be disruptive in class but be a normal child at home, playing Little League baseball, and in church school. This child may have a learning disability without ADD or a specific conflict with the teacher.

Children most likely to be diagnosed correctly with ADD will have many of the following characteristics. They will have a short attention span, particularly for activities that are not fun or entertaining. They will be unable to concentrate because they will be distracted by peripheral stimuli. They will have poor impulse control so that they seem to act on the spur of the moment. They will be hyperactive and usually rather clumsy, resulting in their being labeled "accident-prone." They will certainly have school problems, especially when classwork requires more thinking and planning-often seen about third grade and beyond. They may display attention-demanding behavior and/or show resistant or overpowering social behaviors. Last, children with ADD often act as if they were younger, and "immaturity" is a frequent label. Along with this trait, they have wide mood swings and are seen as very emotional.

Many experts think that ADD is a developmental problem, caused by the failure of the brain and nervous system to grow and mature normally. Thus, while some behavior might be acceptable at earlier ages, when it persists into later ages, it may signal a developmental problem. For an average, normal two-year-old child, a short attention span, impulsivity, distractibility, clumsiness, recklessness, and less-than-perfect planning abilities would not be unexpected or very troublesome. All these characteristics are acceptable for the toddler. When those symptoms persist into and beyond kindergarten, however, they are of greater concern and may signal a need for further evaluation. For some, this slowed development may improve during childhood. For others, however, it may persist into adolescence and create additional problems.

Adolescents who have ADD are usually not hyperactive, although they may have problems with impulsive talking and behavior. They have considerable difficulty complying with rules and following directions. They may be poorly organized, causing problems both with starting projects and with completing them. Their inability to monitor their own behavior leads to problems making and keeping friends and causes them to have conflicts with parents and teachers beyond those normally seen in teenagers. Adolescents with ADD usually have problems in school in spite of average or above-average potential. They may have poor self-esteem and a low frustration tolerance. Because of these and other factors related to ADD, they may also be at greater risk of developing substance use problems and other mental health problems.

Several other neurologic or psychiatric disorders have symptoms that can overlap with ADD, so diagnosis is often difficult. When a child is suspected of having ADD, he or she should have a thorough medical interview with, and physical examination by, a physician familiar with child development, ADD, and related conditions. A psychological evaluation to determine intelligence quotient (IQ) and areas of learning and performance strengths and weaknesses should be obtained. School records need to be reviewed, and teachers may be asked to submit rating forms or similar instruments to document school performance. A thorough family history and a discussion of family problems such as divorce, violence, alcoholism, or drug abuse should be part of the evaluation. Other conditions that might be found to exist along with ADD, or to be the underlying cause of symptoms thought to be ADD, include

oppositional defiant disorder, conduct disorder (usually seen in older children), depression, and anxiety disorder.

Many physicians, teachers, psychologists, and parents do not believe that ADD is a "real" condition, but this disorder is widely accepted as a credible diagnosis for a child who demonstrates many of the above symptoms at home, at play, and at school. ADD was first defined in the third edition of the American Psychiatric Association's *Diagnostic and Statistical Manual of Mental Disorders* (1980), or *DSM-III*, and its definition has evolved since then. In 1998, the National Institutes of Health (NIH) held a Consensus Development Conference on the Diagnosis and Treatment of Attention Deficit Hyperactivity Disorder. While most experts supported the ADD diagnosis, the final report noted a need for further research into the validity of the diagnosis. The fifth edition of the *DSM* (*DSM-5*), published in 2013, updates the definition of ADHD to reflect studies that show that the condition lasts beyond childhood and to help clinicians diagnose and care for adults with ADHD.

Treatment and Therapy

Treatment and therapy for ADD will usually begin with the diagnostic process and involves the family of the child affected. Generally, treatment will consist of some combination of psychotherapy, medication, and education. In some cases, therapy for the child and/or the family may be indicated. This therapy may be help the family learn about ADD. It also may be recommended when things happening in the family are seen as related to the type or severity of symptoms that the child may be experiencing. For instance, if the family is undergoing a stressful event, such as a divorce, serious loss, or death, or other problems such as economic stress, then the symptoms of ADD may worsen. Therefore, treatment may focus on trying to minimize the impact of such stressors on the child.

The medical treatment of ADD is one of the most controversial issues in education and in medicine. Although scientific studies clearly show the value of certain medications, and scores of parents and teachers have noticed remarkable improvement with treatment, some people take issue with using medications to change a child's behavior. Clearly, medications alone are not the answer for ADD. Families and children need guidance and support in the form of counseling, as well as considerable information about the condition. Special accommodations can be arranged with most schools and are mandated by federal law. Once educational adjustments have been made and counseling is in place, however, medications can play an important role.

The most frequently prescribed medications are stimulants; they include dexedrine, methylphenidate (Ritalin), and a combination of dexedrine salts (Adderall). A similar medication, pemoline (Cylert), has been related to side effects, which may limit its usefulness. The stimulant medications may function by influencing chemicals in the brain called neurotransmitters, which help transmit messages among brain and nerve cells. In ADD, it is thought that the medications improve the function of cells that direct the brain to focus attention, resist distraction, control behavior, and perceive time correctly. These medications are generally thought to be safe and effective, although they can have such adverse effects as headache, stomachache, mood changes, heart rate changes, appetite suppression, and interference with going to sleep. All children receiving medication must be monitored at regular intervals by a physician.

Other medications that may be used for ADD include antidepressants and antianxiety medications. Some children are treated with combinations of two medications; in unusual circumstances, there may be even more than two. Some of these medications are Imipramine and Desipramine, antidepressants that act mainly to control impulsiveness and hyperactivity; Bupropion, an antidepressant, and Buspar, an antianxiety medicine, both of which have been used largely in older children and adolescents; and clonidine and guanfacine, which work on brain nerve message transmitters and are sometimes helpful in calming aggressive behavior. Behavior modification and several forms of psychotherapy or counseling are also held to be effective, whether concurrently with or as a replacement for medication. Critics of medication have expressed concerns not only with side effects but also with the potential for contributing to drug abuse, and a belief in the greater long-term effectiveness of psychotherapy alone. The latter view suggests that medication may interfere with promoting true self-control. The 1998 NIH consensus report emphasized the continuing controversies and the need for outcomes research pertaining to these issues.

Costs and risks for adverse effects should be discussed with the physician who has made the diagnosis of ADD before implementing any treatment, to ensure safety and a reasonable expectation of efficacy.

Perspective and Prospects

Attention-deficit disorder remains controversial due to the subjective nature of its symptoms, the possible overdiagnosis and overtreatment of the disorder, and concerns that medications prescribed for the disorder may lead to addiction, anxiety, and psychosis. Historically, experts have estimated that ADD affects between 3 and 7 percent of all children and adolescents. However, in March 2013, the *New York Times* reported that data from the Centers for Disease Control and Prevention showed that approximately 11 percent of children between the ages of four and seventeen have been diagnosed with ADHD, representing a 16 percent increase since 2007 and a 53 percent rise over the last decade. ADHD experts caution against attributing the increase to a single factor, including misdiagnosis and increased treatment of milder forms of the disorder.

For children and adolescents with ADD, the disorder is a real issue that can cause great harm if not recognized and managed correctly. Diagnosis should be based on documentation of the child's and family's history, careful examination, and thorough educational and psychological assessment. Treatment should always include educational accommodations and counseling for the child and the family. When symptoms create problems at home and at school, properly prescribed and managed medications have been shown to offer great relief in most cases. However, in 2013, researchers at Johns Hopkins published the results of a six-year study in which they found that 90 percent of the 186 young children they studied who were treated for ADHD (either with or without medication) continued to have symptoms. The researchers were not sure whether their findings meant that the medications were ineffective, were not being taken as directed, or were being prescribed incorrectly.

Children and parents in the United States can share experiences and resources through organizations that assist families dealing with attention-deficit disorder. The national organization Children and Adults with Attention Deficit/Hyperactivity Disorder (CHADD) has state and local chapters helping families cope with the condition. CHADD chapters often have libraries and provide resources on ADD. Learning Disabilities Association of America (LDA) has state and local chapters helping schools and families cope with a wide range of learning disabilities, including ADD.

In 2013, scientists were able to study real-time images of late-stage fetal brain development. Researchers are hopeful that studies of the development of brain connections in fetuses will lead to improved therapies for ADHD and other disorders.

—Robert W. Block, M.D.;
Nancy E. Macdonald, Ph.D.;
updated by Nancy A. Piotrowski, Ph.D.

See also Anxiety; Brain; Brain disorders; Emotions: Biomedical causes and effects; Learning disabilities; Pediatrics; Psychiatry, child and adolescent; Puberty and adolescence; Stress.

For Further Information:
American Psychiatric Association. *Diagnostic and Statistical Manual of Mental Disorders: DSM-5.* Arlington, Va.: Author, 2013.
Accardo, Pasquale J., ed. *Attention Deficits and Hyperactivity in Children and Adults: Diagnosis, Treatment, Management.* 2d ed. New York: Dekker, 2000.
Barkley, Russell A. *Taking Charge of ADHD.* Rev. ed. New York: Guilford, 2005.
Breggin, Peter R. *Talking Back to Ritalin.* Rev. ed. Cambridge, Mass.: Perseus, 2001.
Children and Adults with Attention Deficit/Hyperactivity Disorder. *CHADD*, 2013.
Dallas, Mary Elizabeth. "HealthDay: ADHD Treatments Not Working for Most Young Children." *MedlinePlus*, Feb. 11, 2013.
HealthDay. "HealthDay: Brains of Fetuses 'Build a Bridge' between Regions, Images Show." *MedlinePlus*, Feb. 20, 2013.
MedlinePlus. "Attention Deficit Hyperactivity Disorder." *MedlinePlus*, May 6, 2013.
Phelan, Thomas W. *All About Attention Deficit Disorder: Symptoms, Diagnosis, and Treatment-Children and Adults.* 2d rev. ed. London: Gardner's, 2006.
Quinn, Patricia O., ed. *ADD and the College Student: A Guide for High School and College Students with Attention Deficit Disorder.* Rev. ed. Washington, D.C.: Magination, 2001.
Quinn, Patricia O., and Judith M. Stern. *Putting on the Brakes: Understanding and Taking Control of Your ADD or ADHD.* 2d ed. Washington, D.C.: Magination, 2008.
Ramsay, J. Russell. *Nonmedication Treatments for Adult ADHD: Evaluating Impact on Daily Functioning and Well-Being.* Washington, D.C.: American Psychological Association Press, 2009.

Rief, Sandra F. *The ADHD Book of Lists: A Practical Guide for Helping Children and Teens with Attention Deficit Disorders*. San Francisco: Jossey, 2003.

Audiology

Specialty

Anatomy or system affected: Ears

Specialties and related fields: Neurology, otorhinolaryngology, speech pathology

Definition: The study of the auditory system and its measurement, including the assessment of the medical, surgical, or rehabilitation implications arising from a number of disorders affecting hearing.

Key terms:

audiologist: one who is specifically trained at an approved institution of learning to provide diagnostic testing and rehabilitative training to those with hearing disorders

audiometer: a calibrated electronic device for the purpose of measuring human hearing to determine the magnitude of loss and the probable rehabilitative course

auditory system: the human hearing mechanism, including the pinna, the external ear canal, the middle ear structures, the cochlea, and the ascending neural pathway that terminates in the auditory cortex of the brain

auditory system disorder: any condition or state that interferes with or alters the normal function of acoustic information transfer from the outer ear to the brain

aural rehabilitation: a program for hearing-impaired individuals that may include auditory prostheses, auditory training, and speech-reading training

communicative skills: those skills required to express thoughts, desires, and feelings effectively through verbal communication

habilitative: referring to the process of creating or teaching a function involving human behavior, thought, and reason

mixed hearing loss: the combined effects of the loss of sensory or neural integrity and the presence of a barrier to the normal transmission of sound (such as wax in the ear, a hole in the eardrum, or some congenital anomaly affecting the transmission pathway of the auditory system)

rehabilitative: referring to the process of re-creating or teaching a function that has been impaired as a result of injury, disease, or aging

retrocochlear hearing loss: any disruption of neural information processing beyond the cochlea

sensorineural hearing loss: the loss of sensory or neural tissue of the auditory system as a result of disease, age, or acquired or congenital factors

Science and Profession

The field of audiology has become an indispensable adjunct in the objective diagnosis of hearing loss and auditory disorders. The scope of audiology practice is rather extensive and includes broad categorical services. According to the US Department of Labor, the audiologist "specializes in diagnostic evaluation of hearing, prevention, habilitative and rehabilitative services for auditory problems and research related to hearing and attendant disorders." Among other functions, the audiologist

determines range, nature, and degree of hearing function...using electroacoustic instrumentation;...coordinates audiometric results with other diagnostic data, such as educational, medical, social, and behavioral information;...differentiates between organic and nonorganic hearing disabilities through evaluation of total response pattern and use of acoustic tests;...[and] plans, directs, conducts, or participates in conservation, habilitative and rehabilitative programs, including hearing aid selection and orientation, counseling guidance, auditory training, speech reading, language rehabilitation, and speech conservation.

Audiologists may have primary affiliations in private practice, clinics and hospitals, military installations, universities and colleges, or public and private school systems.

Because of the significant advances that have been made in providing differential diagnosis of impaired auditory behavior, the number of institutions providing audiology programs increased dramatically in the latter half of the twentieth century. Although the highest degree offered in audiology at many institutions is the PhD, a number of schools offer a professional doctorate of audiology, which stresses clinical diagnosis, auditory prosthetic evaluation, and rehabilitative practice.

A number of professional audiology organizations exist to provide resources and support to those in the field. The membership of the American Speech-Language-Hearing Association (ASHA) consists of speech pathologists and audiologists, with the former having significantly greater numbers. In 1988, James Jerger and other prominent audiologists in the United States formed the American Academy of Audiology. Its members consist exclusively of audiologists holding a master's or PhD degree in that field.

Diagnostic and Treatment Techniques

One of the most common services associated with the practice of audiology is the basic assessment of the auditory system relative to pure-tone air conduction thresholds. This is a procedure in which the patient's ability to detect the presence of a tone delivered through earphones or a speaker is determined. Additionally, speech threshold detection is determined by assessing the patient's ability to identify correctly 50 percent of a list of two-syllable words. Measurements of the acoustic reflex provide information about hearing loss, as do reflex-eliciting auditory tests. The acoustic reflex is the contraction of the stapedial muscle produced by a strong acoustic signal. The strength of the response and the level at which it is elicited are important diagnostic indicators of system malfunction, as is the absence of a reflex response. The degree to which the reflex response deviates in morphology and amplitude from normal is diagnostically significant. Communication handicap inventories also are an essential part of the basic assessment procedure. Such inventories provide useful information as to the degree of social handicap as a concomitant part of hearing impairment. Serial communication inventories serve as indicators of the effectiveness of habilitative or rehabilitative programs designed to enhance communicative skills. The term "basic" is applied to indicate a routine assessment of auditory function. Basic assessment does not provide the preponderance of clinical evidence needed to determine the site of injury or disease or to suggest its medical or surgical management.

Another service associated with audiology is an extended evaluation of the auditory system, which is composed of all anatomical structures that contribute to human hearing. Such an evaluation may include the determination of air conduction, bone conduction, and speech thresholds, as well as the administration of word and sentence recognition tests. Air conduction tests are performed by placing calibrated headphones over the patient's ears and presenting a broad range of discrete frequencies. In practice, that frequency range extends from 250 to 8,000 hertz. Even though the normal human ear is capable of perceiving a much broader frequency range (from 20 hertz to 20,000 hertz), the range between 250 hertz and 8,000 hertz contains all the essential frequencies needed to understand speech. Bone conduction thresholds are determined by placing a vibrator, or bone oscillator, at the mastoid bone and presenting the same frequency range. Often, differences in the patient's response to air-conducted and bone-conducted signals provide essential diagnostic information and suggest the site of injury or disease.

Speech threshold and word or sentence evaluations provide the clinician with performance scores that indicate the degree to which speech understanding has been compromised by the hearing disorder. Such measurements also indicate the probability of understanding connected discourse in communicative situations. There are a number of speech tests that provide information about the status of the auditory system. The most commonly used speech stimuli are two-syllable words to determine an individual's speech reception threshold and one-syllable words to assess the auditory system's discrimination function.

Another standard audiological practice is a comprehensive behavioral evaluation to determine the sensorineural site of lesion, that is, the place in the auditory system from which the hearing disorder originates. For most hearing disorders affecting auditory performance, it is critical that this site be located. It may be found in the peripheral system (the cochlea), which contains specialized sensory tissue that responds to sound pressure changes. The problem could also lie in the ascending auditory pathway, including its terminal projection in the auditory cortex of the brain. To arrive at an accurate diagnosis, the audiologist employs a number of advanced tests, such as sophisticated acoustic reflex tests, tests of frequency discrimination (the ability to detect differences between two or more signals), tests of intensity discrimination, and tests of auditory adaptation. The latter is a clinical procedure in which one determines whether a continuous sound decays over time to the point of inaudibility; such abnormal decay of the test signal indicates possible malfunction of the neural pathway of the auditory system. The results of these several tests increase significantly the probability that the site of lesion can be found.

One of the most promising clinical advances in audiology has been the development of evoked response audiometry (ERA). ERA is best defined as the measurement of neuroelectrical activity generated in the brain stem or of higher orders of brain function elicited by an acoustic signal. Acoustic signals, clicks, and tone pips are submitted to the external auditory ear. If the signals are detected by the auditory system, there is a change in neuroelectrical activity for each signal presented. A computer stores these minute changes in activity. When a sufficient number of acoustic signals have been processed, the computer prints out a response pattern consistent with the transmission of the electrical response from cochlear and subsequent responses as the signal travels to the brain. Response patterns have been classified as first (from the cochlea, zero to two milliseconds), fast (from the acoustic nerve and auditory brain stem, two to ten milliseconds), slow (from the primary and secondary areas of the cerebral cortex, fifty to three hundred milliseconds), and late (from the primary and associated areas of the cerebral cortex, more than three hundred milliseconds). More recent terminology of these time-related events refers to them as early, middle, and late responses.

Evoked potential measurement is significant because it offers a method of auditory assessment for those patients unwilling or unable to give reliable voluntary responses to acoustic stimuli. For example, evoked response audiometry provides a means of detecting hearing impairment in the neonate and very young. It also provides a clinical method of determining normal or abnormal hearing function for those who are mentally retarded. Evoked responses to acoustic stimuli aid in the diagnosis of various types of tumors or neuromas that affect the transmission of auditory signals to the brain. If such lesion sites are detected early, it may be possible to remove them surgically and save the patient's hearing. Certainly, early detection of retrocochlear pathology increases the probability that surgical intervention will preserve auditory system performance.

In 1978, D. T. Kemp published a germinal paper identifying the presence of otoacoustic emissions. Spontaneous emissions are generated within the cochlea and can be measured by a probe microphone assembly inserted into the external ear canal. Not all individuals have spontaneous otoacoustic emissions that can be measured by current probe microphone systems. Evoked otoacoustic emissions can be measured, however, in individuals having normal hearing or hearing loss of no more than forty to forty-five decibels. Such emissions are evoked by presenting a series of clicks or other compatible acoustic stimuli to the patient's auditory system. The cochleomechanical activity induced by these acoustic signals is "picked up" by a probe microphone and processed by a computer. The graphic information obtained has proven to be of significant benefit in the screening of neonates and the very young. The literature would seem to suggest that otoacoustic emission measurement is fast, reliable, and repeatable. Research is under way to assess the range of losses that can be measured and the most appropriate stimuli to be employed in order to gain specific bits of information about cochlear behavior.

Auditory prosthetic evaluations have become common practice in audiology. When tests for hearing function determine that a hearing impairment exists, medical referral is mandatory for appropriate clinical management. For a sizable number of hearing-impaired individuals, however, medical or surgical intervention will not alter the hearing loss. For cases in which hearing impairment is a permanent sensorineural condition, a hearing aid or assistive listening device (or both) is often the preferred treatment modality in the rehabilitative process. To determine the appropriate electroacoustic characteristics of the hearing aid device to compensate best for the hearing deficit, special tests are conducted. Such tests may measure differences in word and speech understanding with and without the hearing aid. Another important test measures the degree of comfort or discomfort resulting from the sound level that is produced by the hearing aid device; if such a test is not performed, the patient may reject the hearing aid because it is too loud and unpleasant. Other tests designed to help determine the appropriate level of amplified sound involve narrow-band noise thresholds and various environmental sounds to which the patient may be periodically exposed during the activities of daily living. The use of environmental sound recordings provides the audiologist with objective indications of the electroacoustic responses that will yield maximum speech discrimination in the presence of specific background noises.

Audiology has helped many children and adults with hearing impairment through the use of hearing aids and the practice of aural rehabilitation. The selection and fitting of hearing aid devices have become important parts of the professional responsibilities of the clinical audiologist. With the many advances in hearing aid technology that have occurred, the audiologist has been given a much broader array of electroacoustic devices from which to select the one that offers the best correspondence with a patient's needs. For example, some commercial hearing aid systems can be digitally programmed to meet the specific acoustic requirements of the hearing-impaired individual. In some cases, programmable hearing aids provide more than one acoustic response at the immediate command of the user. Should the device fail to meet the acoustic requirements of the patient, it can be reprogrammed in a short period of time to achieve a better correlation with the patient's need for amplification.

Auditory (aural) rehabilitation is also of clinical concern to the audiologist, and a major branch of audiological practice is in this field. In this context, rehabilitation refers to the development and conduct of special programs to assist the hearing impaired in using and understanding verbal language (speech) more efficiently. For example, for those children born with a severe auditory deficit, the early introduction of aural rehabilitation programs is of paramount

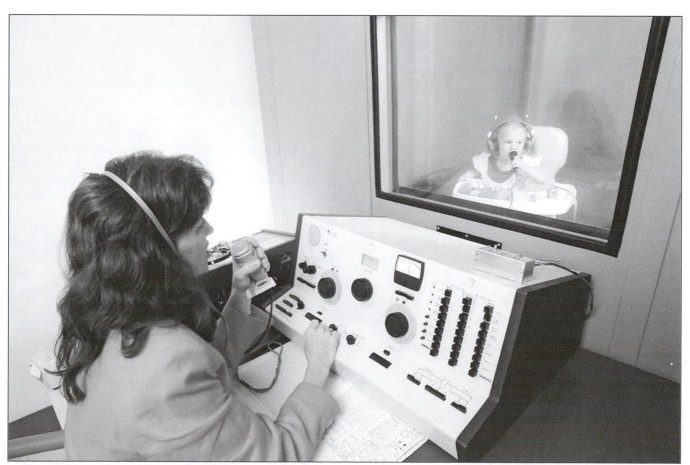

An audiologist administers a hearing test to a child. Routine screening is often used to detect problems in children. (Digital Stock)

importance to the development of verbal language. Consistent with the development of rehabilitation programs is the early detection of hearing impairment that cannot be ameliorated by surgical or medical intervention. From a rehabilitative point of view, early introduction of hearing aid amplification and supportive auditory and speech-reading training programs have been of inestimable value in speech and language development for the hearing-impaired child. In some of the major school systems throughout the United States, there is an "educational audiologist" whose task it is to develop and maintain special programs intended to assist hearing-impaired children.

Equally as important are auditory rehabilitation programs for the hearing-impaired adult. Hearing impairment is a rather insidious phenomenon, gradually worsening over time. Consequently, adult patients are somewhat unaware of hearing loss until they fail to recognize enough of speech sounds to understand intended messages. When speech understanding has been degraded by hearing impairment, rehabilitative programs stress the use of hearing aid amplification and the value of speech reading. Training programs may assist the adult in learning speech-reading skills or in adapting to a hearing aid device. It is important that the audiologist be aware of attitudes or behaviors that may restrict or limit a patient's acceptance of and participation in programs designed to assist the hearing impaired.

Perspective and Prospects

Audiology, as a recognized academic discipline, originated during World War II. At that time, thousands of military personnel needed diagnostic and rehabilitative services for ear injuries incurred during active service. It was essential that an organized program be developed to meet the demand. Several military hospitals and selected universities and colleges undertook the task of developing programs to accomplish these diagnostic and rehabilitative tasks. One of the first textbooks dealing exclusively with audiological practice was authored by Hayes Newby in 1958, while he was teaching at Stanford University. Since that memorable introduction, hundreds of special texts have been published relative to various aspects of audiological practice.

Since the early pioneering days during World War II, the field of audiology and the clinical skills of audiologists have expanded appreciably. Significant advances in auditory disorder diagnosis and in prosthetic and rehabilitative care have been made. Although audiology is a relatively new academic and professional discipline, its contributions to the understanding and treatment of auditory system disorders have greatly advanced the understanding of its role in human communication.

—*Robert Sandlin, Ph.D.*

See also Aging; Aging: Extended care; Biophysics; Deafness; Dyslexia; Ear infections and disorders; Ear surgery; Ears; Hearing; Hearing loss; Hearing tests; Ménière's disease; Motion sickness; Neurology; Neurology, pediatric; Otorhinolaryngology; Sense organs; Speech disorders.

For Further Information:

Alpiner, Jerome G., and Patricia A. McCarthy, eds. *Rehabilitative Audiology: Children and Adults*. 3d ed. Philadelphia: Lippincott Williams & Wilkins, 2000.

Gelfand, Stanley A. *Essentials of Audiology*. 3d ed. New York: Thieme, 2009.

Hall, James W. *Introduction to Audiology*. Boston: Allyn & Bacon, 2013.

Jerger, James, ed. *Pediatric Audiology*. San Diego, Calif.: College-Hill Press, 1984.

Katz, Jack, ed. *Handbook of Clinical Audiology*. 6th ed. Philadelphia: Wolters Kluwer/Lippincott Williams & Wilkins, 2009.

Lubinski, Rosemary, and Carol M. Frattali, eds. *Professional Issues in Speech-Language Pathology and Audiology*. San Diego, Calif.: Thomson/Delmar Learning, 2007.

Madell, Jane R., and Carol Flexer. *Pediatric Audiology Casebook*. New York: Thieme, 2011.

Mendel, Lisa Lucks, Jeffrey L. Danhauer, and Sadanand Singh. *Singular's Illustrated Dictionary of Audiology*. San Diego, Calif.: Singular, 1999.

Newby, Hayes, and Gerald Popelka. *Audiology*. 6th ed. Englewood Cliffs, N.J.: Prentice Hall, 1992.

Roeser, Ross J. *Roeser's Audiology Desk Reference*. 2d ed. New York: Thieme, 2013.

Auras

Disease/Disorder

Anatomy or system affected: Arms, brain, ears, eyes, legs, mouth, nervous system, nose, psychic-emotional system, skin, throat

Specialties and related fields: Internal medicine, neurology, psychiatry, psychology

Definition: Warning sensations of varying kinds received by the patient prior to a seizure, migraine, or psychotic episode.

Causes and Symptoms

Causes of auras include seizures (epilepsy), drug side effects, delirium, dementia, migraines, cerebral palsy, brain cancers, convulsions, hallucinations, and the aging process. General symptoms include skin sensations and motor, vegetative, and psychological phenomena. More specific symptoms include epigastric discomfort, dizziness, faintness, and basic elementary phenomena, such as seeing brilliant dots and lines, hearing nonexistent sounds, and experiencing strange and disagreeable odors. Symptoms occasionally include a "pins-and-needles" feeling on one side of the face or body, followed by numbness, or numbness without tingling. Other symptoms include speech problems, confusion, weakness on one side, mood swings, mental fuzziness, and fluid retention.

Treatment and Therapy

Auras (seizures) are of diagnostic importance because they suggest a cerebral localization. For these sufferers, surgery of the affected brain area may bring some relief, as might the use of appropriate medication.

Migraine aura sufferers benefit from the use of several antimigraine drugs, including Inderal (propranolol) and Sansert (methysergide), as well as analgesics and ergotamines. All of the above are effective drugs in stopping a migraine attack once it has begun. The sufferers of

Information on Auras

Causes: Seizures, migraines, drug side effects, delirium, dementia, cerebral palsy, brain cancers, convulsions, hallucinations, aging process

Symptoms: Skin sensations, dizziness, faintness, seeing brilliant dots and lines, hearing nonexistent sounds, experiencing disagreeable odors, tingling and/or numbness, speech problems, confusion, weakness on one side, mood swings

Duration: Temporary

Treatments: Surgery, medications

auras related to psychosis will also benefit from the use of appropriate psychotropic medications.

Perspective and Prospects

Aura derives from a Greek word for "breeze." The term was introduced by Galen, a Greek physician and writer of the second century BCE, to designate a momentary gasping sensation experienced by some patients before an epileptic attack.

Current US laws permit epilepsy patients with controlled seizures to drive. Factors that significantly decrease the odds of patients with epilepsy having motor vehicle crashes due to seizures are long seizure-free intervals, reliable auras, few prior non-seizure-related accidents, and having had their antiepileptic drugs (AEDs) reduced or switched. Patients who have rare seizures without definite auras should not drive alone.

The majority of current research related to auras is in the area of seizures (epilepsy). Advances have been made in the treatment of auras through surgery and medications. Research and medical advances in the twenty-first century will help health care professionals understand better the causes of auras, refine existing treatment methods, and develop new medications and treatments.

—*Carol A. Heintzelman, D.S.W.*

See also Aging; Brain; Brain disorders; Cerebral palsy; Dementias; Dizziness and fainting; Epilepsy; Hallucinations; Headaches; Migraine headaches; Numbness and tingling; Psychiatric disorders; Psychosis; Seizures; Sense organs; Speech disorders; Synesthesia.

For Further Information:

Collin, P. H., ed. *Dictionary of Medicine.* 3d ed. London: Author, 2001.

Farley, D. "Migraine, Cluster, and Tension: Headache Misery May Yield to Proper Treatment." *FDA Consumer* 26 (September, 1992): 26-32.

Krauss, G. L., et al. "Risk Factors of Seizure-Related Motor Vehicle Crashes in Patients with Epilepsy." *Neurology* 52 (April 22, 1999): 1321-29.

Lindgren, C. E. *Capturing the Aura: Integrating Science, Technology, and Metaphysics.* Nevada City, Calif.: Blue Dolphin, 2001.

MedlinePlus. "Migraine." *MedlinePlus*, May 2, 2013.

National Institute of Neurological Disorders and Stroke. "Seizures and Epilepsy: Hope through Research." *National Institute of Neurological Disorders and Stroke.*, Apr. 8, 2013.

Redlich, F. C., and D. X. Freedman. *The Theory and Practice of Psychiatry.* New York: Basic Books, 1966.

Auscultation
Procedure

Auscultation is the medical term for listening to the sounds inside the body during a medical exam. Auscultation is an important procedure because it provides a non-invasive way for a medical practitioner to identify potential health problems in the cardiac, respiratory, and digestive systems. The most common type of auscultation is that of a medical practitioner using a stethoscope to listen to a patient's heart sounds. However, medical professionals can also listen to the lungs and intestines using a stethoscope. The professional may also listen to the sound of blood flowing through the vessels in an arm or leg, but other devices such as a doppler ultrasound are often used for visualization.

Background

For centuries, medical practitioners have known that listening to the sounds made inside the body could provide clues to a patient's health. Evidence indicates the practice was used by the ancient Egyptians. By directly placing an ear against the patient's body, the healer could listen to the sounds made by the beating heart, appreciate how air flowed in and out of a patient's lungs, and listen to the gurgles of the bowels. Through experience and training, these doctors learned to identify how healthy heart, lungs, and intestines sounded. They also learned which sounds indicated a problem, and what disease or condition was most likely causing the abnormal sound. This allowed the doctor to determine what might be wrong with a patient; thus, how to properly treat the individual.

In 1816, French doctor Rene Theophile Hyacinthe Laënnec (1781-1826) was treating a young woman with suspected heart disease. His ability to diagnose her was complicated by two things. First, the woman was significantly overweight, which made it difficult to accurately hear her heart sounds. Second, the sense of modesty that prevailed during the time period made it difficult for Laënnec to properly listen to her heart as he had to press closely against her chest.

Laënnec solved this problem by applying a principle he had observed in a children's game. He had noticed a child press his ear to a piece of wood and listen to the sounds made when another child scratched against the other end of the wood, and realized sound could be transmitted through an object. Laënnec rolled a piece of paper into a cone shape and pressed one end against the woman's chest and the other to his ear. He discovered that not only could he hear her heart sounds but they were also louder and clearer than the sounds heard when he had placed his ear directly against her chest. Laënnec named his invention "stethoscope;" *stethos* is Greek for "chest" or "breast" and *skopien* is Greek for "explore." He called his new technique *mediate auscultation* after the Latin, *auscultare*, meaning "to listen."

Laënnec would soon devise a more permanent instrument made of wood and refine his technique for use as a diagnostic tool. He spent several years making careful notes of his observations based on body sounds and confirmed his findings by performing autopsies when possible. Three years after he invented the stethoscope, Laënnec published the first comprehensive manual on his findings: *On Mediate Auscultationor Treatise on the Diagnosis of the Diseases of the Lungsand Heart*. Fittingly, he is considered the father of auscultation.

Overview

More than two centuries after Laënnec first established the tools and techniques of mediate auscultation, auscultation remains a standard part of most medical exams. During the most basic exam, a medical practitioner will listen to the sounds made by the heart and lungs. She will follow an established format for doing this, moving the stethoscope around to various regions of the chest and back to listen to the sounds in each area. When possible, the patient will be asked to inhale deeply and exhale through the mouth several times. The patient may be asked to change positioning (such as bending forward and or lying down) to magnify certain sounds. The medical practitioner is listening to learn several things about the sounds, such as how often the sound(s) occur, their volume, duration, and quality of the sounds compared to sounds known to be normal.

During an auscultation examination of the heart, the medical practitioner can determine if the patient has a heart murmur. A murmur is an extra, abnormal sound heard when the heart beats. As the physician listens to the different parts of the heart by moving the stethoscope around on the body, the frequency, intensity, duration, and other characteristics of the murmur can help determine possible causes of the murmur.

While performing an auscultation exam of the respiratory system, the medical practitioner is listening for how easily air flows in and out of the lungs. The frequency, intensity, and length of time for each breath to be taken in and out all provide important clues about the health of the lungs. By having the patient breathe normally, and then more deeply, clinicians determined if the respiratory system is functioning properly or if there is an illness, obstruction, other respiratory problem, or even a heart condition that's affecting the lungs.

Auscultation of the heart and lungs are routine elements of a medical exam. The technique can also be applied to listening to the sounds of the intestines. In this case, the patient is generally lying down while the stethoscope is moved about on the abdomen. The type and quality of sounds heard or the absence of bowel sounds can tell a medical professional a great deal about a person's health. For example, the absence of bowel sounds could indicate constipation or an obstruction.

Interestingly, the technique can also be applied to the unborn in which case the stethoscope is pressed against the mother's abdomen. Other tools can be used for this as well, such as a doppler ultrasound which uses sound waves to detect and visualize on a screen the baby's heartbeat. This doppler ultrasound is also used in the auscultation of limbs to check for impaired blood flow which may indicate a clot or other obstruction in the blood vessel.

—*Lillian Dominguez*

For Further Information:

"Abdominal Sounds." *MedlinePlus*. US National Library of Medicine, "https://medlineplus.gov/ency/article/003137.htm" medlineplus.gov/ency/article/003137.htm. Accessed 6 Sept. 2017.

"Auscultation." *MedlinePlus*. US National Library of Medicine, "https://medlineplus.gov/ency/article/002226.htm" medlineplus.gov/ency/article/002226.htm. Accessed 6 Sept. 2017.

"The Cardiac Exam: Auscultation." *Case Western Reserve University*, "http://filer.case.edu/dck3/heart/listen.html" "Heart_Sounds" Accessed 6 Sept. 2017.

Chandrasekhar, A., MD. "Auscultation of Lungs." *Loyola University Medical Education Network*, INK "http://www.meddean. luc.edu/lumen/MEDED/medicine/pulmonar/pd/pstep29.htm" Accessed 6 Sept. 2017.

Ferguson CM. "Inspection, Auscultation, Palpation, and Percussion of the Abdomen." In: Walker HK, Hall WD, Hurst JW, editors. *Clinical Methods: The History, Physical, and Laboratory Examinations*. 3rd edition. Butterworths; 1990. Chapter 93.

Karnath, Bernard MD and William Thornton, MD. "Auscultation of the Heart." *Hospital Physician*. Sept. 2002 39-43. http://www.turner-white.com/pdf/hp_sep02_heart.pdf. Accessed 6 Sept. 2017.

"Music of the Heart: Rhythms and Murmurs." *Historical Collectives and Archives, Oregon Health & Science University*, http://www.ohsu.edu/xd/education/library/about/collections/historical-collections-archives/exhibits/exhibit-music-of-the-heart.cfm. Accessed 6 Sept. 2017.

Roguin, Ariel, MD PhD. "Rene Theophile Hyacinthe Laënnec (1781-1826): The Man Behind the Stethoscope." *Clinical Medicine & Research*, September 1, 2006, vol. 4 no. 3 230-235, www.clinmedres.org/content/4/3/230.full. Accessed 6 Sept. 2017.

Autism

Disease/Disorder

Also known as: Autistic disorder, autism spectrum disorder, Asperger's syndrome, pervasive developmental disorder

Anatomy or system affected: Brain, psychic-emotional system

Specialties and related fields: Family medicine, genetics, pediatrics, pharmacology, psychiatry, speech pathology

Definition: A neurodevelopmental disorder characterized by impairment in emotional expression and recognition, difficulty with social relationships, delayed and/or abnormal language and communication, and preoccupation with repetitive, stereotyped behaviors or interests.

Key terms:

behavior modification: a type of psychotherapy designed to change specific problematic behaviors through punishment and reward

echolalia: verbal repetitions of the words of others, sometimes modified with each repetition

functional magnetic resonance imaging (fMRI): the use of magnetic radiology to generate fairly detailed images of brain activity during specific functional activities (such as speech or visual imagery)

mental retardation: defined as a score of 70 or less (100 is average) on standardized intelligence quotient (IQ) tests, together with significant difficulties in some or all aspects of daily adaptive functioning (such as self-care, travel, and monetary exchanges) *mirror neuron system*: a network of neurons in the brain that are activated equally when producing an action and when observing the production of that same action by another person; thought to comprise at least part of the neural substrate for empathy and interpersonal understanding

occupational therapy: a form of therapy that focuses on teaching basic life skills

pica: the ingestion of nonfood substances

positron emission tomography (PET): a technique that uses radioactive tracers to produce images of the brain based on metabolism and blood flow

stereotypies: ritualistic, rhythmic, repeated movements of the hands, body, or head

---

Information on Autism

Causes: Unknown

Symptoms: Difficulty with social relationships, language, and communication; preoccupation with repetitive or stereotyped behaviors and interests; general resistance to changes in routine

Duration: Chronic

Treatments: Behavior modification, social skills training, speech/language therapy, occupational therapy, music therapy

---

Causes and Symptoms

Autism is a lifelong neurodevelopmental disorder that is almost always diagnosed in early childhood, though mild presentations may not be diagnosed until middle childhood. According to the handbook of mental health, the American Psychiatric Association's *Diagnostic and Statistical Manual of Mental Disorders: DSM-IV-TR* (4th ed., 2000), autism is diagnosed if there is evidence of qualitative impairment in both social interaction and communication, together with a marked participation or interest in restricted and repetitive behaviors or activities. Autism also typically involves delays or abnormal functioning in imaginative and symbolic play in childhood. At least one of these symptoms must have been observed prior to age three for a diagnosis of autism to be made.

In the *Diagnostic and Statistical Manual of Mental Disorders: DSM-5* (5th ed., 2013), autistic disorder is no longer a separate diagnosis from austism spectrum disorder, which aggregates the formerly separate diagnoses of autism, Asperger syndrome, childhood disintegrative disorder, and pervasive developmental disorder not otherwise specified. According to a 2012 press release from the American Psychiatric Association, these disorders "represent a continuum from mild to severe rather than a simple yes or no diagnosis to a specific disorder." Children with this diagnosis tend to demonstrate a wide range of behavioral, psychological, and physical symptoms at varying levels of severity.

As of 2012, the US Centers for Disease Control and Prevention reports that one in 50 children between the ages of six and seventeen has autism spectrum disorder, with males being four times more likely than females to have these conditions.

Some researchers have argued that autism has become increasingly prevalent, citing studies from the 1950s and 1960s that listed the incidence of autism at four to five cases per 10,000 children. However, it has also been suggested that the apparent rise in the incidence of autism simply reflects a rise in awareness of the disorder and an increase in the accuracy of the diagnostic criteria. Because of such debates, current research is more specifically examining mechanisms by which children may obtain autism, in addition to useful treatment methods.

The social interactions of individuals with autism are strikingly abnormal, ranging from self-imposed social isolation to somewhat engaged but inappropriate social behavior. Typically, those with autism avoid eye contact. They also demonstrate little if any facial expressiveness, and they generally do not produce social gesturing or body language. Individuals with autism generally lack empathy; they do not smile in response to other people's expressions of happiness, nor do they attempt to comfort others in distress. While the majority of children with autism develop attachments to their parents and other caregivers, there is a marked aloofness and lack of social reciprocity in their interactions even with close others. In adults with autism, close friendships and romantic attachments are not common. It is often said that individuals with autism do not relate to other people as people, but rather treat people more like objects. A classic example of this is a child with autism leading an adult by the hand and then placing the adult's hand on a door, rather than verbally or gesturally requesting that the door be opened.

Language development in children with autism is almost always delayed, and between 25 and 30 percent never acquire spoken language, despite having normal hearing abilities. Those individuals with autism who do develop language often show evidence of low-level linguistic disorders such as echolalia, persistent use of neologisms, pronoun reversals, and other grammatical anomalies. The subset of individuals with autism who develop fluent speech typically demonstrate poor conversational skills, related to the general lack of social reciprocity seen in autism. Their speech is often delivered in a monotone, is repetitive, and focuses mainly on their own concerns. Autistic speakers typically show little awareness of the perspectives or interests of their listeners. Individuals with autism also show deficits in receptive communication; there is reduced attention to human voices in general, poor understanding of nonverbal language, including gesture and vocal intonation, and difficulties with nonliteral language such as metaphor and irony.

Individuals with autism demonstrate a preoccupation with restricted and repetitive behaviors, interests, and activities. This focus on repetition can take a range of forms, from performance of stereotypies to compulsive insistence on daily routines to an intense focus upon specific, narrow topics of interest. Common stereotypies seen in autistic individuals are hand flapping, head banging, or more complex whole-body movements. Autistic children sometimes engage in self-injurious behavior patterns, such as self-biting or head banging, and/or self-soothing behaviors, such as rocking or self-stroking. Some children with autism also develop pica, eating such things as paper, paperclips, or dirt. More complex ritualistic behavior patterns might include compulsive hand washing, counting, or arrangement of possessions. This aspect of autism can also include intense preoccupation with highly restricted topics, such as weather patterns, buttons, or television schedules.

Another defining characteristic included in the diagnostic criteria for autism is a lack of imaginative or pretend play in childhood. This symptom may be related to the general literalness seen in autistic communication. The play of children with autism tends to be solitary and to involve the repetitive manipulation of objects. The one-sidedness of autistic children's play and their generally impaired social interactions typically result in failure to develop peer relationships appropriate to their developmental level. Children with autism are therefore often cut off from their peer groups, which can cause feelings of loneliness and depression, especially as they approach adolescence.

Up to three-quarters of children with autism are also mentally disabled, with an intelligence quotient (IQ) below 70. The mental profiles of autistic children can be uneven, however, with particularly low verbal IQ scores but normal or near-normal scores on measures of mathematical and spatial IQ.

As of the early twenty-first century, there is no known cause of autism. Risk factors include genetic relatedness, difficult birth, and comorbid disorders such as attention deficit hyperactivity disorder (ADHD) and obsessive-complusive disorder (OCD). In the 1990s, scientists investigated the claim, initially made by parents and bolstered by apparently rising rates of autism, that the measles, mumps, and rubella (MMR) vaccine, typically given around age eighteen months, caused autism in some cases. A number of thorough epidemiological studies found no evidence for a link between the MMR vaccine and autism, although some researchers suggested that the vaccine could exacerbate already-present autistic symptoms in toddlers.

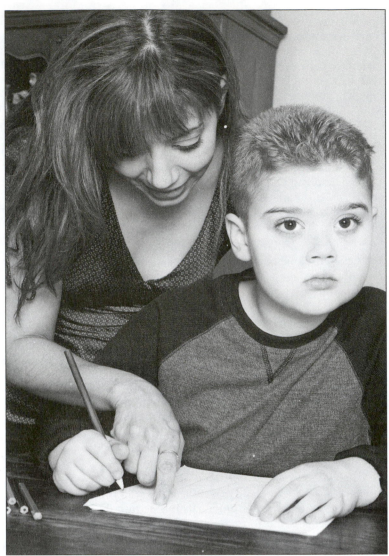

A mom helps her autistic son with his homework. (iStockphoto.com)

Treatment and Therapy

There is no cure for autism, nor is there one single treatment. Because children with autism can display such a wide range of symptoms, the range of available treatments is also wide. Physicians, psychologists, and other health professionals focus on alleviating the symptoms that are the most disruptive to a particular individual with autism. Available treatments include behavior modification, social skills training, speech/language therapy, occupational therapy, play therapy, music therapy, dietary interventions, and medication, among others. Often a combination of these types of treatments will be used to address the therapeutic needs of an autistic individual.

One of the most successful treatments for autism has been intensive behavior modification therapy. In his book *The Autistic Child: Language Development Through Behavior Modification* (1977), O. Ivar Lovaas describes a program of intensive one-on-one behavior modification therapy that can be highly effective in alleviating disturbing symptoms and in engendering positive social behaviors in autistic children. Lovaas's technique is controversial because it involves both rewards for appropriate behaviors, such as making eye contact or maintaining conversation, as well as punishments for inappropriate behaviors, such as self-damaging acts, stereotypies, or pica. In a well-publicized legal case in the 1990s, Massachusetts banned the use of punishment in a school for autistic children. As a result, the children's levels of self-injurious behavior increased, to the extent that the parents petitioned for punishment to be reinstated in the school's behavior modification program.

While the utility of punishment is generally acknowledged, many behavior modification therapists now suggest that the positive reinforcement of rewarding appropriate behavior is effective enough that punishment for inappropriate behavior is not necessary. Despite variations in philosophy and technique, behavior modification aimed at increasing social responsiveness and decreasing inappropriate behaviors is generally an essential component of therapy for autistic children.

Social skills training is used to encourage individuals with autism to adhere to the implicit rules of conversation and social interaction (for example, looking at people's faces when speaking to them). Occupational therapy focuses on teaching skills that allow individuals with autism to participate in daily life: crossing a street, preparing simple meals, making purchases, and answering the telephone. Play therapy involves entering the world of the autistic individual-in the case of children, spending "floor time" with them to break through their aloofness. Music therapy has been used to draw emotional responses from children with autism, with varied levels of success. Dietary interventions have also been found to alleviate some of the symptoms of autism in certain cases.

No drug is specifically prescribed for autism; however, various medications are sometimes used to treat the symptoms of autism. Stimulant drugs may be used to treat the inattentiveness of autistic children who are particularly isolated and unresponsive. Tranquilizing drugs may be prescribed to manage obsessive-compulsive behaviors that are disruptive to normal functioning. Antidepressant drugs are also sometimes prescribed for autistic children to heighten emotional responsiveness and/or to stabilize mood. As many as one-third of children with autism develop seizures, often in adolescence, that are similar to epileptic seizures. These seizures are usually treated with medication.

Outcomes for individuals with autism depend on the severity of their symptoms. Autistic individuals with mild impairments can live at home, participate in family and social life, go to mainstream schools, and eventually take on appropriate paid work. In fact, some highly repetitive occupations, such as shelving books in a library or entering computer data, may fit extremely well with the desires and talents of individuals with autism. Some people with autism are very high-achieving. Those with more profound autistic symptoms or significant mental retardation may go to special schools, participate in remedial programs, or live in special residential facilities. Whatever the setting, individuals with autism respond most positively to a highly structured environment in which the other people are understanding and tolerant of their social and communicative abnormalities.

Parents, siblings, and friends of individuals with autism may also benefit from therapy. Life with an autistic person can be rewarding, especially when progress is made, but it can also be frustrating and depressing. Often the parents, siblings, and friends of children with autism, as well as professionals working with such children, feel rejected by the autistic tendency to avoid close social contact. Most professionals suggest that anyone who spends extended periods of time with an individual with autism will benefit from some form of training and/or emotional support.

Perspective and Prospects

Though it is likely to be an old syndrome, autism was first described in the 1940s. Leo Kanner in the United States and Hans Asperger in Austria independently published papers describing children with severe social and communicative impairments. Both Kanner and Asperger used the term *autism* (meaning "alone") to describe the syndromes they had identified. Kanner described children who had impoverished social relationships from early in life, employed deviant language, and were subject to behavioral stereotypies. Asperger's description identified children with normal IQs and normal language development who suffered from social and some types of communicative impairments. As of the early twenty-first century, there is ongoing controversy as to whether autism and Asperger's syndrome represent two ends of a single spectrum disorder or whether individuals with Asperger's syndrome constitute a distinct clinical group.

In his original report, Kanner observed that the parent-child relationships in cases of children with autism appeared to be somewhat unusual. This suggestion fit with the tenor of the times, in which psychology and psychiatry were dominated by Freudian theories. Thus early explanations of autism, now discredited, suggested that children developed the syndrome as a result of cold, abusive, or confusing home environments (references were made to "refrigerator mothers"), and early treatments of autism focused on improving parent-child relationships or removing children with autism from their home environments.

In the early twenty-first century, work on autism has focused on the physiological and cognitive aspects of the disorder. Brain studies utilizing functional magnetic resonance imaging (fMRI) and positron emission tomography (PET) scanning have uncovered several abnormalities in the brains of individuals with autism, including larger than normal brains, and abnormal functioning in the areas thought to be responsible for social interactions. In particular, the structure and functioning of the mirror neuron system, hypothesized to be the structural substrate for empathy, have been shown to be abnormal in individuals with autism. Cognitive studies into autism have suggested that the perceptual and reasoning proclivities of individuals with autism are abnormal. One hypothesis is that autistic individuals' minds are characterized "weak central coherence," such that they prefer to focus on details and parts rather than on global wholes, leading to the tendency to focus on concrete minutia while avoiding complex and dynamic human interaction. Another hypothesis is that individuals with autism lack a "theory of mind," which results in an inability to consider others' emotions, perspectives, desires, and thoughts.

—*Virginia Slaughter, Ph.D.*

See also Anxiety; Asperger's syndrome; Bonding; Cognitive development; Developmental disorders; Developmental stages; Learning disabilities; Mental retardation; Neuroimaging; Psychiatric disorders; Psychiatry; Psychiatry, child and adolescent; Speech disorders.

For Further Information:

American Psychiatric Association. "*DSM-5* Proposed Criteria for Autism Spectrum Disorder Designed to Provide More Accurate Diagnosis and Treatment." Release No. 12-03. Arlington, Va.: APA, Jan. 20, 2012.

American Psychiatric Association. *Diagnostic and Statistical Manual of Mental Disorders: DSM-5*. 5th ed. Arlington, Va.: APA, 2013.

Autism Society of America. *Autism Society*, n. d.

First Signs. *First Signs*, Jan. 11, 2012.

Frith, Uta. *Autism: Explaining the Enigma*. 2d ed. Malden, Mass.: Blackwell, 2006.

Greenspan, Stanley and Serena Wieder. *Engaging Autism: Using the Floortime Approach to Help Children Relate, Communicate, and Think*. Cambridge, Mass.: Da Capo, 2006.

Happe, Francesca. *Autism: An Introduction to Psychological Theory*. Hove, East Sussex, U.K.: Psychology Press, 2002.

HealthDay. "One in 50 School-Aged Children in the U.S. Has Autism: CDC." *MedlinePlus*, Mar. 20, 2013.

MedlinePlus. "Autism." *MedlinePlus*, May 6, 2013.

Wiseman, Nancy D., and Robert L. Rich. *The First Year: Autism Spectrum Disorders-An Essential Guide for the Newly Diagnosed Child*. Cambridge, Mass.: Da Capo, 2009.

Autoimmune disorders

Disease/Disorder

Anatomy or system affected: circulatory system, lymphatic system, nervous system, skeletal system

Specialties and related fields: immunology

Definition: Damage to the tissues or organs of the body caused by failure of the immune system to distinguish between "self" and "non-self," producing autoantibodies called B cells and autoreactive cells at the request of the T lymphocytes (cells).

Key terms:

alleles: one or more variations of a gene that reflects the genes passed from your parents; usually referred to as dominant and recessive genes; while other genes have more than two more alleles

antibody: a molecule of the immune system, produced by B cells and targeted toward eliminating a specific antigen

antigen: a protein or related molecule that is seen as foreign and therefore induces antibody formation in an individual

autoantibody: an antibody which binds to a protein that is a normal part of the human body from which it originates, as opposed to part of a bacteria, virus, or another human being

B cells: also known as B lymphocytes; the antibody-producing cells of the immune system

multigenetic: referring to a trait or characteristic that requires the product of more than one gene in order to be activated;

selection: the process by which developing immune system cells are either allowed to continue to maturation or destroyed before they can enter the circulation

T cells: also known as T lymphocytes; the immune system cells involved in cellular immunity and regulation of the immune response

tolerance: the ability of the immune system to remain unresponsive to self-antigens

---

> ## Information on Autoimmune Disorders
>
> **Causes:** Unknown, possibly hereditary, environmental, or viral
>
> **Symptoms:** Varies widely; may include pain, fatigue, joint and muscle inflammation, muscle weakness, sleep disturbances, headaches, numbness and tingling, central nervous system disturbances
>
> **Duration:** Often chronic
>
> **Treatments:** Alleviation of symptoms, strengthening the immune system

Causes and Symptoms

Autoimmunity refers to a group of widely varying diseases or disorders that include familiar examples (type 1 diabetes mellitus, myasthenia gravis, multiple sclerosis, rheumatoid arthritis) and many that are not as familiar (idiopathic thrombocytopenic purpura, Graves' disease, Felty syndrome, Hashimoto's thyroiditis). The list is long and growing as researchers continue to ferret out the root causes of many disorders that have been known for one hundred years or more. In many cases, environmental triggers or environmentally controlled flare-ups are common. All autoimmune disorders have one thing in common: the failure of the human immune system to distinguish between self (own) and non-self antigens, thus leading the body to attack itself and damage or destroy tissues or organs. Autoimmunity is not a rare event; it occurs in all people, and it does not necessarily give rise to disease. For instance, aged or damaged cells of the body are normally destroyed by autoantibodies (antibodies directed against the self). However, other autoantibodies, which arise by chance combinations of genes, are normally suppressed during development in the thymus gland. This is referred to as selection. If the thymus fails to do its job, then these autoantibodies may be released into the lymph nodes and into the bloodstream, seeking out tissue or antigens to attack and destroy.

Autoimmune disorders can be classified in several ways. Some diseases affect only one organ system, and some affect multiple systems. Examples of organ-specific disorders are Addison's disease and Graves' disease; non-organ-specific disorders include systemic lupus erythematosus and scleroderma. Alternatively, one can classify autoimmune disorders by the type of immune system cells involved in their onset. Some diseases are caused by the antibody-secreting B cells; they include myasthenia gravis, multiple sclerosis, rheumatic fever, systemic lupus erythematosus, and Graves' disease. Other disorders are the result of the action of the systemic T cells; they include Addison's disease and Hashimoto's thyroiditis.

The onset of an autoimmune disorder hinges on many factors, some of which are still being identified. It is well established, however, that autoimmunity is multifactorial and multi-genic. In other words, many environmental factors and many genes are involved in determining susceptibility to autoimmune disorders. In addition, many environmental factors are thought to be involved in controlling

Figure 1. Partial List of Autoimmune Diseases

Disease	*Organ/Target*
Addison's disease	Adrenal glands
Ankylosing spondylitis	Spine
Antiphospholipid antibody syndrome	Blood clotting
Celiac disease	Small intestine
Crohn's disease	Gastrointestinal tract
Diabetes mellitus type 1 (some forms)	Pancreas islet cell
Felty's disease	Joints and spleen
Goodpasture's syndrome	Kidneys and lungs
Graves' disease	Thyroid gland
Guillain-Barré syndrome	Peripheral nervous system
Hashimoto's thyroiditis	Thyroid gland
Hemolytic anemia	Red blood cells, platelets
Multiple sclerosis	Brain and spinal cord
Myasthenia gravis	Junctions between nerves and muscles
Pemphigus vulgaris	Skin and mucus membranes
Pernicious anemia	Stomach parietal cells
Polymyositis	Skeletal muscle
Poststreptococcal glomerulonephritis	Kidneys
Psoriasis	Skin
Rheumatic fever	Heart
Rheumatoid arthritis	Connective tissue and joints
Scleroderma	Heart, lungs, kidney, gastrointestinal tract
Sjögren's syndrome	Saliva and tear glands
Systemic lupus erythematosus	DNA, platelets, all organs
Thrombocytopenic purpura	Platelets
Wegener's granulomatosis	Lungs and kidneys

remission and flare-ups of autoimmune disorders. Most autoimmune disorders are probably the result of the release of T or B cells that, because they did not properly distinguish between self and non-self, should have been suppressed by the body's immune system.

It is thought that autoimmune conditions are caused by hereditary, the environment, bacteria or viruses, fungi, or drugs. Most of the autoimmune diseases have an unknown cause. There is a theory that there may be a gene that must be turned on for autoimmune diseases to develop.

Symptoms

Varies widely; may include pain, fatigue, joint and muscle inflammation, muscle weakness, sleep disturbances, headaches, numbness and tingling, central nervous system disturbances, kidney damage, and liver damage. They can also affect the skin, red blood cells, connective tissue, blood vessels, nerves, and the endocrine glands. Most of them are chronic conditions.

Treatments/Therapy

A variety of studies have established genetic links in autoimmune diseases, but because most are multi-genetic. There is no simple Mendelian inheritance pattern seen. Nonetheless, there seems to be a clear correlation between certain human leukocyte antigen (HLA) genes and certain autoimmune disorders. For instance, those who have HLA allele B27 have a ninetyfold greater risk than the normal population of developing ankylosing spondylitis. Those with allele DR3 have a twelvefold greater risk of celiac disease and a tenfold greater risk of Sjögren syndrome. In the case of insulin-dependent diabetes, the relative risk factor is fivefold. If one has the DR3 allele and the DR4 allele, then the risk jumps to twentyfold. If the DR3 and DQw8 alleles are present, then the risk factor is one hundredfold. Yet, these alleles themselves do not automatically cause autoimmune disease, as evidenced by several studies on identical twins in which the rate of disease in the twin of an affected person ranged from 25 to 50 percent. Clearly environmental factors can change susceptibility to autoimmune disease into actual manifestation.

Autoimmune disorders are much more common in women than in men. In addition, they are usually more severe in women. This is likely due to the effects of estrogen, which has a role in enhancing the expression of HLA genes and activating macrophages, thus leading to higher tissue destruction. Some autoimmune conditions are noted to flare and subside throughout the menstrual cycle, in conjunction with the rise and fall of estrogen levels. Stress has also been shown to be a contributing factor that can cause an autoimmune disorder to flare. This response is likely mediated through the hypothalamus and pituitary glands, which release hormones that directly stimulate the immune system.

It has been known for many years that the expression of some autoimmune diseases is preceded by infection by a virulent organism. Infections may contribute to autoimmunity in several ways. Some microbes produce antigens that are very close in structure to human antigens.

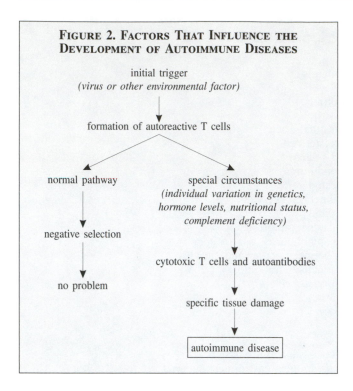

FIGURE 2. FACTORS THAT INFLUENCE THE DEVELOPMENT OF AUTOIMMUNE DISEASES

When antibodies are produced against the invading organism, the antibodies also attack self-antigens because of the chemical similarity. Examples of this response are post-streptococcal glomerulonephritis and rheumatic fever. Other invaders may damage human cells and release proteins that are not normally seen by the immune system (sequestered proteins). These proteins are seen as foreign, and an immune response is set up against these self-antigens. A similar response may be seen when normally sequestered proteins are released through trauma or injury. An example is sympathetic ophthalmia, in which eye lens proteins that are normally not seen in the circulation are released, triggering antibodies that may then attack the opposite (uninjured) eye as well. The symptoms of autoimmune disorders are as varied as the disorders themselves. No one set of symptoms fits all disorders. Symptoms may be systemic or localized, progressive or stable. Symptoms may also be life threatening or simply annoying.

Multiple sclerosis (MS) is an autoimmune disorder involving the central nervous system. Nerve axons of the white matter of the brain are normally surrounded by myelin protein sheaths that protect the nerves and speed the process of transmission. In individuals with MS, these myelin sheath proteins are gradually attacked and destroyed, slowing nerve impulses so that patients develop a loss of control of motor function and vision. This disease often progresses irregularly and unpredictably and is irreversible. It appears to be the result of both B cells, producing antibodies against oligodendroglia, the cells that make myelin protein, and T cells, acting against a peptide product from the myelin protein. Although what triggers the initial response is unclear, it has been suggested that onset may follow infection with either Epstein-Barr or hepatitis B viruses. More than 2.1 million people worldwide are affected

by MS. It is mostly women who are diagnosed between age twenty and fifty.

Systemic lupus erythematosus (SLE), known simply as lupus, is a generalized disorder that occurs predominantly in women. It is clearly linked to B cells and the production of antibodies against parts of the DNA molecule. These DNA antibodies cause tissue damage by combining with free DNA, and form cells that have been damaged through disease or the normal aging process. This may form immune complexes that are deposited in the kidneys and arterioles, leading to tissue destruction and fibrosis, and in the joints, leading to arthritis. Auto antibodies against red blood cells or platelets may also be found in SLE. Antibodies against muscles may be present and contribute to muscle inflammation, while the presence of antibodies to heart muscle may lead to myocarditis and endocarditis. Antibodies against skin components can lead to a characteristic "butterfly rash" on the bridge of the nose and the area around the eyes that is seen in many patients with SLE; this rash worsens in the presence of sunlight.

Rheumatoid arthritis is a common, crippling disease. It is controlled by B cells in the joints that are activated to produce several antibodies, including rheumatoid factor. The result is the formation and deposition of immune complexes in the joint cartilage. Antibodies directed against cartilage may also be seen. The resulting destruction activates chemicals that stimulate T cells to come to the area, and they in turn release destructive enzymes, just as they would if bacteria were invading the joints. All these responses lead to joint damage, inflammation, and pain. As the disease progresses, the synovia swell and extend into the joints, causing further pain and discomfort along with disfigurement of the joints. The cause of antibody activation is unknown and may be quite variable.

Both Hashimoto's thyroiditis and Graves' disease are forms of autoimmune thyroiditis. In Hashimoto's disease, antibodies are formed against a protein within the thyroid cells, leading to attack of the cells and destruction of much of the thyroid tissue. In Graves' disease, antibodies are formed that bind to the receptors for thyroid-stimulating hormone (TSH), the pituitary hormone that stimulates the thyroid gland to produce thyroid hormone. The receptors in turn are stimulated. Thus, the thyroid gland is hyperstimulated, and excess thyroid hormone is turned out, a condition known as thyrotoxicosis.

An individual with myasthenia gravis experiences muscle fatigue and extreme weakness with only mild exercise, such as walking short distances. It is caused by autoantibodies that are directed against the acetylcholine (ACh) receptor molecule. In normal neural cells that control large muscles, ACh is stimulated to be released from the neuron and bind to receptors on the muscle fiber end plate. If that receptor is blocked or destroyed by an antibody, the ACh cannot bind, and therefore the muscle is not stimulated to respond (contract). If a few receptors are blocked, then the muscle may still respond weakly. If enough antibody is present to block a large number of receptors, however, then the threshold limit for muscle response will not be achieved, and the muscle will not respond even in the presence of repeated stimulation from the neuron. Scleroderma, also known as progressive systemic sclerosis, predominantly affects middle-aged women and is caused by collagen deposition in a variety of tissues of the body. Antibodies may be found against the centromere portion of the DNA. Symptoms include calcium deposition in the skin, sensitivity to cold, and decreased esophageal motility. The lungs often experience fibrosis, as do the kidneys.

Most autoimmune disorders cannot be cured; they develop into chronic conditions that require a lifetime of care and monitoring. Treatment is quite varied and depends on the underlying cause and etiology of the disease. Overall, the goals of treatment are to reduce the symptoms and to control the disease or disorder while at the same time allowing the immune system to continue fighting the viruses and bacteria affecting the body on a daily basis. The most generalized treatment is the administration of immunosuppressive drugs. The most commonly used drugs are azathioprine and cyclophosphamide. Corticosteroids are also used to reduce the inflammatory responses seen in many autoimmune disorders. Drugs such as methotrexate have gained wide acceptance in the treatment of rheumatoid arthritis and other autoimmune disorders, but they have systemic side effects that in some cases may be worse than the autoimmune disorder itself, such as suppression of the basic immune responses involved in fighting off everyday viruses and bacteria. While the doses used to fight autoimmunity are much lower than those used to suppress organ graft rejection. These general effects may still be seen, especially in older individuals whose immune systems are declining as a result of age. Thus, a significant amount of effort has been put into finding drugs that will be able to suppress only the self-reactive antibodies and not the entire immune system.

Hormones, proteins, or other substances normally produced or secreted by the cells or organs damaged in autoimmune disease (such as thyroid hormone or insulin) can usually be supplemented to the point that they are within the proper physiologic range. Sometimes this works well. For instance, Graves' disease can be effectively controlled by removing the overactive thyroid gland and then supplementing thyroid hormone in the patient. Treating type 1 diabetes in children by supplementing insulin, however, is a much trickier proposition. The finely controlled release of insulin from the beta cells of the pancreas cannot be duplicated by a single injection.

Many investigators have worked on vaccinations for autoimmune disorders, using animal models of varying types. Some results have been promising, even if the mechanism of action is still mostly unexplained. Vaccinations against autoimmune thyroiditis, encephalitis, and arthritis have been successful in some animal models. Another approach that has been tried experimentally is the use of oral tolerance therapy. Large quantities of the offending autoantigen are given to the patient in the hope that tolerance to the particular protein will develop. This approach is similar to the way in which desensitization is used with allergy sufferers. Oral doses of myelin, for instance, have shown some success as a treatment for patients with multiple sclerosis.

There are new medications that are being used to treat autoimmune conditions. They are called Biologics, and they target certain cells in the immune system. They are also called Monoclonal Antibodies or Tumor Necrosis Factor Inhibitors. Some of these medications are: Rituximab, Infliximab, Tocilizumab, and Belimumab. Rituximab selectively deletes specific B cells that have a particular marker. It is used to treat Rheumatoid arthritis, 2 types of vasculitis, MS, Lupus, and other autoimmune diseases. Some patients have hypersensitivity reactions to Rituximab. Infliximab is an anti-TNF (Tumor Necrosis Factor) drug. This drug is used to treat ulcerative colitis, rheumatoid arthritis, psoriatic arthritis, and plaque psoriasis. Tocilizumab is a cytokine from T cells. It is used to treat rheumatoid arthritis. Belimumab is a B-cell activating factor that can be used to treat lupus, and Sjorgen's Syndrome. These mediations do not cure autoimmune diseases, but they can put them into remission.. These medications are very potent and they have some significant side effects, but they can permit a patient to live a relatively normal life.

Perspective and Prospects

The history of human understanding of autoimmune disorders is quite short. Paul Ehrlich, early in the twentieth century, described a condition of "horror autotoxicus," the attack of the human immune system against the body's own tissues. His studies set the stage for fairly rapid advancement in understanding of the human immune system. Understanding of the genetic and molecular basis for autoimmunity, however, along with the realization that autoimmunity is a normal part of immune system development, began in the 1980s. Even where the cause was well established (such as with insulin-dependent diabetes, established in the 1920s), no significant changes in treatment were made until new genetic tools became available. Indeed, the entire field of immunology, which until the 1970s was in its infancy as a medical field, has grown exponentially as new molecular tools have enabled researchers to elucidate the pathways by which autoimmunity exacts its toll.

There is still plenty to do, both in terms of determining pathways and in developing new therapies aimed at specific targeting of these pathways. With completion of the Human Genome Project, an incredible amount of new knowledge is available that will help researchers produce treatments that are much more targeted and specific than those used in the past. As more is learned about the immune system and pathways of inflammation, new therapies may be designed that may prevent the development of most autoimmune diseases.

—*Kerry L. Cheesman, PhD;*
updated by Christine M. Carroll, RN, BSN, MBA

See also: Antibody, Liver, Blood

For Further Information:

Abbas, Abul K., and Andrew H. Lichtman. *Basic Immunology: Functions and Disorders of the Immune System.* 2d ed. Philadelphia: Saunders/Elsevier, 2006.

A.D.A.M. Medical Encyclopedia. "Autoimmune Disorders." *MedlinePlus*, May 29, 2011.

American Autoimmune Related Diseases Association. http://www.aarda.org. Feldmann, Marc, Fionula M. Brennan, and Ravinder N. Maini. "Rheumatoid Arthritis." *Cell* 85, no. 3 (May 3, 1996): 307-10.

Janeway, Charles A., Jr., et al. *Immunobiology: The Immune System in Health and Disease.* 6th ed.NewYork: Garland Science, 2005.

National Institute of Allergy and Infectious Diseases. National Institutes of Health. http://www.niaid.nih.gov/publications/autoimmune. htm. National Institute of Allergy and Infectious Diseases. "Understanding the Immune System." *National Institutes of Health*, October 26 2012.

National Institute of Arthritis and Musculoskeletal and Skin Diseases. "Understanding Autoimmune Diseases." *National Institutes of Health*, October 2012.

Steinman, Lawrence. "Multiple Sclerosis: A Coordinated Immunological Attack Against Myelin in the Central Nervous System." *Cell* 85, no. 3 (May 3, 1996): 299-302.

Walport, M. J., et al. "Complement Deficiency and Autoimmunity." *Annals of the New York Academy of Sciences* 815 (April, 1997): 267-81.

Zack, Eric, DNP, RN, ACNP, BC, AOCN®. "Emerging Therapies for Autoimmune Disorders". Journal of Infusion Nursing, March/April 2014, volume 37 Number 2, p.109-119.

Roddick, Julie. (19 July 2017) Retrieved on September 10, 2017 from http://www.healthline.com/health/autoimmune-disorders?print=true.

Autopsy

Procedure

Anatomy or system affected: All

Specialties and related fields: Biochemistry, forensic medicine, histology, microbiology, pathology

Definition: The postmortem (after-death) examination of a body in order to determine the cause of death; it involves both a systematic, orderly inspection of the external and internal structures of the body systems and a chemical and microbiological analysis of visceral contents.

Key terms:

anatomic pathologist: a doctor who is especially concerned with the study of the structural and functional changes in tissues and organs that cause or are caused by disease; this doctor performs autopsies

coroner: an officer, often a layperson, who holds inquests in regard to violent, sudden, or unexplained deaths

diener: a person who assists the pathologist in the morgue and at the autopsy

forensic autopsy: a systematic investigation to determine the cause of death, providing the pathologist with information to state an informed opinion about the manner and mechanism of death in cases that are of public interest

gross pathology: that which is visible to the naked eye, or "macroscopic," during inspection

histopathology: the histologic or microscopic description of abnormal pathologic tissue changes; these changes can be seen under the microscope

morgue: a place, usually cooled, where dead bodies are temporarily kept, pending proper identification, autopsy, or burial

The Fundamentals of Pathology

Translated literally, pathology is the study (*logos*) of suffering (*pathos*). As a science, pathology focuses on the study of the structural and functional consequences of injury on cells, tissues, and organs and ultimately the consequences on the entire organism (that is, the patient). Oftentimes, cells and fragments of tissues are obtained surgically from living patients; this procedure, called biopsy, is for the purpose of evaluating the nature and extent of injury. The results of a biopsy help direct the treatment. Autopsy, by contrast, is performed to examine the dead body and the internal organs systematically, in order to determine why the patient died.

Four aspects of a disease process form the core of pathology and are searched for diligently during autopsy studies. These are etiology, or cause; pathogenesis, the mechanism of development of disease; morphologic changes, the structural alterations induced in cells, tissues, and organs of the body; and clinical significance, the functional consequences of these morphologic changes.

There are two major classes of etiologic causation factors: genetic and acquired. Examples of acquired factors are infections, physical trauma, chemical injury and poisoning, nutritional factors, and radiation and solar injury (sunburn). When an autopsy is performed, this etiology is sought, but it has been acknowledged that the classic concept of one cause leading to one disease-developed largely from the discovery of specific infectious agents as the causes of specific diseases-is no longer sufficient. More often than not, multiple factors are acting at once. Genetic factors also affect environmentally induced diseases: for example, not all alcoholic patients develop significant liver disease (cirrhosis). Conversely, environment may have a profound influence on genetically induced disease: for example, not all individuals with the chemical and genetic markers for gout will develop that disease. During autopsies, systematic samplings of blood, body fluids, and tissues are taken in order to test for microbial causes and often chemical causes.

Pathogenesis refers to the sequence of events in the cells and organs that results from injury, from the initial responses to the ultimate expression of disease. It has become clear, for example, that many events at the subcellular and molecular levels are interacting and taking shape long before a disease becomes clinically observable. For example, the virus that causes acquired immunodeficiency syndrome (AIDS) destroys lymphocytes (special white blood cells) and causes a gradual loss of immunity in the body long before AIDS becomes clinically observable as a disease.

Morphologic changes are the structural and associated functional alterations in cells, tissues, and organs that are characteristic of a disease process. They are directly observed at the autopsy table by "gross" or "macroscopic" inspection of the body and organs and later by "microscopic" or histologic study of tissue samples removed from these organs. These morphologic studies can be carried out in extreme detail using the electron microscope (ultrastructural studies) and immunologic or even genetic and molecular analysis. In forensic medicine, deoxyribonucleic acid (DNA) evidence is at times used as a definitive "thumbprint" of specific genetic makeup and can be obtained from even a few hairs.

The nature of these morphologic changes and their distribution in different organs influence normal function and determine the observed clinical features-the signs and symptoms of disease, such as fever and pain-and the disease's course and outcome. Thus, the clinical significance of these alterations can be used to assess the cause of death.

Procedures and Techniques

Autopsies are performed for several generally recognized purposes, which are closely related. Medical autopsies are performed to improve the diagnosis of disease and to help the practicing or treating physician avoid repeating errors in diagnosis and therapy; it has been repeatedly shown that autopsies contribute to improvements in medical care. The College of American Pathologists has stressed the importance and necessity of the autopsy as a service to both the medical community and the public, recognizing it as a useful medical procedure performed by a qualified physician to assess the quality of patient care and evaluate clinical diagnostic accuracy. The autopsy is also a valuable tool for determining the effectiveness and impact of treatment modalities, discovering and defining new and/or changing diseases (as in AIDS), increasing the understanding of biological processes of disease (pathogenesis), and augmenting clinical and basic research. Information gathered from autopsies is used to provide accurate public health and vital statistical information and education as it relates to disease. Finally, the autopsy is used for obtaining legal, factual information.

In the United States, permission to perform an autopsy must be granted. A legal action can arise when the autopsy consent has not been obtained or when it has not been obtained from the proper person. The statutes of individual states usually establish who can consent to the autopsy. In general, a surviving spouse has first priority for authorizing an autopsy, and in the absence of the spouse, the next of kin has legal custody of the body and the right to authorize an autopsy. Some statutes indicate that whoever assumes custody of the body for burial may give permission for autopsy.

At large medical centers, there usually is an autopsy service, the director of which is a qualified anatomic pathologist. At times, there is also a perinatal pathologist, an anatomic pathologist specializing in the pathology of newly born babies. House officers who are medical doctors-in-training often assist in performing the autopsies. The autopsy suite is a well-equipped theater usually in close proximity to the morgue and is served by a diener.

Thus, the usual autopsy is performed by professional pathologists. After carefully examining the body as a whole and recording its various attributes, the pathologist makes a surgical incision to allow for the detailed inspection of the body cavities and the organ systems, looking for gross ab-

normalities. Every organ is thus examined, measured, and weighed and its description recorded. Sampled sections of the organs are then taken for histologic studies, and samples of blood and other body contents may be taken for microbiologic and chemical studies.

The objectives of the autopsy will vary among institutions and even among cases within an institution. For example, an academic institution with a training program in pathology, a private hospital without a training program, and a medical examiner's office might be expected to approach a specific autopsy with very different objectives. Nevertheless, a minimum basic and standard level of examination, description, and tissue sampling is usually done. Photography is also used to document the gross findings.

Histologic study of the tissue samples is completed, and the results of microbiologic and chemical analysis are obtained. After the patient's record is carefully reviewed and all the findings are correlated, often in consultation with the decedent's treating physician, a final document, the autopsy report, is produced.

In many autopsies, the basic gross, histologic, chemical, and microscopic examination will be inadequate to resolve fully all questions raised by the circumstances of the patient's clinical course and death. The ability to carry out additional studies may then become critical to resolving these questions. Ancillary studies to which pathologists may resort include injections of substances into blood vessels to observe blockages (angiography), chromosomal studies, toxicology, x-ray defractions, and histochemical procedures. The results of these studies are also recorded in the final autopsy report.

Two standard techniques are generally used to perform autopsies. They differ from each other in the order in which the organs are removed and in whether single organs or intact organ systems are removed from the body. In Virchow's technique, organs are removed one by one. Originally, the first step was to expose the cranial cavity, the spinal cord, and the thoracic, cervical, and abdominal organs, in that order. This technique, with some modifications, is still widely used. In Rokitansky's technique, the dissection is initially carried out in situ (before the removal) and then combined with en bloc removal. This technique is often modified when used in medical centers, where the en bloc removal of the cervical, thoracic, and abdominal organs is done. Dissection of the various organ systems is performed after removal.

Another technique, Potter's technique, is often used in pediatric autopsies. The external examination, particularly of fetuses and newborns, concentrates on the search for congenital malformations; the face, ears, or hands may reveal characteristic symptoms of a disorder, such as with Down syndrome. The placenta and umbilical cord must be studied in all autopsies for fetuses and newborns. Less invasive autopsy procedures for infants are being developed and put into practice, including MRI scans.

Few autopsies offer more difficulties than postoperative cases, in which death has occurred during or shortly after a surgical operation. The pathologist must evaluate his or her findings in the light of their medicolegal implications, such as complications from surgical intervention, anesthesia, or drug administration. At times, obtaining permission to conduct an autopsy may require certain restrictions in its performance. In such restricted autopsies, access can be confined to only the chest or abdomen, or to the reopening of surgical wounds.

Medicolegal autopsies are best carried out by forensic pathologists, who must first ascertain that death has, in fact, occurred. (Failure to do so has, on occasion, led to embarrassment and serious repercussions.) Not all medicolegal autopsies deal with violent or unnatural deaths. Generally, more than half of all cases investigated by the office of the chief medical examiner in New York are deaths from natural causes that occur suddenly, unexpectedly, or in an unusual manner. Coronary heart disease (heart attacks) and respiratory infections (pneumonias) are the most common causes of death in such cases, and the greatest incidence is in persons forty-five to fifty-five years of age. Strenuous physical or emotional activity may bring about a heart attack in a patient with undetected but severe narrowing of the coronary vessels.

When a crime is suspected, evaluation of the circumstances of death and investigation of the scene where the body was found may be crucial. The position of the body, the distribution of the blood lost by the victim or the assailant, or objects found in the vicinity may offer important clues. Identification of the body can be a complex issue, especially with mutilated or decomposed bodies, and may involve x-ray and dental studies, as well as detailed studies of body contents and hair samples.

Estimation of the time of death is another concern of the forensic pathologist; at times, this can be determined very simply by the circumstantial evidence. For example, when, after a rainy night, the ground under the body is found to be dry, death probably occurred before the onset of rain. More often, however, the time of death is estimated from physical or chemical measurements of values whose rate of postmortem change has been found to be rather constant, such as body temperature or the chemical analysis of certain body and blood constituents. These methods can be useful for short postmortem intervals. For longer intervals, a determination of the level of potassium in the vitreous humor (a gelatinous fluid in the eyeball) is fairly reliable.

Special procedures are used by the forensic pathologist to investigate questions related to criminal abortion, vehicular and aircraft accidents, air embolism, decompression sickness, drowning, exposure to elements, gunshot wounds, rape, and infanticide (in which the main objective is to decide whether the infant was born alive or was a stillbirth).

Toxicologic autopsies, in which poisoning is suspected, are also the responsibility of the forensic pathologist. The sampling of tissues, especially from the brain, liver, lung, kidneys, fat, hair, fingernails, and stomach contents, is done, and samples are also collected from urine, blood, bile, and the vitreous humor of the eyeball. The list of possible poisons and drugs that can be abused is endless, and the investigation of which poison may be the cause of death is both an art and a science.

Perspective and Prospects

The field of pathology is, next to therapeutics (the study of medicinal substances), the oldest division of the healing arts because it is the study of disease itself. Its historical development can be broadly sketched in five different periods, each one highlighted by a fundamental change in the concept of the "seat of disease." An examination of the steps by which pathology has reached its present state provides a useful perspective on the subject.

At the dawn of history, primitive humans believed that there was only a single disease, one that could produce disturbances as varied as headaches, blood vomit, epilepsy, or the death of mother and child during labor. While, in some of those cases, there were apparent causes of death, the real causes were thought to be hidden and supernatural. Thus, the concept of disease was not localized to any specific organ or even to a war wound or broken bone.

The idea of "humors" soon took over. It began in ancient Egypt, was well articulated by the Greeks, and came to dominate medical thought in the Western world up to the Renaissance. The humoral theory of disease proposes that illness is the result of disturbance in the equilibrium between four qualities (hot, cold, wet, and dry) and four elements (air, water, fire, and earth) to affect four body constituents (blood, yellow bile, black bile, and phlegm). This theory was championed by such intellectual giants as Aristotle, Pythagoras, and even Hippocrates and was fine-tuned by Galen in the second century.

The theory of the "equilibrium of humors" implies that disease affects not the entire organism but only such fluids, or humors, indicated by the specific disease. Thus a man has jaundice because of an imbalance of his humors caused by an excess of yellow bile, an excess resulting from the winds blowing in the wrong direction. One disease had become many diseases, with specific seats within the body, but these seats were not subject to anatomic evaluation.

The study of anatomy and gross pathology (that is, autopsy) became generalized in the sixteenth century, and it sounded the death knell for humoral pathology. Antonio Benivieni (1443-1502) is rightfully considered the founder of gross pathology. He is the first physician who performed autopsies, and his medical text appears to be the first to deal with anatomic and gross changes in different organs in relation to clinical symptoms. He worked in the same hospital in Florence, Italy, where the great anatomist Leonardo da Vinci conducted his anatomic dissections. His book contains the protocols for fifteen autopsies performed to ascertain the cause of death, or the seat of disease. Also of great significance in this period is the work of Jean-François Fernel (1497-1558), from Paris, whose book *Medicina* (1554) was divided into three parts: physiology, pathology, and therapeutics. The section on pathology contains 120 chapters and separates diseases into special groups, with brief autopsy presentations for clinical correlation.

The seventeenth century saw the emergence of a small

group of physicians who collected the accounts of all available experiences and published them in enormous volumes. Théophile Bonet (1620-89) is the most important of these reviewers, and his book, *Corps de medecine et de chirurgie* (1679), appearing about two hundred years after Benivieni's, contains summaries of more than three thousand autopsy protocols, including those of Benivieni himself and other masters such as Andreas Vesalius. This book was the stimulus for the monumental contribution of Giovanni Battista Morgagni (1682-1771), whose work marks the official inauguration of anatomic pathology and autopsy as a science. His classic text, *De sedibus et causis morborum per anatomen indagatis* (1761), contains the clinical histories and autopsy protocols of more than seven hundred cases, correlating the morphologic and clinical findings. More important, he committed his autopsy studies to the revelation of the cause of disease, thus establishing the general principle that "seats of disease" are internal body organs, not humors, and that localization in different organs explains different symptoms. This concept served as the basis for the fundamental work of anatomic pathologists-clinicians such as René-Théophile-Hyacinthe Laënnec and Richard Bright.

The next great step in the development of pathology, and establishing the premiership of autopsy as its medium of study, was the French pathologist Marie-François-Xavier Bichat (1771-1802), who established in *Recherches physiologiques sur la vie et la mort* (1800) that organs are formed of elements called tissues. The work of Rudolf Virchow (1821-1902) raised pathology to the premier medical science; he placed the concept of the microscopic cell as the unit of life at the center of medicine and his theory of cellular pathology, thus making cells the unit and "seat" of disease.

Impressive strides in subcellular and molecular pathology have established many morphologic lesions within subcellular structures, even within genes. Such studies can be performed on minute samples of tissues obtained through fine probes. These biopsy techniques and the great technological advances in nuclear and radiologic investigative techniques have allowed the physician to study the cause and extent of disease during the patient's lifetime and with a high level of sophistication. Thus, the role of the autopsy has declined somewhat as an educational tool, but the practice continues to be used in clinical research, medical statistics, public health, and population genetics and to procure organs for tissue transplantation. In fact, many of the functions of autopsy will be extended and improved. For example, the demand for transplantable tissues and organs, procured from cadavers, is likely to increase. Also, recognition of new diseases will occur, aided by postmortem examinations and the application of new technologies and ancillary studies. The autopsy still has much to contribute to education and research, as it constitutes a priceless, continuing, and intimate contact with the natural history of disease.

—*Victor H. Nassar, M.D.*

See also Anatomy; Biopsy; Blood testing; Death and dying; Disease; Forensic pathology; Law and medicine; Malpractice; Pathology; Wounds.

For Further Information:
Burton, Julian, and Guy Rutty, eds. *The Hospital Autopsy*. 2d ed. New York: Arnold, 2001.
Camenson, Blythe. *Opportunities in Forensic Science Careers*. Rev. ed. New York: McGraw-Hill, 2009.
Collins, Kim A., and Grover M. Hutchins, eds. *Autopsy: Performance and Reporting*. 2d ed. Northfield, Ill.: College of American Pathologists, 2003.
Dix, Jay, and Robert Calaluce. *Guide to Forensic Pathology*. Boca Raton, Fla.: CRC Press, 1998.
Gilbert-Barness, E. *Handbook of Pediatric Autopsy Pathology*. Philadelphia: Springer, 2013.
Ludwig, Jurden. *Handbook of Autopsy Practice*. 4th ed. Totowa, N.J.: Springer, 2009.
Patil, Deepa T., Deborah J. Chute, Richard A. Prayson. *Anatomic Pathology*. New York: McGraw-Hill, 2013.
Perez-Tamayo, Ruy. *Mechanisms of Disease: An Introduction to Pathology*. 2d ed. Chicago: Year Book Medical, 1985.
Rutty, Guy N. *Essentials of Autopsy Practice: Innovations, Updates, and Advances in Practice*. Philadelphia: Springer, 2013.
Sheaff, Michael T., and Deborah J. Hopster. *Post Mortem Technique Handbook*. 2d ed. London: Springer, 2005.

Avian influenza

Disease/Disorder

Also known as: Bird flu, avian flu

Anatomy or system affected: Blood, blood vessels, circulatory system, gastrointestinal system, heart, intestines, kidneys, lungs, muscles, musculoskeletal system, nerves, nervous system, nose, reproductive system, respiratory system, stomach, throat, urinary system

Specialties and related fields: Biochemistry, epidemiology, immunology, pathology, virology

Definition: Avian influenza is caused by several virus strains that attack birds; occasionally, a strain develops the ability to attack humans, sometimes triggering an epidemic. There is concern that the H5N1 strain could mutate into a form that is highly contagious among humans and result in a pandemic.

Key terms:

antibody: a specific protein made by an organism in response to one kind of antigen; the antibody attaches to that antigen and deactivates the cell, virus, or chemical to which the antigen is attached, thus protecting the organism

antigen: foreign material that stimulates the host organism to produce antibodies specific to that material

epidemic: the spread of a disease through a population or region

epidemiology: the study of the mechanisms by which diseases spread within and among populations and regions

mutation: a change in the instructions, either deoxyribonucleic acid (DNA) or ribonucleic acid (RNA), of a cell or virus that sometimes changes the characteristics of the cell or virus

pandemic: a disease that spreads around the world

pathogenic: causing disease

reassortment: one means of recombination among viruses; it occurs when two strains are present in the same host, where they may exchange genes to form viruses with new capabilities

RNA virus: a virus that uses RNA as its genetic material, or ultimate instructions for its characteristics *vaccine*: an antigen from a virus or other disease-causing entity that is artificially prepared in a structure not capable of causing disease but which will stimulate the production of antibodies, thus bringing about immunity to the original disease

Causes and symptoms

A group of RNA viruses causes influenza in birds. Most such viruses do not attack humans, although human influenza viruses were probably derived from bird influenza viruses. On the rare occasion that a bird flu strain achieves the ability to enter and reproduce in human cells, the human is unlikely to have effective defenses and the viral attack is likely to be severe. If the virus strain combines its ability to reproduce in humans and its highly pathogenic nature with the ability to transfer from human host to human host efficiently, then it is particularly dangerous. The most deadly human influenza pandemics in history probably began this way. Public health officials have been concerned that the avian influenza A virus strain H5N1 might undergo such a transformation and initiate such a pandemic.

Influenza virus subtypes are named for two types of their surface proteins, hemagglutinin (sixteen subtypes) and neuraminidase (nine subtypes), and all have been identified in avian influenza viruses. Each different protein is assigned a number, so that H5 in H5N1 refers to the hemagglutinin that is assigned the number five. Similarly, N1 refers to the neuraminidase assigned the number one. Hemagglutinins are responsible for attachment of the virus to host cells and entry into those cells. After the production of new viruses in the cell, neuraminidases are used by the new viruses to break out of the cell.

Influenza viruses are notorious for their ability to change their surface antigens and thereby escape host defenses, which are dependent on recognition of those antigens. The H5 and N1 surface proteins characterize the subtype causing severe human disease (since 1997) and are also antigens targeted by host defenses. Both are displayed on the surface of the membranelike coat that surrounds the virus. The hemagglutinin (H5) is the primary target for cell defenses. If an organism has been exposed to a given hemagglutinin, then it will quickly produce antibodies that attach to that hemagglutinin, blocking the site that is normally used to attach to the organism's cells. The virus is rendered harmless if it cannot attach to and enter a cell. If this is the organism's first exposure to the specific hemagglutinin, however, then the response will not be as rapid. The host's immune system will begin making antibodies against the new antigen, but they are made too slowly during this first exposure, and illness results. Most humans have had no exposure to H5 antigens and so are unprotected against H5N1.

Symptoms of avian influenza in humans include the familiar set generally caused by flu viruses. Those symptoms-fever, loss of appetite, clogged sinuses, runny nose, muscle aches, and so forth-pass in three to five days with most influenza strains, and the victim recovers. With H5N1, however, other host systems-such as the circulatory,

---

Information on Avian Influenza

Causes: Virus passed among birds and sometimes to humans

Symptoms: Initially fever, appetite loss, clogged sinuses, runny nose, and muscle aches, progressing to the circulatory, nervous, reproductive, and urinary systems

Duration: From one to five days, often fatal

Treatments: Antiviral drugs

---

nervous, reproductive, and gastrointestinal systems-often become involved. In approximately 60 percent of human cases reported, death occurs, sometimes within a day of the onset of symptoms.

Treatment and Therapy

The major medical solutions to avian flu infection are medications and vaccination. Antiviral medications have been difficult to develop, and few effective drugs are available. Many of the drugs prescribed for viral infections are actually used to combat secondary infections by bacteria attempting to take advantage of the host's weakened condition. Vaccine development against influenza viruses is also problematic. The vaccines target antigens on the surface of the viruses, and the viruses mutate and change their surface antigens so frequently that new vaccines must be developed almost every year to defend against the new strains of influenza. Given these difficulties and the fact that most influenza victims recover in three to five days without treatment, drugs and vaccines against influenza have often not been a high priority compared to those against more deadly diseases such as smallpox. Periodically, however, a particularly pathogenic influenza strain has developed, and effective treatment would have saved many lives. Because the H5N1 strain is feared for its potential to be one of those strains, scientists have sought to develop both drugs and vaccines against this virus.

Four medications that act against flu viruses are available, but the virus has quickly developed resistance to the older pair, amantadine and rimantadine. The H5N1 virus populations in Vietnam and other Southeast Asian countries are already resistant to these drugs. In those countries, the virus has been present in poultry, and occasionally in humans, a bit longer than elsewhere. Two newer drugs, oseltamivir and zanamivir, have shown effectiveness against H5N1, although the virus has sometimes been resistant to oseltamivir. The antiviral resistance of avian flu is being continuously monitored.

Progress in vaccine development has been encouraging, but no 100-percent proven vaccine is available. Even when a vaccine becomes ready for use, production of enough to meet the needs of a pandemic would be challenging. Stockpiling a vaccine in anticipation of a pandemic is possible, but the exact antigen against which it must be directed cannot be known until the virus is in the process of initiating the pandemic. Each year, experts predict the most likely antigens for an approaching flu season, and vaccines are produced in advance against those antigens. Should an influenza virus employ an antigen not anticipated by the experts, then the stockpiled vaccines would be worthless.

Vaccine production technology is also improving, but the improvements have not been fully implemented. In the standard technique, the antigenic virus to be used in the vaccine is grown in fertilized eggs-an expensive, slow, and inefficient method. Tissue culture techniques, in which the antigenic virus is grown in cells in artificial media, promise dramatic improvement in vaccine preparation once they are fully integrated into the production system.

Perspective and Prospects

The history of influenza can be traced much further back in time than the understanding of its cause. Reports describing epidemics and pandemics in which the victims showed symptoms of influenza go back to the early sixteenth century at least, but the first isolation of an influenza virus did not occur until 1933. The worst flu pandemic occurred in 1918 to 1919 (the Spanish flu), when twenty million to one hundred million people died of influenza. It was one of the deadliest diseases in history. Two more recent flu pandemics, the Asian flu (1957) and the Hong Kong flu (1968), were seriously disruptive, but not as deadly. All these pandemics were caused by influenza type A viruses, the type to which strain H5N1 and the other avian influenza viruses belong.

The concern over avian influenza type A H5N1 began in 1997 in Hong Kong, where poultry and humans came under attack. Three events associated with these infections captured the attention of epidemiologists, because together they suggested H5N1's potential as the agent of an influenza pandemic. First, transmission occurred from poultry to humans. Second, H5N1 proved to be highly pathogenic, as six of the eighteen infected humans died. Third, there was some indication of human-to-human transfer of the virus. If the virus maintained its pathogenic nature and its ability to move from poultry to humans, and if it added the ability to transfer efficiently from one human to another, it would almost certainly initiate another deadly pandemic.

Between 1997 and 2006, a number of human cases of

Health officials in Hong Kong collect chickens killed by avian influenza in 2002. (AP/Wide World Photos)

avian influenza type A were documented in a number of countries. Not all were the result of the feared H5N1 strain, but the other strains bear watching as well. Between 2004 and 2006, there were two hundred confirmed cases of human infection with H5N1, most in Southeast Asia (Vietnam, Cambodia, Indonesia, Thailand) but also in Egypt, Iraq, Azerbaijan, and Turkey. Since November 2003, more than six hundred people across fifteen countries in Asia, the Pacific, Europe, Africa, and the Middle East have been infected with H5N1; and more than half of those infected have died. No H5N1 infections have been documented in North America, but avian influenza virus type A H7N2 caused illness in New York, and H7N3 attacked poultry workers in Canada. No North American infection resulted in a human fatality. A new serious strain of avian influenza type A, H7N9, was discovered in China in March 2013. By early May 2013, more than 130 people had been infected, and just over 20 percent of those infected had died. There is concern over H7N9's ability to spread more easily to mammals than other strains of bird flu; health officials have been working on a vaccine against this strain. None of these infections have involved extensive or sustained human-to-human transmission, though a few restricted transfers between humans may have occurred. Most of the human infections were transferred from infected domestic poultry. Some may have been contracted from wild waterfowl (ducks and geese).

Human health is not the only concern regarding the H5N1 strain; there are agricultural and economic concerns as well. Poultry flocks can be destroyed by the virus. There were several poultry outbreaks around the world before 2006, in which an estimated 150 million barnyard birds either died as victims of the virus or were culled to remove the infection focus and prevent further spread of the virus. Although the governments involved often compensated individuals for their culled animals, the compensation was usually well below market value. This practice encourages farmers to hide infections that occur in their flocks, which slows the discovery of potential outbreaks and gives the virus a head start that it does not need. In addition, several governments were suspected of hiding avian flu outbreaks until they were impossible to conceal, in an attempt to protect their countries' economic interests.

The role played by wild birds is an important piece of this puzzle as well. Wild birds, especially waterfowl, act as the reservoir for H5N1. The birds maintain the virus between epidemics. Waterfowl are known to carry the virus, release virus in their feces and oral secretions, and are usually not sickened by the virus infection. These characteristics of the reservoir indicate how easily a pandemic could start from a mutant virus in the reservoir. In Hong Kong in 2002 to 2003 and again in China in 2005, large numbers of wild birds were killed by the virus, emphasizing the virus's tendency to mutate. Experts believe that it may take only a few mutations for the virus to gain the ability to successfully transfer between humans. If they are right, then the waterfowl reservoir is always just a step away from creating a pandemic virus strain.

Given their mobility, especially during migration, wild birds also appear to be good candidates for spreading the virus among countries and continents. However, investigations suggest that, while wild bird migration might play a role in viral geographic expansion, it is probably secondary to the role played by commercial poultry exchanges.

Avian influenza virus type A H5N1 has demonstrated its ability to transfer from wild birds to domestic poultry (and perhaps to humans), to decimate domestic poultry flocks, to be transferred from poultry to humans, and to be highly pathogenic for humans. It has not definitively demonstrated the ability to pass freely from one human to another, although the Centers for Disease Control and Prevention indicates that a limited amount of human-to-human cases may have occured. While for the most part, H5N1 cannot transmit effectively from person to person, if it were to add this last ability successfully to its arsenal, it would be a candidate to initiate a pandemic as deadly as the influenza pandemics of the past. The change required to introduce this ability to the H5N1 virus is not thought to be elaborate. A few simple mutations in the viral RNA might suffice.

Epidemiologists have one special concern, the potential for the H5N1 virus to use pigs for reassortment of its genes. In developing countries, pigs often share living space with chickens and other poultry. Humans often live adjacent to the animals or even share their living space. These associations are troubling because pigs host both human and bird flu viruses-for example, the H1N1 strain that caused a global pandemic between 2009 and 2010 was of swine origin, although the H1N1 virus is endemic to both birds and pigs-and the intimate association of the three species presents the two viral strains with the opportunity to invade the same pig. Together in the same host, they would be expected to exchange RNA strands. Some reassortments might produce a virus with the capability to transfer from human to human. There is no evidence that such a transformation has occurred. However, the possibility is real and the defenses (antiviral drugs and vaccination) are not in place and fully functional, so the concern is understandable.

Some investigators suggest, however, that the concern has been overblown. They point out that no H5 influenza strain has ever caused a pandemic and that successful pandemic-causing influenza strains attach to receptors in the upper parts of the human respiratory tract, while the receptors to which H5N1 viruses attach are in the lower reaches. Some skeptics also argue that if H5N1 went through the changes necessary to achieve efficient transfer among humans, it would invariably lose pathogenic potency in the process, thus minimizing its pandemic potential.

Governments and public health officials are between the proverbial rock and hard place. They would be criticized if they prepared for a threat that did not materialize, but more tragic results would occur if they failed to prepare and a pandemic broke out. Criticism for a perceived lack of preparation is already widespread. While another pandemic is probably inevitable, no one can know when it will materialize or what specific disease organism will be the cause, so there is no easy answer to their conundrum. For the long-term struggle against avian influenza, however, disease patterns in animal populations might be very helpful in predicting which threats have the potential to cause human pandemics and in otherwise understanding the viruses. This possibility calls for close coordination among students of wildlife, veterinary, and human disease. That coordination will not solve all the mysteries of influenza outbreaks but should aid in understanding them, and the influenza viruses will not be controlled until they are more thoroughly understood.

—*Carl W. Hoagstrom, Ph.D.*

See also Epidemics and pandemics; Epidemiology; Immunization and vaccination; Influenza; Viral infections; Zoonoses.

For Further Information:

"Avian Influenza A (H7N9) Virus." *Centers for Disease Control and Prevention*, Apr. 23, 2013.

"Avian Influenza A (H7N9) Virus." *World Health Organization*, May 10, 2013.

"Avian Influenza A Virus Infections in Humans." *Centers for Disease Control and Prevention*, June 21, 2012.

Beigel, John, and Mike Bray. "Current and Future Antiviral Therapy of Severe Seasonal and Avian Influenza." *Antiviral Research* 78 (2008): 91-102.

"Bird Flu." *MedlinePlus*, May 2, 2013.

Carson-DeWitt, Rosalyn. "Avian Influenza." *Health Library*, Dec. 30, 2011.

Clark, Larry, and Jeffrey Hall. "Avian Influenza in Wild Birds: Status as Reservoirs, and Risks to Humans and Agriculture." In *Current Topics in Avian Disease Research: Understanding Endemic and Invasive Diseases*, edited by Rosemary K. Barraclough. Washington, D.C.: American Ornithologists' Union, 2006.

Davis, Mike. *The Monster at Our Door: The Global Threat of Avian Flu*. New York: New Press, 2005.

Green, Jeffrey. *The Bird Flu Pandemic*. New York: Thomas Dunne Books, 2006.

"Highly Pathogenic Avian Infleunza A (H5N1) Virus." *Centers for Disease Control and Prevention*, June 21, 2012.

"Information on Avian Influenza." *Centers for Disease Control and Prevention*, Apr. 12, 2013.

Sfakianos, Jeffrey N. *Avian Flu*. New York: Chelsea House, 2006.

Siegel, Marc. *Bird Flu: Everything You Need to Know About the Next Pandemic*. Hoboken, N.J.: John Wiley & Sons, 2006.

Wehrwein, Peter, ed. "Bird Flu: Don't Fly into a Panic." *Harvard Health Letter* 31, 8 (June, 2006): 1-3.

Babesiosis
Disease/Disorder
Also known as: Human piroplasmosis, Nantucket fever
Anatomy or system affected: Blood, kidneys, liver, respiratory system
Specialties and related fields: Environmental health, hematology, internal medicine, public health, serology
Definition: A parasitic disease that is transmitted to humans by the bite of an infected tick.

Information on Babesiosis

Causes: Parasitic infection
Symptoms: Malaise, fatigue, chills, fever, sweating, muscle and joint pain, jaundice, anemia, shortness of breath
Duration: Days to months
Treatments: Combined antiparasitic and antibiotic therapy, supportive care

---

Causes and Symptoms

Babesiosis is caused by a protozoan parasite that infects livestock and domestic animals and, more rarely, humans. *Babesia microti* (in the United States) and *Babesia divergens* (in certain parts of Europe) are the species more often associated with disease in humans. The parasite, which destroys red blood cells, is spread by the bite of infected deer ticks (in the United States), which also transmit Lyme disease. Ticks become infected with the *Babesia* organism while feeding on infected deer, mice, or voles. The organism can also be transmitted by blood transfusions, although this mode is uncommon.

Many people infected with *Babesia* have no symptoms of illness, even though infection may persist for months to years. Others experience flulike symptoms, such as fatigue, poor appetite, fever, chills, sweating, headaches, body aches, or even nausea. Symptoms usually manifest themselves after a one- to nine-week incubation period and may last for weeks. For people with a weak immune system or who lack a functioning spleen, life-threatening, malaria-like symptoms may develop that include high fevers, severe anemia (as a result of the abnormal breakdown of red blood cells), and jaundice.

Treatment and Therapy

People with no symptoms or only mild symptoms usually recover on their own. Otherwise, the standard treatment has consisted of the antibiotic clindamycin and the antiparasitic drug quinine. More recently, therapy has included the antibiotic azithromycin and the antiparasitic drug atovaquone, which are more easily tolerated.

Transfusions may be given to replace the infected red blood cells in severe cases associated with high levels of parasites in the blood. For complications such as very low blood pressure, breathing difficulties, and kidney failure, supportive care consists of vasopressors (to increase the blood pressure), mechanical ventilation, and dialysis.

Perspective and Prospects

The Romanian scientist Victor Babes was the first to document the symptoms of babesiosis in cattle in 1888. The American scientist Theobald Smith and his colleagues identified a protozoan as the cause of disease and the tick as the agent of transmission in 1893. The first case of babesiosis in humans was reported in 1957 in a person whose spleen had been removed.

In the United States, babesiosis is considered an emerging infection, especially in coastal areas of the northeastern United States and its offshore islands, where the first case was reported in 1969 from Nantucket Island, Massachusetts. No vaccine is available to date. The best prevention is to wear protective clothing to cover the skin and to use insecticides to repel ticks when journeying through wooded, tick-infested areas.

—*Anna Binda, Ph.D.*

See also: Amebiasis; Blood and blood disorders; Environmental diseases; Environmental health; Lice, mites, and ticks; Lyme disease; Parasitic diseases; Protozoan diseases.

For Further Information:
"Babesiosis." *National Institute of Allergy and Infectious Diseases*, Nov. 12, 2010.
Considine, Glenn D., ed. *Van Nostrand's Scientific Encyclopedia*. 10th ed. 3 vols. Hoboken, N.J.: Wiley-Interscience, 2008.
Gelfand, Jeffrey A., and Edouard Vannier. "Babesiosis." In *Harrison's Principles of Internal Medicine*, edited by Anthony Fauci et al. 18th ed. New York: McGraw-Hill, 2012.
Mylonakis, Eleftherios. "When to Suspect and How to Monitor Babesiosis." *American Family Physician* 63 (May, 2001): 1969-1974, 1976.
"Parasites - Babesiosis." *Centers for Disease Control and Prevention*, July 10, 2012.
"Tick Bites." *MedlinePlus*, Apr. 29, 2013.

Bacillus Calmette-Guérin (BCG)
Treatment
Anatomy or system affected: Chest, immune system, lymphatic system, skin
Specialties and related fields: Bacteriology, epidemiology, immunology, internal medicine, microbiology, occupational health, preventive medicine, public health
Definition: An attenuated strain of the tuberculosis bacillus developed by French bacteriologists early in the twentieth century.
Key terms:
attenuation: rendering of a virulent organism less harmful through manipulation or chemical treatment
Mantoux test: screening test for exposure to the tuberculosis bacillus
Mycobacterium bovis: etiological agent of bovine tuberculosis; original source of the BCG strain used for humans
vaccination: induction of immunity in organisms by ingestion or injection of an etiological agent

Indications and Procedures

Tuberculosis is among the most ancient of diseases, with descriptions of the illness dating to at least four thousand years ago. By the late nineteenth century in Europe, an estimated one in three deaths was linked to the disease. In

1882, German physician Robert Koch reported the isolation and laboratory growth of the etiological agent *Mycobacterium tuberculosis*.

The period between the 1870s and the early twentieth century has been called the golden age of microbiology, the result of the unprecedented discovery of the agents of disease and the beginning of vaccine development for their prevention. The passage of bacterial agents associated with human diseases through nonhuman animals or on unusual growth media in the laboratory proved successful in some cases in attenuating these agents. This was the background for development of the BCG vaccine against tuberculosis.

Beginning in 1908 and continuing through the years of World War I, French bacteriologists Albert Calmette and Camille Guérin repeatedly subcultured the bovine strain of the tuberculosis agent *Mycobacterium bovis* in laboratory media, producing an attenuated strain that did not cause disease in either cattle or humans. The first tests of its efficacy in preventing tuberculosis in humans took place in 1921 and proved successful.

BCG vaccine in administered intradermally in a single dose. Anecdotal accounts of raised scar tissue, called keloids, at the site of injection have been largely unfounded.

Uses and Complications

Side effects associated with BCG vaccination are rare, and the vaccine is generally considered to be safe. The primary contraindication is soreness and occasional scarring at the site of injection, a side effect not uncommon with vaccines. Since BCG represents a live agent, the vaccine is not used with patients suffering from immunodeficiency problems, such as those infected with the human immunodeficiency virus (HIV) or suffering from immune-compromising illnesses.

The single major accident associated with the vaccine took place in 1930, when a batch of vaccine was contaminated with the virulent strain and resulted in the death of seventy-two infants during the ensuing year in Luebeck, Germany.

The variable efficacy of BCG vaccination has reduced its use on a more widespread basis. Various studies have shown its effectiveness in long-term protection against the virulent strains of *Mycobacterium tuberculosis* to range from below 10 percent of inoculated persons to greater than 75 percent. No obvious reasons for the variability have been determined. These data as well as the fact the vaccine produces a positive Mantoux test, the primary means of screening for exposure to the tuberculosis bacillus, have resulted in reduced use of BCG as a possible preventive measure.

While the primary use of BCG is in its role as a tuberculosis vaccine, it has also shown promise in the treatment of other conditions. In particular, BCG is commonly used in treatment of early stages (Stage 0 and 1) bladder cancer, as well as an alternative to chemotherapy in the prevention of recurrent bladder cancer following removal of the tumor; BCG has been highly effective in such treatment of noninvasive forms of the disease. In this procedure, the drug is introduced directly into the bladder using a urinary catheter (intravesically). The use of BCG, either directly or as an adjuvant in conjunction with other means of therapy, for treatment of other forms of cancer, such as colorectal cancer, has demonstrated no significant success comparable to that in treating bladder cancer. The mechanism by which BCG acts in treatment of bladder cancer is unclear. It is suspected that localized inflammation may stimulate an effective immune response.

BCG has also been tested as a treatment for other bladder conditions, including interstitial cystitis, commonly known as painful bladder syndrome (PBS). Such patients exhibit bladder and pelvic pain, likely the result of inflammation. The use of BCG as a treatment was based upon the theory that PBS is an autoimmune phenomenon exacerbated by an imbalance in immune function; therefore, BCG, in its effect on the immune response, might ameliorate the condition. While early tests using BCG introduced intravesically showed some promise, follow-up studies demonstrated little benefit beyond that shown by a placebo. There remain few effective treatments for PBS.

Perspective and Prospects

The variation in the efficacy of BCG in providing protection against tuberculosis has limited its use in the United States to those at greatest risk of exposure to mycobacteria: health care workers or persons in intimate contact with tuberculosis patients. A greater understanding of the immune response following exposure to *Mycobacterium* remains a primary focus of research on the disease. It is likely that development of an effective tuberculosis vaccine will utilize newer techniques in gene isolation and subunit vaccines that stimulate cell-mediated immunity; BCG will likely be superseded by this newer generation of vaccines.

BCG, however, has shown significant promise as an adjuvant, a pharmacological agent added to a vaccine that boosts the efficiency of the immune response. Its significant ability to prevent recurrent bladder cancer warrants its testing in the treatment of other localized organ tumors, either replacing some forms of chemotherapy or as a supplement.

See also: Bacterial infections; Bacteriology; Bladder cancer; Cancer; Immunization and vaccination; Lungs; Oncology; Pulmonary diseases; Pulmonary medicine; Tuberculosis; Tumors; Urinary disorders; Urinary system; Urology.

For Further Information:

Baker, Jeffrey, and Samuel Katz. "Childhood Vaccine Development: An Overview." *Pediatric Research* 55, no. 2 (2004): 394.

Feldberg, Georgina. *Disease and Class: Tuberculosis and the Shaping of North American Society.* Piscataway, N.J.: Rutgers University Press, 1995.

Kaufmann S. H. "Fact and Fiction in Tuberculosis Vaccine Research: Ten Years Later." *Lancet Infectious Diseases* 11, no. 8 (2011): 633-640.

Kohnle, Diana. "BCG Vaccine." *EBSCO Health Library*, 2013.

MedlinePlus [Internet]. Bethesda (MD): National Library of Medicine (US); [updated 2013 June 3]. Bacillus Calmette-Guerin (BCG) Vaccine. [updated 2013 June 3; reviewed 2010 Sept. 1; cited 2013 June 19].

Sylvester, R. J., et al. "Bacillus Calmette-Guérin Versus Chemotherapy for the Intravesical Treatment of Patients with Carcinoma In Situ of the Bladder." *Journal of Urology* 174, no. 1 (2005): 86.

Verma, I., and A. Grover. "Antituberculosis Vaccine Development: A Perspective for the Endemic World." *Expert Review of Vaccines* 8, no. 11 (2009): 1547.

Back disorders. *See* Back pain; Spinal cord disorders.

Back pain

Disease/Disorder

Also known as: Backache

Anatomy or system affected: Abdomen, back, bones, hips, joints, legs, ligaments, muscles, musculoskeletal system, nerves, nervous system, spine

Specialties and related fields: Alternative medicine, anesthesiology, emergency medicine, exercise physiology, family medicine, general surgery, geriatrics and gerontology, neurology, nursing, obstetrics, occupational health, orthopedics, osteopathic medicine, physical therapy, preventive medicine, radiology, rheumatology, sports medicine

Definition: Acute or chronic and usually severe pain centered along the spine, usually in the lower back but also common in the neck and upper back.

Key terms:

annular bulge: protrusion of a disk beyond its normal circumference, unusally because of compression caused by gravity, strain on the spine, or aging

cervical spine: the highest of three parts of the spine, consisting of seven vertebrae, named C1 (top of the neck) to C7, in a natural lordosis

herniated disk: prolapse of the nucleus through a rupture or weakness in the annulus

intervertebral disk: the flexible, cylindrical pad between each two vertebrae, consisting of the nucleus pulposis (gelatinous center) and the annulus fibrosis (concentric rings of cartilage); the flexibility, moistness, and thickness of the disk decreases naturally with age

kyphosis: backward curvature of the spine or a section of the spine

lordosis: forward curvature of the spine or a section of the spine

lumbar spine: the lowest of three parts of the spine, consisting of five vertebrae, named L1 to L5 (just above the sacrum), in a natural lordosis

radiculopathy: also called nerve root entrapment or pinched nerve; irritation or compression of the root of a spinal nerve between vertebrae, caused by annular bulge, herniated disk, or spinal injury

referred pain: any pain whose origin is elsewhere in the body from where it is felt; with radiculopathy in the lumbar spine, the pain is typically in the leg

sciatica: intense pain in one buttock and down the back of that leg, caused by inflammation of the sciatic nerve, the largest nerve in the body; in some cases this inflammation is referred pain from radiculopathy where the sciatic nerve originates between L4 and the sacrum

scoliosis: sideways curvature of the spine or a section of the spine

thoracic spine: the middle of three parts of the spine, consisting of twelve vertebrae, named T1 (top of the chest) to T12, in a natural kyphosis

Causes and Symptoms

Most back pain is caused by disk problems, but the disk problems themselves have a wide variety of causes and manifestations. Annular bulge, disk herniation, muscular spasms, and strain from overexertion are just a few of these causes. Among these manifestations are sudden and persistent attacks of sharp, debilitating pain that exaggerate spinal kyphosis, may create scoliosis, and make standing up or bending over without assistance either impossible or very difficult.

The more the lumbar spine approaches either kyphosis or scoliosis, the more out of alignment the natural curvature of the whole spine becomes and the more pain results. Scoliosis or uncontrollable listing to one side is a frequent symptom of disk damage, usually either annular bulge or herniation.

Referred pain may appear from any lumbar radiculopathy, but the two most common presentations are in the thigh, from pinching the femoral nerve between L2 and L4 vertebrae, and as sciatica, from pinching the sciatic nerve between L4 and the sacrum. Shooting pains elsewhere in the leg, genital dysfunction, or incontinence and other urinary or bowel complications may result from radiculopathy of any of several other lumbar, sacral, or lower thoracic nerves. In very severe cases, partial paralysis or constant, intolerable pain may occur.

Treatment and Therapy

Many ways of treating back pain exist, and the program of treatment must be adapted to the particular situation of each patient. Good posture is always essential. Learning to sit up straight, perhaps with a lumbar support roll, or a change of habits, such as learning to lift with the legs rather than the back, may be advised. Sometimes drug therapy with painkillers or muscle relaxants, or physical therapy with manipulation and exercises, is the only additional treatment required. As a last resort and in extreme cases, including emergency cases of incontinence or paralysis, surgery to repair a disk may be indicated.

Treatment options come not only from regular medicine but also from alternative, complementary, or allied systems of health care. The McKenzie method of bending the spine

---

Information on Back Pain

Causes: Usually disk disorders (herniation, muscular spasms, strain from overexertion or poor posture)

Symptoms: Sudden and persistent attacks of sharp, debilitating pain

Duration: Acute or chronic

Treatments: Good posture and habits, painkillers, muscle relaxants, physical therapy; surgery in extreme cases backward, thus emphasizing lumbar lordosis, has proved successful. Techniques drawn from chiropractic, osteopathy, yoga, acupuncture, and other styles of therapy have sometimes provided either temporary or permanent relief.

Perspective and Prospects

Low back pain seems to be equally prevalent in all eras and in all countries. Despite socioeconomic improvements in the lives of physical laborers, and despite the fact that a decreasing proportion of people worldwide make their living from physical labor, no concomitant decrease in new low back pain cases has been observed. If anything, there may be a slight increase in the percentage of low back pain cases in industrialized nations since the mid-twentieth century. People with desk-bound occupations and sedentary habits are at great risk for developing low back pain, especially if they slouch in their chairs or fail to protect the natural lordosis of the lumbar spine.

Physicians no longer consider typical low back pain either an injury or a disease. Since the late twentieth century they have understood it as a natural degenerative condition that can usually be delayed by good posture habits and managed by physical therapy, painkilling drugs, and lifestyle changes.

—*Eric v. d. Luft, Ph.D., M.L.S.*

See also: Aging; Alternative medicine; Bone disorders; Bones and the skeleton; Chiropractic; Disk removal; Kyphosis; Nervous system; Neuralgia, neuritis, and neuropathy; Pain; Pain management; Physical rehabilitation; Sciatica; Scoliosis; Slipped disk; Spinal cord disorders; Spine, vertebrae, and disks; Yoga.

For Further Information:

Borenstein, David G., Sam W. Wiesel, and Scott D. Boden. *Low Back and Neck Pain: Comprehensive Diagnosis and Management*. 3d ed. Philadelphia: W. B. Saunders, 2004.

Brennan, Richard. *Back in Balance: Use the Alexander Technique to Combat Neck, Shoulder, and Back Pain*. London: Watkins, 2013.

Burn, Loic. *Back and Neck Pain: The Facts*. New York: Oxford University Press, 2006.

Cailliet, Rene. *Low Back Pain Syndrome: A Medical Enigma*. Philadelphia: Lippincott Williams & Wilkins, 2003.

Chevan, Julia, and Phyllis A. Clapis. *Physical Therapy Management of Low Back Pain: A Case-Based Approach*. Burlington, Mass.: Jones Bartlett Learning, 2013.

Fishman, Loren, and Carol Ardman. *Back Talk: How to Diagnose and Cure Low Back Pain and Sciatica*. New York: Norton, 1997.

Hodges, Paul W., Jacek Cholewicki, and Jaap H. Van Dieën. *Spinal Control: The Rehabilitation of Back Pain-State of the Art and Science*. New York: Churchill Livingstone/Elsevier, 2013.

Hutson, Michael A. *Back Pain: Recognition and Management*. Boston: Butterworth-Heinemann, 1993.

McGill, Stuart. *Low Back Disorders: Evidence-Based Prevention and Rehabilitation*. Champaign, Ill.: Human Kinetics, 2002.

McKenzie, Robin, and Craig Kubey. *Seven Steps to a Pain-Free Life: How to Rapidly Relieve Back and Neck Pain Using the McKenzie Method*. New York: Dutton, 2000.

Owen, Liz, and Holly Lebowitz Rossi. *Yoga for a Healthy Lower Back: A Practical Guide to Developing Strength and Relieving Pain*. Boston: Shambhala, 2013.

Twomey, Lance T., and James R. Taylor, eds. *Physical Therapy of the Low Back*. New York: Churchill Livingstone, 2000.

Waddell, Gordon *The Back Pain Revolution*. 2d ed. New York: Churchill Livingstone/Elsevier, 2004.

Bacterial infections

Disease/Disorder

Anatomy or system affected: Gastrointestinal system, immune system, intestines, lungs, lymphatic system, respiratory system

Specialties and related fields: Bacteriology, epidemiology, immunology, internal medicine, microbiology

Definition: Infectious diseases caused by bacteria, of which hundreds exist.

Key terms:

antibiotic: a substance that kills microorganisms, including bacteria; antibiotics are used as a primary therapy in combating bacterial diseases

bacteria: small, single-celled organisms with a very simple structure; they live virtually everywhere and most varieties are harmless, although some types are capable of causing disease

cell: the smallest unit of a living thing; a bacterium consists of one cell, whereas humans are made of billions

immune system: the natural defenses of the body, which kill invading organisms such as harmful bacteria

immunity: resistance to infection by a particular disease-causing microorganism, often acquired by vaccination

infectious disease: diseases that can be passed from person to person through direct or indirect contact; many bacterial diseases are infectious

inflammation: signs and symptoms of the body's immune response to some bacterial infections; may include redness, swelling, heat, pain, and the production of pus

metabolism: the chemical reactions in an organism that sustain life and lead to growth and reproduction

microorganism: any small organism, including bacteria, protozoans, mold, fungi, and viruses; in this context, refers to those which cause disease

vaccination: the process of injecting into an individual a substance that provides immunity to a particular disease

Causes and Symptoms

Bacteria are very small, one-celled organisms (the cell being the smallest unit of a living organism) with an average size of thousandths of a millimeter. Based on their relatively simple structure, they are classified as prokaryotic cells. Prokaryotic cells have a rigid outer cell wall, very simply organized hereditary material (deoxyribonucleic acid, or DNA) floating free within the cell, and only a few other structures necessary for their survival, growth, and reproduction. Eukaryotic cells, such as those found in humans, plants, and other animals, have highly organized DNA and many more internal structures. Despite the fact that bacteria are relatively "simple," they are still very

---

Information on Bacterial Infections

Causes: Exposure to bacteria

Symptoms: Localized pain, fever, inflammation, production of pus

Duration: Ranging from one to several days or weeks

Treatments: Antibiotics, vaccinations for prevention

complex living organisms.

The many types of bacteria can be divided into three categories based on their shape: coccus (round), bacillus (rod-shaped), or spirillum (spiral). Another major distinction between types of bacteria is based on the sugar and lipid (fat) composition of their cell walls. This difference can be identified through Gram staining, the result of the stain determining whether the organism is gram-positive or gram-negative. Various types of bacteria may have additional structures that are useful in their identification. Capsules and slime layers are water-rich sugary materials secreted by the bacteria that cling to their surfaces and form halolike structures. Flagella are long, thin, whiplike structures found in one location on the bacterium or occasionally covering its entire surface. These structures are used to enhance the motility, or movement, of the bacteria.

Some bacteria are normal, harmless inhabitants of human bodies, such as those on the surface of the skin. Others, such as those that live in the human intestinal tract, aid in digestion and are essential for good health. The warm, moist, nu-

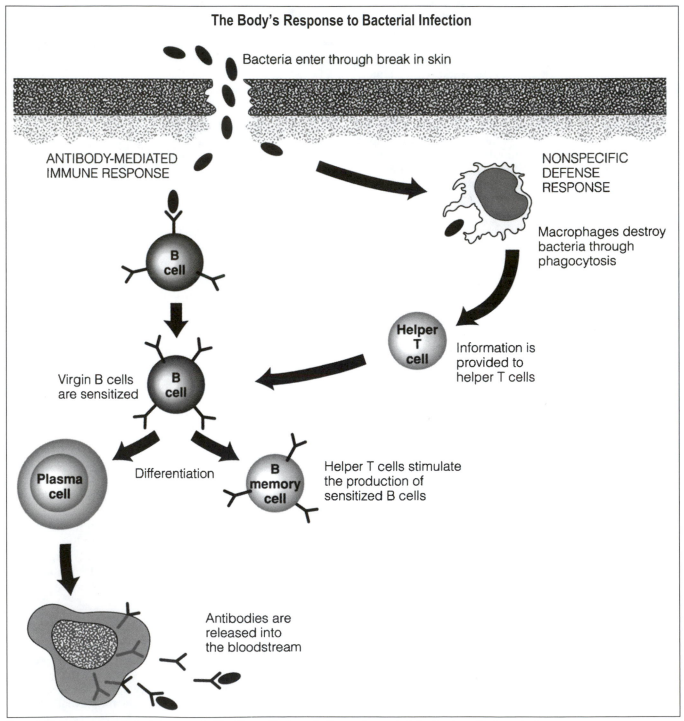

The Body's Response to Bacterial Infection

Bacteria enter through break in skin

ANTIBODY-MEDIATED IMMUNE RESPONSE

NONSPECIFIC DEFENSE RESPONSE

Macrophages destroy bacteria through phagocytosis

B cell

Helper T cell

Information is provided to helper T cells

Virgin B cells are sensitized

B cell

Plasma cell

Differentiation

B memory cell

Helper T cells stimulate the production of sensitized B cells

Antibodies are released into the bloodstream

Bacterial infections cause the body to respond with either antibody production or phagocytosis leading to antibody production.

trient-rich human body also provides an excellent breeding ground for numerous harmful bacterial invaders. For bacteria to cause infectious disease, several stages must occur. The bacteria must enter the person, they must survive and multiply on or in the person, they must resist the natural defenses of the human body, and they must damage the infected person. Most bacterial diseases are infectious because of the ease with which they can be transmitted from individual to individual by physical contact with the person, a contaminated object, or bacteria expelled into the air, such as by coughing or sneezing. A few bacterial diseases, such as food poisoning, are not classified as infectious.

Bacterial infections cause disease by a variety of mechanisms. Many of them produce chemical compounds that are toxic to human beings. For example, *Salmonella* and *Staphylococcus aureus* are two types of bacteria that are capable of causing food poisoning. *Clostridium botulinum* produces the deadly botulism toxin. In each case, ingestion of the toxin in contaminated food can lead to serious illness. *Clostridium tetanii* can enter the body through puncture wounds and will multiply rapidly deep in tissue where there is little exposure to the air. The toxin that it produces acts on the central nervous system and causes severe muscle spasms, which can lead to death from respiratory failure. Water that has been contaminated with raw sewage is a potent source of disease-causing bacteria. *Vibrio* cholera produces a potent toxin that causes severe diarrhea leading to death if it is not vigorously treated. Certain varieties of *Escherichia coli* and *Shigella* found in contaminated water can also cause severe intestinal disorders. Toxic shock syndrome is associated with the production of toxins by *Staphylococcus aureus*.

Another common cause of disease from bacterial infections is the result of the physical destruction of tissue by the invading organisms. Leprosy (also called Hansen's disease), caused by *Mycobacterium leprae*, if left untreated, can lead to severe deterioration and disfiguration of large areas of a person's body. If a wound interrupts the blood supply to an area of the body such as a hand or foot, the tissues begin to decay, thereby providing nutrients for many bacteria, especially *Clostridium perfringens*. These bacteria can greatly accelerate the destruction of the tissue, which causes the condition known as gas gangrene.

In many cases, disease results when the infecting bacteria are recognized by the body's natural defense system (the immune system) as "nonself," that is, as invaders. Certain cells within the body are designed to attack intruders and eliminate them. During this process, disease symptoms that are consequences of the immune system's response may be evident: inflammation (redness and swelling), the production of pus, and fever, among other symptoms. In some cases, certain components of the bacteria, such as capsules and slime layers, may protect them from being eliminated by the immune system. The bacteria may also multiply exceedingly rapidly, producing increasing amounts of toxins that overwhelm the capacity of the immune system to eliminate them. In these cases, continued and increasingly elevated disease symptoms such as fever can cause severe,

even fatal, damage unless an alternate method for eliminating the infection is found. Failure to eliminate the bacterial invaders can also lead to a long-term, chronic infection that damages body tissues.

Many respiratory diseases are associated with the body's immune response to bacterial invasion. *Streptococcus pyogenes* is the causative agent of strep throat, whose features include severe redness, inflammation, pain, and the production of pus in throat tissue. In a small percentage of cases, strep throat can also lead to an infection of and potential permanent damage to the heart valves in a disease called rheumatic fever. In tuberculosis, *Mycobacterium tuberculosis* enters the lungs through inhalation. The body's defense system walls off the intruders and forms a nodule called a tubercle deep in the lung tissue. Nevertheless, the bacteria continue to multiply in the nodule and can travel to new sites in the lung. Tubercle formation occurs at these new sites. Eventually, this repeated cycle of infection and nodule formation becomes a chronic disease and leads to the destruction of lung tissue. Bacterial pneumonia can be caused by several different organisms, including *Klebsiella pneumoniae* and *Mycobacterium pneumoniae*. A pneumonia-like disease, Legionnaires' disease, was first identified in 1976 after twenty-nine delegates to an American Legion convention died from a mysterious respiratory disorder. The lengthy process of identifying a causative agent led to the discovery of a type of bacteria not previously known, *Legionella pneumophila*.

The human urinary and genital tracts are also potential havens for invading bacteria. Cystitis (bladder infections) are caused by many different types of bacteria. Kidney infections can be acquired as corollaries of urinary tract infections. Sexually transmitted diseases (STDs) are contracted through sexual contact with an infected partner, and two common STDs have a bacterial origin. Gonorrhea is caused by *Neisseria gonorrhoeae* and leads to a severe inflammatory response and rapid spread of the organisms throughout the body. If not treated, it can lead to sterility as well as to diseases of the joints, heart, nerve coverings, eyes, and throat. Syphilis, caused by *Treponema pallidum*, can also have serious consequences if left untreated, including dementia and death. In addition, it can be passed to a fetus developing inside an infected mother in a condition known as congenital syphilis.

Treatment and Therapy

The medical management of the many bacterial infections and the diseases they cause begins with diagnosis. Diagnosis relies on a variety of biochemical tests that are analyzed in conjunction with the signs and symptoms exhibited by the infected individual. Treatment is then designed so that it not only eliminates the disease symptoms but also eradicates all invading bacterial organisms, thereby minimizing the chance of a recurrence of the disease. Prevention involves steps that the individual takes to avoid potential contact with infectious diseases, as well as the use of medical procedures that protect against specific bacterial diseases.

To treat a bacterial disease properly, the invading organism must be identified correctly. In some cases, symptomology can be specific enough to identify the offending bacterium, but since there are literally thousands of different types of disease-causing organisms, a systematic approach using a variety of tests is undertaken to make a definitive diagnosis. First, a specimen from the infected person is collected. This may be a blood or urine sample; a swab of the infected area, such as the throat or another skin surface; or a secretion, such as sputum, mucus, or pus. Since human bodies are normally inhabited by a variety of harmless bacteria, the individual types of bacteria are isolated in pure cultures, in which each bacterium present is of the same type. The pure cultures are then tested to determine the identity of the organisms. Staining procedures, such as Gram staining, and microscopic examination of the stained bacteria to determine the Gram reaction and the shape of the bacteria can narrow down the identity of the organisms considerably.

Based on these results, a standard series of tests is performed, continually narrowing down the possible identities until only one remains. One test measures the organisms' growth requirements. Many identifications are aided by analyzing the types of sugars and proteins that the organisms can use as food sources. The by-products of their metabolism (chemical reactions occurring inside the bacteria), such as acids and gas, are identified. Oxygen requirements, motility, and the presence of a capsule are three other common characteristics that are examined. For cases in which the identification of a particular variety of one type of bacteria is necessary, more complex tests may be undertaken, such as an analysis of the particular sugars and proteins on the surface of the organism or tests for the production of specific toxins. Once the bacterium's identity is confirmed, treatment may begin.

The most common type of treatment for bacterial infection is antibiotic therapy. Antibiotics are chemical compounds that kill bacteria. Originally discovered as antibacterial compounds produced by bacteria, molds, and fungi (such as penicillin from bread mold), many more are synthetically produced. Antibiotics work in a variety of fashions. Some, such as penicillin and the cephalosporins, interfere with the synthesis of cell walls by bacteria, thus preventing the organisms from multiplying. Other commonly used antibiotics prevent the bacteria from synthesizing the proteins that they need to survive and multiply. These include the tetracyclines (a class of antibiotics that act against a large range of bacteria), erythromycin, and streptomycin. A host of other antibiotics target a variety of bacterial functions, including specific chemical reactions and the propagation of genetic material, and the structural components of the bacteria. Each class of antibiotics works best on certain types of bacteria. For example, penicillin is most efficient in killing cocci (such as *Streptococcus* and *Staphylococcus*) and Gram-positive bacilli.

Frequently, the symptoms of a bacterial disease may disappear rapidly after the beginning of antibiotic therapy. This reaction is attributable to the inhibition of bacterial multiplication and the destruction of most of the microorganisms. A small number of the bacteria may not be killed during this initial exposure to antibiotics, however, and if antibiotic therapy is ended before all are killed, a recurrence of the disease is likely. A full prescription of antibiotics should be taken to avoid this situation. For example, effective treatment and eradication of all bacteria in tuberculosis may take six months to a year or more of antibiotic treatment, despite the fact that the symptoms are alleviated in a few weeks.

Upon repeated exposure to a type of antibiotic, some bacteria develop the capacity to degrade or inactivate the antibiotic, thus rendering that drug ineffective against the resistant microorganism. In these cases, other antibiotics and newly developed ones are tested for their effectiveness against the bacteria. Such situations have arisen in the bacteria that cause gonorrhea and tuberculosis.

While antibiotics exist to combat infections of most types of bacteria, in some cases the human immune system is capable of clearing the infection without additional intervention. In these instances, the symptoms of the infection are treated until the body heals itself. This is the common treatment path in mild cases of food poisoning, such as those caused by some *Salmonella* and *Staphylococcus* varieties. Diarrhea and vomiting are treated by replacing water and salts, by drinking large volumes of fluids, and perhaps by using over-the-counter remedies to ease some of the symptoms.

Many bacterial diseases can be easily prevented through good hygiene. Foods, such as eggs and meats, that are not thoroughly cooked may become quickly contaminated by the rapid growth of food-poisoning organisms present on their surfaces. Proper cooking kills these organisms. Similarly, foods that are not properly stored but left out in warm places can also provide a potent breeding ground for toxin-producing bacteria. Picnic food not properly refrigerated is a common source of food poisoning. Similarly, questionable water sources should never be used for drinking or cooking water without proper treatment. Filtering with an ultrafine filter specifically designed to remove bacteria is one safeguard, as is boiling for the required time period based on altitude. Food that may have been washed with contaminated water sources should always be cooked or peeled before consumption.

Many diseases can be prevented with vaccinations. A bacterial vaccine is a mixture of a particular bacterium, its parts, or its inactivated toxins. When this solution is injected into an individual, it provides immunity (resistance to infection) to the particular organism contained in the vaccine. Some vaccines provide lifetime immunity when enhanced with an occasional booster shot, while some are relatively short-acting. Many types of vaccines that are directed against specific diseases are part of standard preventive care given to children. For example, the DTaP vaccine (or Tdap for adults) confers immunity to diphtheria, pertussis (whooping cough), and tetanus. Some vaccines are useful for individuals who are living, working, or traveling in areas where certain diseases are endemic, or for those who regularly come into contact with infected individuals. Examples of these sorts of vaccines include those for plague (*Yersinia pestis*), typhoid fever (Salmonella typhi), cholera, and tuberculosis.

Perspective and Prospects

Bacteria were first described as "animalcules" by the Dutch scientist Antoni van Leeuwenhoek in 1673 after he observed them in water-based mixtures with a crudely designed microscope. In 1860, Louis Pasteur recognized that bacteria could cause the spoiling of wine and beer because of the by-products of their metabolism. Pasteur's solution to this problem was heating the beverages enough to kill the bacteria, but not change the taste of the drink-a process known as pasteurization, which is used today on milk and alcoholic beverages. In addition, Pasteur settled a long-standing debate on the origin of living things that seemed to arise spontaneously in fluids exposed to the air. He demonstrated that these life-forms were seeded by contaminating bacteria and other microorganisms found in the air, in fluids, and on solid surfaces. Pasteur's work led to standard practices in laboratories and food processing plants to prevent unwanted bacterial contamination; these practices are referred to as aseptic techniques.

Prior to the late nineteenth century, deaths from wounds and simple surgeries were quite common, but the reason for these high mortality rates was unknown. In the 1860s, Joseph Lister, an English surgeon, began soaking surgical dressings in solutions that killed bacteria, and the rate of survival in surgical and wound patients was greatly improved. In 1876, Robert Koch, a German physician, discovered rod-shaped bacteria in the blood of cattle that died from anthrax, a disease that was devastating the sheep and cattle population of Europe. When he injected healthy animals with these bacteria, they contracted anthrax, and samples of their blood showed large numbers of the same bacteria. By these and other experiments, Koch, Lister, and others proved the "germ theory of disease"-that microorganisms cause disease-and appropriate measures were instituted to protect against the transmission of bacteria to humans through medical procedures and food.

A milestone in the prevention of infectious diseases was the development of vaccinations. The first vaccine was developed in 1798, long before the germ theory of disease was proven. The British physician Edward Jenner first used vaccination as a preventive step against the contraction of deadly smallpox, a viral disease. How vaccinations work and their use as a protection against bacterial diseases were discovered around 1880 by Pasteur.

The first antibiotic, penicillin, was discovered by Alexander Fleming in 1928. Since then, scores of others, produced both naturally and synthetically, have been analyzed and used in the treatment of bacterial diseases. All these discoveries have made bacterial disease a much less deadly category of illness than it was in the late nineteenth century. Yet bacterial diseases are by no means conquered. Overuse of antibiotics in medical practice and in cattle feed results in the appearance of new varieties of bacteria that are resistant to standard antibiotic therapy. Research will continue to develop new means of controlling and destroying such infective organisms. Bacteria also play an important role in synthesizing new antibiotics and other pharmaceuticals in the laboratory through recombinant DNA technology. These organisms will continue to provide challenges and opportunities for human health in the years to come.

—*Karen E. Kalumuck, Ph.D.;*
updated by Matthew Berria, Ph.D.

See also: Anthrax; Antibiotics; Bacteriology; Botulism; *Campylobacter* infections; Childhood infectious diseases; Cholecystitis; Cholera; *Clostridium difficile* infections; Cystitis; Diphtheria; Drug resistance; *E. coli* infection; Endocarditis; Enterocolitis; Epiglottitis; Gangrene; Gonorrhea; Gram staining; Hemolytic uremic syndrome; Impetigo; Infection; Laboratory tests; Legionnaires' disease; Leprosy; *Listeria* infections; Lyme disease; Mastitis; Methicillin-resistant *Staphylococcus aureus* (MRSA) infections; Microbiology; Microscopy; Necrotizing fasciitis; Osteomyelitis; Pelvic inflammatory disease (PID); Plague; Pneumonia; Pyelonephritis; Quinsy; Salmonella infection; Scarlet fever; Serology; Shigellosis; Staphylococcal infections; Strep throat; Streptococcal infections; Styes; Syphilis; Tetanus; Tonsillitis; Toxic shock syndrome; Tropical medicine; Tuberculosis; Tularemia; Typhoid fever; Typhus; Whooping cough.

For Further Information:

"Bacterial Infections." *MedlinePlus*, May 2, 2013.

Biddle, Wayne. *A Field Guide to Germs*. 3d ed. New York: Anchor Books, 2010.

Brachman, Philip S., and Elias Abrutyn. *Bacterial Infections of Humans: Epidemiology and Control*. 4th ed. New York: Springer Science, 2009.

Forbes, Betty A., Daniel F. Sahm, and Alice S. Weissfeld. *Bailey and Scott's Diagnostic Microbiology*. 12th ed. St. Louis, Mo.: Mosby/Elsevier, 2007.

Frank, Steven A. *Immunology and Evolution of Infectious Disease*. Princeton, N.J.: Princeton University Press, 2002.

Hart, C. A. *Microterrors: The Complete Guie to Bacterial, Viral, and Fungal Infections that Threaten Our Health*. Buffalo, New York: Firefly Books, 2004.

Joklik, Wolfgang K., et al. *Zinsser Microbiology*. 20th ed. Norwalk, Conn.: Appleton and Lange, 1997.

US Department of Health and Human Services. National Institute of Allergy and Infectious Diseases. *Understanding Microbes: In Sickness and in Health*. NIH Pub. No. 09-4914, Sept. 2009.

Pelczar, Michael J., Jr., E. C. S. Chan, and Noel R. Krieg. *Microbiology: Concepts and Applications*. New York: McGraw-Hill, 1993.

Schlegel, Hans G. *General Microbiology*. 7th ed. New York: Cambridge University Press, 2003.

Shaw, Michael, ed. *Everything You Need to Know About Diseases*. Springhouse, Pa.: Springhouse Press, 1996.

Willey, Joanne M., et al. *Microbiology*. 8th ed. New York: McGraw-Hill, 2011.

Wilson, Michael, Brian Henderson, and Rod McNab. *Bacterial Disease Mechanisms: An Introduction to Cellular Microbiology*. New York: Cambridge University Press, 2002.

Bacteriology

Specialty

Anatomy or system affected: Cells, immune system
Specialties and related fields: Biochemistry, epidemiology, microbiology, pathology, pharmacology, public health
Definition: The study of bacteria.
Key terms:

anaerobic: free of oxygen
fermentation: a chemical reaction that splits complex

organic compounds into relatively simple substances
infection: the invasion of healthy tissue by a pathogenic microorganism, resulting in the production of toxins and subsequent injury of tissue

Science and Profession

Bacteriology is the study of bacteria, unique life-forms that maintain the basic physiological and genetic processes of all other types of cellular life but that have the unusual characteristic of chemicophysiological diversity. Many bacteria live in totally anaerobic environments, converting carbohydrates to acids and alcohol by fermentation, nitrate to nitrogen gas, sulfate to hydrogen sulfide, and hydrogen and carbon dioxide to methane gas. Some bacteria live by photosynthetic processes similar to those of plants, while others survive by using energy obtained through the oxidation of sulfur, hydrogen, ammonia, or ferric minerals.

The Culturing of Bacteria

Bacteriologists use culturing techniques to identify types of bacteria and to develop and test antibiotics to destroy them; some bacteria are either harmless or helpful to humans, but harmful bacteria can cause a number of diseases, such as syphilis, typhoid fever, streptococcal infections, and staphylococcal infections.

The history of life on Earth is closely linked to the presence of bacteria. Geologic evidence suggests the early increase in Earth's atmospheric oxygen more than two billion years ago was the direct result of bacteriological activity. Throughout time, bacteria have continued to play a crucial role in recycling materials necessary for the survival of plants and animals. In the biosphere, bacteria are responsible for degrading and converting complex substances into useful products. Bacteria break down carbohydrates, proteins, and lipids to form carbon dioxide, and they convert ammonia to nitrate and nitrogen gas to amino acids, all of which are essential to the life cycle of plants. Bacteria are the basis of many industrial processes. Bacteria colonies are involved in producing cheeses and fermented foods such as pickles, sausage, and sauerkraut. Bacteria thriving in sewage and landfills produce methane gas, which is used as an alternative energy source by humans. The exploitation of bacteria as a detoxifying agent of environmental pollutants is becoming widespread. Almost all medically important antibiotics are produced by bacteria cultures.

Many types of bacteria live in association with animals. Most bacteria associated with humans live on the surface of the skin, in the mouth, or in the intestinal tract; the majority are harmless, and many are quite beneficial. Some bacteria, known as pathogens, are opportunistic and able to establish themselves in the body of a host, multiply, and produce local or systemic infections. Many pathogens are the causes of severe diseases in humans; most notable are anthrax, tuberculosis, bubonic plague, typhoid fever, pneumonia, gonorrhea, syphilis, gangrene, meningitis, botulism, diphtheria, scarlet fever, tetanus, streptococcal infections, and pertussis (whooping cough).

Medical bacteriology involves the study of infectious diseases produced by bacteria. Medical bacteriologists isolate bacteria suspected of being infectious, relate their role to the disease in question, study the life cycle of the bacteria colony, and seek means to provide therapy to infected victims and prevent further spread of the infectious pathogen.

Bacteriologists are highly skilled scientists who have undergone advanced studies in the fields of biology, microbiology, and chemistry; many have additional training in medical specialties such as pathology, epidemiology, and serology.

Diagnostic and Treatment Techniques

The way in which bacterial infections develop usually follows a consistent pattern. Transmission may occur by one of four pathways: direct contact, such as sneezing or sexual intimacy; inhalation; common source contacts, such as food, water, or blood; and vector-borne spreading by insects or parasites. Bacteria first invade the body through some opening, such as a wound or the skin, nose, throat, lung, intestine, urethra, or bloodstream. The bacteria then target specific cells and begin to reproduce, establishing a primary infection. If the infection remains unchecked, it may spread to the lymphatic system or bloodstream, and multiple sites of infection may develop. The resulting infection destroys local tissue by producing toxins that damage cells or by producing compounds that interfere with body metabolism.

The control of bacterial infections is accomplished by breaking the links in the chain of transmission. This can be done by altering the behavior of potential hosts through education programs, quarantine, health inspections of common source contacts, and pest eradication programs. Other efforts to control infections involve altering the defensive capability of the host. The most effective means has been through vaccination. Vaccination immunizes individuals so that they are no longer susceptible to the targeted infection. Additionally, many bacterial infections can be treated with injections or topical and oral applications of antibiotics.

Perspective and Prospects

During the mid-nineteenth century, studies by Louis Pasteur into undesirable fermentation of beers and wines led him to the conclusion that infections in animals might be the result of some type of fermentation process. Pasteur experimented with the microbiological cause of infections by studying the characteristics of anthrax and cholera bacilli. Pasteur noted that the introduction of dead bacterial pathogens into a healthy host did not result in disease. Furthermore, if the host was injected with a virulent supply of the subject bacteria, the host did not contract the disease. The result of this work was the discovery of a method for acquired immunity to disease.

Working during the same period, German physician Robert Koch provided proof that anthrax and tuberculosis are caused by bacteria. Earlier in his career, Koch developed methods for isolating pure cultures of bacteria and then identifying, staining, and cataloging bacilli. This en-

The Culturing of Bacteria

Bacteria are introduced onto a nutrient plate and incubated at body temperature.

Any bacteria present multiply rapidly to form visible colonies.

Clear areas around a disk indicate that the bacteria are being killed by that antibiotic.

Disks of different antibiotics are placed within the colonies of bacteria.

Streptococcus (causes sore throat)

Staphylococcus (causes boils)

Salmonella typhosa (causes typhoid fever)

Spirochaeta (causes syphilis)

Bacteriologists use culturing techniques to identify types of bacteria and to develop and test antibiotics to destroy them; some bacteria are either harmless or helpful to humans, but harmful bacteria can cause a number of diseases, such as syphilis, typhoid fever, streptococcal infections, and staphylococcal infections.

abled Koch and other investigators to view infected blood samples and then quickly isolate and cross-reference noted bacilli with previously identified pathogens.

The groundwork that Pasteur and Koch provided helped to establish the role that microorganisms play in the development of infectious disease and ushered in a golden age of discovery into the cause of infectious diseases and their control by immunization.

—*Randall L. Milstein, Ph.D.*

See also: Antibiotics; Bacterial infections; Cells; Cholecystitis; Cys-
titis; Cytology; Cytopathology; Drug resistance; *E. coli* infection; Gangrene; Gram staining; Immunology; Immunopathology; Infection; Laboratory tests; Mastitis; Microbiology; Microscopy; Pathology; Pharmacology; Staphylococcal infections; Strep throat; Streptococcal infections; Tropical medicine.

For Further Information:

Alcamo, I. Edward. *Microbes and Society: An Introduction to Microbiology*. 2d ed. Sudbury, Mass.: Jones and Bartlett, 2008.
Graumann, Peter. *Bacillus: Cellular and Molecular Biology*. 2d ed. Norfolk: Caister Academic, 2012.

Madigan, Michael T., et al. *Brock Biology of Microorganisms*. 13th ed. Boston: Benjamin Cummings, 2012.

Shnayerson, Michael, and Mark J. Plotkin. *The Killers Within: The Deadly Rise of Drug Resistant Bacteria*. Boston: Little, Brown, 2003.

Snyder, Larry, and Wendy Champness. *Molecular Genetics of Bacteria*. 3d ed. Washington, D.C.: ASM Press, 2007.

Topley, W. W. C. *Topley and Wilson's Microbiology and Microbial Infections*. Edited by Leslie Collier, Albert Ballows, and Max Sussman. 10th ed. 6 vols. New York: Oxford University Press, 2005.

Volk, Wesley A. *Essentials of Medical Microbiology*. 5th ed. Philadelphia: Lippincott-Raven, 1996.

Wassenaar, Trudy M. *Bacteria: The Benign, the Bad, and the Beautiful*. Hoboken: Wiley-Blackwell, 2012.

Wilson, Michael, Brian Henderson, and Rod McNab. *Bacterial Disease Mechanisms: An Introduction to Cellular Microbiology*. New York: Cambridge University Press, 2002.

Balance disorders

Disease/Disorder

Anatomy or system affected: Nervous system

Specialties and related fields: Neurology

Definition: Problems with balance that may be described by sufferers as dizziness or vertigo and usually are associated with the inner ear; balance disorders may result in falls and other accidents.

Causes and Symptoms

Being able to stand upright and walk with a steady gait is the result of a complex of body systems. For example, sight and hearing provide information about an individual's location and movement, and proprioceptors in muscles and joints help evaluate the individual's position in the environment. Age affects many of these systems, and age-related changes often impair the sense of balance.

Balance disorders include light-headedness, unsteadiness, or imbalance in walking. Such disorders also include vertigo, the feeling that a person's surroundings are moving or spinning around or that the person is spinning. Vertigo is sometimes accompanied by nausea. Because the ears often are involved, dizziness or vertigo may also be accompanied by tinnitus, a hissing, buzzing, or ringing sound in one or both ears.

Balance disorders often involve the labyrinth, a membrane-lined inner-ear chamber filled with fluid. The labyrinth consists of three canals, each at right angles to the other two. Any head movement-shaking, nodding, or tilting-is sensed by the canals, and the information is transmitted to the brain. Sometimes the labyrinth becomes inflamed, often from a viral infection, thus interfering with the signals relating to movement. Interference also occurs in motion sickness, in which the eyes see one kind of movement while the body, via the labyrinth, senses another kind of movement. The result is a confusion of signals and, often, the familiar sensations of dizziness, nausea, and vomiting.

Other causes of balance problems include neural dysfunctions and restrictions on the supply of blood to the brain. Light-headedness, for example, may be the result of changes in the flow of blood to the brain; if the flow is di-

---

Information on Balance Disorders

Causes: Age-related changes, viral infection in inner ear, motion sickness

Symptoms: Light-headedness, unsteadiness, imbalance in walking, vertigo, nausea, tinnitus

Duration: Temporary or chronic

Treatments: Antibiotics, neurological assessment

---

minished, the result often is a "graying out," or darkening of vision. In extreme cases, the sufferer faints.

A balance disorder such as unsteadiness in walking may be the result of a dysfunction in the cerebellum, the back part of the brain. If the condition persists or worsens, it may be a symptom of a serious neurological disorder. Also, as part of the aging process, fine hairs in the inner ear may be reduced in number or size and thus function imperfectly. This frequently results in balance dysfunctions. Ear pain, nasal congestion, or discharge from the ears may result from middle-ear disorders and accompanying balance problems. Other causes include some medications, poor sleep habits, and vision problems.

Treatment and Therapy

Balance disorders may be symptomatic of serious physical problems and are best dealt with by a physician. If a balance

---

In the News: Epley Manuever for Benign Paroxysmal Positional Vertigo

In 1980, John Epley, an otolaryngologist from Portland, Oregon, first discussed the basis for the maneuver now commonly used to treat benign paroxysmal positional vertigo. The theory behind this procedure was first described that year in an article published in volume 88 of journal *Otolaryngology and Head and Neck Surgery*. Also known as canalith repositioning, the Epley maneuver consists of four positions, performed sequentially and each maintained for thirty seconds. In the first step, the individual is placed in a reclining position with his or her head extending off the table at a forty-five-degree angle. Second, the individual turns the head to a ninety-degree angle. After thirty seconds in this position, the individual rolls onto the side, angling the head toward the unaffected ear and looking at the floor. To complete the procedure, the individual sits up, tilting the head to look downward. The intent of the Epley maneuver is to shift calcium crystals (canaliths) out of the semicircular canals in the ear into a portion of the inner ear where they generally will cause no harm. Repositioning of the head causes the shifting of these calcium crystals out of the semicircular canals and makes the vertigo disappear. This result will generally occur with only one treatment, although occasionally additional sessions are required. A follow-up study, conducted by U. M. Rashad in 2009, as described in volume 123 of the *Journal of Laryngology and Otology*, examined more than one hundred patients five years after their treatment with the Epley maneuver. According to this study, 65 percent of patients treated had no follow-up instances of vertigo during that period. Thus, the Epley maneuver is considered to be an effective means to treat benign paroxysmal positional vertigo.

—Robin Kamienny Montvilo, R.N., Ph.D.

problem is occasional and of short duration, relief may be gained simply by lying down for a brief while in a darkened room.

—*Albert C. Jensen, M.S.*

See also: Batten's disease; Brain; Brain disorders; Dizziness and fainting; Eye infections and disorders; Hypotension; Ménière's disease; Vision disorders.

For Further Information:

American Medical Association. *American Medical Association Family Medical Guide.* 4th rev. ed. Hoboken, N.J.: John Wiley & Sons, 2004.

Aminoff, Michael J., David A. Greenberg, and Roger P. Simon. *Clinical Neurology.* 7th ed. New York: McGraw-Hill Medical, 2009.

"Balance Disorders." *National Institute on Deafness and Other Communication Disorders*, Dec. 2009.

"Balance Problems" *Health in Aging*, Mar. 2012.

"Balance Problems." *MedlinePlus*, Apr. 24, 2013.

Bannister, Roger. *Brain and Bannister's Clinical Neurology.* 7th ed. New York: Oxford University Press, 1992.

Brandt, Thomas. *Vertigo: Its Multisensory Syndromes.* 2d ed. New York: Springer, 2003.

Parsons, Malcolm, and Michael Johnson. *Diagnosis in Color: Neurology.* New York: Mosby, 2001.

Baldness. *See* Hair loss.

Bariatric surgery

Procedure

Also known as: Gastric bypass, stomach stapling, weight loss surgery

Anatomy or system affected: Abdomen, endocrine system, gallbladder, gastrointestinal system, intestines, psychic-emotional system, skin, stomach

Specialties and related fields: Endocrinology, gastroenterology, general surgery, internal medicine, nutrition, orthopedics, plastic surgery, psychiatry, psychology

Definition: Any surgical procedure changing the structure of the digestive system in order to achieve weight reduction.

Key terms:

bariatrics: the medical management of obesity and related conditions

body mass index (BMI): a calculation using an individual's weight in kilograms divided by height in meters squared; a BMI of 30 or more is considered obese

duodenum: the first segment of the small intestine, attached to the stomach

gallstones: solid deposits of cholesterol or calcium salts found in the gallbladder or bile ducts

ileum: the last and usually longest segment of the small intestine

jejunum: the middle segment of the small intestine

laparoscopic surgery: surgery performed with a laparoscope, a slender, tubular instrument with a tiny video camera attached; enables smaller incisions

malabsorption: the abnormal utilization of nutrients from food

sleep apnea: breathing irregularities during sleep

Indications and Procedures

Candidates for bariatric surgery are the severely obese, with a body mass index (BMI) of 40 or more, or a BMI of 35 to 39 with serious medical conditions, such as diabetes mellitus, heart disease, hypertension, and sleep apnea. Typically, to qualify for surgery patients must first have tried other methods of weight loss (dietary modification, exercise, and/or drug therapy) and must be seriously impaired in their ability to perform routine activities. In addition, patients should undergo extensive psychiatric evaluation to ensure that they understand the risks of the procedure and are motivated enough to cope with its dramatic effects and permanent lifestyle changes.

There are two types of procedures. Restrictive surgery-including vertical banded gastroplasty, gastric banding, or laparoscopic gastric banding (lap band)-uses bands or staples near the top of the stomach to create a small pouch that restricts food intake to no more than one-half to one cup. The stoma, a tiny gap in the pouch that opens into the lower stomach, slows the emptying of the pouch to prolong fullness, thus reducing hunger.

Malabsorptive surgery involves surgical rearrangement of the digestive system to bypass parts of the stomach and small intestine, where most nutrients are absorbed. Roux-en-Y gastric bypass is the most commonly performed operation, derived from a procedure developed in 1966 by Edward E. Mason and named after the Y-shaped connection it creates. Roux-en-Y combines restriction with malabsorption, bypassing the lower stomach and the duodenum to connect the stomach pouch directly to the jejunum, or (less frequently) the iliem. In biliopancreatic diversion, sometimes performed on patients with a BMI of 50 or more, a portion of the stomach is actually removed, with the remaining section attached directly to the ileum, thus shortening the small intestine drastically to produce greater weight loss.

Uses and Complications

To lose weight and keep it off, surgery alone is not enough; strict diet and exercise regimens must be maintained. On average, bypass patients lose 66 percent of their excess weight after two years but gain some back as a result of stretching of the pouch over time. At five years, the loss of excess weight typically stabilizes at 33 to 50 percent. Restrictive procedures tend to result in comparatively less weight loss because there is no malabsorption. Diabetes, hypertension, and high cholesterol may improve significantly after surgery, often before marked weight loss occurs. Arthritis, sleep apnea, and other obesity-related conditions may gradually improve as weight is lost. In addition, patients often experience improved mobility and stamina and may report enhanced self-esteem and social acceptance.

Patients with very severe obesity, heart disease, diabetes, or sleep apnea and those who have inexperienced surgeons are at greater risk of developing complications. Gastric bypass patients face a 0.5 to 1.0 percent fatality rate; restrictive surgery patients fare better at 0.1 percent. Follow-up operations are required in 10 to 20 percent of patients. Most lap band patients experience at least one side effect, including abdominal pain, heartburn, nausea, vomiting, and band slippage to the extent that up to 25 percent may have the bands removed. If staples are used, then the risk of developing a leak or rupture is around 1.5 percent, leading to serious infection and often requiring further surgeries; laparoscopic patients appear to be at higher risk. Because 30 percent of patients develop gallstones after surgery as a result of rapid weight loss, the gallbladder is often removed as well. In 2 percent of cases, the spleen may be injured, necessitating its removal.

Other complications include blood clots, gaseous distention, infection, bowel or esophageal perforation, bowel strangulation, hernias, strictures, ulcers, late staple breakdown, menstrual irregularities, and hair loss. Patients undergoing malabsorptive procedures by definition will suffer from nutritional deficiencies, including anemia and metabolic bone disease resulting in osteoporosis, unless supplements are taken daily; regular vitamin B_{12} shots are necessary for some patients. Many patients will require further cosmetic surgery to remove large, sagging folds of skin.

All patients may experience vomiting from eating too much or too quickly. Pain behind the breastbone can result from insufficient chewing, causing large food particles to lodge in the stoma. About 70 percent of gastric bypass patients will develop dumping syndrome, a condition caused by eating too much fat or sugar, which can result in severe dizziness or weakness, abdominal cramps, nausea, vomiting, and diarrhea. Biliopancreatic bypass is further associated with chronic diarrhea and other long-term complications such as liver disease.

Perspective and Prospects

Surgical treatment for obesity began in the early 1950s with dangerous intestinal bypass procedures. As techniques have improved, the number of surgeries performed has mushroomed. The American Society for Bariatric Surgery reports that its member surgeons performed 28,800 operations in 1999 and 63,100 in 2002. During the same period, however, many more of the lucrative surgeries were performed by nonmembers. As of 2007, no regulatory body oversaw bariatric surgical practices, and board certification was voluntary. Evolving surgical practices and long-term outcomes remain difficult to evaluate as clinical trial data are lacking, and proof of overall improvements in health and longevity is scanty. According to the American Medical Association (AMA), the long-term consequences of weight loss surgery remain uncertain. To establish the overall safety and efficacy of such surgery, more research and stringent clinical trials are needed.

—*Sue Tarjan*

See also: Digestion; Eating disorders; Gastrectomy; Gastroenterology; Gastrointestinal system; Hyperadiposis; Liposuction; Malabsorption; Malnutrition; Nutrition; Obesity; Obesity, childhood; Plastic surgery; Weight loss and gain; Weight loss medications.

For Further Information:

American Society for Bariatric Surgery. http://www.asbs.org.

Davis, Garth, and Laura Tucker. *The Expert's Guide to Weight-Loss Surgery*. New York: Hudson Street Press, 2009.

Flancbaum, Louis, Erica Manfred, and Deborah Flancbaum. *The Doctor's Guide to Weight Loss Surgery: How to Make the Decision That Could Save Your Life*. New York: Bantam Books, 2004.

Hart, Dani. *I Want to Live: Gastric Bypass Reversal*. Fort Collins, Colo.: Mountain Stars, 2002.

Inabnet, William B., Eric J. DeMaria, and Sayeed Ikramuddin, eds. *Laparoscopic Bariatric Surgery*. Philadelphia: Lippincott Williams & Wilkins, 2005.

Kothari, Shanu N. *Bariatric and Metabolic Surgery*. Philadelphia: Saunders, 2011.

Mitchell, James E., and Martina de Zwaan, eds. *Bariatric Surgery: A Guide for Mental Health Professionals*. New York: Routledge, 2005.

Nussbaum, Michael S. *Gastric Surgery*. Philadelphia: Lippincott Williams and Wilkins, 2013.

Rogers, Jennifer T. *Gastric Bypass: Surgical Procedures, Health Effects, and Common Complications*. New York: Nova Science, 2010.

U.S. Department of Health and Human Services. Public Health Service. National Institutes of Health. Office of Medical Applications of Research. *Gastrointestinal Surgery for Severe Obesity: A Consensus Development Conference*. Bethesda, Md.: Author, 1991.

Basal cell carcinoma. *See* Skin cancer.

Batten's disease

Disease/Disorder

Also known as: Neuronal ceroid lipofuscinoses (NCLs), Spielmeyer-Vogt-Sjögren-Batten disease, Santavouri-Haltia disease, Jansky-Bielchowsky disease, Spielmeyer-Vogt disease, Kufs' disease, Parry's disease

Anatomy or system affected: Brain, cells, eyes, nervous system, skin

Specialties and related fields: Genetics, neurology, ophthalmology, pediatrics

Definition: A progressive neurological disruption and deterioration of intellectual and physical development caused by mutated genes.

Causes and Symptoms

An umbrella term for neuronal ceroid lipofuscinoses (NCLs), Batten disease occurs in four types that are distinguished by the patient's age when symptoms first appear. Batten disease is associated with defective genes and usually is transmitted as a recessive trait. The prevalence of this disease in the United States is approximately 1 per 25,000 births. Variations of the disease share similar symptoms associated with lipopigment accumulation in tissues. These excess proteins and fats disrupt cellular functioning, particularly in the brain and eyes. Abnormal enzyme activity alters metabolism and body chemistry.

Infantile type, sometimes referred to as Finnish or Santavouri-Haltia type, usually is evident when children are between six months and two years old. A defective palmitoyl protein thioesterase (PPT) gene on chromosome 1 causes this type of Batten disease. The patient's physical and mental development and growth, particularly head size, cease to follow normal patterns. Most patients with

---

Information on Batten's Disease

Causes: Genetic mutation leading to excess proteins and fats in tissues

Symptoms: Seizures, sight impairment, diminished motor skills and intellect, behavioral extremes, unbalanced movement, dementia

Duration: Lifelong

Treatments: Medications to prevent seizures and minimize motor difficulties, institutionalization

---

this type die by age six.

Children with late infantile type, or Jansky-Bielchowsky type, seem normal until two to four years of age. They then suffer seizures, sight impairment, and diminished motor skills and intellect. Death often occurs by age twelve. This type is linked to the ceroid-lipofuscinosis, neuronal 2 (CLN2) gene on chromosome 11.

Juvenile NCL, or Spielmeyer-Vogt, type appears in children at approximately five to ten years of age. The ceroid-lipofuscinosis, neuronal 3 (CLN3) gene on chromosome 16 is associated with this type. Symptoms occur at a slower rate than with the first two types. Patients sometimes become paralyzed.

Kufs or Parry disease is the rare adult type of Batten disease. Sometimes this type is inherited as a dominant disease, and people with one defective gene are affected. Unlike with other types, adult patients do not have convulsions or impaired eyesight. Behavioral extremes and unbalanced movement characterize this type. Progressive mania can result in dementia.

Physicians diagnose Batten disease by studying the patient's skin tissues for lipopigment deposits. An eye examination may reveal the cell depletion associated with Batten disease. Additional tests, imaging, X-rays, and electroenceph-alograms can verify the diagnosis.

Treatment and Therapy

Because Batten disease cannot be prevented or cured, treatment focuses on the alleviation of symptoms. Physicians prescribe medications to prevent seizures and to minimize motor difficulties and loss of balance. Nutritional strategies and various therapies can also ease symptoms. Sometimes, patients need to be institutionalized as a result of their mental and visual incapacities.

Perspective and Prospects

Christian Stengel's 1826 medical article is credited as the first clinical report of patients with Batten disease symptoms. Frederick E. Batten observed several types of this disease in patients in 1903, differentiating it from Tay-Sachs disease. Karl Sjögren initiated genetic investigations. By the 1990s, researchers linked specific genes to Batten disease.

The Batten Disease Support and Research Association distributes information, while the National Batten Disease Registry and designated tissue banks compile data.

—*Elizabeth D. Schafer, Ph.D.*

See also: Balance disorders; Brain; Brain disorders; Eyes; Genetic diseases; Intellectual disability; Nervous system; Neuralgia, neuritis, and neuropathy; Neuroimaging; Neurology; Neurology, pediatric; Seizures; Vision disorders.

For Further Information:
Alan, Rick, and Kari Kassir. "Batten Disease." *Health Library*, Nov. 26, 2012.

"Batten Disease Fact Sheet." *National Institute of Neurological Disorders and Stroke*, Oct. 18, 2012.

Batten Disease Support and Research Association. "Juvenile Batten Disease." *Genetics Home Reference*, May 6, 2013.

Mole, Sara E. "Batten's Disease: Eight Genes and Still Counting?" *The Lancet* 354, no. 9177 (August 7, 1999): 443-445.

Opitz, John M., ed. *Ceroid-Lipofuscinoses: Batten Disease and Allied Disorders*. New York: A. R. Liss, 1988.

U.S. Department of Health and Human Services. Public Health Service. National Institutes of Health. *Batten Disease*. Bethesda, Md.: Author, 1992.

Wisniewski, Krystyna E., and Nanbert Zhong, eds. *Batten Disease: Diagnosis, Treatment, and Research*. San Diego, Calif.: Academic Press, 2001.

Bed-wetting

Disease/Disorder

Also known as: Enuresis

Anatomy or system affected: Bladder, muscles, musculoskeletal system, urinary system

Specialties and related fields: Family medicine, pediatrics, psychology, urology

Definition: A condition characterized by an inability of the bladder to contain the urine during sleep, often a developmental condition in children.

Key terms:

alarm therapy: the practice of utilizing mechanical or electronic devices to detect bed-wetting as it occurs

bladder: a membranous sac in the body that serves as the temporary retention site of urine

diaphragm: a body partition of muscle and connective tissue separating the chest and abdominal cavities

enuresis: an involuntary discharge of urine; incontinence of urine

nervous system: the bodily system that receives and interprets stimuli and transmits impulses to the organs

neurophysiological: pertaining to the nervous system in the human body

phrenic: of or relating to the diaphragm

sphincter: a muscle surrounding and able to contract or close a bodily opening (such as the opening to the bladder)

Causes and Symptoms

Primary enuresis is defined medically as the inability to hold one's urine during sleep. The condition is quite common and occurs most often in children; between 15 and 20 percent of children under the age of six suffer from the condition. These percentages decrease to about 5 percent at age ten, 2 percent at age fifteen, and only about 1 percent of adults. Secondary enuresis is bed-wetting in a child who had previously achieved bladder control. (These terms do not apply, however, to urination problems caused by physical illness, disease, or anatomical defect.) The condition is more common in boys than in girls. Bed-wetting usually occurs during the first third of sleep, although it can occur during all sleep stages and without relation to awakening periods.

It is important to realize that enuresis is considered to be a developmental concern rather than an emotional, behavioral, or physical one. Donald S. Kornfeld and Philip R. Muskin report in *The Columbia University College of Physicians and Surgeons Complete Home Medical Guide* (rev. ed., 1989) that "enuresis is due to a lag in development of the nervous system's controls on elimination." Many parents fail to understand this neuropsychological element and thus punish the child for a wet bed. Punishing, ridiculing, or shaming the child does not correct the situation; in fact, in many cases, it may prolong the problem as well as cause other unnecessary and undesirable psychological problems. Emotional problems have resulted from enuresis, as the child may be too embarrassed to partake in normal childhood activities such as camping or sleepovers.

Treatment and Therapy

Techniques for helping the enuretic child achieve dryness range from withholding liquids near bedtime to alarm systems to medical intervention. Generally, restriction of liquid intake after dinner is the first course of action. This treatment method, however, does not have a very high success rate. Should this treatment fail after a trial period of a few weeks, other methods may be employed.

Alarm therapy can help a child achieve control within four months, sometimes in only a few weeks. A beeper- or buzzer-type alarm sounds when moisture touches the bedding or underwear; the desired result is that the child, while sleeping, will eventually recognize the need to urinate and awaken in time to get to the bathroom. Electronic alarms are generally of two types. The first is a wired pad, consisting of two screens, which is placed under the sheets to detect wetness; when the child wets, the moisture activates the battery-operated alarm. The second is a device worn on the body, either in the underpants and connected by a wire to an alarm or a wristwatch-type alarm; the underwear serves as a separating cloth for the contact points. In either case, as wetness occurs, the alarm sounds, thus wakening the child; the child can then be directed to the bathroom to complete urination.

Barry G. Powell and Lynda Muransky cite several case histories in which alarm therapy proved to be effective in stopping enuresis. For example, a six-year-old who never had a dry bed achieved dryness within a week through the use of an alarm. In another case, a fifteen-year-old had been trying to overcome his bed-wetting problem for ten years. Several trips to the doctor showed that he had no physical cause for enuresis. His parents labeled him "lazy, inconsiderate, and difficult." His desire to join his hockey team in overnight travel gave him the impetus to seek help. Powell and Muransky found his problem to be primary enuresis aggravated by family ridiculing. Through the use of his alarm, he achieved dryness within two weeks.

A case involving secondary enuresis is described as well.

> ### Information on Bed-Wetting
> **Causes:** Immature development of the phrenic reflex, physical illness, disease, anatomical defect
> **Symptoms:** Passage of urine during sleep
> **Duration:** Often chronic until phrenic reflex matures
> **Treatments:** Alarm therapy, chiropractic manipulation, drug therapy

A child who had suffered through primary enuresis, then achieved dryness, was found to be wetting again. This second bout of bed-wetting seems to have been the result of his parents' marital separation. After a medical examination revealed no physical problems, it appeared the problem was psychological, caused by emotional upset. He resumed dryness in three weeks (although an alarm system on his bed for six months gave him more confidence). It is important to note, however, that alarms can take up to several months' time before a child feels comfortable in stopping its use. Also, parental supervision is imperative for this type of therapy to work properly.

Chiropractic spinal manipulation has been found to be effective in the treatment of some cases of enuresis. Some believe that a spinal reflex is involved in bed-wetting. As nighttime breathing slows down (a normal reaction), carbon dioxide builds up in the body. When the carbon dioxide buildup reaches a certain level, a breathing mechanism called the phrenic reflex is triggered. This mechanism normally causes the diaphragm to return breathing to its normal pattern. If the mechanism does not work properly, however, the carbon dioxide continues to increase, resulting in an involuntary relaxation of the sphincter muscle at the opening to the bladder. Fluid (urine) is released and leaks out of the bladder. A child in a deep state of sleep does not recognize that the bed has been wet. Generally, chiropractors believe that the bed-wetting child sleeps in a state of high carbon dioxide intoxication.

While immature development of the phrenic reflex is the most common cause of bed-wetting, in some children a misalignment of the bones in the neck and spine (referred to as "subluxation" by chiropractors) is thought to cause pressure on the nerves that are related to the phrenic reflex. Through chiropractic adjustments, it is argued, the subluxation can be corrected, thus relieving pressure on the nerves. With the spine realigned and bodily functions working normally, enuresis can be eliminated. One child had never had a dry bed in his first ten years of life; after only two spinal adjustments by a licensed chiropractor, the child stopped wetting immediately. Chiropractors usually recommend a series of adjustments in order to realign the spine and nerves and keep them in the proper position.

Drug therapy solely for the treatment of enuresis is controversial. However, when an illness such as diabetes mellitus is the underlying cause of the bed-wetting, the use of drugs may be indicated. The drug imipramine hydrochloride (an antidepressant agent) has been studied to assist in contraction of the sphincter; however, because of the high toxicity and limited effectiveness of such antidepressants, its use is not widespread. Relapse rates are high, and cure rates are relatively low. More success has been achieved with desmopressin acetate, an antidiuretic drug. There is an immediate improvement in 70 percent of treated children. Relapse rates are lower than those associated with imipramine but higher than with the use of bed-wetting alarms, probably because the sphincter muscle is not fully developed in the enuretic child. In general, drug therapy yields a final success rate of about 25 percent.

Perspective and Prospects

The history of bed-wetting is probably a lengthy one. The term "enuresis" was coined around 1800, and the condition has plagued children from every ethnic background and socioeconomic level around the world. It continues to be a problem for many children today and probably will be so in the future as well.

Most enuretics are deep sleepers who are usually quite active during their waking hours. This sleeping pattern, combined with urinary systems that are not yet fully developed, is generally the main cause of bed-wetting. There are some indications that enuresis is hereditary; many children who suffer from the condition have a parent who was enuretic as a child. It is reassuring to know that almost all affected children outgrow the problem by adulthood. While no immediate cure is available, continued experiments with alarm systems and drugs will certainly alleviate the discomfort and embarrassment until the body's lag in development corrects itself.

—*Carol A. Holloway*

See also: Anxiety; Incontinence; Psychology; Sleep disorders; Stress; Urinary disorders; Urinary system; Urology; Urology, pediatric.

For Further Information:

A.D.A.M. Medical Encyclopedia [Internet]. Atlanta (GA): A.D.A.M., Inc.; (c) 2005. Bedwetting; [updated 2011 Aug. 2; cited 2013 Aug. 29]; about 3 p.

"Alarm Bells for Enuresis." *The Lancet* 337 (March 2, 1991): 523.

American Medical Association. *American Medical Association Family Medical Guide*. 4th rev. ed. Hoboken, N.J.: John Wiley & Sons, 2004.

"Defining Enuresis." *FDA Consumer* 23 (May, 1989): 10.

Hurl, C. "Urine Trouble: A Social History of Bedwetting and Its Regulation." *History of the Human Sciences* 24.2 (2011): 48-64.

Kemper, Kathi J. *The Holistic Pediatrician: A Pediatrician's Comprehensive Guide to Safe and Effective Therapies for the Twenty-five Most Common Ailments of Infants, Children, and Adolescents*. 2d ed. New York: Quill, 2007.

Kornfeld, Donald S., and Philip R. Muskin. "Enuresis, or Bed-Wetting." In *The Columbia University College of Physicians and Surgeons Complete Home Medical Guide*, edited by Donald Tapley et al. Rev. 3d ed. New York: Crown, 1995.

Morison, Moya J. "Living with a Young Person Who Wets the Bed: The Families" Experience." *British Journal of Nursing* 9, no. 9 (May 11-24, 2000): 572.

Rogers, June. "Child Centered Approach to Bed-Wetting." *Community Practitioner* 76, no. 5 (May, 2003): 163-65.

Ronen, T., L. Hamama, and M. Rosenbaum. "Enuresis: Children's Predictions of Their Treatment's Progress and Outcomes." *Journal of Clinical Nursing* 22 no. 1-2 (January, 2013): 222-32.

Bedsores

Disease/Disorder

Also known as: Decubitus ulcers, pressure sores, pressure ulcers

Anatomy or system affected: Blood vessels, immune system, muscles, skin

Specialties and related fields: Dermatology, internal medicine, nursing, nutrition, surgery

Definition: Sores caused by sustained pressure with restricted blood flow to the skin.

Causes and Symptoms

Bedsores are caused by sustained pressure on the skin, blocking blood flow. Impaired circulation causes the skin tissue to die and tear.

Persons at risk for bedsores include the bedridden, wheelchair-bound, immobile, or unconscious. Paraplegics and others with spinal cord disease or neuromuscular injuries are at risk because of their inability to sense pain in affected limbs or because of sitting in a wheelchair. Bed-bound persons who lie in one position for extended lengths of time may develop bedsores. The malnourished may experience bedsores as a result of little padding over bony areas. The elderly prove more vulnerable to bedsores because of thin skin, decreased circulation, and restricted mobility. Chronic diseases such as diabetes, urinary incontinence, or vascular disease can increase the risk of bedsores.

Bedsores typically occur in the skin over bony areas such as the elbows, heels, ankles, back, lower spine or tailbone, hips, shoulders, and back of the head. In the early stage, the skin becomes red, soft, and warm to the touch. If pressure is relieved by changing body position, then the skin will heal. If the pressure continues, however, then the skin may blister and then break down, leaving an open wound. Without intervention, the bedsore can progress to skin cell death, with damage to deeper levels of skin or muscle. An advanced bedsore smells odorous and becomes infected without proper treatment. Unattended, the bedsore can result in infection leading to fever, confusion, and death.

Treatment and Therapy

Certain measures can prevent or minimize the development of bedsores in persons at risk. Relief from pressure on the skin by frequently changing body position is critical. Other approaches include keeping the skin clean and dry, minimizing friction against the skin, and maintaining healthy nutrition. Treatment for bedsores includes moni-

---

Information on Bedsores

Causes: Sustained pressure to the skin around bony areas

Symptoms: Redness, blistering, skin ulceration, fever

Duration: Acute or chronic

Treatments: Repositioning, clean dry skin, good nutrition, dressing changes, debridement, antibiotics, wound VAC toring the skin for redness and taking immediate measures to minimize further breakdown. The bedsore should be cleansed and covered with a dressing as prescribed by the health-care provider. Dead tissue can be removed to prevent infection and encourage healing through surgical debridement or mechanical debridement by gentle scrubbing or wound irrigation. Enzyme preparations are available to dissolve dead tissue. Antibiotic solutions can be applied to the bedsore and oral antibiotics can be taken to decrease the risk of secondary infections. Negative pressure therapy, which is also called vacuum assisted therapy (wound VAC), uses a device that is applied over the wound that clears bacteria and drainage with suction. (Mayo Clinic, Bedsores (Pressure Ulcers), 2017).

—Marylane Wade Koch, RN, MSN;
updated by Mary Dietmann Ed. D. APRN CNS and
Geraldine Marrocco

See also: Aging: Extended care; Blisters; Canker sores; Circulation; Dermatology; Dermatopathology; Healing; Hospice; Lesions; Necrotizing fasciitis; Palliative*medicine; Paralysis; Rashes; Sepsis; Skin; Skin disorders; Skin lesionremoval; Terminally ill: Extended care; Ulcers; Wounds.*

For Further Information:

Brown, Pamela. *Quick Reference to Wound Care.* Sudbury, Mass.: Jones and Bartlett, 2009.

MedlinePlus [Internet]. Bethesda (MD): National Library of Medicine (US); [updated 2005 Aug 12]. *PressureSores*; updated 2013 Aug. 26; reviewed 2013 June 5; cited 2013 Aug. 29; about 2 p.

Ousey, Karen. *PressureArea Care.* Malden, Mass.: Blackwell, 2005.

Pieper, Barbara. *PressureUlcers: Prevalence, Incidence, and Implications for the Future.*Washington, D.C.: National Pressure Ulcer Advisory Panel, 2012.

Webster, J. G. *Prevention ofPressureSores: Engineering and Clinical Aspects.* New York: Taylor & Francis, 1991.

Behçet's disease

Disease/Disorder

Also known as: Mucocutaneous ocular syndrome, Silk Road disease

Anatomy or system affected: Eyes, genitals, mouth, nervous system, skin

Specialties and related fields: Internal medicine, ophthalmology, rheumatology

Definition: A multisystem disease characterized by recurrent oral and genital ulcers.

Causes and Symptoms

Behçet's disease, or Behçet's syndrome, usually appears in early adulthood with painful aphthous ulcers (similar to canker sores) in the mouth and genitals. These ulcers generally subside after one to two weeks, but they recur throughout the course of the disease. Some patients also have painful skin nodules known as erythema nodosum. Brief periods of joint pain are also common. Rarely, the ulcers of Behçet's disease are found in the gastrointestinal tract. Involvement of the central nervous system causes a variety of symptoms ranging from mild confusion to paralysis. However, the most serious complication of Behçet's disease is involvement of the eyes, since this may progress to blindness. Patients also have an increased predisposition

---

> ### Information on Behçet's Disease
>
> **Causes:** Unknown
>
> **Symptoms:** Inflammation of small blood vessels, oral and genital ulcers, painful skin nodules, joint pain; complications may include mild confusion, paralysis, blindness, blood clots
>
> **Duration:** Chronic, with episodes lasting one to two weeks
>
> **Treatments:** Topical glucocorticoids, thalidomide, oral steroids (prednisone), immunosuppressive agents (azathioprine, cyclosporine)

for the formation of blood clots, usually in the venous system. These clots can be life-threatening if they migrate to the lungs.

The common factor underlying these diverse manifestations of Behçet's disease is inflammation of the small blood vessels, but it remains unclear what environmental or genetic factors trigger this inflammation. Rare reports have been made of familial forms of the disease, raising the possibility of a genetic basis, but this remains under investigation. Diagnosis is made on clinical grounds.

Treatment and Therapy

Behçet's disease is a chronic condition, but the severity of the disease generally lessens over time. Ulcers are first treated with topical glucocorticoids, in the form of either mouthwash or paste. Refractory cases may require thalidomide, a drug that must be used with extreme caution because of its ability to cause birth defects. Because of the risk of blindness, ocular and central nervous system disease is managed more aggressively with oral steroids (such as prednisone), along with azathioprine or cyclosporine.

Apart from the above complications, the long-term prognosis of Behçet's disease is quite good, and the life expectancy of patients is comparable with that of the general population.

Perspective and Prospects

The first description of Behçet's disease appears in the writings of Hippocrates in the fifth century BCE, but it was first recognized in the modern era by the Turkish physician Hulusi Behçet in 1937. Although Behçet's disease is seen throughout the world, the highest prevalence is in countries along the ancient Silk Road, a trading route extending from the Far East to the Mediterranean Sea.

—Ahmad Kamal, M.D.

See also: Blindness; Eyes; Genital disorders, female; Genital disorders, male; Nervous system; Neurology; Ophthalmology; Rheumatology; Thrombosis and thrombus; Ulcers; Vascular medicine; Vascular system; Vision disorders.

For Further Information:

"Behçet's Disease." *National Institute of Arthritis and Musculoskeletal and Skin Diseases*, Apr. 2012.

"Behçet's Syndrome." *MedlinePlus*, Mar. 14, 2013.

"Common Symptoms and Signs of Behçet's Disease." *American Behçet's Disease Association.*

Lee, Sungnack, et al., eds. *Behçet's Disease: A Guide to Its Clinical Understanding*. New York: Springer, 2001.

Parker, James N., and Philip M. Parker, eds. *The Official Patient's Sourcebook on Behcet's Disease*. San Diego, Calif.: Icon Health, 2002.

Plotkin, Gary R., John J. Calabro, and J. Desmond O'Duffy, eds. *Behçet's Disease: A Contemporary Synopsis*. Mount Kisco, N.Y.: Futura, 1988.

Zeis, Joanne. *Essential Guide to Behçet's Disease*. Uxbridge, Mass.: Central Vision Press, 2002.

Bell's palsy

Disease/Disorder

Anatomy or system affected: Ears, eyes, head, mouth, muscles, nerves

Specialties and related fields: Family medicine, neurology, nutrition

Definition: A weakening or paralysis of facial muscles caused by damage to the seventh cranial nerve.

Causes and Symptoms

The most likely cause of Bell's palsy is a weakened immune system produced by the common cold virus or herpes viruses. The condition has also been associated with chronic middle ear infection, sarcoidosis, Lyme disease, high blood pressure, tumors, and trauma to the head. A diagnosis of Bell's palsy is made from facial appearance and weakness, blood tests, electromyography to confirm nerve damage, and magnetic resonance imaging (MRI) or computed tomography (CT) to assess any pressure on the facial nerve.

In 99 percent of cases, Bell's palsy produces paralysis on only one side of the face. Other symptoms may include an inability to close the eye on the affected side, frequent tear-

Bell's palsy results in a temporary sagging and paralysis of one side of the face; dashed lines show the main neural pathways affected.

> ### Information on Bell's Palsy
>
> **Causes:** Damage to seventh cranial nerve, immune system weakness from common cold or herpes, chronic middle ear infection, sarcoidosis, Lyme disease, high blood pressure, tumors, head trauma
>
> **Symptoms:** Weakening or paralysis of facial muscles on one side, with inability to close eye, frequent tearing and dryness of eye, drooping eyelid and mouth, drooling, increased sensitivity to sound, ringing in ear, taste impairment, jaw pain, impaired speech, headache, dizziness
>
> **Duration:** Improvement within two weeks, total recovery within three to six months
>
> **Treatments:** Antiviral drugs (acyclovir, famciclovir, valacyclovir), prednisone, moist heat, facial massage and exercise, B vitamins

ing from that eye, dryness of the affected eye, drooping of the eyelid and mouth, drooling, increased sensitivity to sound and ringing in the affected ear, impairment of taste, jaw pain, impaired speech, headache, and dizziness. Typically, the symptoms appear rather suddenly and peak within the first forty-eight hours after onset. Most patients experience dramatic improvement within two weeks, and most recover totally within three to six months after onset.

Treatment and Therapy

Various treatments can be effective if administered within seven days after onset. Antiviral drugs such as acyclovir, famciclovir, or valacyclovir cause the virus to run its course faster by binding viral enzymes so that the harmful cells cannot replicate. Prednisone, a synthetic hormone that mimics the natural steroid cortisol produced by the body, is also administered to help reduce swelling and the inflammation compressing the seventh cranial nerve.

The application of moist heat can help reduce pain and discomfort. The affected eye should be kept moist to protect it from debris and injury. Facial massage and exercise may help prevent the permanent shrinkage of facial muscles. Since vitamins B_1, B_6, and B_{12} are essential for proper nervous system functioning, a B-complex vitamin is often prescribed. Ample rest is necessary to restore the immune system.

Perspective and Prospects

First described in the nineteenth century by Scottish surgeon Sir Charles Bell, Bell's palsy affects approximately forty thousand Americans each year. It can occur at any age but is less common before age fifteen and after age sixty. Diabetics are particularly susceptible to the condition, as are pregnant women, particularly during the last trimester.

No cure has been found for Bell's palsy. Research focuses on achieving a better understanding of how the nervous system works, developing methods of repairing damaged nerves and restoring full use of injured areas, and finding ways to prevent nerve damage. Methylcobalamin, an essential component in the process of building nerve tissue, shows promise for treating Bell's palsy.

—*Alvin K. Benson, Ph.D.*

See also: Muscle sprains, spasms, and disorders; Muscles; Nervous system; Neuralgia, neuritis, and neuropathy; Neuroimaging; Neurology; Neurology, pediatric; Palsy; Paralysis.

For Further Information:
"Bell's Palsy." *MedlinePlus*, Apr. 23, 2013.
"Bell's Palsy Fact Sheet." *National Institute of Neurological Disorders and Stroke*, Sept. 4, 2012.
Matthews, Gary G. *Cellular Physiology of Nerve and Muscle*. 4th ed. Hoboken, N.J.: John Wiley & Sons, 2009.
Standring, Susan, et al., eds. *Gray's Anatomy*. 40th ed. New York: Churchill Livingstone/Elsevier, 2008.
Waxman, Bruce. *Electrotherapy for Treatment of Facial Nerve Paralysis (Bell's Palsy)*. Rockville, Md.: Department of Health and Human Services, 1984.
Wood, Debra, and Rimas Lukas. "Bell's Palsy." *Health Library*, Oct. 11, 2012.

Benign prostatic hyperplasia. *See* Prostate enlargement.

Beriberi
Disease/Disorder

Also known as: Thiamine deficiency, vitamin B_1 deficiency

Anatomy or system affected: Gastrointestinal system, heart, muscles, nervous system

Specialties and related fields: Family medicine, pediatrics

Definition: A nutritional disease resulting from thiamine deficiency.

Causes and Symptoms

Thiamine, one of the B vitamins, plays an important role in energy metabolism and tissue building. When there is not enough thiamine in the diet, these basic energy functions are disturbed, leading to problems throughout the body. There are two major manifestations of thiamine deficiency, cardiovascular disease (wet beriberi) and nervous system disease (dry beriberi). Each can be caused by chronic alcoholism, malnutrition, diuresis, dialysis, and high carbohydrate intake.

The accompanying symptoms of thiamine deficiency may include weakness, irritability, nausea, vomiting, tingling, or loss of sensation in the hands and feet (peripheral neuropathy). Progressed symptoms include mental confusion and difficulties speaking or walking; these are often the precursor symptoms leading to coma and/or death.

Treatment and Therapy

Thiamine hydrochloride is the initial treatment of choice for beriberi. Successful treatment reverses the deficiency and alleviates most of the symptoms. Severe deficiencies may be treated with high doses of thiamine given by muscular injection.

Alternative treatments stress a diet rich in foods that provide thiamine and other B vitamins, such as brown rice, whole grains, raw fruits and vegetables, legumes, nuts and seeds, and yogurt. Additional supplements of B vitamins, a multivitamin and mineral complex, and vitamin C are also recommended. A balanced diet containing all essential nutrients will prevent thiamine deficiency and the development of beriberi. People who consume large quantities of soda, pretzels, chips, candy, and high-carbohydrate foods made with unenriched flours may also need vitamin supplements to avoid thiamine deficiency.

Perspective and Prospects

The first clinical descriptions of beriberi were conducted by the Dutch physician Nicolaes Tulp around 1652. Tulp treated a young Dutchman who, upon returning from the East Indies, suffered from what the natives of the Indies called beriberi, or "the lameness." Not until the early twentieth century did scientists discover that rice bran, the outer covering of white rice, actually contains something that prevents the disease, thiamine. In the 1920s, extracts of rice polishings were used to treat the disease.

Beriberi is fatal if left untreated. Most symptoms can be reversed, and full recovery is possible when thiamine levels are returned to normal and maintained with a balanced diet and vitamin supplements as needed.

—*Jason A. Hubbart, M.S.*

See also: Alcoholism; Malnutrition; Nutrition; Vitamins and minerals.

For Further Information:
Anderson, Jean, and Barbara Deskins. *The Nutrition Bible*. New York: William Morrow, 1997.
Kliegman, Robert, and Waldo E. Nelson, eds. *Nelson Textbook of Pediatrics*. 19th ed. Philadelphia: Saunders/Elsevier, 2011.
Johnson, Larry E. "Thiamin." *Merck Manual Home Health Handbook*, Feb. 2013.
Rivlin, Richard. "Vitamin Deficiency." In *Conn's Current Therapy*, edited by Robert E. Rakel and Edward T. Bope. Philadelphia: Saunders/Elsevier, 2007.
"Thiamin (Vitamin B1)." *MedlinePlus*, Sept. 19, 2012.
Vorvick, Linda J., and David Zieve. "Beriberi." *MedlinePlus*, Aug. 10, 2012.
Williams, Sue Rodwell, and Eleanor D. Schlenker. *Essentials of Nutrition and Diet Therapy*. 9th ed. St. Louis, Mo.: Mosby/Elsevier, 2007.

Information on Beriberi

Causes: Thiamine deficiency from chronic alcoholism, malnutrition, diuresis, dialysis, high carbohydrate intake

Symptoms: Weakness, irritability, nausea, vomiting, tingling, loss of sensation in hands and feet, confusion, difficulty speaking or walking; may progress to coma and death

Duration: Chronic, sometimes fatal

Treatments: Thiamine hydrochloride, dietary changes

Bile
Biology
Also known as: Gall

Anatomy or system affected: Blood vessels, gallbladder, immune system, liver, muscles

Specialties and related fields: Dermatology, gastroenterology, internal medicine, nutrition, surgery

Definition: Bile has an important role in digestion, but it is not an enzyme; that is, on its own it does not break down molecules. Bile is an emulsifier, increasing the surface area of fat globules to provide a greater area on which lipase, an enzyme that digests fat, can act. Bile, by acting as an emulsifier, also has a role in the absorption of fat-soluble vitamins such as vitamins A, D, E, and K.

Structure and Function

Bile is a yellow or green fluid that is secreted by hepatocytes or liver cells. Bile is composed of several materials, including water, cholesterol, pigments (bilirubin, produced by the breakdown of red blood cells), acid, lecithin, and bicarbonate. Bile is produced in the liver, but it is stored in the gallbladder, a small saclike organ that is tucked into the liver. The human liver is able to produce almost 1 liter of bile a day.

The bile produced by the hepatocytes moves along canaliculi, small passageways in the liver. The canaliculi join at the common hepatic duct, which then meets with the cystic duct of the gallbladder and forms the common bile duct; bile then empties into the gallbladder. The gallbladder concentrates the bile by removing some of the water. After a meal is eaten, the gallbladder discharges bile by way of the pancreatic duct into the small intestine (specifically, the duodenum) to assist in the digestion of lipids (fats). Like many structures in the digestive system, a sphincter, in this case called the sphincter of Oddi, controls the passage of materials. Before meals, the sphincter is closed so that bile flows from the liver to the gallbladder for storage. When food is sensed in the small intestine, the sphincter opens and releases bile.

Disorders and Diseases

The most common problem associated with bile is the formation of gallstones, which occur when the cholesterol in the bile forms lumps or stones. Gallstones can block bile ducts, which can lead to liver failure. The risk factors for the formation of gallstones include genetics, obesity, aging, pregnancy, diabetes, liver disease, and rapid weight loss as a result of "crash dieting" or gastric bypass surgery. Gallstones take many years to form, so it is often difficult to pinpoint their exact cause. They range in size from sand-like crystals to large pebbles.

—*M. A. Foote, Ph.D.*

See also: Acid reflux disease; Enzymes; Food biochemistry; Gallbladder; Gallbladder diseases; Gastroenterology; Gastrointestinal disorders; Gastrointestinal system; Heartburn; Indigestion; Liver; Stone removal; Stones; Vitamins and minerals.

For Further Information:

Choi, Young, and William B. Silverman. "Biliary Tract Disorders, Gallbladder Disorders, and Gallstone Pancreatitis." *American College of Gastroenterology*, July 2013.

Chwistek, Marcin. "Conditions InDepth: Gallstones." *Health Library*, October 11, 2012.

Feldman, Mark, Lawrence S. Friedman, and Lawrence J. Brandt, eds. *Sleisenger and Fordtran's Gastrointestinal and Liver Disease: Pathophysiology, Diagnosis, Management*. 9th ed. Philadelphia: Saunders/Elsevier, 2010.

Johnson, Leonard R., ed. *Gastrointestinal Physiology*. 7th ed. Philadelphia: Mosby/Elsevier, 2007.

Scanlon, Valerie, and Tina Sanders. *Essentials of Anatomy and Physiology*. 6th ed. Philadelphia: F. A. Davis, 2011.

Bilirubin

Biology

Anatomy or system affected: digestive system, circulatory system, liver

Specialties and related fields: gastroenterology, hepatology

Definition: a metabolic product of heme metabolism

Key terms:

bile: a compound secreted by the liver that aids in digestion

heme: an iron containing compound that carries oxygen in myoglobin, hemoglobin and other biological molecules

jaundice: the condition of yellowing of the skin, sclera of the eye and other tissues caused by the accumulation of bilirubin

urobilin: the yellow pigment derived from bilirubin and found in urine

stercobilin: a brown pigment derived from bilirubin and found in feces

Structure and Functions

Old or damaged red blood cells collect in the liver which digests them releasing hemoglobin. Liver enzymes metabolize the heme molecules into bilirubin, a yellow-brown compound. The liver adds glucuronic acid, a sugar, to some of the bilirubin making it soluble in water. Conjugated bilirubin (also known as direct bilirubin) is released by the liver with bile which is stored in the gallbladder. Unconjugated bilirubin is referred to as indirect bilirubin. Bile containing conjugated bilirubin is released into the small intestine from the gallbladder. The salts in the bile are used to emulsify fats to facilitate their digestion. The conjugated bilirubin moves along the digestive system into the colon where bacteria de-conjugate the bilirubin and further metabolize it into urobilinogen which is subsequently oxidized to urobilin and stercobilin. Urobilin, a yellow compound, is absorbed into the blood and is excreted in the urine whereas stercobilin, a brown compound, is eliminated via the feces. Some urobilinogen may normally appear in urine.

Diseases and Disorders

Several physiological conditions including bile duct obstruction, liver malfunction, hemolysis, Gilbert's syndrome (a genetic defect in bilirubin metabolism) and hepatitis among other conditions can lead to the release of bilirubin into the blood resulting in *hyperbilirubinemia*. Sex steroids can also lead to mild *hyperbilirubinemia*. Conjugated bilirubin released in *hyperbilirubinemia* is excreted in the urine making the urine an amber color. With *hyperbilirubinemia*, bilirubin may be deposited in tissues and organs especially in the sclera of the eyes causing a yellow color known as jaundice. Some physiological conditions such as bile duct obstruction release conjugated bilirubin while others such as hemolysis release unconjugated bilirubin. The determination of which type of bilirubin is in the blood can be diagnostic as to the cause. Tests can determine the levels of conjugated and unconjugated bilirubin in the blood and urine. Other blood and liver function tests can aid in the diagnosis of the cause of *hyperbilirubinemia* and other liver disorders.

Newborns sometimes have *hyperbilirubinemia* because the red blood cells are breaking down at a high rate. Too much bilirubin in infants can cause serious problems, including brain damage or *kernicterus*. Usually newborns who experience jaundice within the first few days after birth are not affected, and it disappears quickly.

Persistent hyperbilirubinemia must be treated. A variety of treatments are available including intense phototherapy, blood transfusions, plasmapheresis, hemoperfusion, calcium phosphate and cholestyramine.

—*Josephine Campbell;*
updated by Charles L. Vigue, PhD

For Further Information:

"Bile -Higher Tier." *GCSE Bitesize/BBC*, www.bbc.co.uk/schools/gcsebitesize/science/add_edexcel/common_systems/digestion rev4.shtml. Accessed 3 Oct. 2016.

Case-Lo, Christine. "Bilirubin Blood Test." *Healthline*, 5 July 2016, www.healthline.com/health/bilirubin-blood. Accessed 3 Oct. 2016.

"Facts about Jaundice and Kernicterus." *Centers for Disease Control and Prevention*, 23 Feb. 2015, www.cdc.gov/ncbddd/jaundice/facts.html. Accessed 3 Oct. 2016.

Healthwise Staff. "Bilirubin." *WebMD*, 21 Aug. 2015, www.webmd.com/digestive-disorders/bilirubin-15434#1. Accessed 3 Oct. 2016.

Lightner, David A. *Bilirubin: Jekyll and Hyde Pigment of Life*. Springer, 2013.

"Liver Function Tests." *WebMD*, www.webmd.com/a-to-z-guides/liver-function-test-lft#1. Accessed 3 Oct. 2016

MacGill, Marcus. High Bilirubin Levels: Symptoms and Tests. *Medical News Today*. January 9, 2017. http://www.medicalnewstoday.com/articles/315086.php

Rodak, Bernadette F., George A. Fritsma, and Kathryn Doig, editors. *Hematology: Clinical Principles and Applications*. Saunders Elsevier, 2007.

Weisiger, Richard A. "Conjugated Hyperbilirubinemia." *Medscape*, 5 Jan. 2016, emedicine.medscape.com/article/178757-overview. Accessed 3 Oct. 2016.

Biofeedback

Procedure

Anatomy or system affected: Brain, circulatory system, endocrine system, glands, heart, muscles, musculoskeletal system, nerves, nervous system, psychic-emotional system

Specialties and related fields: Alternative medicine, cardiology, exercise physiology, family medicine, internal medicine, neurology, occupational health, physical therapy, preventive medicine, psychology, sports medicine, vascular medicine

Definition: The learned self-regulation of the autonomic nervous system through monitoring of the physiological activity occurring within an individual.

Key terms:

biodisplay: audio or visual information about the physiological activity within an organism displayed by various instruments and processes

biofeedback: the provision of information about the biological or physiological processes of an individual to him or her, with the objective of empowering the individual to make conscious changes in the processes being monitored; it can be instrumental (using devices that monitor physiological or biological processes) or noninstrumental (using bodily sensations)

biofeedback instrument: a device (usually electronic) that is capable of measuring and displaying information about a physiologic process in a way that allows an individual to monitor the physiologic activity through his or her own senses

electrodermal response (EDR) biofeedback: the monitoring and displaying of information about the conductivity of the skin; used for anxiety reduction, asthma treatment, and the treatment of sleep disorders

electroencephalographic (EEG) biofeedback: the monitoring and displaying of brain wave activity; used for the treatment of substance abuse disorders, epilepsy, attention-deficit disorders, and insomnia

electromyograph (EMG): an instrument that is capable of monitoring and displaying information about electrochemical activity in a group of muscle fibers

neuromuscular rehabilitation: the process of employing electromyographic biofeedback to correct physiological disorders that have both muscular and neurological components, such as the effects of strokes and fibromyalgia; also called myoneural rehabilitation

physiological autoregulation: the process by which an individual utilizes information about a physiological activity to effect changes in that activity in a direction that contributes to normal (or desirable) functioning

Indications and Procedures

Biofeedback has been utilized in both research and clinical applications. The term itself denotes the provision of information (feedback) about a biological process. It has been found that individuals (laboratory animals included), when given feedback that is reinforcing, are able to change physiological processes in a desired direction; homeostatic processes being what they are, these changes are in a positive direction. In the case of humans, the feedback is provided about a physiological function of which the individual would not otherwise be aware were it not for the provision-via a biodisplay-of information about that process.

Human maladies range from the purely structural to the purely functional, with various gradations. An example of a structural disorder is a broken bone, while an example of a functional disorder might be a person who manifests symptoms of blindness for which there is no known or identifiable organic cause. Looking at the spectrum of human maladies, one can consider the continuum as "structural," "psychophysiological," "mental-emotional," "hysterical," and "feigned." The category of psychophysiological lies midway between structural and mental-emotional. A psychophysio-logical disorder has elements of both mind and body interactions; it is a physiological disorder brought about by thoughts, feelings, and emotions. There are those who take the position that all human maladies and disorders have a mental-emotional component to them, that there can be no change in the mental-emotional state without a corresponding change in the physiological state and no change in the physiological state without a corresponding change in the mental-emotional state.

It is currently the preference of many scientifically and technologically oriented practitioners to deal with the more structural disorders (or to treat the disorder as if it were mostly structural). It is also the case that many mental health practitioners prefer to deal with disorders that fall more into the mental-emotional category. A growing number of practitioners, however, have an interest in and training for dealing with psychophysiological disorders. This emerging field is referred to as behavioral medicine, and a large percentage of the practitioners in this field employ biofeedback as a modality.

A classic example of biofeedback being used to correct a physiological problem would be the employing of electromyograph (EMG) biofeedback for the correction of a simple tension (or psychophysiologic) headache. The headache is caused by inappropriately high muscle tension in the neck, head, or shoulders. In surface electromyographic biofeedback, the biofeedback practitioner attaches electronic sensors to the muscles of the forehead, neck, or shoulders of the patient. The electronic sensors pick up signals from electrochemical activity at the surface of the skin in the area of the involved muscle groups. The behavior of the muscles being monitored is such that minute changes in the electrochemical activity in the muscles-tension and relaxation-occur naturally.

The sensitivity of the biofeedback instrument (the magnification of the signal may be as high as one thousand times) and the display of the signal make the individual aware of these changes via sound or visual signals (biodisplays). When the biofeedback signal indicates that the muscle activity is in the direction of relaxation, the individual makes an association between that muscle behavior and the corresponding change in the strength of the signal. The individual can then increase the duration, strength, and frequency of the relaxation process. Having learned to relax the involved muscles, the individual is able to prevent or abort headache activity.

It is axiomatic that any physiological process (behavior) that is capable of being quantified, measured, and displayed is appropriate for biofeedback applications. The following are some of the more commonly used biofeedback instruments.

An electromyograph is an instrument that is capable of monitoring and displaying information about electrochemical activity in a group of muscle fibers. Common applications of surface electromyography (in which sensors are placed on the surface of the skin, as opposed to the insertion of needles into the muscle itself) include stroke rehabilitation. Surface electromyography is also used in the treatment of tension headaches and fibromyalgia.

An galvanic skin or electrodermal response (EDR) biofeedback instrument is capable of monitoring and displaying information about the conductivity of the skin. An increase in the conductivity of the skin is a function of moisture accumulating in the space recently occupied by blood. The rate of blood flow depends on the amount of autonomic nervous system arousal present within the organism at the time of measurement. The higher the level of autonomic nervous system arousal, the greater the amount of skin conductivity. Common applications of EDR biofeedback are the reduction of anxiety caused by phobic reactions, the control of asthma (especially in young children), and the treatment of sleep disorders. For example, many insomniacs are unable to drop off to sleep because of higher-than-appropriate autonomic nervous system activity.

An instrument that is capable of monitoring and displaying the surface temperature of the skin, as correlated with an increase in vascular (blood flow) activity in the area of the skin in question, can also be used for biofeedback. Such an instrument is helpful in treatment for high blood pressure and migraine headaches.

Electroencephalographic (EEG) biofeedback involves the monitoring and displaying of brain wave activity as a correlate of autonomic nervous system activity. Different brain waves are associated with different levels of autonomic nervous system arousal. Common applications of EEG biofeedback are in the treatment of substance abuse disorders, epilepsy, attention-deficit disorders, and insomnia.

Heart rate variability (HRV) biofeedback monitors and displays the changing intervals between heart beats. Studies have indicated that HRV biofeedback may be beneficial in treating cardiovascular, respiratory, and emotional conditions.

Uses and Complications

Biofeedback is gaining in popularity because of a number of factors. One of the principal reasons is a growing interest in alternatives to the lifetime use of medications to manage a disorder.

To understand the rationale for biofeedback in a clinical setting, it is essential to discuss the types of disorders for which it is commonly employed. As pointed out in the National Institute of Mental Health's publication *Biofeedback*, the more common usages of biofeedback treatment techniques include "migraine headaches, tension headaches, and many other types of pain; disorders of the digestive system; high blood pressure and its opposite, low blood pressure; cardiac arrhythmias (abnormalities, sometimes dangerous, in the rhythm of the heartbeat); Raynaud's disease (a circulatory disorder that causes uncomfortably cold hands); epilepsy; paralysis and other movement disorders."

Thus, biofeedback can be safely and effectively employed in the alleviation of numerous disorders. One example worth noting-in terms of the magnitude of the problem-is the treatment of cardiovascular disorders. Myocardial infarctions, commonly known as heart attacks, are one of the major health problems in the industrialized world and an area of special concern to those practitioners with a psychophysiological orientation.

One of the principal causes of heart attacks is hypertension (high blood pressure). Emotions have much to do with the manifestation of high blood pressure (hypertension), which places this condition in the category of a psychophysiological disorder. Researchers have demonstrated that biofeedback is an effective methodology to correct the problem of high blood pressure. The data reveal that many individuals employing biofeedback have been able to decrease (or eliminate entirely) the use of medication to manage their hypertension. Studies also show that these individuals maintain normal blood pressure levels for as long as two years following the completion of biofeedback training.

Because of its noninvasive properties and its broad applicability in the clinical setting, biofeedback is also increasingly becoming one of the more commonly utilized modalities in many fields, such as behavioral medicine. Researchers have provided documented evidence showing that biofeedback is effective in the treatment of so-called stress-related disorders. Research has also shown that biofeedback has beneficial applications in the areas of neuromuscular rehabilitation (working with stroke victims to help them develop greater control and use of afflicted muscle groups) and myoneural rehabilitation (working with victims of fibromyalgia and chronic pain to help them obtain relief from debilitating pain).

Research in the 1960s pointed to the applicability of EEG biofeedback for seizure disorders, such as epilepsy. Advanced technology and later research findings have demonstrated EEG biofeedback to be effective in the treatment of attention-deficit disorder, hyperactivity, and alcoholism as well.

Biofeedback appears to have particular applicability for children. Apparently, there is an innate ability on the part of the young to learn self-regulation skills, such as the lowering of autonomic nervous system activity, much more quickly than older persons. Since this activity is highly correlated with respiratory distress, biofeedback is often used in the treatment of asthma in prepubescent children. Biofeedback is also being successfully used as an alternative to prescription medications (such as Ritalin) for youngsters with attention-deficit disorder.

The use of biofeedback is also found in the field of athletics and human performance. Sports psychologists and athletic coaches have long recognized that there is an inverted U pattern of performance where autonomic nervous system activity and performance are concerned. In the field of sports psychology, this is known as the Yerkes-Dobson law. The tenets of this law state that as the level of autonomic nervous system arousal rises, performance will improve-but only to a point. When autonomic nervous system arousal becomes too high, a corresponding deterioration in performance occurs. At some point prior to an athletic competition, it may be desirable for an athlete to experience an increase (or a decrease) in the level of autonomic nervous

system activity (the production of adrenaline, for example). Should adrenaline levels become too high, however, the athlete may "choke" or become tense.

To achieve physiological autoregulation (often referred to in this athletic context as "self-regulation"), athletes have used biofeedback to assist them with establishing better control of a variety of physiologic processes. Biofeedback applications have ranged from hand-warming techniques for cross-country skiers and mountain climbers to the regulation of heartbeat for sharpshooters, such as biathletes and archers, to the lowering of adrenaline levels for ice-skaters, gymnasts, and divers.

Biofeedback, apart from empirical studies or research on both animal and human subjects, is seldom used in isolation. In most treatment protocols, it is employed in combination with such interventions as behavioral management, lifestyle counseling, exercise, posture awareness, and nutritional considerations. In most biofeedback applications, the individual is also taught a number of procedures that he or she is encouraged to use between therapy sessions. The conscientious and effective practice of these recommended procedures has been proven to be a determining factor in the success rate of biofeedback. The end aim of biofeedback is self-regulation, and self-regulation must extend to situations outside the clinical setting.

Biofeedback (when employed as a part of a behavioral medicine program) is usually offered as a component of a treatment team approach. The biofeedback practitioner commonly interfaces with members of other disciplines to design and implement a treatment protocol to correct the presenting problem (for example, fibromyalgia) for which the referral was made.

One commonly found model of biofeedback is for the patient, the biofeedback practitioner, and the primary medical care provider to constitute a team. The team concept applies even to the extent that the biofeedback practitioner (in many ways acting as a coach) will give the patient a number of procedures to follow between treatment sessions and will then evaluate, with the patient and the medical practitioner, the effectiveness of the procedure. Modifications in the modalities and in the interventions follow from these evaluations. Biofeedback interventions are dynamic and measurable so that the effectiveness of the protocol can be adjusted to meet the needs of the patient.

Perspective and Prospects

Biofeedback, as a treatment modality, is relatively new. The history of biofeedback as a research tool, however, dates back to early attempts to quantify physiological processes. From the time of Ivan Pavlov and his research on the salivary processes in canines, both psychologists and physiologists have long been interested in the measurement of human behavior (including physiological processes).

Early in the twentieth century, the work of Walter B. Cannon, with his book *The Wisdom of the Body* (1932), helped to set the stage for the field of self-regulation. Another landmark was the 1929 publication of Edmund Jacobson's *Progressive Relaxation*. More recently, the work of such pioneers as John V. Basmajian, Neal Miller, Elmer Green, Joseph Kamiya, and many others spawned research and development efforts that by 1975 produced more than twenty-five hundred literature references utilizing biofeedback as a part of a study.

The evolution of biofeedback as a treatment modality has its historical roots in early research in the areas of learning theory, psychophysiology, behavior modification, stress reactivity, electronics technology, and biomedical engineering. The emerging awareness-and acceptance by the general public-that individuals do in fact have the potential to promote their own wellness and to facilitate the healing process gave additional impetus to the development of both the theory and the technology of biofeedback treatment. Several other factors have combined to produce the climate within which biofeedback has gained recognition and acceptance. One of these was widespread recognition that many of the disorders that afflict humankind have, as a common basis, some disruption of the natural feedback processes. Part of this recognition is attributable to the seminal work of Hans Selye on stress reactivity.

Developments in the fields of electronics, physiology, psychology, endocrinology, and learning theory produced a body of knowledge that spawned the evolution and growth of biofeedback. Further refinement and an explosion of technology have resulted in procedures and techniques that have set the stage for the use of biofeedback as an effective intervention with wide applications in the treatment of numerous disorders.

A number of devices have been designed for home biofeedback use. Some are computer-based while others are stand-alone, handheld devices. Consumers interested in such equipment should consult with their biofeedback team regarding the safety and reputability of the products under consideration.

A new version of biofeedback has promising hope for people with brain damage due to injury, paralysis, or stroke. Known as "neuroprosthetics," "nanobiotechnology," or occasionally, "brain interface chips," this technology is in the early stages of research but is enabling people to control machinery with their thoughts.

Some research and clinical trial studies have shown that quadriplegic people can learn to operate a computer, manipulate a robotic arm, or play video games through the use of an implanted electrode. Signals from the chip are sent to an analog-to-digital converter, which processes the simultaneous firings of neurons into digital data. For example, if a person thinks about turning off a computer, the analog information translates this into an actual motion, controlling the cursor on the computer screen. Other research has utilized noninvasive methods of assimilating neuronal activity. In some research studies, quadriplegic persons and persons with no neuromuscular impairment could control a cursor by controlling their EEG patterns. Participants are able to do this by learning to identify, over time, feedback from brain-wave activity.

Both electrode implants and EEG methods have their positives and negatives. EEGs are a bit cumbersome, due to the wires and electronic equipment; however, wireless EEG technology in the future may be possible. Implanted electrodes may provide more precise information, but this approach requires surgery and is expensive and potentially risky.

Neither method directly affects actual movement; that is, it does not read minds but instead enables the mind to act directly on an external object. The futuristic prospect of controlling machinery with thoughts has many psychological, medical, and ethical implications that will need to be uncovered as research progresses.

—Ronald B. France, Ph.D.;
updated by LeAnna DeAngelo, Ph.D.

See also: Alternative medicine; Anxiety; Arrhythmias; Asthma; Attention-deficient disorder; Brain; Cardiac rehabilitation; Cardiology; Electrocardiography (ECG or EKG); Electroencephalography (EEG); Epilepsy; Exercise physiology; Headaches; Heart attack; Hypertension; Hypnosis; Meditation; Nervous system; Neurology; Pain management; Paralysis; Phobias; Physical rehabilitation; Physiology; Preventive medicine; Respiration; Sleep disorders; Sports medicine; Stress; Stress reduction.

For Further Information:
A.D.A.M. Medical Encyclopedia. "Biofeedback." *Medline Plus*, October 30, 2011.

"Biofeedback: Using Your Mind to Improve Your Health." *Mayo Foundation for Medical Education and Research*, January 26, 2013.

Blumstein, Boris, et al., eds. *Brain and Body in Sport and Exercise: Biofeedback Applications in Performance Enhancement*. New York: Wiley, 2002.

Constans, A. "Mind Over Machines." *Scientist* 19, no. 3 (2005): 27.

Olton, David S., and Aaron R. Noonberg. *Biofeedback: Clinical Applications in Behavioral Medicine*. Englewood Cliffs, N.J.: Prentice Hall, 1980.

Phillips, Nelson, et al., eds. *Handbook of Mind-Body Medicine for Primary Care*. Thousand Oaks, Calif.: Sage, 2003.

Robbins, Jim. *A Symphony in the Brain: The Evolution of the New Brain Wave Biofeedback*. Rev. ed. New York: Grove Press, 2008.

Schwartz, Mark S., and Frank Andrasik, eds. *Biofeedback: A Practitioner's Guide*. 3d ed. New York: Guilford Press, 2003.

Underhill, Linda H., and Brian Randall. "Understanding Biofeedback." *Health Library*, December 28, 2011.

Bioinformatics

Specialty

Anatomy or system affected: None

Specialties and related fields: Genetics

Definition: A rapidly growing area of quantitative, mathematical, and computational biology that is coming to resemble physics and chemistry in the detail and rigor of the science.

Key terms:

genomics: the study of genetic material, such as the deoxyribonucleic acid (DNA) sequences of chromosomes

microarray: a technique used to measure the amount of ribonucleic acid (RNA) that each gene makes

molecular evolution: how genomes and regulatory networks change over time

phylogenetics: the building of evolutionary trees, such as to describe accurately the base-by-base changes in a particular protein from different species *proteomics*: studying the results after RNA translation, such as the amounts of protein in different forms

sequence alignment: lining up (with gaps if necessary) the same sites in the same gene from different species or different genes

structural biology: the study of how proteins fold into a three-dimensional shape and how they interact with one another to form larger complexes

systems biology: the study of how systems of molecules, subcellular structures, and cells work together

Introduction

The answer to the question "What is bioinformatics?" is not straightforward, yet in addressing this question the richness and extent of the field become clear. Part of the reason that it is difficult to give a concise definition of bioinformatics is that, as researchers publishing in the field realize, the definition is somewhat artificial and its boundaries are still expanding. This is not surprising, as bioinformatics might also be called mathematical/computational molecular biology, which points to large parts of biology taking on the aspects of a "hard" science such as physics or chemistry.

The creation of bioinformatics was triggered by a combination of factors in the 1990s. Key elements were progress in computing power, the existence of much larger data sets, and increasingly quantitative approaches to molecular biology, including molecular evolutionary studies. The large data sets came from a number of sources, including long individual DNA sequences (for example, genomes), large between-species comparative or evolutionary alignments, microarray-generated gene expression data, proteomics data from two-dimensional gel electrophoresis and mass spectroscopy techniques, and structural information-broadly speaking, the fields of comparative, functional, and structural genomics. It was also increasingly recognized that quantitative molecular biology required vast amounts of computer power not only to assemble genomes but also to complete fundamental analyses, such as aligning related DNA sequences or building a tree from such an alignment. For example, with just twenty sequences there are more different trees relating these sequences than Avogadro's number (approximately 6×10^{23}), and every tree must be checked to ensure that the optimal solution has been found.

The Scope of Research

Bioinformatics itself touches on other areas of science such as biomedical informatics, computer science, statistical analysis, molecular biology, and mathematical modeling. In turn, each of these fields contributes uniquely to the progress of bioinformatics toward a mature science. Equally definitive of bioinformatics is recognizing those areas wholly or partly subsumed by an approach mixing computing power with mathematical and statistical modeling to solve biological questions based on molecular data. These areas include genomics, evolutionary biology, population genetics, structural biology, microarray gene expression analysis, proteomics, and the modeling of cellular processes plus systems biology (for example, modeling a neurological pathway in which individual neurons respond to molecular events).

In bioinformatics, as in chemistry and physics, there is a fundamental split between empirical/experimental and theoretical science. At one extreme may be a laboratory focusing on generating large amounts of microarray data with relatively little analysis, and at the other extreme may be a mathematician working alone to solve a theorem with an application to better analyze that microarray data. It is clear that both approaches are needed for science to develop. However, it is not uncommon to find researchers actively tackling both problems (for example, gathering large data sets and seeking better methods to analyze them). Increasingly, the scale and cost of major bioinformatics projects call for a new model of interdisciplinary biological research in which biologists, statisticians, computer scientists, chemists, mathematicians, physicians, and physicists interact closely together.

The nature of bioinformatics research highlights the need for interdisciplinary skills in modern biology. Some universities issue bioinformatics degrees based on their own formulas. A more direct approach is to require a quadruple major in statistics, computer science, mathematics, and biology. The importance of such a background is that, for example, someone who is not the best mathematician still needs to know how to ask the best mathematicians for help with the problems that inevitably crop up in research in this area. A good example of this interdependence arose in the Celera Genomics effort to complete the human genome, in which mathematicians with a specialty in tiling algorithms were essential to reassembling the millions of sequenced fragments.

In the future, bioinformatics will be increasingly involved with projects, the magnitude of which are technically and intellectually as challenging as anything previously faced in science. For example, a key problem might be a complete computer model of a single cell. Perfection would be achieved only when a biologist could not tell the difference between real and experimental data when the cell experienced a change internally or externally.

Perspective and Prospects

The implications of bioinformatics for medicine are enormous. The strictly informatics side is already central to medical genetics. Databases of human characteristics, including detailed medical histories and biochemical profiles, are matched up with millions of genetic markers within each individual. Only through such enormous databases can statistical sleuths uncover the basis of most diseases that are caused by multiple genes. This is the population genetics of humans on a vast scale. Elsewhere, medical research such as cancer modeling is rapidly becoming a branch of bioinformatics, driven by the fact that cancer is caused by many interacting genes.

The overall prospect is that bioinformatics will make possible a different sort of medicine in the twenty-first century in which fundamental research leads to pharmaceutical intervention, which leads to treating a disease at its root cause in a way that avoids the need for surgical intervention. Treatments of tomorrow, from diagnosis to cure, will involve processing large amounts of data via computers, with doctors remaining the key to ensuring an appropriate treatment regime with the consent and comfort of the patient foremost.

In short, one answer to the question "What is bioinformatics?" is the development of virtual molecular biology. As time passes, this scientific endeavor will propagate upward and outward to meet other major areas of biology, such as physiology and ecology. Eventually, much of biology and medicine may come to rest solidly on the same principles as chemistry and physics, yet require major computational resources because of the complexity of the models needed to approximate reality reliably.

—Peter J. Waddell, Ph.D.

See also: Biophysics; Biostatistics; DNA and RNA; Genomics.

For Further Information:

Campbell, A. Malcolm, and Laurie J. Heyer. *Discovering Genomics, Proteomics, and Bioinformatics*. 2d ed. San Francisco: Pearson/Benjamin Cummings, 2007.

Davidson, Eric H. *The Regulatory Genome: Gene Regulatory Networks in Development and Evolution*. Boston: Academic Press/Elsevier, 2006.

Higgs, Paul G., and Teresa K. Attwood. *Bioinformatics and Molecular Evolution*. Malden: Wiley-Blackwell, 2013.

International Human Genome Sequencing Consortium. "Initial Sequencing and Analysis of the Human Genome." *Nature* 409, no. 6822 (2001): 860-921.

National Institute of Allergy and Infectious Disease. "Bioinformatics." *National Institutes of Health*, May 24, 2013.

Pevsner, Jonathan. *Bioinformatics and Functional Genomics*. 2d ed. Malden: Wiley-Blackwell, 2013.

Biological therapies

Treatment

Also known as: Biological agents, biological response modifiers, biotherapy, immunotherapy

Anatomy or system affected: Blood, cells, immune system, lymphatic system

Specialties and related fields: Alternative medicine, biotechnology, genetics, hematology, immunology, oncology, pathology

Definition: Treatments that use natural substances from the immune system to fight disease or infections or to overcome side effects from other treatments.

Key terms:

cancer: any malignant cellular tumor

cytokine: small proteins released by cells that have specific effects on cell-cell interactions, communication, and behavior of other cells

immunotherapy: therapy using antibodies or other immune system components or using antigens designed to stimulate an immune response to a tumor

Indications and Procedures

Biological therapies are treatments designed to improve or restore the ability of the immune system to fight disease and infection and to help in protecting the body from side effects of other treatments. The immune system includes different types of cells that are used to fight diseases such as cancer, diabetes, rheumatoid arthritis, and Crohn's disease. The immune system consists of organs and structures that include the spleen, lymph nodes, bone marrow, tonsils, and white blood cells. The different types of white blood cells play an especially important role in fighting disease. They include B and T lymphocytes and natural killer (NK) lymphocytes. B cell lymphocytes produce antibodies that attack other cells, and T cell lymphocytes directly attack diseased cells and signal other immune system cells to defend the body. The NK cells make chemicals that bind to and kill foreign invaders in the body.

In addition to B, T, and NK cells, the immune system has white blood cells called monocytes that engulf and digest foreign invaders. Dendritic cells of the immune system are used to transport and deliver foreign cells to other immune system cells. Lymphocytes and monocytes are produced in the bone marrow and are later distributed into the bloodstream to be available to every part of the body. They allow for the protection from cancer and other diseases and invaders to the body. The immune system secretes two types of substances to fight disease: antibodies and cytokines. Antibodies respond to foreign invaders that they recognize, called antigens. An antibody is found to match or recognize a specific antigen and attach itself to the antigen to give an immune response. Cytokines are proteins produced by the immune system to directly attack cells and are considered messenger cells, as they communicate with other cells to form a response. This type of therapy, therefore, is designed in part to boost the immune response, both directly and indirectly, in order to make the immune system respond to diseased or cancer cells.

There are four goals of biological therapy. The first is to make the immune system better able to recognize diseased or cancer cells in order to destroy them, prevent them from spreading, or make them more like healthy cells. The second is to stop the process that converts normal cells to cancer cells. The third is to improve the body's ability to repair or replace damaged cells. The fourth is to stop side effects caused by other forms of cancer treatments, such as chemotherapy and radiation.

Uses and Complications

There are different types of biological therapies whose method of treatment will vary depending on what type of cancer or other disease is involved, how far the disease has spread, and what other treatments are used. The types of biological therapies that are utilized today are predominately for treating cancer patients. These therapies include monoclonal antibodies, cancer vaccines, growth factors, cancer growth inhibitors, anti-angiogenics, interferons and interleukins, and gene therapy.

Monoclonal antibodies are specific antibodies developed in a laboratory that recognize only a single type of antigen or foreign invader in the body. Antigens are typically found on the surface of various cancer cells, and by producing specific antibodies for these antigens, one can selectively attack cancer cells of interest. A monoclonal antibody can also be programmed to act against cell growth factors, thereby interfering with the growth of cancer cells. Monoclonal antibodies can be developed to react with anticancer drugs or other toxins by attaching to the cancer cell and aiding in the destruction of that cell. Monoclonal antibodies can also be established to carry radioisotopes that, when attached to a cancer cell, will identify that cell and can then be used to identify the specific cancer type. Examples of monoclonal antibodies approved by the Food and Drug Administration (FDA) include rituximab (Rituxan) and trastuzumab (Herceptin). Rituxan is used for the treatment of non-Hodgkin's lymphomas, and Herceptin is used to treat breast cancer that involves an overproduction of the HER2 (ERBB2) gene and protein product.

Vaccines are another type of biological therapy that is widely used to prevent diseases, such as influenza, mumps, measles, and other infectious diseases. Vaccines are defined as substances that are used to help protect individuals from infection or disease. Cancer vaccines are currently being developed and are in use for only a few cancer types, such as human papillomavirus (HPV), which may give rise to cervical cancer, and Bacillus Calmette-Guérin (BCG), which is a vaccine typically used for tuberculosis but is being developed for bladder cancer. The advantage of a vaccine is that it has the ability to trigger an immune response in the body. White blood cells in the body can make antibodies that will recognize the proteins in the vaccine, whether the vaccine is from a virus, bacterium, or cancer cell. The antibodies will then be available to fight those antigens and prevent or decrease the impact of disease.

Growth factors are considered biological therapies because they are natural substances in the body that are used to stimulate the bone marrow to produce blood cells. Growth factors are used in conjunction with other types of cancer treatments, since chemotherapy devastates both the normal and the diseased population of blood cells in a cancer patient as its means of killing the cancer cells, thus depleting the blood cells needed for health. After chemotherapy is completed, growth factors can be given to a patient to boost blood counts and help fight infection and further disease. Examples of growth factors are filgrastim (Neupogen) and pegylated G-CSF (Neulsta).

Cancer growth inhibitors or blockers are natural substances that can block a growth factor that will otherwise trigger a cancer cell to divide and grow. Growth factors that reside on the surface of cancer cells include epidermal growth factor (EGF) and fibroblast growth factor (FGF), which control cell growth, and platelet-derived growth factor (PDGF), which controls blood vessel development and cell growth. Each of these growth factors has a specific receptor molecule on the cell surface of the cancer cell, such as epidermal growth factor receptor (EGFR). Most cancer cell inhibitors currently used will block the signaling pathway of receptors, such as tyrosine kinase inhibitors and proteosome inhibitors. Examples of tyrosine kinase inhibitors are iminitab (Gleevac), used to treat chronic myeloid leukemia (CML), and bortezomib (Velcade), used to treat melanoma.

Anti-angiogenics are substances that block cancer blood vessel growth. Angiogenesis is the process of growing new blood vessels. Anti-angiogenic drugs are used to stop tumors from growing their own blood vessels. Since cancer cells need a blood supply to continue their growth and division process, blocking blood vessel growth will eventually kill the cancer cell. Anti-angiogenic drugs can block the growth factor from reaching the cell, block the signaling within a cell, or affect the signal between cells. One example of an anti-angiogenic drug is thalidomide, which affects the chemicals that cells use to signal one another. This drug has proven helpful in treating melanoma and other cancers.

Interferons and interleukins are substances that are part of the body's immune response, called cytokines. These cytokines work by interfering with the growth and cell division of cancer cells, by stimulating an immune response and enhancing the ability of killer T cells and other cells to attack and kill cancer cells, and by encouraging the cancer cell to produce chemicals that attract the immune system to them. Interferons and interleukin-2 are used to treat cancers such as melanoma, multiple myeloma, and some types of leukemia.

Gene therapies are currently experimental, but they have potential in the treatment of cancers and other diseases. Genes are made up of strands of deoxyribonucleic acid (DNA), which are coded messages for various functions in the body. Normal cells have a set of genes that are needed for normal growth, development, and maintenance of the body's systems and functions. Cancer cells differ from normal cells in that a genetic mutation has occurred that gives rise to uncontrolled cell growth and division. The advantage of gene therapy is that it targets specific cancer cells, thereby not affecting normal cells that would otherwise be destroyed by conventional therapies.

Side effects are associated with each type of biological therapy. They vary depending on the individual's medical history, diagnosis, and type of therapy. Each person may react differently to specific treatments. Biological therapies often cause flulike symptoms, such as chills, fever, muscle aches, nausea, vomiting and diarrhea, bone pain, loss of appetite, and fatigue. Other side effects may include rashes, bleeding or bruising easily, and low levels of blood cells. Swelling at the injection site is also common. Side effects may be severe, mild, or absent. If they are severe, then patients may need to stay in the hospital during treatment. Side effects do not often last long, and they usually go away after treatment is completed. Allergic reactions may have additional symptoms.

Certain treatments can be given to control side effects, such as Neupogen or G-CSF to increase white blood cell counts and help prevent infection in patients who use chemotherapy; Procrit, Epogen, or erythropoietin to increase red blood cell counts in patients who develop anemia; and IL-11, interleukin-11, Oprelvekin, or Neumega to increase platelet counts. Paracetamol or antihistamine may be given before the first treatment to prevent an allergic reaction.

Perspective and Prospects

Biological therapies have been investigated for many years as an important advance in the treatment of cancer and other diseases. It could be said that biological therapies have been in use for more than two hundred years with the discovery of immunization by Edward Jenner to treat a disease called vaccinia, or cowpox. Around the beginning of the twentieth century, William B. Coley began treating cancer patients with bacteria to build an immune response. This approach, which became known as Coley toxins, was used for decades with great success. In 1908, Paul Ehrlich received the Nobel Prize in Physiology or Medicine for his work on biotherapies by discovering receptor molecules (antigens) that reside on cell surfaces that can attach to antibodies, triggering the release of antitoxins to fight disease. Work on biological therapies continued in the 1980s when interferon came to be used for the treatment of a blood disorder called hairy-cell leukemia. This treatment became FDA approved for this and other cancer disorders such as chronic myeloid leukemia, AIDS-related Kaposi's sarcoma, and genital warts. Further work on cytokines gave rise to interleukin treatment for kidney cancer, metastatic cancer, and AIDS.

Further developments have led to many treatments for cancer, viral diseases, and autoimmune disorders. With current technologies in genetics, more information about the genetic basis of cancer has led to advances in biological therapies for more than two hundred types of cancer. Most therapies to date are not targeted to a specific genetic makeup. However, new therapies are arising that can target specific genetic mutations that have become known. For example, Herceptin can treat HER2-positive metastatic breast cancer and MabThera can be used for particular genetic mutations in non-Hodgkin's lymphoma. This individualized type of therapy will not only improve the management of different diseases but also decrease the toxicity of treatment that results from an individual's genetic makeup. Most of what is used today for biological therapies is just the beginning, with the future holding tremendous promise for continued success with these treatments.

—*Susan M. Zneimer, Ph.D.*

See also: Antibodies; Autoimmune disorders; Bacillus Calmette-Guérin (BCG); Bionics and biotechnology; Breast cancer; Cancer; Cells; Chemotherapy; Clinical trials; DNA and RNA; Gene therapy; Genetics and inheritance; Genomics; Human papillomavirus (HPV); Immune system; Immunization and vaccination; Immunology; Leukemia; Lymphadenopathy and lymphoma; Malignancy and metastasis; Oncology; Pharmacology; Radiation therapy; Tumors.

For Further Information:

Black Jacquelyn G., and Laura J. Black. *Microbiology*. Hoboken, N.J.: Wiley, 2013.

Danquah, Michael K., and Mahato, Ram I., eds. *Emerging Trends in Cell and Gene Therapy*. New York: Humana Press, 2013.

De Vita, Vincent T., Jr., Samuel Hellman, and Steven A. Rosenberg, eds. *Principles and Practice of Oncology*. 9th ed. Philadelphia: Lippincott Williams & Wilkins, 2011.

European Oncology Nursing Society. http://www.cancer nurse.eu/education/biological_therapies.html.

Fischer, David S., et al. *The Cancer Chemotherapy Handbook*. 6th ed. St. Louis: Mosby, 2003.

Hawkins Robert E. *Cellular Therapy of Cancer: Development of Gene Therapy Based Approaches*. New York: World Scientific, 2013.

Lattime, Edmund C., and Stanton L. Gerson. *Gene Therapy of Cancer: Translational Approaches from Preclinical Studies to Clinical Implementation*. Amsterdam: Academic Press, 2013.

Rosenberg, Steven A., ed. *Principles and Practice of the Biologic Therapy of Cancer*. 3d ed. Philadelphia: Lippincott Williams & Wilkins, 2000.

Stern, Peter L., Peter C. L. Beverley, and Miles W. Carroll, eds. *Cancer Vaccines and Immunotherapy*. New York: Cambridge University Press, 2000.

Williams, J. "Principles of Genetics and Cancer." *Seminars in Oncology Nursing* 13, no. 2 (1997): 68-73.

Biomarker

Procedure

Anatomy or system affected: All
Specialties and related fields: Genetics

A *biomarker* is a characteristic of a biological system that can be measured, compared, and evaluated to determine the health of a living being. Biomarkers can also be used to help determine the progress of an illness or the success of a treatment and to predict the course of an illness in an individual or a group of individuals. Sometimes biomarkers are easy to measure and interpret, while other times more advanced means must be used. Health care providers would have a very difficult time diagnosing and treating a patient for any condition without the assistance of biomarkers.

Background

Biomarker is short for *biological marker* and can refer to any of a host of different aspects of a biological organism that can be measured, compared, and evaluated. Some-for example, taking a pulse measurement to determine heart rate-have existed for nearly as long as humans have attempted to tend to the health of others. Common biomarkers that are assessed at almost every visit to a Health care provider include heart rate, blood pressure, body temperature, weight, and height. A Health care provider assessing the overall health of an individual may also order tests of biomarkers that are detectible in bodily fluids such as blood and urine. These include tests for cholesterol, triglycerides, and blood glucose.

Health care providers can use changes in these biomarkers to assess the patient's relative health as well as their health progress over time. For instance, a Health care provider will chart the height and weight of a child at successive visits and match these to a chart that shows the height and weight of many other children of the patient's same age. By comparing the child's growth to the patterns seen in the examinations of many other children, the Health care provider can help to determine if the child's height and weight are appropriate for their age or indicate a possible problem.

Sometimes one of these biomarkers or another procedure will indicate that the patient has a disease. In such cases, the Health care provider can use other biomarkers to determine the status of the illness. For example, if a person's blood pressure reading indicates that the person might have heart disease, the Health care provider can order blood tests and other procedures such as an electrocardiogram. The biomarkers from these tests can help the Health care provider assess the patient's condition and determine what treatment, if any, is needed.

Biomarkers also have uses far beyond routine health care. Scientists have identified markers that can be used to detect or track the status or progression of diseases such as diabetes, heart disease, cancer, multiple sclerosis, Parkinson's disease, Alzheimer's disease, schizophrenia, thyroid disease, and many others. Ways have also been found to test how well a condition is responding to a drug or other therapy.

In some cases, biomarkers can also be used to determine the effects of something in the environment, such as measuring the level of lead or another contaminant in a person's blood to determine if they have been exposed to the substance. A biomarker can also be a substance placed inside the body as an aid to measuring some aspect of its function, such as the use of radioactive iodine to determine how well the thyroid is working. However, the most common usage for the term refers to measuring and evaluating some existing aspect of a biological system to determine its health and/or function.

Overview

Biomarkers that are effective in helping a Health care provider measure health have several characteristics. They are generally easy to measure and do not place either the Health care provider or patient at any significant risk. They perform in a consistent manner regardless of the patient's gender or ethnic background. They show the effects of treatment, improving or worsening depending on medications, diet, etc. Another sign of a good biomarker is that improving it provides a good, cost effective way to better the patient's health. For example, the effects of a lower blood glucose level are so beneficial to the treatment of diabetes that it is worth the cost of treatment to achieve that lower level.

Biomarkers are also objective. This is a key difference between a biomarker and a symptom, although biomarkers can present as symptoms as well. A patient who is having chest pains may take their blood pressure at home. Finding it high, the patient calls the Health care provider and reports that he or she is not feeling well and is experiencing chest pains and high blood pressure. The patient is presenting both as symptoms. However, the chest pains are only a symptom because they cannot be measured in objective terms. People experience pain at different intensities; what some people find bearable is excruciating to others. Pain is therefore a symptom, not a biomarker. A blood pressure reading, on the other hand, meets the requirements of a biomarker because of its consistency (a common baseline number is considered good and deviations from that are generally bad), it is easily measurable, and improvements in blood pressure generally accompany improvements in a patient's health.

These properties of biomarkers also make them useful in developing drugs and other therapies to treat illnesses. For example, for many years, treatments for cancer were aimed at killing the cells in the part of the body where the cancer was located. These treatments would kill indiscriminately, affecting healthy cells as well as those with cancer and often creating additional health concerns for the patient. By identifying certain biomarkers that appear in cancer cells but not in healthy cells, scientists have been able to develop anti-cancer drugs that target the cancer cells but leave the healthy cells alone. Researchers have also identified biomarkers for cancer and other health conditions that allow them to identify these conditions earlier, possibly even before the patient develops symptoms, so preventive treatments can be used. In some cases involving infectious diseases such as influenza, researchers can use these biomarkers to determine how the disease might affect the population and develop immunizations or more effective treatments for the disease.

—*Janine Ungvarsky;*
updated by Nancy Banasiak

For Further Information:

"Biomarkers." *University of Washington Alzheimer's Disease Research Center,* http://www.pathology.washington.edu/research/adrc/research-101/biomarkers/. Accessed 3 Nov. 2017.

"Biomarkers and Human Biomonitoring." *World Health Organization,* Oct. 2011, http://www.who.int/ceh/capacity/biomarkers.pdf. Accessed 3 Nov. 2017.

"Defining Pesticide Biomarkers." *US Environmental Protection Agency,* http://www.epa.gov/pesticide-science-and-assessing-pesticide-risks/defining-pesticide-biomarkers. Accessed 3 Nov. 2017.

Mandal, Anaya. "What Is a Biomarker?" *News in Medical and Life Sciences,* 7 Oct. 2014, http://www.news-medical.net/health/What-is-a-Biomarker.aspx. Accessed 3 Nov. 2017.

"Role of Biomarkers in Medicine." *Coriell Institute for Medical Research,* http://www.coriell.org/research-services/biomarkers/role-of-biomarkers-in-medicine. 3 Nov. 2017.

Strimbu, Kyle and Jorge A. Tavel. "What Are Biomarkers?" *Current Opinions in HIVAIDS,* Nov. 2010, http://www.ncbi.nlm.nih.gov/pmc/articles/PMC3078627/. Accessed 3 Nov. 2017.

"What Exactly Is a Biomarker and Why Is It so Essential?" *The University of Chicago Medicine Celiac Disease Center,* Feb. 2013, http://www.cureceliacdisease.org/faq/what-exactly-is-a-biomarker-and-why-is-it-so-essential/. Accessed 3 Nov. 2017.

Bionics and biotechnology

Procedures

Anatomy or system affected: All

Specialties and related fields: Biotechnology, cytology, genetics, immunology, microbiology

Definition: The integration and application of biological and engineering knowledge to the medical sciences; bionics applies this knowledge to the design of artificial systems that act in the place of natural systems, while biotechnology applies this knowledge at the molecular and genetic levels of these natural systems in order to diagnose, treat, cure, or learn more about diseases.

Key terms:

bioengineering: the combination of biological principles and engineering concepts and/or methodology to improve knowledge in both areas *biological principles*: knowledge concerned with living organisms and their natural systems, particularly at the cellular, molecular, and genetic levels

biological systems: any of several levels of life, from that of the individual organism to the functional level (for example, the circulatory system, respiratory system, or musculoskeletal system), the organ level (such as the heart or liver), the cellular level, and the molecular level; also called natural systems

cybernetics: a field of study, closely associated with bionics, which is concerned with communication and control in living systems and their application to artificial systems

engineering concepts and methodology: an analysis of how systems work (in particular, the step-by-step processes involved) and how these systems can be duplicated

gene: a segment of deoxyribonucleic acid (DNA) that provides information to make a protein

genomic DNA: the complete sequence of an organism's DNA

monoclonal antibodies: antibodies (proteins that protect the body against disease-causing foreign bodies such as bacteria and viruses) produced in large quantities from cloned cells

protein: a biological macromolecule that performs a specified function within a living cell

recombinant DNA technology: manipulation of the genetic material DNA whereby pieces are separated and interchanged in order to obtain a desired result

Indications and Procedures

Bionics and biotechnology are part of the larger arena of bioengineering. This broad interdisciplinary field integrates the many disciplines of biology, physics, and engineering for use in the medical sciences, as well as in other areas such as agriculture, chemical manufacturing, environmental studies, and mining. Because of the interdisciplinary nature of these studies, an often-confusing array of terms may be used, such as biochemical engineering, bioelectronics, biofeedback, biological modeling, biomaterials, biophysics, biomechanics, environmental health engineering, genetic engineering, human engineering, and medical engineering. When applied to the medical sciences, these various areas of knowledge can be integrated under the headings of bionics and biotechnology when considering the diagnosis, investigation, prevention, or treatment of diseases and damaged biological systems.

Within the medical sciences, bionics is concerned with applying physics and engineering concepts and methodology to constructing artificial systems, such as organs or limbs, in order to replace damaged or diseased natural systems. To duplicate biological systems and replace them successfully, knowledge of how these systems function biologically, chemically, and mechanically is required. Creating artificial systems has evolved from the making of crude imitations, such as an artificial kidney machine, to the making of sophisticated replicas of the natural system, with the replacement being made in the living organism. While it is necessary to apply physics and engineering

knowledge to duplicate these natural systems, the fact that these are natural systems requires the application of biological knowledge to the engineering effort. Some animals have the ability to regenerate lost or destroyed limbs; humans, however, must rely on their ingenuity. Biotechnology is an interdisciplinary field that seeks to replace, if not re-create, nature.

Within the medical sciences, biotechnology is concerned with the manipulation and study of biological systems at the molecular and genetic level. In addition to a basic understanding of how these systems function at these levels, biotechnology is used for practical purposes as well, including noninvasive diagnostic methods, cardiovascular measurements, bio-optics, medical imaging, modeling in physiology, and microsurgical techniques. A significant application is the synthesis of biological products, such as antibiotics, biochemicals used in diagnostic tests, drugs, enzymes, vaccines, and vitamins. This field is also concerned with the manipulation of genetic material to improve this synthetic process, as well as the study of genetic diseases and the manipulation of the associated genes to prevent or cure these diseases. These kinds of syntheses and studies involve the use of molecules, cells, or genes as raw materials in biological processes that are duplicated under artificial conditions in order to improve or increase the quantities of needed biological products. The techniques and methodologies used to achieve these results are the basis of the technology. Thus, once again, a thorough knowledge of biology and engineering is needed to understand the natural system and to improve the process by which the natural system works in order to accomplish an imposed artificial result.

Much of this work has been carried out through the use of recombinant DNA technology. Since genes provide the instructions controlling those processes by which biological products are made, it is possible to change the processes, or the rate of the processes, by changing the genes. Through genetic engineering, cell cloning, and other techniques, it is possible to make naturally produced antibiotics, vaccines, vitamins, and other needed biological products rather than duplicating these products with artificial materials using artificial means. Also, the rate at which these products are naturally produced can be increased so that large quantities can be obtained (under natural conditions, these products are produced in extremely small amounts). Another aspect of recombinant DNA technology has to do with diseases that result from biological processes that are improperly controlled by genes at critical points. Genetic engineering is used to replace or correct the genetic structure in order to replace or correct the instructions used to guide the biological process.

There is still much to be learned about biological processes and about the genetic material. It is estimated that there are about 100,000 genes constructed from some 3 billion base pairs. Discovering how these genes interact and the biological processes that each controls is a formidable task. By 2003, the Human Genome Project had successfully mapped the entire human genetic structure from

In the News: Nanobots

Through the technology of nanorobotics, robots the size of the period at the end of this sentence are being developed to capture and transport single cells and bacteria. These minuscule robots, also known as microbots, nanorobots, or nanobots, are fewer than seven hundred millionths of a meter tall and approximately two hundred millionths of a meter wide. Some of these tiny robots are being constructed from layers of polymers and gold. Resembling a human arm, the nanobots have flexible elbow and wrist joints. They are being made in a variety of forms with "hands" containing two to four digits.

Because nanobots are being constructed to work while submerged in liquids, including blood, urine, and cell-culture media, they have many biotechnical applications. Because the joints contain conducting polymers, the nanobots can either absorb ions from the surrounding liquid or lose ions to the liquid. The resulting swelling or shrinking of the robot joints causes them to bend. As they do so, the nanobot arm flexes, causing the wrist to bend and the fingers to open and close.

Future nanobots might be able to repair the human body by picking up cells and moving them around for detailed analysis or assemblage into needed microstructures. By placing nanobots at the end of a catheter, surgeons may be able to probe deeper inside the human body. Other possible applications include using nanobots to create images directly on the human retina and implanting nanobots in the brain to substitute for brain functions in the event of a stroke.

—*Alvin K. Benson, Ph.D.*

which all biological processes are controlled, including the flawed ones that cause diseases. Eventually, studies of other genomes, such as those of bacteria and viruses, will treat or prevent diseases and illnesses caused by them as well. This study of genetic material and the use of the tools of proteomics, whereby proteins produced from this genetic material are identified and their functions are elucidated, along with the ongoing study of genetic diseases and of other diseases at the molecular level, will have an increasingly important impact on the overall diagnosis, prevention, and treatment of diseases.

Biotechnology has contributed much to the medical sciences in a relatively short time. It has provided a better understanding of human physiology and an improved fundamental knowledge of disease itself. Knowledge has been gained about the physiological control networks (in part resulting from related studies in cybernetics), the key regulatory agents and processes, the target molecules needed for therapeutic intervention, and the molecular and genetic causes of disease.

With rapid advances in biotechnology, however, the scientific and medical professions are entering sensitive and controversial areas that have raised legal and regulatory concerns. The alteration of genes, the creation of modified organisms, the development of new drugs, the safety and side effects of new biochemicals, the detection of genetic diseases in the fetus, experimental therapies, the ability to clone, the ability to enhance brain functions, and the na-

tional and international competition to produce pharmaceuticals are some of the concerns facing medical practitioners, the biomedical industry, government, society, and the individual. These concerns will escalate as biotechnological advances delve even deeper into the molecular and genetic basis of life in order to achieve improved health benefits.

Uses and Complications

Most of the applications of bionics have been centered on replacing damaged or diseased natural systems. Bionic implants, either in development or commercially available, include retinal implants, urinary implants, cochlear implants, hippocampus replacements, larynx implants, and advanced hand replacements.

The learning retinal implant system includes an implant that replaces the function of a defective retina in individuals with retinal degeneration, including, for example, those with retinitis pigmentosa and macular degeneration. A normal retina includes cells that are stimulated by light to produce a signal that is transmitted to the brain and converted into a visual perception. When such cells do not function, vision is affected. A relatively system includes a retinal stimulator implanted in the eye, a pocket processor, and glasses that contain a small camera. The processor includes a microcomputer responsible for translating image data into retinal stimulation commands. Initial studies with four patients using a prototype system, which included all the above components except the camera, have been positive in that the patients were able to see light as well as simple patterns.

The urinary implant is an implantable pacemaker for the bladder. It will be marketed for bladder dysfunctions caused by spinal cord injury. The device allows for urine storage and full bladder control without the use of catheters.

The cochlear implant is commercially available and consists of an implant that delivers electrical signals to an electrode array. Unlike hearing aids, which act to amplify sound, the cochlear implant sends sound signals directly to the auditory nerve, thus bypassing the damaged portion of the ear.

A neural interface system is being developed that allows severely motor-impaired individuals to communicate with a computer through their thoughts. The system includes a sensor that attaches to a portion of the brain and a device that analyzes brain signals. The signals are translated and allow an individual to control a computer cursor. In the future, it is hoped that the device will allow an individual to control other devices, including lights, telephones, and television sets.

Yet another brain implant being developed is a hippocampus replacement. The hippocampus is a portion of the brain that is important, among other things, in learning and memory; it is the first portion of the brain damaged in Alzheimer's disease. The silicon hippocampus replacement is considered the first prosthesis to replace a damaged area of the brain. In 2007, it was tested in rats, and tests in humans were projected to take place sometime in the near future.

A further application being developed is the implantable artificial electrolarynx communication system. The system is designed for patients who have had a complete laryngectomy. Approaches will be used to attempt to approximate normal voice and speech production.

The Cyberhand Project is developing a cybernetic prosthesis that is controlled by brain signals. Therefore, the hand will allow amputees to use their thoughts to move it and use it to grasp objects naturally. Additionally, the user will also be able to feel objects with which the device comes in contact.

While there are many applications of biotechnology, some of the more significant ones include the production of pharmaceuticals and biochemicals, the production of monoclonal antibodies, the improved understanding and control of complex diseases such as cancer and acquired immunodeficiency syndrome (AIDS), and the improved understanding of genetic diseases. Many of the biotechnology techniques and methodologies are still experimental, as are the resulting products (for example, antibodies, drugs, enzymes, vaccines, vitamins, cloned cells, and recombinant DNA). Some are considered useful and practical, but are not yet approved for use.

The production of pharmaceuticals and biochemicals has been one of the most practical outgrowths of biotechnology research. It has produced both the knowledge of what needs to be done to correct a certain disease process and the ability to make the needed corrections. Some diseases result from deficiencies in particular proteins, as is the case with diabetes, hemophilia, and dwarfism. Others result from deficiencies in enzymes that would normally break down other chemicals, thus resulting in an accumulation of these chemicals, such as in Fabry's, Gaucher's, and Tay-Sachs disease. Still others result from a lack of cellular control, such as cancers.

It has been possible to produce proteins (insulin for diabetes, factor VIII for hemophilia, and growth hormone for dwarfism), enzymes, and bioregulatory proteins (interferon for cancer). This is done by learning how these proteins are produced naturally and then engineering the cells or biochemical processes that can produce these proteins in quantity. In addition to these various kinds of proteins, other biochemical products can be made, including antibiotics, vaccines, and vitamins. Scientists may produce natural, unaltered biochemicals; altered biochemicals (for improved results); or synthetic versions of the biochemicals.

Monoclonal antibodies are a significant group of naturally produced, unaltered biochemicals. They are highly specific biochemicals used for the diagnosis of infectious diseases, for monitoring cancer therapy, for determining the blood concentrations of therapeutic drugs and hormones, for use in some pregnancy tests, for suppressing immune responses, and, to some extent, for disease therapy (for example, to kill cancer cells). Examples of monoclonal antibodies that have been approved by the Food and Drug Administration (FDA) include those used to treat transplant rejection, macular degeneration, multiple sclerosis,

inflammatory diseases (including inflammatory bowel disease, rheumatoid arthritis, psoriasis, and allergy-related asthma), and a wide variety of cancers (including non-Hodgkin's lymphoma, breast cancer, acute myelogenous leukemia, chronic lymphocytic leukemia, colorectal cancer, head and neck cancers, and non-small-cell lung cancer). While much of this work is still experimental, there is a great potential for the development of highly specific vaccines and for reagents used in diagnostic tests. In addition to being highly specific, these vaccines and reagents would be free of any biological contamination and tend to be reliably stable at room temperature. The vaccines would also be safer since their production would not require the handling of large quantities of the pathogenic agent (which is how vaccines have traditionally been obtained). Possible uses could involve immunological protection against hepatitis B, herpes simplex, polio myelitis, rabies, and malaria.

Molecular pharmacologists also develop biochemicals from nonhuman sources. In fact, the diversity of animal and plant life in the world is a natural pharmacy of potentially useful biochemicals. Many medicinal plants are already known, and systematic studies of other species are under way. Animals also contribute useful biochemicals. For example, excretions from the skin of tropical frogs have been used to treat skin diseases, diabetic ulcers, eye infections, and cancers. Through the study of fifty species of poison arrow frogs, scientists have discovered more than three hundred chemicals. Biotechnology has made it possible to study natural biochemicals in small amounts and at the molecular level and has provided the necessary techniques and methodologies for using these biochemicals in the study of diseases.

Cancers form a complex group of diseases that continue to defy the best attempts to understand them. A cancer is composed of cells that have proliferated uncontrollably. This response may be caused by a mutated gene, by carcinogenic agents (for example, chemicals or ultraviolet light), or by viruses. Cancers develop in multiple stages that involve different physiological mechanisms. Understanding these mechanisms and the genes and biochemicals that are involved has been possible in large part because of the techniques and methodologies of biotechnology research. Gene therapy is showing great promise for curing some types of cancer.

The same can be said of the efforts to study AIDS. This syndrome is caused by a virus that infects and kills certain kinds of T lymphocytes that are needed to initiate and maintain normal immune system responses; therefore, AIDS is characterized by the occurrence of unusual infections or by Kaposi's sarcoma (a rare cancer). The nucleotide sequence of the viral genome has been determined through recombinant DNA technology, and the functions of the genes are being characterized. Diagnostic tests to determine if blood is contaminated by the virus have been developed, and efforts are under way to develop a vaccine. The proteins used in these immunological investigations are made in large quantities by genetically engineered microorganisms. Other vaccine studies are concerned with using recombinant DNA technology to disable the AIDS virus genetically (by removing or altering its genes) so that it will infect and generate protective immunity without actually causing the disease.

Genetic diseases are also beginning to be understood as a result of biotechnology. Many of these diseases are caused by gene mutations that cause the absence of a protein or the production of a defective protein, affecting biochemical processes. Recombinant DNA technology is providing methods of detecting these defects, as well as providing therapies for correcting or replacing them. Many of these defects can even be diagnosed in the fetus and in previously undetectable carriers. Some of the commonly known genetic diseases include Alzheimer's disease, cystic fibrosis, hemophilia, Huntington's disease, muscular dystrophy, sickle cell disease, and thalassemia. There are approximately three thousand genetic diseases resulting from single-gene mutations. In addition to studying these numerous mutations, efforts are being made to study diseases associated with specific normal genes (such as the susceptibility for heart attacks by individuals with genes producing specific cholesterol-carrying proteins) and to cure genetic disorders by replacing the mutated gene with a normal gene. This normal DNA acts as a template for production of a certain type of ribonucleic acid (RNA), messenger RNA (mRNA), which acts as a template for production of the normal protein.

One advantage of learning more about common genetic diseases is that more can be learned about normal genomes by comparing them with mutated genomes. These diseases are few in number, however, and much remains to be done. With a map of the human genome (as well as the genome of other animals, plants, bacteria, and viruses), biotechnology, and its usefulness to the medical sciences, will advance significantly. The Human Genome Project has essentially produced a map of the entire human genetic structure, including every gene in the twenty-three chromosome pairs. This accounts for about 100,000 genes with about 3 billion base pairs. In addition, there are about 3 million differences per genome from one individual to another. These differences are responsible for such things as personality differences and inherited diseases. To find and understand some of the rarest disease-causing genes, it is estimated that the differences between the genomes of some 4 billion individuals will need to be studied. This resulting database would strain even state-of-the-art computers, not to mention the researchers who will compile the database.

Study of the differences between the genomes of individuals, and in particular the differences in genes involved in drug metabolism, will be a starting place to provide researchers with a way to overcome adverse reactions to drugs from selected portions of the population by applying the tools of pharmacogenomics, the study of how a person's genetic makeup (genotype) affects the response to drug treatment. After correlating the differences in the genes with a specific negative response, researchers will then need to determine the genotype of a specific individual and use that information to determine the treatment regime that will be most effective for that individual. Alternatively, such information will allow drugs to be developed that are customized for the population to which the individual belongs.

Although many therapeutic strategies involve replacing a mutated gene with a normal gene, other strategies that are currently being developed use short pieces of DNA, called oligonucleotides, to correct the underlying mutation in the DNA of an individual. For example, single-stranded oligonucleo- tides that include the correct sequence of nucleotides (the basic components of DNA) are introduced into a living cell and, through a process known as homologous recombination, are exchanged with the defective portion of the genomic DNA. Other methods include use of RNA of the proper sequence to substitute for defective RNA formed from defective DNA. Although these methods ensure a properly functioning protein will be produced, in some cases it is advantageous to stop production of selected proteins in various disease states, such as in various viral infections, cardiovascular disease, or cancer.

RNA may be used to prevent production of specified proteins. For example, using antisense technology, single-stranded RNA or DNA (called the antisense strand) is administered to an individual and binds to a portion of the mRNA that will produce a specified protein. Once bound, it will physically block production of the protein, and the double-stranded molecule formed will then be degraded. Other methods to prevent protein synthesis utilizing RNA include RNA interference. In this method, double-stranded RNA is administered to an individual and it ultimately causes the target mRNA to be degraded, thereby preventing protein production, by a different mechanism than found in antisense technology. Vitravene (fomivirsen) is the first, and presently the only, antisense drug that the FDA has allowed to be marketed. It is used to treat a particular viral infection, cytomegalovirus retinitis, in individuals with AIDS. Many other antisense drugs are currently in various stages of development to treat a variety of other viral infections, cardiovascular diseases, or cancers, including cancer of the colon, skin, lung, and prostate.

Perspective and Prospects

Artificial limbs have been in use for centuries, but no attempt was made to duplicate natural limbs except in the crudest sense. The use of microorganisms for the production of fermented beverages (such as beer, wine, and vinegar) and food (such as bread) goes back many centuries. Likewise, folk medicine made use of natural biochemicals to treat diseases for many centuries. These traditional processes, however, did not involve an understanding of what was occurring and may only be considered biotechnology by default. The knowledge needed for biotechnology required the development of several scientific disciplines, all of which only occurred after the 1950s, when scientifically understood and controlled processes were developed to produce biological products. It was not until the 1970s that recombinant DNA technology allowed significant advances in the understanding of many molecular and genetic processes.

The advancement of bionics and biotechnology after the 1950s was the result of advances made in related scientific fields during earlier decades, primarily after 1900. These developments included the discovery that enzymes were proteins and the theory of enzyme action; the discovery of the structure and function of vitamins; the discovery of the composition of nucleic acids; the discovery of the structure of carbohydrates; the development of a better understanding of the cellular infrastructure; work on natural and experimentally induced mutation; the study of hereditary metabolic errors; a better understanding of immunology, viral and bacterial diseases, tumors, and cell pathology; the realization that genes were found in the chromosomes; early studies concerning chromosome recombinations and the mechanisms of genetic expression; the ultraviolet analysis of DNA and RNA; the increased use of electron microscopy; the development of the technology involved in the large-scale production of penicillin; and the further development and integration of studies in genetics, biochemistry, and physiology.

The 1950s and 1960s saw important advances in the discovery of the structure of DNA, the breaking of the genetic code, the discovery of how gene actions were regulated, the structure of the gene and of numerous proteins, the discovery and study of numerous hereditary diseases, the development of medical procedures for organ transplants, the evolution of the branch of science known as molecular biology, and the continuing synthesis of discoveries and theories from a variety of scientific disciplines. The 1970s saw the development of technologies that further developed these areas of study, in particular recombinant DNA technology and monoclonal antibody technology. The future will see an increased refinement of these technologies and further developments resulting from the success of the Human Genome Project.

—*Vernon N. Kisling, Jr., Ph.D.;*
updated by Jason J. Schwartz, Ph.D., J.D.

See also: Amputation; Biofeedback; Biophysics; Cloning; Computed tomography (CT) scanning; Dialysis; DNA and RNA; Electrocardiography (ECG or EKG); Electroencephalography (EEG); Gene therapy; Genetic engineering; Genetics and inheritance; Heart transplantation; Heart valve replacement; Magnetic resonance imaging (MRI); Mutation; Pacemaker implantation; Pharmacology; Physical rehabilitation; Plastic surgery; Positron emission tomography (PET) scanning; Prostheses.

For Further Information:

Albertini, Alberto, Claude Lenfant, and Rodolfo Paoletti, eds. *Biotechnology in Clinical Medicine*. New York: Raven Press, 1987.
Borem, Aluizo, et al. *Understanding Biotechnology*. Upper Saddle River, N.J.: Prentice Hall, 2003.
Glick, Bernard R., Jack J. Pasternak, and Cheryl L. Patten. *Molecular Biotechnology: Principles and Applications of Recombinant DNA*. 4th ed. Washington, D.C.: ASM Press, 2010.
Hodge, Russ. *The Future of Genetics: Beyond the Human Genome Project*. New York: Facts On File, 2010.
McElheny , Victor K. *Drawing the Map of Life: Inside the Human Genome Project*. New York: Basic Books, 2010.
Murray, Thomas H., and Maxwell J. Mehlman, eds. *Encyclopedia of Ethical, Legal, and Policy Issues in Biotechnology*. New York: John Wiley & Sons, 2000.
Vasil, Indra K. *Biotechnology: Science, Education, and Commercialization*. New York: Elsevier, 1990.
Walker, Sharon. *Biotechnology Demystified*. New York: McGraw-Hill, 2007.

Biopsy

Procedure

Anatomy or system affected: Cells

Specialties and related fields: Cytology, dermatology, general surgery, gynecology, histology, oncology, pathology, radiology

Definition: The removal and examination of tissue and cells from the body, which is performed to establish a precise diagnosis and to determine proper treatment and prognosis.

Key terms:

cytology: the study of cells, their morphologic changes, and pathology

endoscopy: the visual inspection of body cavities and hollow structures and organs through the use of a tubelike instrument that can be introduced through any body orifice (for example, the mouth or anus) or through small cuts into the skin leading to a cavity

excisional biopsy: biopsy by incision to excise and completely remove an entire lesion, including adjacent portions of normal tissue

frozen section: an extremely thin tissue section cut by a specially designed instrument called a microtome from tissue that has been rapidly frozen, for the purpose of microscopic evaluation and rendering a diagnosis

incisional biopsy: biopsy of a selected sample of lesion

needle biopsy: the obtaining of tissue fragments by the puncture of a tumor, through a larger caliber needle, syringe, and plunger; the tissue within the lumen of the needle is obtained through the rotation and withdrawal of the needle

oncology: the branch of medicine concerned with the study and treatment of cancer

pathology: the branch of medicine that treats the essential nature of disease, especially of the structural and functional changes in cells, tissues, and organs of the body that cause or are caused by disease

staining: the artificial coloring of tissue sections and cells to facilitate their microscopic study

surgical pathology: the branch of pathology that deals with the interpretation of biopsies

Indications and Procedures

Biopsy is one of the most common diagnostic tools in medicine. Illness or disease can be caused by biological agents (such as viruses, bacteria, fungi, and parasites), by physical agents (such as radiation, heat, extreme cold, and trauma), by genetic and metabolic abnormalities (such as diabetes), or by cancer, which is a new, abnormal growth commonly called a tumor. Often, however, the cause of an illness or disease may not be known. Nevertheless, the structural changes caused by the disease are characteristic enough so that the study of these alterations can give a clear picture of the nature and course of the disease. Diseases may primarily affect one organ at a time, such as hepatitis (the inflammation of the liver), or may involve many organ systems at once, as in acquired immunodeficiency syndrome (AIDS).

The signs and symptoms of disease are not specific and are often shared by many conditions. For example, all diseases of the liver can result in jaundice, or yellowing of the skin, and abnormal blood tests. The clinician, who may be an expert in liver disease, may not be able to tell for certain whether the underlying liver condition is caused by a virus, by a toxic substance such as alcohol, or by both. A needle biopsy of the liver may then be obtained. The sample is examined by an expert surgical pathologist, and a specific diagnosis is rendered.

Similarly, a lump in the breast may be innocuous (benign) or cancerous (malignant). Only a biopsy of such a lesion can determine this conclusively. Such a biopsy can be obtained by fine needle aspiration, which is a simple procedure that can be performed in a clinic, or by excision in the operating room. A frozen section is then made for the purpose of rapid diagnosis and management.

Once a biopsy is obtained, it is placed in a special fixative, such as formalin. This solution will preserve-or fix-the internal structure of the tissue and its cells. Expert technicians in histology, called histotechnologists, will then embed the tissue in waxlike paraffin to obtain a "block." The tissue block is then placed in a microtome, and extremely thin pieces (about 5 micrometers thick in width) are cut from it. The slices are placed on glass slides and stained with different dyes, the most common of which is hematoxylin and eosin (H & E), to delineate the cellular substructures. The slides are examined by a surgical pathologist, who renders a pathology report in which the gross and microscopic features are described, and a diagnosis is made. A differential diagnosis may also be made, in which other possible causes of disease that may give a similar histologic picture are discussed. In addition to the routine study described above, a much more extensive and expensive workup of the biopsy may be done, depending on the anticipated complexity of the condition and organ.

The study of a biopsy requires diligent preparation and staining of the tissue, which is the realm of histotechnologists. Staining refers to the application of artificial dyes to tissue sections and cells to facilitate their microscopic study. Certain tissues and cell parts have different chemical and biological affinities for dyes which, when properly applied, help demarcate and differentiate the properties of these cells. A huge battery of special stains exists that can be used to examine every aspect of cell function in both health and disease. For example, specific enzymes can be evaluated; this technique is called enzyme histochemistry.

Immunologic stains, which help evaluate the status of immune system cells, are expensive and extremely tedious, and their proper interpretation requires considerable expertise. Many antibodies are commercially available for such testing. When directed against specific antigenic cell markers, they form immune complexes that can be targeted with

A biopsy is performed when diagnosis requires a sample of cells, tissue, or fluid for further analysis in the laboratory. The gathering of such a sample can be done with a scalpel (shown here), needle, curette, or syringe. (PhotoDisc)

immunological stains. Such stains can then be evaluated by immunofluorescence or immunoperoxidase techniques. Both types employ as their principle of action the forming of complexes between antigens and antibodies and the staining of these complexes. Immunofluorescence staining techniques involve the use of special stains that cause the tissue to shine when it is viewed under a fluorescent microscope; such procedures are performed on frozen section tissues. With immunoperoxidase stains, fixed tissues are used, and the stains are permanent.

Tissue samples can also be studied with an electron microscope, in which electron beams greatly magnify subcellular structures. In this way, the alterations of specific cellular components such as cell membranes, mitochondria, and intracellular viruses can be visualized and analyzed. This ultrastructural study is especially valuable in needle biopsies of the kidneys, as well as in the study of certain unusual cancer cells.

Another highly sophisticated method used to evaluate tissue and cell function in a biopsy is the application of molecular genetics and molecular biopsy techniques. The polymerase chain reaction (PCR) involves the splitting (splicing) of a specific section of genetic material in a cell and its amplification through a chemical chain reaction into innumerable folds, so that it can be visualized through a light microscope. This type of evaluation allows for the examination of specific microorganisms in a cell and can determine the presence of certain genetic markers of unusual diseases or cancer.

Another way to study the properties of cells is by examining their genetic makeup. Karyotyping is a technique in which the actual chromosomes in a cell are photographed during mitotic divisions; the chromosomes appear as patterns of bands. Genetic abnormalities can be identified by the number of chromosomes and their appearance. This procedure is often used in the study of cancer cells. An even more sophisticated study of cellular genetic makeup is called gene rearrangement, in which the order of gene stacking is examined for specific markers of certain cancerous growths, especially of white blood cells. Other techniques that are used to evaluate cell functions and morphology are cellular imaging, in which the contours of cell membranes and surfaces are compared using computers, and the use of flow cytometers, in which cells are targeted immunologically and then counted. Both techniques are employed in cancer studies, and the second is also used for patients with abnormal immune systems, such as those with AIDS.

The aforementioned studies are expensive and available only at large medical centers and research institutes. The diagnostic workup in most hospitals, however, does not require the use of these sophisticated methods. Usually, routine H & E stains are applied. The Papanicolaou stain is commonly used with fine needle aspiration biopsies.

A department of pathology in a large medical center usually has one or more surgical pathologists, who are closely affiliated with the clinical and surgical departments and with their many branches and specialties. Interpreting biopsies obtained by any of the surgical or medical specialties is the most important duty of the surgical pathologist, and it requires great expertise and diligence. Because of the complexity of this task, specialized experts in pathology are becoming the norm. For example, a dermatopathologist is a surgical pathologist trained to interpret skin biopsies. Similarly, hematopathologists, neuropathologists, and nephropathologists are experts in the interpretation of blood-related, nerve- and brain-related, and kidney-related biopsies, respectively.

In incisional biopsies, only a portion of the lesion is sampled, and the procedure is strictly of a diagnostic nature. In excisional biopsy, the entire lesion is removed, usually with a rim of normal tissue, and therefore the procedure serves both a diagnostic and a therapeutic function. The decision whether to perform an incisional or an excisional biopsy depends primarily on the size and location of the lesion; the smaller the lesion, the more logical it is to remove it completely. It is preferable, however, to sample a deeply seated large tumor first because the type and extent of the excision varies considerably depending on the tumor type. For example, a small skin mole is usually excised completely, whereas a large soft tissue or bone tumor should be sampled.

Biopsies are also classified according to the instrument used to obtain them: cold knife versus cautery, needle, or endoscope. Of these the one usually least suitable for microscopic study is that obtained with a cautery, which uses a hot knife that burns, chars, and distorts tissue.

An endoscope is a tubelike fiber-optic instrument that is inserted into an orifice or small incision in order to view the contents of a body cavity. The instrument can be rigid or flexible and is equipped with a light source (usually a laser) and a small cutting tool at its tip to allow for the removal of small samples of tissue. Endoscopic biopsies are frequently used to obtain tissue and cell samples from the lungs and the airways, mainly to diagnose laryngeal and lung cancers; this procedure is usually done by a lung specialist. The endoscope is also used to sample lesions in the esophagus, stomach, intestines, and the rest of the intestinal tract,

including the rectum. Such procedures are usually performed by a gastroenterologist, a specialist in the stomach and the gastrointestinal tract. Endoscopic biopsies of the urinary bladder and the prostate are done by urologists.

Needle biopsies are commonly used to obtain samples from superficial or deep-seated lumps. A slender, cylindrical core of tissue, corresponding to the open diameter of the needle, is obtained. The needle biopsy is commonly used to obtain tissue samples from kidneys, bone, and the deep viscera such as the liver. The modified technique of aspiration cytology, commonly called fine needle aspiration, employs a fine-caliber needle (0.6 to 0.9 millimeter in open diameter) and is widely used to obtain cytologic and minute tissue samples, especially for lesions of the lymph glands, breasts, thyroid gland, salivary glands, lungs, and prostate. Fine needle aspiration is often inexpensive, safe, quick, and, when performed and interpreted by experienced workers, quite accurate. Because of the ready availability and relative inexpense of the endoscopic and fine needle aspiration biopsy techniques, they have become popular; almost every part of the body is now within reach of one or another of these two techniques.

Frozen section biopsy requires great expertise because this biopsy is usually a form of consultation done during surgery. A tissue sample is instantly frozen, sectioned, stained, and examined-all within about fifteen minutes-in order to render a specific diagnosis. The implications of this diagnosis are far reaching and will influence the surgical procedure and the long-term therapy and outcome for the patient. A frozen section report, for example, may determine whether an organ such as a breast, lung, or kidney must be removed and whether long-term radiation therapy or chemotherapy will be administered; such would be the case if the diagnosis is read as malignant.

There are two indications, other than establishing a diagnosis, for performing a frozen section: determining the adequacy of the margins of surgical excision (for example, to remove a malignant tumor completely) and establishing whether the tissue obtained contains an ample diagnosable sample to carry out other specialized tissue studies.

Uses and Complications

The following examples illustrate the practical use of the various biopsy techniques.

An excisional biopsy is performed on a pigmented dark lesion on a sun-exposed surface of the body of a young man and is diagnosed as malignant melanoma, which is a tumor of the pigment-producing cells of the body. This diagnosis is confirmed through the use of specialized immunological stains employing specific antibodies against melanin. The pathologist also comments that surgical margins of excision of that tumor are safe and do not contain tumor, and that the tumor is only superficial in nature and does not show deep invasion into the tissue. These two points imply that the patient will probably have a complete cure.

A fine needle aspiration biopsy is applied on a lump on the breast of a young woman. The material obtained is spread on slides, stained with a Papanicolaou stain, and evaluated within hours of its removal. The lump is diagnosed as a fibroadenoma, which is a benign tumor that is completely innocuous and of no further consequence to the young patient.

An elderly patient has an endoscopic biopsy of a visualized mass in the colon, which proves to be cancer. The patient is taken to the operating room, and the colon is resected. A frozen section is performed on the margin on the surgical excision to make sure that it contains no tumor. The stains used in this example are the simple and routine H & E stains.

A liver biopsy is performed on a patient with jaundice (yellowing of the skin), and a diagnosis of viral hepatitis B is made. This diagnosis is made following the study of the liver biopsy by routine stains and by stains that use immunological antibodies against the viral antigen. This is a specific and highly accurate diagnostic study.

A lymph gland excisional biopsy is performed on a patient who feels lumps all over his body. The biopsy is examined with routine and special stains, immunological marker studies, and gene rearrangement. Such extensive studies are performed to make sure that his condition is completely benign and is not neoplastic-that is, that he does not have malignant lymphoma (cancer of lymph tissue).

The biopsy, in its varied forms and techniques, has become an essential component of quality medical care. The biopsy report is both a medical and a legal document. Tissue slides and blocks are often stored for many years, in some places indefinitely. Peer slide reviews and consultations are common and are used as gauges for quality control and management. There are some limitations with histologic diagnosis, which mainly revolve around recognizing a specialist's own limitations and the need to seek a consultation by another expert pathologist as needed.

Perspective and Prospects

The first attempts to affirm the role of biopsy in medical practice were made by Carl Ruge and Johann Veit of the University of Berlin, who in the 1870s introduced surgical biopsy as an essential diagnostic tool. Despite the inevitable controversies that followed, Johann F. A. von Esmarch, a professor of surgery and a leading military surgeon of his time, presented forceful arguments at the German Surgical Congress of 1889 on the need to establish a microscopic diagnosis before operating in suspected cases of malignant tumors requiring extensive mutilating procedures. Shortly thereafter, the freezing microtome was introduced for the purpose of creating frozen sections, which hastened the acceptance of this recommendation. In the United States, the specialty of surgical pathology, which deals with biopsy interpretations, was created by a collaboration between surgeons and a gynecologist.

It is said that the first full-fledged American surgical pathologist was Joseph Colt Bloodgood, in the division of surgical pathology created by W. S. Halsted of Johns Hopkins Hospital in Baltimore. The founders of modern American surgical pathology and biopsy interpretation are Arthur Purdy Stout of Columbia Presbyterian Hospital in New York, James Ewing and his successors Fred Stewart and Frank Foote of Memorial Hospital in New York City, and Pierre Masson of the University of Montreal.

The biopsy remains the cornerstone for modern medical management, especially in cancer therapy. It will continue to enjoy that role in diagnostics as more venues become established to obtain, study, and evaluate minute tissue and cytologic samples.

—*Victor H. Nassar, M.D.*

See also: Breast biopsy; Breast cancer; Colorectal cancer; Colorectal polyp removal; Cyst removal; Cysts; Cytology; Cytopathology; Dermatology; Dermatopathology; Endometrial biopsy; Endoscopy; Histology; Immunopathology; Invasive tests; Laboratory tests; Lesions; Mastectomy and lumpectomy; National Cancer Institute (NCI); Oncology; Pap test; Pathology; Skin; Skin cancer; Skin disorders; Skin lesion removal; Tumor removal; Tumors.

For Further Information:

Bancroft, John D., and Marilyn Gamble, eds. *Theory and Practice of Histological Techniques*. 6th ed. New York: Churchill Livingstone/Elsevier, 2008.

Dubowitz, Victor, Caroline A. Sewry, and Anders Oldfors. *Muscle Biopsy: A Practical Approach*. Oxford: Saunders, 2013.

Fisher, Cyril, Elizabeth A. Montgomery, and Khin Thway. *Biopsy Interpretation of Soft Tissue Tumors*. Philadelphia: Wolters Kluwer/Lippincott, Williams and Wilkins, 2011.

Koss, Leopold G., StanisÅ,aw Woyke, and WÅ,odzimierz Olszewski. *Aspiration Biopsy: Cytologic Interpretation and Histologic Basis*. 2d ed. New York: Igaku-Shoin, 1992.

Mills, Stacey E., et al., eds. *Sternberg's Diagnostic Surgical Pathology*. 5th ed. 2 vols. Philadelphia: Wolters Kluwer Health/Lippincott Williams & Wilkins, 2010.

Rosai, Juan. *Rosai and Ackerman's Surgical Pathology*. 9th ed. 2 vols. New York: Mosby, 2004.

Shah, Rajal B., and Ming Zhou. *Prostate Biopsy Interpretation: An Illustrated Guide*. New York: Springer-Verlag, 2012.

Sloan, John P. *Biopsy Pathology of the Breast*. 2d ed. New York: Oxford University Press, 2001.

Taxy, Jerome B., Aliya N. Husain, and Anthony G. Montag. *Biopsy Interpretation: The Frozen Section*. Philadelphia: Wolters Kluwer/Lippincott, Williams and Wilkins, 2010.

Yazdi, Hossein M., and Irving Dardick. *Diagnostic Immunocytochemistry and Electron Microscopy: Guides to Clinical Aspiration Biopsy*. New York: Igaku-Shoin, 1992.

Biostatistics

Procedure

Anatomy or system affected: None

Specialties and related fields: All

Definition: The application of statistical concepts to biology and medicine in order to summarize the characteristics of samples and to test predictions about the populations from which the samples were taken.

Key terms:

correlation: a number between −1 and +1 that describes the strength of the relationship between two variables

descriptive statistics: the use of numbers to summarize the characteristics of samples

inferential statistics: the making and testing of numerical statements about populations

null hypothesis: a statement about a population that can be tested numerically

population: all the people, research animals, or other items of interest in a particular study *probability*: a number varying between 0 (for an impossible event) to 1 (for an absolutely certain event)

random sample: a sample in which every member of the population has the same probability of being included

regression: an equation that allows one variable to be predicted from another

sample: the members of a population that are actually studied or whose characteristics are measured

variable: any quantity that varies, such as height or cholesterol level

The Methodology of Statistics

The aim of every study in the field of biostatistics is to discover something about a population-all patients with a particular disease, for example. Populations are usually much too large to be studied in their entirety: It would be impractical to round up all the patients with diabetes in the world for a study, and the researcher would still miss those who lived in the past or who have yet to be born. For this reason, most research focuses on a sample drawn from the population of interest-for example, those diabetics who were studied at a particular hospital over a two-year period. Ideally, the sample would be a random sample, one in which each member of the population has an equal chance of being included. In practice, a random sample is hard to achieve: The patients with diabetes at a hospital in Chicago, for example, will differ in various ways from those at hospitals in London, Hong Kong, or rural Mexico.

Descriptive statistics are statistics that describe samples. The most commonly used statistics are mean, median, mode, and standard deviation. The mean of *n* values is simply the sum of all the values divided by *n*, or, symbolically, $\overline{X}=\sum x/n$, where $\overline{X}$ (pronounced "*x*-bar") stands for the mean, *n* stands for the number of observations, and $\sum x$ (pronounced "sum of x") stands for the sum obtained when all the different values of *x* (*n* of them) are added together. The median of a series of values is the middle value; it must always be the case that half of the values are above the median and half are below. The mode is simply the most common value, the value that occurs most often.

The mean, median, and mode are all "typical" values that characterize the center of distribution of all the values. The standard deviation, which is always positive, is a measure

Normal Distribution

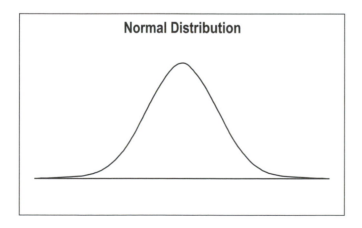

Table 1. A Comparison Between Diabetics and Non-diabetics

Diabetics		Nondiabetics
Height (cm)	Weight (kg)	Height (cm)
166	78	172
171	90	180
157	72	184
161	82	187
179	92	166
186	82	173

of variation that describes how close all the values cluster about a central value.

The numerator is calculated by subtracting the mean (X) from each value, squaring the difference, and adding together all these squared differences. After the sum is divided by *n* -1, the square root of the entire quantity is taken to determine the standard deviation. A small standard deviation indicates that the values differ very little from one another; a large standard deviation indicates greater variability among the values.

When two quantities vary, such as height and weight, correlation and regression coefficients are also calculated. A correlation coefficient is a number between -1 and +1. A correlation near +1 shows a very strong relationship between the two variables: When either one increases, the other also increases. A correlation near -1 is also strong, but when either variable increases, the other decreases. A correlation of 0 shows independence, or no relationship, between the variables: An increase in one has no average effect on the value of the other. Correlations midway between 0 and 1 show that an increase in one variable corresponds only to an average increase in the other, but not a dependable increase in each value. For example, taller people are generally heavier, but this is not true in every case.

Regression is a statistical technique for finding an equation that allows one variable to be predicted from the value of the other. For example, a regression of weight on height allows a researcher to predict the average weight for persons of a given height.

Inferential statistics, the statistical study of populations, begins with the study of probability. A probability is a number between 0 and 1 that indicates the certainty with which a particular event will occur, where 0 indicates an impossible occurrence and 1 indicates a certain occurrence. If a certain disease affects 1 percent of the population, then each random sampling will be subject to a .01 probability that the next person sampled will have the disease. For a larger sample than only one individual, the so-called binomial distribution describes the probability that the sample will include no one with the disease, one person with the disease, two people with the disease, and so on.

Table 2. A Contingency Table Comparing Pet Owners and Non-owners

	Pet owners	Non-owners	Totals
Arthritis	22	58	80
Heart Disease	11	29	40
Cancer	21	9	30
Other	36	54	90
TOTALS	90	150	240

A variable such as height is subject to so many influences, both genetic and environmental, that it can be treated mathematically as if it were the sum of thousands of small, random variations. Characteristics such as height usually follow a bell-shaped curve, or normal distribution (see figure on next page), at least approximately. This means that very few people are unusually tall or unusually short; most have heights near the middle of the distribution.

Each study using inferential statistics includes four major steps. First, certain assumptions are made about the populations under study. A common assumption, seldom tested, is that the variable in question is normally distributed within the population. Second, one or more samples are then drawn from the population, and each person or animal in the population is measured and tested in some way. Most studies assume that the samples are randomly drawn from the populations in question, even though true randomness is extremely difficult to achieve. Third, a particular assumption, called the null hypothesis, is chosen for testing. The null hypothesis is always an assumption that can be expressed numerically and that can be tested by known statistical tests. For example, one might assume that the mean height of the population of all diabetics is 170 centimeters (5.5 feet). Fourth, each statistical procedure allows the calculation of a theoretical probability, often a calculated value from a table. If the calculated probability is moderate or high, the null hypothesis is consistent with the observed results. If the calculated probability is very small, the observed results are very unlikely to occur if the null hypothesis is true; in these cases, the null hypothesis is rejected.

Some common types of inferential statistics are t-tests, chi-square tests, and the analysis of variance (also called ANOVA).

The Application of Statistics to Medicine

Nearly all medical research studies include biostatistics. Descriptive statistics are often presented in tables of data or in graphic form.

In the following example, height and weight data were gathered from a sample of six diabetic patients, and height was also measured in a sample of six nondiabetic patients (see Table 1). The mean height of these diabetic patients is

$(166 + 171 + 157 + 161 + 179 + 186) \div 6 = 1,020 \div 6 = 170$ centimeters. In order to calculate the standard deviation, this mean is subtracted from each of the six values, to yield differences of -4, 1, -13, -9, 9, and 16. Squaring these differences and adding them up gives a numerator of $16 + 1 + 169 + 81 + 81 + 256 = 604$. Dividing this by $n - 1 = 5$ (n is 6) and taking the square root reveals that the standard deviation is 11.0 centimeters (rounded to the nearest tenth). Similar calculations show that the mean height of the nondiabetic sample is 177 centimeters, with a standard deviation of 8.0 centimeters.

In this example, the nondiabetic sample averaged 7 centimeters taller than the diabetic sample. Inferential statistics can be used to find out if this difference is a meaningful one. In this case, a technique known as a t-test can compare the means of two samples to determine whether they might have come from the same population (or from populations with the same mean value). The assumptions of this test (not always stated explicitly) are that the six diabetic patients were randomly drawn from a normally distributed population and that the six nondiabetic patients were randomly drawn from another normally distributed population. The null hypothesis in this case is that the populations from which the two samples were drawn have the same mean height. The value of t calculated in this test is 1.141; this value is looked up in a table to reveal that the probability is larger than .1 (or 10 percent). In other words, if the null hypothesis is true, then this value of t (or a larger value) is expected to arise by chance alone more than 10 percent of the time. Under the usual criterion of a test at the 5 percent level of significance, one would keep or accept the null hypothesis. This means that the difference between the above sample means is not large enough to demonstrate a difference

between the two populations from which these samples are derived. There may in fact be an average difference in height between diabetic and nondiabetic populations, but samples this small cannot detect such a difference reliably. In general, when differences between populations are small, larger sample sizes are required to demonstrate their existence.

A t-test similar to the one above can also be used in drug testing. A drug is given to one set of patients, and a placebo (a fake medicine lacking the essential drug ingredient being tested) is given to a second group. Some relevant measurement (such as the drug's level of an important chemical that the patients normally lacked) is then compared between the two groups. The null hypothesis would be that the groups are the same and that the drug makes no difference. Rejection of the null hypothesis would be the same as demonstrating that the drug is effective.

For the diabetic patients in the above sample, a correlation coefficient of .60 can be calculated. This moderate level of correlation shows that, on the average, the taller among these patients are also heavier and thus the shorter patients are also lighter. Despite this average effect, however, individual exceptions are likely to occur. The square of the correlation coefficient, .36, indicates that about 36 percent of the variation in weight can be predicted from height. The equation for making the prediction in this case is "weight = 13.99 +.404 (height)," where the numbers 13.99 and .404 are called regression coefficients. The variable being predicted (weight in this example) is sometimes called the dependent variable; the variable used to make the prediction (in this case, height) is called the independent variable. A high positive correlation signifies that the regression equation offers a very reliable prediction of the dependent variable; a correlation near zero signifies that the regression equation is hardly better than assigning the mean value of the dependent variable to every prediction.

To illustrate another type of inferential statistics, consider the following data on the diseases present among elderly patients who own pets, compared to a comparable group who do not. This type of table is called a contingency table.

As illustrated in Table 2, $90 \div 240$, or three-eighths of the patients sampled, are pet owners. Thus, if there were no relationship between the diseases and pet ownership (which is the null hypothesis), one would expect three-eighths of the eighty arthritis patients (or 30) to be pet owners and five-eighths of the eighty (or 50) to be nonowners. Calculating all the expected frequencies in this way, one can compare them with the actual observations shown above.

The result is a statistic called chi-square, which in this problem has a value of 18.88. A table of chi-square values shows that, for a 2 x 4 contingency table, a chi-square value this high occurs by chance alone much less than 1 percent of the time. Thus, something has been observed (a chi-square value of 18.88) that is extremely unlikely under the null hypothesis of no relationship between disease and pet ownership, so the null hypothesis is rejected and one must conclude that there is a relationship. This conclusion applies only to the population from which the sample was drawn, however, and it does not reveal the nature of the relationship. Further investigation would be needed to discover whether pet ownership protected people from arthritis, whether people who already had arthritis were less inclined to take on the responsibility of pet ownership, or whether people who had pets gave them up when they became arthritic. All these possibilities (and more) are consistent with the findings.

The analysis of variance (also called ANOVA) is a very powerful technique for comparing many samples at once. Suppose that overweight patients were put on three or four different diets; one diet might be better than another, but there is also much individual variation in the amount of weight lost. Analysis of variance is a statistical technique that allows researchers to compare the variation between diets (or other treatments) with the individual variation among the people following each diet. The null hypothesis would be that all the diets are the same and that individual variation can account for all the observed differences. Rejecting the null hypothesis would demonstrate that a consistent difference existed and that at least one diet was better than another. Further tests would be required to pinpoint which diet was best and why.

Perspective and Prospects

The historical foundations of biostatistics go back as far as the development of probability theory by Blaise Pascal (1623-62). Karl Friedrich Gauss (1777-1855) first outlined the characteristics of the normal (also called Gaussian) distribution. The chi-square test was introduced by Karl Pearson (1857-1936). The greatest statistician of the twentieth century was Ronald A. Fisher (1890-1962), who clearly distinguished descriptive from inferential statistics and who developed many important statistical techniques, including the analysis of variance.

Although medicine existed long before statistics, it has become a nearly universal practice for every research study to use statistics in some important way. New medical procedures and new drugs are constantly being evaluated by using statistical techniques to compare them to other procedures or older drugs.

—*Eli C. Minkoff, Ph.D.*

See also: Bioinformatics; Epidemiology; Screening.

For Further Information:
Brase, Charles Henry, and Corrinne Pellillo Brase. *Understandable Statistics*. 10th ed. Boston: Brooks/Cole, 2012.

Daniel, Wayne W. *Biostatistics: A Foundation for Analysis in the Health Sciences*. 9th ed. Hoboken, N.J.: John Wiley & Sons, 2009.

Glaser, Anthony N. *High-Yield Biostatistics, Epidemiology, and Public Health*. Philadelphia: Lippincott, Williams and Wilkins, 2013.

Hebel, J. Richard, and Robert J. McCarter. *A Study Guide to Epidemiology and Biostatistics*. 7th ed. Burlington, Mass.: Jones and Bartlett, 2012.

Le, Chap T. *Health and Numbers: Problems-Based Introduction to Biostatistics*. Malden, Mass.: Blackwell, 2009.

Merrill, Ray M. *Fundamentals of Epidemiology and Biostatistics: Combining the Basics*. Burlington, Mass.: Jones and Bartlett, 2013.

Phillips, John L. *How to Think About Statistics*. 6th ed. New York: Henry Holt, 2002.

Sokal, Robert R., and F. James Rohlf. *Biometry*. 4th ed. San Francisco: W. H. Freeman, 2012.

Walpole, Ronald E. *Elementary Statistical Concepts*. New York: Macmillan, 1976.

Zar, Jerrold H. *Biostatistical Analysis*. 5th ed. Englewood Cliffs, N.J.: Pearson, 2010.

Biotechnology. *See* Bionics and biotechnology.

Bipolar disorders

Disease/Disorder

Anatomy or system affected: Psychic-emotional system

Specialties and related fields: Psychiatry, psychology

Definition: Affective (mood-related) illness characterized by periods of depressed and elevated mood.

Key terms:

anticonvulsants: drugs typically used to manage conditions involving brain seizures and sometimes used to treat bipolar disorders

bipolar I: less formally known as manic-depressive disorder; a condition that involves both severe symptoms of mania and depression and includes at least one episode of mania

bipolar II: a condition that involves both hypomania (milder symptoms of mania) and severe symptoms of depression and includes at least one episode of hypomania

dual diagnosis: a broad term used among professionals to indicate that an individual has two disorders needing integrated care and often used in psychiatry to indicate that an individual has received the diagnosis of a substance use disorder and another major clinical syndrome, such as a bipolar disorder

lithium: a drug composed of lithium carbonate used in the treatment of bipolar disorders

mood disorders: a group of disorders characterized by disturbance of mood and including symptoms of depression and/or mania that are not caused by any other physical or mental disorder

mood stabilizers: drugs that decrease the frequency and intensity of mood fluctuation, including drugs such as lithium and anticonvulsants

psychosis: a symptom associated with a variety of mental disorders and characterized by faulty perceptions and thinking that may be short-lived or enduring, being out of touch with reality, and lacking awareness of these problems; often includes hallucinations and delusions

unipolar depression: a term used by professionals to indicate that a person has the condition of depression with no evidence of having experienced a manic or hypomanic episode

unipolar mania: a very rare condition in which a person experiences periods of mania but has no experience of depression; is not caused by another disorder or condition

Causes and Symptoms

Although the causes of bipolar disorders are not known definitively, research indicates that some persons may be genetically predisposed to respond readily with manic or depressive episodes to internal and external influences. While changes in brain metabolism are thought to be significant in the development of bipolar disorders, both psychological and nonpsychological stresses are known to precipitate the onset of problems. It is often not possible to find one precipitating factor, however, because there is presumably a complex interaction between the effects of internal and external influences in persons suffering from this illness.

Bipolar disorders are illnesses that often occur in attacks, or episodes, lasting several days to a week or longer. They may be attacks of mania (periods of extreme elation and increased activity), hypomania (notably elevated mood and heightened activity), or depression (periods of abnormal sadness and melancholy). Recent work indicates that many variants of this disorder exist. Bipolar I is a variant of bipolar disorder in which individuals experience at least one episode of depression and one episode of mania. Bipolar II is a variant in which individuals experience at least one episode of depression and one episode of hypomania. For some individuals, these episodes signifying the presence of a disorder may be time limited and singular occurrences. For others, there may be repeated bouts of depression, mania, and hypomania or even times when symptoms appear

---

Information on Bipolar Disorders

Causes: Unknown; possibly genetic factors, changes in metabolism of brain, stress

Symptoms: Episodes of mania (increased mental activity, heightened emotions, excessive self-confidence and feelings of invincibility, sleeplessness) and depression (extreme sadness, lack of self-confidence, decreased mental activity, feeling tired and emotionally drained, fear of social interaction, anxiety and agitation)

Duration: Chronic

Treatments: Medications (lithium, antidepressants, neuroleptics), psychotherapy, electroconvulsive therapy

---

to be a mix of all three. Further, these episodes may be interspersed with periods of normal behavior, with no mood problems at all, which can vary in

length from brief amounts of time to years. In addition, a condition called cyclothymia refers to the presence of hypomania and a milder form of depression than is seen in bipolar disorders. These disorders are distinguished from unipolar depression (in which there is no mania or hypomania), the very rare condition of unipolar mania, and a more chronic but less severe form of depression known as dysthymia.

Bipolar disorders occur in about 1 percent of the population as a whole. They may occur in both adults and children and are diagnosed more often in women than in men. For persons over the age of eighteen, they are diagnosed in about two to three persons out of every one hundred. They also may occur in adolescence and childhood.

The onset of the disease frequently occurs between the ages of twenty and fifty, but it may appear for the first time in childhood or in later life, even beyond age sixty. Bipolar episodes manifest themselves differently in different persons. They can also vary within a particular person from one time to another. Further, although depression, mania, and hypomania have characteristic features, not all features are present during each episode.

Prominent features of manic episodes are elation, easily aroused anger, and increased mental activity. The elation varies from unusual vigor to uninhibited enthusiasm. The anger most often takes the form of irritability. Manic patients become annoyed if other people are unable to keep up with their racing thoughts. Intellectual activity takes place with lightning speed, ideas race through the mind, and speech flows with great rapidity and almost uninterruptedly.

During a manic episode, individuals are often excessively self-confident and lacking in self-criticism and insight into their behavior. This accompanies previously unknown energy, and when that energy is combined with racing thoughts, indefatigability, and lack of inhibition, the consequences are often disastrous. During manic episodes, individuals may destroy their relationships, ruin their reputations, create financial disasters, and engage in behavior that is not characteristic for them, such as indiscriminate sexual behavior, substance use, or even criminal activity. They may even demonstrate signs of psychosis. Despite reduced sleep, they also rarely feel tired and are usually kept awake by the rapid flow of ideas. Sexual activity may be greatly increased. Manic individuals may neglect to eat, and so they may lose considerable weight. The combination of activity, decreased food intake, and an inadequate amount of sleep may lead to dangerous physical exhaustion.

Hypomanic episodes are distinguished from manic episodes primarily in terms of being less intense, having fewer symptoms, and being less disruptive. The elevated mood also never reaches the point where psychosis is present. In fact, individuals may be highly functional during hypomanic episodes and may experience these times as pleasant and productive. The primary disruption is likely to be related to the driven nature of the behavior and how it may affect social interactions. Generally, though, any problems caused are not severe in nature.

Depressed episodes are in many respects the opposite of manias. They are characterized by sadness, a lack of self-confidence, and decreased mental activity. The sadness may vary from a slight feeling of being "down" to the bleakest despair. Ideas are few, thoughts move slowly, and memory function is impaired. Frequently, depressed individuals feel tired and emotionally drained; they feel the need to cry but are unable to do so. Weighed down by feelings of guilt and self-reproach, they may contemplate or even commit suicide. The depressed individual's self-confidence often is eroded, and, as a result, they may withdraw socially, lack initiative and energy, feel that obstacles are insurmountable, and have difficulty making even trivial decisions. Because of accompanying low self-esteem and feelings of inadequacy, individuals suffering from depression often fear social interaction and become anxious, agitated, and restless in a crowd. Sleep disturbances are also frequent. Occasionally, there is an increased need for sleep, and often individuals have difficulty sleeping, such as with insomnia. Some individuals find it difficult to fall asleep, others wake up frequently during the night, and others wake up early with feelings of anxiety. Depressed individuals also often experience variations in mood over the course of a day. The desire to stay in bed is overwhelming, and during the first hours of the day, they may experience basic daily activities as an extraordinary challenge.

Depressive episodes are often accompanied by physical transformations. The muscles may give the impression of being slack, the facial expression static, and movement slowed. There may be constipation, menstruation may stop, and sexual interest and activity may decrease or disappear completely for a time. Appetite may decrease and may result in loss of weight. Alternatively, eating may increase or remain the same, but because of decreased activity, weight gain may be experienced.

In addition to manic, hypomanic, and depressed episodes, bipolar disorders may manifest as mixed states during which signs of mania, hypomania, and depression are present concurrently. Individuals who experience mixed states may be sad and without energy but also irritable, or they may be manic and restless yet feel an underlying melancholy. Mixed states may occur as independent episodes, but they are seen more often during transitions between episodes. During these periods of transition, the condition may alternate between mood states several times a day.

Treatment and Therapy

Lithium is the drug frequently used for the treatment of bipolar disorders. A metallic element discovered by a Swedish chemist in 1818, lithium is produced from minerals such as spodumene, amblygonite, lepidolite, and petalite. As a drug, lithium is always used in the form of one of its salts-for example, lithium carbonate or lithium citrate. It is the lithium portion of these salts that is effective medically. Lithium was introduced into medicine in 1850 for the treatment of gout, and during the following century many medical uses of the element were proposed. It was used as a stimulant, as a sedative, for the treatment of diabetes, for the treatment of infectious diseases, as an additive to toothpaste, and for the treatment of malignant growths. The efficacy of lithium in these conditions was not proved, however, and lithium treatment never became widespread.

In 1949, an Australian psychiatrist, John Cade, published an article that forms the basis of all later lithium treatment. The prophylactic action of lithium in manic-depressive type illnesses was debated in the psychiatric literature for some years, but extensive trials in many countries have fully documented the efficacy of the drug. Its prophylactic action is exerted against both manic and depressive relapses. One of the characteristic features of lithium is that it removes manic symptoms without producing sedation, unlike treatment with neuroleptics, which are also effective in the treatment of mania but which exert sedative action. Lithium may occasionally produce side effects, such as nausea, stomachache, tremor of the hands, and muscle weakness, but these symptoms are usually neither severe nor incapacitating. The greatest drawback of the treatment is that the full antimanic effect is usually not seen until after six to eight days of treatment, and sometimes it is necessary to supplement lithium with a neuroleptic drug.

Until the 1950s, the condition commonly described as manic depression, and now known as the varied conditions of bipolar disorders, had remained intractable, frustrating the best efforts of clinical practitioners and their predecessors. This long history ended abruptly with the discovery of the therapeutic effects of lithium. In an ironic turn of events, the pharmacological revolution then initiated a renaissance in the psychotherapy of manic-depressive patients. Substantially freed from the severe disruptions of mania and the profound withdrawal of depression, these individuals, with the help of their therapists, focused on the many psychological issues related to the illness and confronted what was needed for them to maintain health. Unfortunately, lithium and the psychotherapy approaches available at that time did not help everyone every time, and so the search for helpful treatments continued. Part of this was because not all individuals who need to take lithium will adhere to their prescribed drug regimen. Also, some individuals cannot take lithium because of its toxicity to the body or because of physical conditions they may have.

Electroconvulsive therapy (ECT) is one alternative to medications in treating bipolar disorders. This therapy is particularly useful for individuals who have failed to respond to drugs, who may not be able to tolerate drugs such as lithium because of other physical conditions, or who need immediate relief from their mood symptoms in order to avoid suicide or life-threatening conditions. In ECT, following narcosis (an unconscious state induced by narcotics), certain parts of the patient's brain are stimulated electrically through electrodes placed on the skin. This stimulation elicits a seizure, but since the drug relaxes the muscles, the seizure manifests as muscle twitching only. The individuals do not feel the treatment, but during the hours following the treatment, they may have headaches and feel tenderness of the muscles. Short-term memory impairment may also occur. Treatment often occurs two to four times a week for three to four weeks at a hospital or on an outpatient basis and leads to amelioration of symptoms in most patients.

For treatment of symptoms such as agitation related to bipolar conditions, drugs referred to as antipsychotic medications, or neuroleptics, are often used. These are sedative drugs such as chlorpromazine (Largactil, Thorazine) and haloperidol (Haldol). Neuroleptics exert a powerful tranquilizing effect on anxiety, restlessness, and tension. They also attenuate or relieve hallucinations and delusions. Neuroleptics are not specific for any single disease. They may be used, possibly in conjunction with lithium, in the treatment of mania, and they may be used in depressions that are accompanied by delusions. Neuroleptics may, however, produce side effects involving the muscles and the nervous system.

Antidepressants act, as the name indicates, on depression, but only on abnormal depression. They do not affect the normal ups and downs that people without these conditions might experience, and they do not make people experience a "drug high" or become happy. They instead work to bring individuals back from a depressed state to a more normal state. Drugs that fit in this group have included substances such as imipramine (Tofranil), amitriptyline (Elavil, Tryptizol), and fluoxetine (Prozac), among others. The side effects of antidepressants may include tiredness, mouth dryness, tremor, constipation, difficulty in urinating, and a tendency to faint. Changes in heart rate and rhythm may also occur, and careful evaluation is necessary in patients with cardiac disease. As new drugs are developed, drug makers often work hard to reduce such side effects. Also, some of these side effects may lessen over time as the person's body becomes habituated to the drug.

Where antidepressants do work, however, treatment is often continued for some time after disappearance of the symptoms. For example, continuing treatment for three, six, twelve, or even twenty-four months would not be uncommon.

Bipolar disorder is treated most effectively with a combination of lithium or other medications and adjunctive psychotherapy. Drug treatment, which is primary, relieves most patients of the severe disruptions of mood episodes. Psychotherapy can assist them in coming to terms with the repercussions of past episodes and in comprehending the practical implications of living with bipolar disorder. It may also be useful for helping to identify life stressors that may cause or exacerbate their mood-related symptoms.

Although not all patients require psychotherapy, most can benefit from individual, group, and/or family therapy. Moreover, participation in a self-help group is often useful in supplementing or supplanting formal psychotherapy. Psycho-therapeutic issues are dictated by the nature of the illness for the specific individual. What this means is that the way in which their therapy will progress depends on what other issues of importance may be present. Additional problems related to suicide, violence, alcohol and drug use, and other mental health concerns may be present. It is also important to remember that although reactions vary widely, some individuals will feel angry and ambivalent about both the illness and its treatment. They may deny its existence, its severity, or its consequences, and they are often concerned about issues such as relationships and the possibility of genetically transmitting the illness to their children.

No one technique has been shown to be superior in the psychotherapy of individuals with bipolar disorder. The therapist is guided by knowledge of both the illness itself and its manifestation in the individual patient. In style and technique, the therapist must remain flexible in order to adjust to the patient's fluctuating levels of dependency and mood change, cognition, and behavior. The therapist must be especially alert to their reactions to working with these types of individuals, which may pose special challenges for the therapist. In addition, educating patients and their families is essential because it helps them to recognize new episodes.

Perspective and Prospects

Bipolar disorders are among the most consistently identifiable of all mental disorders and among the oldest. They are discernible in descriptions in the Old Testament, and they were recognized in clinical medicine almost two thousand years ago. The medical writers of ancient Greece (the Hippocratic school) conceived of mental disorders in terms that sound remarkably modern. They believed that melancholia was a psychological manifestation of an underlying biological disturbance-specifically, a perturbation in brain function. Early conceptions of "melancholia" and "mania" were, however, broader than those of modern times. These two terms, together with "phrenitis," which roughly corresponds to an acute organic delirium, comprised all mental illnesses throughout most of the ancient period.

As they did with other illnesses, the Hippocratic writers argued forcefully that mental disorders were not caused by supernatural or magical forces, as primitive societies had believed. Their essentially biological explanation for the cause of melancholia, which survived until the Renaissance, was part of the prevailing understanding of all health as an equilibrium of the four humors-blood, yellow bile, black bile, and phlegm-and all illness as a disturbance of this equilibrium. First fully developed in the Hippocratic work *On the Nature of Man* (ca. 400 BCE), the humoral theory linked the humors with the seasons and with relative moistness. An excess of black bile was seen as the cause of melancholia, a term that literally means "black bile." Mania, by contrast, was usually attributed to an excess of yellow bile.

Reflections on the relationship between melancholia and mania date back at least to the first century BCE. and Soranus of Ephesus. Aretaeus of Cappadocia, who lived in the second century CE., appears to have been the first to suggest that mania was an end-stage of melancholia, a view that was to prevail for centuries to come. He isolated "cyclothymia" as a form of mental illness with phases of depression alternating with phases of mania. Though this term is no longer used in this way, he provided an early record of problems similar to bipolar disorders. Although Aretaeus included syndromes that in the twentieth century would be classified as schizophrenia, his clear descriptions of the spectrum of mood conditions involving depression and mania are impressive even in modern times.

The next significant medical writer, Galen of Pergamum (ca. 129-ca. 199 CE), firmly established melancholia as a chronic condition. His few comments on mania included the observation that it can be either a primary disease of the brain or secondary to other diseases. His initial contribution was his all-encompassing elaboration of the humoral theory, a system so compelling that it dominated medical thought for more than a millennium.

Medical observations in succeeding centuries continued to subscribe to the conceptions of depression and mania laid down in classical Greece and Rome. Most authors wrote of the two conditions as separate illnesses yet suggested a close connection between them. Yet where mania and depression are considered in the historical medical literature, they are almost always linked.

The explicit conception of manic-depressive illness as a single disease entity dates from the mid-nineteenth century. Jean Pierre Falret and Jules Baillarger, French "alienists," independently and almost simultaneously formulated the idea that mania and depression could represent different manifestations of a single illness. In 1854, Falret described a circular disorder that he expressly defined as an illness in which the succession of mania and melancholia manifested itself with continuity and in an almost regular manner. That same year, Baillarger described essentially the same thing, emphasizing that the manic and depressive episodes were not two different attacks, but two different stages of the same attack. Despite the contributions of Falret, Jeanne-Étienne-Dominique Esquirol, and other observers, however, most clinical investigators continued to regard mania and melancholia as separate chronic entities that followed a deteriorating course.

It was left to the German psychiatrist Emil Kraepelin (1856-1926) to distinguish psychotic illnesses from one another and to draw the perimeter clearly around manic-depressive illness. He emphasized careful diagnosis based on both longitudinal history and the pattern of current symptoms. By 1913, in the eighth edition of Kraepelin's textbook of psychiatry, virtually all of melancholia had been subsumed into manic-depressive illness.

Wide acceptance of Kraepelin's broad divisions led to further explorations of the boundaries between the two basic categories of manic-depressive illness and dementia praecox, the delineation of their similarities, and the possibility that subgroups could be identified within two basic categories. Kraepelin's synthesis was a major accomplishment because it formed a solid and empirically anchored base for future developments.

During the first half of the twentieth century, the views of Adolf Meyer (1866-1950) gradually assumed a dominant position in American psychiatry, a position that they maintained for several decades. Meyer believed that psychopathology emerged from interactions between an individual's biological and psychological characteristics and his or her social environment. This perspective was evident in the label "manic-depressive reaction" in the first official American Psychiatric Association diagnostic manual, which was published in 1952. When the Meyerian focus, considerably influenced by psychoanalysis, turned to manic-depressive illness, the individual in the environment became the natural center of study, and clinical descriptions of symptoms and the longitudinal course of the illness were given less emphasis.

Eugen Bleuler (1857-1939), in his classic contributions to descriptive psychiatry, departed from Kraepelin by conceptualizing the relationship between manic-depressive (affective) illness and dementia praecox (schizophrenia) as a continuum without a sharp line of demarcation. Bleuler also broadened Kraepelin's concept of manic-depressive illness by designating several subcategories and using the term "affective illness." His subcategories of affective illness anticipated the principal contemporary division of the classic manic-depressive diagnostic group-the bipolar-unipolar distinction. The bipolar-unipolar distinction represents a major advance in the classification of affective disorders primarily because it provides a basis for evaluating genetic, pharmacological, clinical, and biological differences rather than representing a purely descriptive subgrouping. As research on this disorder continues, it is likely that the relationship of bipolar disorder to substance use disorders will increase. In 1997, it was estimated that at least 50 percent of individuals affected by one are affected by the other. As such, common mechanisms of problems related to these two types of disorders may lead to more specific treatments designed to address situations when there are co-occurring disorders.

—Genevieve Slomski, Ph.D.;
updated by Nancy A. Piotrowski, Ph.D.

See also: Antianxiety drugs; Antidepressants; Anxiety; Depression; Psychiatric disorders; Psychiatry; Psychiatry, child and adolescent; Psychiatry, geriatric; Psychoanalysis; Psychology; Shock therapy; Sleep disorders.

For Further Information:
"Bipolar Disorder." *MedlinePlus*, March 29, 2013.

Castle, Lana R., and Peter C. Chybrow. *Bipolar Disorder Demystified: Mastering the Tightrope of Manic Depression*. New York: Avalon, 2003.

Coryell, William H. "Psychotic Features in Major Depressive and Manic Episodes." In *Clinical Guide to Depression and Bipolar Disorder: Findings from the Collaborative Depression Study*, edited by Martin B. Keller. Arlington, Va.: American Psychiatric Publishing, 2013.

Geller, Barbara, and Melissa P. DelBello, eds. *Bipolar Disorder in Childhood and Early Adolescence*. Rev. ed. New York: Guilford, 2006.

Goodwin, Frederick K., and Kay Redfield Jamison. *Manic-Depressive Illness*. 2d ed. New York: Oxford University Press, 2007.

Jamison, Kay Redfield. *An Unquiet Mind: A Memoir of Moods and Madness*. New York: Knopf, 1998.

Kellner, Charles H. *Brain Stimulation in Psychiatry: ECT, DBS, TMS, and Other Modalities*. Cambridge: Cambridge University Press, 2012.

Leonard, Basia, and Joann Jovinelly. *Bipolar Disorder*. New York: Rosen, 2012.

Mondimore, Francis M. *Depression: The Mood Disease*. 3rd ed. Baltimore: Johns Hopkins University Press, 2006.

Rosenthal, Norman E. *Winter Blues: Everything You Need to Know to Beat Seasonal Affective Disorder*. New York: Guilford, 2006.

Birth. *See* Childbirth; Childbirth complications.

Birth defects

Disease/Disorder

Anatomy or system affected: All bodily tissues

Specialties and related fields: Embryology, genetics, neonatology, obstetrics, pediatrics, perinatology

Definition: Congenital malformations or structural anomalies and their accompanying functional disorders that originate during embryonic development; they are involved in up to 6 percent of human live births.

Key terms:

deletion: the loss of a portion of a chromosome as a result of induced or accidental breakage

multifactorial inheritance: the interaction of genetic and environmental factors, which leads to certain congenital malformations

mutation: a change in the deoxyribonucleic acid (DNA), which may lead to the occurrence of congenital malformations

nondisjunction: the failure of chromosomes to separate during cell division, resulting in new cells that either lack a chromosome or have an extra chromosome

organogenetic period: the period of embryonic development, from approximately fifteen to sixty days after fertilization, during which most body organs form

spina bifida: a birth defect involving malformation of vertebrae in the lower back, often resulting in paralysis and lower-body organ impairment

teratogen: an environmental factor that can induce the formation of congenital malformations

teratology: the study of congenital malformations

translocation: the structural chromosomal defect that occurs when a piece of one chromosome attaches to another

Causes and Symptoms

As the human embryo develops, it undergoes many formative stages from the simple to the complex, most often culminating in a perfectly formed newborn infant. The formation of the embryo is controlled by genetic factors, external influences, and interactions between the various embryonic tissues. Because genes play a vital role as the blueprint for the developing embryo, they must be unaltered and the cellular mechanisms that allow the genes to be expressed must also work correctly. In addition, the chemical and physical communications between cells and tissues in the embryo must be clear and uninterrupted. The development of the human embryo into a newborn infant is infinitely more complex than the design and assembly of the most powerful supercomputer or the largest skyscraper. Because of this complexity and the fact that development progresses without supervision by human eye or hand, there are many opportunities for errors that can lead to malformations.

Errors in development can be caused by both genetic and environmental factors. Genetic factors include chromosomal abnormalities and gene mutations. Both can be inherited from the parents or can occur spontaneously during gamete formation, fertilization, and embryonic development. Environmental factors, called teratogens, include such things as drugs, disease organisms, and radiation.

Chromosomal abnormalities account for about 6 percent of human congenital malformations. They fall into two categories, numerical and structural. Numerical chromosomal abnormalities are most often the result of nondisjunction occurring in the germ cells that form sperm and eggs. During the cell division process in sperm and egg production, deoxyribonucleic acid (DNA) is duplicated so that each new cell receives a complete set of chromosomes. Occasionally, two chromosomes fail to separate (nondisjunction), such that one of the new cells receives two copies of that chromosome and the other cell none. Both of the resulting gametes (either sperm or eggs) will have an abnormal number of chromosomes. When a gamete with an abnormal number of chromosomes unites with a normal gamete, the result is an individual with an abnormal chromosome number. The missing or extra chromosome will cause confusion in the developmental process and result in certain structural and functional abnormalities. For example, persons with an extra copy of chromosome number 21 suffer from Down syndrome, which often includes mental deficiency, heart defects, facial deformities, and other symptoms and can be caused by nondisjunction in one or more cells of the early embryo. Abnormal chromosome numbers may also result from an egg's being fertilized by two sperm, or from failure of cell division during gamete formation.

Structural chromosomal abnormalities result from chromosome breaks. Breaks occur in chromosomes during normal exchanges in material between chromosomes (crossing over). They also may occur accidentally at weak points on the chromosomes, called fragile sites, and can be induced by chemicals and radiation. Translocations occur when a broken-off piece of chromosome attaches to another chromosome. For example, an individual who has the two usual copies of chromosome 21 and, as the result of a translocation, carries another partial or complete copy of 21 riding piggyback on another chromosome will have the symptoms of Down syndrome. Deletions occur when a chromosome break causes the loss of part of a chromosome. The cri du chat syndrome is caused by the loss of a portion of chromosome number 5. Infants affected by this disorder have a catlike cry, are intellectually and developmentally disabled, and have cardiovascular defects. Other structural chromosomal abnormalities include inversions (in which segments of chromosomes are attached in reverse order), duplications (in which portions of a chromosome are present in multiple copies), and isochromosomes (in which chromosomes separate improperly to produce the wrong configuration).

Gene mutations (defective genes) are responsible for about 8 percent of birth defects. Mutations in genes occur spontaneously because of copying errors or can be induced by environmental factors such as chemicals and radiation. The mutant genes are passed from parents to offspring; thus certain defects may be present in specific families and geographical locations. Two examples of mutation-caused defects are polydactyly (the presence of extra fingers or toes) and microcephaly (an unusually small cranium and brain). Mutations can be either dominant or recessive. If one of the parents possesses a dominant mutation, there will be a 50 percent chance of this mutant gene being transmitted to the offspring. Brachydactyly, or abnormal shortening of the fingers, is a dominantly inherited trait. Normally, the parent with the dominant gene also has the disorder. Recessive mutations can remain hidden or unexpressed in both parents. When each parent possesses a single recessive gene, there is a 25 percent chance that any given pregnancy will result in a child with a defect. Examples of recessive defects are the metabolic disorders sickle cell disease and hemophilia.

Environmental factors called teratogens are responsible for about 7 percent of congenital malformations. Human embryos are most sensitive to the effects of teratogens during the period when most organs are forming (organogenetic period), that is, from about fifteen to sixty days after fertilization. Teratogens may interfere with development in a number of ways, usually by killing embryonic cells or interrupting their normal function. Cell movement, communication, recognition, differentiation, division, and adhesion are critical to development and can be easily disturbed by teratogens. Teratogens can also cause mutations and chromosomal abnormalities in embryonic cells. Even if the disturbance is only weak and transitory, it can have serious effects because the critical period for the development of certain structures is very short and well defined. For example, the critical period for arm development is from twenty-four to forty-four days after fertilization. A chemical that interferes with limb development, such as the drug thalidomide, if taken during this period, may cause missing arm parts, shortened arms, or complete absence of arms. Many drugs and chemicals have

---

Information on Birth Defects

Causes: Genetic factors (chromosomal abnormalities, gene mutations), environmental factors (drugs, disease, radiation)

Symptoms: Vary widely; can include missing limbs or body parts, reduced mental capacity, developmental delays, speech impediments, metabolic disorders

Duration: Vary widely; some temporary and treatable in utero or shortly after birth, others lifelong

Treatments: Preventive measures (genetic counseling, healthy diet during pregnancy), specialized and intense medical treatment (surgery, drug therapy)

---

been identified as teratogenic, including alcohol, aspirin, and certain antibiotics.

Other environmental factors that can cause congenital malformations include infectious organisms, radiation, and mechanical pressures exerted on the fetus within the uterus. Certain infectious agents or their products can pass from the mother through the placenta into the embryo. Infection of the embryo causes disturbances to development similar to those caused by chemical teratogens. For example, German measles (rubella virus) causes cataracts, deafness, and heart defects if the embryo is infected early in development. Exposure to large doses of radiation-such as those released by the accident at the Chernobyl nuclear power plant in 1986 or by the atomic bombs dropped on Hiroshima and Nagasaki, Japan, during World War II-can result in death and damage to embryonic cells. There was an increase of about 10 to 15 percent in birth defects in children born to pregnant women exposed to atomic bomb radiation in Japan. Diagnostic X-rays are not known to be a cause of birth defects. Some defects such as hip dislocation may be caused by mechanical forces inside the uterus; this could happen if the amnion is damaged or the uterus is malformed, thus restricting the movement of the fetus. About 25 percent of congenital defects are caused by the interaction of genetic and environmental factors (multifactorial), and the causes of more than half (54 percent) of all defects are unknown.

Treatment and Therapy

Because many birth defects have well-defined genetic and environmental causes, they often can be prevented. Preventive measures need to be implemented if the risk of producing a child with a birth defect is higher than average. Genetic risk factors for such defects include the presence of a genetic defect in one of the parents, a family history of genetic defects, the existence of one or more children with defects, consanguineous (same-family) matings, and advanced maternal age. Prospective parents with one or more of these risk factors should seek genetic counseling in order to assess their potential for producing a baby with such defects. Also, parents exposed to higher-than-normal levels of drugs, alcohol, chemicals, or radiation are at risk of producing gametes that may cause defects, and pregnant women exposed to the same agents place the developing embryo at risk. Again, medical counseling should be sought by such prospective parents. Pregnant women should maintain a well-balanced diet that is about 200 calories higher than normal to provide adequate fetal nutrition. Women who become anemic during pregnancy may need an iron supplement, and the U.S. Public Health Service recommends that all women of childbearing age consume 0.4 milligram of folic acid (one of the B vitamins) per day to reduce the risk of spina bifida and other neural tube defects. Women at high risk for producing genetically defective offspring can undergo a screening technique whereby eggs taken from the ovary are screened in the laboratory to select the most normal appearing ones prior to in vitro fertilization and then returned to the uterus. Some couples may decide to use artificial insemination by donor if the prospective father is known to carry a defective gene.

The early detection of birth defects is crucial to the health of both the mother and the baby. Physicians commonly use three methods for monitoring fetal growth and development during pregnancy. The most common method is ultrasound scanning. High-frequency sound waves are directed at the uterus and then monitored for waves that bounce back from the fetus. The return waves allow a picture of the fetus to be formed on a television monitor, which can be used to detect defects and evaluate the growth of the fetus. In amniocentesis, the doctor withdraws a small amount of amniotic fluid containing fetal cells; both the fluid and the cells can be tested for evidence of congenital defects by growing the cells in tissue culture and examining their chromosomes. Amniocentesis generally cannot be performed until the sixteenth week of pregnancy. Another method of obtaining embryonic cells is called chorionic villus sampling and can be done as early as the fifth week of pregnancy. A tube is inserted into the uterus in order to retrieve a small sample of placental chorionic villus cells, identical genetically to the embryo. Again, these cells can be tested for evidence of congenital defects. The early discovery of fetal defects and other fetal-maternal irregularities allows the physician time to assess the problem and make recommendations to the parents regarding treatment. Many problems can be solved with therapy, medications, and even prenatal surgery. If severe defects are detected, the physician may recommend termination of the pregnancy.

Children born with defects often require highly specialized and intense medical treatment. For example, a child born with spina bifida may have lower-body paralysis, clubfoot, hip dislocation, and gastrointestinal and genitourinary problems in addition to the spinal column deformity. Spina bifida occurs when the embryonic neural tube and vertebral column fail to close properly in the lower back, often resulting in a protruding sac containing parts of the spinal meninges and spinal cord. The malformation and displacement of these structures result in nerve damage to the lower body, causing paralysis and the loss of some neural function in the organs of this area. Diagnostic procedures including X-rays, computed tomography (CT) scans, and urinalysis are carried out to determine the extent of the disorder. If the sac is damaged and begins to leak cerebrospinal fluid, it needs to be closed immediately to reduce the risk of meningitis. In any case, surgery is done to close the opening in the lower spine, but it is not possible to correct the damage done to the nerves. Urgent attention must also be given to the urinary system. The paralysis often causes loss of sphincter muscle control in the urinary bladder and rectum. With respect to the urinary system, this lack of control can lead to serious urinary tract infections and the loss of kidney function. Both infections and obstructions must be treated promptly to avoid serious complication. Orthopedic care needs to begin early to treat clubfoot, hip dislocation, scoliosis, muscle weakness, spasms, and other side effects of this disorder.

The medical treatment of birth defects requires a carefully orchestrated team approach involving physicians and specialists from various medical fields. When the abnormality is discovered (before birth, at birth, or after birth), the primary physician will gather as much information as possible from the family history, the medical history of the patient, a physical examination, and other diagnostic tests. This information is interpreted in consultation with other physicians in order to classify the disorder properly and to determine its possible origin and time of occurrence. This approach may lead to the discovery of other malformations, which will be classified as primary and secondary. When the physician arrives at a specific overall diagnosis, he or she will counsel the parents about the possible causes and development of the disorder, the recommended treatment and its possible outcomes, and the risk of recurrence in a subsequent pregnancy. Certain acute conditions may require immediate attention in order to save the life of the newborn.

In addition to treating the infant with the defect, the physician needs to counsel the parents in order to answer their questions. The counseling process will help them to understand and accept their child's condition. To promote good parent-infant bonding, the parents are encouraged to maintain close contact with the infant and participate in its care. Children born with severe chronic disabilities and their families require special support. When parents are informed that their child has limiting congenital malformations, they may react negatively and express feelings of shock, grief, and guilt. Medical professionals can help the parents deal with their feelings and encourage them to develop a close and supportive relationship with their child. Physicians can provide a factual and honest appraisal of the infant's condition and discuss treatments, possible outcomes, and the potential for the child to live a happy and fulfilling life. Parents are encouraged to learn more about their child's disorder and to seek the guidance and help of professionals, support groups, family, and friends. With the proper care and home environment, the child can develop into an individual who is able to interact positively with family and community.

Perspective and Prospects

Birth defects have been recognized and recorded

throughout human history. The writer of the Old Testament book of 2 Samuel (21:20) describes the defeat of a giant with six fingers and six toes. Defects were recorded in prehistoric art, and the cuneiform records of ancient Babylon considered birth defects to be omens of great significance. Aristotle described many common human birth defects such as polydactyly. Superstitions about birth defects abounded during the Middle Ages. People believed that events occurring during pregnancy could influence the form of the newborn; for example, deformed legs could be caused by contact with a cripple. Mothers of deformed children were accused of having sex with animals. In a book written about birth defects in 1573, *Monstres et prodiges*, Ambroise Paré describes many human anomalies and attempts to explain how they occur. Missing body parts such as fingers or toes were attributed to a low sperm count in the father, and certain characteristics such as abnormal skin pigmentation, body hair, or facial features were said to be influenced by the mother's thoughts and visions during and after conception.

With advances in science and medicine these superstitions were swept aside. Surgery for cleft palate was performed as early as 1562 by Jacques Honlier. William Harvey, a seventeenth-century English physician, recognized that some birth defects such as cleft lip are normal embryonic features that accidentally persist until the time of birth. The study of embryology, including experiments on bird and amphibian embryos, blossomed as a science during the nineteenth century, leading to a better understanding of how defects arise. At the same time, physicians were developing improved ways to treat birth defects. By 1816, Karl von Graefe had developed the first modern comprehensive surgical method for repairing cleft palate. The modern technique for repairing congenital pyloric stenosis (narrowing of the junction between the stomach and small intestine) was developed by Conrad Ramstedt in 1912. The principles of genetic inheritance developed by Gregor Mendel in the mid-nineteenth century were rediscovered by biologists at the beginning of the twentieth century and soon were applied to the study of human heredity, including the inheritance of birth defects. Geneticists realized that defects such as hemophilia and Down syndrome are inherited diseases. Beginning in the 1930s, other scientists began to show that congenital defects could be induced in experimental animals by such factors as dietary deficiencies, hormone imbalances, chemicals, and radiation. In some cases, a lack of complete testing of environmental factors such as drugs has led to tragedies but also a better understanding of the nature of birth defects. The tranquilizer thalidomide caused limb malformations in more than seven thousand children in Europe before it was withdrawn from the market in 1961. Pregnant women treated for cervical cancer in the 1960s with large doses of radiation bore children with defects and developmental disabilities.

Indeed, much of the medical and environmental health research today centers on the effects of drugs, toxic chemicals, radiation, and other factors on human health and development. Genetic counseling and testing of parents at risk for inherited defects has become an accepted part of medical practice. In addition, there have been many advances in the treatment of congenital defects since the 1950s. Modern orthopedic and plastic surgery is used to correct such problems as clubfoot and cleft palate. Transplants are used to correct deficiencies of the liver, kidneys, and other organs. Biomedical engineers have developed improved prosthetic devices to replace lost limbs and to aid in hearing, speaking, and seeing. An understanding of metabolic disorders such as phenylketonuria (PKU) has led to better treatment that utilizes special diets and medications. Because it is difficult to undo the damage of congenital defects fully, the most promise seems to be in the areas of prevention and protection. Prospective parents and their medical care providers need to be alert to potential hereditary problems, as well as to exposure to hazardous environmental agents. Pregnant women need to maintain a healthy diet and check with their physicians before taking any drugs. With advances in preventive medicine, diagnosis, and treatment, the future is much brighter for reducing the health toll of congenital malformations.

—*Rodney C. Mowbray, Ph.D.;*
updated by Alexander Sandra, M.D.

See also: Amniocentesis; Cardiology, pediatric; Cerebral palsy; Chiari malformations; Childbirth; Childbirth complications; Chorionic villus sampling; Cleft lip and palate; Cleft lip and palate repair; Color blindness; Congenital disorders; Congenital heart disease; Cornelia de Lange syndrome; Cystic fibrosis; Developmental disorders; Diabetes mellitus; DiGeorge syndrome; DNA and RNA; Down syndrome; Dwarfism; Embryology; Endocrinology, pediatric; Enzymes; Fetal alcohol syndrome; Fetal surgery; Gene therapy; Genetic counseling; Genetic diseases; Genetics and inheritance; Gigantism; Hemophilia; Hydrocephalus; Intellectual disability; Metabolic disorders; Muscular dystrophy; Mutation; Obstetrics; Phenylketonuria (PKU); Polydactyly and syndactyly; Porphyria; Pregnancy and gestation; Premature birth; Rubinstein-Taybi syndrome; Screening; Sickle cell disease; Spina bifida; Tay-Sachs disease; Teratogens; Thalassemia; Thalidomide.

For Further Information:
"Birth Defects." *MedlinePlus*, May 2, 2013.
"Birth Defects: Overview." *National Institute of Child Health and Human Development*, Apr. 3, 2013.
"Birth Defects: What They Are and How They Happen." *March of Dimes*, 2013.
"Facts about Birth Defects." *Centers for Disease Control and Prevention*, Feb. 24, 2011.
Heyman, Bob, and Mette Henriksen. *Risk, Age, and Pregnancy: A Case Study of Prenatal Genetic Screening and Testing.* New York: Palgrave, 2001.
Moore, Keith L., and T. V. N. Persaud. *The Developing Human.* 8th ed. Philadelphia: Saunders/Elsevier, 2008.
Nixon, Harold, and Barry O'Donnell. *The Essentials of Pediatric Surgery.* 4th ed. Boston: Butterworth Heinemann, 1992.
Sadler, T. W. *Langman's Medical Embryology.* 12th ed. Philadelphia: Lippincott Williams & Wilkins, 2012.
Sherwood, Lauralee. *Human Physiology: From Cells to Systems.* 8th ed. Pacific Grove, Calif.: Brooks/Cole/Cengage Learning, 2013.
Stray-Gundersen, Karen, ed. *Babies with Down Syndrome.* Rev. ed. Kensington, Md.: Woodbine House, 1995.

Bites and stings

Disease/Disorder

Anatomy or system affected: Heart, immune system, skin
Specialties and related fields: Emergency medicine, immunology, toxicology
Definition: Injuries from animals or insects.

Bites and stings cause four major types of damage to the victim's body: physical damage, the introduction of disease-causing organisms, the introduction of poisons (toxins, venoms), and allergic responses, including anaphylactic shock. Often, more than one form of damage is associated with a bite or sting. Alone or in combination, they can be life-threatening, but usually the damage from a bite or sting is minor. A wide variety of organisms can bite or sting, but the most important among them are mammals, reptiles (snakes and lizards), some fish (sharks, rays, moray eels), arthropods (including insects, centipedes, spiders, mites, ticks, and scorpions), and cnidarians (jellyfish, Portuguese man-of-wars, and their relatives).

Bites causing physical damage. Bites delivered by a mammal (most often a dog or cat) are likely to cause the most extensive physical damage. The specialized teeth of mammals, especially carnivores, in combination with powerful jaw muscles, can produce a serious wound. If wounding is in a vulnerable spot or is very extensive, or if the bleeding is not stopped, the physical damage can be fatal. A bite that causes physical damage is almost certain to introduce bacteria, viruses, or other infectious agents. An important example is the rabies virus, but many kinds of organism are dangerous if introduced into the bloodstream, or into the bone marrow of bones broken by the bite. Most mammalian bites do not introduce toxins into the victim. Some shrews have a venom in their saliva, but their small size and secretive habits minimize their threat to human health. Bites from mammals are also of minimal concern with respect to dangerous allergic responses. Physical damage is also the most serious problem in shark and moray eel bites.

Prevention, by avoiding animals prone to bite, is usually readily accomplished. Treatment involves stopping the bleeding, repairing the damage, and preventing infection.

Bites introducing infectious agents. Bites that cause serious physical damage are not the only ones that can introduce infectious agents. Any bite or sting can introduce infection to the victim because it penetrates the first line of defense, the skin. The arthropods are the most important disease vectors. Malaria is caused by a parasitic protozoan (single-celled, animal-type organism) transferred from one host to another by mosquitoes. Lyme disease is caused by a bacterium and is transported between hosts by ticks. Viruses cause yellow fever, and mosquitoes transport the virus to new hosts. Insects and ticks are vectors for a number of other diseases, most of which are introduced to the victim by a bite (including the stabs of blood-sucking arthropods such as mosquitoes).

Prevention of these diseases involves avoiding and/or eliminating the vectors; neither is always possible. Active immunization (stimulating the host to form antibodies

---

Information on Bites and Stings

Causes: Bite or wound from an organism
Symptoms: Bleeding, swelling, infection, allergic response
Duration: Temporary or acute
Treatments: Immunization, drug therapy (antivenin, adrenaline, antihistamines)

---

against the disease-causing organism) is also used when available. Treatment involves drugs that destroy the disease organism or the use of passive immunization (the injection of preformed antibodies against the disease organism).

Bites and stings introducing toxins. Toxins or poisons are introduced to the victim most often by arthropods (scorpion stings, spider bites), cnidarians (stings), or reptiles (bites). Some mollusks-the cone shell snails, for example-can also inject toxins into a victim. The chemicals involved include enzymes that destroy tissue, neurotoxins that interfere with appropriate nerve cell responses (blocking or stimulating nerve cell signals), and others that interfere with the normal functions of the victim's body chemistry. Rattlesnakes and their relatives, coral snakes, and the Gila monster (a large lizard) are examples of poisonous reptiles. The brown recluse and black widow spiders are dangerous examples of their group. The sea wasp (a jellyfish) and the Portuguese man-of-war are the best known, but by no means the only, dangerous cnidarians in coastal waters off North America.

Prevention involves avoiding the animals that inject the toxin, which is easily accomplished much, but not all, of the time. Treatment involves injection of antivenin, a solution of antibodies that neutralize a specific toxin. Research on snake antivenin indicates that it might be possible to create a single antivenin that inactivates several snake venoms.

Bites and stings causing allergic reactions. Any bite or sting can cause an allergic response in the victim, because all introduce large foreign molecules, called antigens. These are often proteins, and they stimulate a response in the victim's immune system. If the response is more than that needed to destroy the antigen, it is called an allergic response and the foreign protein is called an allergen. The allergic response may simply be a nuisance causing minor inflammation, but it is exceptionally dangerous if it escalates into anaphylaxis. Anaphylaxis is a hyperreaction to a foreign substance in which the heart rate increases; bronchioles in the lungs constrict, making breathing difficult; and blood pressure drops. If symptoms continue, the victim may go into shock and even die. The toxins introduced by venomous arthropods, reptiles, cnidarians, and mollusks are often allergenic, even causing anaphylaxis, but even nonpoisonous or minimally toxic materials such as the venom introduced in a bee or wasp sting can cause life-threatening anaphylactic shock in sensitive people. A painful sting for people not sensitized to the foreign material becomes a threat to the life of a sensitized, hypersensitive person.

Prevention, by avoiding the allergen, is the preferred defense against allergic reactions. If avoidance is not possible or cannot be assured, the injection of small amounts of the substance to which an individual is hypersensitive, followed by increasingly larger doses, is sometimes effective in desensitizing the individual. Treatment of severe anaphylactic reactions involves the injection of adrenaline. Antihistamines, taken orally or injected, are used in less severe situations.

—*Carl W. Hoagstrom, Ph.D.*

See also: Allergies; Chagas' disease; Dengue fever; Emergency medicine; Encephalitis; Epidemiology; First aid; Immune system; Infection; Insect-borne diseases; Leishmaniasis; Lice, mites, and ticks; Lyme disease; Malaria; Parasitic diseases; Plague; Poisoning; Rabies; Rocky Mountain spotted fever; Shock; Sleeping sickness; Snakebites; Toxicology; Tropical medicine; Yellow fever; Zoonoses.

For Further Information:

Dossenbach, Hans D. *Beware! We Are Poisonous! How Animals Defend Themselves*. Woodbridge, Conn.: Blackbirch Press, 1999. Dossenbach examines some of the world's most poisonous animals and shatters some myths about creatures long perceived as dangerous. Includes a bibliography.

Foster, Steven, and Roger A. Caras. *A Field Guide to Venomous Animals and Poisonous Plants: North America, North of Mexico*. Boston: Houghton Mifflin, 1994. Containing excellent information and bright color pictures, and written for an easy understanding, this book should be in any nature enthusiast's library.

Halstead, Bruce W., and Paul S. Auerbach. *Dangerous Aquatic Animals of the World: A Color Atlas*. Princeton, N.J.: Darwin Press, 1992. Spectacular gallery of animals as diverse as polar bears and sea anemones. A natural history of the envenomation, or wounding apparatus, with slight detail on range, and none on life cycles. The excellent color photos are augmented by fine drawings of the anatomy of the dangerous parts of animals.

Harvey, Alan L., ed. *Snake Toxins*. New York: Pergamon Press, 1991. Discusses various topics, such as immunology of snake toxins, dendrotoxins, the structure and pharmacology of elapid cytotoxins, the influence of snake venom proteins on blood coagulation, and amino acid sequences and toxicities of snake venom components. Includes an index.

Krohmer, Jon R., ed. *American College of Emergency Physicians First Aid Manual*. 2d ed. New York: DK, 2004. A comprehensive guide that details the treatment and techniques, in text and photographically, of a range of emergencies. Bites and stings are covered specifically.

Nagami, Pamela. *Bitten: True Medical Stories of Bites and Stings*. New York: St. Martin's Press, 2004. Nagami describes strange and often gruesome true cases of bites and stings, resulting infections, and treatments.

Silverstein, Alvin, et al. *Bites and Stings*. New York: Scholastic, 2002. A young adult book that covers information about bites and stings from insects, pets, wild animals, sea creatures, and plants. Body reactions, transmittable diseases, treatment, and protection are also covered.

Spiders and Other Arachnids. http://spiders.ucr.edu. Site provides links to information about the spider, scorpion, bee, wasp, and ant species worldwide whose bites cause morbidity and mortality.

Tu, Anthony T., ed. *Reptile Venoms and Toxins*. New York: Marcel Dekker, 1991. In twenty-four contributed chapters, thirty-seven international specialists describe the latest developments in research on snake venom-including different types of venoms and toxins, actions, antidotes, and applications-and summarize what is known to date on Gila monster and frog toxins.

Bladder cancer
Disease/Disorder

Also known as: Bladder malignancy, bladder carcinoma, urothelial cancer, urothelial carcinoma

Anatomy or system affected: Bladder, urinary system

Specialties and related fields: Oncology, urology

Definition: Cancer that forms in tissues of the bladder, including transitional cell carcinomas (cancers that form in cells in the innermost tissue layer of the bladder), which account for about 90 percent of all bladder cancer cases; squamous cell carcinomas (cancers that begin in flat cells lining the bladder); and adenocarcinomas (cancers that begin in cells that release fluids). In 2002, 357,000 new cases and 145,000 deaths were attributed to the disease worldwide.

Key terms:

Bacillus Calmette-Guérin (BCG): an inactive strain of *Mycobacterium bovis* that stimulates the immune system in nonspecific ways

bladder: the muscular, membranous, hollow organ that stores urine and is located in the front of the pelvic cavity; also called the vesica urinaria

cystoscope: a thin, tubelike instrument used to look inside the bladder and urethra; has a light and a lens for viewing and usually equipped with a tool to remove tissue

cystoscopy: examination of the bladder and urethra using a cystoscope inserted through the urethra and into the bladder

urothelial: pertaining to a layer of cells that line the bladder and some other organs of the urinary system

Causes and Symptoms

The symptoms of bladder cancer are the presence of blood in the urine, pain and burning during urination, frequent urination, and pelvic pain. Urinary tract infections create the same symptoms, but the presence of a tumor or tumors distinguishes bladder cancer from an infection. Tumors can be imaged by cystography, ultrasound, computed tomography (CT) or magnetic resonance imaging (MRI) scans, and cystoscopy. Occasionally, a mass is conspicuous upon manual examination. If any of these procedures suggest the presence of a tumor, then cystoscopy can confirm the diagnosis. During cystoscopy, a doctor looks inside the bladder with a cystoscope passed through the urethra and removes material for biopsy to determine whether malignant cells, which are diagnostic for cancer, are present. Frequently, malignant cells can be seen by microscopic examination of urine from patients with bladder cancer.

Although the precise cause of bladder cancer is not known, age, gender, and several environmental factors contribute to its occurrence. Bladder cancer affects mainly elderly people, with an average age at diagnosis of sixty-five to seventy years, and males are three to four times more likely to have this cancer than women. Cigarette smoking is reported to be the primary risk factor for the disease, and exposure to other carcinogens such as radiation, aromatic amines, and polycyclic aromatic hydrocarbons also increases risk. Chronic or frequent bladder infections can increase the risk of bladder cancer. Additionally, it appears that diets high in meat and fat increase the risk of bladder cancer. All these risk factors taken together suggest that irritations of the interior walls of the bladder play an important role in the development of this disease.

Treatment and Therapy

Appropriate treatment of bladder cancer depends on the severity of the disease. In the vast majority of cases, the tumors are superficial and can be removed completely by cystoscopic procedures. Even with complete removal, recurrences are likely, so patients are usually given an anticancer agent, which is instilled directly into the bladder. This can be a chemotherapeutic agent such as mitomycin C or doxorubicin, but often Bacillus Calmette-Guérin (BCG) is used. This inactivated bacterium stimulates the immune system and is thought to be the most effective preventative for future occurrences. Some studies have indicated, however, that high doses of vitamins A, B_6, and C and zinc are more effective at delaying recurrences than BCG treatment.

Patients with tumors that have invaded the muscles of the bladder wall usually require partial or total surgical removal of the bladder. A patient without a bladder will be provided with an alternate means of storing and removing urine. Some patients are given an external bag connected by a piece of intestine. Increasingly, patients whose bladders have been removed are provided with a neobladder, an internal reservoir built from intestinal tissue. These patients learn how to control the shape of this reservoir with their abdominal muscles in order to regulate the flow of urine. In this way, the neobladder works almost like a normal bladder.

Patients with inoperable cancers or whose cancer has spread to other parts of the body may benefit from chemotherapy, depending on their ability to tolerate the toxicity of the treatments. Doctors and patients evaluate the probable benefits to each individual before starting such a drug regimen.

Perspective and Prospects

The introduction of the cystoscope in 1877 by the German scientist Maximilian Nitze, who is called the founder of urology, initiated the first scientific studies of bladder cancer. This instrument allowed the first accurate morphological descriptions of tumors within the bladder and led directly to the ability to remove bladder tumors without invasive surgery. Although the yearly number of new cases of bladder cancer has increased in the late twentieth and early twenty-first centuries, the number of deaths has declined. This is in part a tribute to Nitze's genius.

Studies with bladder cancer in the 1890s were the first to show an association between environmental toxins and any cancer. These studies showed that people who worked with aniline dyes were more likely to develop bladder cancer.

Although smoking may be the primary risk factor for bladder cancer, and although the number of smokers is declining, the number of new cases of bladder cancer continues to increase. This leaves researchers with the idea that

---

Information on Bladder Cancer

Causes: Unknown; factors include advanced age, carcinogens (smoking, radiation), chronic or frequent bladder infections

Symptoms: Blood in the urine, pain and burning during urination, frequent urination, pelvic pain, and the presence of tumor(s)

Duration: Chronic

Treatments: Depends on severity; may include tumor removal, chemotherapy, Bacillus Calmette-Guérin bacterium, bladder removal

---

other environmental risk factors are becoming more important.

This increase in new cases of bladder cancer while treatment continues to improve has motivated an increasing emphasis on prevention. Many studies are under way to look at ways of preventing both the initial occurrence and recurrences of bladder cancer. Various studies have suggested that selenium supplementation and high-fiber diets, as well as megadoses of the vitamins mentioned above, may be beneficial. Other studies have pointed to environmental assaults to be avoided.

—*Lorraine Lica, Ph.D.*

See also: Bacillus Calmette-Guérin (BCG); Bladder removal; Cancer; Carcinogens; Chemotherapy; Cystoscopy; Hematuria; Oncology; Tumor removal; Tumors; Urinalysis; Urinary disorders; Urinary system; Urology.

For Further Information:
"Bladder Cancer." *American Cancer Society*, Jan. 17, 2013.
"Bladder Cancer." *MedlinePlus*, Apr. 10, 2013.
"Bladder Cancer Treatment." *National Cancer Institute*, 2013.
Calvagna, Mary, and Mohei Abouzied. "Bladder Cancer." *Health Library*, Nov. 15, 2012.
Dunetz, Gary N. *Bladder Cancer: A Resource Guide for Patients and Their Families*. Bloomington, Ind.: AuthorHouse, 2006.
Gillenwater, Jay Y., et al., eds. *Adult and Pediatric Urology*. 4th ed. Baltimore: Lippincott Williams & Wilkins, 2002.
Grossman, H. Barton, ed. "Contemporary Diagnosis and Management of Urothelial Carcinoma." *Urology* 67, no. 3, supp. S1 (March, 2006): 1-72.
Schoenberg, Mark P. *The Guide to Living with Bladder Cancer*. Baltimore: Johns Hopkins University Press, 2000.
Walsh, Patrick C., et al., eds. *Campbell-Walsh Urology*. 4 vols. 9th ed. Philadelphia: Saunders/Elsevier, 2007.

Bladder infections. *See* Urinary disorders.

Bladder removal

Procedure

Anatomy or system affected: Abdomen, bladder, urinary system

Specialties and related fields: General surgery, gynecology, proctology, urology

Definition: The surgical removal of the bladder and accompanying structures or organs.

Indications and Procedures

Cystectomy (bladder removal) is often the treatment of

Bladder Removal

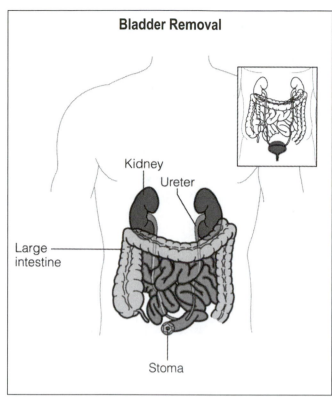

Kidney

Ureter

Large
intestine

Stoma

The removal of the bladder, usually as a result of cancer, necessitates the creation of a stoma, in which the ureters are connected to a section of small intestine, through which urine is voided from the body.

choice in cases of bladder cancer, which may be treated with chemotherapy or radiation in combination with surgery. The procedure, usually performed under general anesthesia, is carried out by making an incision in the abdomen, after which the ducts that carry urine from the bladder, called ureters, are cut and tied. The affected bladder is removed and, in men, the prostate gland is also excised. In women, the uterus, Fallopian tubes, and ovaries are removed along with the diseased bladder.

If an external bag will be used for urine storage, then a permanent opening is made in the abdomen. The two ureters are joined to a tiny section of small intestine that has been removed from the rest of the intestines, formed into a loop, and inserted through the abdominal wall. Urine is excreted through this opening, called a stoma. If an internal reservoir, called a neobladder, is to be created, then intestinal tissue will be used.

Uses and Complications

A cystectomy has serious consequences. In men, the result is usually impotence because the nerve tracts that permit penile erections are usually damaged severely by the surgery. In women, the outcome is infertility as a result of the combination of cystectomy and hysterectomy. Because most women who undergo the procedure have already experienced menopause, however, this consequence usually does not affect them adversely.

In addition to the complications from infection and systemic shock that can accompany any major surgery, cystectomy poses another problem: Following surgery and

for the remainder of a patient's life, either urine must be collected in a pouch that is worn externally or patients must learn to control the internal neobladder with their abdominal muscles. It takes some patients considerable time to adapt to such complications. Enterostomy therapists teach patients how to care for a stoma; patients are usually referred to these specialists following a cystectomy.

Some patients also experience problems with proper intestinal function in the days immediately following a cystectomy. This difficulty is overcome through the regular administration of a solution of saline fluids and glucose intravenously beginning soon after the surgery.

—*R. Baird Shuman, Ph.D.*

See also: Bladder cancer; Cancer; Cystoscopy; Hysterectomy; Oncology; Prostate gland removal; Urinalysis; Urinary disorders; Urinary system; Urology.

For Further Information:
Chalker, Rebecca, and Kristene E. Whitmore. *Overcoming Bladder Disorders*. New York: HarperCollins, 1990.
Droller, Michael J. *Bladder Cancer: Current Diagnosis and Treatment*. Totowa, N.J.: Humana Press, 2001.
Droz, Jean-Pierre, and Riccardo A. Audisio. *Management of Urological Cancers in Older People*. London: Springer, 2013.
Ellsworth, Pamela, and Brett Carswell. *One Hundred Questions and Answers About Bladder Cancer*. Sudbury, Mass.: Jones and Bartlett, 2006.
Guyton, Arthur C., and John E. Hall. *Guyton and Hall Textbook of Medical Physiology*. 12th ed. Philadelphia: Saunders/Elsevier, 2011.
Humes, H. David, et al., eds. *Kelley's Textbook of Internal Medicine*. 4th ed. Philadelphia: Lippincott Williams & Wilkins, 2000.
Lokeshwar, Vinata B., Axel S. Merseburger, and Stefan H. Hautmann. *Bladder Tumors: Molecular Aspects and Clinical Management*. New York: Humana Press, 2011.
Nilsson, William E. *Bladder Cancer: Etymology, Diagnosis, and Treatments*. Hauppauge, N.Y.: Nova Science, 2010.
Schoenberg, Mark P., et al. *The Guide to Living with Bladder Cancer*. Baltimore: Johns Hopkins University Press, 2001.
Wallace, Robert A., Gerald P. Sanders, and Robert J. Ferl. *Biology: The Science of Life*. 4th ed. New York: HarperCollins, 1996.
Walsh, Patrick C., et al., eds. *Campbell-Walsh Urology*. 4 vols. 9th ed. Philadelphia: Saunders/Elsevier, 2007.

Bladder stones. *See* Stone removal; Stones.

Bleeding
Biology/Anatomy

Anatomy or system affected: Blood, blood vessels, circulatory system

Specialties and related fields: Emergency medicine, family medicine, hematology, internal medicine, vascular medicine

Definition: Damage or disruption to hemostasis (the natural process of the body to stop bleeding) resulting in loss of blood or abnormal clotting.

Key terms:

coagulation: the sequential process by which multiple, specific factors (predominantly proteins in plasma) interact, ultimately resulting in the formation of an insoluble clot made of fibrin

fibrin: the insoluble protein that forms the essential portion of a blood clot; the soluble protein in plasma converted to fibrin is called fibrinogen

fibrinolysis: the process of dissolving clots; the fibrinolytic system dissolves fibrin through enzymatic action

hemostasis: the arrest of bleeding from injured blood vessels, confining circulating blood to those vessels; blood vessels, platelets, the coagulation system, and the fibrinolytic system contribute to the process of hemostasis

plasma: the fluid portion of blood in which the particulate components are suspended; the majority of coagulation factors are proteins in plasma

platelets: disk-shaped structures in blood that are vital for the maintenance of normal hemostasis

vitamin K: a group of fat-soluble vitamins that play an integral role in the production of multiple, properly functioning coagulation factors by the liver

Causes and Symptoms

Patients with bleeding abnormalities are commonly encountered in medicine. Such patients may be evaluated because of previous episodes or a family history of bleeding disorders. Often these abnormalities are detected during preliminary studies before surgery or other invasive procedures. Bleeding manifestations can be described as local or generalized. It is important to distinguish between these two possibilities because the causes and treatment may be different. The evaluation of patients with suspected bleeding disorders includes a detailed medical history, a thorough physical examination, and appropriate screening tests for hemostatic functioning. Bleeding may result from disruption in the appropriate interactions among blood cells (platelets), proteins (clotting factors), and blood vessels.

Inherited disorders. There are numerous inherited disorders of hemostasis. Fortunately, most are quite rare. The two most common inherited bleeding disorders are von Willebrand's disease and hemophilia A. Inherited bleeding disorders usually become evident in infancy or early childhood. There is often a family history of abnormal bleeding, and abnormal bleeding may have been experienced in association with surgery or trauma. Bleeding from the umbilical cord at birth or bleeding following circumcision may provide evidence of inherited hemostatic disorders. There are, however, some exceptions. For example, Ehlers-Danlos syndrome or hereditary hemorrhagic telangiectasia may not become evident until later in life.

Family history is helpful in the evaluation of hemostatic disorders because a pattern of bleeding among family members may be revealed. If only male members of a family are affected, this suggests an X-linked recessive pattern of inheritance (transmitted by the X sex chromosome). Such diseases are usually transmitted from females who are carriers of the trait. Hemophilia A, hemophilia B, and Wiskott-Aldrich syndrome are transmitted as X-linked recessive traits. Inherited bleeding disorders such as von Willebrand's disease occur in both sexes through non-sex-linked, or autosomal, transmission. Some bleeding disorders occur because of a gene mutation. Some individuals, therefore, are the first members of their family to have an inherited bleeding disorder.

Information on Bleeding

Causes: Injury, disease, inherited disorders, medications, nutritional deficiency

Symptoms: Local (bleeding pinpointed to specific body part) or generalized (abnormal bleeding at multiple, distinct sites)

Duration: A few minutes to chronic

Treatments: Surgery, drug therapy

Acquired disorders. These may first become evident in adulthood; however, there are also some exceptions. For example, Idiopathic thrombocytopenic purpura (ITP) is an acquired hemostatic abnormality that may occur in childhood usually as a result of an infection. Some medical conditions such as kidney and liver disease may be associated with bleeding abnormalities for numerous reasons such as decrease in plasma coagulation factors or abnormal platelet function. Vitamin K is necessary for the production of numerous functional plasma coagulation factors in the liver. A deficiency of vitamin K as seen in cases of poor nutrition may lead to abnormal bleeding. Another source of vitamin K is bacteria located in the gastrointestinal (GI) tract. Antibiotic use can cause bacteria to die leading to vitamin K deficiency as well. Oral anticoagulant therapy (warfarin therapy), which is used in the treatment of blood clots in the legs, causes a reduction of functional vitamin K dependent coagulation factors and is a common cause of drug-induced bleeding.

Diagnosis by type of bleeding. In diagnosis, the type of abnormal bleeding may provide important clues. In vascular or platelet abnormalities, bleeding typically occurs in the skin or mucous membranes.

Petechiae, small, red spots about the size of a pinhead, represent tiny hemorrhages from small blood vessels, such as capillaries. These spots are a sign of platelet or vascular abnormalities.

Ecchymoses (bruises) are larger lesions caused by the leakage of blood into tissue of the skin or mucous membranes, usually as the result of trauma. Ecchymoses can be seen with all hemostatic disorders. Spontaneous ecchymoses, bruises appearing in the absence of prior trauma, may be a sign of a hemostatic problem.

Hematomas are collections of blood that accumulate in organs, body spaces, or tissues. They produce deformity of the area in which they develop and may be quite painful. Hematomas tend to be associated with abnormalities in the coagulation mechanism, such as hemophilia. Bleeding into joint spaces is known as hemarthrosis and it may be seen in hemophilia.

Telangiectases and angiomata, caused by vascular malformations, are red spots or patches caused by the presence of blood in abnormally dilated vessels. Unlike the other lesions previously discussed, these vascular lesions blanch with pressure.

Epistaxis (nose bleeding) is most frequently caused by mild trauma (for example, nose blowing) to dilated vessels of the nose in individuals with normal hemostasis.

First Aid for Trauma-Related Bleeding

1. Press hard over the wound. If necessary, pinch the wound edges together with fingers and thumb. Maintain pressure for at least 10 minutes.

2. Lay the patient down to elevate the bleeding area (this reduces the area blood flow).

Never move a part which may be fractured.

3. Replace the hand pressure with pressure from a pad held firmly in place by a tight bandage or by whatever is at hand: stockings, belts, socks, handkerchiefs, ties.

4. If blood appears to be oozing through, do not investigate by removing the bandage already applied; instead apply additional pressure with more padding and bandage. Continue this procedure until control is achieved.

5. Apply antishock measures, as necessary. Get medical aid.

Epistaxis in the setting of bleeding disorders is often associated with low platelet counts, the vascular abnormality called hereditary hemorrhagic telangiectasia, and von Willebrand's disease. Epistaxis consistently occurring on one side may be the result of a local abnormality, as opposed to a generalized hemostatic defect.

Laboratory tests. Laboratory evaluation of hemostatic functioning consists of screening tests, to aid in the detection of abnormalities, and confirmatory tests, to characterize the disorders. Microscopic examination of a blood smear is a simple screening procedure that may provide valuable information.

The automated platelet count and bleeding time are screening tests for the evaluation of platelets. A representative normal range for the platelet count is 150,000 to 400,000 platelets per microliter of blood; however, the risk of life-threatening hemorrhage does not markedly increase until the platelet count drops below 10,000 per microliter. A representative normal range for the bleeding time is four to seven minutes. A prolonged bleeding time may be a sign of a platelet or vascular abnormality.

The plasma coagulation system is composed primarily of a set of proteins that interact to produce clotting of blood. Most plasma coagulation factors are identified by a roman numeral (for example coagulation factor VIII). For ease of analysis, the plasma coagulation system has been divided into groups of proteins known as the intrinsic pathway, the extrinsic pathway, and the final common pathway. Screening tests for the plasma coagulation system include the thrombin time (TT), the prothrombin time (PT), and the activated partial thromboplastin time (aPTT). The screening tests detect significant deficiencies or abnormalities of plasma coagulation factors and help localize the defects within the pathways.

Specific, and often more complex, laboratory studies of hemostasis are performed based on information derived from the medical history, physical examination, and screening laboratory tests. The goal of specific tests is to pinpoint the diagnosis of hemostatic abnormalities.

Platelet disorders. Thrombocytopenia, a low platelet count in the blood, has numerous causes. Platelets are produced in the bone marrow and subsequently released into the blood. Bone marrow damage may result in inadequate numbers of platelets. Drugs, toxins, radiation, and infections may damage the bone marrow. Certain diseases, such as leukemia or other cancers, may lead to the replacement of bone marrow cells with abnormal cells or fibrous tissue. Some diseases result in inadequate release of platelets from the bone marrow. Inadequate platelet release may be the result of nutritional deficiencies, such as vitamin B12 or folic acid deficiencies, or it can be seen in some rare hereditary disorders, such as May-Hegglin anomaly or Wiscott-Aldrich syndrome. Individuals with an enlarged spleen may develop thrombocytopenia because of the pooling of platelets within the organ. Massive transfusion may result in thrombocytopenia when the blood volume is replaced with transfused solutions that do not contain platelets.

Certain disorders result in the rapid destruction or con-

Arterial Pressure Points

sumption of platelets. If the production of platelets by the bone marrow does not compensate for the rate of destruction, thrombocytopenia occurs. Platelet consumption with resultant thrombocytopenia is a component of disseminated intravascular coagulation (DIC). Thrombocytopenia caused by accelerated destruction may also occur with prosthetic heart valves, blood infections (sepsis), and vascular defects called hemangiomas. The development of antibodies against one's own platelets (such as with ITP) causes platelet consumption. ITP can be a self-limited disorder with a complete return to normal (acute ITP) or a prolonged thrombo- cytopenic condition (chronic ITP). Acute ITP is seen most frequently in children between two and six years of age. The disease is preceded by a viral infection in about 80 percent of cases. The platelet count returns to normal within six months in more than 80 percent of patients; the usual period of thrombocytopenia is four to six weeks. Mortality from acute ITP occurs in about 1 percent of cases. Chronic ITP typically occurs in young and middle-aged adults, and the disorder is about three times more common in females than in males. As many as 50 percent of children born to mothers with ITP have thrombocytopenia at birth as a result of the transfer of antiplatelet antibodies across the placenta. Isoimmune neonatal thrombocytopenia and posttransfusion purpura are other conditions in which thrombocytopenia is caused by antiplatelet antibodies.

Numerous drugs have been associated with thrombocytopenia. Examples of such drugs include gold salts, quinine, quinidine, sulfonamide drugs, and heparin. Thrombocytopenia may occur within twenty-four hours following exposure to an offending drug. All nonessential medications should be discontinued in patients suspected of having drug-induced thrombocytopenia.

Platelet function defects may be inherited or acquired. They may occur without evidence of an associated disease or be secondary to a recognizable clinical disorder. Platelet function defects are suspected when there is abnormal skin or mucous membrane bleeding, a prolonged bleeding time, and a normal platelet count. Bleeding disorders caused by the inability of platelets to stick to damaged blood vessel walls in a normal manner are called platelet adhesion defects; Bernard-Soulier syndrome and von Willebrand's disease are examples of such defects.

Certain molecules necessary for normal platelet function are contained within platelets (that is, in the storage pool). Deficiencies or defects of these molecules lead to platelet dysfunction and are called storage pool defects. Examples of storage pool defects include gray platelet syndrome and dense granule deficiency. Platelet release defects occur when there is a failure to release storage pool contents normally. Hereditary deficiency of the enzymes cyclo-oxygenase or thromboxane synthetase causes platelet release defects. Aspirin causes a platelet release defect by inactivating cyclo-oxygenase.

Disorders that render platelets unable to interact with one another to form large clumps at the site of vascular injury are known as platelet aggregation defects. Ganzmann's thrombasthenia and hereditary afibrinogenemia are examples of such defects.

Platelets also play a key role in secondary hemostasis by providing a surface on which many coagulation factors can interact. A bleeding disorder results if the platelet surface is incapable of supporting secondary hemostasis. Hereditary bleeding disorders caused by this type of platelet defect are quite rare.

Acquired platelet dysfunction is quite common. Renal failure (uremia) may cause acquired platelet dysfunction. Liver disease can cause multiple bleeding abnormalities, including platelet dysfunction. A vast number of drugs and medications, such as aspirin and penicillin, cause platelet dysfunction. Acquired platelet function defects are seen with cardiopulmonary bypass procedures and in association with numerous blood diseases.

Coagulation disorders. The overall incidence of inherited coagulation factor disorders is about 1 in 10,000. In such conditions, either there is a failure to make a sufficient amount of a coagulation factor (quantitative disorder), or a dysfunctional factor is made (qualitative disorder). An inherited disorder exists for every coagulation factor, although most are quite rare. Symptoms range from serious spontaneous bleeding, which occurs in the severe forms of hemophilia A (factor VIII disorder) or hemophilia B (factor IX disorder), to an absence of abnormal bleeding in other inherited conditions (factors XII, prekallikrein, and high molecular weight kininogen). In general, for disorders which cause bleeding, the more profound the coagulation factor defect, either quantitatively or qualitatively, the more severe the bleeding. Severe disorders are usually easily identified. Moderate or mild disorders are more common and may go undetected until there is a significant hemostatic challenge, such as surgery.

Von Willebrand's disease is probably the most common inherited bleeding disorder. It is caused by deficiencies or defects in a vital group of hemostatic proteins known collectively as von Willebrand factor. Manifestations include epistaxis, menorrhagia, prolonged bleeding after trauma or surgery, frequent ecchymoses, and persistent gum bleeding. Severe episodes of epistaxis may occur during childhood, and such episodes may cease during puberty. In women, epistaxis may recur after menopause. Important diagnostic clues include a family history of abnormal bleeding, affected members in every generation (males and females), and marked worsening of bleeding following the ingestion of aspirin or other drugs that impair platelet function. Von Willebrand's disease consists of a very diverse spectrum of abnormalities: At least twenty-one distinct subtypes of von Willebrand's disease have been recognized.

Hemophilia A and hemophilia B are clinically indistinguishable; laboratory testing is required for their diagnosis. Hemophilia A is described here. Hemophilia A is an inherited disorder of a portion of coagulation factor VIII. Hemophilia A is typically seen in males, while females are carriers of the abnormal gene and can transmit the disease. Twenty percent of affected individuals have a negative family history and likely developed their disease because of a mutation of the factor VIII gene. Once the abnormal gene is established in a family, the severity of the disease is the same for all affected males. Hemophilia A is divided into severe, moderate, and mild subtypes based on the amount of functional factor VIII present. Bleeding in hemophiliacs may be spontaneous or posttraumatic. Spontaneous bleeding tends to occur only in severe hemophilia. It characteristically affects joints and muscles, and it may lead to crippling injury without prompt and adequate treatment. Posttraumatic bleeding may occur in mild, moderate, or severe hemophilia A. Such episodes are often prolonged and dangerous. Bleeding into the head (intracranial bleeding) remains a common cause of severe disability and death in hemophilia A. Modern treatment, however, has reduced the incidence of this severe complication. Antibodies (inhibitors) directed against factor VIII develop in approximately 12 to 15 percent of patients who require transfusions to provide factor VIII. The development of inhibitors is a serious complication that may compromise the effectiveness of therapy. Factor VIII inhibitors may occur in nonhemophiliacs, leading to serious bleeding in affected males and females.

Acquired coagulation factor disorders may be caused by reduced or absent factor production (for example, in liver disease), the production of defective or inactive factors (such as in liver disease or vitamin K deficiency), factor inhibitors, or accelerated consumption or clearance of factors. Examples in the latter group include DIC (accelerated consumption), kidney disease (factors lost in the urine), and the attachment of factors to abnormal tissue, which occurs in a disease called amyloidosis.

DIC is a hemostatic disorder that arises as part of a disease or medical condition. Examples of associated conditions include obstetrical accidents, abnormal destruction of red blood cells within blood vessels, infections, malignancies, burns, severe injuries, liver disease, and diseases of blood vessels. DIC may be an explosive, life-threatening syndrome (high-grade DIC) or a troublesome, less dramatic feature of a disease (low-grade DIC). Conditions associated with DIC cause abnormal activation of the hemostatic response, resulting in the widespread formation of blood clots in the vascular system. The clots obstruct the blood supply to vital organs (the kidneys, heart, lungs, and brain), leading to impaired organ function. Abnormal bleeding may develop if coagulation factors and platelets become depleted because of their incorporation into widespread blood clots. The breakdown of blood clots may also become inadequately controlled and contribute further to abnormal bleeding.

Perspective and Prospects

The existence of bleeding disorders has been known for many centuries. Abnormal bleeding observed in the males of certain families was described in the Jewish Talmud in the second century. Interest in such disorders increased markedly with the discovery of hemophilia in the royal families of Europe. In 1853, Queen Victoria gave birth to her fifth son, Leopold. She was a carrier of hemophilia, and Leopold had the disease. He died of a brain hemorrhage following a minor blow to the head at the age of thirty-one. Two of Victoria's daughters gave birth to affected sons. Her granddaughter, Alexandra, became the czarina of Russia, and Alexandra's only son, Alexis, suffered from hemophilia.

The transformation of fluid blood to a solid mass has fascinated investigators since ancient times. Aristotle noted that blood contained fibers and, upon cooling, solidified. He also observed that "diseased" blood did not solidify.

The realization that blood clotting minimized blood loss from wounds occurred in the early eighteenth century. In the late eighteenth century, William Hewson described the clotting time of whole blood. He found it to be shortened in some diseases and infinite in one woman after delivering a baby. In 1863, work published by Lord Joseph Lister laid the foundation for the discovery of the intrinsic pathway of coagulation. In 1905, Paul Morawitz, aided by the discoveries of such investigators as Alexander Schmidt and Olof Hammarsten, proposed what is now called the classic theory of blood coagulation. This led to the characterization of the extrinsic pathway of coagulation. In 1964, the "cascade" (by Robert Macfarlane) and "waterfall" (by Earl Davie and Oscar Ratnoff) hypotheses of coagulation were proposed. These discoveries paved the way for much of the current understanding of coagulation.

Alfred Donné is credited with the first description of platelets, reported in 1842. In 1881, Giulio Bizzozero became the first author to use the term "blood platelets." Shortly thereafter, discoveries in the late nineteenth century highlighted the importance of platelets in normal hemostasis. In recent times, the study of platelets has intensified. A large volume of information on platelets and platelet function has accumulated since the 1960s.

The study of hemostasis is a relatively young discipline. Better understanding of interrelationships of endothelium, platelets, and coagulation factors in normal and abnormal hemostasis has also helped in designing medical treatments to prevent blood from clotting. Clots may form in venous or arterial vessels; however, there are significant differences between them. We already know that platelets are an important component of arterial clots (white clots). This explains why antiplatelets are used in combination with anticoagulants in the treatment of medical conditions characterized by the formation of clots in the arterial system such as in the case of myocardial infarction (MI) whereas they are not indicated in the treatment of deep venous thrombosis (DVT). Aspirin is a widely used antiplatelet. Plavix (Clopidrogrel) can be used as a substitute for aspirin in cases of allergy or intolerance. However, Plavix has also proved to be helpful in patients with coronary artery disease (CAD) undergoing stenting.

—*James R. Stubbs, M.D.;*
updated by Rupinder P. Kaur, D.O. and Angel Perez, M.D.

See also: Anemia; Blood and blood disorders; Blood vessels; Circulation; Concussion; Disseminated intravascular coagulation (DIC); Ebola virus; Emergency medicine; First aid; Healing; Hematology; Hematology, pediatric; Hematomas; Hematuria; Hemophilia; Hemorrhage; Intraventricular hemorrhage; Nosebleeds; Shock; Thrombocytopenia; Transfusion; Vascular medicine; Viral hemorrhagic fevers; Von Willebrand's disease; Wiskott-Aldrich syndrome.

For Further Information:
Bick, Roger L. *Disorders of Thrombosis and Hemostasis: Clinical and Laboratory Practice.* 3rd ed. Philadelphia: Lippincott Williams & Wilkins, 2002. An excellent introduction to the diagnosis and management of clotting and bleeding disorders.

Colman, Robert W., et al., eds. *Hemostasis and Thrombosis: Basic Principles and Clinical Practice*. 5th ed. Philadelphia: Lippincott Williams & Wilkins, 2006. This is the bible in the study of hemostasis. An extensive and comprehensive reference textbook that deserves a spot on the bookshelf of all those involved with hemostasis.

Dahlback, Bjorn. "Blood Coagulation." *The Lancet* 355, no. 9215 (May 6, 2000): 1627-1632. Discusses the coagulation pathway and the role of thrombin in the clotting cascade. Also covers disturbances of the natural balance between the procoagulant and anticoagulant systems due to genetic or acquired factors.

Grogan, Tracy A. "Bringing Bloodless Surgery into the Mainstream." *Nursing* 29, no. 11 (November, 1999): 58-61. Grogan discusses how bloodless surgery can benefit a patient who objects to transfusions for religious reasons. Bloodless surgery means that surgeons use all available alternatives to minimize blood loss, salvage as much of the patient's blood as possible, and treat the patient with pharmaceuticals to maximize blood production.

Harmening, Denise M., ed. *Clinical Hematology and Fundamentals of Hemostasis*. 5th ed. Philadelphia: F.A. Davis, 2009. A technical work designed for professionals in the field.

Lichtman, Marshall, et al., eds. *Williams Manual of Hematology*. 7th ed. New York: McGraw-Hill, 2006. An accessible handbook that covers the pathogenetic, diagnostic, and therapeutic essentials of blood cell and coagulation protein disorders.

Owen, Charles A., E.J. Walter, and John H. Thompson. *The Diagnosis of Bleeding Disorders*. 2nd ed. Boston: Little, Brown, 1975. A classic in the field of hemostasis. Although this is a somewhat older work, much vital information on hemostasis can still be obtained from the text. The extensive chapter on the history of hemostasis is interesting reading.

Portyansky, Elena. "Drug Offers New Clotting Factor for Hard-to-Treat Hemophilia." *Drug Topics* 143, no. 9 (May 3, 1999): 25. A recently approved product, Novoseven (recombinant coagulation factor VIIa) from Novo Nordisk, holds promise for hemophilia A or B patients with inhibitors to coagulation factors VIII or IX.

Ratnoff, Oscar D., and Charles D. Forbes, eds. *Disorders of Hemostasis*. 3rd ed. Philadelphia: W. B. Saunders, 1996. A comprehensive textbook edited by two giants in the field of hemostasis. Although this is a detailed textbook, the authors cover various aspects of hemostasis in an organized and understandable manner.

Rodak, Bernadette, ed. *Hematology: Clinical Principles and Applications*. 3rd ed. St. Louis: Saunders/Elsevier, 2007. A comprehensive textbook covering all aspects of hematology and hemostasis.

Voet, Donald, and Judith G. Voet. *Biochemistry*. 3rd ed. Hoboken, NJ: John Wiley & Sons, 2004. An excellent general biochemistry book that contains a few sections on blood and blood components, their properties, and functions.

Blepharoplasty. *See* Face lift and blepharoplasty.

Blindness

Disease/Disorder
Anatomy or system affected: Eyes
Specialties and related fields: Geriatrics and gerontology, ophthalmology
Definition: The absence of vision, or its extreme impairment to the extent that activity is limited; about 95 percent of all blindness is caused by eye diseases, the rest by injuries.
Key terms:
glaucoma: excessive pressure inside the eye that can damage the optic nerve
laser: an intense light beam used in eye surgery

Information on Blindness

Causes: Eye injury, disease (especially glaucoma), aging process
Symptoms: Tunnel vision, black spots, pain, eventual loss of sight
Duration: Temporary to chronic
Treatments: Laser therapy, medication, surgery

---

macular degeneration: a deterioration of vision in the most sensitive, central region of the retina
retina: a paper-thin membrane lining the inside surface of the eyeball, where light is transformed into nerve impulses
trachoma: a contagious eye infection primarily found in the developing world

Causes and Symptoms

The major cause of blindness among older adults in the Western world is glaucoma. The aqueous fluid produced inside the eye fails to drain properly and causes pressure to build up. In extreme cases, the eyeball becomes hard. Without prompt treatment, the outer layer of the optic nerve starts to deteriorate. The patient can still see straight ahead but not off to the side. When the cone of forward vision has narrowed to less than 20 degrees (called tunnel vision), the patient is considered legally blind.

Cataracts are another common defect of vision among the elderly. The lens of the eye develops dark spots that interfere with light transmission. Cataracts are not caused by an infection or a tumor but instead are a normal part of the aging process, like gray hair. There is no known treatment to retard or reverse the growth of cataracts, though they may be surgically removed.

Macular degeneration and diabetes mellitus can cause blindness as a result of hemorrhages from tiny blood vessels in the retina. The macula is a small region in the middle of the retina where receptor cells are tightly packed together to obtain sharp vision for reading or close work. With aging, blood circulation in the macula gradually deteriorates until the patient develops a black spot in the center of the field of view. Advanced diabetes also causes blood vessel damage in the eye. In serious cases, fluid can leak behind the retina, causing it to become detached. The resulting visual effect resembles a dark curtain that blacks out part of the scene.

Trachoma is a blinding eye disease that afflicts millions of people in poor parts of the world. It is a contagious infection of the eyelid similar to conjunctivitis (commonly known as pinkeye). If untreated, it causes scarring of the cornea and eventual blindness. Trachoma is caused by a virus that is spread by flies, in water, or by direct contact with tears or mucus.

Many kinds of injuries may cause blindness. Car accidents, sports injuries, chemical explosions, battle wounds, and small particles that enter the eye all can result in a serious loss of vision.

In the News:
New Drugs for Age-Related Macular Degeneration and Other Visual Impairments

At the annual meeting of the Association for Research in Vision and Ophthalmology (ARVO) held in May, 2003, several research groups reported their research findings for promising new drugs being tested as possible treatments for neovascular macular degeneration (also called wet macular degeneration), a condition that has previously been resistant to drug therapy. Visual impairment occurs when new blood vessels grow into regions of the eye where they are normally absent. This growth process is known as angiogenesis.

Abnormal blood vessel growth specifically has been implicated in neovascular macular degeneration, diabetic retinopathy, neovascular glaucoma, and the retinopathy of prematurity. Angiogenesis is a multistep process with many regulatory points, and it thus provides many possible targets for drug action. Several different approaches that take advantage of recent advances in the understanding of the process of angiogenesis are being used to devise anti-angiogenesis drugs to treat wet macular degeneration.

One treatment approach makes use of an antibody that binds specifically to a growth factor called vascular endothelial growth factor (VEGF), which is required for blood vessel formation. One such antibody, called rhuFAB, has been tested on humans by injecting it into the vitreous. When it binds to VEGF, it should theoretically inactivate it and thus stop the growth of blood vessels that would interfere with vision. At the ARVO annual meeting, researchers from Genentech, where rhuFAB was developed, reported that in their clinical trials, rhuFAB was well tolerated and effective at improving vision or stabilizing vision loss in approximately 90 percent of patients with newly developed wet macular degeneration.

Other approaches that treat impaired vision caused by new blood vessel formation include inhibiting the action of VEGF with RNA molecules called aptamers; inhibiting the production of VEGF by antisense RNA; inhibiting enzymes required for angiogenesis, such as matrix metalloproteinases; preventing cell-cell interactions needed for angiogenesis; inhibiting angiogenesis with thalidomide; and making use of steroids, such as anecortave acetate, that block blood vessel formation.

—*Lorraine Lica, Ph.D.*

Treatment and Therapy

An indispensable tool in the treatment of serious eye problems is the laser. Its intense light focused into a tiny spot, the laser's heat can burn away a ruptured blood vessel or weld a detached retina back into place. For glaucoma patients, medication to reduce fluid pressure in the eye may be effective for a while. Eventually, a laser can be used to burn a small hole through the iris in order to improve fluid drainage. The laser can be used only to prevent blindness, however, and not to restore sight.

Cataracts formerly were a major cause of blindness among older people. Once the eye lens starts to become cloudy, nothing can be done to clear it. Cataract surgery to remove the defective lens and to insert a permanent, plastic replacement has become common. In the United States,

more than a million cataract surgeries are performed annually, with a success rate that is greater than 95 percent.

The infectious eye disease called trachoma has been known for more than two thousand years. Effective modern treatment uses sulfa drugs taken orally, combined with antibiotic eyedrops or ointments. Unfortunately, reinfection is common in rural villages where most people have the disease and sanitation is poor. The World Health Organization has initiated a public health program to teach parents about the importance of cleanliness and frequent eye washing with sterilized water for their children.

Perspective and Prospects

Various techniques have been developed for helping sightless people to live a self-reliant lifestyle. Using a white cane or walking with a trained dog allows a blind person to get around. Biomedical engineers have designed a miniature sonar device built into a pair of glasses that uses reflected sound waves to warn the wearer about obstacles.

The Braille system of reading, using patterns of raised dots for the alphabet, was invented in 1829 and is still widely used. For blind students, voice recordings of textbooks, magazines, and even whole encyclopedias are available on tape. A recent development is an optical scanner connected to a computer with a voice simulator that can read printed material aloud.

The National Federation of the Blind was founded in 1940. Its goals are to assist the blind to participate fully in society and to overcome the still-prevalent stereotype that the blind are helpless. Blind men and women hold jobs as engineers, teachers, musical performers, ministers, insurance agents, computer programmers, and school counselors. As society becomes more sensitive to all forms of disability, opportunities for blind people continue to expand.

—*Hans G. Graetzer, Ph.D.*

See also: Behçet's disease; Blurred vision; Cataract surgery; Cataracts; Color blindness; Diabetes mellitus; Eye infections and disorders; Eye surgery; Eyes; Glaucoma; Macular degeneration; Refractive eye surgery; Trachoma; Vision; Vision disorders.

For Further Information:

American Foundation for the Blind (AFB). *AFB*, 2013.

Buettner, Helmut, ed. *Mayo Clinic on Vision and Eye Health: Practical Answers on Glaucoma, Cataracts, Macular Degeneration, and Other Conditions*. Rochester, Minn.: Mayo Foundation for Medical Education and Research, 2002.

Johnson, Gordon J., et al., eds. *The Epidemiology of Eye Disease*. 2d ed. New York: Oxford UP, 2003.

Maurer, Marc. "Reflecting the Flame." *Vital Speeches of the Day* 57 (Sept. 1, 1991): 684-90.

MedlinePlus. "Cataract." *MedlinePlus*, Mar. 20, 2013.

MedlinePlus. "Vision Impairment and Blindness." *MedlinePlus*, Apr. 2, 2013.

Morrison, John C., and Irvin P. Pollack. *Glaucoma: Science and Practice*. New York: Thieme, 2003.

National Federation of the Blind. *NFB*, 2013.

Peninsula Center for the Blind. *The First Steps: How to Help People Who Are Losing Their Sight*. Palo Alto, Calif.: Peninsula Center, 1982.

Sardegna, Jill, et al. *The Encyclopedia of Blindness and Vision Impairment*. 2d ed. New York: Facts On File, 2002.

Westcott, Patsy. *Living with Blindness*. Austin, Tex.: Raintree, 2000.

Blindsight

Disease/Disorder

Anatomy or system affected: Visual perception, consciousness

Specialties and related fields: Neuroscience, psychology, cognitive neuroscience, neurology, optometry, ophthalmology

Definition: The ability of some patients with occipital cortex damage to respond at above chance levels to stimuli presented in their blind visual field.

Key terms:

forced-choice alternative paradigms: experimental methodology for demonstrating blindsight; patients must "guess" from a range of options (i.e., make a forced choice from a range of alternatives) regarding a specific stimulus property (e.g., location, direction of motion, etc.)

geniculostriate pathway: primary pathway for vision from the retina via the lateral geniculate nucleus of the thalamus and optic radiations to primary visual cortex (occipital cortex)

homonymous hemianopia: blindness in one half of visual space due to unilateral occipital cortex damage; hemianopic field defects occur in contralesional space; homonymous refers to the uniform nature of the field defect seen in some patients

implicit processing: demonstration of altered behavioral responses to a stimulus in the absence of conscious reportage

occipital cortex: posterior portion of the cortex with a retinotopic representation of visual space

retinotopic map: a one-to-one representation of visual space mapped onto the occipital cortex, i.e., specific portions of the retina that respond to specific regions of space are then mapped to a correspondingly specific region of the occipital cortex

Causes and Symptoms

Blindsight itself is not really a "symptom," but a residual ability in individuals who have suffered damage to the occipital cortex leading to a corresponding region of blindness. That is, the occipital cortex is organized retinotopically with specific regions of space being represented in specific portions of the occipital cortex and beyond (often referred to as the striate and extrastriate cortex). Damage to left hemisphere occipital cortex will lead to blindness for the right visual space and vice versa. The most common cause of such blindness is stroke, but any process that damages the occipital cortex will lead to blindness in a corresponding region of retinotopic space.

There are perhaps two common symptoms in cortically blind individuals that would hint at the presence of blindsight. The first is known as Riddoch's phenomenon in which the patient reports having a "sense" of motion in their blind field. It is important to note that the patient does not routinely report "conscious" perception of motion, but rather has a sense or "feeling" that something is moving in the blind field. Two-alternative forced choice testing can then demonstrate the veracity of such blind field motion

processing. Second, cortically blind patients may show themselves to be adept at obstacle avoidance even for stimuli appearing in their blind field. Casual observation of such obstacle avoidance does not represent proof of blindsight, as in an uncontrolled environment the patient could simply be utilizing learned strategies and eye movements to compensate for their blindness. As such, detailed testing controlling for a variety of factors, including eye movements, is needed to demonstrate true obstacle avoidance in the blind field.

Treatment and Therapy

Blindsight is not considered a "deficit" but rather a residual function. It has been used to demonstrate the presence of secondary visual pathways in the primate brain that transmit visual information from the retina to the extrastriate cortex without the need to first go through the occipital cortex. A variety of treatments have been tried for those suffering hemianopic field defects (with or without blindsight). These include the use of optical prisms intended to expand the patient's functional field of view and training to encourage patients to use intact abilities such as eye movements to compensate for their visual field loss. Finally, and more controversially, there have been attempts at restitution of vision following stimulation of the blind field. Here the patient is presented with repetitive visual stimuli at the border of their sighted and blind fields with the assumption that neuroplasticity will expand the functional visual fields of neurons in this "transition" region. Research on restitution of this kind has been mixed.

Perspective and Prospects

Blindsight was first demonstrated by Weiskrantz and colleagues in the early 1970s with a patient who could localize, by pointing or eye movements, targets presented to his blind field at better than chance levels. Since then, a wealth of research has demonstrated above chance responses to a wide range of blind field stimuli, although it should be noted that these demonstrations have been evident in a relatively small number of patients. Residual capacities range from target localization, motion, form and color discrimination, to semantic priming and even affective responses to nonconscious stimuli. These results have been taken to reflect the fact that there are multiple pathways for visual information to reach the cortex, some of which bypass the primary cortical target of the geniculostriate pathway-the primary occipital cortex (V1).

The notion that blindsight provided evidence for secondary visual pathways was initially challenged by Gazzaniga and colleagues as instead reflecting the activity of spared "islands" of intact cortex within the damaged hemisphere. In addition, Campion and colleagues suggested that light scatter-light from a blind field stimulus scattering into the sighted field, or light within the orbit scattering to regions of the retina that process sighted field stimuli-provided a more likely explanation for blindsight. However, more recent work using structural MRI (magnetic resonance imaging) and diffusion tensor imaging (which highlights white matter tracts in the human brain), as well as behavioral studies with appropriate controls for light scatter, have conclusively shown that blindsight does indeed rely upon secondary visual pathways that bypass V1.

Clearly, the geniculostriate visual pathway-or *primary visual pathway*-provides us with the rich mental representation of our visual world. What blindsight allows us to explore is the functionality of secondary pathways that rapidly transmit information to the cortex with little need for conscious processing. Our ability to rapidly respond to moving stimuli, avoid obstacles in our periphery, or even formulate a rapid response to emotionally valenced stimuli, may depend on these secondary networks to give a quick "first pass" neural analysis that can then be fed back to the slower acting primary visual pathway.

—*James Danckert, Ph.D.*

See also: Vision; Vision disorders

For Further Information:

Cowey, Alan. "The Blindsight Saga." *Experimental Brain Research* 200 (2010): 3-24.

Danckert, James, and Yves Rossetti. "Blindsight in Action: What Can the Different Sub-types of Blindsight Tell Us about the Control of Visually Guided Actions?" *Neuroscience and Biobehavioral Review* 29 (2005): 1035-1046.

Grunda, T., P. Marsalek, and P. Sykorova. "Homonymous Hemianopia and Related Visual Defects: Restoration of Vision after a Stroke." *Acta Neurobiologiae Expermentalis* 73 (2013): 237-249.

Striemer, C.L., C.S. Chapman, and Melvyn A. Goodale. "'Real-time' Obstacle Avoidance in the Absence of Primary Visual Cortex." *Proceedings of the National Academy of Sciences, USA* 106 (2009): 15996-16001.

Weiskrantz, Larry. "Blindsight Revisited." *Current Opinion in Neurobiology* 6 (1996): 215-220.

Blisters

Disease/Disorder
Also known as: Vesicles (small), bullae (large)
Anatomy or system affected: Skin
Specialties and related fields: Dermatology, family medicine, pediatrics
Definition: A local swelling of the skin that contains watery fluid and is usually caused by burning or irritation.

Causes and Symptoms

Blisters are fluid-filled lesions that can be caused by a variety of medical conditions or problems. They can be viral in origin, as in the case of chickenpox (also known as varicella), or they can arise because of irritants such as hot water or oil splashing on the skin. Blisters can also be caused by the friction of something rubbing against the skin, as in the case of an improperly fitting shoe.

A blister can range from painless to very painful. An individual with a blister will notice an area of the skin that is raised and filled with a clear liquid. The liquid inside the blister is typically sterile, which means that it does not contain bacteria. In some instances, as in chickenpox, the fluid may carry a virus. If the blister contains a virus, the virus spreads once the blister has ruptured or opened. Blisters can also contain blood, generally as the result of trauma that has

---

Information on Blisters

Causes: Viruses (varicella, herpes), irritation (hot liquids, friction), insect or spider bites, poisonous plants, trauma (heat or electrical burns), allergic contact (hives)
Symptoms: Raised area of skin filled with clear liquid and sometimes blood; may become red, warm, and painful
Duration: Acute
Treatments: None; if rupture occurs, topical antibiotic

---

caused a blood vessel to break. A blister can be singular, or they can occur in groups or clusters. If a group of blisters forms one larger blister, it is often referred to as a bulla.

Blisters are commonly located on the arms or legs. However, depending on the cause, they can be found on any part of the body.

Blisters that are very painful are usually associated with herpes 1 (cold sores), herpes 2 (genital herpes), and shingles (varicella-zoster virus). Other common causes of blisters are insect or spider bites, improperly fitting shoes, exposure to plants such as poison ivy or poison oak, trauma from heat or electrical burns, and hives resulting from allergic contact.

Impetigo is a staphylococcal (bacterial) infection of the skin that occurs commonly in children and is highly contagious. When the fluid within a blister becomes cloudy, this means that there is most likely a bacterial infection that needs to be treated with an antibiotic (by mouth or topical).

Treatment and Therapy

Prevention is the first step in the management of blisters. Blisters on the feet can be prevented by wearing properly fitting shoes and all-natural fiber (cotton or wool) socks, which minimizes friction. Since the fluid inside blisters is generally sterile, the best management is not to open the blister and instead to let it reabsorb into the skin. If the blister spontaneously opens, then it is best to keep the area clean and dry. A topical antibiotic can be used. If infection develops, then the area will become red, warm, and painful. Medical treatment, such as the administration of an antibiotic, should be sought. In the case of insect bites, an anti-itch medicine such as caladryl and/or an oral antihistamine (Benadryl) is useful to alleviate the itch. Scratching blisters or lesions can lead to a secondary infection, which may require an oral and/or topical antibiotic. Keeping the area clean and dry is another component of ensuring that the lesion will heal.

—*Rosslynn S. Byous, D.P.A., PA-C*

See also: Abscess drainage; Abscesses; Acne; Antibiotics; Bacterial infections; Boils; Burns and scalds; Chickenpox; Cold sores; Cysts; Dermatitis; Dermatology; Dermatopathology; Eczema; Frostbite; Gangrene; Hand-foot-and-mouth disease; Herpes; Impetigo; Insect-borne diseases; Lesions; Lice, mites, and ticks; Plague; Poisonous plants; Rashes; Scabies; Skin; Skin disorders; Smallpox; Staphylococcal infections; Sunburn.

For Further Information:

Graedon, Joe, and Theresa Graedon. *The People's Pharmacy Guide to Home and Herbal Remedies*. New York: St. Martin's Press, 2002.

Lanternier, Matthew L., and Karen Brannon. "Dermatology." In *University of Iowa: The Family Medicine Handbook*, edited by Mark A. Graber, Jennifer L. Jones, and Jason K. Wilbur. 5th ed. Philadelphia: Saunders/Elsevier, 2006.

Wolff, Klaus, Richard Allen Johnson, and Dick Suurmond. *Fitzpatrick's Color Atlas and Synopsis of Clinical Dermatology*. 6th ed. New York: McGraw-Hill Medical, 2009.

Blood and blood disorders

Disease/Disorder

Anatomy or system affected: Blood vessels, circulatory system, immune system, liver, lymphatic system

Specialties and related fields: Hematology, immunology, serology

Definition: The fluid that circulates in veins and arteries, carries oxygen and nutrients throughout the body, transports waste materials to excretory channels, and participates in the body's defense against infection.

Key terms:

blood: the fluid that circulates through the cardiovascular system; composed of a fluid and a cellular fraction that consists of erythrocytes, leukocytes, and thrombocytes

blood group system: a classification of individuals into groups based on the presence or absence of blood group antigens found on the surfaces of red blood cells

blood group antigen: glycolipid surface markers on the outer surface of red blood cell membranes that determine an individual's blood group; two main groups of blood surface antigens are called ABO (blood type A, B, AB, and O) and Rh (Rh-positive or Rh-negative)

blood typing: identification of surface blood group antigens of an individual for classification into specific blood groups

erythrocytes: red blood cells; non-nucleated, disk-shaped blood cells that contain hemoglobin

hemoglobin: oxygen-carrying red pigment present in red blood cells that is responsible for oxygen exchange in cells and tissues

leukocytes: white blood cells; any of the white or colorless nucleated cells that occur in blood

plasma: the protein-containing fluid portion of the blood in which blood cells are suspended

serum: the clear, yellowish fluid obtained from blood after it has been allowed to clot

thrombocytes: platelets; small, irregularly shaped cells in the blood that participate in blood clotting

Structure and Functions

Blood provides a common communication channel for all organs in the body. It is responsible for the transport of oxygen, enzymes, hormones, drugs, and many other substances, as well as for transfer of heat produced by chemical reactions in the body. The average-sized adult has about ten pints (~4.7 L) of blood. At rest, ten pints a minute (and up to forty pints during exercise) are pumped by the heart via the arteries to the lungs and other tissues, and returns to the heart through veins in a continuous circuit.

The Components of Blood

Blood consists of cells floating in a fluid called plasma. The cells that comprise blood include red blood cells, platelets, and white blood cells, with cells comprising about half the volume of whole blood. The remainder of the blood volume is comprised of plasma, which contains dissolved proteins, sugars, fats, and minerals. Red blood cells, also known as erythrocytes, contain hemoglobin, a protein that carries oxygen. Platelets are involved in blood clotting mechanisms. White blood cells, which are divided into

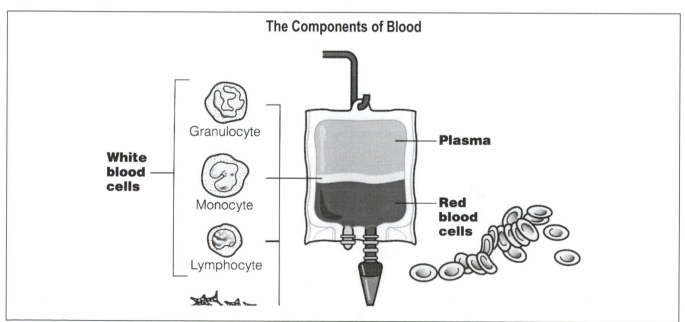

The Components of Blood

Blood consists of cells floating in a fluid called plasma. Red blood cells contain hemoglobin, an important substance that carries oxygen; platelets are involved in clotting mechanisms; and white blood cells, which are divided into granulocytes, monocytes, and lymphocytes, are responsible for the immune response to foreign matter.

granulocytes, monocytes, and lymphocytes, are the cells primarily responsible for the immune response.

All types of blood cells are formed in the bone marrow by divisions of a single cell called a hematopoietic stem cell. Red blood cells, or erythrocytes (from the Greek *eruthros*, "red"), are very small, have no nucleus, and require very little oxygen for survival. Red blood cells have a large surface area relative to their volume, which allows oxygen and carbon dioxide to diffuse in and out of the cell rapidly. This large surface also allows the cell to swell and shrink and to squeeze through narrow capillaries without shearing or bursting. Red blood cells cannot repair themselves, and after three or four months (roughly 120 days) in the circulation, they are eliminated by stationary phagocytic cells in the liver, spleen, and bone marrow, and replaced by the bone marrow. The main function of red blood cells is to transport oxygen by means of their enriched hemoglobin content; as such, they are among the most highly specialized cells in the body.

Hemoglobin, the red, iron-containing pigment responsible for the color of blood, has a great affinity for oxygen. It will release oxygen in a situation where free oxygen is scarce, such as in working tissues. Hemoglobin gives blood an oxygen-carrying capacity eighty times greater than if the oxygen were merely dissolved in plasma. When hemoglobin releases oxygen, it becomes capable of taking up carbon dioxide, which it carries back to the lungs. Hemoglobin occupies 33 percent of the red blood cell volume and accounts for 90 percent of its dry weight.

Leukocytes, or white blood cells (from the Greek *leukos*, meaning "clear" or "white"), are larger and less plentiful than red blood cells and can also be found in tissues. The purpose of white blood cells is to remove foreign material and to defend against microorganisms. Leukocytes travel through the circulatory system and can pass through the walls of blood vessels to carry out specific effector functions in surrounding tissues. White blood cells play an important role in defense against infection by viruses, bacteria, fungi, and parasites. There are three main populations of leukocytes: granulocytes, monocytes, and lymphocytes. Granulocytes, also known as polymorphonuclear (PMN) leukocytes, contain granules and have a segmented nucleus. There are three types of granulocytes: neutrophils, basophils, and eosinophils. The most abundant are the neutrophils, which are responsible for killing invading bacteria (pus consists largely of neutrophils). They are also called phagocytes ("engulfing cells") because of their ability to ingest bacteria and other foreign materials. In the absence of activation, neutrophils reside in the blood for only six to nine hours, but upon activation, they can move to sites of infection, or travel to tissues where they may survive a few more days. Eosinophils are involved in allergic reactions. Monocytes are also a type of phagocyte important in the immune system.

Lymphocytes participate in the adaptive immune response, such as the production of antibodies and rejection of tissue grafts. They play important roles in directing the activity of other cells involved in the immune response.

Lymphocytes become specialized against specific antigen in the lymph nodes. Lymphocytes live for longer periods of time, with their lifetime ranging between three months to several years. Unlike granulocytes and monocytes, lymphocytes do not engulf solid particles, or phagocytose, but instead play a part in producing antibodies and important immune hormones known as cytokines. An antibody is a protein that may be soluble in blood plasma or lymph and may affix to other cells. There are many different types of lymphocytes, each of which has a different function. T lymphocytes are responsible for delayed hypersensitivity phenomena and produce substances called lymphokines, a type of cytokine that affects the function of many cells. They also moderate the activity of other lymphocytes called B lymphocytes, cells which produce antibodies. Antibodies help kill or specifically mark foreign material so that it is more readily detected and eliminated by scavenger cells. Most B lymphocytes are in a state of surveillance to create an early warning system to detect foreign material. If these cells encounter foreign material that binds to specific molecular pattern detection receptors (known as Toll-like Receptors or TLRs) in their membranes, or receive such material from another cell, they move to a lymph node where they divide to produce daughter cells that manufacture antibodies specifically active against that foreign material. Natural killer, or NK cells, are also a type of lymphocyte with roles in direct killing of virus-infected cells.

Platelets are the smallest cells in blood; they can survive there for about nine days. They circulate in the blood in an inactive state, but under certain circumstances they begin to adhere to blood vessels and to each other, producing and releasing chemicals that initiate blood clotting. Platelets are critical in hemostasis, or stopping blood flow.

Plasma is the straw-colored fluid in which blood cells are suspended. It is composed mainly of water (95%), with a salt content similar to salt water. Other constituents comprising plasma include nutrients, waste products, proteins, and hormones. Nutrients, such as sugars, fats, vitamins, minerals, and amino acids, are transported to tissues after absorption from the intestinal tract or following release from storage in the liver. Among the proteins in plasma are substances such as fibrinogen (involved in coagulation), immunoglobulins and complement proteins (bacteria fighters that are part of the immune system), carrier proteins known as globulins, and albumin.

The term *blood group* refers to classification of blood according to differences in the makeup of its red blood cells. The ABO system consists of three blood group substances, the A, B, and H antigens (substances that induce production of an antibody when injected into an animal), which are components of erythrocyte surface substances. Individuals with type-A red blood cells carry anti-B antibodies in their serum; those with type-B red blood cells carry anti-A antibodies; those with type AB red blood cells (which bear both A and B antigens) carry neither anti-A nor anti-B antibodies; and type O individuals, whose red blood cells bear neither antigen, carry both anti-A and anti-B antibodies.

The transfusion of type A blood into a type B individual, for example, clumps together the transfused erythrocytes and results in an often-fatal blockage of blood vessels, which indicates the importance of blood typing before a transfusion is performed.

Another blood group system is based on the rhesus (or Rh) factor. The system involves several antigens, but the most important is called factor D. It is found in 85 percent of the population; those individuals are called Rh positive. If it is not present, the person is classified as Rh negative. Based on this system, individuals are therefore classified as O positive or AB negative, for example, based on their ABO and Rh blood groups. The main importance of the Rh group is during pregnancy. A Rh-negative woman who is pregnant with a Rh-positive baby may form antibodies against the baby's blood. Such women are given antibodies directed against factor D after delivery to prevent the development of anti-D antibodies, which would cause hemolytic disease of the newborn in successive Rh-positive infants. The transfusion of Rh-positive blood into a Rh-negative patient can cause a serious reaction if the patient has had a previous blood transfusion that contained the Rh antigen.

About four-hundred other antigens have been discovered, but they are widely scattered throughout the population and rarely cause transfusion problems. Only the ABO and the Rh blood group systems have major clinical importance. Blood typing is used to categorize blood for transfusion. Knowledge of blood group substances and of their inheritance has been useful for legal, historical, and medical purposes. The ABO blood groups are found in all people, but the frequency of each group varies with race and geographical distribution. This fact can aid anthropologists who are involved in investigating, for example, early population migrations. The blood group of an individual is determined by the genes inherited from his or her parents. Identification of a blood group can be used in a paternity case to establish that a man could not have been the father of a particular child, although it cannot be shown positively that a man is the father by blood grouping. Blood found at the scene of a crime can be typed and used to exclude suspects if the type does not match. Some blood groups are associated with particular disorders. For example, blood group A has been found to be more common in people suffering from cancer of the stomach, while group O is found more often in people suffering from peptic ulcers.

Disorders and Diseases

Blood tests can be used to ascertain on the health of major organs as well as respiratory functions, hormonal balance, the immune system, and metabolism. They can reveal not only blood cell abnormalities characteristic of some diseases but also healthy variations in blood induced by response to infections. Blood tests can be classified into three categories: hematological, biochemical, and microbiological tests. Hematological tests involve studying the components of blood itself by looking at the number, shape, size, and appearance of its cells, as well as by testing the function of clotting factors. The most important tests of this type are the blood count, blood smear, and blood-clotting tests. Biochemical tests examine at chemicals in the blood such as sodium, potassium, uric acid, urea, vitamins, gases, and drugs. In microbiological tests, blood is examined for microorganisms, such as bacteria, viruses and viral particles, fungi, and parasites, and for antibodies against them.

Known causes of blood disorders include genetic factors (an inherited or acquired abnormality in the production of some blood component), nutritional disorders (i.e., vitamin deficiency), infections by microorganisms, over- or under-production of certain immune cell types or immune factors; tumors (such as bone marrow cancer), poisons (carbon monoxide, lead, snake and spider venoms), drugs (which can produce blood abnormalities as a side effect), and radiation.

Abnormalities can occur in any of the blood components. Leukemias are disorders in which the number of white blood cells is abnormally high, and can arise from multiple cell types. Leukemias can arise from lymphocytes, such as acute or chronic lymphocytic leukemias, or from cells of the granulocyte lineage, such as acute or chronic myeloid leukemias. Overproduction of red blood cells can also occur and result in diseases such as polycythemia vera, an acquired blood disorder in which there is a defect in signaling that results in overproduction of red blood cells. Lymphomas are cancers of the lymph nodes or lymphatic system, and include Hodgkin's and non-Hodgkin's lymphomas. These types of cancers vary in their severity, available treatment options, and prognosis. In acquired immunodeficiency syndrome (AIDS), T lymphocytes are infected by the Human Immunodeficiency Virus (HIV), which results in immune dysfunction and increased risk for certain types of infections and cancers. Abnormal platelet numbers, or the lack of platelets, can lead to some types of bleeding disorders, such as hemophilia (inability of the blood to clot properly) or von Willebrand disease in which there is disruption of normal clotting processes. Unwanted clot formation (thrombosis) can occur from circumstances that over-activate the blood's clotting mechanisms. Probably the most common blood disorder is anemia, which results from a deficiency of hemoglobin and includes a corresponding reduction in the blood's oxygen-carrying capacity. Deficiencies of blood plasma proteins include hypoalbuminemia (albumin deficiency), and may indicate malnutrition or liver disease. Thalassemia is an inherited blood disorder characterized by less hemoglobin and fewer red blood cells than normal, resulting in anemia and fatigue and may require blood transfusions. Sickle cell anemia is an inherited condition in which there aren't enough healthy red blood cells to adequately distribute oxygen; in this condition, red blood cells are sticky and crescent shaped and don't flow easily through vessels.

Perspective and Prospects

Blood is a liquid of complex structure and vital functions

that has been considered the essence of life for centuries. There is no shortage of irrational or unscientific ideas about the supposed properties of human blood-one can speak of "blood brotherhood," "blood feuds," "blood relations," and of someone being "bloodthirsty."

The present medical understanding of blood has developed over the past two or three thousand years. The study of blood began in Egypt and Mesopotamia, around 500 BCE, and it moved to countries around the Mediterranean that had become intellectually active. Ancient Greek thinkers noted differences between arteries and veins and that blood moved through them. According to whether the heart, the liver, or the brain was thought to be the prime organ controlling the rest of the body, various functions were tentatively ascribed to blood, such as its relation to sleep, distribution of heat, and animation of the body. The Greek school of medicine became personified in Hippocrates who denied the widely accepted theory of the existence of spirits and proposed that the body followed natural laws. He presented the concept of body juices, or humors. There were four of them: blood, lymph or phlegm, yellow bile (or choler), and black bile (or melancholy), with blood being the most important one. The philosopher Aristotle accepted the humoral hypothesis. One of his pupils was Alexander the Great, whose military conquests spread Greek influence widely. A notable medical school developed in Alexandria, Egypt, and the ideas of Hippocrates and Aristotle were taught there. There was, however, a variation regarding blood; namely, the theory of plethora, in which it was postulated that an excess of blood in the circulatory system or one organ caused illness.

Four hundred years later, Galen, a product of the Alexandria School of Medicine, denied the doctrine of plethora and returned to the humoral approach. Health and disease were thought to occur because of an upset in the equilibrium of these humors. Bloodletting to restore the balance of the humors by purging the body of its contaminated fluids was practiced from the time of Hippocrates until the nineteenth century. During Galen's time, animal dissection was widely practiced and provided a better concept of blood and its functions. It was proposed that the liver changed food to blood, which was distributed to the body along the veins. At the same time, impurities from the body were thought to be absorbed into venous blood and returned to the liver and then to the right side of the heart, where they supposedly ascended in the pulmonary artery to the lungs to be exhaled. The weakening of medieval ideas set the stage for English doctor William Harvey's discovery of blood circulation. He used the analogy of the heart as a pump and veins and arteries as pipes, where blood is moving around and is being driven in a continuous circuit. Four years after Harvey died in 1661, the Italian anatomist Marcello Malpighi observed the capillary blood vessels with the aid of the microscope. The cellular composition of blood was also recognized using a microscope, as Antoni van Leeuwenhoek, a Dutch naturalist, accurately described and measured red blood cells. The discovery of white blood cells and platelets followed after microscope lenses were improved. William Hewson first observed leukocytes in the eighteenth century. He thought that these cells came from nucleated cells in the lymph and that they eventually emerged from the spleen as red blood cells. In the nineteenth century, interest in leukocytes intensified with studies on inflammation and microbial infection.

In 1852, Karl Vierordt published the first quantitative results of blood cell analysis after several attempts were made to correlate blood cell counts with various diseases. In 1865, Felix Hoppe-Seyler discovered the oxygen carrying capacity of the red pigment (hemoglobin) in cells. The early history of protein chemistry is essentially that of hemoglobin, because it was one of the first molecules to have its molecular weight accurately determined and the first to be associated with a specific physiological function, i.e., carrying oxygen.

In 1900, the German pathologist Karl Landsteiner began mixing blood taken from different people and found some mixtures were compatible and others were not. This incompatibility resulted in illness and sometimes death after transfusions. He discovered two types of marker proteins, or antigens, on the surface of red blood cells, which he called A and B. According to whether a person's blood contains one or the other antigen, both, or neither, it is classified as type A, B, AB, or O. He also discovered the Rh factor in 1940 during experiments with rhesus monkeys. Improved methods of blood examination in the 1920s and the growth of knowledge of blood physiology in the 1930s allowed anemias and other blood disorders to be studied. Modern hematology recognizes that alterations in the components of blood are a result of disease, and research is conducted continually for a better understanding of this relationship and of blood itself.

Currently, there are many advances in what we know about the immune system and its function. We also are continuing to learn about many blood disorders, including leukemias and lymphomas, and defects in regulation of production of immune production and signaling. Blood continues to be an area of emerging science and vital to maintenance and function of all life processes.

—*Cathy Walsh*

For Further Information:

American Medical Association. *American Medical Association Complete Encyclopedia of Medicine*. New York: Random House Reference, 2003. A medical encyclopedia written by the American Medical Association and lists medical terms and definitions, explains surgical procedures and tests, includes descriptions of benefits and side effects of treatments, and provides general information about blood disorders.

Bick, Roger L. *Disorders of Thrombosis and Hemostasis: Clinical and Laboratory Practice*. 3rd ed. Philadelphia: Lippincott Williams & Wilkins, 2002. This book provides current data on antithrombotic therapy, information for diagnosis and treating bleeding and clotting disorders, and etiology, pathophysiology, clinical, laboratory diagnosis and management of disorders of thrombosis and hemostasis.

Lichtman, Marshall, et al., eds. *Williams Manual of Hematology*. 9th ed. New York: McGraw-Hill, 2016. A quick-access summary of epidemiology, etiology, pathogenesis, diagnostic criteria, differential diagnosis, and therapy of blood cell and coagulation protein disorders.

Rodak, Bernadette, ed. *Hematology: Clinical Principles and Applications*. 4th ed. St. Louis, Mo.: Elsevier Saunders, 2012. This text explores essential aspects of hematology including identification of cells, understanding hemostasis and thrombosis, normal hematopoiesis, and diseases of erythroid, myeloid, lymphoid and megakaryocytic origins.

Saba, Hussain I., and Harold R. Roberts, ed. *Hemostasis and Thrombosis: Practical Guidelines in Clinical Management*. 1st edition. Hoboken, NJ: John Wiley & Sons, Ltd, 2014. A handbook summarizing current understanding of hemostasis and thrombosis, with emphasis on clinical diagnosis, treatment, and daily management of thrombotic and bleeding disorders.

Zucker-Franklin, D., et al. *Atlas of Blood Cells: Function and Pathology*. 3rd ed. Philadelphia: Lea & Febiger, 2003. Updated with biomolecular advances, including apoptosis, and advances in detect methods including immune-electron microscopy and fluorescent in situ hybridization for detecting chromosomal abnormalities.

Blood banks

Organizations

Definition: Temporary storehouses of blood, kept at reduced temperatures, for transfusions into persons needing an additional supply; such transfers are vital in surgery and in unexpected emergency procedures.

Key terms:

antigens: proteins, carbohydrates, or other substances on the surface of cells that bind to their respective antibodies

cardiology: the study of the heart and its action, as well as the diagnosis and treatment of its diseases

cardiovascular: relating to or involving the heart and blood vessels

corpuscle: a minute particle; a protoplasmic cell floating free in the blood

erythrocyte: a red blood cell

hematosis: the formation of blood

hemophilia: a tendency (usually hereditary) to profuse bleeding, even from slight cuts

leukocyte: a white or colorless blood corpuscle

phagocyte: any leukocyte active in ingesting and destroying waste and harmful material

phlebotomy: the act or practice of opening a vein for letting blood

serology: the science of serums, their reactions, preparation, and use

The Study of Blood Throughout History

For centuries, blood was thought to be a simple liquid, but it is actually a bodily tissue. The cells, instead of being joined together as in solid bodily tissues, are suspended in a fluid called plasma, which comprises more than half of blood composition. The cellular portion of blood is largely red blood cells, with smaller numbers of white blood cells and platelets also present. Blood itself is the final functioning tool of the circulatory system, which helps to transport the blood to where it is needed in the body. Blood is an extremely complicated substance, and more things are being learned about it every year.

Some ancient civilizations, such as that of the Greeks, recognized that blood was an important fluid in the body, but they thought that it was motionless in certain areas. Between 300 and 250 BCE, some Egyptians were studying the anatomy of corpses. About 300 BCE, the Greek physician Praxagoras showed that there were tubes connected to the heart. Some were filled with blood; others were empty, filled with air. One of the physician's students, Herophilus, found that arteries gave a beat or pulse. When dissection was outlawed in Egypt and the library of Alexandria was burned, progress in learning about blood was stopped for a thousand years.

Galen, the Greek physician who served five Roman emperors over thirty years to 200 CE, believed that the arteries originated in the heart and pumped blood. Contrary to later Egyptian medical thought, Galen theorized that the heart was one pump, not two. Around 1300, doctors in Italy began to dissect bodies again-in 1316, Mondino de Luzzi wrote the first book dealing entirely with anatomy, in which he supported Galen's teachings. In 1543, Belgian anatomist Andreas Vesalius wrote a much-improved book on anatomy. However, it did not improve upon Galen's theories about the heart.

In 1242, a Syrian surgeon named Ibn an-Nafīs had written a book in which he theorized about how blood moved from the right ventricle to the left and that a double pump was involved in moving it. Ironically, Europeans did not discover his writings until 1924.

Meanwhile, Spanish physician Michael Servetus published a treatise in 1553 describing how circulation of blood to the lungs and back (often called the lesser circulation) might occur. Unfortunately, because he also included religious views, all copies of his writings that could be found were destroyed, and he was burned at the stake. Eventually, in 1694, a copy of his book was found, and it showed that his circulation theory matched later findings.

In 1559, an Italian anatomist, Realdo Colombo, also thought of lesser circulation and published a book on it. Colombo's work was so widely read that he is credited with discovering lesser circulation. In 1574, another Italian, Girolamo Fabrici, observed little valves on veins that opened in only one direction. The importance of this discovery was deduced by a student of Fabrici, the English doctor William Harvey, when Harvey determined that blood in the leg veins could move only to the heart. His laboratory work proved that the heart pumped blood into the arteries and that the blood returned by way of the veins. Furthermore, Harvey showed that the blood had a double circulation, returning to both ventricles. His continued experimentation showed that the same blood had to circulate and be used repeatedly.

All these medical pioneers were hampered by the inability to see more than the human eye would permit, until the development of lenses and microscopes. In 1661, Italian anatomist Marcello Malpighi was able to see, with the aid of a microscope, very fine blood vessels that connected the smallest arteries and veins: capillaries. With the discovery of capillaries, the concept of the circulation of blood was complete. In the eighteenth century, the English scientist Stephen Hales was the first to measure blood pressure.

The microscope also enabled scientists to observe the

components of blood. Malpighi saw reddish objects in a clear, faintly yellow fluid. Dutch scientist Jan Swammerdam, with the aid of a microscope, was able to describe them further. In 1674, the renowned Dutch scientist Antoni van Leeuwenhoek, using the best of these early microscopes, was able to describe the red cells as flat disks with depressions in the center. He even tried to measure them-in 1852, his calculations were refined by German scientist Karl Vierordt. Leeuwenhoek was able to study the path of red blood cells in tadpoles, frogs, and other animals and determined that, without doubt, blood traveled in an entirely closed circle, proving Harvey's contention. Soon, in 1669, English doctor Richard Lower noted that blood coming through arteries was red and that blood flowing toward the heart in veins was bluish.

English chemist Joseph Priestley discovered the gas oxygen in 1774, and French chemist Antoine-Laurent Lavoisier was able to show in 1778 that air consisted (mainly) of two gases, oxygen (one-fifth) and nitrogen (four-fifths). A German chemist, Julius Lothar Meyer, showed in 1857 that oxygen did not generally mix with the liquid part of the blood, combining instead with red blood cells.

The scientific detective work on blood continued with the aid of improved microscopes. It was learned that the cells of the body contained complicated substances called proteins, each of which was made up of groups of atoms called molecules. German scientists were among the first to examine the composition of blood. Otto Funke obtained a protein from red blood cells in 1851. Then Felix Hoppe-Seyler purified it, studied it, and named it hemoglobin ("blood protein"). The secrets of this precious commodity continued to unfold. In 1747, Italian chemist Vincenzo Antonio Menghini found that there was a small quantity of iron in blood, apparently stored in red blood cells.

Gradually, these findings led to the transfusion of blood from one person to another. In the seventeenth century, blood transfusions were attempted between animals. In 1666, Richard Lower unsuccessfully tried to transfuse blood from an animal to a human being. Sometimes the operation helped, but occasionally people died after such a transfusion, so doctors largely abandoned the practice. Then, in 1818, James Blundell, an English physician who theorized that the blood of a particular kind of animal would help only that particular kind, transfused blood from healthy human beings to other human beings who needed blood. While often successful, the procedure sometimes caused agglutination, a process in which red blood cells clumped together and would not function properly.

In 1901, an Austrian doctor named Karl Landsteiner solved the problem by observing that there were four kinds of blood cells. Depending on the chemical content, the blood was named as types A, B, AB, and O. Continuing practice showed that not all blood types worked well with one another; some tended to agglutinate when introduced to the wrong type.

Although red blood cells are by far the most numerous objects that float in the bloodstream, they are not the only ones. In 1850, French physician Casimir-Joseph Davaine noticed cells, pale and uneven in shape, that were much larger than red blood cells. By 1869, he noticed that these cells would absorb bits of foreign matter in the blood. In 1875, German doctor Paul Ehrlich, interested in using dyes on these white cells, found that he was able to classify them into different types.

In the late nineteenth century, Russian scientist Élie Metchnikoff (also known as Ilya Ilich Mechnikov), while studying bacteria, noticed that whenever there was a cut, white cells were carried to it in great numbers by the blood. So much blood went to the injured part that it grew red and inflamed and was painful from the pressure exerted by the blood on the vessel walls. Metchnikoff called the bacteria-eating cells phagocytes. He had become interested in the study of bacteria following the pioneering work of France's Louis Pasteur in the 1860s.

The clotting of wounds became more interesting to the medical community. In 1842, French scientist Alfred Donne had reported a new type of object floating in the bloodstream. An Italian physician, Giulio Cesare Bizzozero, concluded that the foreign objects had something to do with clotting. He called them platelets because their shape resembled tiny plates. What was to be learned about them much later is that they have a life span of about nine days and that they break down when exposed to air after bleeding starts. As they begin to break down, platelets release a substance that starts a long chain of chemical changes that ends in clotting.

While many scientists were concentrating on the study of red blood cells, white blood cells, and platelets, attention was also being paid to plasma, the colorless liquid that serves as a transport mechanism for objects floating in it. Eventually, it was learned that plasma carries red blood cells to the lungs to take up oxygen and then to the rest of the body to deliver the oxygen. Plasma carries white blood cells to any part of the body where they are needed to fight bacteria. It also carries platelets to any part of the body where blood loss must be stopped. Furthermore, the watery plasma absorbs heat at the liver and delivers it to the skin so that the body stays warm.

More recent studies show that about 8 percent of plasma is composed of dissolved substances that are important in keeping conditions in the body even. Some chemicals in the plasma neutralize acids and bases, which could threaten cells. The plasma also carries glucose molecules and fatty acids to specific destinations in order to produce energy in the body. Furthermore, it dissolves wastes such as carbon dioxide and delivers urea to the kidneys for disposal. Hormones, which were first discovered in 1902, are also carried by the plasma to any part of the body where they are needed.

More than half the weight of substances dissolved in plasma are proteins. Proteins fall into two groups, albumins and globulins. Some proteins combine easily with substances that the body needs in small amounts. Gammaglobulins have the capacity to neutralize foreign substances, such as viruses or the poisonous toxins produced by bacteria, by combining with them. Gammaglobulins that act in this way are called antibodies.

All these discoveries and many others (such as the existence of fibrinogen, fibrin, the Rh factor, and enzymes) have combined to improve the procedures for storing and transfusing blood. Safeguarding blood for transfusion has always been a problem. The precious liquid is unstable, and a fresh supply has always been needed in any emergency.

In the late 1930s, Russian scientists discovered that citrated blood can be stored if refrigerated at a temperature of about 4.5 degrees Celsius (40 degrees Fahrenheit). Then, in 1936, a Canadian doctor, Norman Bethune, made large-scale use of a blood bank with antifascist forces during the Spanish Civil War. During World War II, the noted American blood bank pioneer Charles Drew, who had made a special study of ways to store and ship blood plasma, organized a nationwide "Blood for Britain" campaign in which thousands of lives were saved.

Before blood banks could evolve, a number of additional discoveries had to be made. Before the discovery of agglutinins and blood typing, blood was transfused directly from donor to patient. The two lay side by side, and the blood flowed from the artery of the donor to the vein of the recipient. There was no way of measuring the amount of blood being transfused. It became dangerous for the donor if he or she changed from rosy-colored and talkative to pale or unconscious. There was also the danger that a blood clot in the tube might enter the patient's blood vessels. In addition, the blood might be flowing too fast and overload the patient's heart.

A new tube to facilitate blood transfusion more safely was developed in 1909. Then, in 1914, Argentine doctor Luis Agote discovered that sodium citrate could stop the clotting of blood, permitting blood to be kept in a bottle while it was slowly directed into a patient's vein. Physicians could finally control the quantity and speed of transfusions.

The use of stored blood began in 1918 by Oswald H. Robertson, a World War I physician, who found it could be kept virtually intact for several days by storing it at low temperatures, from 2 to 4 degrees Celsius. The first large blood bank was established at the Cook County Hospital in Chicago in 1937.

The Role of Blood Banks

A blood bank is an organizational unit responsible for collecting, processing, and storing blood to be used for transfusion and other purposes. It is usually a subdivision of a laboratory in a hospital and is often charged with the responsibility for all serologic testing. Although blood can be withdrawn from one person and transfused directly into another, the usual practice is for hospitals and authorized agencies to select donors, draw blood (phlebotomy), screen the specimens, arrange them into blood groups, and store the blood until it is needed.

Each unit of donated blood, referred to as whole blood, is approximately 1 pint. After it is drawn, the blood separated into its constituent parts, which consist primarily of red blood cells, plasma, and platelets. The components can then be transfused to different patients depending on their individual needs.

The storage of blood was once short-lived because of clotting and inadequately low temperature levels. A blood bank can now store blood for much longer periods of time, sometimes a year or two. It is stored with an anticoagulant, generally an acid-citrate-dextrose (ACD) solution composed of trisodium citrate, citric acid, dextrose, and sterile water. Red blood cells from blood stored in an ACD solution will survive in the recipient for one hundred days. All chemical changes in blood are slowed by cold temperatures. Red blood cells can be stored for a maximum of 42 days via refrigeration. Platelets, on the other hand, are stored at room temperature and can only be stored for a maximum of five days. It has been found that more prolonged storage of blood can be achieved by freezing and maintaining it at extremely low temperatures-below -70 degrees Celsius (-94 degrees Fahrenheit). While freezing and thawing of whole blood does not harm plasma, it can damage red blood cells unless glycerol or dimethyl sulfoxide solutions are used to minimize the damage and permit red cells to be maintained in a frozen state for months without significant injury. Red blood cells may be frozen for up to ten years, while plasma can only be frozen for one year.

After Karl Landsteiner discovered that blood could be classified into four major blood groups, safer transfusions could be attempted. Landsteiner also worked with the American pathologist Alexander S. Wiener to discover another system of blood grouping known as the Rh system. The name was derived from the rhesus monkeys with which the scientists experimented.

It was found that a person with type A blood (having "A" antigens in the red blood cells and "b" antibodies in the blood plasma) cannot successfully give blood to a person with type B blood (having "B" antigens and "a" antibodies) because the clumping of blood cells would occur.

Successful blood transfusions depend on the type of antigens in the donor's red blood cells, not on the type of antibodies in the plasma, because the recipient's blood cells greatly outnumber the antibodies in the donor's blood, and serious clumping could not occur. A donor's red blood cells, however, are few enough in number that all of them can be agglutinated by the recipient's antibodies. These clumps could then plug the capillaries, reducing and eventually cutting off the flow of blood. This reaction is serious and can cause death.

A person with type AB blood, who has both "A" and "B" antigens in the red blood cells and no agglutinins in the plasma, can receive the red blood cells of any other group. A type O person (a universal donor) has no antigens and can donate blood to any person but can receive only type O blood. Therefore, type O is the most requested blood type by hospitals.

The ABO system of grouping blood types has led to further refinements. Ten major and minor blood groupings have been identified from the variety of proteins also found in blood cells. The most important is the Rh system. There are two Rh blood types: Rh positive and Rh negative. A person with the Rh-positive factor has the protein, while a person with Rh-negative blood does not have the protein. Infusing an Rh-negative person with Rh-positive blood causes special antibodies to be formed in the blood of the recipient. A later transfusion of Rh-positive blood would result in the agglutination of the red blood cells received.

This reaction is especially important when incompatibility occurs between the blood of a pregnant woman and her baby. This happens only if the mother has Rh-negative blood and the baby has Rh-positive blood because it has inherited Rh-positive genes from the father. When such a baby is born, some of the baby's blood enters the mother's circulatory system, causing her body to produce antibodies to combat the "foreign material." Since this intrusion of blood almost always happens as a delayed reaction after the baby is born, the first baby is probably unharmed. However, a subsequent baby could be the victim of these antibodies, which the mother's body continues to produce. Such a developing baby could suffer the destruction of its red blood cells if it has Rh-positive blood, unless preventive steps such as a blood transfusion for the baby are taken. Another medical development is a medicine known as Rho(D) immune globulin, which provides protective immunization and has almost eliminated the dangers of Rh incompatibility. Blood transfusions are regularly used in crises such as accidents or life-threatening illnesses. Most commonly, they are used to restore the volume of circulating blood lost by acute hemorrhaging. They are also used to restore the large volume of plasma that is often lost after severe burns. In acute or chronic anemia cases, such as with acquired immunodeficiency syndrome (AIDS) or leukemia, they are used to maintain hemoglobin and red blood cells at adequate levels. Transfusions are also used to provide platelets for coagulation in order to counteract various bleeding disorders or acute hemorrhaging.

Blood transfusions are being used more extensively-and more safely-than ever before. Many more surgeries are possible with transfusions including organ implants, heart repair, limb reconstruction, grafting for severe burn cases, and bone grafts.

Perspective and Prospects

Five million patients a year receive blood, largely in emergency cases. Many are in need of emergency surgery for an internal disorder, but many others are victims of social

---

In the News:
Blood Banks and Antigerm Screening

Blood banks in the early twenty-first century faced growing challenges as new diseases threatened the purity of their blood supplies. In response to such threats, researchers attempted to design improved methods for blood banks to screen donors and blood for protection against contamination.

West Nile virus, a mosquito-borne disease, was first identified in the United States in 1999. In the fall of 2002, health officials discovered that organ transplant recipients had become infected with the virus through blood transfusions. The majority of West Nile victims displayed no visible symptoms and had unintentionally donated contaminated blood. In November of that year, the Food and Drug Administration (FDA) called for the development of a test before the outbreak of the 2003 mosquito season. Although some experts doubted that a screening method could be produced so quickly, two tests that detected minute fragments of the West Nile virus genes were in use by July 1. The tests also revealed the presence of viruses responsible for Japanese, St. Louis, and Murray encephalitis, permitting blood banks to reject blood contaminated with these diseases as well.

Although no conclusive evidence proved that either Creutzfeldt-Jakob disease (the human form of mad cow disease) or severe acute respiratory syndrome (SARS) were in fact transmissible through blood transfusions, blood banks used verbal screening of potential donors to defend against these recent disease outbreaks. FDA guidelines mandated rejection or deferral of blood donations from people who might have been exposed to either disease.

In 2002, the FDA approved nucleic acid amplification tests (NAT) for the hepatitis C virus (HCV) and the human immunodeficiency virus 1 (HIV-1). Unlike existing tests for the presence of antibodies, which do not develop in the earliest stages of a disease, the NAT reacts to small fragments of virus deoxyribonucleic acid (DNA) and can detect infections before the appearance of symptoms. The West Nile virus tests use similar methods.

Ongoing research into improved techniques for detecting bacteria and other blood pathogens, and into ways of using physical or chemical methods to destroy these organisms, may further improve blood supply safety.

—Milton Berman, Ph.D.

---

violence, earthquakes, and hurricanes. Large-scale devastation often comes close to depleting the blood supply in an area. New and repeat donors, therefore, are always in demand. New ways of storing blood safely and for longer periods of time are constantly being researched. In the United States, the work of blood banks comes under the ultimate supervision of the Food and Drug Administration (FDA) and federal agencies, as well as the Oversight and Investigations Subcommittee of the House Energy and Commerce Committee. Also interested in their function are the congressionally funded Public Health Service and the Centers for Disease Control (CDC). The largest United States blood bank is that of the Red Cross, which provides, through its local affiliates, about half of the 16 million units of blood donated each year in the United States. The Red Cross, as well as individual nonprofit and commercial agencies, is striving for improved health and safety procedures in blood donation.

The American Association of Blood Banks gathers and interprets data each year. It has found that there have been relatively few transfusion-induced cases of viral infection. Almost all the transfusion-related AIDS cases, for example, developed in 1985, before tighter screening of donors, safer procedures, and strict testing were instituted. Only fifteen cases of AIDS from blood transfusion were reported between 1985 and 1992. This contrasts with the pre-1985 figure of 3,425 transfusion-associated cases of AIDS reported to the Centers for Disease Control.

Concern about other viral infections transmitted through blood transfusions has increased vigilance against blood impurities and has improved sanitary procedures. Governmental agencies, the Red Cross, and private corporations have intensified their efforts to protect the quality of the blood supply. The International Society of Blood Transfusion continues to examine new threats.

Steps are continually reviewed to improve record keeping, blood collection, tracking, and distribution by all organizations. The FDA has a comprehensive inspection program that focuses on all phases of the collection-dispersal program of all blood banks, as well as on their training of workers and updating of procedures. It looks closely at procedures for donor screening, the testing for hepatitis and AIDS virus antibodies, and the quarantine and destruction of unsuitable blood products.

The American Red Cross complies with these regulations and works with the FDA to create the safest blood supply possible. It has a state-of-the-art computerized information system. It keeps track of all its donors and retains files on all persons disqualified from giving blood. This information is available throughout the United States. The computerized program is also being expanded internationally because there is a growing import-export business between countries in need of new supplies. The American Red Cross database lists would-be donors, types and quantities of blood in storage, location of hospitals and distribution centers, and other information vital to the prompt, efficient, and safe distribution of blood.

In 2010, the CDC launched a national public health surveillance known as the Hemovigilance Module. Its purpose is to monitor and record adverse reactions resulting from blood transfusions. By collecting a large pool of data in a national system, the CDC will be able to amass this information and develop new methods to prevent the adverse incidents that can come with transfusion.

Blood safety begins with screening. Only healthy individuals are allowed to give blood. Blood samples undergo extensive screening designed to detect any blood-borne infectious agent. Some collection agencies are developing lists of unwanted donors, including persons with a high risk of having been exposed to the AIDS virus or to other dangerous viruses or bacteria, such as those that cause hepatitis or syphilis. The goal is to reduce the chance of obtaining infectious blood as much as possible.

According to the CDC, there are currently seven infectious disease pathogens that all donated blood must be screened for. These include bacterial contamination, Hepatitis B and C viruses, Human Immunodeficiency Virus (HIV) types 1 and 2, Human T-Lymphotropic Virus (HTLV) types I and II, Treponema pallidum (syphilis), and West Nile Virus. Cytomegalovirus and Trypanosoma cruzi (Chagas disease) are often tested by blood centers but are not among the required tests. The various pathogens are tested through different means including cultures and anti-

body detection. It is an expensive set of procedures, and hospitals, clinics, and other medical institutions are working on how to reduce these costs.

Many viruses are elusive, including the dreaded HIV, which takes time to develop. To hasten its identification, scientists have developed the technique of "pooling" by combining blood known to contain infected cells with samples of blood with uninfected normal lymphocytes in an effort to stimulate HIV replication and make the HIV come to light faster. It has been found that the most reliable mix is a pool of fifty donors. The concept of pooling is scientifically valid and economically feasible.

While the risk of acquiring a transfusion-related infection is extremely low, there is still concern among the public that individuals might be susceptible to specific blood diseases.

—Walter Appleton;
updated by Andrea Sarchi, OMS-IV

See also: Bleeding; Blood and blood disorders; Blood testing; Cytology; Emergency medicine; Hematology; Hematology, pediatric; Rh factor; Screening; Serology; Transfusion

For Further Information:
Hillier, Christopher D., et al., eds. *Blood Banking and Transfusion Medicine: Basic Principles and Practice.* 2nd ed. Philadelphia: Churchill Livingstone/Elsevier, 2007. Draws data from basic, transnational, and clinical studies; explores the latest advances in the use of blood products, new methods of disease treatment, and stem cell transplantation; and addresses a range of controversies in practice.
McCullough, Jeffrey. *Transfusion Medicine.* 2nd ed. Philadelphia: Churchill Livingstone/Elsevier, 2005. Transfusion medicine, a young science, is continuously growing and changing. The result is a great body of knowledge about the practical aspects of blood collection and transfusion, and an incomparably better understanding of the blood groups and of the unintended effects of transfusion at the molecular level.
Schaub Di Lorenzo, Marjorie, and Susan Strasinger. *Blood Collection: A Short Course.* 2nd ed. Philadelphia: F.A. Davis, 2009. Details all phlebotomy issues important in collecting a quality blood specimen and includes excellent photographs that clearly demonstrate the preferred techniques, supplies, and collection procedures.
Starr, Douglas P. *Blood: An Epic History of Medicine and Commerce.* New York: Perennial, 2002. Starr reflects on the societal role of blood as it transformed from a mythical enigma to a scientific entity to a product of industry. He examines the past racism of blood banks, the spread of the AIDS epidemic among hemophiliacs, and the role of blood in helping the Allies win World War II.
Wailoo, Keith. *Drawing Blood: Technology and Disease Identity in Twentieth-century America.* Baltimore: Johns Hopkins University Press, 1999. The author, a medical historian, traces the way in which physicians throughout the twentieth century used medical technology to define disease, establish medical specialties, and shape political agendas.

Blood poisoning. *See* Septicemia.

Blood pressure
Biology
Anatomy or system affected: Blood, blood vessels, circulatory system, heart
Specialties and related fields: Cardiology, exercise physiol-

ogy, family medicine, geriatrics and gerontology, vascular medicine

Definition: The force exerted by blood upon the walls of blood vessels as the heart pumps blood through the circulatory system.

Key terms:

diastolic pressure: the minimum blood pressure as the heart relaxes

hypertension: high blood pressure; a systolic pressure of at least 140 or a diastolic pressure of at least 90

hypotension: low blood pressure, diagnosed by symptoms of low blood flow

sphygmomanometer: an instrument for measuring blood pressure; commonly called a blood pressure cuff

systolic pressure: the maximum blood pressure as the heart contracts

Structure and Functions

When the left ventricle of the heart beats, it pumps five liters of blood per minute to the aorta, through the arteries, and into the arterioles. As these blood vessels decrease in diameter, they create resistance to blood flow and the pressure of the blood against their walls increases. This blood pressure is expressed as two numbers measured in millimeters of mercury (mmHg) by a sphygmomanometer. The first number, called the systolic pressure, is the maximum pressure that occurs when the heart contracts and the ventricle is emptying its blood. The second number, called the diastolic pressure, is the minimum pressure that occurs when the heart relaxes and the ventricle is filling with blood before the next contraction.

Blood pressure depends on the strength of the heart muscle, the volume and thickness of blood being pumped, and the diameter and flexibility of the blood vessels, all of which may vary with age, health, and physical condition. Blood pressure is also affected by activity, diet, hydration (including caffeine and alcohol), emotional stress, physical pain, tobacco use, weight (including pregnancy), abrupt changes in body position, and medication.

Blood pressure is a commonly measured indicator of the body's state of health, along with body temperature, pulse rate (number of heartbeats per minute), and respiratory rate (number of breaths per minute). It can be measured noninvasively using a sphygmomanometer,, which may be electronic and automatic or mercury-based and require manual inflation and deflation. With the patient seated or lying down, an inflatable cuff is wrapped firmly around the upper arm at the level of the heart with the lower edge of the cuff 1 inch above the crease in the elbow. The arm should be bare and any sleeve should be pushed or rolled up without constricting circulation. If the meter is electronic, then the cuff will automatically inflate and deflate when activated and a digital reading will be displayed. If the meter is manual, then a health care provider will place the bell of a stethoscope over the large artery on the inside of the elbow, just below the cuff. The cuff is then inflated by quickly squeezing a rubber bulb until the gauge reads 10-30 mmHg higher than the expected systolic pressure but no higher than 210 mmHg. No sound should be heard through the stethoscope. A valve is opened so that the cuff deflates slowly; the pressure reading should drop 2-3 mmHg per second. When the sound of pulsing blood is first heard through the stethoscope, the reading on the gauge is the systolic pressure. As the cuff continues to deflate, this sound will disappear and the reading on the gauge at that point is the diastolic pressure. Blood pressure should be checked at least every year or two. It should be checked more often during illnesses and medical treatments.

Disorders and Diseases

The average blood pressure for healthy adults is 120 over 80 mmHg (written as 120/80). A systolic pressure of 120 to 139 mmHg or a diastolic pressure of 80 to 89 mmHg is considered to be slightly elevated, a condition called prehypertension. A systolic pressure of at least 140 mmHg or a diastolic pressure of at least 90 mmHg is considered to be elevated, a condition called hypertension. In most cases, hypertension has no known direct medical cause; however, in some cases, it is secondary to other health conditions such as kidney disease. Four groups of people are predisposed to hypertension: obese people, elderly people, people with diabetes, and African Americans. Chronic hypertension is a risk factor for heart attack, stroke, and aortic aneurysm.

The goal of hypertension treatment is to get the resting blood pressure below 140/90. In some cases, this may be accomplished solely with lifestyle changes, which should be tried before drug therapy is begun. These lifestyle changes include discontinuing alcohol consumption and tobacco use, reducing dietary salt and sugar intake, eating foods low in saturated fat, performing regular low-intensity exercise such as walking, and getting sufficient sleep and stress relief. When these changes alone are insufficient, one or more medications may be prescribed, such as diuretics, beta-blockers, calcium-channel blockers, or angiotensin-converting enzyme (ACE) inhibitors.

While hypertension is diagnosed from specific elevated blood pressure measurements, hypotension is diagnosed by symptoms of low blood flow rather than solely by blood pressure numbers. These symptoms include light-headedness, weakness, visual disturbance, and fainting.

To increase the volume and thickness of blood being pumped, patients with hypotension are typically instructed to drink more liquids (excluding caffeinated and alcoholic beverages) and ingest more salt. They must also avoid dehydration from excess sweating and hot showers or baths. To improve the resistance in blood vessels, patients may wear compression stockings and should regularly perform moderate exercise. Little is known about the causes of hypotension and few medications are available to raise low blood pressure safely.

Perspective and Prospects

Direct measurement of arterial blood pressure was first reported by Reverend Stephen Hales in 1733. He inserted a glass tube in a horse's artery and found that the column of blood rose to a vertical height of more than 8 feet. Pressures were later measured with columns of water and saline, but they still required an unwieldy length of tube. Eventually, a mercury column was used because mercury is more than thirteen times as dense as water and the column length was more manageable. Sphygmomanometers today no longer use mercury, but the standard unit of mmHg remains.

—*Bethany Thivierge, M.P.H., E.L.S.*

See also: Arteriosclerosis; Blood and blood disorders; Blood vessels; Cardiology; Circulation; First aid; Heart; Heart attack; Hypertension; Hypotension; Physical examination; Preeclampsia and eclampsia; Pulmonary hypertension; Strokes; Vascular medicine; Vascular system.

For Further Information:

Fortmann, Stephen P., and Prudence E. Breitrose. *The Blood Pressure Book: How to Get It Down and Keep It Down.* 3d ed. Boulder, Colo.: Bull Publishing Company, 2006.

Gatzoulis, Michael A. *OCL Pulmonary Arterial Hypertension.* Oxford: Oxford University Press, 2011.

Humbert, Marc, et al. *Pulmonary Vascular Disorders.* Basel, Switz.: Karger, 2012.

Kowalski, Robert E. *The Blood Pressure Cure: Eight Weeks to Lower Blood Pressure Without Prescription Drugs.* Hoboken, N.J.: John Wiley & Sons, 2008.

Rubin, Alan L. *High Blood Pressure for Dummies.* Hoboken, N.J.: John Wiley & Sons, 2010.

Shibao, Cyndya, et al. "Evaluation and Treatment of Orthostatic Hypotension." *Journal of the American Society of Hypertension* 7, no. 4 (July-August, 2013): 317-324.

Blood testing

Procedure

Anatomy or system affected: Blood, blood vessels, circulatory system, skin

Specialties and related fields: Cytology, forensic medicine, hematology, pathology, public health, serology, toxicology

Definition: The withdrawal of blood from an individual and its analysis for one of many purposes, including blood typing and a search for acquired or genetic disease indicators.

Key terms:

antibody: a protein synthesized in response to a specific antigen; antibodies physically combine with antigens as part of the immune process

antigen: a molecule which induces the production of antibodies

antiserum: the fluid portion of blood that contains specific antibodies

Rh factor: a specific antigen present on 85 percent of an individual's red blood cells; also called Rhesus factor

Indications and Procedures

Most blood tests require a substantial sample of blood. A sample of several milliliters or more is withdrawn from a vein using a syringe. The sample is transported to a diagnostic laboratory for the appropriate analysis.

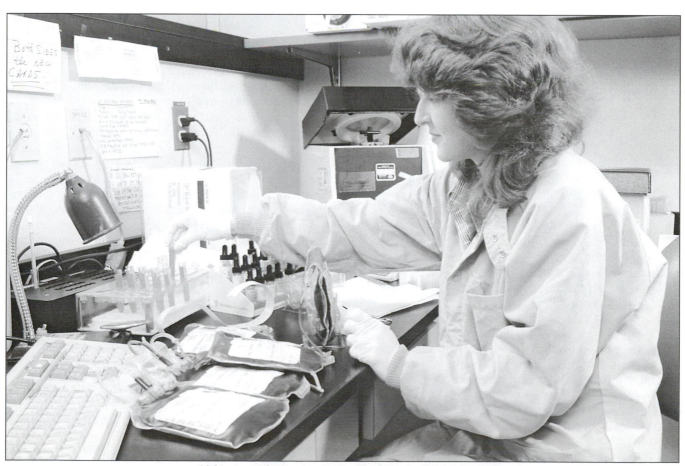

A laboratory technician runs tests on blood samples. (Digital Stock)

In blood typing, red blood cells are marked on their surface with the protein antigens designated A, B, AB (both A and B), or O (no antigen). Individuals possess antibodies, found in the liquid or serum portion of the blood, to the antigens that they themselves do not possess. In ABO typing, red blood cells are isolated from the blood sample and mixed with antiserum with a known antibody type. Cells marked with antigen A will clump when mixed with antibody A, cells with B antigen will clump when exposed to antibody B, AB antigens clump with either, and O clumps with neither. The type of positive clumping reaction determines blood type. Rh type is determined in the same manner, with Rh-positive blood exhibiting a clumping reaction with Rh antibodies. Histocompatibility leukocyte antigen (HLA) typing is performed similarly but uses white blood cells as the antigenic material. HLA typing is more complex and time consuming because more than forty different HLAs are known to exist.

Deoxyribonucleic acid (DNA) analysis requires isolating DNA from white blood cells and amplifying certain regions with a procedure called "polymerase chain reaction (PCR)." The amplified DNA is cut with enzymes and run through an electric field in a gel matrix, thus separating the pieces of DNA by size. Specific patterns are visually analyzed. When this technique is repeated across many different regions of a person's DNA, a pattern unique to that individual can be obtained. This information can be used to answer questions of paternity and relatedness or to help convict or exonerate suspects in murder and rape cases. A similar analysis is used to determine the presence of certain genetic diseases or the possibility of transmitting a genetic disease.

The use of blood tests to diagnose diseases covers a wide range, and the test is matched to the analysis requested. Abnormal levels of red blood cells can indicate anemia, while abnormal white cell counts may suggest a severe infection. Inappropriate enzyme levels could signal organ malfunction, and abnormal hormone levels indicate an endocrine disease. High levels of particular antibodies herald an infection with the corresponding antigenic agent.

Uses and Complications

Blood testing may be performed for a variety of reasons, including monitoring of organ function and blood clotting, evaluation of medication effectiveness, and diagnosis of and/or risk assessment for specific diseases or conditions. If an individual has suffered a large loss of blood and/or requires surgery that may necessitate a blood transfusion, ABO and Rh factor blood typing is performed. Pregnant women need to know their own Rh status and that of their fetus in order to prevent gestational complications from Rh incompatibility. If an organ transplant is required, the HLAs present on all cells except red blood cells must be matched as closely as possible to prevent graft rejection. In the event of paternity determination or forensic analysis, the DNA sequences found in white blood cells can be analyzed for proper identification. Some genetic diseases in an affected individual, a fetus, or unaffected individuals who

may transmit the genetic disease to their offspring can be detected with blood DNA analysis. Many types of disorders and diseases are diagnosed through a determination of the presence of abnormal levels of blood cell types, enzymes, hormones, and electrolytes (sodium, potassium, phosphate, magnesium, and calcium) or the presence of infectious agents in the blood, such as bacteria and viruses. Not all genetic diseases can be tested using DNA analysis. A partial list of those that can be detected includes hemophilia, Huntington disease, cystic fibrosis, and sickle cell disease. Others, such as Tay-Sachs disease, can be detected with an enzyme test of the blood.

Should proper ABO typing not be performed and an individual be given an incompatible blood transfusion, the antibodies in the individual's blood would destroy the newly transfused cells, causing a life-threatening condition. Failure to diagnose and treat an Rh-incompatible pregnancy could result in death of the fetus or a baby born with severe hemolytic disease and jaundice because of the destruction of fetal blood cells by the mother's immune system.

In modern hospitals with standard precautions, there are only minor side effects to blood withdrawal with a syringe. Some pain from puncturing the vein wall and localized bruising may occur. If the procedure is done under unsanitary conditions or if needles are used repeatedly, the risk of transmitting bacterial infections or viral infections, such as hepatitis and human immunodeficiency virus (HIV), increases dramatically.

Perspective and Prospects

DNA analysis is rapidly providing new and better diagnostic tools for the identification of genetic disease and its carriers as well as for the prediction of an individual's tendency to develop heart disease and certain cancers, such as those of the breast and colon. Such predictive tests could save millions of lives through close monitoring and early treatment.

Such advances of technology, however, are not without consequences. Since genetic testing became routine in the 1980s, there has been great concern about the access of employers and insurance companies to such potentially damaging information. For many years, lack of regulation of DNA testing laboratories frequently resulted in incorrect or ambiguous test results. Movements toward regulation and licensing of these laboratories are alleviating these problems.

—*Karen E. Kalumuck, Ph.D.*

See also: Acquired immunodeficiency syndrome (AIDS); Anemia; Blood and blood disorders; Blood banks; Cholesterol; Circulation; Dialysis; DNA and RNA; Endocrine disorders; Ergogenic aids; Forensic pathology; Genetic counseling; Genetic diseases; Genetics and inheritance; Grafts and grafting; Hematology; Hematology, pediatric; Hormones; Human immunodeficiency virus (HIV); Immune system; Laboratory tests; Pathology; Pregnancy and gestation; Rh factor; Screening; Serology; Transfusion.

For Further Information:

A.D.A.M. Medical Encyclopedia. "Blood Typing." *MedlinePlus*, February 5, 2010.

A.D.A.M. Medical Encyclopedia. "Histocompatibility Antigen Test." *MedlinePlus*, February 2, 2011.

Feldman, Eric A., and Ronald Bayer. *Blood Feuds: AIDS, Blood, and the Politics of Medical Disaster.* New York: Oxford University Press, 1999.

Hillier, Christopher D., et al., eds. *Blood Banking and Transfusion Medicine: Basic Principles and Practice.* 2d ed. Philadelphia: Churchill Livingstone/Elsevier, 2007.

Lab Tests Online. "Blood Typing." *American Association for Clinical Chemistry*, September 24, 2012.

Lab Tests Online. "Tips on Blood Testing." *American Association for Clinical Chemistry*, December 9, 2011.

National Heart, Lung, and Blood Institute. "Explore Blood Tests." *National Institutes of Health, US Department of Health and Human Services*, January 6, 2012.

Pagana, Kathleen Deska, and Timothy J. Pagana. *Mosby's Diagnostic and Laboratory Test Reference.* 9th ed. St. Louis, Mo.: Mosby/Elsevier, 2009.

Rodak, Bernadette, ed. *Hematology: Clinical Principles and Applications.* 3d ed. St. Louis, Mo.: Saunders/Elsevier, 2007.

Schaub Di Lorenzo, Marjorie, and Susan Strasinger. *Blood Collection in Healthcare.* Philadelphia: F. A. Davis, 2002.

Youngson, Robert M. "Blood Transfusion." In *The Surgery Book: An Illustrated Guide to Seventy-three of the Most Common Operations.* New York: St. Martin's Press, 1993.

Blood transfusion. *See* Transfusion.

Blood vessels

Biology/Anatomy

Anatomy or system affected: Blood, blood vessels, circulatory system, heart, lymphatic system

Specialties and related fields: Cardiology, hematology, internal medicine, vascular medicine

Definition: Elastic tubes that circulate blood from the heart throughout the body represented by arteries, capillaries, and veins.

Key terms:

aorta: a large artery from the left ventricle of the heart that supplies oxygenated blood to the body

atherosclerosis: fatty deposits that collect along the walls of arteries

intermittent claudication: pain that comes and goes in the leg due to poor circulation in the arteries of the lower extremities

thrombolytic: able to break up or dissolve a blood clot

vena cava: a large vein that carries deoxygenated blood into the right atrium of the heart from the lower half of the body

Structure and Functions

The circulatory system is comprised of the heart and blood vessels. Under this closed system, oxygen and nutrients present in blood are provided to muscles and organs. The heart works as a pump. The circulatory system consists of three main types of blood vessels: arteries, capillaries, and veins. The walls of a blood vessel are made up of three layers known as the tunica intima, tunica media, and tunica adventitia. The tunica intima, the innermost and thinnest layer, is made up of endothelial cells and connective tissue. The middle layer, tunica media, is composed of smooth muscle along with elastic fibers and is the thickest layer.

The outermost layer, the tunica adventitia, is composed of connective tissue. Generally speaking, arteries have a narrow lumen with more muscle and elastic tissue, while veins have a larger lumen with less muscle and elastic tissue.

The path by which blood is pumped from the heart is as follows; aorta to arteries, arterioles to capillaries, venules to veins, and back to the heart via the superios and inferior vena cava. Arteries contract and relax based upon responses from the sympathetic nervous system. The main function of arteries is to transport oxygenated blood away from the heart. Arteries branch into arterioles, which regulate blood flow and pressure. Arterioles then empty into capillaries. Capillaries are extremely narrow vessels that supply blood to major organs and tissue structures within the body. It is at the capillary networks where oxygen, carbon dioxide, and other nutrients (that is, water and salt) are exchanged. Capillaries also collect waste products from surrounding cells. Blood then drains from capillaries into venules. Venules are microscopic vessels that merge into veins. Veins transport deoxygenated blood back toward the heart. Valves are present inside veins to prevent blood from flowing in the reverse direction.

Blood flow through blood vessels is regulated by many factors. Blood flows from areas of high pressure to lower pressure. Neural and hormonal negative feedback systems and autoregulation are also responsible for maintaining blood flow and pressure. Vasomotor nerves (sympathetic) allow for dilation and constriction of vessels. Baroreceptors (pressure-sensitive receptors), chemoreceptors (oxygen, carbon dioxide, and hydrogen sensitive receptors), and several hormones (angiotension II, aldosterone, epinephrine, and norepinephrine) communicate with the brain to control blood pressure as well.

Disorders and Diseases

Heart disease or cardiovascular disease can affect the blood vessels and/or the heart muscle. Heart disease is the number one killer of men and women worldwide. In fact, in the United States heart disease is responsible for 40 percent of all deaths.

Typically, diseases of the blood vessels involve the narrowing or blockage of a vessel. When a blood vessel hardens or becomes blocked, the blood supply to vital organs, including the heart and brain, is impaired. One of the processes by which arteries become blocked is known as atherosclerosis. Fatty deposits accumulate in the arteries, restricting blood flow and thus leading to coronary heart disease. Risk factors for developing atherosclerosis are an unhealthy diet, physical inactivity, being overweight, and smoking.

Patients may experience symptoms such as shortness of breath, chest pain, and/or numbness, pain, weakness of the extremities which may represent heart attacks, angina, or strokes.

The main goal in the treatment of atherosclerotic disease is to reopen the arteries, thereby improving blood flow. The treatment options include lifestyle changes, medications, and/or cardiac procedures or surgery. Lifestyle changes consist of a low-sodium and low-fat diet, at least thirty minutes of exercise per day, quitting smoking, and limiting alcohol intake. Several types of medications can help slow the progression of atherosclerosis. Blood pressure-lowering drugs (diuretics; angiotensin-converting enzyme, or angiotensin converting enzyme (ACE) inhibitors; and beta-blockers), cholesterol-lowering drugs (statins and fibrates), and blood thinners (aspirin) offer some benefit in patients with heart disease. Lastly, coronary angioplasty is a procedure that requires the use of a catheter (usually from the groin area) with a small balloon at the tip. The catheter is threaded up to the blocked artery. When the balloon is inflated, the artery is reopened. A metal coil, known as a stent, is then used to keep the artery open and allow for blood flow. Coronary artery bypass surgery is an invasive procedure in which a vein from the patient's leg is used to replace a blocked artery of the heart.

Atherosclerosis can also cause peripheral vascular disease (PVD), which is the narrowing of blood vessels outside the brain and heart. Peripheral artery disease (PAD) occurs when this disorder affects arteries. In this case, cell and tissue death occur due to lack of oxygen-rich blood being provided by blood vessels. Typically, the result is pain in the lower extremities upon exertion that resolves upon rest. Intermittent claudication triggers leg pain, leg cramps, and coldness of the extremities. Treatment for PVD includes lifestyle changes such as quitting smoking, exercising, and increasing omega-3 fatty acid intake. Medications that control blood pressure, blood sugar, and cholesterol are often prescribed. In addition, drugs used to widen the blood vessels and prevent blood clots can be beneficial. Angioplasty, bypass surgery, and thrombolytic therapy are invasive treatment options.

Vasculitis or arteritis is the inflammation of a blood vessel. Blood vessels affected by vasculitis are thickened, narrow, and weak. As a result, vital organs do not receive sufficient blood and nutrients, leading to tissue and organ damage. There are many types of vasculitis, each classified by the size of the vessel(s) affected. An autoimmune response attacking the body's blood vessels causes fever, fatigue, and weight loss in many patients. Although some types of vasculitis may resolve spontaneously, other types require the use of steroids or immunosuppressive drugs.

Perspective and Prospects

The discovery of blood vessels was preceded by the finding of capillary circulation as early as 1628 by William Harvey. Harvey was first to theorize that blood circulates peripherally via capillaries. His findings also suggested that there was a system of arteries and veins fueled by a muscle pump. It was not until 1661 that Marcello Malpighi confirmed the passing of blood from arteries to veins through the use of a double convex lens. After about ten years and a very primitive microscope, Antoni van Leeuwenhoek realized that there was continuity in arteries and veins. Significant strides in vascular circulation did not take place until technology improved. In 1832, Marshall Hall was able to distinguish capillaries, arterioles, and venules with the use of a Dollond's microscope. This point seemed to be the catalyst to further understanding of capillary blood flow, concept of resistance, and location and function of capillary networks.

In 2009, scientists used high-resolution vascular biology research. This technique allows the study of clinical tissue material with cell-specific resolution. Blood vessels can potentially be taken from a patient and evaluated for certain diseases. Identification of the blood vessels in human tissue is then examined for genome-wide screening. Since blood vessels are essential components of many diseases, the implications of such research in cancer and chronic wounds is being questioned. Gene transfer to blood vessels is another potential therapy for various cardiovascular diseases. This method utilizes gene therapy to alter the nerves and muscles of blood vessels. Hypertension and the slowing of atherosclerosis are candidates for this novel approach. Gene transfer may replace pharmacological agents in the treatment of some cardiac diseases.

—*Jigna Bhalla, Pharm.D;*
updated by Rupinder P. Kaur

See also: Angiography; Angioplasty; Arteriosclerosis; Blood and blood disorders; Blood pressure; Bypass surgery; Cardiology; Carotid arteries; Circulation; Claudication; Embolism; Heart; Heart attack; Heart disease; Hypertension; Hypotension; Stents; Strokes; Vascular medicine; Vascular system; Vasculitis

For Further Information:
Kuntzman, Andrew J., and Gerard J. Tortora. "The Cardiovascular System: Blood Vessels and Circulation." *Anatomy and Physiology for the Manual Therapies,* 594-626. Hoboken, NJ: John Wiley & Sons, 2010.
McCann, A.B., and M.R. Jaff. "Treatment Strategies for Peripheral Artery Disease." *Expert Opinion on Pharmacotherapy* 10, no. 10 (July, 2009): 1571-1586.
Spittel, Peter C. "Peripheral Vascular Disease." *Mayo Clinic Cardiology Concise Textbook,* edited by Joseph G. Murphy and Margaret A. Lloyd. Rochester, MN: Scientific Publications, 2007.
Wennberg, Paul W. "Vasculitis." *Mayo Clinic Cardiology Concise Textbook,* edited by Joseph G. Murphy and Margaret A. Lloyd. Rochester, MN: Scientific Publications, 2007.

Blue baby syndrome

Disease/Disorder
Also known as: Tetralogy of Fallot
Anatomy or system affected: Circulatory system, heart
Specialties and related fields: Cardiology, embryology, neonatology
Definition: A congenital heart disease consisting of four distinct defects that result in poorly oxygenated blood being delivered to the tissues, thereby causing a bluish discoloration of the skin and mucous membranes upon birth.

Causes and Symptoms

Most congenital heart defects are thought to arise from maternal infections or the intake of certain drugs during pregnancy. The developing fetal heart is particularly susceptible to these effects during the second month of pregnancy, when major developmental changes are taking place.

Four distinct defects, called the tetralogy of Fallot, occur in infants suffering from blue baby syndrome. The first is a narrowing (stenosis) of the pulmonary trunk that takes

---

Information on Blue Baby Syndrome

Causes: Congenital heart defects resulting in poorly oxygenated blood delivered to body tissue
Symptoms: Bluish discoloration of skin and mucous membranes upon birth, breathlessness after exertion
Duration: Temporary, once corrected
Treatments: Surgery

---

blood to the lungs, where it is oxygenated. Narrowing of the pulmonary trunk is accompanied by a narrowing of the pulmonary semilunar valve, which resides in the pulmonary trunk. These two defects decrease blood flow to the lungs, resulting in a decreased oxygenation of the blood. Second, the wall that separates the left and right ventricles of the heart fails to form completely, thereby allowing the poorly oxygenated blood in the right ventricle to mix with the well-oxygenated blood in the left ventricle and decreasing oxygen delivery to tissues. Third, the aorta, which typically opens from the left ventricle and carries oxygenated blood to the tissues, is misaligned such that it opens from both the left and right ventricle. Fourth, the right ventricular muscle is thickened, as this muscle must work harder to push blood through the narrowed pulmonary semilunar valve and pulmonary trunk.

The first three defects result in poorly oxygenated blood being delivered to tissues, causing the skin and mucous membranes to appear bluish within minutes after birth, a condition called cyanosis. Children with uncorrected blue baby syndrome suffer from breathlessness after any form of exertion.

Treatment and Therapy

The tetralogy of Fallot is relatively rare, occurring in about one in every 1,500 births. Most defects can be corrected surgically. Successful correction of these defects early in the child's life prevents delayed growth and other complications of poor oxygen delivery.

—David K. Saunders, Ph.D.

See also: Apgar score; Birth defects; Cardiology, pediatric; Cardiovascular system; Circulation; Congenital disorders; Congenital heart disease; Cyanosis; Heart; Neonatology; Surgery, pediatric.

For Further Information:

Gersh, Bernard J., ed. *The Mayo Clinic Heart Book*. 2d ed. New York: Morrow, 2000.

Koenig, Peter, Ziyad M. Hijazi, and Frank Zimmerman, eds. *Essential Pediatric Cardiology*. New York: McGraw, 2004.

Levin, Daniel L., and Frances C. Morriss, eds. *Essentials of Pediatric Intensive Care*. 2d ed. New York: Churchill, 1997.

MacDonald, Mhairi G., Mary M. K. Seshia, and Martha D. Mullett, eds. *Avery's Neonatology: Pathophysiology and Management of the Newborn*. 6th ed. Philadelphia: Lippincott, 2005.

Neill, Catherine A., Edward B. Clark, and Carleen Clark. *The Heart of a Child: What Families Need to Know about Heart Disorders in Children*. 2d ed. Baltimore: Johns Hopkins UP, 2001.

Nixon, Harold, and Barry O'Donnell. *The Essentials of Pediatric Surgery*. 4th ed. Boston: Butterworth, 1992.

Park, Myung K. *The Pediatric Cardiology Handbook*. 4th. New York: Mosby, 2010.

Rosenblum, Laurie. "Tetralogy of Fallot." *Health Library*, Sept. 12, 2012.

Schumacher, Kurt R. "Tetralogy of Fallot." *MedlinePlus*, Dec. 1, 2011.

Blurred vision

Disease/Disorder
Anatomy or system affected: Eyes
Specialties and related fields: Emergency medicine, environmental health, family medicine, geriatrics and gerontology, gynecology, internal medicine, occupational health, ophthalmology, optometry, pediatrics, pharmacology, preventive medicine, sports medicine
Definition: A decrease in clarity of vision (visual acuity).

Causes and Symptoms

Blurred vision can result from any disturbance in the pathway of light as it travels from the cornea (the front of the eye) to the retina. By far the most common causes, however, are myopia (nearsightedness), hyperopia (farsightedness), astigmatism (failure of the eye to focus light evenly), and presbyopia (age-related difficulty in keeping near objects in focus). With nearsightedness and astigmatism, distance vision tends to be blurred. With farsightedness, near vision is blurred. Presbyopia is first noticed as middle-aged persons find difficulty in reading small type, such as that in telephone directories. Common, too, are incidents of blurred vision caused by improper prescription lenses or by improperly fitted or misused contact lenses.

Viral conjunctivitis (pinkeye) may produce blurred vision. It may be a symptom of infections of the retina by viruses, fungi, or parasites (often seen in AIDS patients) and of many other eye disorders including cataracts, glaucoma, and macular degeneration.

Blurred vision may also be a symptom of an underlying disease or disorder. Diabetes is a common cause; blurred vision can also result from the fluctuations in blood sugar level common to women in pregnancy. Blurred vision has been connected with kidney and nerve disease and with hypertension; it may be a warning sign or symptom of a stroke. Blurred vision has been associated with migraine headaches and brain tumors.

Environmental factors may also produce blurred vision. The most common environmental cause is extended exposure to the glare of computer monitors. Blurred vision can also result from injuries to the eye and head, exposure to chemical spills, and reactions to pollen, wind, sunlight, soaps, lotions, or cosmetics. Welders' exposure to ultraviolet radiation can produce blurred vision. Many prescription

---

Information on Blurred Vision

Causes: Myopia, hyperopia, astigmatism, presbyopia, viral conjunctivitis, retinal infections, disease, injury, environmental factors, medications
Symptoms: Difficulty reading small type, lack of visual acuity or focus
Duration: Temporary to chronic
Treatments: New or corrected lens prescription, medications, surgery

---

medicines, including some antibiotics, antihistamines, antidepressants, appetite suppressants, hormonal supplements, and blood pressure medications can cause difficulty in focusing. Steroids, which can lead to glaucoma, may also cause a swift rise in blood sugar, producing blurred vision.

Treatment and Therapy

Therapy and treatment depend on quick and reliable diagnosis of the cause, so examination by an ophthalmologist is advisable; adults should regularly schedule such examinations. Injuries to the eye or head and blurred vision in conjunction with any other symptom of retinal detachment require emergency care. Problems with prescription lenses may be taken either to opticians or ophthalmologists. Persons suffering from computer-screen glare may benefit from antireflective coatings on eyeglasses or glare-cutting filters that fit over computer monitors.

—*Betty Richardson, Ph.D.*

See also: Astigmatism; Brain disorders; Cataracts; Conjunctivitis; Diabetes mellitus; Eye infections and disorders; Eye surgery; Eyes; Glaucoma; Hypertension; Macular degeneration; Migraine headaches; Myopia; Occupational health; Ophthalmology; Optometry; Optometry, pediatric; Sense organs; Sjögren's syndrome; Steroids; Strokes; Vision; Vision disorders.

For Further Information:

Buettner, Helmut, ed. *Mayo Clinic on Vision and Eye Health: Practical Answers on Glaucoma, Cataracts, Macular Degeneration, and Other Conditions*. Rochester, Minn.: Mayo Foundation for Medical Education and Research, 2002.

Cassel, Gary H., Michael D. Billig, and Harry G. Randall. *The Eye Book: A Complete Guide to Eye Disorders and Health*. Baltimore: Johns Hopkins UP, 2001.

Komaroff, Anthony, ed. *Harvard Medical School Family Health Guide*. New York: Free Press, 2005.

National Foundation for Eye Research. *National Foundation for Eye Research*, 2004.

Porter, Robert S., et al., eds. *The Merck Manual Home Health Handbook*. Whitehouse Station, N.J.: Merck Research Laboratories, 2009.

Sardegna, Jill, et al. *The Encyclopedia of Blindness and Vision Impairment*. 2d ed. New York: Facts On File, 2002.

Vorvick, Linda J. "Vision Problems." *MedlinePlus*, Sept. 3, 2012.

Body dysmorphic disorder

Disease/Disorder

Also known as: Dysmorphobia, imagined ugliness syndrome

Anatomy or system affected: Brain, psychic-emotional system, skin

Specialties and related fields: Dermatology, family medicine, internal medicine, plastic surgery, psychiatry

Definition: A psychiatric somatoform disorder resulting in exaggerated preoccupation with an imagined or minor defect in physical appearance that causes significant impairment of social functioning.

Key terms:

cognitive behavior psychotherapy: talk therapy consisting of cognitive interaction between a patient and a mental health professional

dysmorphic: abnormal in shape or appearance

neurotransmitter: a chemical that carries messages between cells in the brain or nervous system

selective serotonin reuptake inhibitor (SSRI): a class of antidepressant medications effective in the treatment of anxiety disorders

somatoform disorder: a mental disorder whose symptoms focus on the physical body

Causes and Symptoms

Body dysmorphic disorder (BDD) may be related to, though distinct from, other psychiatric disorders such as obsessive-compulsive disorder, eating disorders, and depression. No definitive cause has been identified, though proposed models suggest an interaction of societal overemphasis on physical appearance, low self-esteem, and brain neurotransmitter abnormalities. There is increasing evidence of a genetic predisposition to anxiety-related disorders.

Patients have an overblown concern about one or more perceived body defects, commonly of the face, hair, or skin. Some patients may fixate on muscles, penis, breasts, or buttocks. Individuals suffer extreme distress as a result, which interferes with social and occupational functioning. Diagnostic criteria determined by the American Psychiatric Association include preoccupation with an imagined or minor defect in physical appearance that causes significant interruption of social functioning and is not explained by another mental disorder, such as anorexia nervosa.

Patients are often embarrassed or ashamed of the problem. They may become housebound and have difficulty maintaining interpersonal relationships. They may spend hours each day checking their appearance in mirrors and attempting to correct or hide the defect with excessive grooming rituals. Poor school and job performance are common, and approximately three-quarters of patients are unmarried.

Sufferers will often seek help from plastic surgeons or dermatologists to correct their perceived defect. This approach is most often unsuccessful, as the change in appearance is rarely enough to satisfy the patient. This may lead to repeated attempts at corrective surgery, which continue to result in disappointment, as they address only a symptom rather than the underlying disordered thinking.

Approximately 1 percent of the general adult population is thought to suffer from body dysmorphic disorder, with men and women being equally affected. The typical onset is in late adolescence or early adulthood. Patients are at increased risk for major depression. It is estimated that 60 percent of these patients also suffer from depression, and this combination places them at significant risk of suicide. Coexisting obsessive-compulsive disorder is also common.

Treatment and Therapy

The disorder is not uncommon, but it is frequently missed or misdiagnosed. Patients are most likely to be identified during visits to family practitioners, internists, dermatologists, or plastic surgeons where they describe physical features that they wish to change. Often they are seeking referral to a specialist for correction of the imagined defect.

When BDD is suspected, referral to a psychiatrist for evaluation and treatment is most appropriate. Definitive treatment is unknown, but pharmacologic treatment with high-dose selective serotonin reuptake inhibitors (SSRIs) combined with nonpharmacologic cognitive behavior psychotherapy is the most effective approach currently. It is important to avoid attempted cosmetic correction, which does not treat the underlying disorder and is rarely effective.

SSRIs are thought to reduce symptoms by regulating neurotransmitters in the brain. Their use has been shown to decrease the frequency of disturbing thoughts and ritualistic behaviors related to the perceived physical flaw. This treatment is more effective when combined with cognitive behavior psychotherapy to address the patient's low self-esteem and negative body image. Therapy that educates and includes family members, spouses, and other close individuals may improve outcome.

Body dysmorphic disorder is typically a chronic condition requiring ongoing care. Relapse following discontinuation of therapy is common. The prognosis is good with continued treatment and follow-up.

Perspective and Prospects

Italian physician Enrique Morselli coined the term *dysmorphobia* in 1891 to describe patients who were tortured by their fear of an imagined physical deformity that was not noticeable to others. The condition was recognized by the American Psychiatric Association in 1987, renamed body dysmorphic disorder, and classified as a distinct somatoform disorder in the *Diagnostic and Statistical Manual of Mental Disorders, Fourth Edition* (DSM-IV; 1994). Among other updates, the *DSM-5*, published in 2013, adds the diagnostic criterion of repetitive behavior, feelings, or thoughts in response to a preoccupation with a perceived flaw.

The disorder has received significant attention and is now the subject of ongoing clinical research. Additional data are needed to pinpoint causes and evaluate new treatment approaches.

—*Rachel Zahn, M.D.*

See also: Antidepressants; Anxiety; Breast surgery; Breasts, female; Delusions; Dementias; Depression; Dermatology; Dermatology, pe-diatric; Ear surgery; Face lift and blepharoplasty; Gender reassignment surgery; Liposuction; Obesity; Obsessive-compulsive disorder; Otoplasty; Phobias; Plastic surgery; Psychiatric disorders; Psychiatry; Psychosomatic disorders; Ptosis; Rhinoplasty and submucous resection; Skin; Skin lesion removal; Surgical procedures; Varicose vein removal; Varicose veins; Warts.

For Further Information:

American Psychiatric Association. *Diagnostic and Statistical Manual of Mental Disorders: DSM-5*. 5th ed. Arlington, Va.: Author, 2013.

American Psychiatric Association. "Highlights of Changes from DSM-IV-TR to DSM-5." Arlington, Va.: Author, 2013.

Anxiety and Depression Association of America. "Body Dysmorphic Disorder (BDD)." *ADAA*, 2010-13.

Hunt, T. J. "The Mirror Lies: Body Dysmorphic Disorder." *American Family Physician* 104.7 (July, 2008): 1204-17.

Phillips, K. A. *The Broken Mirror: Understanding and Treating Body Dysmorphic Disorder*. New York: Oxford UP, 2005.

Slaughter J. R., and A. M. Sun. "In Pursuit of Perfection: A Primary Care Physician's Guide to Body Dysmorphic Disorder." *American Family Physician* 60.6 (October, 1999): 1738-42.

Bonding

Development

Anatomy or system affected: Psychic-emotional system

Specialties and related fields: Neonatology, psychiatry, psychology

Definition: The formation of an attachment; specifically, the developing relationship between infants and their parents that begins immediately after birth.

Key terms:

attachment: the development of a nurturing relationship between an infant and its caretaker(s)

failure to thrive: a lack of healthy growth that may result from the absence of a nurturing presence and support, both emotionally and physically

Physical and Psychological Factors

Bonding is usually associated with neonates (newborns), but it is an ongoing relationship that occurs between infants, toddlers, or children and their caretakers.

After the initial cry, the neonate calms down and uses its first touch with the mother to relax. This experience may occur in a brightly lit hospital room with medical attendants or in a semidark birthing room at home with nurses or midwives attending. Usually, the infant is placed on the mother's abdomen for contact to begin. The initial moments of connection may include the parents touching, rubbing, and stroking the baby's cheeks, fingers, toes, abdomen, and back. Research reports that even in these early moments, an infant may engage in limited imitations of the parents by moving the head, opening and closing the mouth, and responding to their facial gestures.

These first touches begin the relationship that may initiate a successful bonding attachment with the primary caregivers and the extended family. Some circumstances, however, may start a process that does not lead to successful attachment. The process of bonding between a newborn and caregivers is an essential part of normal development. The care that the infant receives at this point, as well as through the subsequent early stages of life, is vital to his or

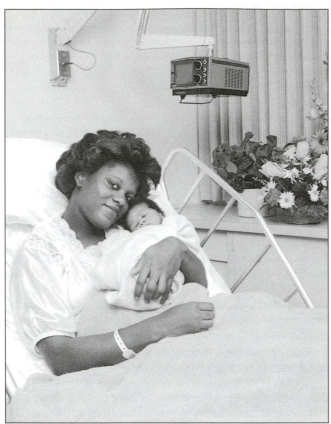

Bonding is an emotional and physiological process that begins at birth. (Digital Stock)

her healthy development. Some infants, however, may need ancillary medical care that removes the child from the mother's touch and postpones connecting immediately after birth.

As the infant begins to grow, the early stages of development should be supported, sharpened, and enhanced during the continuing developmental and bonding process. Babies actively seek stimulation, and the first week of life involves hearing, seeing, smelling, and touching. Distinguishing sounds is a learning process. Soft noises, lullabies, and soft music are soothing. Basic visual powers exist that are important for communication and learning. Infants are sensitive to the intensity of light. They can discriminate shapes and patterns. Feeding involves smelling food, distinguishing tastes, and becoming aware of the presence of the mother or primary caregiver. The infant can feel changes in temperature and respond to skin contact and touch.

While bonding tends to be associated with the mother-infant relationship, the attachment and bonding process also includes the relationship with the other parent, siblings, and other relatives who come into frequent contact with the developing baby. The interaction within this social network creates a variety of relationships and opportunities for positive and responsive stimulation, support, and encouragement. Connections with grandparents, aunts, uncles, and cousins can provide strong supportive bonds that help infants thrive. The strength of these relationships can make up for limitations with the primary caregivers.

Disorders and Effects

The relationship between some caregivers and infants may encounter serious problems as they try to establish attachment. Bonding disorders such as failure to thrive can occur with infants who are abused or neglected. One of the major reasons that babies in institutions do not do well is the infrequent handling and touching that they receive.

Infants exhibiting failure to thrive show a variety of symptoms. They are usually quite small. They appear ill, listless, and immobile and may be unable to digest food. Other symptoms of failure to thrive include low birth weight, eye contact avoidance, and evidence of delayed development. Improvements can occur with appropriate feeding and care. Failure to thrive may also occur due to purely physical causes, such as congenital genetic disorders. Such disorders are generally not reversible, unless the specific defect can be corrected medically.

If a mother had early developmental experiences of abuse and neglect, these experiences may appear as obstacles to the development of her own infant. The mother of a failure-to-thrive infant may be using drugs or alcohol. She may be depressed, physically or mentally ill, or unable to cope well enough to provide a positive bonding experience for her child. She may have recently been involved in a significant crisis that was emotionally draining.

Significant variables may precede the attachment phase, or environmental forces may impede the infant's maternal attachment as the bonding process proceeds. If the infant does not have a positive experience with the mother during the first months of life, developmental problems may begin. When the mother or infant must remain in a hospital for a prolonged period of time, the mother may be unavailable; nurturing can be delayed or occur only for short periods. A mother may be psychologically unable to be close to her infant because of other young children or her own psychological problems or disorders. Some mothers experience postpartum depression as a result of hormonal imbalances and overwhelming demands. Economic and social circumstances may also impede the bonding process.

Establishing warm, comforting relationships through interactions between babies, parents, caregivers, and other family members in the earliest weeks is critical to forming secure attachments and developing successful bonding.

—Gwenelle S. O'Neal, D.S.W.;
updated by Alexander Sandra, M.D.

See also: Breast-feeding; Cognitive development; Developmental stages; Failure to thrive; Psychiatry, child and adolescent.

For Further Information:

A.D.A.M. Medical Encyclopedia. "Infant-Newborn Development." *MedlinePlus*, January 17, 2011.

Caplan, Theresa. *The First Twelve Months of Life: Your Baby's Growth Month by Month*. New York: Bantam, 1995.

Cohen, Lawrence. *Playful Parenting*. New York: Random House, 2002.

Craig, Grace J., Marguerite D. Kermis, and Nancy Digdon. *Children Today*. 2d ed. Toronto, Ont.: Prentice Hall, 2002.

Kids Health. "Bonding with Your Baby." *Nemours Foundation*, January 2012.

Leach, Penelope. *Your Baby and Child: From Birth to Age Five*. London: Dorling Kindersley, 2003.

MedlinePlus. "Infant and Newborn Care." *MedlinePlus*, June 17, 2013.

Mercer, Jean. *Understanding Attachment: Parenting, Child Care, and Emotional Development*. Westport, Conn.: Praeger, 2006.

Parker, DeAnsin Goodson, and Karen W. Bressler. *Yoga Baby: Exercises to Help You Bond with Your Baby, Physically, Emotionally, and Spiritually*. New York: Broadway Books, 2000.

Sears, William, and Martha Sears. *The Attachment Parenting Book: A Commonsense Guide to Understanding and Nurturing Your Baby*. New York: Little, Brown, 2001.

Bone cancer

Disease/Disorder

Anatomy or system affected: Bones, musculoskeletal system

Specialties and related fields: Immunology, oncology, orthopedics, radiology

Definition: Cancer of the bone, which may have originated there or have spread from another site in the body.

Key terms:

adjuvant therapy: the use of multiple treatments for cancer, such as chemotherapy and/or radiation, following surgery to prevent metastasis

biopsy: the removal of tissue from a suspected cancer site in order to identify abnormal cells under microscopic examination by a pathologist

bone scan: a diagnostic technique using a radioactive tracer that is strongly absorbed by a tumor, whose location then can be detected by radiation counters

computed tomography (CT) scanning: a method of displaying the outline of a tumor, utilizing a computer to combine information from multiple X-ray beams

magnetic resonance imaging (MRI): a diagnostic technique used to see the outline of an internal organ or a tumor without using X rays

medullary cavity: the interior of a bone, where new blood cells are formed by the bone marrow, surrounded by a hard outer cortex

metastasis: the spread of cancer cells from an original tumor site to other parts of the body

palliative treatment: the use of drugs or radiation to suppress a tumor and to provide relief from pain when a cure is not possible

sarcoma: a malignant tumor originating in bone or connective tissue

staging: a numerical classification system used by physicians to describe how far a cancerous growth has advanced

Causes and Symptoms

Out of about one million new cancers that are diagnosed annually in the United States, less than 0.2 percent are primary bone cancer. The American Cancer Society estimates that approximately 3,010 new cases of bone cancer will be diagnosed in 2013. Most of these cases arise in children under the age of twenty. If diagnosis is made before the bone cancer has spread to the lungs or other sites in the body, prompt treatment by surgery, radiation, or chemotherapy can provide a good prognosis for recovery.

In older adults, most cases of so-called bone cancer actually are secondary tumors that have spread from other parts

> ### Information on Bone Cancer
> **Causes:** Gene mutations in bone cells, metastasized tumors from other sites
> **Symptoms:** Localized swelling followed by persistent, dull pain; fatigue, fever, loss of appetite, other signs of general illness
> **Duration:** Acute or long-term
> **Treatments:** Surgery, radiation, chemotherapy

of the body, especially from the breast, prostate, thyroid, lung, or kidney. Such metastasized tumors consist of cells that are characteristic of their original, primary site. Secondary bone cancers are far more common than those which start in the bone.

The first symptom of bone cancer in children usually is a localized swelling followed by persistent, dull pain. It is easily mistaken for a sprain or a bruise that might come from a minor injury. Additional symptoms are fatigue, fever, loss of appetite, and other signs of general illness. Unfortunately, early symptoms may be ignored until the disease has already spread to other parts of the body. Before chemotherapy became available in the 1970s, the spread of bone cancer to the lungs occurred within two years for about 80 percent of patients.

A variety of diagnostic techniques are available to the physician if the examination of a patient arouses the suspicion of bone cancer. Blood tests, including a study of liver and kidney functions, have become increasingly useful because of improvements in analytical procedure. X-ray photography and computed tomography (CT) scanning will give pictorial evidence of any lesions or excess bony growth. Magnetic resonance imaging (MRI) provides the best visualization of tumors extending into soft tissue. Finally, the most important diagnostic procedure is biopsy. Usually, the bone is opened surgically and a sample of tissue is taken. Sometimes, a hollow needle inserted through the bone cortex can be used to withdraw a small sample. A pathologist who specializes in oncology examines the tissue under a microscope to confirm if cancer cells are present and to identify their type.

Magnetic resonance imaging as a diagnostic technique was developed in the 1980s, giving remarkable picture clarity for soft tissue. A strong magnetic field and radio waves are used to determine the concentration of hydrogen in a region of the body. Since tissue is mostly water (which contains hydrogen) and bone is dry, the image will show bright areas for tissue or soft organs against a dark background. Also, MRI shows contrast between normal tissue and a denser, tumorous mass.

Another diagnostic technique, the bone scan, is used to investigate whether a tumor has metastasized to other bones in the body. A small amount of radioactive tracer, usually technetium, is injected into the patient. It circulates in the bloodstream and gradually accumulates in the bone marrow. After several hours, radiation counters are used to scan the entire skeleton from head to foot. Regions of rapid cell growth, which may signal a tumorous mass, are indicated by a relatively high counting rate. If secondary tumors are detected by the bone scan, their shape and size can be investigated further using MRI.

Several kinds of bone cancer have been identified. One type is called osteosarcoma. It occurs most frequently during puberty, when a child's bones are growing rapidly. The tumor is likely to develop inside the long bones of the arms, in the legs near the knee, or in the pelvis. As its size increases and the surrounding bone material becomes soft, the bone may fracture because of internal pressure in the bone. Osteosarcomas also may grow on the exterior surface of bones, producing hard spikes that radiate outward. Another type of bone cancer is called Ewing's sarcoma. MRI and CT scans commonly exhibit a "moth-eaten" appearance where bone destruction has taken place. Both the inner (medullary) cavity and the outer cortex of the bone can be affected. Subsequently, a tumorous mass develops within the covering of tissue that surrounds the bone. This abnormal growth tends to form concentric layers, like the skin of an onion. The localized swelling expands in size, causing soreness and eventually impeding motion at the joints.

Bone cancer can take a variety of other forms. For example, a tumor may invade the bone from the outside and then penetrate into the medullary cavity. To make an accurate diagnosis and institute the best possible treatment for bone cancer, particularly for children, it is important for patients and their families to find an oncologist and supporting staff with specialized experience in this relatively rare condition. In general, the orthopedic surgeon who does the biopsy should be a specialist who is trained to do the ultimate bone surgery, so that any cancer cell contamination at the site of the biopsy will be completely removed.

Treatment and Therapy

To develop an appropriate treatment plan for a patient with bone cancer, all the relevant diagnostic information must be brought together. A medical team consisting of a radiologist, pathologist, radiation therapist, orthopedic surgeon, and medical oncologist will assess how far the cancer has advanced. This is called staging, that is, classifying its stage of growth.

Three designations commonly are used to characterize a cancer: G for its grade (based on the microscopic tissue analysis), T for tumor size and penetration, and M for evidence of metastasis. For example, (G1) (T2) (M0) would describe a low-grade tumor (G1) that has broken out of its bone compartment (T2) but has not metastasized (M0) to the lungs or elsewhere.

Before 1970, treatment of a cancerous bone normally meant amputation. The prognosis for recovery was less than 20 percent, however, because microscopic, invisible metastases to the lungs and other organs usually were already present. The experimental search for drugs that can fight cancer cells started in the 1930s. Charles B. Huggins discovered that the female sex hormone estrogen could halt the growth of prostate cancer in men. He received the Nobel Prize in Medicine in 1966 for his work. Since that pioneering success, several hundred thousand drugs have been tested, with less than a hundred showing any substantial benefit. The anticancer drugs also can have severe side effects on healthy cells. Fortunately, a rapidly growing tumor has a higher rate of metabolism, so drugs will kill the cancer cells at a lower dose and spare most normal cells.

An effective method of treating bone cancer in children is to use chemotherapy or radiation even before surgery, in order to shrink the size of a tumor. Instead of complete amputation, the surgeon may need to remove only part of a bone, thus saving the limb. Even when a bone joint must be amputated, it may still be possible to salvage the limb by inserting an artificial joint or one from an organ donor.

In older adults, cancer of the bone almost invariably is caused by metastasis from another location in the body. The tumor in the bone may be very painful. Radiation to the affected area can provide palliative treatment, while more aggressive action is taken against the primary cancer site.

A wide range of medications is available to help control pain and to counteract the disagreeable side effects of radiation or chemotherapy. Special attention is given to the diet of cancer patients to prevent weight loss and to maintain body strength. Loss of appetite and digestion problems are common symptoms during therapy. Strong painkilling drugs such as codeine and morphine sometimes are necessary. The dose should be limited, however, so that the patient's ability to interact socially is not completely lost.

Vigorous research to find more effective therapies for cancer is widely supported. The goal is to find procedures that are less mutilating, less expensive, and less painful for the patient. Promising new drugs must be tested to determine how large a dose is needed and how serious the side effects are. Therefore, patients may be asked to become volunteers in a clinical trial of an experimental treatment. Although people have a justified sense of reluctance to become "guinea pigs" in an untested therapy, clinical trials with human subjects have been essential in the development of successful medical procedures. Firm guidelines have been established for testing new therapies, such as the requirement to obtain the informed consent of patients and their families. In addition, doctors in the United States are responsible to a medical oversight committee and are obligated to submit their results for professional review. Cancer treatment can make progress through willing participation by patients in the carefully planned clinical trials.

Perspective and Prospects

Bone cancer first came to the attention of the public in the 1920s through a notorious case of industrial poisoning. A manufacturing company in New Jersey was utilizing radioactive radium to make watch dials that would glow in the dark. The women workers who were hired to apply the luminous paint would twirl the paint brushes between their lips to make a fine tip. The ingested radium, being chemically similar to calcium, became concentrated in bones, especially of the jaw and neck. Eventually, more than forty workers died of bone cancer, including the company's chief chemist.

After this incident, it became clear that radiation has a particularly damaging effect on bone marrow. In fact, any rapidly dividing cells in the body are especially radiosensitive. This would include hair, skin, and the reproductive system. It is unfortunate that it took until the 1950s before X-ray fluoroscopes were removed from shoe stores. Parents were fascinated to see the bones of their child's foot inside a new shoe without realizing that the radiation was harmful.

Until 1970, the outlook for a child who developed bone cancer was very poor. In spite of amputation of the affected limb, 80 percent of the young patients died within two years. In 1972, Norman Jaffe and Emil Frei in Boston made a major breakthrough in therapy by giving their patients large doses of a drug called methotrexate after limb surgery. It was a new approach in chemotherapy to stop the cancer from spreading even though no metastasis was visible yet. The experimental drug was so powerful that other antidote drugs were given to control side effects. The first trial with seventeen children was very successful, with all of them still surviving after twenty-one months.

However, an article written in 1994 by Tim Beardsley summarizing the status of cancer in the United States came to a rather pessimistic conclusion. The cancer rate was higher and the likelihood of cure had not improved for most types of adult cancer since the "war on cancer" was initiated by President Richard M. Nixon in 1971. The cumulative effects of smoking, poor diet, and continuing exposure to harmful chemicals may help to explain this lack of progress. The good news was that the death rate from childhood cancer fell by almost half in that period. Early diagnosis and improved therapy have helped greatly. The family of a child with cancer can now look forward with substantial hope for a cure without recurrence.

—*Hans G. Graetzer, Ph.D.*

See also: Bone disorders; Bones and the skeleton; Cancer; Chemotherapy; Ewing's sarcoma; Fracture and dislocation; Fracture repair; Malignancy and metastasis; National Cancer Institute (NCI); Nuclear radiology; Oncology; Orthopedic surgery; Orthopedics; Orthopedics, pediatric; Palliative medicine; Radiation therapy; Sarcoma; Stem cells; Tumors.

For Further Information:
American Cancer Society (ACS). "What Are the Key Statistics about Bone Cancer?"*American Cancer Society*, Jan. 22, 2013.
Cady, Blake, ed. *Cancer Manual*. 7th ed. Boston: American Cancer Society, 1986.
Dollinger, Malin, et al. *Everyone's Guide to Cancer Therapy*. 5th ed. Kansas City, Mo.: Andrews, 2008.
Dorfman, Howard D. and Bogdan Czerniak. *Bone Tumors*. St. Louis, Mo.: Mosby, 1998.
Eyre, Harmon J., Dianne Partie Lange, and Lois B. Morris. *Informed Decisions: The Complete Book of Cancer Diagnosis, Treatment, and Recovery*. 2d ed. Atlanta: American Cancer Society, 2002.
Janes-Hodder, Honna, and Nancy Keene. *Childhood Cancer: A Parent's Guide to Solid Tumor Cancers*. 2d ed. Cambridge, Mass.: O'Reilly, 2002.
MedlinePlus. "Bone Cancer." *MedlinePlus*, Apr. 10, 2013.

Bone disorders

Disease/Disorder

Anatomy or system affected: Back, bones, feet, hands, legs, musculoskeletal system, ribs, vertebral column

Specialties and related fields: Geriatrics and gerontology, oncology, orthopedics, rheumatology

Definition: The various traumatic events or inherited conditions that can affect bones and the tissues surrounding them, such as fractures, dislocations, degenerative processes, infections, osteoporosis, and cancer.

Key terms:

acute: referring to the sudden onset of a disease process

cartilage: connective tissue between bones that forms a pad or cushion to absorb weight and shock

chronic: referring to a lingering disease process

osteoblast: bone-forming cells that secrete the matrix that mineralizes into bone

osteoclast: large, multinucleated cells that resorb bone

pathogen: any disease-causing microorganism

Causes and Symptoms

Bones are usually studied together with their surrounding structures because many of the disorders to which bones are subjected also involve the muscular, connective and cartilaginous tissues to which they are joined. Hence, a common term for this medical category is "musculoskeletal and connective tissue disorders."

There are 206 bones in the human body that serve three functions. Some form protective housing for body organs and structures; these include the skull, which encloses the brain, and the rib cage, which encloses the heart and lungs. Some support the body's posture and weight, including the spine and the bones of the hips and legs. The third function is motion: most of the bones in the body are involved in movement. These bones include those of the hands, wrists, arms, hips, legs, ankles, and feet.

Bone consists of three sections: an outer layer called the periosteum; the hard, bony tissue itself, composed of widely mineralized networks of collagen and other proteins that form rigid skeletal structures; and the interior, a spongy mass of cancellous (chambered) tissue, where blood marrow and some fat cells are stored. Bone is living tissue. It is a depository for calcium, phosphate, and other minerals that are vital to many body processes. Calcium and phosphate are constantly being deposited in and withdrawn from bone tissue to be used throughout the body.

Skeletal dysplasias: Inherited bone disorders are collectively known as *skeletal dysplasias*. These genetic diseases constitute a highly heterogeneous group of conditions. Skeletal dysplasias are estimated to occur in 15.7 per 100,000 births.

Achondroplasia is the most common skeletal dysplasia in humans and results from mutations in the *FGFR3* (fibroblast growth factor receptor 3) gene. Achondroplasia causes short statue (dwarfism) due to long-bone shortening that affects both the upper and lower extremities.

Dysostosis multiplex results from storage metabolic disorders in which the body cannot degrade complex macromolecules like complex carbohydrates,

Information on Bone Disorders

Causes: Fractures, dislocations, degenerative processes, infections, cancer

Symptoms: Varies widely; may include porous and brittle bones, impaired movement, pain, inflammation, numbness and tingling

Duration: Acute to chronic

Treatments: Setting and immobilization of bones in cast or splint, surgery, medications (antirheumatic drugs, corticosteroids), supplements (vitamin D, calcium, hormone therapy), orthopedic support, lifestyle changes

glycoproteins, or glycolipids. The progressive accumulation of these waste products affects cartilage and bones and the vertebrae flatten and the ribs show "paddle rib deformities." The long bones are affected as are the bones of the hands.

Disorders that cause low bone density include osteogenesis imperfecta and hypophosphatasia. Osteogenesis imperfecta results from mutations that cause abnormal deposition, formation, and/or secretion of bone-specific collagen (type I collagen) Because type I collagen is both a highly complex protein with three polypeptide chains wound about in a triple-helical structure that is cross-linked to form tight, strong cable-like structures, and the major organic component of bone, mutations in either the type I collagen structural genes (*COLA1* and *COLA2*), or genes that encode proteins necessary for processing, folding, synthesis, or secretion (*FKBL10, CRTAP, LEPRE1, PPIB, SERPINF1, SERPH1,* and *IFITM5*) of type I collagen result in various forms of osteogenesis imperfecta. Hypophosphatasia is caused by mutations in the tissue-nonspecific alkaline phosphatase gene (*TNSALP*), which starves the forming bones for phosphate and inhibits bone mineralization.

Other skeletal dysplasias cause excessively high bone density. Bone equilibrium relies on bone deposition by cells called osteoblasts and bone resorption by cells called osteoclasts. Skeletal dysplasias that cause high bone densities, known as osteopetroses, are usually caused by poor osteoclast activity. Pyknodysostosis is caused by mutations in the *CTSK* gene, which encodes the cathepsin K protein, an enzyme used by osteoclasts to degrade bone. This condition causes short statue, abnormal teeth, skull, face, and hand structure. Infantile malignant osteopetrosis is caused by mutations in the carbonic anhydrase type II (*CA2*) gene and is associated with early mortality. Autosomal dominant osteopetrosis type II (also known as Albers-Schönberg disease) is caused by mutations in the *CLCN7* gene, which encodes a chloride channel, and results in deformities to the base of the skull, spine, and pelvis.

Finally, metaphyseal dysplasias cause disproportionately short statues with short limbs. These include cartilage-hair hypoplasia (caused by mutations in the *RMRP* gene), Schmid metaphyseal chondroplasia (caused by mutations in the *COL10A1* gene), Jansen type metaphyseal chondroplasia (caused by mutations in the *PTHR1* gene), and Schwachman-Diamond syndrome (caused by mutations in the *SBDS* gene).

Bones can be attacked in many other ways as well: They can be broken or dislocated; the processes by which they form, grow, and maintain themselves can be compromised; they can be attacked by pathogens; they can be subject to a series of degenerative diseases that impede function and even destroy bone tissue; and they can become cancerous.

Dislocations take place when the bones of a joint are forced out of alignment. They may occur in the elbows of young children whose arms are forcibly pulled. Fractures are more common. They arise from sports activities, accidents, falls, or hundreds of possible causes, including various disease conditions.

Bone infection is called osteomyelitis; it occurs most often in children. Infection can be introduced to the bone by fracture or other exposure, or it can be carried to the bone in the blood. By far the most prevalent long-term bone disorders are those in the general class of diseases called arthritis. Osteoarthritis, a common form, is sometimes called "wear and- tear arthritis" because it usually surfaces in older people after years of work have constantly challenged certain joints. It occurs often in contact sports such as football, where its progression can be accelerated by years of rough-and-tumble activity. Joints are cushioned by pads of cartilage. Eventually, this cartilage can wear down and become rough. It cannot protect the bones of the joint, and little nodes form at the ends of the bones. Bones of the neck and back are often affected, as are the hips and knees.

Osteoarthritis is painful and debilitating, but it is rarely crippling. More painful and far more serious is rheumatoid arthritis, a progressive disease. It often starts with inflammation in the joints of the hands or feet and is usually bilateral, for example affecting both hands, both feet, or both knees. While rheumatoid arthritis may start with relatively mild inflammation, it can progress to severe deformity and even complete destruction of the joint. Fingers and toes can become grossly twisted; the joint can become completely fused and immobile. There are other relatively common forms of arthritis. People with the skin condition psoriasis can develop psoriatic arthritis. Reiter's syndrome is a form of arthritis that can be transmitted through sexual contact. Ankylosing spondylitis is a form of arthritis that can affect any of the joints in the torso, such as the shoulders and hips, but is most often found in the neck and spine. Patients with inflammatory bowel disease (IBD) may also develop a concomitant arthritis in the joints of the hands or feet.

The bone condition called gout can affect many joints, but it appears most often in the big toe. The body produces a substance called uric acid. If, for any reason, too much is produced, or if it is not properly eliminated, uric acid crystals can form around joints and trigger inflammation. Gout is extremely painful, and an attack may last for weeks. The spine is subject to a wide range of disorders. One of the most common is the prolapsed (slipped) disk. The individual vertebrae of the spine are separated and cushioned by pads of cartilage called disks. For various reasons, a disk can bulge out and impinge on the nerves of the spinal column. The result can be severe pain, numbness, and loss of movement. In some individuals, the spine fails to grow correctly or becomes misaligned, or curved. This condition is called scoliosis. The curvature of the spine can cause the ribs on one side of the body to separate as those on the other side are pushed together. Over time, this separation can cause severe heart and lung problems.

Many cases of joint pain are attributable to inflammation of the tissues surrounding the bony structures. An example is bursitis, in which the bursa, a saclike membrane enclosing many joints, becomes inflamed. Repetitive activities, such as throwing a baseball, hitting a tennis ball, or scrubbing the floor on one's knees, can irritate the membrane and cause inflammation.

Osteomalacia is a disorder of bone mineralization that occurs at newly formed bone sites. This disorder causes bone pain and tenderness, higher rates of fractures, difficulty walking and changes in gait, and muscle weakness, spasms, cramps and numbness and tingling. Poor bone mineralization results from inadequate calcium, phosphate, or alkaline phosphatase levels, severe vitamin D deficiencies, hyperthyroidism, and inherited kidney conditions that cause excessive phosphate loss (type 2 renal tubular acidosis).

Paget disease of bone occurs in about three percent of patients of 40 and up to nine percent of older patients. Paget disease is characterized by localized overgrowth of bone at various sites. Most of these overgrowths cause no symptoms (asymptomatic), but some impinge on nearby organs and cause pain, or compromise the function of compressed organs. Paget disease results from osteoclast malfunction.

Bone cancers or tumors can be benign or malignant. Cancer rarely begins in the bone; it usually spreads there from a tumorous site elsewhere in the body. Of the cancers that arise directly within bone tissue, the most common are multiple myeloma, in which cancer originates in plasma (white) cells and affects the body's ability to produce proteins and fight infection, and osteosarcoma, in which the cancerous tumor originates on the bone itself.

Treatment and Therapy

In treating a fractured bone, the most important thing is to realign the segments and keep them immobile until they can fuse. Most often, the physician will X-ray the fracture, set the bones correctly, and immobilize the limb in a cast. If injury to the spinal column is suspected, the physician may also order computed tomography (CT) scanning. Surgery is sometimes required to set the bones, and the surgeon may join the bone segments together with pins, plates, or screws. In some cases, it is possible to cement bone fragments together with a special glue. Broken arms, legs, fingers, and toes can usually be easily immobilized with appropriate casts or splints. In cases of accidents, falls, or other trauma, if there is any suspicion of injury to the spinal column, it is critical not to move the patient. Movement can worsen the injury and even cause permanent paralysis.

Dislocations, like fractures, should be X-rayed. If the spinal column appears to be involved, CT scanning may be required. The misaligned bones are put back in their proper positions, and the joint is immobilized, often with a splint. Osteoporosis requires both preventive and therapeutic care. If the physician recognizes that an individual, usually a postmenopausal woman, is at high risk for osteoporosis, supplementary calcium will be prescribed and, in some patients, estrogen replacement therapy. When osteoporosis has begun, supplementary calcium, vitamin D, and hormone therapy may check the progress of the disease. Drugs called bisphosphonates, which inhibit osteoclast activity, can stabilize bone density and reduce the risk of osteoporotic fractures of the spine, wrist, hip, humerus, and pelvis. Unfortunately, these drugs do not help increase bone density. To increase bone density, teriparatide (*Forteo*), a shortened, recombinant form of parathyroid hormone, recombinant salmon calcitonin (*Miacalcin*), or denosumab (*Prolia*, *Xgeva*) can increase bone density in patients with osteoporosis or decrease bone loss in patients with bone cancer. Teriparatide and calcitonin tend to increase osteoblast activity, but denosumab inhibits the maturation of pre-osteoblasts into mature osteoblasts. A disadvantage of these drugs in that once they are discontinued, the patient tends to steadily lose bone density anew.

A patient may suffer from acute back pain because of crushed vertebrae in the spine. Pain relievers such as aspirin may be required, and the patient may need orthopedic support. Gentle exercise is recommended to strengthen back muscles. In osteomalacia, vitamin D, phosphorus, and calcium supplements are the mainstays of therapy. In osteomyelitis, antibiotics will usually eradicate the infection, but in some cases, surgery is required to remove infected tissue. In other cases, amputation is the only option. The first line of therapy for osteoarthritis and rheumatoid arthritis is the relief of pain and inflammation. The physician may recommend rest and immobilization of the joint; heating pads and hot baths may give some relief. Exercise can maintain motility in the joints and help the patient avoid stiffness. Most patients are given over-the-counter pain relievers such as aspirin, ibuprofen, or acetaminophen. In many patients, however, these drugs are either not adequate to manage the pain or, as in the case of aspirin, ibuprofen, and others, may be irritating to the gastrointestinal tract. Gastrointestinal disturbances are also common with the drugs proscribed for arthritis. Gastric and duodenal ulcers are often reported and are sometimes so severe that the patient requires surgery. In a small but significant number of patients who develop such ulcers, the outcome is fatal.

Because rheumatoid arthritis is a crippling disease that worsens over the years, the physician has an additional goal: to prevent the progress of the disease, avoiding bone deterioration and degeneration. In these patients, a group of drugs called disease-modifying antirheumatic drugs (DMARDs) may be used in conjunction with pain relievers. Corticosteroids are also used to alleviate acute episodes of pain and inflammation. They can be very effective, but they cannot be used over the long term and may have severe side effects.

Surgery is often required for arthritis patients. Synovectomy is a procedure in which part or all the synovial membrane that surrounds the diseased joint is removed. It gives temporary relief in inflammation and may help preserve joint function. When a joint has deteriorated severely, the physician may recommend joint replacement therapy. In this procedure, the degenerated bone and joint structures are surgically removed and replaced with an orthopedic device of metal and/or plastic. This procedure is most effective in hip replacement, although it is also used in the knee. Relief of pain is the main goal of therapy in other arthritic conditions such as psoriatic arthritis and Reiter's syndrome. In ankylosing spondylitis, exercise is also an important facet of treatment, to help avoid stiffening of the spine. Gout tends to recur. Therefore, there are medications for acute episodes, such as pain relievers, and others to control levels of uric acid and prevent attacks. Benign bone tumors sometimes require surgery. Malignant tumors can be treated surgically and may also require radiation and chemotherapy.

Perspective and Prospects

Radical new therapies for bone disorders are evolving, with exciting possibilities: bone regeneration, bone cements, and glues to knit fractures and replace bone destroyed by disease. Osteoarthritis, rheumatoid arthritis, and other forms of arthritis continue to afflict vast populations around the world. Current medical treatment is significantly flawed by the incidence of side effects, especially gastrointestinal effects, from the medications used. The search for safer medications is ongoing, as is the search for treatment modalities that will halt the degenerative processes of rheumatoid arthritis. Orthopedic implants are now quite successful in the hip, sometimes successful in the knee, but otherwise not universally useful in elbows, fingers, toes, and other joints that can be destroyed by disease. This is an area that is being addressed. Operating techniques and instrumentation improve constantly. Many procedures are now done with the aid of arthroscopic instruments. Rather than an extensive incision to reveal the joint and surrounding tissues, the surgeon works through a tiny hole, through which he or she can inspect the inflamed joint and even perform minor surgery. Operations on prolapsed spinal disks once entailed long incisions and laborious, careful removal of disk tissue. Fusion of the involved vertebrae was often necessary, limiting spinal movement. Healing time could be extensive. Today, simpler, less painful procedures may be as successful and far less traumatic. In one procedure, an enzyme is injected into the prolapsed disk, causing it to shrink and reducing pressure on nearby nerves. In another procedure, disk material is removed with a needle inserted through the skin into the disk. Overall, progress in the treatment of bone disorders has been significant: Many people who would have lived with deformities and disability are being helped with modern medical and surgical techniques, medications, and instrumentation.

—*C. Richard Falcon;*
updated by Michael A. Buratovich

See also: Amputation; Arthritis; Bone cancer; Bone grafting; Bone marrow transplantation; Bones and the skeleton; Bowlegs; Bunions; Cartilage; Casts and splints; Cerebral palsy; Chiropractic; Ewing's sarcoma; Feet; Flat feet; Foot disorders; Fracture and dislocation; Fracture repair; Hammertoe correction; Hammertoes; Head and neck disorders; Heel spur removal; Hip fracture repair; Hip replacement; Jaw wiring; Joints; Kneecap removal; Knock-knees; Kyphosis; Lower extremities; Orthopedic surgery; Orthopedics; Orthopedics, pediatric; Osgood-Schlatter disease; Osteochondritis juvenilis; Osteogenesis imperfecta; Osteomyelitis; Osteonecrosis; Osteoporosis; Paget's disease; Pigeon toes; Rheumatology; Rickets; Sarcoma; Scoliosis; Slipped disk; Spina bifida; Spinal cord disorders; Spine, vertebrae, and disks; Upper extremities.

For Further Information:

"Bone Diseases." *MedlinePlus*, May 6, 2013.

"Bone Health Basics." *OrthoInfo*. American Academy of Orthopaedic Surgeons, May 2012.

"Bone Infections." *MedlinePlus*, April 1, 2013.

Hodgson, Stephen F., ed. *Mayo Clinic on Osteoporosis: Keeping Bones Healthy and Strong and Reducing the Risk of Fractures*. Rochester, Minn.: Mayo Clinic, 2003.

Hunder, Gene G. *Mayo Clinic on Arthritis*. Rev. ed. Rochester, Minn.: Mayo Clinic, 2002.

Lane, Nancy E., and Daniel J. Wallace. *All About Osteoarthritis: The Definitive Resource for Arthritis Patients and Their Families*. New York: Oxford University Press, 2002.

Lenarz, Michael, and Victoria St. George. *The Chiropractic Way*. New York: Bantam, 2003.

Osteoporosis and Related Bone Diseases National Resource Center. National Institutes of Health, 2013.

Nelson, Miriam E., and Sarah Wernick. *Strong Women, Strong Bones: Everything You Need to Know to Prevent, Treat, and Beat Osteoporosis*. Rev. ed. New York: Berkley Books, 2006.

Neuwirth, Michael, and Kevin Osborn. *The Scoliosis Sourcebook*. 2d ed. New York: McGraw-Hill, 2001.

Rosen, Clifford J., Julie Glowacki, and John P. Bilezikian. *The Aging Skeleton*. San Diego, Calif.: Academic Press, 1999.

Schommer, Nancy. *Stopping Scoliosis: The Whole Family Guide to Diagnosis and Treatment*. Rev. ed. New York: Putnam, 2002.

Yates, George, and Michael B. Shermer. *Meeting the Challenge of Arthritis*. Los Angeles: Lowell House, 1990.

Bone grafting

Procedure

Anatomy or system affected: Bones, immune system, musculoskeletal system

Specialties and related fields: Hematology, immunology, orthopedics

Definition: The transplantation of a section of bone from one part of the body to another, or from one individual to another.

Indications and Procedures

Ideally, the grafting procedure involves the transfer of bone tissue from one site to another on the same individual, which is termed an autogenous graft. This method eliminates the chance of rejection, allowing the transplantation of entire functional units of tissue: arteries, veins, and even nerves, as when a toe is used to replace a finger or thumb (toe-digital transfer). Autogenous rib or fibula grafts may be utilized for the reconstruction of the face or extremities.

Bone grafts are often used in situations in which a bone fracture is not healing properly. A fracture that fails to heal in the usual time is considered to be a delayed union.

Cancellous material from the bone (the spongy inner material), usually obtained from the iliac crest of the pelvis or from the ends of the long bones, is placed around the site. The fracture must then be immobilized for several months, allowing the grafted material to infiltrate and repair the fracture.

Uses and Complications

The grafting of bone tissue is carried out to correct a bone defect, to provide support tissue in the case of a severe fracture, or to encourage the growth of new bone. The source of the skeletal defect may be congenital malformation, disease, or trauma. For example, reconstruction may be necessary following cancer surgery, particularly for the jaw or bones elsewhere in the face.

If the autogenous bone supply is inadequate to fill the need, allogeneic bone grafts, the transplantation of bone from an individual other than an identical twin, may be necessary. Such foreign tissue is more likely to undergo rejection, reducing the chance of a successful procedure; the more closely the tissues of the two persons are matched, the less likely rejection will be a problem.

If the graft is able to vascularize quickly and to synthesize new tissue, the procedure is likely to be successful. The graft itself may provide structural support, or it may gradually be replaced by new bone at that site, completing the healing process.

—*Richard Adler, Ph.D.*

See also: Amputation; Bone cancer; Bone disorders; Bones and the skeleton; Fracture and dislocation; Fracture repair; Grafts and grafting; Lower extremities; Oncology; Orthopedic surgery; Orthopedics; Osteonecrosis; Transplantation; Upper extremities.

For Further Information:

Aho, OM. "The mechanism of action of induced membranes in bone repair." *Journal of Bone and Joint Surgery.* 95, 7. (April 2013): 597-604.

Bentley, George, and Robert B. Greer, eds. *Orthopaedics.* 4th ed. Oxford, England: Linacre House, 1993.

Callaghan, John J., Aaron Rosenberg, and Harry E. Rubash, eds. *The Adult Hip.* 2d ed. Philadelphia: Lippincott Williams & Wilkins, 2007.

Doherty, Gerard M., and Lawrence W. Way, eds. *Current Surgical Diagnosis and Treatment.* 12th ed. New York: Lange Medical Books/McGraw-Hill, 2006.

Dowthwaite, SA. "Comparison of fibular and scapular osseous free flaps for oromandibular reconstruction: a patient-centered approach to flap selection." *JAMA Otolaryngol Head Neck Surgery.* 139, 3. (March 2013): 285-292.

Eiff, M. Patrice, Robert L. Hatch, and Walter L. Calmbach. *Fracture Management for Primary Care.* 2d ed. Philadelphia: W. B. Saunders, 2003.

Lindholm, T. Sam. *Advances in Skeletal Reconstruction Using Bone Morphogenetic Proteins.* London: World Scientific, 2002.

Tapley, Donald F., et al., eds. *The Columbia University College of Physicians and Surgeons Complete Home Medical Guide.* Rev. 3d ed. New York: Crown, 1995.

Tierney, Lawrence M., Stephen J. McPhee, and Maxine A. Papadakis, eds. *Current Medical Diagnosis and Treatment 2007.* New York: McGraw-Hill Medical, 2006.

Wood, Debra. "Bone graft." *Health Library*, December 21, 2011.

Bone marrow

Anatomy/Biology

Anatomy or system affected: All systems

Specialties and related fields: Hematology, immunology, oncology

Definition: The spongy, flexible tissue on the inside of bones that contains stem cell populations that generate all the cells that circulate through the bloodstream.

Key terms:

cytokines: Small proteins secreted by certain cells of the immune system that signal to other immune cells and induce specific biological responses.

hematopoiesis: The process that produces all types of blood cells in our bodies. This process involves the formation, development, and differentiation of blood cells that originate from hematopoietic stem cells.

hematopoietic stem cells: Multipotent, self-renewing progenitor cells that reside in bone marrow and give rise to all blood cells.

mesenchymalstem cells: Multipotent, adult stem cells found in almost all tissues. These cells can be divided into into bone-making cells (osteoblasts), cartilage-making cells (chondrocytes), fat cells (adipocytes), and muscle cells (myocytes).

stem cells: Undifferentiated cells capable of self-renewal through-division and copying processes-whose progeny can be differentiated into other types of cells.

Structure and Functions

Confined to the inside of bones, bone marrow is the primary residence of hematopoietic stem cells (HSCs), which form all the "formed elements," or cellular components of blood. Bone marrow also consists of blood vessels, immature red and white blood cells in various stages of differentiation, phagocytic cells that gobble up any cell debris or damaged tissue, bone-making osteoblasts, bone-destroying osteoclasts, and supporting cells known as *stromal cells*. Adults have two types of bone marrow: (1) Red or active bone marrow, also called myeloid tissue, and (2) yellow or inactive bone marrow, which tends to have a yellowish color because it also contains fat. In adults, active marrow is found in the proximal parts of the humerus and the femur and in the flat bones of the mandible, cranium, sternum, ribs, vertebrae, and pelvis. During emergencies that require the replacement of large quantities of blood cells, yellow marrow can be converted back to red marrow.

The primary arteries of the bones penetrate the bones and vascularize them. These bone-based arteries branch extensively in the bone to establish a network of capillaries that form large venous sinuses. This labyrinth of sinuses is surrounded by hematopoietic tissue or fat. Newly formed blood cells squeeze between the endothelial cells that line these sinuses to enter circulation. Under normal circumstances, blood cells do not enter circulation until they have undergone complete cellular differentiation because they must express the appropriate cell surface receptors to bind to the endothelial cells that line the venous sinuses in the bone marrow and pass between them. Under pathological conditions, however, premature release of immature blood cells can occur.

The hematopoietic tissue in bone marrow consists of various nooks and crannies known as "niches" that provide different microenvironments that regulate HSC function. Many different cells occupy these niches and secrete a host of signaling molecules called "cytokines" that influence HSC activity. HSCs constitute a true stem cell population, since they can self-renew throughout the lifetime of the individual. There are two distinct niches in bone marrow: (1) niches centralized around osteoblasts (osteoblastic niche), and (2) niches organized around the endothelial cells that line the bone marrow sinuses (vascular niche). Another common denizen of these niches are mesenchymal stem cells, which are a population of stromal cells that play important supportive roles. In the osteoblastic niches, the HSCs are in direct contact with osteoblasts and mesenchymal stem cells, and these interactions keep the HSC in a dormant state. In the vascular niches, the HSCs are in direct contact with sinusoidal endothelial cells and mesenchymal stem cells, and these interactions activate the HSC to divide and produce new red and white blood cells. Dormant HSCs can be moved to vascular niches and become active. Active HSCs in vascular niches can be moved to osteoblastic niches where they will become quiescent and held in reserve.

HSCs divide to form a replacement HSC, and a progenitor cell that senses the microenvironment of the bone marrow and the combination of growth factors and cytokines presented to it. This symphony of different signals drives the progenitor to form either lymphoid cells, which consist of B and T lymphocytes and natural killer cells, or myeloid cells, which consist of red blood cells, platelet-making megakaryocytes, macrophages, neutrophils, eosinophils, or basophils. Progenitor cells initially possess the ability to divide, but as they differentiate into specific blood cell lineages, they begin to lose their ability to divide. Exposure to the cytokine erythropoietin, which is made by the kidney, drives progenitor cells into the red blood cell program. Exposure to granulocyte-monocyte colony stimulating factor (GM-CSF) moves the progenitor cell into the granulocytes/monocyte lineage. The progenitor cells differentiate and mature into red or white blood cells that are eventually released into the blood.

Disorders and Diseases

Because of the absolute dependence of our bodies on a constant supply of blood, and since under normal circumstances bone marrow is the only source of blood cells for our bodies, diseases that compromise bone marrow function can have severe consequences. Bone marrow abnormalities can cause anemias (red blood cell deficiencies), leukopenias (leukocyte deficiencies), or pancytopenia (deficiencies of red and white blood cells). Anemias cause pallor and weariness and leukopenias increase susceptibility to infection.

A group of disorders known as bone marrow failure syndromes are caused by a decrease of or damage to HSCs or

their niches, defects in blood cell maturation (e.g., vitamin B12 or folate deficiencies), or defects in progenitor cell differentiation (e.g., myelodysplastic syndromes). Damage to HSCs can be either acquired or congenital. Causes of HSC damage include (1) exposure to radiation, viruses, toxins, or chemicals, such as chloramphenicol, benzene, fungicides, herbicides, insecticides, or anticancer drugs like alkylating agents, topoisomerase II inhibitors, and antimetabolites; (2) alterations to the HSC niche; (3) suppression of hematopoiesis by the immune system, as in the case of pure red cell aplasia, immune panleukopenia, systemic lupus erythematosus, atypical cases of aplastic anemia and other diseases; and (4) mutations in genes that cause inherited bone marrow failure syndromes. Inherited bone marrow failure syndromes include Fanconi anemia, dyskeratosis congenita, Diamond-Blackfan anemia, Shwachman-Diamond syndrome, amegakaryocytic thrombocytopenia, and congenital neutropenia. Some bone marrow abnormalities may only affect the production of one type of blood cell (single cytopenias). For example, pure red cell aplasia only affects the production of red blood cells. Some abnormalities may affect the production of all types of blood cells (pancytopenia), as in the case of aplastic anemia.

Myelodysplastic syndrome (MDS) describes a group of closely related hematopoietic disorders that usually result from aberrant blood cell maturation. The bone marrow fills with poorly differentiated and immature cells devoid of function. MDSs can either cause persistent, refractory anemias or they can transition to acute myeloid leukemia (AML) or chronic myelomonocytic leukemia (CMML).

Primary tumors of HSCs are some of the most important diseases that interfere with bone marrow function. Leukemias, for example, are malignant diseases of the bone marrow in which precursor cells proliferate and displace normal HSCs in the bone marrow. Such diseases cause a host of symptoms, but one of the most pronounced symptoms is anemia, with its accompanying signs and symptoms. Polycythemia vera (PV) is a neoplastic disorder of HSCs that causes uncontrolled red blood cell production. The blood contains radically elevated numbers of red blood cells in combination with increased white blood cell and platelet production. PV is caused by mutations in the *Janus kinase 2* (*JAK2*) gene. The JAK2 gene encodes a protein kinase that mediates the response of cytokines. The mutant version of the JAK2 protein causes highly exaggerated responses to cytokines and can be activated even in the absence of cytokines. Increased blood cell production thickens the blood, and slowed blood flow causes chest pain, vertigo, headache, visual disturbances, tinnitus, enlarge liver and spleen (hepatomegaly and splenomegaly), hypertension, and pain in the legs (intermittent claudication).

Over the past 50 years, bone marrow transplantation and HSC transplantation have been used with increasing frequency to treat a wide range of malignant and nonmalignant diseases. Improvements in transplantation techniques and supportive therapies have improved survival rates and decreased patient morbidity. Bone marrow transplantation is usually reserved for patients with life-threatening conditions. Bone marrow transplants can be *autologous* procedures, in which stem cells are removed from a person's marrow and then frozen to be kept until the original donor needs it for a transplant, or *allogenic* procedures, in which bone marrow cells are taken from another person whose cells would be compatible, often someone closely related to the patient. Donor bone marrow is taken from the donor's pelvic bones under anesthesia in a procedure called a bone marrow harvest. Recovery from bone marrow donation takes about three weeks on average.

To prepare the patient for a bone marrow transplant, the diseased cells in the existing bone marrow are killed by means of chemotherapy or radiation treatments. However, there are two types of pretreatment regimens for bone marrow and HSC transplant recipients: (1) myeloablative regimens that kill all residual cancer cells in autologous or allogenic transplantation and cause immunosuppression for engraftment in allogenic transplantation; and (2) nonmyeloablative regimens in which the immune system of the recipient is suppressed, but not destroyed, since the immune response against the tumor elicited by the donor lymphocytes effect is relied upon to kill tumor cells. In either case, the immune system of the recipient is suppressed long enough for the donor cells to be adopted into the body, but this renders the patient vulnerable to numerous infections. The transplant itself is not invasive but relies on injecting the new cells into the blood. The new marrow is vulnerable to infection and rejection and full recovery can take as long as a year.

Over the past decade, the use of umbilical cord blood as a source of transplantable HSCs has rapidly expanded, and more than 2000 cord blood transplants have been performed. Cord blood has been used in transplants for any diseases in which a bone marrow transplant could be used. The five-year survival rate for umbilical cord blood recipients in children with leukemia is similar to those who received bone marrow transplants. The limited number of cells in cord blood has traditionally restricted its use to children and small adults. Techniques studied for making this source available to a wider range of patients have included transfusion of multiple units, ex vivo expansion of the cord blood unit before transplantation, and exposure of the cord blood graft to compounds intended to improve homing and engraftment.

An alternative procedure that utilizes peripheral blood stem cells (PBSCs) has gained popularity as a source of stem cells since its initial introduction in the 1980s. Although HSCs circulate in blood, they do so at very low concentrations. Nevertheless, circulating HSCs can be identified and quantified using a technique called flow cytometry. Administration of recombinant cytokines G-CSF and GM-CSF releases HSCs into the peripheral blood, which can be collected through a procedure called apheresis.

Perspective and Prospects

The first bone marrow transplant from a donor who was not related to the patient took place in 1979. The first successful umbilical cord blood transplantation occurred in 1988. A young boy with Fanconi anemia was treated with umbilical cord blood collected at the birth of his sibling, and this patient remains alive and well to date. In 1992, a patient was successfully transplanted with cord blood instead of bone marrow for the treatment of leukemia.

In the United States, there is a national bone marrow registry called Be the Match that is designed to find compatible cells for patients if no close relative is available. Be the Match is operated by the National Marrow Donor Program, a nonprofit agency founded in 1986 and located in Minneapolis. Other countries have similar programs. Bone Marrow Donors Worldwide, located in Leiden, Netherlands, coordinates tissue matches and donations from national programs on a global basis. Many donor-recipient relationships take place across national lines.

Shyni Varghese and her colleagues at the University of California, San Diego created a synthetic bone filled with donor HSCs that was successfully implanted into a mouse. This artificial bone marrow functions properly in mice and this may be the beginning of exciting new developments in regenerative medicine for patients with bone marrow diseases.

The scientific and medical uses of stem cells are expanding rapidly, and marrow is the major source of adult stem cells in the human body. Adult stem cells are particularly popular because they do not raise the religious and ethical issues of stem cells derived from embryos and fetal tissue. Stem cells are extracted from bone marrow for research and other uses by bone marrow aspirations—a procedure similar to that used for marrow donation. Stem cells offer the possibility of treatments for cell-based diseases by creating replacement cells.

—William E. Burns, PhD;
updated by Michael A. Buratovich, PhD

For Further Information:
Anton, Joseph H., and Deborah Yolin Raley. *Manual of Stem Cell and Bone Marrow Transplantation.* Cambridge: Cambridge UP, 2013. Print.

Cherry, Daniel A. *Bone Marrow: A Practical Manual.* N. p.: CRC, 2011. Print.

Gatter, Kevin, and David Brown. *Bone Marrow Diagnosis: An Illustrated Guide.* Chichester: Wiley, 2014. Print.

Hoffman, Ronald, et al. *Hematology: Basic Principles and Practice.* Philadelphia: Elsevier Saunders, 2013. Print.

Islam, Anwarul. *Manual of Bone Marrow Examination.* Bloomington: Trafford, 2013. Print.

Passweg, J. R., et al. "European Society for Blood and Marrow Transplantation EBMT. Hematopoietic SCT in Europe: Data and Trends in 2012 with Special Consideration of Pediatric Transplantation." *Bone Marrow Transplant* 49 (2014): 744-50. Print.

Shih, Yu-Ru, Kang, Heemin, Rao, Vikram, Chiu, Yu-Jui, Kwon, Seong Keun, and Shyni Varghese. (2017). In vivo engineering of bone tissues with hematopoietic functions and mixed chimerism. *Proceedings of the National Academy of Sciences USA*, 114(21): 5419-5424.

Stewart, Susan. *Bone Marrow and Blood Stem Cell Transplants: A Guide for Patients.* BMT Infonet.org. 6 June 2015. Web. 30 Dec. 2015. http://www.bmtinfonet.org/books/transplants-2012.

Bone marrow transplantation

Procedure

Anatomy or system affected: Back, blood, bones, immune system, musculoskeletal system

Specialties and related fields: General surgery, genetics, hematology, immunology, oncology

Definition: The replacement of diseased or inadequate bone marrow with healthy marrow.

Key terms:

bone marrow: the material inside bones that produces red blood cells (which carry oxygen), platelets (which stop bleeding), and white blood cells (which are the functional units of the immune system).

genetic locus: a fixed position on a chromosome that contains a specific set of DNA sequences that encode a gene or set of genes that are inherited as a discrete unit.

graft-versus-host disease: a condition that complicates the transplantation of tissue from a genetically different person.

human leukocyte antigen(HLA): a complex of cell surface proteins used by the immune system to distinguish self from non-self.

stem cell: a master cell from which other blood cells develop; these cells are primarily located in the bone marrow.

Indications and Procedures

Bone marrow transplantation is used when the immune and blood-forming systems of the body are malfunctioning or have been severely damaged. Without adequate white blood cells from the bone marrow, a person will soon die from infection—therefore, transplantation is needed. Transplantation is an attempt to cure or arrest diseases such as leukemia, cancer, and sickle cell disease and conditions such as brain tumors and hereditary diseases. Bone marrow transplantation is used when all other methods of treatment have failed. The procedure is usually performed on patients who are younger than fifty years old, with the greatest success rates found in children. Before the procedure can be performed, a suitable donor must be found. The donor can be the patient (autologous transplantation) or someone else (allogeneic transplantation). Once the donor is identified, the bone marrow is harvested. This procedure is usually done under general anesthesia and takes one to two hours. A needle is inserted in the hip, and marrow is sucked out from different locations in the pelvic bone. Approximately 1 to 3 pints of marrow are taken. The donor usually stays overnight in the hospital and may be sore for one or two weeks following the operation.

The marrow, which contains the stem cells necessary to reestablish the blood-producing and immune systems of the patient, is processed and stored until the patient is prepared for the transplantation. During the hospital stay, the patient is kept in a sterile room to prevent infection. If the surgery is being performed on a cancer patient, the patient receives extensive chemotherapy and/or radiation before the donor marrow is transplanted; this action destroys any cancer cells in the patient, as well as his or her immune system.

The patient then receives the bone marrow transplantation in a manner similar to a blood transfusion: The donor cells are introduced through the veins and into the bloodstream. Until the transplanted cells begin to function (usually two to four weeks), the patient receives blood and platelet transfusions, as well as antibiotics to fight infection. The patient is usually discharged from the hospital in a month but must take antibiotics and antiviral medications for six months to two years after the transplantation because the recovery of the immune system is slow.

Uses and Complications

Bone marrow transplantation is a risky procedure with a

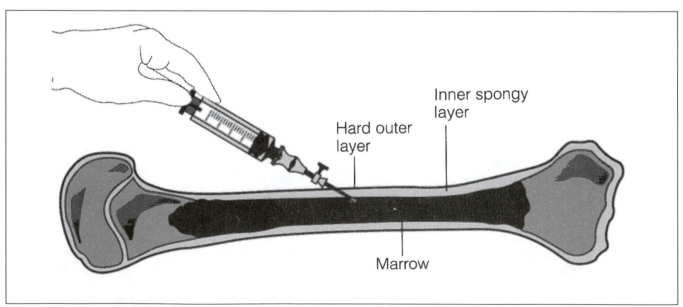

Bone marrow transplantation is used to treat several types of cancer. Marrow can be extracted from a donor or from the patient and reintroduced at a later time, usually after chemotherapy or radiation therapy.

success rate that ranges from 10 to 90 percent. One of the greatest obstacles is finding a suitable donor. The best possible match is between siblings, but even here the probability of a correct match is only 25 percent. Unrelated donor and patient matches made with marrow from donor banks increase the risk of a mismatch.

Bone marrow donors and recipients are matched according to their human leukocyte antigens (HLAs). HLAs are cell surface proteins that serve as molecular bar codes for the body's cells. The immune system encounters all foreign substances through the context of the HLA proteins and if the specific HLA proteins on the surfaces of cells do not match those of all the other cells, such mismatched cell is treated as a foreign interloper and is destroyed. There are two types of HLA proteins; class I, which are on the surface of every nucleated cell in the body (including platelets), and class II, which are on certain white blood cells (dendritic cells, B lymphocytes, and macrophages). There are three genes that encode class I HLAs (HLA-A, -B, and -C) and three genetic loci that encode the alpha and beta subunits of class II HLAs (HLA-DR, -DQ, and -DP). Because humans have two copies of each gene, there are 12 different genes to compare between donors and recipients. When searching among siblings, potential donors and recipients should match at least six of six of these HLA alleles (HLA-A, -B, and HLA-DRB1), but if a six of six match is not available, then the transplant center proceeds with an unrelated donor search. For unrelated donors, an eight of eight match is desirable (genetic matches at HLA-A, -B, -C, and DRB1). If an eight of eight donor is not available, then single mismatches at HLA-B and -C are the most preferable.

Finding a suitable donor is imperative because of the risk of graft-versus-host disease (GVHD). GVHD occurs when the donor white blood cells recognize the host's body as foreign and react against it. This reaction may occur within a hundred or more days after the transplant and can vary in severity from a mild rash to the fatal destruction of tissue and organs. For correctly matched donors and recipients, the risk of life-threatening GVHD is 10 to 20 percent. For mismatched donors and recipients, the risk rises to 80 percent. Nonpermissive mismatches of the HLA-DPB1 gene seems to play a significant role in the risk of developing GVDH. In some cases, especially with leukemia and cancerous blood diseases, patients who suffer mild GVHD have an improved chance of survival because part of GVHD is a graft-versus-leukemia (GVL) effect. In these cases, the transplanted immune system acts against any remaining leukemia cells.

When the patient does not have a condition that damages the bone marrow, transplantation can be performed with his or her own marrow. After marrow has been collected from the patient, radiation and/or chemotherapy can be used to destroy the remaining immune system. Autologous transplantation eliminates the need to find a compatible donor and the risk of GVHD. This method can be used for treating solid tumors and has shown promise in curing brain tumors that were once considered fatal, with a success rate of 20

percent. In April 2013, scientists at the Abramson Cancer Center of the University of Pennsylvania published a study of 300,000 bone marrow transplant recipients. Although the transplants were successful, the study concluded that transplant recipients are at increased risk for suicide and accidental death.

Perspective and Prospects

Research on bone marrow transplantation began in the early 1950s, with the first successful transplantations performed on children in 1968. By the 1990s, more than five thousand bone marrow transplantations were being performed worldwide every year. The development of drugs that work to suppress the immune system has increased the chances for survival for these patients.

Several areas of research promise even better results in the future. A growing understanding of disease at the genetic level offers the possibility of separating unhealthy bone marrow cells from healthy ones. Methods of growing cells outside the body for use in transplantation are being developed. Progress has also been made in increasing the donor pool. National and international programs actively seek potential donors. Healthy people may begin storing their own bone marrow for a possible need in the future.

Perhaps one of the most promising potential sources of donor bone marrow is umbilical cord blood, which is rich in stem cells. Transplants using umbilical cord blood were first used in 1989 and have proven very successful. If established, umbilical cord blood banks could greatly increase the quantity of available donor marrow. Also, because of inherent immaturity of the white blood cells in umbilical cord blood, lower-quality HLA matches are often better tolerated in cord blood transplantations than with bone marrow transplantations.

—*Virginia L. Salmon;*
updated by Michael A. Buratovich PhD

See also: Blood and blood disorders; Blood banks; Bones and the skeleton; Cancer; Chemotherapy; Immune system; Immunology; Immunopathology; Leukemia; Oncology; Radiation therapy; Sickle cell disease; Stem cells; Transfusion; Transplantation.

For Further Information:
"After-transplant problems that may show up later." *cancer.org*, October 24, 2012.
Blood and Marrow Transplant Information Network. http://www.bmtinfonet.org.
Bolwell, Brian J., ed. *Current Controversies in Bone Marrow Transplantation*. Totowa, N.J.: Humana Press, 2000.
Marget, Madeline. *Life's Blood*. New York: Simon & Schuster, 1992.
Marshak, Daniel R., David Gottlieb, and Richard L. Gardner, eds. *Stem Cell Biology*. Cold Spring Harbor, N.Y.: Cold Spring Harbor Laboratory Press, 2002.
National Research Council. *Stem Cells and the Future of Regenerative Medicine*. Washington, D.C.: National Academy Press, 2002. Stewart, Susan K. *Autologous Stem Cell Transplants: A Handbook for Patients*. Highland Park, Ill.: Blood and Marrow Transplant Information Network, 2000.
Seaman, Andrew M. "Suicide, accidents linked to bone marrow transplant." *Medline Plus*, April 12, 2013.
Swerdlow, Joel L. "A New Kind of Kinship." *National Geographic* 180, no. 3 (September, 1991): 64-92.
"The transplant process." *cancer.org*, October 24, 2012.

U.S. Department of Health and Human Services, National Institutes of Health. *Bone Marrow Transplantationand PeripheralBlood Stem Cell Transplantation*. Rev. ed. Bethesda, Md.: Author, 1994.

Bones and the skeleton

Anatomy

Anatomy or system affected: Back, feet, hips, legs, musculoskeletal system

Specialties and related fields: Exercise physiology, orthodontics, orthopedics, osteopathic medicine, podiatry, sports medicine

Definition: Bones are hard tissues that form the skeleton, the structure underlying the softer tissues of the body; they provide support while allowing flexibility.

Key terms:

calcitonin: a hormone made and released by the thyroid gland that lowers the level of calcium in the blood by stimulating the formation of bone

collagen: a protein found in bone and other connective tissues; collagen fibers are well suited for support and protection because they are sturdy, flexible, and resist stretch

hormones: molecules made in the body and released into the blood that act as chemical messengers for the regulation of specific body functions

matrix: in bone, the matrix is a solid nonliving material that is a composite of protein fibers and mineral crystals

osteoblast: a bone cell that can produce and form bone matrix; osteoblasts are responsible for new bone formation

osteoclast: a large bone cell that can destroy bone matrix by dissolving the mineral crystals

osteocyte: the primary living cell of mature bone tissue

tissue: a collection of similar cells that perform a specific function

Structure and Functions

Bones are active throughout life: the 206 bones of the skeleton establish the size and proportions of the body and interact with all other organ systems. Disorders of the skeleton can have profound effects on the other organ systems and serious health consequences for the organism.

Bone, or osseous tissue, contains specialized cells and a solid, stony matrix. The unique hardened quality of the matrix results from layers of calcium salt crystals such as calcium phosphate, which is responsible for about two-thirds of a bone's weight, and calcium carbonate. The living cells found in bone account for less than 2 percent of the total bone mass.

Despite the great strength of the calcium salts, their inflexible nature means that they can fracture when exposed to sufficiently great bending or twisting forces, or to sharp impacts. Because the calcium crystals exist as minute plates positioned on a framework of collagen protein fibers, the resulting composite structure does lend a certain degree of flexibility to the bone matrix.

Based on the internal organization of its matrix, bone is classified as either compact (dense) bone or cancellous (spongy) bone. Compact bone is internally more solid, while cancellous bone is made from bony filaments (trabeculae) whose branching interconnections form a three-dimensional network. The cavities of the cancellous bone network are filled usually by bone marrow, the primary location for blood cell formation in adults.

Both types of bone contain bone cells (osteocytes) living in small chambers called lacunae, found periodically between the plates of the matrix. Microscopic channels (canaliculi) connect neighboring lacunae and permit the exchange of nutrients and wastes between osteocytes and accessible blood vessels. Osteocytes provide the collagen fibers and the conditions for proper maintenance of the mineral crystals of the matrix.

A typical skeletal bone has a central marrow cavity that is bordered by cancellous bone. This is enclosed by compact bone, and the outer surface is covered by periosteum. Periosteum consists of a fibrous outer layer and a cellular inner layer. The periosteum plays an important part in the growth and repair of bone, and it is the attachment site for muscles. Collagen protein fibers from the periosteum interconnect with the collagen fibers of the bone.

The marrow cavity inside the bone is lined by endosteum. Endosteum is an incomplete layer covering the trabeculae of cancellous bone and contains a variety of different types of cells. The endosteum also plays important roles during bone growth and repair.

The bone matrix is not an unchanging, permanent structure. During a person's life, the bone matrix is being constantly dissolved while new matrix is synthesized and deposited. Approximately 18 percent of the protein and mineral constituents of bone are replaced each year. Such bone remodeling can result in altered bone shape or internal rearrangement of the trabeculae. It may also result in a change in the total amount of minerals stored in the skeleton. These processes of bone demineralization (osteolysis) and new bone production (osteogenesis) are precisely regulated in the healthy individual.

The type of bone cell responsible for dissolving the mineralized matrix is called an osteoclast. The cells that produce the materials that later become the bony matrix are called osteoblasts. The activities of these cells are influenced by several hormones as well as by the physical stress forces to which a bone may be exposed, such as when a particular muscle becomes stronger as the result of weight training and pulls more strongly on the bones to which it is attached. Increased stress forces on a bone result in that bone becoming thicker and stronger, thereby allowing the bone to withstand the stresses better and reducing the risks of bone fracture. When bones are not subjected to ordinary stresses, such as in persons confined to bed or in astronauts living in microgravity conditions during space flight, there is a corresponding loss of bone mass, with the unstressed bones becoming thinner and more brittle. After several weeks in an unstressed state, a bone can lose nearly a third of its mass. Following the resumption of normal loading stresses, the bone can regain its mass just as quickly.

The skeleton has five major functions: support for the body; protection of the soft tissues and organs; leverage to change the direction and size of the muscular forces; blood cell production, which occurs within the red marrow residing in the marrow cavities of many bones; and storage of both minerals (to maintain the body's important reserves of calcium and phosphate) and fats (in yellow marrow to serve as an important energy reserve for the body).

The human skeleton contains 206 bones. These are distributed between two subdivisions of the skeleton: the axial skeleton and the appendicular skeleton. The axial skeleton contains 80 bones distributed among the skull (29 bones), the chest (25 bones), and the spinal (vertebral) column (26 bones). The remaining 126 bones are found in the appendicular skeleton's components: 4 bones in the shoulder (pectoral) girdles, 60 bones in the arms (including the 54 bones located in both of the hands and wrists), 2 bones in the hip (pelvic) girdle, and 60 bones in the legs (including the 52 bones found in the ankles and feet).

Skeletal bones are classified according to their shape. Long bones occur in the upper arm, the forearm, the thigh, the lower leg, the palm, the fingers, the sole of the foot, and the toes. Short bones are cuboid in shape and are found in the wrist and the ankle. Flat bones form the top of the skull, the shoulder blade, the breastbone, and the ribs. Sesamoid bones are typically small, round, and flat. They are found near some joints, such as the kneecap on the front of the knee joint. Irregular bones have shapes that are difficult to describe because of their complexity. Examples of irregular bones are found in the spinal column and the skull.

Learning to name the bones solely by their appearance is made somewhat easier by the fact that each one has a definitive form and distinctive surface features. The places where blood vessels and nerves enter into a bone, or lie along its surface, are commonly discernible as indentations, grooves, or holes. The locations where muscles are connected to bones by tendons, or where a bone is tethered to another bone by ligaments, are often clearly visible as elevations, projections, or ridges of bony matrix, or as roughened areas on the surface of the bone. Finally, the areas of the bone that are involved in forming joints (articulations) with other bones have characteristic shapes that impart particular properties to the joint. Various specialized terms are used to name these features.

Articulations are found wherever one bone meets another. The amount of motion permitted between the bones forming an articulation ranges from none (for example, between the skull bones) to considerable (as at the shoulder joint). The anatomy of the joint determines its functional capability, and the parts of the bones that form the joint have distinctive structural features.

Disorders and Diseases

Among the disorders of the skeleton, a number of them

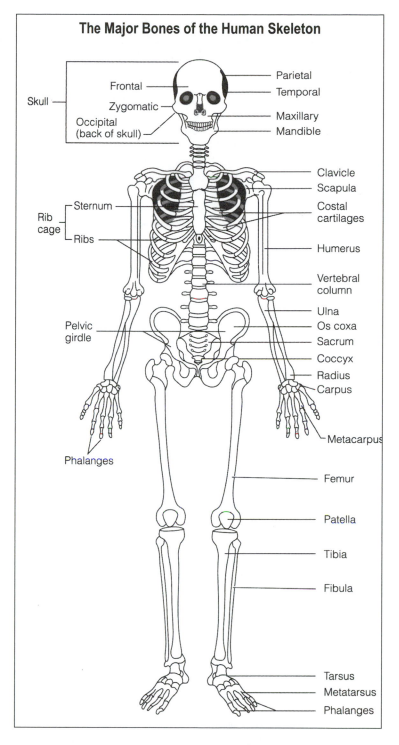

The Major Bones of the Human Skeleton

occur during the growth and development of the bones. The problems usually result in abnormal (most often decreased) stature or abnormal shape of the bones. The aberrations may alter the entire skeleton or be restricted to a portion of it. The basis of the pathology is to be found in a disruption of the normal, orderly sequence of events that take place during the growth and remodeling of the bones.

Osteopetrosis belongs to this class of disturbance. It is an inherited condition in which abnormal remodeling results in increased bone density. This seems to result from a reduced level of activity by the cells responsible for dissolving the bone matrix-the osteoclasts. In healthy, normal individuals, there is a precisely regulated relationship between osteoclast and osteoblast activity. Depending on the current needs of the body, or merely those of a single bone, the rate of bone matrix formation by osteoblasts may be greater than, equal to, or less than the rate of bone resorption by osteoclasts.

Osteoclasts are derived from cells that are made in the bone marrow. For this reason, bone marrow transplantation has been tried as a treatment for osteopetrosis; however, this approach is risky and not always successful. There has also been improvement in the condition of some osteopetrosis patients following treatment with a hormone related to vitamin D. This particular hormone can increase bone resorption and thereby may prevent the increase in bone density that characterizes this condition.

Another member of this category of disturbance is congenital hypothyroidism. The basic problem in this condition is underactivity of the thyroid gland during the development of the fetus, resulting in a decrease in the production of thyroid hormones in the fetus. This condition can be caused by an insufficient supply of the element iodine in the pregnant mother, or it may result from inherited errors in the production of the thyroid hormones.

Among the organ systems seriously affected by this condition is the skeleton. The bones do not develop correctly; consequently, the bones are shorter and thicker than nor-

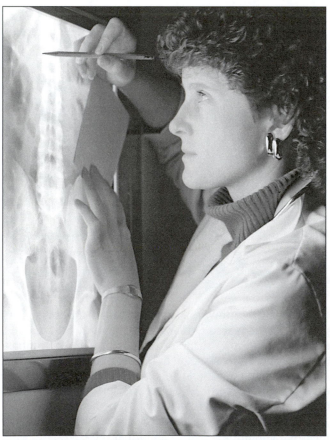

X rays are one of the best ways to evaluate the health and structure of the skeleton. (Digital Stock)

mal, with corresponding changes in the appearance of the child. Early diagnosis of the condition and timely treatment with drug forms of the thyroid hormones can halt the disease. Otherwise, the adult skeleton has stubby arms and legs, a somewhat flattened face, and disproportionately large chest and head.

A disorder of the pituitary gland can result in skeletal development abnormalities that are opposite to those observed in congenital hypothyroidism: namely, excessive growth in the length of bones. This condition is called giantism (or gigantism) and results from the overproduction of growth hormone by the pituitary gland before normal adult stature has been achieved. The most common cause of this situation is a tumor in the pituitary gland. Cases are known of people attaining heights of more than eight feet tall. Unfortunately, because of complications involving other organ systems as a result of the excessive production of growth hormone, the persons suffering from this disorder usually die before the age of thirty.

Surgical removal of the pituitary tumor is often attempted. If the tumor is successfully removed, then the overproduction of growth hormone will be stopped. In other cases, radiation treatments are used to destroy the tumor. It is also possible to combine both of these treatment techniques. Drug therapy is also possible. Because of the high doses necessary and the accompanying side effects of high drug dosages, however, the reduction of growth hormone levels through drug treatment is usually applied only in conjunction with one or both of the other therapies.

There are also disorders that afflict adult bone. Most of the remodeling disorders involve a loss of bone mass. The group of disorders known as osteoporosis (porous bone) is a rather common example; according to the International Osteoporosis Foundation, by 2013, osteoporosis affected more than 200 million people worldwide. The reduction in bone mass is sufficient to result in increased fragility and ease of breakage. There is also slower healing of bone fractures. In advanced cases, bones have been known to break when the person sneezes or simply rolls over in bed.

Loss of bone mass is a normal feature of aging, becoming quite marked after the age of seventy-five, particularly in the hip and leg bones. Because of the normal decrease in bone mass with aging, there is not a clear distinction to be made between normal, age-related skeletal changes and the clinical condition of osteoporosis. The occurrence of excessive fragility at a relatively early age is an indication that osteoporosis is developing. Normally, between the ages of thirty and forty, the activity of the osteoblast cells (those that form bone matrix) begins to decrease while the osteoclast cells (those that dissolve the matrix) maintain their previous level of activity. This results in the loss of about 8 percent of the total bone mass each decade for women and about 3 percent for men. Because of unequal loss in the different regions of the skeleton, the outcome is a gradual reduction in height, the loss of teeth, and the development of fragile limbs.

Osteoporotic bones are indistinguishable from normal bones with respect to their bone composition. The problem is simply too little of the strength-imparting matrix, with both compact and spongy bone being affected.

There are multiple causes of osteoporosis. Some cases have no known cause (idiopathic osteoporosis), some are inherited, and others are brought about as a result of hormonal (endocrine) disorders, vitamin or mineral deficiency, or effects of the long-term use of certain drugs.

The fact that women are more often affected than men, and that the process is most conspicuous in women beyond the age of the menopause, has implicated the female sex hormones (and, specifically, their decreased production) in the initiation of the osteoporotic process. One form of therapy is the administration of certain female sex hormones (specifically estrogens) to postmenopausal women (who have decreased production of estrogens). This treatment slows their loss of bone mass. While hormone therapy has been the mainstay of osteoporosis treatment for many years, controversy regarding the risks of hormone therapy has caused many women to stop using this treatment altogether. In 2002, two major studies found that the risks associated with hormone therapy outweigh the benefits. Following these studies, doctors began to look closer at the roles that high-impact exercise and the use of calcium and vitamin D play in decreasing bone density loss.

Other treatments of osteoporosis include administering the hormone calcitonin and increasing the dietary intake of the mineral calcium. The hormone calcitonin, produced by the thyroid gland, is sometimes used to treat osteoporosis because it stimulates the production of bone matrix by increasing the activity of the osteoblasts. At the same time, calcitonin inhibits the breakdown of bone by decreasing the activity of osteoclasts. Although this treatment theoretically should produce the desired result of preventing the accelerated loss of bone mass characteristic of osteoporosis, actual clinical results are not always positive.

For those cases of osteoporosis that are the result of endocrine gland disturbances, the appropriate treatment depends on the specific glandular disorder that is present. In some instances, hormone therapy can produce improvement in the patient's condition.

Regular exercise is a means both of preventing the onset of osteoporosis and of slowing its progression. Because muscular activity is critical for the maintenance of bone mass, extended periods of inactivity or immobilization can actually induce osteoporosis. For women, it is known that the amount and regularity of their exercise during the teenage years is strongly associated with their chances of developing osteoporosis thirty and more years later. The exercise need only be of moderate intensity in order to decrease significantly the risk of developing osteoporosis. Indeed, exercise that is at a level of intensity so high that it interferes with the normal female menstrual cycle (stopping the occurrence of menstruation completely or causing irregular cycle lengths) can actually increase the risk of developing osteoporosis later in life.

Perspective and Prospects

One of bone's primary functions is the protection of softer, more vulnerable tissues and organs. The physical properties of bone-it is as strong as cast iron but only weighs as much as an equally large piece of pine wood-make it ideally suited for this job. This combination of strength and lightness derives from the bony matrix of mineral crystals and the architecture of the bone, which unites compact and spongy bone.

The physical and chemical properties of the mineral crystals also result in the permanency of bone following death. Often the only trace of a dead body is the skeleton. Because of the resistance of bone to the processes of decomposition that befall the other tissues of the body following death, investigators are often able to determine the sex of the person whose skeleton has been found even though all other tissues have long since disappeared. This is possible because of the characteristic differences between male and female adult skeletons. Racial differences in the detailed structure of the skull and pelvis, age-related changes in the skeleton, signs of healed bone fractures, and the prominence of ridges where muscles attach (giving clues about the degree of muscular development) are also valuable sources of information when attempting to identify skeletal remains.

The sexual differences in the human skeleton are most obvious in the adult pelvis. These are genetically determined differences that are structural adaptations for childbearing. For example, the pelvis is smoother and wider in the female than in the male. Other differences include a lighter and smoother female skull, a more sloping male forehead, a larger and heavier male jawbone, and generally heavier male bones that also typically possess more prominent markings.

Among the common age-related changes found in skeletons are a general reduction in the mineral content and less prominent bone markings, both of which become more obvious after about age fifty. Various bones in the skull fuse together at characteristic ages ranging from one to thirty years of age. Other bones throughout the body can also be examined to achieve more accurate estimates of the age of a skeleton at the time of death.

Another consequence of the permanent nature of bone is that it provides a record of the changes in the skeletal anatomy of humans that have occurred during the hundreds of thousands of years of human evolution. Expert examination of skeletal remains can actually reveal an amazing wealth of information concerning the health and even the lifestyle of the deceased.

—*John V. Urbas, Ph.D.*

See also: Amputation; Anatomy; Arthritis; Arthroplasty; Arthroscopy; Bone cancer; Bone disorders; Bone grafting; Bone marrow transplantation; Bowlegs; Bunions; Cartilage; Casts and splints; Cerebral palsy; Chiropractic; Cleft lip and palate; Cleft lip and palate repair; Congenital hypothyroidism; Disk removal; Dwarfism; Ewing's sarcoma; Feet; Flat feet; Foot disorders; Fracture and dislocation; Fracture repair; Gigantism; Hammertoe correction; Hammertoes; Head and neck disorders; Heel spur removal; Hip fracture repair; Hip replacement; Jaw wiring; Joints; Kneecap removal; Knock-knees; Kyphosis; Laminectomy and spinal fusion; Lower extremities; Orthopedic surgery; Orthopedics; Orthopedics, pediatric; Osgood-Schlatter disease; Osteochondritis juvenilis; Osteogenesis imperfecta; Osteomyelitis; Osteonecrosis; Osteopathic medicine; Osteoporosis; Paget's disease; Physical rehabilitation; Pigeon toes; Podiatry; Polydactyly and syndactyly; Rheumatology; Rickets; Sarcoma; Scoliosis; Slipped disk; Spinal cord disorders; Spine, vertebrae, and disks; Sports medicine; Temporomandibular joint (TMJ) syndrome; Tendon disorders; Tendon repair; Upper extremities.

For Further Information:

Ballard, Carol. *Bones*. Chicago: Heinemann Library, 2002.

Currey, John D. *Bones: Structures and Mechanics*. Princeton, N.J.: Princeton University Press, 2002.

International Osteoporosis Foundation. "Facts and Statistics." *International Osteoporosis Foundation*, 2013.

Joyce, Christopher, and Eric Stover. *Witnesses from the Grave: The Stories Bones Tell*. Boston: Little, Brown, 1991.

KidsHealth. "Bones, Muscles, and Joints." *Nemours Foundation*, 2013.

Marieb, Elaine N., and Katja Hoehn. *Human Anatomy and Physiology*. 9th ed. San Francisco: Pearson/Benjamin Cummings, 2010.

NIH Osteoporosis and Related Bone Diseases National Resource Center. "Bone Health for Life." *National Institutes of Health*, November 2011.

OrthoInfo. "Bone Health Basics." *American Academy of Orthopaedic Surgeons*, May 2012.

Seeley, Rod R., Trent D. Stephens, and Philip Tate. *Anatomy and Physiology*. 7th ed. New York: McGraw-Hill, 2006..

Van De Graaff, Kent M., and Stuart Ira Fox. *Concepts of Human Anatomy and Physiology*. 5th ed. Dubuque: Iowa: Wm. C. Brown, 2000.

Botox

Treatment

Also known as: Botulinum toxin

Anatomy or system affected: Eyes, head, muscles, neck

Specialties and related fields: Neurology, ophthalmology, plastic surgery

Definition: A neurotoxin produced by bacteria that causes botulism in very high doses and is also used as a therapeutic agent for a variety of conditions.

Indications and Procedures

Botulinum toxin has found wide applications as an effective treatment for a variety of conditions associated with excessive muscle contractions. A protein produced by the bacterium *Clostridium botulinum*, botulinum toxin is a potent neurotoxin, causing botulism in very high doses. Botulism is a syndrome of paralysis associated with gastrointestinal symptoms including abdominal cramps and ultimately with respiratory failure from the paralysis of respiratory muscles. As a therapeutic agent, botulinum toxin is injected into muscles and blocks the release of the neurotransmitter acetylcholine from nerve terminals, thus causing paralysis. There are seven different types of botulinum toxin. Two types, botulinum A and B, are available in the United States for clinical use. Botulinum A is also known under the brand name Botox.

Botulinum toxin is available as a purified, vacuum-dried toxin and is reconstituted by the addition of sterile, preservative-free saline. The toxin is then injected into targeted muscles to produce a localized muscle paralysis effect.

Uses and Complications

The utility of botulinum toxin was first demonstrated clinically for the treatment of strabismus, a disorder of abnormal alignment of the eyes. Other disorders treated with botulinum toxin include blepharospasm, a condition of forceful eyelid closure, and focal dystonias, which are syndromes of sustained muscle contractions associated with abnormal postures. Examples of focal dystonias treated with botulinum toxin include cervical torticollis (involuntary neck turning), laryngeal dystonia (abnormal movements of the vocal cords), and oromandibular dystonia (abnormal muscle spasms of the jaw and lower facial muscles). Hemifacial spasm, a disorder of involuntary contractions of the face, also responds well to toxin treatment. Botulinum toxin is also used to treat spasticity, which refers to an excessive increase in muscle tone in the extremities.

Hyperhidrosis (excessive sweating) and sialorrhea (hypersalivation) have also been treated with botulinum toxin, with good results reported. Botulinum toxin has achieved much public attention for its cosmetic use as a treatment for facial wrinkles.

The onset of effect of the injection occurs within several days and generally causes weakness and muscle atrophy for approximately several months, with the effect wearing off gradually. Side effects of botulinum toxin treatment are generally transient and may be the result of a local effect of injection, such as bruising, or related to diffusion of the toxin to nearby muscles. The potential side effect encountered depends on the location of injection. For example, injection into neck muscles has the potential side effects of excessive weakness or dysphagia (difficulty swallowing). Over time, some patients may develop resistance to the effects of the medication, which may be associated with the development of neutralizing antibodies.

—*Winona Tse, M.D.*

See also: Botulism; Collagen; Face lift and blepharoplasty; Head and neck disorders; Hyperhidrosis; Muscle sprains, spasms, and disorders; Muscles; Nervous system; Neuralgia, neuritis, and neuropathy; Neurology; Neurology, pediatric; Paralysis; Plastic surgery; Skin; Strabismus; Sweating; Torticollis; Wrinkles.

For Further Information:

Aaron, Shara. "Botulinum Toxin Injections-Cosmetic." *Health Library*, October 31, 2012.

Aaron, Shara. "Botulinum Toxin Injections-Medical." *Health Library*, May 24, 2013.

"Botulinum Rejuvenation" *AgingSkinNet*, June 13, 2013.

Blitzer, Andrew, and Lucian Sulica. "Botulinum Toxin: Basic Science and Clinical Uses in Otolaryngology." *Laryngoscope* 111 (2001): 218-226.

Childers, Martin K., Daniel J. Wilson, and Diane Simison. *The Use of Botulinum Toxin Type A in Pain Management*. New York: Demos Medical, 1999.

Klein, Arnold W., ed. *The Clinical Use of Botulinum Toxin*. Philadelphia: W. B. Saunders, 2004.

Thant, Zin-Soe, and Eng-King Tan. "Emerging Therapeutic Applications of Botulinum Toxin." *Medical Science Monitor* 9, no. 2 (2003): RA40-48.

Botulism

Disease/Disorder

Anatomy or system affected: Nervous system

Specialties and related fields: Bacteriology, critical care, emergency medicine

Definition: A paralytic illness caused by a powerful neurotoxin produced by the bacterium *Clostridium botulinum*.

Causes and Symptoms

Clostridium botulinum is a bacillus that produces spores. Both bacteria and spores can be found in the intestines of humans and other animals as well as in contaminated soil and water. The spores are highly resistant to heat and can survive boiling and other measures employed to kill bacteria and destroy toxins for safe food preparation. Under appropriate anaerobic conditions (those lacking oxygen), the spores germinate into the toxin-producing vegetative bacilli. The exotoxin is a protein synthesized within the bacteria and released only after the death and lysis (disintegration) of the bacteria. When ingested, the toxin resists the acid and enzymes of the stomach by creating complexes with other bacterial proteins. This allows the toxin to reach the intestines, where it is absorbed into the bloodstream and carried to nerve endings. The toxin is bound and internalized into the presynaptic nerve endings, preventing release of the neurotransmitter acetylcholine. The binding is irreversible, and recovery can occur only after nerve endings regenerate.

Human illness is caused by toxin ingestion or the entry of toxin-producing bacteria into the host. Improper processing of food, especially home canning, can result in the germination of contaminating spores, with subsequent toxin production. Food poisoning occurs when toxin-containing food is ingested, unless it has has been heated sufficiently to denature the protein toxin.

The symptoms of descending paralysis usually begin twelve to thirty-six hours after ingestion. Blurred vision, slurred speech, and difficulty swallowing are followed by labored breathing and weakness of the upper and then the lower extremities. Spores may also contaminate a wound and then germinate and form toxin within the host, producing symptoms similar to food poisoning. Botulism is diagnosed by identification of the toxin and/or bacteria in the patient's serum, stool, or wound, or in ingested food. The specific type of botulinum toxin is verified using the mouse neutralization test.

Treatment and Therapy

The outcome of botulism has improved with the development of critical care and supportive measures. Intubation and mechanical ventilation is vitally important until neuromuscular control of breathing is regained. Specific treatment with botulism antitoxin may be used in severe or progressive cases. Because this antitoxin is of equine origin, however, a high incidence of hypersensitivity reactions (9 to 20 percent) occurs in human patients.

Perspective and Prospects

In 1820, a German named Justinus Kerner first noted the association between sausage consumption and paralytic disease. The term *botulism* is derived from *botulus*, the Latin word for "sausage." Wound botulism was first recognized in 1943. Infant botulism, which is caused by swallowed spores rather than preformed toxin, was first noted in 1976. The most common form of human botulism in the United States, infant botulism can be contracted from exposure to honey, but most cases seem to be related to spores found in soil and dust.

Despite these insights, however, the epidemiology of many botulism cases remains obscure. A diagnostic test more rapid and widely available than the mouse neutralization test, which takes forty-eight hours, is needed. Antitoxin, perhaps from deoxyribonucleic acid (DNA) hybridization technology, would improve therapy over the scarce and dangerous equine product.

—*H. Bradford Hawley, M.D.*

See also: Bacterial infections; Bacteriology; Biological and chemical weapons; Botox; Food poisoning; Nervous system; Neuralgia, neuritis, and neuropathy; Neurology; Neurology, pediatric; Paralysis; Poisoning; Toxicology.

For Further Information:

Brachman, Philip S., and Elias Abrutyn, eds. *Bacterial Infections of Humans: Epidemiology and Control.* 4th ed. New York: Springer, 2009.

Mandell, Gerald L., John E. Bennett, and Raphael Dolin, eds. *Mandell, Douglas, and Bennett's Principles and Practice of Infectious Diseases.* 7th ed. New York: Churchill, 2010.

MedlinePlus. "Botulism." *MedlinePlus*, Apr. 23, 2013.

Pommerville, Jeffery C. *Alcamo's Fundamentals of Microbiology.* 9th ed. Sudbury, Mass.: Jones, 2010.

Wood, Debra. "Botulism." *Health Library*, Nov. 11, 2012.

Bowlegs

Disease/Disorder

Also known as: Genu varum

Anatomy or system affected: Bones, feet, hips, joints, knees, legs, ligaments, muscles

Specialties and related fields: Orthopedics, pediatrics, physical therapy

Definition: A deformity of the legs that can be temporary or persistent, depending on causation.

Causes and Symptoms

Bowlegs describes a condition in which a person standing with ankles and feet together has knees that do not touch and tibias and femurs that curve away from the body's axis. Because of the compression of limbs in the uterus, babies are born with flexed hips and knee capsules with contracted fibers. Infants have rotated feet and legs, with tibias curving inward and femurs outward. As children mature, knee

---

Information on Botulism

Causes: Infection with bacterial spores through ingestion or wound contamination

Symptoms: Descending paralysis, with blurred vision, slurred speech, difficulty swallowing, labored breathing, weakness in extremities

Duration: Acute

Treatments: Antitoxin, intubation and mechanical ventilation

Information on Bowlegs

Causes: Compression of limbs in uterus, bone diseases, genetic diseases, injuries, tumors, deformities, rickets, repetitive motions
Symptoms: Curving leg bones
Duration: Temporary or chronic
Treatments: Muscle exercises, vitamin D supplements, orthotic braces and shoes, surgical straightening

---

angles gradually acquire normal alignment because ligament fibers stretch and bones rotate to correct positions. If the legs do not straighten, a child's movement will be hindered. These children may be susceptible to falling and walking pigeon-toed. Some children exhibit a single bowleg, with the other leg appearing straight.

Bone diseases, genetic conditions, injuries, tumors, and deformities can cause bowlegs to persist beyond childhood. Some babies are born with misshapen leg bones that curve. Blount's disease (tibia vara) alters tibia growth in the plate adjacent to the knee, causing bowing. Environmental factors include inadequate nutrition resulting in rickets and conditions associated with deficient vitamins and minerals that are essential to healthy bone growth. Weak bones are more vulnerable to curve unnaturally. Repetitive motions such as kicking can change the strength and length of leg muscles. As a result, muscles can become uneven. When movement exerts pressure on knees and imbalanced legs, curvature is exacerbated.

Treatment and Therapy

Physicians assess the degree of a patient's bowlegs by measuring the space between the legs while standing. They also observe the patient's movement. Most mild cases occurring temporarily during normal childhood development do not require treatment. Legs can be manipulated to stretch fibers and rotate bones gradually to desired angles. Muscle exercises can prevent imbalances that make people susceptible to bowlegs. Vitamin D supplements can resolve bowlegs caused by rickets.

Doctors use X rays to detect knee and leg bone structural flaws in older children whose bowlegs have not naturally straightened or have worsened. Braces and shoes are sometimes used to correct bowlegs. Most Blount's disease patients constantly wear a corrective knee-ankle-foot orthosis (KAFO) to aid normal bone growth by reducing joint pressure. Surgical bone straightening occasionally is required for extreme cases of bowlegs. Pins are used to inhibit leg bone growth where it is abnormal. The osteotomy procedure adjusts the upper tibia. Some Blount's disease patients require osteotomy if the KAFO does not alleviate their condition.

Perspective and Prospects

Philipp Erlacher documented Blount's disease by 1922. Fifteen years later, Walter Blount differentiated between the infantile and adolescent types of that condition. Later researchers expanded knowledge of this condition and

bowlegs, and using radiographic images, Anders Langenskiold and E. B. Riska classified six stages of Blount's disease deformity.

—*Elizabeth D. Schafer, Ph.D.*

See also: Birth defects; Bone disorders; Bones and the skeleton; Braces, orthopedic; Growth; Lower extremities; Orthopedic surgery; Orthopedics; Orthopedics, pediatric; Rickets; Vitamins and minerals.

For Further Information:
England, Stephen P., ed. *Common Orthopedic Problems*. Philadelphia: W. B. Saunders, 1996.
Hensinger, Robert N., ed. *The Pediatric Lower Extremity*. Philadelphia: W. B. Saunders, 1987.
Herring, John A., ed. *Tachdjian's Pediatric Orthopaedics*. 4th ed. 3 vols. Philadelphia: Saunders/Elsevier, 2008.
Kaneshiro, Neil K. "Bowlegs." *MedlinePlus*, Nov. 12, 2012.
Morrissy, Raymond T., and Stuart L. Weinstein, eds. *Lovell and Winter's Pediatric Orthopaedics*. 6th ed. Philadelphia: Lippincott Williams & Wilkins, 2006.

Braces, orthodontic

Treatment
Also known as: Dental braces, orthodontic treatment
Anatomy or system affected: Mouth, teeth
Specialties and related fields: Dentistry, orthodontics
Definition: A system, usually consisting of brackets and wires, placed in the mouth to move teeth by applying steady pressure. Orthodontic braces are used to straighten teeth, to correct their spacing, and to correct the contact between the teeth of the upper and lower jaws.
Key terms:
malocclusion: a condition in which the teeth of the upper and lower jaws do not fit together properly
mandible: the lower jaw, which is hinged to the skull
maxilla: the upper jaw, which is fixed to the skull
occlusion: the alignment of the teeth of the upper and lower jaws when a person bites down

Indications and Procedures

Orthodontic braces are designed to correct cosmetic and structural imperfections of the teeth and jaw, such as crooked teeth and malocclusions. Braces apply constant, even pressure to move teeth into position for optimal spacing and alignment.

Dentists describe three types of malocclusion using the Angle Classification Method. Class 1 cases have an appropriate relationship between the upper and lower teeth, but the teeth may be crowded or rotated. In class 2 cases, the mandible is especially recessed relative to the maxilla; this is called an overbite. In class 3 cases, the mandible is more forward than the maxilla; this is called an underbite.

Malocclusions may result from physiological conditions such as early or late loss of baby teeth, tumors of the mouth or jaw, and jaw fracture. They may also result from habits such as nail biting, lip biting, and long-term sucking on thumbs, fingers, or pacifiers.

Dentists typically recognize malocclusions when a child's permanent teeth erupt, between the ages of six and twelve. Orthodontic treatment is most effective while the

Orthodontic braces. (© Alexkalina/Dreamstime.com)

child's jaw and teeth are still growing, between the ages of eight and fourteen.

Orthodontic treatment is most commonly performed by an orthodontist, a dentist with specialized training in the diagnosis and treatment of malocclusions. The orthodontist gathers data on a patient from which to make a diagnosis, customize a treatment plan, and measure treatment progress. These data come from a clinical examination, complete medical and dental histories, X rays of the teeth (including those that have not yet erupted), X rays of the face, impressions of the upper and lower teeth from which to make models, and photographs of the teeth and face. From the diagnosis and treatment plan, the orthodontist designs appropriate braces to correct the position and alignment of the teeth.

Braces that are attached to the teeth apply more pressure on the teeth than braces that are removable, and these fixed braces are used to achieve more difficult results. Braces consist of wires and springs that are positioned by brackets cemented onto the teeth or metal bands that wrap around individual molars. Elastic ties hold the wires to the brackets. Every four to six weeks, the nickel-titanium wires must be modified to keep the teeth moving and the elastic ties are replaced. This adjustment is likely to cause temporary discomfort.

Braces are generally worn for two years, although treatment can range from six months to three years. This period is dependent upon the severity of the malocclusion being corrected, the growth of the teeth and face, and the health of the mouth.

Uses and Complications

When the size of the mouth is small relative to the size of the adult teeth, the teeth become crowded and may overlap, grow crooked (tipped forward or backward or twisted), erupt in the wrong position, or become trapped in the bone and not erupt.

Crowding also occurs when baby teeth fall out earlier or later than usual, interfering with the normal eruption of the adult teeth. Crowded teeth are difficult to keep clean by brushing, increasing the risk of tooth decay and gum dis-

ease. Therefore, relieving the crowding as the result of orthodontic treatment promotes oral health.

Orthodontic braces may also be used to correct other conditions that result from malocclusions, such as clicking, popping, and pain in the temporomandibular joint (where the lower jaw is hinged to the skull), difficulty chewing, speech impediments, and mouth breathing that can contribute to snoring and sleep apnea. In addition, straight, evenly spaced teeth improve a smile, which can increase a person's self-confidence.

Untreated malocclusions can lead to additional problems such as chipped or broken teeth, inadvertent biting of the lips, cheeks, and tongue, abnormal wear on tooth surfaces, trauma to the teeth and jaw muscles, bone loss, and loosening or loss of teeth.

Braces create spaces that easily trap food and bacteria, so it is especially important for a person wearing braces to brush regularly with a fluoride toothpaste, floss carefully, rinse with a fluoride mouthwash, and continue with regular dental visits.

Patients commonly feel discomfort when the braces are first attached and after each adjustment. This may interfere with eating. The lips, cheeks, and tongue may become irritated during the initial adaptation.

Foods that are sticky or especially hard may damage the braces. Sticky foods to be avoided include taffy, caramel, toffee, and bubble gum. Hard foods to be avoided include raw carrots, ice, nuts, and popcorn. If a bracket or wire comes loose, then the orthodontist needs to repair or replace it promptly.

Patients who wear braces and participate in contact sports should wear an appropriate protective mouth guard while playing.

Perspective and Prospects

Orthodontics as a specialty of dentistry arose in the 1880s, although people have long sought methods for straightening teeth. Norman W. Kingsley, J. N. Farrar, and Edward H. Angle are considered to be founders of this field.

Traditional braces with metal brackets and rugged metal wires are highly visible, which may make children self-conscious. Some orthodontists now offer thin metal wires and ceramic brackets that are translucent and approximate the color of the natural teeth for a less noticeable appearance. Children who are not adverse to attention, however, may now choose colored elastic ties for a more noticeable appearance.

Increasing numbers of adults are choosing to wear braces. Orthodontic treatment usually takes longer in adults because their teeth and bones are no longer growing, but many cosmetic and functional problems may still be corrected.

—*Bethany Thivierge, M.P.H., E.L.S.*

See also: Bones and the skeleton; Dentistry; Jaw wiring; Orthodontics; Periodontal surgery; Teeth; Tooth extraction.

For Further Information:
Gill, Daljit S. *Orthodontics at a Glance.* Malden, Mass.: Wiley-Blackwell, 2008.

Graber, Lee W. *Orthodontics: Current Principles and Techniques.* 5e. Maryland Heights, Missouri: Mosby, 2011.

Mitchell, Laura. *An Introduction to Orthodontics.* 3d ed. New York: Oxford University Press, 2007.

Nanda, Ram S. *Biomechanics in Orthodontics: Principles and Practics.* Hanover Park, Illionois: Quintessence Publishing, 2010.

Proffit, William R. *Contemporary Orthodonics.* 5e. Maryland Heights, Missouri: 2012.

Singh, Gurkeerat, ed. *Textbook of Orthodontics.* 2d ed. New Delhi, India: Jaypee Brothers, 2007.

Braces, orthopedic

Treatment

Anatomy or system affected: Back, bones, joints, knees, musculoskeletal system, neck

Specialties and related fields: Orthopedics, sports medicine

Definition: A device to aid a joint by immobilization, restriction of movement, movement assistance, weight-bearing support or postural maintenance.

Indications and Procedures

Orthopedic braces have been developed for virtually any joint of the human body. Braces are used to prevent injury, maintain function, or enhance rehabilitation. They are often used in sports-related activities. Individuals who are considered susceptible to a specific injury are be given a brace to reduce the chances of injury. Some individuals may have had a previous injury that affects performance or the ability to perform day-to-day activities. These people would be given braces to help them function normally or obtain closer-to-normal function. People who are recovering from an injury may also use braces to help speed up the recovery process and protect against further injury.

When professionals choose a specific brace, several factors must be considered, including type of shoes worn, type of playing surface, type of activity, previous injuries, weather, and the individual's attitude about wearing braces. Selecting the appropriate brace is critical for protecting the body part or decreasing recovery time.

For orthopedic braces to perform well, they must be positioned properly, securely fastened, easy to put on, comfortable, and durable. Improper placement may increase the chances of injury. Adjustments to the brace during activity may also be necessary if the brace becomes loose and moves around. Many athletes do not like wearing braces because they find them uncomfortable, do not like to spend time putting them on, and believe they can negatively affect performance. Therefore, good braces generally are easy to apply and are made of comfortable, light materials. Durability of materials used in brace construction is also important because braces are often exposed to sweat, environmental elements, and impact with other objects during normal use.

Uses and Complications

Braces fall into one of two broad types, prophylactic and rehabilitative. Prophylactic braces are used to protect joints from injuries during various activities, many of which fall in the category of competitive sports. These braces

An orthopedic brace can be used to support the knee after injury. (© Suzanne Tucker/Dreamstime.com)

stabilize the joint to protect it against contact forces, lateral movements, falls, or repetitive movements. Rehabilitative braces are used after an injury or surgery to support joints or limit movements and assist the healing process.

The most commonly injured joint is the ankle. There are numerous ankle braces on the market, such as lace-up braces, elastic braces, and semirigid braces. Still, it is common to see standard ankle taping as an injury prevention technique. Despite these numerous options, professionals do not agree about which method of ankle bracing is best.

Another common joint injury is to the knee, especially the anterior cruciate ligament (ACL). Many different knee braces have been designed, ranging from simple neoprene to more elaborate hinged braces. Although these braces cannot completely protect the knee, they do help to stabilize the joint.

Upper extremity braces are also used. Specialized braces are made for the shoulder, elbow, wrist, hand, and fingers. These braces include casts, cuffs, and splints as well as basic taping. By limiting some movements at specific joints, the joints are protected from some injuries or reinjuries.

Braces can be used to protect the core of the body as well, as with neck, back, abdominal, and rib braces. Neck or cervical collars are used to stabilize the neck and in some cases to limit movement. Back braces help to reduce back pain by supporting the back and abdominal muscles. Abdominal binders are generally used to compress the abdominal muscles, which may have been weakened by incisions from surgery or childbirth. Rib belts are used to compress the chest area and restrict the expansion of the rib cage. This is beneficial for individuals with chest injuries such as broken ribs or chest infections.

In general braces are noninvasive and present few complications to the individual as long as they are put on appropriately. They have been successfully used to prevent injuries and assist in rehabilitation without major risks to the individuals using them.

Perspective and Prospects

Advances in orthopedic braces are due in part to better materials and enhanced designs. A common brace many years ago was the plaster cast. These casts are very effective at immobilizing body parts, but they are not commonly used for athletes because of its greater weight, limited durability, and hardness, which poses a danger to other athletes. Silicone rubber splints are used in competitive contact sports because they are rigid enough to stabilize the body part but soft enough that the injured athlete or opponents or are not put at risk of injury from contact with the device.

Thermoplastics are materials that can be shaped when heated to fit a specific body part. Upon cooling, the material hardens to the shape of the limb and helps to protect it. However, the thickness is less than other braces, and thermoplastics cannot be used for recent fractures. One of the more common materials used in the construction of orthopedic braces is neoprene. Neoprene works well because it compresses the joint, which reduces pain, helps warm the joint (which aids healing), and helps train the body to react to external forces. Since neoprene is soft and light, it is comfortable to wear.

By combining new materials with better designs, orthopedic braces will continue to improve. They will be lighter, stronger, softer, easy to put on, and more durable. Most important, they will better protect the body parts from injury.

—*Bradley R. A. Wilson, Ph.D.*

See also: Back pain; Bone disorders; Bones and the skeleton; Exercise physiology; Fracture and dislocation; Fracture repair; Head and neck disorders; Kinesiology; Muscle sprains, spasms, and disorders; Muscles; Orthopedic surgery; Orthopedics; Orthopedics, pediatric; Physical rehabilitation; Preventive medicine; Rotator cuff surgery; Spine, vertebrae, and disks; Sports medicine; Tendinitis; Tendon disorders; Tendon repair; Whiplash.

For Further Information:

Perrin, David H. *Athletic Taping and Bracing*. 3d ed. Champaign, Ill.: Human Kinetics, 2012.

Prentice, William E. *Arnheim's Principles of Athletic Training*. 14th ed. New York: McGraw-Hill, 2011.

Street, Scott, and Deborah Runkle. *Athletic Protective Equipment: Care, Selection, and Fitting*. New York: McGraw-Hill, 2000.

Brain

Anatomy

Anatomy or system affected: Head, nerves, nervous system, psychic-emotional system

Specialties and related fields: Neurology, psychiatry, psychology

Definition: The most complex organ in the body, which is used for thinking, learning, remembering, seeing, hearing, and many other conscious and subconscious functions.

Key terms:

action potential: an electrochemical event that nerve cells use to send signals along their cellular extensions in the nervous system

axon: a nerve cell extension used to carry action potentials from one place to another in the nervous system

dendrite: a branching nerve cell extension that receives and processes the effects of action potentials from other nerve cells

dyskinesia: a neurologic disorder causing difficulty in the performance of voluntary movements

nucleus: in reference to brain structure, a collection of nerve cell bodies separable from other groups by their cellular form or by surrounding nerve cell extensions

soma: the body of a cell, where the cell's genetic material and other vital structures are located

synapse: an area of close contact between nerve cells that is the functional junction where one cell communicates with another

tract: a collection of nerve fibers (axons) in the brain or spinal cord that all have the same place of origin and the same place of termination

Structure and Functions

The human brain is a complex structure that is composed of two major classes of individual cells: nerve cells (or neurons) and neuroglial cells (or glial cells). It has been estimated that the adult human brain has around one hundred billion neurons and an even larger number of glial cells. An average adult brain weighs about 1,400 grams and has a volume of 1,200 milliliters. These values tend to vary directly with the person's body size; therefore, males have a brain that is typically 10 percent larger than that of females. There is no correlation of intelligence with brain size, however, as witnessed by the fact that brains as small as 750 milliliters or larger than 2,000 milliliters still show normal functioning.

Neurons process and transmit information. The usual structural features of a neuron include a cell body (or soma), anywhere from several to several hundred branching dendrites that are extensions from the soma, and a typically longer extension known as the axon with one or several synaptic terminals at its end.

The information that is processed and transmitted in the brain takes the form of very brief electrochemical events, with a typical duration of less than two milliseconds, called action potentials or nerve impulses. These impulses most often originate near the point at which the axon and soma are joined and then travel at speeds of up to 130 meters per second along the axon to the synaptic terminals.

It is at the synaptic terminals that one neuron communicates its information to other neurons in the brain. These specialized structural points of neuron-to-neuron commu-

The Anatomy of the Brain

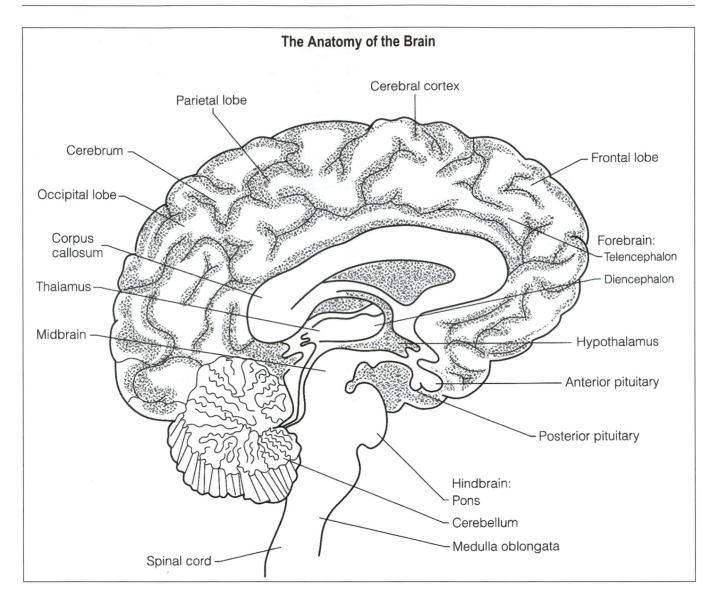

nication are called synapses. Most synapses are found on the dendrites and soma of the neuron that is to receive the nerve signal. A neuron may have as many as fifty thousand synapses on its surface, although the average seems to be around three thousand. It is thought that as many as three hundred trillion synapses may exist in the adult brain.

The neuroglia function as supporting cells. They have a variety of important duties that include acting as a supporting framework for neurons, increasing the speed of impulse conduction along axons, acting as removers of waste or cellular debris, and regulating the composition of the fluid environment around the neurons in order to maintain optimal working conditions in the brain. Neuroglia actually make up about half of the brain's total volume.

The brain can be divided into two major components: gray matter and white matter, both named for their general appearance. The gray matter is composed primarily of neural soma, dendrites, and axons that transmit information at relatively slow speeds. The white matter is made of collections of axons that have layers of specialized glial cells wrapped around them. This enables much faster informa-

tion transfer along these axons.

The brain has six major regions. Beginning from the top of the spinal cord and moving progressively upward, these regions are the medulla oblongata, the pons, the cerebellum, the mesencephalon (or midbrain), the diencephalon, and the cerebrum.

The initial lower portion of the medulla oblongata resembles the spinal cord. The medulla has a variety of functions besides the simple relaying of various categories of sensory information to higher-brain centers. Within the medulla there are a number of centers that are important for the execution and regulation of basic survival and maintenance duties. These duties are called visceral functions and include jobs such as regulating the heart rate, breathing, digestive actions, and blood pressure.

The term *pons* comes from the Latin word meaning "bridge." The pons serves as a bridge from the medulla oblangata to the cerebellum, which is actually situated on the backside of the brain stem. The pons contains tracts and nuclei that permit communication between the cerebellum and other nervous system structures. Some pontine nuclei facilitate the control of such voluntary and involuntary muscle actions as chewing, breathing, and moving the eyes; other nuclei process information related to the sense of balance.

The cerebellum is a small brain in itself. The two main functions of the cerebellum are to make adjustments, quickly and automatically, to the muscles of the body that assist in maintaining balance and posture and to coordinate the activities of the skeletal muscles involved in movements or sequences of movements, thereby promoting smooth and precise actions. These functions are possible because of the input of sensory information to the cerebellum from position sensors in the muscles and joints; from visual, touch, and balance organs; and even from the sense of hearing. There are also many communication channels to and from the cerebellum and other brain areas concerned with the generation and control of movements. While the cerebellum is not the origin of commands that initiate movements, it does store the memories of how to perform patterns of muscle contractions that are used to execute learned skills, such as serving a tennis ball.

The mesencephalon, or midbrain, is located just above the pons. The midbrain contains pathways carrying sensory information upward to higher-brain centers and transmitting motor signals from higher regions down to lower-brain and spinal cord areas involved in movements.

Two important pairs of nuclei, the inferior and superior colliculi, are found on the backside of the mesencephalon. They coordinate visual and acoustic reflexes involving eye and head movements, such as eye focusing and orienting the head and body toward a sound source. The nucleus known as the substantia nigra operates with nuclei in the cerebrum to generate the patterns and rhythms of such activities as walking and running. Additional mesencephalic nuclei are important for the involuntary control of muscle tone, posture maintenance, and the control of eye movements.

The diencephalon, located above the midbrain, contains the two important brain structures known as the thalamus and hypothalamus. The thalamus is the final relay for all sensory signals (except the sense of smell) before they arrive at the cerebral cortex (the cerebrum's outer covering of gray matter). The hypothalamus is important for regulating drives and emotions, and it serves as a master link between the nervous and endocrine systems.

The thalamus is a collection of different nuclei. Some cooperate with nuclei in the cerebrum to process memories and generate emotional states. Other nuclei have complex involvement in the interactions of the cerebellum, cerebral nuclei, and motor areas of the cerebral cortex.

The relatively small hypothalamus plays many crucial roles that help to maintain stability in the body's internal environment. It regulates food and liquid intake, blood pressure, heart rate, breathing, body temperature, and digestion. Other significant duties encompass the management of sexual activity, rage, fear, and pleasure.

The final major brain region is the cerebrum, which is the largest of the six regions and the seat of higher intellectual capabilities. Sensory information that reaches the cerebrum also enters into a person's conscious awareness. Voluntary actions originate in the cerebral neural activities.

The cerebrum is divided into two cerebral hemispheres, each covered by the gray matter known as the cerebral cortex. Below the cortex is the white matter, which consists of massive bundles of axons carrying signals between various cortical areas, down from the cortex to lower areas, and up into the cortex from lower areas. Embedded in the white matter are also a number of cerebral nuclei.

The cerebral cortex has areas that are the primary sensory areas for each of the senses and other areas whose major duties deal with the origin and planning of motor activities. The association areas of the cortex integrate and process sensory signals, often resulting in the initiation of appropriate motor responses. Cortical integrative centers receive information from different association areas. The integrative centers perform complex analyses of information (such as predicting the consequences of various possible responses) and direct elaborate motor activities (such as writing).

The cerebral nuclei, also called the basal nuclei or basal ganglia, form components of brain systems that have complex duties such as the regulation of emotions, the control of muscle tone and the coordination of learned patterns of movement, and the processing of memories.

The electrochemical signal that constitutes an action potential in a neuron, and that is sent along the neuron's axon to the synaptic contacts formed with other neurons in the brain, is the basic unit of activity in neural tissue. Although the electrical voltage generated by a single action potential is very small and difficult to measure, the tremendous number of neurons active at any moment results in voltages large enough to be measured at the scalp with appropriate instruments called electroencephalographs. The recorded signals are known as an electroencephalogram (EEG).

Although interpreting an EEG can be compared to standing outside a football stadium filled with screaming fans and trying to discern what is happening on the playing field by listening to the crowd noises, it still provides clinically useful information and is used regularly in clinics around the world each day. The typical EEG signal appears as a series of wavy patterns whose size, length, shape, and location of best recording on the head provide valuable indications concerning the conditions of brain regions beneath the recording electrodes placed on the scalp.

Disorders and Diseases

One of the most useful applications of the EEG is in the diagnosis of epilepsy. Epilepsy is a group of disorders originating in the brain. There are multiple possible causes. Epilepsy is characterized by malfunctions of the motor, sensory, or even psychic operations of the brain, and there are often accompanying convulsive movements during the attack.

The most common type is known as idiopathic epilepsy, so called because there is no known cause of the attacks. The usual episode occurs suddenly as a large group of neurons begins to produce action potentials in a very synchronized fashion (called a seizure), which is not the typical mode of action in neural tissue. There may be no impairment of consciousness or a complete loss of consciousness, and the seizure may be restricted to a localized area of brain tissue or may spread over the entire brain. When areas of the brain that generate or control movements become involved, the patient will exhibit varying degrees of involuntary muscle contractions or convulsions.

Some cases of epilepsy can be traced to definite causes such as brain tumors, brain injuries, drug abuse, adverse drug reactions, or infections that have entered the brain. Regardless of the cause, the diagnosis is often made through examination of the EEG, whereby a trained examiner can quickly identify the EEG abnormalities characteristic of epilepsy.

The usual treatment is directed toward preventing the synchronized bursts of neural activity. This is most often achieved by administering anticonvulsive drugs such as phenobarbital or phenytoin. These agents block the transmission of neural signals in the epileptic regions and thereby suppress the explosive episodes of synchronized neuronal discharges that induce the seizures. Many epileptics are successfully treated by this approach and are able to lead normal, productive lives, free from the uncontrollable seizures. In some cases, the medication can eventually be discontinued and the patient will never again suffer a seizure.

Unfortunately, there are also cases where even the strongest medications do not prevent the seizures, or only do so with debilitating side effects. In the most severe cases, the patients may have dozens of seizures each day, making any form of normal existence impossible. In addition, the large number of seizures eventually can lead to permanent brain damage. For some of these patients, the most drastic form of treatment has been used: surgical removal of the brain tissue responsible for the seizures. This technique is accompanied by great risk because of the danger that removing a portion of brain tissue may leave the patient unable to speak or to speak intelligently, unable to understand spoken words, unable to interpret visual information, or suffering from any of a wide variety of behavioral disturbances, depending on the precise area of the brain that has been removed.

Although this approach is not appropriate in all cases, it has been successful in many. For these patients, success is usually defined as the possibility, following surgery, to control or prevent future seizures through the use of anticonvulsive drugs and to resume a normal life or a life that is much more normal than it was before surgery.

A varied group of disorders known as dyskinesias causes difficulty in the performance of voluntary movements. The movements actually look like normal body movements or portions of normal movements. Dyskinesia often results from problems involving the basal nuclei. When the basal nuclei are affected, the dyskinesic movements usually do not occur during sleep and are reduced during periods of emotional tranquillity. Anxiety, emotional tension, and stressful conditions, however, cause the dyskinesia to become worse. These observations can be explained by the fact that neural pathways are known to connect the brain centers involved with the generation of emotional states to the basal nuclei.

One example of a dyskinesia affecting the basal nuclei is the inherited condition of Huntington's disease (or Huntington's chorea), for which no cure exists. A chorea is a dyskinesia in which the patient's movements are quick and irregular. Huntington's chorea first makes its appearance when the patient is in middle age. It results in the progressive degeneration of the basal nuclei, known as the corpus striatum, that are located in the cerebrum. Some of the common symptoms are involuntary facial grimacing, jaw and tongue movements, twisting and turning movements of the torso, and speaking difficulties. As the brain atrophy (degeneration) progresses, the patients become totally disabled. Death usually results ten to fifteen years following the appearance of the first symptoms.

A category of generalized disturbances of higher-brain function is known as dementia. Dementia is characterized by a generalized deficiency of intellectual performance, mental deterioration, memory impairment, and limited attention span. These are often accompanied by changes in personality such as increased irritability and moodiness.

Various diseases can cause dementia. One of the most frequently observed is known as Alzheimer's disease; it is progressive and usually develops between the ages of forty and sixty. The disease is marked by the death of neurons in the cerebral cortex and the deep cerebral regions known as the nucleus basalis and the hippocampus. The exact cause of neural death in Alzheimer's disease is unknown. While some cases are inherited, other instances seem to appear without any family history of the disease. Death usually occurs within ten years after the appearance of the first symptoms, and no cure exists.

The areas of the brain showing neural degeneration also have abnormal collections of a specific type of protein. The appearance of this protein in the blood and the fluids that surround the brain is a clinical sign of Alzheimer's disease. The areas of the brain that deteriorate during the progression of this disease illustrate the functional roles played by these regions. The hippocampus, in particular, is crucial for learning, the storage of long-term memories, memory of recent events, and the sense of time. Therefore, the death of hippocampal neurons helps to explain the memory disturbances and related behavioral changes seen in Alzheimer's disease patients.

Perspective and Prospects

Given the complexity of the human brain, understanding its structure and function is the ultimate challenge to medical science. The challenge exists because in order to treat brain disorders rationally, it is necessary to know how a normal brain functions. An appreciation of this can be gleaned by studying the history of some approaches used through the ages to treat brain disorders.

For example, in the Middle Ages it was a common practice to treat people with epilepsy by cutting open the patient's scalp and pouring salt into the wound (all of which was performed without anesthesia, since anesthetics were not yet known). The purpose of this treatment was to poison the spirits possessing the patient, forcing them to leave.

As modern science discovered the cellular basis of life, such measures were gradually replaced with treatments directed toward the biochemical imbalances, infections, or interruptions of blood flow that were found to be the cause of many brain disorders. The development of nonsurgical techniques permitting the visualization of the brain regions that are active, or inactive, during various tasks or illnesses greatly advanced the understanding of brain function and improved diagnosis, the planning of effective treatments, and the tracking of either the improvement or the deterioration of patients.

Late in the 1970s, the disease known as acquired immunodeficiency syndrome (AIDS) attracted the attention of the world's scientists. AIDS is caused by the human immunodeficiency virus (HIV). A significant portion of AIDS patients experience various neurological problems, including difficulties of movement, loss of memory, and cognitive disturbances. In some cerebral cortical areas, as many as half of the neurons may die. To understand how the virus causes these effects, it is necessary to analyze how the brain's components function when infected by the virus and then form a clear explanation of the consequences of viral infection.

HIV actually infects certain classes of neuroglial cells. Infection of these glial cells causes them to release distinct types of chemicals that can be toxic to neurons. One type of glial cell, known as the astrocyte, can begin to appear in abnormally large numbers as a result of these chemicals being released. In turn, the presence of large numbers of astrocytes provokes the release of even more of the toxic chemicals. This sort of effect is referred to as a positive feedback loop. The significance of this cascade of mutually stimulating events (neurotoxic chemicals causing astrocytes to appear in greater numbers, and increased numbers of astrocytes causing more production of neurotoxic chemicals) is that only a few HIV-infected cells can trigger extensive neural damage.

Additionally, a protein part of the virus, called gp120, can stimulate release of the same neurotoxic chemicals and can disrupt the normal functioning of the astrocytes. One important function of astrocytes is to regulate the chemical environment of neurons by removing certain types of chemicals. One of these chemicals, called glutamate, is normally present and used by some neurons to send signals to other neurons at their synaptic contacts. When glutamate is not promptly removed from the environment of the target neurons, however, it becomes toxic to the neurons and kills them. The HIV protein gp120 disrupts the ability of astrocytes to remove glutamate, thereby increasing the death of neurons in the brain as they become exposed to toxic levels of glutamate.

—*John V. Urbas, Ph.D.*

See also: Abscess drainage; Abscesses; Addiction; Alcoholism; Alti-

tude sickness; Alzheimer's disease; Amnesia; Anatomy; Aneurysmectomy; Aneurysms; Angiography; Aphasia and dysphasia; Biofeedback; Brain damage; Brain disorders; Brain tumors; Chiari malformations; Chronic wasting disease (CWD); Cluster headaches; Coma; Computed tomography (CT) scanning; Concussion; Craniotomy; Creutzfeldt-Jakob disease (CJD); Dementias; Dizziness and fainting; Dyslexia; Electroencephalography (EEG); Embolism; Emotions: Biomedical causes and effects; Encephalitis; Endocrinology; Endocrinology, pediatric; Epilepsy; Fetal tissue transplantation; Frontotemporal dementia (FTD); Hallucinations; Head and neck disorders; Headaches; Huntingdon's disease; Hydrocephalus; Hypnosis; Hypothalamus; Intellectual disability; Intraventricular hemorrhage; Learning disabilities; Leukodystrophy; Light therapy; Memory loss; Meningitis; Migraine headaches; Narcolepsy; Narcotics; Neuroimaging; Neurology; Neurology, pediatric; Neurosurgery; Parkinson's disease; Positron emission tomography (PET) scanning; Psychiatric disorders; Psychiatry; Psychiatry, child and adolescent; Psychiatry, geriatric; Psychology; Seizures; Shock therapy; Shunts; Sleep disorders; Strokes; Subdural hematomas; Systems and organs; Thrombosis and thrombus; Toxicology; Transient ischemic attacks (TIAs); Tremors; Tumor removal; Tumors; Unconsciousness.

For Further Information:

Bear, Mark F., Barry W. Connors, and Michael A. Paradiso. *Neuroscience: Exploring the Brain*. 3d ed. Philadelphia: Lippincott Williams & Wilkins, 2007.

Bloom, Floyd E., M. Flint Beal, and David J. Kupfer, eds. *The Dana Guide to Brain Health*. New York: Dana Press, 2006.

Davis, Joel. *Mapping the Mind: The Secrets of the Human Brain and How It Works*. Bridgewater, N.J.: Replica Books, 1999.

Edelman, Gerald M. *Bright Air, Brilliant Fire*. New York: Basic Books, 1992.

Epilepsy Foundation. "The Brain." *Epilepsy Foundation*, 2012.

Horstman, Judith. *The "Scientific American" Day in the Life of Your Brain: A Twenty-four-Hour Journal of What's Happening in Your Brain*. New York: Jossey-Bass, 2009.

Marieb, Elaine N., and Katja Hoehn. *Human Anatomy and Physiology*. 9th ed. San Francisco: Pearson/Benjamin Cummings, 2010.

MedlinePlus. "Brain Diseases." *MedlinePlus*, June 21, 2013.

National Institute of Neurological Disorders and Stroke. "Brain Basics: Know Your Brain." *National Institutes of Health*, March 20, 2013.

Nolte, John. *Human Brain: An Introduction to Its Functional Anatomy*. 6th ed. Philadelphia: Mosby/Elsevier, 2009.

Scientific American 267 (September, 1992).

Seeley, Rod R., Trent D. Stephens, and Philip Tate. *Anatomy and Physiology*. 7th ed. New York: McGraw-Hill, 2006.

Van De Graaff, Kent M., and Stuart Ira Fox. *Concepts of Human Anatomy and Physiology*. 5th ed. Dubuque, Iowa: Wm. C. Brown, 2000.

Woolsey, Thomas A., Joseph Hanaway, and Mokhtar Gado. *Brain Atlas: A Visual Guide to the Human Central Nervous System*. 3d ed. Hoboken, N.J.: Wiley, 2008.

Brain banks

Organizations

Definition: An institution that acquires, preserves, stores, and distributes normal and diseased brain tissue for medical research.

Key terms:

formalin: an aqueous solution that contains formaldehyde and is used for the preservation of tissue

histology: a branch of biology that studies the microscopic structure of tissue

morphology: a branch of biology that studies form and structure, independent of function

neuropathology: the study of diseases associated with the nervous system

postmortem: after the death of an individual

Science and Profession

Brain banks employ a variety of people. There are nontechnical staff who handle the database and donation paperwork, as well as administrative personnel who handle things like public relations. Once a human brain has been acquired, technicians dissect and preserve the tissue, and then neuroanatomists and neuropathologists study the brain morphology and histological characteristics to diagnose it. Research scientists help sort through the requests to use the tissue for research. Usually, the director of the brain bank, along with collaborating scientists, will have an earned doctorate in medicine (MD) or a specialist's doctoral degree (PhD) in neuroscience or a related field.

Perspective and Prospects

While brain banks got their initial start at the end of the nineteenth century, it was not until the 1960s that formalized practices were instituted and eventually widely adopted. The number of brain banks has grown exponentially over the past 30 years. There were just three brain banks in the early-to-mid-1970s, but now, they number in the several hundreds. Most collections are small, with fewer than twenty brains. Smaller banks most often result from a focus on only one type of pathology (e.g., Alzheimer's disease, schizophrenia, posttraumatic stress disorder, etc.). It has been suggested that these smaller banks seek out relationships with each other for the purpose of forming tissue-sharing networks.

One exception to this trend of small, specialized banks would be the Harvard Brain Tissue Resource Center. It is one of the world's oldest brain banks and the repository of over 6,000 brains from individuals diagnosed with several different pathological disorders. It is important to note that brain banks also collect nondiseased brains for use as normal controls in studies. Nondiseased brains are more difficult to acquire since donors are less motivated to turn the organ over for scientific study.

The recent rise of brain banks results from their ability to fill several niches in the world of clinical research. Their development grew out of the need for investigators to study human tissue as opposed to tissue from nonhuman species (e.g., mice, rats, monkeys) because in many instances, animal models of specific kinds of pathology are not available. Even today, current brain imaging technologies (e.g., functional magnetic resonance imaging [fMRI] and positron emission tomography [PET]) and genetics methods are often unsuitable for the research of brain pathology. Therefore, as a means of acquiring the human tissue necessary to study the cellular lesions of brain diseases, brain banks are vital. Even though brain tissue is vital to certain kinds of research, it is not easy to procure. So, brain banks provide the legal, ethical, and scientific expertise to manage the acquisition, storage, and distribution of human brains to responsible investigators for study. The alternative would be for individual laboratories to bear the considerable burden of acquiring and managing their own tissue. Even in instances where this would be possible, it would be prohibitively expensive and inefficient.

In conjunction with the fact that autopsy rates are declining worldwide, meaning there is less clinically relevant tissue to observe, brain banks are key to gaining access to brain tissue. A third, bigger-picture role involves the urgency to understand how the brain functions. It has been estimated that one-third of all human disease is attributed to neurological illness. Acquiring a more comprehensive understanding of the inner workings of the brain could help neuroscientists develop treatments that would alleviate horrific symptoms associated with brain pathology and even open up the door to possible cures. Brain banks are central to facilitating these kinds of investigations conducted in labs around the world.

Procedures and Ethics

Once a brain bank acquires a brain, it must quickly process and preserve the tissue. A typical protocol begins with removal of some key structures, like the cerebellum. One hemisphere is then immersed in a 10 percent formalin solution, which preserves the tissue. It is then stored at room temperature. The other is sliced up into segments. The sections are photographed and stored in a database along with any information known about the donor. The slices are vacuum-packed and frozen to approximately -80° Celsius. These cold storage techniques preserve the properties of the tissue-including enough detail for genetic analyses-for years.

Brain banks, similar to other organ procurement organizations (e.g., heart, lung, etc.), need consistent procedures to address the inevitable ethical challenges. Foremost is the need to obtain premortem informed consent from the donor or postmortem consent from next of kin. This procedure was mandated by the American Department of Health and Human Services in 2001. Other regulation forbids selling human brains in general, while still allowing brain banks the ability to recover some of the costs associated with diagnostics, storage, and transportation.

Brain banks also need strict guidelines regarding tissue dissemination. It is imperative that agencies who request brain tissue be vetted to ensure they have appropriate training and scientific credentials as well as suitable facilities for safe handling of the tissue. As it is the defining human organ, dealing with the brain carries a heightened ethical sensitivity, so banks must conduct their collection practices responsibly.

—Bryan C. Auday, Ph.D., and Trevor Hinshaw

See also: Neuroethics; Neuroscience; Psychiatry

For Further Information:
Abbott, Alison. "Brain Child." *Nature* 478 (2011): 442-443.
Benes, Francine M. "Deserving the Last Great Gift." *Cerebrum* (July 2003): 61-73.
Kretzschmar, Hans. "Brain Banking: Opportunities, Challenges and Meaning for the Future." *Nature Reviews Neuroscience* 10 (2009): 70-77.
Ravid, Rivka, and Isidro Ferrer. "Brain Banks as Key Part of Biochemical and Molecular Studies on Cerebral Cortex Involvement in Parkinson's Disease." *The FEBS Journal* 279 (2012): 1167-1176.

Brain damage

Disease/Disorder
Anatomy or system affected: Brain, nervous system
Specialties and related fields: Neurology, psychiatry, psychology
Definition: Mild, moderate, or traumatic brain injury, which occurs when cells that make up the brain die.
Key terms:

closed headinjury: an injury to the brain that arises from a problem within the cranium

cognitive functions: mental functions such as reasoning, language, memory, and problem-solving

computed tomography(CT) scan: a visual diagnostic technology using X rays that can detect brain abnormalities

glucose: a simple sugar that is the primary source of fuel for brain cells

magnetic resonance imaging(MRI): a visual diagnostic technology that can create high-resolution pictures of brain structures

paralysis: inability to move a particular part of the body

stroke: temporary loss of blood flow to the brain

traumatic brain injury: an injury to the brain caused by blunt force

---

Information on Brain Damage

Causes: Accidents (automobile collisions, falls, sports injuries); strokes
Symptoms: Motor control problems, paralysis, balance and sensory problems; often speech and language difficulties, memory loss, concentration and attention problems; if extensive, loss of consciousness, coma, and death
Duration: Acute
Treatments: Depends on cause; may include surgery (hemorrhage, tumor) or drug therapy (swelling, blockage, infection)

Causes and Symptoms

Brain damage can occur as a result of several causes such as neurological illness or disease, stroke, and traumatic brain injury. Therefore, physicians have found it helpful to categorize the types of injuries that most often lead to the death of brain cells. The most common type that leads to brain damage is the closed head injury. It occurs when a problem, such as the disruption of blood flow to the brain, prevents vital oxygen and nutrients from reaching the cells that make up the brain. If the brain is deprived of oxygen and glucose for more than six or seven seconds, then a person usually becomes unconscious and brain cells begin to die.

Accidents such as automobile collisions, falls, and sports injuries can lead to brain damage by causing the brain to bleed inside the cranium. This kind of closed head injury frequently results in brain swelling that puts pressure on delicate structures, preventing them from working properly and sometimes leading to permanent damage. Strokes also result in brain damage either by blocking normal blood flow within the arteries that feed the brain or by causing a blood vessel to break and leak blood into surrounding tissue.

When brain damage occurs, symptoms may include motor control problems, paralysis, and difficulty with balance and the integration of sensory information. In the case of an accident that leads to brain damage, it would not be uncommon to see cognitive functions affected, creating speech and language difficulties, memory loss, and problems with concentration and attention. Problems with motivation and the expression of emotions may develop, and to some degree a person's personality can be altered because of brain damage. In cases of extensive damage, the result could be loss of consciousness, coma, and even death.

Treatment and Therapy

Treatment for brain damage begins with an assessment of the cause and extent of the injury. Several distinct technologies can be used to image not only the structures of the brain but the functioning of specific areas as well. If bleeding or swelling of the brain is suspected, then a computed tomography (CT) scan can be used to provide pictures of the brain to assess which structures are implicated. If a tumor or areas of localized damage is suspected, then magnetic resonance imaging (MRI) is more helpful because of its ability to create a clear, well-defined image.

Specialized neuropsychological tests are used to determine the extent of deficits in thinking-such as language processing, memory, and decision making-as well as in sensory perception and motor functioning. Visual diagnostics alone usually cannot determine the specific impact on mental processes and specific functions. Neuropsychological procedures, often administered in a particular array, or test battery, along with visual imaging, provide the best appreciation for how the damage affects brain function.

Since there are several different causes of brain damage, treatments can vary. Drug therapy can be used in instances where the brain is being damaged by swelling or when an artery inside the brain is partially blocked. High doses of antibiotics can be used when damage occurs as a result of a bacterial infection. If a weakened artery is found that is leaking blood into the brain or a tumor is detected using an MRI, then surgery could be recommended. In instances where no immediate treatment can be performed, specific rehabilitation therapies are used to stimulate surviving brain tissue that is near the injury to take over some of the functioning of the damaged tissue.

Perspective and Prospects

Although brain injuries have occurred since the beginning of humankind, the question of what the brain does and how it contributes to behavior has only been partially answered. There is evidence from human skull remains that small holes were drilled as a form of crude brain surgery as far back as 2000 BCE. The purpose of the procedure is unknown; however, it could have helped an injured person by relieving brain swelling. Prior to the first century CE, it was not widely accepted that the brain was the center for reasoning, emotions, and movement. During early human history, the heart was believed to control the thoughts and emotions. Galen of Pergamum (130-201 CE), a Roman physician, was influential in bringing forth the notion that the brain, and not the heart, gave rise to behavior. He learned much about the brain and its impact on behavior by observing injured gladiators who survived fierce battles in the Roman coliseum. Prospects for future therapies to compensate for brain damage include stem cell tissue transplantation to stimulate new brain cell development. Better drugs are being developed for stroke victims whose blood has leaked into the brain and had begun killing nearby cells. Also, brain imaging technologies are continuing to be refined to produce clearer pictures that allow practitioners to make more accurate diagnoses.

—*Bryan C. Auday, PhD*

See also: Accidents; Brain; Brain disorders; Chiari malformations; Coma; Computed tomography (CT) scanning; Concussion; Craniotomy; Critical care; Critical care, pediatric; Dizziness and fainting; Emergency medicine; Emergency medicine, pediatric; Emotions: Biomedical causes and effects; Fetal tissue transplantation; Head and neck disorders; Intraventricular hemorrhage; Magnetic resonance imaging (MRI); Memory loss; Neuroimaging; Neurology; Neurology, pediatric; Neurosurgery; Sports medicine; Strokes; Subdural hematomas; Unconsciousness.

For Further Information:

Brain Injury Association of America. "Diagnosing Brain Injury." *Brain Injury Association of America*, 2013.

Dallas, Mary Elizabeth. "HealthDay: Brain Imaging Detects Tiny Lesions Related to Mild Injury: Study." *MedlinePlus*, Mar. 12, 2013.

Landau, Elaine. *Headand Brain Injuries*. Berkeley Heights, N.J.: Enslow, 2002.

Zasler, Nathan D., Douglas I Katz and Ross D. Zafonte. *Brain Injury Medicine*. 2nd ed. New York: Demos Medical Publishing, 2013.

Zollman, Felise S. *Manual of Traumatic Brain Injury: Assessmentand Management*. 2d ed. New York: Springer Publishing, 2016.

Brain death

Disease/Disorder

Also known as: Cerebral death, End of life

Anatomy or system affected: Nervous System, Endocrine system

Specialties and related fields: Neurology, End of life care, organ transplantation

Definition: Brain death refers to the absence of function in all parts of the brain including the brain stem. It appears in an EEG as the complete absence of any electrical activity in the brain (flat EEG).

Key terms:

encephalogram: measurement of the electrical activity in the brain shown as brain waves. It is one of the key components assessed in brain death.

flat(isoelectric) EEG: absence of electrical activity in the brain as measured by an EEG.

tissue and organ procurement: procedures used for obtaining tissues or organs for transplant after brain death has been declared.

Causes and Criteria

Brain death occurs when there is total, irreversible damage to the entire brain including the brain stem. This could occur after a traumatic event to the head, or due to disease and loss of blood flow/oxygen to the brain. It should be noted that although brain death is often used synonymously with cerebral death, it truly encompasses more than death of the cerebrum. True brain death occurs when there is absolutely no electrical activity in any part of the brain. This includes the cerebrum, cerebellum, and brain stem. When there is no electrical activity in any part of the brain, there will be no heartbeat, respiration or blood pressure. This should be the actual definition of brain death. Such an individual can be "kept alive" by artificial means such as a ventilator. This individual will demonstrate no response to pain and no reflexes under the control of the twelve cranial nerves. If they are kept alive by artificial means, a brain dead individual may occasionally demonstrate movement as a result of reflexes that are controlled by the spinal cord. It should also be noted that brain death is different than a persistent vegetative state as well. When an individual is in a persistent vegetative state, they appear unconscious, but continue to have electrical activity of the brain and show some cranial nerve reflexes. They typically still have brainstem function and may breathe on their own.

Historically, death had been defined by absence of heart beat and respiration. However, with the advent of cardiopulmonary resuscitation (CPR) it was found that many people who lacked vital signs could be brought back to life. It was then realized that perhaps absence of pulse and respiration was not adequate to define clinical death. This became especially important with the development of organ transplant procedures. In order for organ procurement for transplants to proceed smoothly, there needed to be a more rigorous definition of death (of the donor). This has been an issue for the past 50 years. During this time, brain death has been the most acceptable determinant of the death of the individual. However, different countries throughout the world are still using different definitions of brain death, and there is a lack of agreement on the criteria that are used to define brain death. *Beyond Brain Death: The Case Against Brain Based Criteria for Human Death (2000)* presents a review of the first 40 years of debate on the definition and criteria that have been used internationally. While the debate continues, the American Academy of Neurology has published guidelines for the determination of brain death that are the most consistently followed.

The guidelines for determination of brain death set forth by the American Academy of Neurology include the following. An attempt should be made to find the immediate cause of the lack of consciousness (trauma or disease) making sure that it is not due to the ingestion of a drug or alcohol, a chemical imbalance, or decreased body temperature. While the individual is on life support, his or her blood pressure should be slowly increased to a normal level. Following these guidelines will help to ensure that results of any neurologic exam are accurate. The neurologic examination should be performed by a physician and should be carried out twice. In the assessment, the patient must be totally unresponsive even to the most noxious of stimuli. Additionally, the patient must demonstrate absence of all brainstem reflexes (e.g., gag reflex). When these reflexes are all shown to be absent, the patient is disconnected from the ventilator, and given an apnea test. If no breathing is noted in an 8-minute period and the patient's arterial blood gas shows an increase in carbon dioxide, the apnea test is deemed positive and supports the "diagnosis of brain death." Following a diagnosis of brain death, confirmatory tests are often carried out. Often in countries outside of the United States, such confirmatory tests are mandatory for a diagnosis of brain death. Within the U.S., these confirmatory tests are optional. Confirmatory tests fall into two categories, those which measure blood flow to the brain (e.g., cerebral angiography) and hose which measure electrical activity of the brain (e.g., EEG). It is now felt that these confirmatory tests are not necessary since the definition and diagnosis of brain death have become more widely used, accepted, and accurate.

Perspective and Prospects

The definition and diagnosis of death has been controversial over the course of history. For the past 50 years, the diagnosis has seemed to hinge on the notion of brain death, while there was still controversy over how that was diagnosed. Currently, within the U.S. the guidelines for diagnosis of brain death have been set forth by the American Academy of Neurology. As organ transplantation has become more common, the accurate diagnosis of brain death has become more important allowing for more efficient procurement of organs from deceased donors. Since brain death is irreversible this seems to be the best indicator of organs that are truly available for transplant.

—*Robin Kamienny Montvilo, RN, PhD*

For Further Information:

American Academy of Neurology. *Guidelines for Brain Death Determination.* May, 2017.

De Georgia, M. A. "History of brain death as death: 1968 to the present." *Journal of Critical Care, (29),* 673-678. August, 2014.

Jennett, B. "The Definition of death: Contemporary controversies." *Brain, 123*(2), 408-411. February, 2000.

Potts, M., P. A. Byrne, and R. G. Nilges. (Eds.) *Beyond Brain Death: The Case Against Brain Based Criteria for Human Death.* New York: Springer, 2000.

Wijdicks, E. F. "The case against confirmatory tests for determining brain death in adults." *Neurology, 75*(1), 77-83. July, 2010.

Brain disorders

Disease/Disorder

Anatomy or system affected: Brain, head, central nervous system, psycho-social-emotional system

Specialties and related fields: geriatrics and gerontology, neurology, neuropsychology, psychiatry

Definition: Disorders of the brain can interfere with its role in the control of body functions, behavior, learning, and expression, while defects can also threaten life itself.

Key terms:

anencephaly: a fatal congenital condition in which tissues that should have differentiated to form the brain failed to do so

coma: a condition of unconsciousness that may or may not be reversible; various degrees of coma are assessed by the presence or absence of reflex responses, such as pupil dilation when a light is shone into the eyes

dementia: a diseased state in which intellectual ability is ever decreasing; personality changes, decreased interest or ability to care for one's self, and long-term and short-term memory loss can indicate dementia

embolus: a clot or other piece of matter that may travel through the circulatory system to tiny blood vessels (as in the brain) and block the path that normally allows blood flow

hydrocephalus: a condition caused by excess cerebrospinal fluid within the confines of the cranium

ischemia: an inadequate blood flow to a region; may be caused by an incomplete blockage in or constriction of a blood vessel (as may occur with atherosclerosis or a blood clot)

seizure: a misfiring of cortical neurons that alters the patient's level of consciousness; the seizure may or may not involve changes in emotion and muscular convulsions

stroke: a loss of blood flow to a region of the brain that is of sudden onset

thrombus: a blood clot that is attached to the interior wall of a blood vessel

Causes and Symptoms

The cerebral cortex acts as a processor for sensory information and as an integrator of memory, interpretation, creativity, intellect, and passion. Disorders of the brain or brain defects can disrupt these processing or integrating functions. Disorders of the brain include such commonly heard terms as stroke, ischemia, dementia, seizure, and coma. Brain disorders may also occur as a result of infection, various tumors, traumas leading to blood clots (hematomas) or lack of oxygen (hypoxia), and cancer. Brain defects include anencephaly, a congenital defect in which a newborn lacks a brain, and hydrocephaly, commonly called "water on the brain."

A stroke is any situation in which the blood supply to a region of the brain is lost. This can occur as a result of a cerebral hemorrhage, during which blood escapes from blood vessels to surround and compress brain tissue; cerebral thrombosis, whereby a clot attached to the wall of a blood

---

Information on Brain Disorders

Causes: Congenital disorders, age-related degeneration, traumas leading to blood clots or restricted blood flow to brain, disease, infection, seizure, stroke, psychological disorders

Symptoms: Varies widely; may include forgetfulness, sudden sharp pain, impaired movement, dementia, lethargy, headache, dullness, blurred vision, nausea, vomiting

Duration: Acute to chronic

Treatments: Surgery, medications, neurorehabilitation

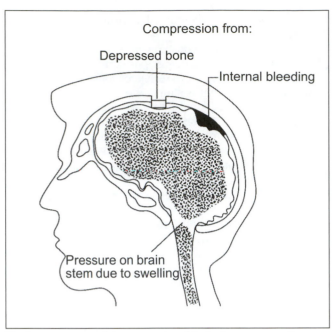

Compression from:

Depressed bone

Internal bleeding

Pressure on brain stem due to swelling

Head trauma may result in compression of the brain, consequent distortions, and severe neurological reactions.

vessel restricts the amount of blood flowing to a particular region; or an embolus, a foreign substance which may be a clot that migrates in the bloodstream, often to lodge in a smaller vessel in the brain. The embolus will block blood flow to some area. An embolus can originate from substances other than a blood clot, which is why health care staff often squirt fluid out of a needle before administering a shot or other therapy: to ensure that no air embolus, which could induce a stroke or prove fatal if it enters the brain, is injected.

Transient ischemic attacks (TIAs) are often thought of as small strokes, but, technically, ischemia simply means that oxygen is not reaching the cells within a tissue. Basically, the mechanism is similar to a stroke, in that blood flow to a portion of the brain is compromised. Although blood actually reaches the brain tissue during ischemia, there is not a sufficient flow to ensure that all cells are receiving the oxygen necessary to continue cellular life. This condition is called hypoxia (low oxygen). If hypoxia is sustained over a sufficient period of time, cellular death occurs, causing irreversible brain damage.

The important differences between a stroke and a TIA are the onset and duration of symptoms, as well as the severity of the damage. Persons with atherosclerosis actually have fat deposits along the interior walls of their blood vessels. These people are vulnerable to experiencing multiple TIAs. Many TIAs are small enough to be dismissed and ignored; others are truly unapparent, causing no symptoms. This is unfortunate because TIAs often serve as a warning of an impending full-scale stroke. Action and treatments could be implemented, if medical advice is sought early, to decrease the likelihood of a stroke. Repeated TIAs also contribute to dementia.

Dementia is not the normal path for the elderly, nor is it a sign of aging. Dementia is a sign of neurological chaos and

can be caused by diseases such as Alzheimer's disease or acquired immunodeficiency syndrome (AIDS). Although most elderly are not afflicted with dementia, nearly all have a slowing of reaction and response time. This slowing is believed to be associated with chemical changes within nerve cell membranes as aging occurs; slowing of reaction times is not necessarily indicative of the first steps on a path to dementia. In addition, forgetfulness may not be a sign of dementia, since it occurs at all ages. Forgetfulness is such a sign, however, if it is progressive and includes forgetting to dress or forgetting one's name or date of birth.

While it is incorrect to say that dementia is caused by aging, it is correct to say that dementia is age-related. It may first appear in a person any time between the late thirties and the mid-nineties, but it usually begins to appear in the late seventies. Patients with Alzheimer's disease are believed to account for about 60-70% percent of all cases of dementia. Other diseases cause dementia, including an autosomal-dominant genetic disease called Huntington's disease. Huntington's disease manifests itself with a distinct chorea, or dance, of the body that is neither solicited nor controlled. This genetic disease is particularly cruel in that its symptoms appear in midlife, often after the adult has had offspring and passed on the gene. The disease continues to alter the intellect and personality of the afflicted one and progresses to the point of complete debilitation of the body and mind.

A seizure occurs when a collection of neurons misfires, sending nerve impulses that are neither solicited nor controllable. In the everyday use of the term, seizure describes a condition of epilepsy or convulsion. Medically speaking, a seizure is a sign of an underlying problem within the gray matter of the brain; it is the most common neurological disorder. Epilepsy is a term used to describe a condition of repeated seizures, while convulsion is a term generally applied to describe an isolated seizure. A seizure may occur as a consequence of extreme fever or a violent blow to the head. Seizures are also associated with metabolic disorders, such as hypoglycemia (low blood sugar); trauma causing a loss of blood or oxygen to a region, such as in a newborn after a traumatic birth; toxins, as seen in drug abuse or withdrawal; or bacterial or viral encephalitis or meningitis. In addition, about one-third of those persons who survive a gunshot wound to the head will experience seizures afterward. In closed head trauma, which can occur in a sporting or automobile accident, there is a 5 percent chance of post trauma seizures.

Loss of consciousness can be caused by a violent impact to the head, a lack of oxygen or blood flow to the head, a metabolic imbalance, or the presence of a toxin such as alcohol. Usually, this is a transient event, but it may become a condition that could last weeks or months. When this happens, a person is said to be in a coma initially, then after approximately 30 days the person is classified as being in a persistent vegetative state. A person in a persistent vegetative state exists in a nonresponsive state and may be assessed for brain death. Brain death is a legally defined term which means that no electrical activity in the brain is seen on an electroencephalogram (EEG). Thus some comatose patients may be determined to be brain-dead, particularly if the condition is deemed irreversible.

Brain defects are not common, but they do occur. One particularly tragic defect is the absence of a brain in a newborn, called anencephaly. Death usually occurs within a few hours of birth. Although anencephaly is rare and generally associated with a genetic factor, there have been cases in population clusters, such as one in the Rio Grande area of south Texas, suggesting that an environmental factor may contribute to these defects.

Another defect that may appear in newborns or in an infant's first months of life is hydrocephalus. Although the descriptive term "water on the brain" is often used, the condition does not involve a collection of water in the cranium; rather, it involves an accumulation of cerebrospinal fluid (CSF). CSF is the fluid that insulates the brain and allows it to "float" under the bony cranial encasement. As the ventricles, or spaces, in the brain fill with CSF, bulging occurs and pressure builds to the point of compressing the surrounding brain tissue. This can be very painful and is fatal if untreated. Hydrocephalus can be caused by an overproduction of CSF or a blockage of the CSF drainage from the ventricles of the brain. The symptoms often include a protrusion or abnormal shape of the cranium. In newborns, the skull bones have not yet sutured (fused) to one another, so the soft bones are pushed apart, causing unusual head shapes. This is a warning sign. Another sign is observed if a newborn's head has a circumference greater than 35.5 centimeters (14 inches); if that is the case, the newborn must be immediately checked for hydrocephalus. Adolescents and adults may also experience hydrocephalus. This can be a response to head trauma, infection, or the overproduction of CSF. The symptoms include lethargy, headache, dullness, blurred vision, nausea, and vomiting.

Treatment and Therapy

TIAs can progress to strokes. In fact, about 30 percent of those diagnosed with TIA will have a major stroke within the subsequent four years. One of the most prevalent causes of TIAs is hypertension. Hypertension is known as the "silent killer" because many persons with this problem ignore the subtle symptoms of fatigue, headache, and general malaise. Hypertension is also known as a good predictor of major strokes if left untreated. Thus, hypertensive persons need to be diagnosed as such in order to control their blood pressure. This allows them to avoid or delay either a major stroke or multiple TIAs. Management for hypertensive blood pressure may include taking diuretics and hypotensive drugs (to lower the blood pressure). If taken diligently, these drugs offer longevity and quality of life to the sufferer. Aside from hypertension, TIAs may be induced in some metabolic disorders, which should be corrected if possible, or by constricted blood vessels. Sometimes, surgery on such vessels can stop the ischemic attacks and prevent or delay the onset of a stroke.

Although TIAs lead to strokes, strokes are not necessarily preceded by a TIA. Nearly 90 percent of all major

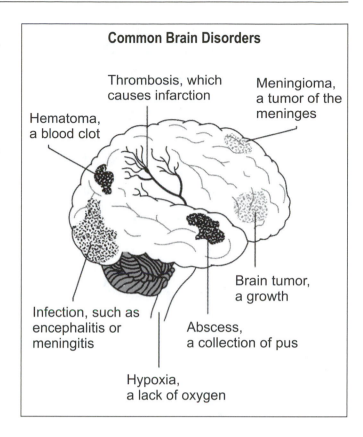

Common Brain Disorders

Hematoma, a blood clot

Thrombosis, which causes infarction

Meningioma, a tumor of the meninges

Brain tumor, a growth

Infection, such as encephalitis or meningitis

Abscess, a collection of pus

Hypoxia, a lack of oxygen

strokes occur without warning. Sadly, hypertension is the main contributor to this number. Measures can be taken to avoid strokes. This includes maintaining cardiovascular health by exercising, not smoking, and managing hypertension, diabetes mellitus, or other problems that may place stresses on the body's chemical balance.

Dementia is so poorly understood in terms of causes that a rational probe of drug therapy or a cure is nearly impossible. The drugs most often used in dementia treatment, the ergoloid mesylates, are used to manage the symptoms; namely, the confused mind. These drugs, however, do not stop or prevent the unexplained cellular degeneration associated with dementia. It is interesting to note that a tiny subgroup within those persons suffering from Alzheimer's disease have greatly improved in mental status with the drug tacrine. It is unfortunate that all patients are not responsive to this drug-a fact which suggests that Alzheimer's disease is a complex condition.

Seizures are treated pharmacologically according to type. Carbamazepine, phenobarbital, phenytoin, and valproate are some of the drugs available to treat seizure disorders. Barbiturates may also be used in certain cases. Most of these drugs are highly effective when taken as prescribed, and patient noncompliance is the main cause of drug failure. Sometimes, two drugs are combined in therapy. It should be mentioned that pregnant women with epilepsy are urged to continue taking anti-epilepsy drugs during pregnancy since a maternal seizure may be more damaging to the fetus than the drug itself. Some forms of hydrocephalus can be corrected surgically by performing a CSF shunt from the cranium to the peritoneal (abdominal) region, where the fluid can be eliminated from the body as waste. This is not without risk, and the introduction of infection into the brain is a major concern.

Perspective and Prospects

The therapies in use for brain diseases and disorders have been derived from the practical experience of physicians, the laboratory research of scientists, and the hopes of multitudes of doctors, patients, families, and friends. Medical science has done much to improve the lives of those who suffer with seizures, to reduce the risk of strokes to the hypertensive person and those with TIAs, and is making great progress in treating certain kinds of dementia. Yet much remains to be done. While one can argue that much is known about the human brain, it would be erroneous to argue that the human brain is fully understood. Despite centuries of research, the brain, as it functions in health, remains largely a mystery. Since the healthy brain is yet to be understood, it is not surprising that the medical community struggles to determine what goes wrong in dementia, seizure, or mental illness or to discover drug therapies that can cross the blood-brain barrier. Thus, the human brain is the uncharted frontier in medicine. As technology improves to support researchers and medical practitioners in their pursuits of cures and treatments for brain diseases and disorders, one can only remain hopeful for the future ability to restore health to the damaged human brain. In April 2013, US president Barack Obama announced the launch of the Brain Research through Advancing Innovative Neurotechnologies (BRAIN) Initiative, a research initiative tasked with finding new ways to prevent, treat, and cure brain disorders and injuries. The Defense Advanced Research Projects Agency, National Institutes of Health, and National Science Foundation will fund approximately $100 million in research starting in fiscal year 2014.

—*Mary C. Fields, MD;*
updated by Bryan C. Auday, PhD

See also: Abscess drainage; Abscesses; Alzheimer's disease; Amnesia; Aphasia and dysphasia; Brain; Brain damage; Brain tumors; Cerebral palsy; Chiari malformations; Chronic wasting disease (CWD); Cluster headaches; Concussion; Creutzfeldt-Jakob disease (CJD); Dementias; Dyslexia; Embolism; Encephalitis; Epilepsy; Frontotemporal dementia (FTD); Guillain-Barré syndrome; Hallucinations; Headaches; Hemiplegia; Huntington's disease; Hydrocephalus; Intraventricular hemorrhage; Lead poisoning; Learning disabilities; Leukodystrophy; Memory loss; Meningitis; Migraine headaches; Motor neuron diseases; Multiple sclerosis; Nervous system; Neuralgia, neuritis, and neuropathy; Neuroimaging; Neurology; Neurology; Neurorehabilitation; Neurosurgery; Numbness and tingling; Palsy; Paralysis; Parkinson's disease; pediatric; Pick's disease; Seizures; Shock therapy; Tics; Unconsciousness.

For Further Information:

American Medical Association. *American Medical AssociationFamily Medical Guide*. 4th rev. ed. Hoboken, N.J.: Wiley & Sons, 2004.

Bloom, Floyd E., M. Flint Beal, and David J. Kupfer, eds. *The Dana Guide to Brain Health*. New York: Dana, 2006.

Dana Foundation. *Dana Foundation*, 2013.

Lewis, Steven L. Ed. *NeurologicalDisorders Due to Systemic Disease*. Oxford: Wiley-Blackwell, 2013.

Office of the Press Secretary. "Fact Sheet: BRAIN Initiative." *White House*, Apr. 2, 2013.

Weiner, William J., Christopher G. Goetz, Robert K. Shin, Steven L. Lewis. Eds. *Neurologyfor Non-neurologists*. 6th ed. New York: Lippincott Williams & Wilkins, 2010.

Woolsey, Thomas A., Joseph Hanaway, and Mokhtar Gado. *Brain Atlas: A Visual Guide to the Human Central Nervous System*. 3d ed. Hoboken, N.J.: Wiley, 2008.

Brain tumors

Disease/Disorder

Anatomy or system affected: Brain, head, nervous system, spine

Specialties and related fields: General surgery, neurology, oncology, radiology

Definition: An abnormal growth in or on the brain.

Key terms:

glioma: a cancer arising from and in brain substance

hydrocephalus: excessive cerebrospinal fluid within the cranial cavity; commonly called water on the brain

metastasis: the spread of cancer cells

Causes and Symptoms

The earliest symptom of a brain tumor may be a persistent headache, although this symptom does not necessarily stem from a brain tumor. Nevertheless, when headaches occur regularly, it is essential that the cause be investigated as early as possible and a diagnosis made.

As brain tumors continue to grow and crowd the brain, other symptoms become evident. Even though such tumors are frequently benign, they can become disabling. As brain tissue and the nerve tracks inside the skull are compressed by the incursion that such tumors make on them, patients may suffer muscle weakness, dizziness, loss of vision, reduction of hearing, nausea, speech problems, emotional problems, disorientation, and sometimes seizures.

Brain tumors can, but rarely, enhance mental functioning. Nearly always, they cause impairment across a range of mental aptitudes. Memory loss is common, as are unexplained mood swings. A tumor that grows so that it restricts the flow of cerebrospinal fluid will cause an additional condition, hydrocephalus. Hydrocephalus, also known as "water on the brain," is when the cerebrospinal fluid flows into brain tissue itself. This swelling quickly becomes painful and is lethal if not reduced.

The incidence of brain tumors is small, representing about 1.3 percent of cancers diagnosed in the United States in a given year. Two age groups are at greater risk than the general population. Adult males between fifty-five and sixty-five years of age seem to be vulnerable to primary brain tumors, and children between three and twelve years of age also have a higher incidence of this condition.

The causes of brain tumors have not been fully determined. It has been noted that genetic factors may play a role in the development of such tumors in young people, particularly those with a parent who has had colon cancer or cancer of the salivary glands or nervous system. Children exposed to high energy radiation applied to the head in the treatment of leukemia or who develop neck or facial cancers suffer an increased risk of developing brain tumors.

Among adults, those whose work exposes them to vinyl

chloride have a high incidence of brain tumors, as do those whose work involves exposure to lead in such industries as mining, printing, and chemical industries. Those who suffer from epilepsy are at higher risk of developing gliomas, tumors arising from brain substance, some 60 percent of which are malignant. The risk seems less in people whose diets include little fat and refined sugar and plentiful fresh fruits and vegetables.

Many brain tumors develop from tissues within the skull, but others result from the metastasis, or spread of cancer cells from malignancies elsewhere in the body, often the lungs or breasts. Of the 170,000 Americans who develop lung cancer annually, about 55,000 will also develop brain tumors. Adults who have had organ transplants are also at increased risk.

Treatment and Therapy

Where a brain tumor-malignant or benign-exists, the preferred treatment is surgical removal by opening the skull. Such delicate surgery is performed by a neuro-oncological surgeon who understands the brain's contours and their relationship to the nervous system and spinal cord.

Such diagnostic tools as computed tomography (CT) scanning and magnetic resonance imaging (MRI) can determine the extent of a brain tumor before a decision is made about how to treat the condition. Sometimes surgery is not indicated because the tumor is embedded in vital areas of the brain that would be irreparably damaged by removal.

In such cases, radiation may be used initially to shrink the tumor, sometimes to the point that eventually it can be removed surgically. In other cases, it may be possible to remove part of the tumor, thereby releasing the pressure that it exerts on the brain. Partial removal is usually followed by a course of radiation and/or chemotherapy, generally with the expectation that additional surgical removal will occur if the tumor decreases in size.

Corticosteroids have in some cases succeeded in controlling the swelling of tumors so that pressure on the brain is reduced and symptoms are mitigated.

Perspective and Prospects

In the United States, brain tumors do not occur frequently. The American Cancer Society estimates that in 2013 there will be about twenty-three thousand new cases of primary brain and other nervous system cancers, and about fourteen thousand deaths related to such cancers. The life of one child in every three thousand in the population ends before age ten because of a primary brain tumor. Some fifteen hundred children are diagnosed every year with brain tumors, most located in the cerebellum, the midbrain, or the optic nerve.

There has been an increase in primary brain tumors among the elderly since 1980, while the percentage of resulting deaths has decreased. In viewing such statistics, one must remember that with advances in medical technology, more people are achieving old age and are developing diseases when, fifty years ago, they would not have still been living.

Advances in cell research and in the development of drugs that control and, in some cases, eliminate specific cancer cells provide encouragement that medical progress is being made consistently. Neuro-oncological surgery has undergone great advances and will likely substantially reduce the threat of human error as sophisticated robotic surgical procedures are developed. Although cancer is still a scourge, recent medical research offers realistic hope of controlling it.

—*R. Baird Shuman, Ph.D.*

See also: Brain; Brain disorders; Cancer; Chemotherapy; Head and neck disorders; Headaches; Hydrocephalus; Imaging and radiology; Malignancy and metastasis; Neuroimaging; Neurology; Neurology, pediatric; Neurosurgery; Oncology; Plastic surgery; Radiation therapy; Tumor removal; Tumors.

For Further Information:

American Cancer Society. *Cancer Facts & Figures 2013*. Atlanta, Ga.: American Cancer Society, 2013.

Jasmin, Luc. "Brain tumor-Primary-Adults." *MedlinePlus*, Nov. 2, 2012.

Register, Cheri. *The Chronic Illness Experience: Embracing the Imperfect Life*. City Center, Minn.: Hazelden, 1999.

Roloff, Tricia Ann. *Navigating Through a Strange Land: A Book for Brain Tumor Patients and Their Families*. 2d ed. Minneapolis, Minn.: Fairview, 2001.

Shiminski-Maher, Tania, Patsy Cullen, and Maria Sansalone. *Childhood Brain and Spinal Cord Tumors: A Guide for Families, Friends, and Caregivers*. Sebastopol, Calif.: O'Reilly, 2002.

Stark-Vance, Virginia, and M. L. Dubay. *One Hundred Questions and Answers About Brain Tumors*. 2d ed. Sudbury, Mass.: Jones, 2011.

Wood, Debra. "Brain Tumor and Brain Cancer-Adult." *Health Library*, Jan. 18, 2013.

Zeltzer, Paul M. *Brain Tumors: Leaving the Garden of Eden*. Encino, Calif.: Shilysca, 2004.

Breast biopsy

Procedure

Anatomy or system affected: Breasts (female)

Specialties and related fields: General surgery, gynecology

Definition: The surgical removal of a lump or tissue from the breast to determine whether it is malignant.

Indications and Procedures

Among women, breast cancer is the most common malignancy. (While men can have breast cancer, such cases are relatively rare.) Women have learned the importance of regular clinical breast examinations and the need to report any suspicious lumps and other breast changes they find to a physician. Mammography (an x-ray of the breasts) is used as a breast cancer screening tool, and suspicious findings on a mammogram are the most common indication for biopsy. A woman finding a suspicious lump often leads to biopsy as well. Some physicians use breast ultrasound to determine whether biopsy is needed.

Many techniques are used to conduct a breast biopsy. The physician can use a thin needle and syringe to collect cells from suspicious areas (fine needle aspiration). Often, draining a cyst (a fluid-filled sac) is the only treatment needed. Surgeons can conduct a core needle biopsy, using a needle with a cutting edge to cut out a small piece of tissue. Ultrasound, magnetic resonance imaging (MRI), or mammography equipment may be used during a core needle biopsy to help the clinician locate the suspicious tissue. Small lumps are often removed in an excisional biopsy (lumpectomy). When lumps are larger, the surgeon may do an incisional biopsy to remove part of the lump for further examination. When no lump is present but suspicious tissue has been revealed by mammography, the surgeon can use the x-ray to place small needles in order to remove tissue samples. A vacuum device is used in some biopsies to assist with the collection of multiple samples. Following a breast biopsy, a patient may experience bleeding, bruising, or localized pain. Infections can also occur.

Pathologists examine the lump, tissue, or cells that are removed from the breast to determine whether cancer is present. If cancer is found, the patient has several treatment options, including removal of part or all of the breast, lumpectomy with radiation therapy, chemotherapy, and hormone therapy. If cancer is not found or biopsy results are inconclusive, patients are typically encouraged to have a repeat imaging test within six to twelve months of the biopsy.

—*Russell Williams, M.S.W.*

See also: Biopsy; Breast cancer; Breast disorders; Breast surgery; Breasts, female; Cancer; Cyst removal; Cysts; Gynecology; Mammography; Mastectomy and lumpectomy; Mastitis; Oncology; Pathology; Plastic surgery; Tumor removal; Tumors; Women's health.

For Further Information:

"Breast Biopsy." *Mayo Foundation for Medical Education and Research*, August 9, 2011.

"Breast Cancer: Prevention and Control." *World Health Organization*, 2013.

"Breast Needle Biopsy." *Health Library*, January 22, 2013.

Carter, Darryl. *Interpretation of Breast Biopsies*. 4th ed. Philadelphia: Lippincott Williams & Wilkins, 2003.

DeVita, Vincent, Jr., Samuel Hellman, and Steven A. Rosenberg, eds. *Cancer: Principles and Practice of Oncology*. 7th ed. Philadelphia: Lippincott Williams & Wilkins, 2005.

Elk, Ronit, and Monica Marrow. *Breast Cancer for Dummies*. New York: Wiley, 2003.

Health News. "Longer Wait for Mammogram After Benign Breast Biopsy May Be Warranted." *HealthDay*, May 2, 2013.

Mulholland, Michael W., et al., eds. *Greenfield's Surgery: Scientific Principles and Practice*. 4th ed. Philadelphia: Lippincott Williams & Wilkins, 2006.

Sloane, John P. *Biopsy Pathology of the Breast*. 2d ed. New York: Oxford University Press, 2001.

Sloane, Michael P., and Catherine Beckman. "Methods of Biopsy." In *Illustrative Handbook of General Surgery*, edited by Herbert Chen. London: Springer-Verlag, 2010.

U.S. Department of Health and Human Services, Public Health Service, and National Institutes of Health. *Breast Biopsy: What You Should Know*. Bethesda, Md.: Author, 1990.

Breast cancer

Disease/Disorder

Anatomy or system affected: Breasts, cells, glands, lymphatic system

Specialties and related fields: General surgery, genetics, gynecology, histology, oncology, pathology, preventive medicine, radiology

Definition: A general term for a group of solid tumor malignancies arising in the tissues of the breast.

Key terms:

carcinoma: a solid tumor malignancy occurring in cells of the epithelium or tissues surrounding the major organ systems of the body

metastasis: the unique property of cancer cells that permits them to spread to multiple sites within the body

mutation: a change in gene structure that disrupts the normal functions of the encoded protein

Causes and Symptoms

Breast cancer is the most common malignancy in women (besides skin cancer) and the second leading cause of cancer deaths in women (behind lung cancer). More than 200,000 new cases are diagnosed each year in the United States alone, and approximately 40,000 deaths occur yearly as a consequence of this disease. A diagnosis of breast cancer may strike a profound sense of fear in a patient, but this fear can be alleviated somewhat through a better understanding of its causes and the treatment options and preventive strategies that show promise in countering this disease.

To understand breast cancer, it is first necessary to know the anatomy and structures that constitute the breast tissue from which cancer arises. Breast tissue consists of fatty tissue and the functional tissue of the breast: the lobes and ducts that are involved in the production and secretion of milk. The arrangement of the lobes and ducts of the breast resembles the spokes of a wheel around the nipple area. Inside each lobe are multiple lobules in which the milk is produced. The milk then travels down the ducts and is released through the nipple. Most important, the growth and development of the breast tissue is under hormonal control and begins at the time of puberty. The sex hormones progesterone and estrogen, produced by the ovaries, are largely responsible for the development of breast tissue.

This information is important to an understanding of how cancer arises in the breast. The majority of breast cancers occur in the ductal tissue (80 percent), and most of the remaining breast cancers originate in the lobular tissue (10 to 15 percent). Moreover, many cancers are hormonally responsive, meaning that the sustained growth of the abnormal tissue is stimulated by the presence of the female sex hormones. Cells of the breast may undergo growth changes during the process of tissue renewal and differentiation that ultimately may give rise to cancer.

Thus, in many ways tumor formation in the breast may reflect aspects of the normal proliferation of newly forming ductal or lobular cells, including hormonal sensitivity. In breast cancer, however, the process goes awry to produce abnormal cells with proliferative and invasive properties that may become life-threatening. Thus, to understand how breast cancer arises it is necessary to understand the developmental pathways of the tissue and its responses to the hormones and growth factors that regulate tissue development.

The nature of the cellular abnormalities responsible for the development of breast cancer has been the object of intense research for many years. Although the process by which malignant tumors of the breast develop remains unclear, scientists have learned a great deal about the profound cellular transformation that results in breast cancer. Tumors originate in the individual cells within the breast tissue that begin to proliferate abnormally as a direct result of genetic changes within the breast cells and/or in response to abnormal proliferative stimuli, such as hormones or other growth factors in the local environment of the breast.

Approximately 5 to 10 percent of women who develop breast cancer have mutations in genes that are inherited and predispose them to develop this disease. The first gene to be identified was *BRCA1*. Carriers of mutations in this gene have a markedly increased risk of developing breast cancer or ovarian cancer during their lifetime. Inherited mutations in a second gene, *BRCA2*, also produce significantly greater risks for the development of this disease. Mutations in *BRCA1* and *BRCA2* appear to promote the development of cancer as a result of their growth-promoting effects on breast tissue.

In the vast majority of women, however, breast cancer develops in the absence of any known predisposing genetic factor. The original lesion in those cases may involve a spontaneous mutation that alters the cells' proliferative capacity and/or sensitivity to hormonally induced signals. For patients without a family history (approximately 90 percent of women), a number of risk factors have been identified. The disease is linked to advancing age, with 77 percent of cases occurring in women over age fifty. Additional factors that may increase the risk of developing breast cancer are first menstruation before age twelve, first childbirth after age thirty-five, and menopause after age fifty-five. These risk factors are linked to the exposure of breast tissue to the circulating reproductive hormones estrogen and progesterone. In fact, breast cancers can generally be divided into two groups depending on whether they display sensitivity to hormonal stimulation of tumor cell growth.

To understand further this process of malignant cell transformation, it is necessary to follow the fate of a cell along the path of malignancy. Cancer begins at the level of individual cells within a tissue that proliferates abnormally

---

Information on Breast Cancer

Causes: Hormonal, genetic, environmental, and lifestyle factors
Symptoms: Tumor, which may or may not be palpable
Duration: Chronic
Treatments: Surgical removal of tumor and sometimes surrounding tissues and structures, radiation, chemotherapy (selective estrogen receptor modulators, aromatase inhibitors, monoclonal antibodies, etc.)

---

as a direct result of genetic changes and/or in response to abnormal proliferative stimuli. Abnormal cells arise in the ductal tissue of the breast in ductal carcinoma in situ (DCIS). This condition may progress to invasive infiltrating ductal carcinoma if the tumor breaks through the lining of the milk ducts and invades the fatty tissue of the breast. In the normal process of development during puberty, the ductal tissue develops in response to the hormone estrogen that is produced by the ovaries. Similarly, the growth of lobular tissue in the breast is stimulated by the hormone progesterone. Tumors that arise in this tissue are called lobular carcinoma in situ (LCIS). This type of cancer begins in the lobules that produce milk and may progress to infiltrating invasive lobular carcinoma.

Cells of the breast may undergo genetic changes during the process of development or tissue renewal that ultimately give rise to cancer. Breast cancer may take years to develop, silently progressing from a small group of abnormal cells that are no longer responsive to the "rules" governing normal cell cycle proliferation. Over a long period, these cells may accumulate added mutations that render them even more capable of unrestricted proliferation. Target genes that frequently appear to be involved in this process include members of the epidermal growth factor receptor (EGFR) family and the estrogen receptor (ER).

By the time that a tumor is palpable and can be detected as a lump by breast self-examination, the tumor may be defined as malignant based on the results of a number of diagnostic procedures. The vast majority of breast cell abnormalities are benign, meaning that the abnormal tissue is localized in the breast and will not spread further. For example, fluid-filled cysts represent benign breast lesions, as do the cysts characteristic of fibrocystic breast disease. Mammography, a procedure involving radiography of the soft tissue of the breast, and ultrasonography, which uses sound waves to explore tissue structure, are common diagnostic tests useful in detecting the presence of small tumors in the breast and distinguishing between benign and malignant lesions. The definitive test for malignancy is the microscopic examination of affected breast tissue. This examination requires a biopsy, a procedure that involves the removal of a small amount of tissue from the breast.

Cells comprising a benign tumor generally appear very similar in morphology and appearance to normal cells of the same tissue type. In contrast, malignant cells may deviate significantly in structure, morphology, and staining properties, to the extent that the tissue of origin may not

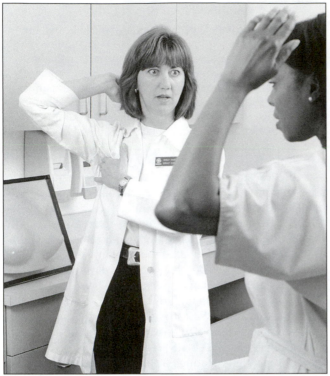

A doctor shows a woman how to perform a breast self-examination. Combined with periodic mammograms, such screening procedures can catch many cases of breast cancer. (PhotoDisc)

even be identifiable in tumors designated "high grade."

At the time of diagnosis, a malignant tumor may be restricted to its site of origin, defined as a carcinoma in situ, or may have spread within the breast or possibly to other tissues and organs of the body, such as the lungs or bones, by a process termed metastasis. Metastasis occurs when tumor cells travel first to the local lymph nodes in the area of the breast and then are disseminated to other sites within the body, where secondary tumors may develop. The diagnosis of metastatic tumor spread, made through lymph node analysis, is of concern since breast cancer is significantly more difficult to treat once it has spread to other sites within the body.

Treatment and Therapy

The hallmarks of malignancy-tumor size, appearance, local invasiveness, and lymph node involvement as evidence of possible metastasis-are all critical components of treatment recommendations and long-term prognosis. Although much research has been directed toward a more molecular diagnostic and therapeutic approach to breast cancer, few genetic lesions have been definitively linked to the occurrence of this disease.

Surgical removal of the tumor is the primary treatment for breast cancer. For small, localized tumors that show no evidence of spread within the tissue or lymph node involvement, simple removal of the tumor and surrounding tissues by a procedure termed lumpectomy is the general treatment choice. Even for more advanced breast malignancies, radical mastectomy, a procedure that involves complete removal of the breast, associated lymph nodes, and underlying chest muscles, is seldom performed any longer, since the operation causes disfigurement and similar results can usually be obtained using less extensive surgery. For example, for tumors that have spread within the breast, a portion of the breast may be removed without significant disfigurement. In cases where complete breast removal is required for tumor resection, simultaneous breast reconstruction often accompanies the surgical procedure in order to reduce the physical and psychological effects of mastectomy.

If any evidence exists that a cancer has spread, either locally within the breast tissue or lymph nodes or systemically to other sites within the body, then radiation and chemotherapy may be useful adjuvants to surgical removal of the tumor. Localized treatment involves the use of external beam high-energy radiation that is directed locally to the target tissue to avoid damaging other organs and tissues in the body. The principle underlying the use of radiation to treat cancer involves the fact that high-energy ionizing radiation damages deoxyribonucleic acid (DNA) and destroys dividing cells within the body.

Similarly, conventional chemotherapy involves the use of drugs that interfere with the process of DNA duplication or replication in dividing cells by producing changes in the structure or integrity of the DNA molecule. Unlike radiation, chemotherapy is a systemic form of cancer treatment that is directed at metastatic tumors and cancer cells that may have spread to various sites within the body. Many chemotherapeutic drugs have been used in the treatment of breast cancer. Some of the more commonly used are cyclophosphamide, methotrexate, 5-fluorouracil, and cisplatin. These drugs may be administered intravenously, either individually or in combinations, over a period of weeks to months in an attempt to destroy any remaining cancer cells following surgery or radiation. Another chemotherapeutic drug that has been used successfully to treat breast cancer is paclitaxel, better known as Taxol, a drug originally obtained from the Pacific yew tree that blocks the process of cell division. Taxol targets a specific stage in the cell division cycle involving the separation of chromosomes by threadlike fibers called microtubules in newly forming cells. Taxol binds to the microtubules, thereby arresting the cell division process.

Both radiation and chemotherapy may produce significant side effects, such as anemia, hair loss, nausea and vomiting, fatigue, weight loss, and mouth sores. These side effects occur because radiation and chemotherapeutic drugs target not only cancer cells but also all cells within the body that are actively dividing.

In many patients, chemotherapy and radiation may block the progress of disease within the body, resulting in long-term survival. However, each year many women continue to die of breast cancer despite aggressive treatment. The reasons that cancer treatments fail are as mysterious as the disease process itself. Tumor cells may not respond to chemotherapy and radiation even at very high doses as a result of the phenomenon of drug resistance, which is characteristic of many cancers, especially at advanced stages. For example, very high dose chemotherapy, which removes cells of the immune system, followed by stem cell replacement therapy has been shown to have negligible benefits in patients with advanced metastatic disease. Though the molecular basis of drug resistance remains unclear, mutations in certain genes, such as the multidrug resistance gene 1 (*MDR1*), have been identified. Moreover, the complexities of tumor structure and behavior may overwhelm the potential cytotoxic (cell-killing) effects of drugs commonly used to treat this disease.

New treatments for breast cancer have been developed as a consequence of an increased understanding of the biology of breast cancer neoplasms. For example, a significant percentage of breast cancers have been shown to be hormonally responsive, meaning that their growth is stimulated by the female sex hormones estrogen or progesterone. These tumors are classified as estrogen-responsive (ER) or progesterone-responsive (PR). A class of drugs that targets the estrogen receptor in ER-positive breast cancers, called selective estrogen receptor modulators (SERMs), has shown great clinical promise in the treatment of breast cancer as well as in preventing recurrences of the disease.

Tamoxifen is the oldest and most prominent member of this group; this drug specifically targets the estrogen receptor in breast tissue and blocks the growth-promoting effects of estrogen in estrogen-sensitive breast cancers. Tamoxifen has been used therapeutically to treat metastatic breast disease and also to prevent breast cancer recurrences, with significant success. A number of clinical studies have shown that patients receiving this drug have dramatically lower recurrence and mortality rates than patients who do not receive this drug. For example, a major study conducted in 1998 by the National Cancer Institute demonstrated a 50 percent reduction in breast cancer occurrence in high-risk women treated with tamoxifen. Moreover, the study showed that this drug also arrested the progression of DCIS and LCIS to invasive disease. These clinical trials have shown significant benefits from tamoxifen taken over periods of up to five years to prevent the recurrence of breast cancer in high-risk patients. It is not surprising, however, that this drug is ineffective against breast cancers that are not estrogen-responsive. Tamoxifen has also been used in combined chemotherapy with conventional chemotherapeutic drugs such as cyclophosphamide, methotrexate, and 5-fluorouracil, with varying results.

Unfortunately, tamoxifen does have significant side effects, including an increased risk of developing uterine

---

In the News:
Breast Cancer Treatments

According to the National Cancer Institute, the results of a twenty-year follow-up to the British Columbia randomized radiation trial indicated that when radiation therapy is used in addition to chemotherapy after surgery, breast cancer survival rates increase by nearly one-third. Patients involved in this study were women who had lymph node involvement, prompting the American Cancer Society to state that the use of radiation to the breast and the lymph nodes after surgery (mastectomy or lumpectomy) should improve the survival rates of breast cancer patients who either had lymph node involvement or a tumor larger than five centimeters.

Radiation therapy, which today exists in many different forms, typically is not begun until about a month after surgery in order to allow the tissue to heal. The most common type of radiation used to treat breast cancer is external beam radiation. With this approach, the entire breast (and chest wall) receives radiation. A newer technique undergoing clinical trials is partial breast irradiation. With this technique, the patient receives radiation to only part of the breast and for a shorter period of time (five days). Results from this study are eagerly awaited.

The alternative to external radiation therapy is brachytherapy or internal (interstitial) radiation. With this technique, radioactive isotopes are implanted in the breast tissue next to the cancer site. Another method of internal radiation used following lumpectomy is mammosite. This involves the insertion of a balloon filled with saltwater solution into the lumpectomy space. Over a period of five days, a radioactive material is inserted and removed twice a day and then treatment is terminated. Additional evaluation of internal radiation is ongoing. Newer radiation techniques also minimize side effects. Since radiation is avoided with these techniques, no increase in heart disease is seen. Remaining side effects are fatigue, decreased sensation in the radiated tissue, and dermatological problems in the treated area.

Just as chemotherapy paired with radiation has led to increased survival, so have two new chemotherapy techniques. "Dose dense" chemotherapy involves chemotherapy administered with a reduced time period between successive doses. Patients can tolerate this dose-dense schedule because of a new drug, filgrastin, which helps prevent the decrease in white blood cells (neutropenia) that usually accompanies chemotherapy. A second technique, involving the use of Herceptin (a genetically engineered drug) along with individual chemotherapy to advanced breast cancer patients, also leads to increased survival.

—Robin Kamienny Montvilo, R.N., Ph.D.

---

cancer, since the drug stimulates the growth of ER-positive endometrial cells in the uterus. For this reason, patients taking this drug should be monitored carefully by a physician. Tamoxifen use has also been linked to vascular disease, including blood clots and strokes in some patients.

Another SERM called raloxifene hydrochloride, marketed under the name Evista, is an antiestrogen that has also shown significant clinical benefit, with results similar to those obtained using tamoxifen. For example, clinical trials have indicated that raloxifene use decreases the risk of breast cancer in high-risk postmenopausal women by as much as 70 percent. An important difference between these two drugs, however, is that raloxifene blocks estrogen receptors in both the breast and the uterus, thereby decreasing the risk of developing uterine cancer for patients taking this drug.

A newer class of antiestrogens are the aromatase inhibitors (AI). These drugs block the formation of estrogen within the body and are especially beneficial to older, postmenopausal women. This class of drugs works by blocking the conversion, or aromatization, of androgens produced by the adrenal glands to estrogen. This reaction is carried out by enzymes called aromatases and occurs in fatty tissues throughout the body, significantly contributing to estrogen production in postmenopausal women. These aromatase inhibitors, marketed under the names Arimidex and Femara, have shown clinical promise in the treatment of postmenopausal women with advanced breast cancer. However, clinical studies on the combined use of AIs with SERMs such as tamoxifen have shown no significant clinical benefit so far over the use of these drugs individually.

As a means of reducing the potential side effects associated with tamoxifen, clinical studies published since 2002 have demonstrated the increased effectiveness of adjuvant chemotherapy in treating certain forms of breast cancer in postmenopausal women. For example, anastrozole (Arimidex), an aromatase inhibitor, when used in conjuction with tamoxifen during long-term treatment, produced fewer side effects and was as effective in reducing metastasis.

In addition to hormone therapy, drugs that target abnormal genes in breast cancer cells have also been used successfully to treat breast cancer and to prevent its recurrence. For example, approximately 25 percent of breast cancer patients show overexpression of the *HER2/neu* gene product as a consequence of genetic rearrangements that increase the number of copies of this gene by a process called gene amplification in the tumor cells. The *HER2/neu* gene is a member of a family of genes that encode cell surface receptors for epidermal growth factor, a growth-promoting protein that stimulates cell cycle proliferation. The overexpression of the *HER2/neu* receptor in breast cancer cells therefore renders these cells inordinately sensitive to growth factor stimulation of cell division, which directly contributes to the growth of the malignant breast tissue. The drug trastuzumab, better known as Herceptin, is a humanized monoclonal antibody that specifically targets and binds to the *HER2/neu* receptor, thereby blocking its interaction with epidermal growth factor and the resulting stimulation of cell proliferation. Herceptin has shown positive clinical benefit in patients with *HER2/neu*-positive tumors, both in the treatment phase and in long-term use in the prevention of breast cancer recurrence.

Perspective and Prospects

The ultimate goal of breast cancer research is prevention. To achieve this goal, it will be necessary to identify more clearly the risk factors that contribute to the development of this disease and to design preventive strategies for counteracting genetic changes and/or hormonal changes within the body that may ultimately give rise to malignant tumors of the breast tissue. Women with an inherited genetic predisposition to breast cancer, such as mutations in the *BRCA1* and *BRCA2* genes, would receive the greatest benefit from these preventive approaches. Some women who carry *BRCA1* or *BRCA2* mutations undergo preventive

bilateral mastectomy, as precancerous lesions that cannot be detected might exist.

Early detection methods aimed at identifying and removing precancerous breast lesions such as DCIS and LCIS represent an important preventive strategy whose benefits have not yet been fully realized. Currently, mammography and breast self-examination are the most common means of breast cancer detection. Although useful, these methods may fail to detect small tumors before they have become invasive. Ultrasonography and magnetic resonance imaging (MRI), used in conjunction with other detection methods, may improve the likelihood of detecting premalignant lesions and early-stage cancers. Better methods of breast cancer detection need to be developed, a goal that may become increasingly possible given the increased understanding of the molecular basis of breast cancer. Molecular methods may also be useful in the development of diagnostic tests that identify additional genetic predispositions to the development of breast cancer, so that aggressive preventive approaches can be taken in women identified as higher risk that may prevent the occurrence of this disease.

Clinical studies using hormone therapy approaches have shown that, under certain conditions, breast cancer can be prevented by drugs that target hormone and growth factor receptor signal pathways in tumor cells. These data provide further evidence in support of many epidemiological studies suggesting that the lifetime exposure of breast tissue to estrogen is associated with an increased risk of developing breast cancer. For this reason, women who take oral estrogen/progesterone in the form of oral contraceptives or hormone therapy need to be aware of potential risks associated with the use of these drugs. Many studies have shown that oral contraceptive use in women under age thirty-five who do not smoke does not appear to produce a significantly elevated risk of breast cancer or other complications. However, recent well-documented clinical data on hormone therapy in perimenopausal or postmenopausal women suggest that its use may contribute to a significantly elevated risk of aggressive breast cancers that are difficult to detect by mammography. In addition, it has been associated with side effects that may result in an increased risk of blood clots, strokes, and heart attacks. Despite these risks, there are clear benefits to using hormone therapy. Thus, it should be used under the careful supervision of a physician.

Many studies have been carried out to assess the role of diet in breast cancer prevention. For example, epidemiological studies have shown repeatedly that Japanese women have a far lower incidence of breast cancer than do American women. This decreased incidence in Japanese women has been attributed in part to dietary differences in the amount of fat consumption, as well as to the extensive use of soy products in Japanese cooking. Soy contains an estrogen receptor binding substance called genistein. It is believed that the genistein in soy binds to estrogen receptors to block their binding to the growth-promoting hormone estrogen. However, studies have shown mixed results as to whether an increase in one's soy intake will help lower one's risk of breast cancer or increase the risk of breast cancer recurrence. The role of diet in the prevention of breast cancer is unclear, as study results range from reduced risk associated with low-fat diets to no effects at all. Some of the confusion may be the result of the complexity of breast cancer. Low-fat, high-fiber (vegetarian) diets have been demonstrated to reduce the levels of estrogen and other reproductive hormones, and it may be in this manner that the risk of certain forms of cancer is reduced.

Although the goal of eliminating breast cancer still remains elusive, those who conduct breast cancer research and those whose lives have been touched by this disease may find it comforting to realize that so much progress has been made in understanding the cellular and molecular basis of this disease.

—Sarah Crawford, Ph.D.;
updated by Richard Adler, Ph.D.

See also: Breast biopsy; Breast disorders; Breast surgery; Breasts, female; Cancer; Chemotherapy; Fibrocystic breast condition; Gynecology; Hormone therapy; Malignancy and metastasis; Mammography; Mastectomy and lumpectomy; Oncology; Radiation therapy; Women's health.

For Further Information:
Arnot, Bob. *Breast Cancer Prevention Diet*. Boston: Little, Brown, 1999.
"Breast Cancer." *American Cancer Society*, Feb. 26, 2013.
"Breast Cancer." *Centers for Disease Control and Prevention*, Mar. 25, 2013.
"Breast Cancer." *MedlinePlus*, May 3, 2013.
"Breast Cancer Treatment." *National Cancer Institute*, Apr. 5, 2013.
Canfield, Jack, et al. *Chicken Soup for the Soul-Healthy Living Series: Breast Cancer*. Deerfield Beach, Fla.: Health Communications, 2005.
LaRusso, Laurie, and Mohei Abouzied. "Breast Cancer." *Health Library*, Jan. 21, 2013.
Link, John. *Breast Cancer Survival Manual*. Rev. 5th ed. New York: Henry Holt, 2012.
Love, Susan, and Karen Lindsey. *Dr. Susan Love's Breast Book*. Rev. 5th ed. Cambridge, Mass.: Da Capo Press, 2010.
Narod, Steven, and William Foulkes. "BRCA1 and BRCA2: 1994 and Beyond." *Nature Reviews/Cancer* 4 (September, 2004): 665-676.

Breast disorders

Disease/Disorder

Anatomy or system affected: Breasts, glands, lymphatic system

Specialties and related fields: Cytology, general surgery, gynecology, histology, neonatology

Definition: A variety of benign breast conditions, including fibrocystic disease and mastitis, which cause discomfort and anxiety and can make self-examination and diagnosis of cancer difficult.

Key terms:

biopsy: the removal of sample tissue for microscopic inspection and analysis by a pathologist

cyst: a fluid-filled, enclosed sac in the body

fine needle aspiration: a surgical procedure in which a thin, hollow needle is used to withdraw tissue from the body

necrosis: cell death, usually involving the rupture of the cell membrane and the release of cell contents into the surrounding tissue

---

> **Information on Breast Disorders**
>
> **Causes:** Hormones, bacterial infection, trauma
> **Symptoms:** Swelling and tenderness, lumps or cysts, pain, infection and inflammation, nipple discharge, fibroadenomas
> **Duration:** Acute to chronic
> **Treatments:** Surgery, antibiotics, hormonal treatment

Causes and Symptoms

Because of fear of breast cancer and discomfort, noncancerous breast disorders often cause women a great deal of anxiety and distress. The most common breast concern of women is the presence of fibrocystic breasts, which can feel nodular and tender. Other, less common breast conditions include mastitis, fat necrosis, nipple discharge, and a variety of benign breast tumors.

Common symptoms of fibrocystic breast condition include a dense and lumpy texture, which is usually more evident in the upper and outer quadrants of the breast. Intermittent or persistent dull pain, tenderness, and itching of the nipples often occur premenstrually, lessening after menstruation begins. This condition is so common, occurring in an estimated 60 percent of women between thirty and fifty years old, that it is considered a variation of normal. The lumpy tissue often causes significant discomfort, and its presence can terrify women checking for cancer during breast self-examination and make the diagnosis of cancer more difficult.

The cause of fibrocystic breasts is unknown, although the associated discomfort fluctuates with the menstrual cycle and rarely occurs after menopause, so ovarian hormones are likely involved. A family history of fibrocystic breasts increases risk, and excessive dietary fat and caffeine intake may exacerbate the condition.

After breast lumps and pain, nipple discharge is the third most common breast complaint. Clear, milky, yellow, or green discharge occurring from both nipples does not usually indicate cancer, and a significant percentage of women will experience such discharge at some point while performing a self-examination. Women should see a doctor if the nipple discharge is bloody, watery, sticky, persistent, occurs on one side, or appears spontaneously without squeezing the nipple, although only about 10 percent of such discharges are the result of cancer.

Mastitis is an infection caused when the *Staphylococcus aureus* bacteria found normally on the skin enters the breast and causes swelling in the fatty breast tissue. It is most common in breast-feeding women. The symptoms include pain; lumps; irregular breast enlargement; breast swelling, redness, or warmth; nipple discharge and itching; enlarged lymph nodes; and fever. In rare cases, severe infections may cause abscesses.

Four types of benign tumors commonly occur in the breast. Galactoceles are noncancerous cysts filled with breast milk that occur in pregnant and lactating women. Fibroadenomas are round tumors comprised of connective and glandular breast tissue that develop in young adult

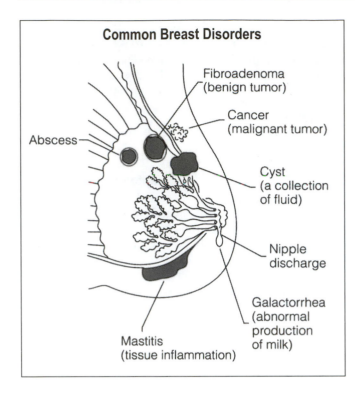

Common Breast Disorders

Fibroadenoma (benign tumor)

Cancer (malignant tumor)

Abscess

Cyst (a collection of fluid)

Nipple discharge

Galactorrhea (abnormal production of milk)

Mastitis (tissue inflammation)

women, most commonly African Americans. They occur singly and in clusters, are marblelike, and are diagnosed by needle biopsy. Intraductal papillomas are branching, stalklike growths in the milk ducts near the nipple. They can cause bloody nipple discharge. Duct ectasia, which typically affects women aged forty to sixty, is a hardening of the milk duct that can cause a thick, dark green discharge. A lump can develop around the duct and be mistaken for cancer.

Fat necrosis often occurs after the breast has been injured and the injured area is replaced with firm scar tissue or oil-filled cysts.

Treatment and Therapy

The diagnosis of fibrocystic breast condition is made by physical examination. Fibrocystic lumps are usually rounded, smooth, and malleable, although they can mimic hard and stationary cancerous lumps. The density of fibrocystic tissue makes physical examinations and mammography less effective, and ultrasound scans and needle biopsies are often necessary to rule out cancer. Although synthetic androgen (male) hormone therapy can be prescribed in severe cases and oral contraceptives can lessen symptoms, reducing dietary fat and caffeine intake are good first steps. Homeopathic treatments such as soy, vitamin E, vitamin B_6, and evening primrose oil are controversial.

For mastitis, application of a hot, moist compress to the infected area can relieve symptoms, and the infection usually responds well to antibiotics. Lactating women should continue to breast-feed or pump while undergoing treatment. For women who are not breast-feeding, mastitis should be differentiated from a rare form of breast cancer through mammography or biopsy.

Galactoceles are generally left untreated unless they cause discomfort. They can be drained by fine needle aspiration if necessary. Fibroadenomas usually stop growing without treatment, but they need to be surgically removed if they continue to grow. Intraductal papillomas are treated by removing the affected duct. Duct ectasia can be treated with heat compresses, by antibiotics, or, in severe cases, by removal of the duct.

For fat necrosis, fine needle aspiration, often used for diagnosis, usually relieves the symptoms and serves as the primary treatment.

Perspective and Prospects

Like most disorders that primarily affect women and are associated with sex differentiation, noncancerous breast disorders were rarely discussed and were not well understood before the mid-twentieth century. In the nineteenth century, breast disorders were surrounded by myth and social stigma, and mastitis often went untreated for weeks, causing tremendous discomfort. The invention of mammography in the mid-1960s, as well as that decade's increased sexual openness, made it easier to talk about breast disorders as well as to diagnose them accurately. Fibrocystic breast condition, originally called fibrocystic disease, is now accepted as normal for many women, and testing procedures are beginning to adapt to this norm. Over time, mammography, the collection of data from two generations of women, and the generally increased awareness of women's health issues have improved the diagnosis and treatment of these disorders.

—*Caroline M. Small*

See also: Breast biopsy; Breast cancer; Breast-feeding; Breasts, female; Cyst removal; Cysts; Fibrocystic breast condition; Gynecomastia; Mammography; Mastitis.

For Further Information:
"Breast Diseases." *MedlinePlus*, May 3, 2013.
Chinyama, Catherine N. *Benign Breast Disease: Radiology, Pathology, Risk Assessment*. New York: Springer, 2004.
Dixon, J. Michael, ed. *ABC of Breast Diseases*. 4th ed. Hoboken, N.J.: BMJ Books-Wiley, 2012.
Love, Susan, and Karen Lindsey. *Dr. Susan Love's Breast Book*. 5th ed. Cambridge, Mass.: Da Capo Press, 2010.
McCoy, Krisha, and Andrea Chisholm. "Mastalgia." *Health Library*, Oct. 12, 2012.
McGinn, Kerry Anne. *The Informed Woman's Guide to Breast Health: Breast Changes That Are Not Cancer*. 3d ed. Palo Alto, Calif.: Bull, 2001.
Polsdorfer, Ricker, and Andrea Chisholm. "Fibrocystic Disease." *Health Library*, Sept. 28, 2012.

Breast-feeding
Biology

Anatomy or system affected: Breasts, glands, reproductive system

Specialties and related fields: Gynecology, nutrition, obstetrics, perinatology

Definition: The preferred feeding method for infants, providing optimal nutrition for the infant (including immunologic protection), mother-infant bonding, and enhanced maternal health.

Key terms:

alveoli: the milk-producing cells of the mammary gland

bifidus factors: factors in colostrum and breast milk that favor the growth of helpful bacteria in the infant's intestinal tract

bonding: a process in which a mother forms an affectionate attachment to her infant immediately after birth

colostrum: the secretion from the breast before the onset of milk

foremilk: the milk released early in a nursing session, which is low in fat and rich in nutrients

hindmilk: the milk released late in a nursing session, which is higher in fat content

lactoferrin: a breast milk factor that binds iron, preventing it from supporting the growth of harmful intestinal bacteria; it may also promote the ability to absorb dietary iron

let-down reflex: the reflex that forces milk to the front of the breast

oxytocin: the hormone secreted from the posterior pituitary gland that stimulates the mammary glands to eject milk; it also stimulates the uterus to contract after birth

prolactin: a hormone secreted from the anterior pituitary gland that signals the breast to start and sustain milk production

Process and Effects

The terms *breast-feeding*, *nursing*, and *lactation* all refer to the best method of infant feeding. Although there are a few rare exceptions, almost every mother can breast-feed and thereby provide low-cost nutritional support for her infant. Although it is often thought otherwise, the size of the mother's breast has no relationship to successful lactation. In fact, the physiology of successful lactation is determined by the maturation of breast tissue, the initiation and maintenance of milk secretion, and the ejection or delivery of milk to the nipple. This physiology is dependent on hormonal control, and all women have the required anatomy for successful lactation unless they have had surgical alteration of the breast.

Hormonal influence on breast development begins in adolescence. Increased estrogen causes the breast ducts to elongate and duct cells to grow. (The ducts are narrow tubular vessels that run from the segments of the breast into the tip of the nipple.) More fibrous and fatty tissue develops, and the nipple area matures. As adolescence progresses, regular menstrual cycle hormones cause further development of the alveoli, which are the milk-producing cells.

The elevated levels of estrogen present during pregnancy promote the growth and branching of milk ducts, while the increase in progesterone promotes the development of alveoli. Throughout pregnancy and especially during the first three months, many more milk ducts are formed. Clusters of milk-producing cells also begin to enlarge, while at the same time placental hormones promote breast development.

Shortly before labor and delivery, the hormone prolactin is produced by the pituitary gland. Prolactin, which is necessary for starting lactation and sustaining milk produc-tion, reaches its peak at delivery. Another hormone, oxytocin, which is also produced by the pituitary, stimulates the breast to eject milk. This reaction is called the letdown reflex, which causes the milk-producing alveoli to contract and force milk to the front of the breast. Oxytocin serves an important function after delivery by causing the uterus to contract. Initially, the letdown reflex occurs only when the infant suckles, but later on it may be initiated simply by the baby's cry. An efficient letdown reflex is critical to successful breast-feeding. Emotional upset, fatigue, pain, nervousness, or embarrassment about lactation can interrupt this reflex; these psychological factors, rather than breast size or physiology, are predictive of successful lactation.

Breast-feeding is a natural response to childbirth, and the nutrient content of breast milk is ideal for the human infant. More than one hundred constituents of breast milk, both nutritive and nonnutritive, are known. Although the basic nutrient content is a solution of protein, sugar, and salts in which fat is suspended, those concentrations vary depending on the period of lactation and even within a given feeding.

Colostrum, often called first milk, is produced in the first few days after birth. It is lower in fat and calories (kilocalories) and higher in protein and certain minerals than is mature breast milk. Colostrum is opaque and yellow because it contains a high concentration of the vitamin A-like substances called carotenes. It also has a high concentration of antibodies and white blood cells, which pass on immunologic protection to the infant.

Within a few days after birth, the transition is made from colostrum to mature milk. There are two types of mature milk. Foremilk is released first as the infant begins to suckle. It has a watery, bluish appearance and is low in fat and rich in other nutrients. This milk accounts for about one-third of the baby's intake. As the nursing session progresses, the draught reflex helps move the hindmilk, with its higher fat content, to the front of the breast. It is important that the nutrient content of breast milk be determined from a sample of both types of milk in order to make an adequate assessment of all nutrients present.

Breast milk best meets the infant's needs and is the standard from which infant formulas are judged. Several nutrient characteristics make it the ideal infant food. Lactose, the carbohydrate content of breast milk, is the same simple sugar found in any milk, but the protein content of breast milk is uniquely tailored to meet infant needs. An infant's immature kidneys are better able to maintain water balance because breast milk is lower in protein than cow's milk. Most breast milk protein is alpha-lactalbumin, whereas cow's milk protein is casein. Alpha-lactalbumin is easier to digest and provides two sulphur-containing amino acids that are the building blocks of protein required for infant growth.

The fat (lipid) content of breast milk differs among women and may even vary day to day in milk from the same woman. The types of fatty acids that make up most of the fat component of the milk may vary in response to maternal diet. Mothers fed a diet containing corn and cottonseed oil produce a milk with more polyunsaturated fatty acids, which are the predominant fatty acids in those oils. Breast milk is higher in the essential fatty acid called linoleic acid than is cow's milk, and it also contains omega-3 fatty acids. About 55 percent of human milk calories come from fat, compared to about 49 percent of calories found in infant formulas. In addition, enzymes in breast milk help digest fat in the infant's stomach. This digested fat is more efficiently absorbed than the products that result from digesting cow's milk.

Breast milk contains more cholesterol than cow's milk, which seems to stimulate development of the enzymes necessary for degrading cholesterol, perhaps offering protection against atherosclerosis in later life. Cholesterol is also needed for proper development of the central nervous system.

The vitamin and mineral content of breast milk from healthy mothers supplies all that is needed for growth and health except for vitamin D and fluoride, and these are easily supplemented. Breast milk and the infant's intestinal bacteria also supply all the necessary vitamin K, but since no bacteria are present at birth, an injection of vitamin K should be given to prevent deficiencies.

Breast milk mineral content is balanced to promote growth while protecting the infant's immature kidneys. Breast milk has a low sodium content, which helps the immature kidneys to maintain water balance. No type of milk is a good source of iron. Although breast milk contains relatively small amounts of iron, about 50 percent of this iron can be absorbed by the body, compared to only 4 percent from cow's milk. This phenomenon is called bioavailability. Because of the high bioavailability of breast milk iron, the introduction of solids, which are given to replace depleted iron stores, can be delayed until six months of age in most infants; this delay may help to reduce the incidence of allergies in susceptible infants. There is also evidence that zinc is better absorbed from breast milk.

The vitamin content of milk can vary and is influenced by maternal vitamin status. The water-soluble vitamin content of breast milk (the B vitamins and vitamin C) will change more because of maternal diet than the fat-soluble vitamin content (vitamins A, E, and K). If women have diets that are deficient in vitamins, their levels in breast milk will be lower. Yet even malnourished mothers can breast-feed, although the quantity of milk is decreased. As the maternal diet improves, the level of water-soluble vitamins in the milk increases. There is a level, however, above which additional diet supplements will not increase the vitamin content of breast milk.

There are many nonnutritive advantages to breast-feeding. A major advantage is the immunologic protection and resistance factors that it provides to the infant. Bifidus factors, found in both colostrum and mature milk, favor the growth of helpful bacteria in the infant's digestive tract. These bacteria in turn offer protection against harmful organisms. Lactoferrin, another resistance factor, binds iron so that harmful bacteria cannot use it. Lysozyme, lipases,

Breast-feeding involves a hormonal feedback loop that encourages milk production.

and lactoperoxidases also offer protection against harmful bacteria.

Immunoglobulins are present in large amounts in colostrum and in significant amounts in breast milk. These protein compounds act as antibodies against foreign substances in the body called antigens. Generally, the resistance passed to the infant is from environmental antigens to which the mother had been exposed. The concentration of antibodies in colostrum is highest in the first hour after birth. Secretory IgA is the major immunoglobulin that provides protection against gastrointestinal organisms. Breast milk also contains interferon, an antiviral substance that is produced by special white blood cells in milk. Protection against allergy is another advantage of breast-feeding. It is not known, however, whether less exposure to the antigens found in formula or some substance in the breast milk itself provides this protection. Normally, a mucous barrier in the intestine prevents the absorption of whole proteins, the root of an allergic reaction. In the newborn, this barrier is not fully developed to allow whole immunologic proteins to be absorbed. The possibility that whole food proteins will be absorbed as well is greater if cow's milk or early solids are given, and this absorption increases the potential for allergic reactions.

Other possible benefits of breast-feeding are protection against the intestinal disorders Crohn's disease and celiac sprue, and insulin-dependent diabetes. The reasons for this protection are not clear.

Breast-feeding also encourages infant bonding, a process in which the mother and baby form an attachment. It is a matter of controversy whether breast-feeding mothers bond better than bottle-feeding mothers. If a mother has early and prolonged contact with her baby, however, the mother is more likely to breast-feed and to nurse her baby for more months.

Milk from mothers delivering preterm infants is higher in protein and nonprotein nitrogen, calcium, IgA, sodium, potassium, chloride, phosphorus, and magnesium. It also has a different fat composition and is lower in lactose than mature milk of mothers delivering after a normal term. These concentrations support more rapid growth of a preterm infant.

Breast-feeding is not only good for the baby but also good for the mother. There is an association between reduced breast cancer rates and breast-feeding, although the reason is not known. In addition, the hormonal influences caused by suckling the infant help to contract the uterus, returning it to prepregnancy size and controlling blood loss. Breast-feeding also helps to reduce the mother's weight. Calories required to make milk are drawn from the fat stores that were deposited during pregnancy. Nevertheless, breast-feeding should be viewed not as a quick weight loss program but as a healthy, natural weight loss process.

If a woman breast-feeds completely, which means that no supplements or solid foods are given until the baby is six months of age, often she will not menstruate. Many women find this lack of menstrual periods psychologically pleasant while not realizing the physiological benefit of restoring the iron stores that were depleted during pregnancy and delivery. An important advantage to breast-feeding in developing countries is that it can help to space pregnancies naturally. Most infant malnutrition occurs when the second child is born, because breast-feeding is stopped for the first child. The first child is weaned to foods that do not supply enough nutrients. By spacing pregnancies out, the first child has a chance to nurse longer.

Breast-feeding is very convenient and does not require time to mix and prepare formula or sterilize bottles. Breast milk is always sterile and at the proper temperature. The money needed for the extra food required to produce breast milk is much less than that required to purchase commercial formula. This can be a major benefit for women with low incomes and is critically important for the health of those babies born in developing countries.

Complications and Disorders

Some special problems or circumstances can make breast-feeding difficult. The breasts may become engorged-so full of milk that they are hard and sore-making it difficult for the baby to latch onto the nipple. Gentle massaging of the breasts, especially with warm water or a heating pad, will allow release of the milk and reduce pain in the breast. This situation is common during the first few weeks of nursing but will occasionally recur if a feeding is missed or a schedule changes.

Sometimes a duct will become plugged and form a hard lump. Massaging the lump and continuing to nurse will remedy the situation. If influenza-like symptoms accompany a plugged duct, the cause is probably a breast infection. Since the infection is in the tissue around the milk-producing glands, the milk itself is safe. The mother must apply heat, get plenty of rest, and keep emptying the breast by frequent feedings. Stopping nursing would plug the duct further, making the infection worse.

Of concern to many mothers are reports of contaminants in breast milk. Drugs, environmental pollutants, viruses, caffeine, alcohol, and food allergens can be passed to the infant through breast milk. Drug transmission depends on the administration method, which influences the speed with which it reaches the blood supply to the breast. Whether that drug can remain functional after it is subjected to the acid in the baby's digestive tract varies. Large amounts of caffeine in breast milk can produce a wakeful, hyperactive infant, but this situation is corrected when the mother stops her caffeine consumption. Large amounts of alcohol produce an altered facial appearance that is reversible; however, some psychomotor delay in the infant may remain even after the mother's drinking has stopped. Nicotine also enters milk, but the impact of secondhand smoke may pose more of a health threat than the nicotine content of breast milk. Since the human immunodeficiency virus (HIV), the virus that causes acquired immunodeficiency syndrome (AIDS), can also pass through breast milk, HIV-positive mothers should not breast-feed their infants.

Of greater concern is the presence of contaminants that cannot be avoided, such as pesticide residues, industrial waste, or other environmental contaminants. Polychlorinated biphenyls (PCBs) and the pesticide DDT have received the most attention. Long-term exposure to contaminants promotes their accumulation in the mother's body fat, and the production of breast milk is one way to rid the body of these contaminants. Concentrations present in the breast milk vary. Ordinarily, these substances are in such small quantities that they pose no health risk. Women who have consumed large amounts of fish from PCB-contaminated waters or have had occupational exposure to this chemical, however, need to have their breast milk tested. It is also possible for these substances to enter the infant's food supply from other sources.

Perspective and Prospects

Although breast-feeding is the best method of infant feeding, many women choose not to breast-feed. Before the eighteenth century, human milk was the only source for infant feeding. If a mother did not breast-feed, a woman called a wet nurse fed her baby. At the end of the nineteenth century, formula feeding became popular when bottles were developed and water sanitation improved. In the United States, breast-feeding rates declined to only about 20 percent by 1970 but increased to more than 75 percent by 2009, according to the Centers for Disease Control and Prevention. More than 47 percent of mothers in the United States continue breast-feeding until their infants are at least six months of age.

Breast-feeding used to be more prevalent among more-educated, higher-income mothers. Increased employment of women outside the home, however, has dramatically altered trends in breast-feeding. Although mothers may opt to breast-feed in the hospital, many quit because they are returning to work and believe that it would be too difficult to continue. A working mother needs four to six weeks at home to establish successful breast-feeding. Mothers who are unable to maintain a regular breast-feeding schedule because of work or other obligations often use pumps to collect milk that can then be stored, thus allowing infants to benefit from nutritious milk even when their mothers are absent and enabling women to return to their normal schedules.

Formula use has increased in developing countries. Because formula is very expensive, it is often diluted with water and therefore does not provide enough nutritional support to the infant. The quality of water is often poor, which causes the infant to be exposed to disease-causing organisms. In addition, formula-fed infants do not receive the immunologic protection of breast milk. The result is a higher infant mortality rate.

There are very few instances in which a woman should not breast-feed her infant. Babies with a rare genetic disorder called galactosemia cannot nurse, since they lack the enzyme to metabolize milk sugar. Phenylketonuria (PKU), another genetic disorder, requires close monitoring of the infant's blood phenylalanine level, but the infant can be totally or at least partially breast-fed. Breast-feeding is contraindicated for women suffering from AIDS, alcoholism, drug addiction, malaria, active tuberculosis, or a chronic disease that results in maternal malnutrition. The presence of other conditions, from diabetes to the common cold, is not a reason to avoid breast-feeding.

—*Wendy L. Stuhldreher, Ph.D., R.D.*

See also: Breast disorders; Breasts, female; Glands; Hormones; Mastitis; Nutrition; Perinatology; Phenylketonuria (PKU); Pregnancy and gestation.

For Further Information:

A.D.A.M. Medical Encyclopedia. "Breastfeeding." *MedlinePlus*, September 13, 2011.

A.D.A.M. Medical Encyclopedia. "Breast Milk-Pumping and Storing." *MedlinePlus*, September 9, 2012.

Bennett, Peter N., ed. *Drugs and Human Lactation*. 2d ed. New York: Elsevier, 1996.

Centers for Disease Control and Prevention. "Breastfeeding Report Card-United States, 2012." *Centers for Disease Control and Prevention*, June 6, 2013.

Hillis, Anne, and Penelope Stone. *Breast, Bottle, Bowl: The Best Fed Baby Book*. Rev. ed. Pymble, N.S.W.: HarperCollins, 2008.

Huggins, Kathleen. *The Nursing Mother's Companion*. 5th ed. Boston: Harvard Common Press, 2005.

La Leche League International. *The Womanly Art of Breastfeeding*. Rev. ed. New York: Ballantine Books, 2010.

Mason, Diane, and Diane Ingersoll. *Breastfeeding and the Working Mother*. Rev. ed. New York: St. Martin's Griffin, 1997.

Meek, Joan Younger, and Sherill Tippins, eds. *American Academy of Pediatrics New Mother's Guide to Breastfeeding*. New York: Bantam, 2006.

Riordan, Jan, ed. *Breastfeeding and Human Lactation*. 4th ed. Sudbury, Mass.: Jones and Bartlett, 2010.

Rolfes, Sharon Rady, Linda Kelly DeBruyne, Eleanor Noss Whitney. *Life Span Nutrition: Conception Through Life*. 2d ed. St. Paul, Minn.: West, 1998.

South Dakota Department of Health. "Feeding Your Infant: Ages 0 to 4 Months." *Health Library*, September 12, 2012.

Stanway, Penny, and Andrew Stanway. *Breast Is Best*. 4th rev. ed. London: Pan Books, 2005.

Breast surgery

Procedures

Anatomy or system affected: Breasts, glands

Specialties and related fields: General surgery, plastic surgery, psychiatry

Definition: Procedures performed on the breast to diagnose or treat benign and malignant breast disease or for reconstructive and cosmetic purposes.

Key terms:

abscess: a collection of infected fluid, which may be treated with antibiotics and drainage

areola: the pigmented tissue immediately surrounding the nipple

augmentation: an increase in the volume or size of the breast

axillary dissection: removal of lymph nodes found in the armpit (also known as axilla) to determine the spread of breast cancer; this procedure helps in planning therapy and in preventing spread of the cancer

lumpectomy: removal of a breast mass without removal of the noninvolved areas of the breast

mastectomy: surgical removal of the breast

reduction: a decrease in the total volume or mass of breast tissue

Indications and Procedures

The indications for breast surgery can be grouped into benign disease, malignant disease, reconstructive purposes, and cosmetic purposes. Indications for breast surgery in benign disease include persistent breast cysts which are not responsive to aspiration, such as in fibrocystic breast disease. In women who have a solid breast mass, excision of the lump to determine whether it is cancerous would be another indication for breast surgery. In this situation, the breast surgery would be diagnostic as well as potentially curative (for example, if the mass is benign). Another indication for breast surgery would be a breast abscess refractory to drainage; in this situation, excision of the abscess would offer the best chance of a cure.

Breast cancer is another indication for breast surgery. The surgery is usually performed after clinical breast examination, mammogram, and biopsy have confirmed the

Gel and smooth saline breast implants. (SIU School of Medicine)

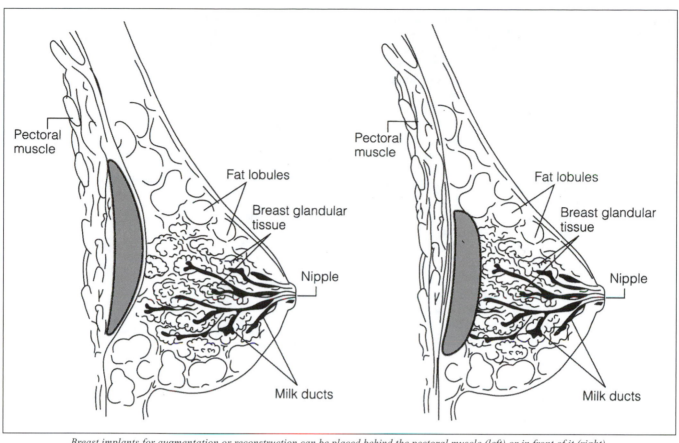

Breast implants for augmentation or reconstruction can be placed behind the pectoral muscle (left) or in front of it (right).

malignancy. The extent of disease and its aggressiveness determine to a large extent the type of breast surgery performed. In early-stage breast cancer, a modified radical mastectomy may be performed. This involves removal of the entire breast and the axillary lymph nodes. Alternatively, a lumpectomy with axillary node dissection (followed by radiation therapy) may be performed. Which procedure a patient receives also depends on the tumor size, tumor location, and the patient's breast size.

When a breast is completely removed, the patient may opt for reconstructive surgery. One common type of reconstructive surgery involves fashioning a new breast using a saline implant and a piece of the rectus abdominis muscle (a muscle on the anterior abdominal wall) called a transverse rectus abdominis myocutaneous (TRAM) flap. The areola may be reconstructed using a darker piece of skin taken from another part of the body, and tattooing may also be performed to give the nipple a more natural appearance.

Cosmetic breast surgery is indicated in cases where the patient is not satisfied with the appearance or size of her breasts. Most commonly, this cosmetic surgery takes the form of breast augmentation or breast reduction. In breast augmentation, implants are introduced under or over the pectoralis major muscle that lies underneath the existing breast. This is accomplished through an incision under the armpit, from the underside of the breast, or in the margin around the areola. The procedure may be done under local anesthesia as an outpatient procedure or under general anesthesia. The latter option is generally used when the implants are placed underneath the pectoralis muscle.

Breast reduction surgery, also called reductive mammoplasty, can be indicated when the patient suffers from back, shoulder, or neck pain from large breasts. It is also indicated when the patient is not satisfied with the appearance of her breasts. A patient with large breasts often suffers from ptosis, or drooping of the breasts (which can also occur with aging or pregnancy and lactation). Reductive mammoplasty will correct the ptosis as well as reduce the overall size of the breasts. Commonly, tissue is removed from the most dependent (lowest) portion of the breast using vertical incisions, preserving the nipple and the underlying structures (nerves and lactic ducts). After the excess breast tissue is removed, the incision is then closed, with care taken for optimal cosmetic appearance. The breasts are wrapped in bandages to support the tissue while they heal. General anesthesia is almost always used, and blood loss can be greater than for breast augmentation. Drains may be placed temporarily in the breasts to prevent infection and the buildup of fluid. The patient is usually hospitalized for several days.

Uses and Complications

The uses of breast surgery include the diagnosis and treatment of benign and malignant breast disease, reconstruction after trauma or mastectomy, and the alteration of breast size and appearance for cosmetic or functional purposes.

Potential complications of all breast surgery include infection, scarring, and bleeding. Infections are infrequent but must be treated aggressively with antibiotics when they occur. If a prosthesis is involved, then it may be removed and reinserted three to six months later. Scarring is of concern because breast surgery is most often undertaken for cosmetic or aesthetic reasons. The placement of incisions along skin folds and careful skin closure help to minimize scarring. Restricting immediate postoperative activities, especially those that require stretching, also reduces scarring. As with all surgical procedures, bleeding is a risk of breast surgery. Blood loss from breast surgery can be minimized with careful inspection prior to closing incisions and the cauterization of any bleeding areas.

Although most patients who receive breast augmentation maintain normal breast function and can breast-feed after the surgery, many patients who have undergone breast reduction have difficulty with lactation. In addition, a larger number of women who have undergone breast reduction report loss of sensation than do women who have undergone breast augmentation. Also, scarring in women who have undergone breast reduction tends to be more extensive than in women who have undergone breast augmentation.

When implants are used, complications such as contracture and leakage may occur. Contracture occurs when the tissue immediately surrounding the prosthesis scars and shrinks, leading to an unnatural breast appearance. In rare cases, saline implants may leak. In the past, implants filled with silicone leaked, and a number of patients claimed that these leaks led to a number of medical problems. Although the connection between silicone leakage and medical disease remains controversial, the legal climate led to the withdrawal of silicone breast implants in North America until 2006, when the US Food and Drug Administration began approving them for use in women aged twenty-two years or older.

Perspective and Prospects

The number of breast surgeries performed in the United States continues to rise. In particular, cosmetic breast augmentation was the most frequently performed cosmetic surgical procedure between 2006 and 2010. According to the American Society of Plastic Surgeons, 296,203 augmentation mammoplasties were performed in the United States in 2010, and the total number of women with implants in the United States is in the millions. As the number of women who have had breast augmentation grows, health care providers will probably deal more with the problems particular to breast implants, such as the increased difficulty in detecting breast masses and breast cancers.

—*L. Fleming Fallon, Jr., M.D., Ph.D., M.P.H.; updated by Anne Lynn S. Chang, M.D.*

See also: Breast biopsy; Breast cancer; Breast disorders; Breasts, female; Gender reassignment surgery; Grafts and grafting; Mammography; Mastectomy and lumpectomy; Oncology; Plastic surgery; Women's health.

For Further Information:
American Society of Plastic Surgeons. *American Society of Plastic Surgeons Report of the 2010 Plastic Surgery Statistics*. [N. p.]: ASPS National Clearinghouse of Plastic Surgery Procedural Statistics, 2011.
Berger, Karen, and John Bostwick III. *A Woman's Decision: Breast Care, Treatment, and Reconstruction*. 3th. ed. St. Louis, Mo.: Quality Medical Publishing, 2011.
Bostwick, John, III. *Plastic and Reconstructive Breast Surgery*. 2d ed. St. Louis, Mo.: Quality Medical Publishing, 2000.
Doherty, Gerard M., and Lawrence W. Way, eds. *Current Surgical Diagnosis and Treatment*. 13th ed. New York: Lange Medical Books/McGraw-Hill, 2010.
Georgiade, Nicholas G., Gregory S. Georgiade, and Ronald Riefkohl, eds. *Aesthetic Surgery of the Breast*. Philadelphia: W. B. Saunders, 1990.
Guthrie, Randolph, and Doug Podolsky. *The Truth About Breast Implants*. New York: John Wiley & Sons, 1994.
Health Library. "Mastectomy." *Health Library*, October 31, 2012.
Stewart, Mary White. *Silicone Spills: Breast Implants on Trial*. Westport, Conn.: Praeger, 1998.
Tanne, Janice Hopkins. "FDA Approves Silicone Breast Implants 14 Years after Their Withdrawal." *British Medical Journal*333, no. 7579 (December, 2006): 1139.

Breasts, female

Anatomy

Anatomy or system affected: Endocrine system, glands, muscles, musculoskeletal system, reproductive system
Specialties and related fields: Endocrinology, gynecology, obstetrics, oncology, plastic surgery
Definition: The female mammary glands and their surrounding muscles and tissues.
Key terms:
alveolar cell: also known as an acinar cell; the fundamental secretory unit of the mammary glandular tissue
colostrum: thin, yellow milky secretions of the mammary gland just a few days before and after childbirth; it contains more proteins and less fat and carbohydrates than does milk
Cooper's ligament: projections of breast parenchyma covered by fibrous connective tissue that extend from the skin to the deep layer of superficial fascia
lactiferous duct: a single excretory duct from each lobe of mammary glandular tissue that converges yet opens separately at the tip of the nipple; the mammary gland has fifteen to twenty lactiferous ducts
milkline: a line that originates as a primitive milk streak on each front side of the fetus; it extends from axilla to vulva, where rudimentary breast tissues or nipples could be located
myoepithelial cell: a cell that is anatomically located next to the alveolar cells and contractile in nature to aid in the movement of milk from the alveoli into the ducts

Structure and Functions

Mammogenesis-the growth and differentiation of the mammary gland-begins early in fetal life. By the sixth week of fetal development, the primitive milk streak can be identified as an ectodermal thickening along the ventrolateral aspect on each side of the fetus. In the ensuing weeks, this milk streak regresses, leaving normally only one pair of mammary glands in the thoracic region; however, multiple nipples and breast tissue may occasionally continue to develop anywhere along the milk line, extending from the armpit to the groin.

During the second trimester, projections of the ectoderm from the primary sprouts-usually between fifteen and twenty-will eventually elongate and arborize (branch out) to form the lactiferous ducts. Canalization of the ducts occurs late in fetal life and requires placental hormones for stimulation. Once the ducts canalize, two layers of epithelial cells are identified: the inner layer of cells, which forms the secretory component, and the outer layer of cells, which forms the myoepithelium, constituting the contractile elements for the expulsion of milk.

Between approximately four and seven days after birth, 80 to 90 percent of newborns have breast secretions (so-called witches' milk). Such secretions have been noted with equal frequency in male and female infants, and they usually last for three or four weeks. After the first neonatal month, the breast tissue reverts to an undifferentiated state and remains quiescent until puberty. Minimal ductal growth occurs during childhood, and there is no lobuloalveolar development.

At puberty, the surge of female hormones initiates lactiferous duct proliferation, along with deposition of fat and connective tissue. These changes produce a rapid increase in the size and density of the breast and are coordinated by the action of multiple hormones (prolactin, cortisol, growth hormone, insulin, and thyroxin) in addition to estrogen and progesterone. Estrogen encourages ductal proliferation and maturation, while progesterone stimulates lobuloalveolar growth. Ovarian steroids appear necessary for mammary development, as breast enlargement fails to occur at puberty in girls with gonadal dysgenesis. By the time of breast enlargement, the areola becomes more pigmented and the nipple enlarges.

In adult women, size, density, and nodularity of the breast are dependent on the build of the individual, because much of the breast tissue consists of fat. During the menstrual cycle, the breasts undergo a cyclic change. The rising estrogen and progesterone levels cause an increase in blood flow and interlobular edema. The engorgement, along with increase in density and nodularity, is particularly noticeable late in the menstrual cycle. The week preceding menstruation, hormonal changes can bring about breast discomfort, tenderness, and a sensation of fullness. This increased sensitivity, often accompanied by marked nodularity, makes the clinical breast examination difficult. It is therefore important to examine the breasts seven to ten days following the onset of menstruation, as only during this time can tumors be differentiated from physiological nodularity. At menses, the breast decreases in size, the result of a reduction in the number and size of glandular cells with loss of edema.

During pregnancy, the breast undergoes final maturation in preparation for lactation. In the early weeks, the breast begins to enlarge, and marked histological changes take place. There is concurrent enlargement, pigmentation, and increased vascularity of the nipple. The earliest

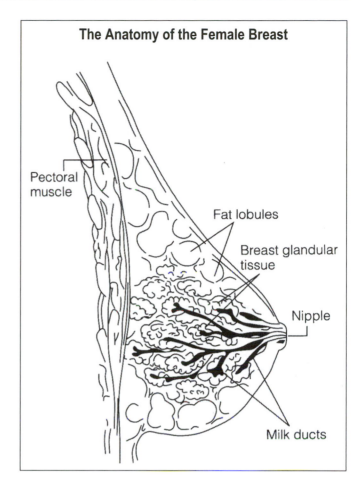

The Anatomy of the Female Breast

Pectoral muscle

Fat lobules

Breast glandular tissue

Nipple

Milk ducts

histological change within the acinar epithelial cells is cytoplasmic vacuolation. Lymphocytes, plasma cells, and eosinophils collect in the interstitial spaces. During the second trimester, the lobules enlarge and there is increase in the number and size of the constituent acini. The mammary blood supply is enhanced by increasing vascular luminal diameters and by formation of new capillaries around the lobules. During the last trimester, the secretory cells fill with fat droplets, and the alveoli are distended with a proteinaceous secretion termed colostrum.

Within three to four days postpartum, estrogen and progesterone levels rapidly decline. Prolactin can now, unrepressed by estrogen and progesterone, activate lactation, which is maintained by the infant's suckling. This stimulates further release of prolactin and oxytocin, which activate the myoepithelial cells, leading to expulsion of the alveolar secretion. During the first few days of lactation, only colostrum is produced. Once the colostrum has been expelled, normal production of milk ensues. Prolactin sustains milk production. Each nursing episode makes prolactin increase fivefold to tenfold, but, as weeks go by, prolactin levels gradually return to normal until even the nursing-induced rise is negligible. For unknown reasons, however, successful lactation can be maintained for months.

Changes of involution occur in the breast with increasing age and also after lactation. Between the ages of thirty-five and forty-five, the glandular tissue begins to disappear and alveoli and lobules shrink. These changes are not uniform throughout the breast; some lobules remain prominent, while others become more atrophic. At menopause, the breasts decrease in size and become less dense. There is an increase in the elastic tissue component of the breast.

Anatomically, the extent of the normal female breast is approximately from the second to the sixth rib. The medial border touches the sternum, and the lateral border extends to the mid-portion of the armpit (axilla). The majority of the glandular tissue is in the upper outer quadrant and often extends deep into the axilla. The most important factor controlling the variation in breast size, shape, and density is obesity. The mammary gland is enclosed between the superficial and deep layers of the superficial fascia. The superficial layer is a thin and delicate structure that is thicker at the inferior portion of the breast and becomes thinner as it approaches the clavicle. The deeper layer splits off the superficial fascia and extends deep into the mammary gland. Between this deep layer and the pectoral fascia, there is a well-defined space, termed retromammary space, that contains loose tissue, allowing the breast to glide freely over the chest wall. Portions of the deep layer of the superficial fascia form connective tissue extensions that pass through the retromammary space and join with the pectoral fascia. These extensions help support the breast. The breast is firmly fixed to the skin in the area of the nipple, and the remainder of the lobules are attached to the skin by dense fibrous bands termed Cooper's ligaments. Involvement of these ligaments with cancer gives rise to the physical sign of skin dimpling.

The breast is composed of glandular tissue, blood vessels, nerves, lymphatics, and varying amounts of fat. The glandular tissue is composed of between fifteen and twenty lactiferous ducts radially arranged around the nipple, each separated by fibrous septa. The terminal portion of the lactiferous duct dilates, forming the lactiferous sinus before it empties into the nipple. The functional unit of the breast is the terminal duct lobular unit, which consists of between ten and one hundred alveoli with the intralobular terminal duct and extralobular terminal duct. The arteries supplying the breast are derived from the thoracic branches of the internal mammary artery, the axillary artery, and the intercostal arteries. The chief blood supply to the breast is from perforating branches of the internal mammary artery. The venous drainage of the breast is through the superficial subcutaneous veins, which drain either through the superficial veins into the lower neck or via medial connections into the internal mammary veins. There are also three groups of deep venous drainage. Although there appears to be some cross-drainage from one breast to the other, it is highly unlikely that this is a significant route for metastatic spread of carcinoma to the opposite breast.

Innervation of the breast skin is separated by quadrants. The upper quadrants receive their innervation from the third and fourth branches of the cervical plexus, while the lower quadrants are supplied by the thoracic intercostal nerves. The nipple's sensitivity is derived from the lateral cutaneous branch of the fourth intercostal nerve.

Lymphatic drainage of the breast can be divided into a superficial system draining the skin and a deeper system draining the lobules. The drainage from the upper quadrants passes to the axilla, as does drainage from the lower medial quadrant and adjacent abdominal wall. The breast's lymphatic drainage is primarily to the axilla, with lesser drainage occurring along the internal mammary chain.

Disorders and Diseases

Congenital anomalies of the breast are relatively rare. The most common are accessory breast tissue (polymastia) and accessory nipples (polythelia) along the milk line. A complete lack of one or both breasts (amastia) or nipples (athelia) is very rare; however, underdeveloped rudimentary breasts are not uncommon. Accessory breasts or nipples occur in approximately 2 percent of the population. Their most frequent location is just below the normal breast. This accessory breast tissue is of little clinical significance, although it is subject to the same disease processes that occur in normal breasts. Hypertrophy, or overgrowth, of the breast is another development variation that affects young women, especially adolescents. The most frequent type of true hypertrophy of the breast occurs in adolescence following a normal puberty. The breasts fail to cease enlargement as they reach their normal limits. The excessive growth is the result of increased deposition of fibrous and adipose tissue. Little abnormality is to be found in the glandular elements of the breast. The breasts may gain massive size and require surgical reduction.

The inflammatory conditions of the breast may be acute or chronic and can be caused by various factors, including infectious agents, foreign bodies, or trauma. Acute mastitis is usually the result of spread of microorganisms from the nipple, particularly during lactation. The breast shows acute inflammation with swelling, warmness, and redness. An abscess, or collection of pus, may form in the subareolar or deep glandular tissue. Diffuse cellulitis occasionally develops as the infection spreads into the adjacent soft tissue. Acute mastitis usually resolves following appropriate antibiotic treatment. Chronic mastitis may follow acute mastitis, or its onset may be insidious. The causative organisms are similar to those responsible for acute mastitis.

Fat necrosis within the breast tissue may follow trauma or a breast augmentation procedure using silicone or other materials. It may also be associated with necrosis developing in a malignant tumor. A history of trauma with surrounding bruises and pain is found in only about half the cases. Fat necrosis often manifests itself as a small, firm nodular mass of insidious onset. The consistency, adhesion to skin, and lack of pain, as well as the presence of calcifications on mammography, add to the confusion with carcinoma. In chronic cases, extensive fibrosis is seen. Careful microscopic sampling of different areas of the lesion is necessary, since malignant tumors could be associated with the foci of fat necrosis.

Almost all women are affected by a benign condition called fibrocystic change of breast at some time in their lives. Many other terms have been used for fibrocystic change in the medical literature, such as mammary dysplasia, fibrocystic disease, and chronic cystic mastitis, but these terms are no longer considered appropriate. This condition primarily affects women between twenty and forty-five years of age. Symptoms include nodularity in the breasts that may be associated with pain and tenderness, particularly around menses. Although the pathogenesis is not clear, fibrocystic changes appear to be the result of a hormonal imbalance of estrogen and progesterone. Oral contraceptives reduce the incidence of some types of fibrocystic changes. Genetic makeup, age, parity, and lactational history may also play a role. The majority of fibrocystic changes are not premalignant.

The most common benign neoplasm of the breast is fibroadenoma, with most cases occurring between fifteen and thirty years of age. Thought to be of lobular origin, these neoplasms are estrogen-dependent, are often associated with menstrual irregularities, and can enlarge significantly during pregnancy. Clinically, fibroadenomas are usually well-defined, rounded lesions that have a firm or rubbery consistency. They are freely mobile, since there are no attachments between the tumor and the adjacent tissue. Fibroadenomas vary in size, with the majority being between one and three centimeters in diameter. Some tumors, however, can be as large as ten to twelve centimeters and are termed giant fibroadenoma; these are more common in adolescents, particularly people of African descent in their second decade of life. The large size of these tumors may be intimidating, but they have no malignant potential. Local excision with nipple preservation is adequate and allows subsequent normal development of the breast.

Breast cancer is a major cause of death among women worldwide. The World Health Organization estimates that in 2011, breast cancer was responsible for more than 508,000 deaths in women (Global Health Estimates, WHO, 2013). The initial physical signs and symptoms of breast carcinoma are varied. The most common clinical manifestation is a discrete lump. Swelling, nipple retraction, skin dimpling, axillary lumps, and occasionally bloody nipple discharge make up the remainder of the local physical signs. In general, nipple discharge is not often associated with cancer. When it is, it is usually a persistent, spontaneous bloody discharge. In women younger than fifty years of age, the presence of a bloody discharge is usually associated with an intraductal papilloma, which is not a malignant breast lesion. Skin retraction is caused by shortening of the Cooper's ligaments; its presence classically raises strong suspicion of a breast carcinoma. Other benign breast lesions can produce similar changes, however, the most common of which are plasma cell mastitis, fat necrosis, and Mondor's disease. Women with distant metastasis may experience general malaise, weight loss, bone pain, and headaches.

The site of the breast lump in most cases is in the upper outer quadrant or in the retroareolar area, just beneath the nipple. This is likely attributable to the fact that the majority of mammary glandular tissue occupies the upper outer quadrant of the breast. Approximately 5 percent of breast cancers occur in both breasts.

There are several different histopathological subtypes of breast cancer. Their recognition by the pathologist is crucial, since some have different prognostic implications. Most breast malignancies are primarily epithelial in origin, with only a small number of sarcomas and metastatic tumors reported. Although the terminal duct lobular unit is probably the location of origin of almost all cancers, neoplasms are traditionally classified into ductal and lobular carcinomas.

The most common malignant neoplasm of the breast is a nonspecific type of infiltrating ductal carcinoma, which is reported in 75 percent of breast cancer cases. It is presumed to be ductal in origin, and there may be coexistent areas of intraductal carcinoma, although this component is not always obvious. There is a poorly defined area of firmness that can often be palpated within the breast. At the time of surgical biopsy, most of these cancers range between one and three centimeters in diameter. Tumors less than one centimeter in diameter are not usually detected, although the increased use of screening mammography has brought some of these early lesions to light. Other tumors may reach a massive size, greater than ten centimeters, before the patient seeks medical advice, often because of the patient's denial or lack of knowledge. The mass has a hard consistency and gives a gritty resistance when the specimen is cut. The outer margin of the mass is irregular with numerous fibrous bands, which can cause retraction of the nipple and dimpling of the overlying skin. The neoplasm may also be fixed to the underlying chest wall. Ulceration of the nipple or other parts of the skin is uncommon, except in advanced cases.

Invasive lobular carcinoma is the second most common breast malignancy. These tumors tend to be multifocal and bilateral. When the opposite, or uninvolved, breast is sampled, about one-third show areas of carcinoma. Nodules of invasive lobular carcinoma are frequently difficult to localize, and occasionally no masses are encountered.

Perspective and Prospects

Breast cancer has been described in many cultures and can even be found recorded in early Egyptian hieroglyphics. In recent years, the investigation of breast diseases has blossomed. The normal physiological conditions of the breast, various benign diseases, and breast cancer have been clearly separated. The significance, prognosis, relation to breast cancer, and treatment of these diseases have been elucidated. Epidemiological studies have shown marked differences in the incidence of breast cancer within populations. These findings have suggested hypotheses as to the etiology and natural history of breast cancer. Increased patient awareness and continued advancement of screening mammography have resulted in earlier diagnosis of the disease.

Throughout the nineteenth century and in the early twentieth century, the prognosis for breast cancer was dismal because of the advanced stage of the disease at the usual time of its initial manifestation. In 1894, William Halsted and Willy Meyer each published, independently and for the first time, a description of the radical mastectomy procedure, including the resection of the entire breast, pectoral muscles, axillary lymph nodes, and associated skin and subcutaneous tissue. It was not until the late 1930s, however, that the Halsted radical mastectomy was beginning to be questioned by other surgeons. Enthusiasm for more conservative management-simple mastectomy with adjuvant radiation therapy-was ignited. In the early 1950s, newer concepts emerged for the management of benign and malignant breast diseases. For example, the concept that breast cancer was a systemic disease and potentially unaffected by local treatment had risen. For the first time, a staging system was devised. Several studies confirmed that the most important prognostic indicator was the presence or absence of axillary nodal metastasis. In the 1960s and 1970s, hormonal therapy and adjuvant chemotherapy gradually gained acceptance.

Developments in the understanding of breast diseases and the variety of treatments available have provided major roles for the surgeon, medical oncologist, radiation oncologist, diagnostic radiologist, and pathologist. The multidisciplinary approach necessitates a coordinated, multidisciplinary team of experts to achieve the most optimal outcome of patient care.

—*Stan Liu, MD, and Lawrence W. Bassett, MD; updated by Mary Dietmann Ed. D. APRN CNS and Geraldine Marrocco*

See also: *Anatomy; Biopsy; Breastbiopsy; Breastcancer; Breastdisorders; Breast-feeding; Breastsurgery; Cancer; Cystremoval; Cysts; Fibrocystic breastcondition; Genderreassignment surgery; Glands; Gynecology; Mammography; Mastectomyand lumpectomy; Mastitis; Muscles; Oncology; Pathology; Plastic surgery; Reproductive system; Systems and organs; Tumorremoval; Tumors; Women's health.*

For Further Information:

American Cancer Society. (2016). "Non-cancerous Breast Conditions." *Cancer.org*

Centers for Disease Control and Prevention. "Breast Cancer." *Division of CancerPrevention and Control,* April 14, 2016.

MedlinePlus. "Breast Diseases." *MedlinePlus*, May 19, 2013.

Susan G. Komen for the Cure. "Benign Breast Conditions." *Susan G. Komen*, 2013.

World Health Organization. "Breast Cancer: Prevention and Control." *World Health Organization*, 2013.

Bronchi

Anatomy
Anatomy or system affected: Lungs, respiratory system
Specialties and related fields: Pulmonary medicine
Definition: The large, rigid breathing tubes that connect the trachea to the inside of the lungs.

Structure and Functions

The bronchi are a direct continuation of the trachea, which separates into the right and left mainstem bronchi at the level of the fifth thoracicvertebra of the spinal column. They are composed of rings of cartilage supported by thick muscle fibers with a mucous membrane interior coating. This structure renders the bronchi rigid and not easily collapsible. The left bronchus is about 5 centimeters in length and enters the lung at the level of the sixth thoracic vertebra. The right bronchus is shorter, measuring about 2.5 centimeters in length, and enters the lung at the level of the fifth thoracic vertebra. The right bronchus also differs in that it is wider and runs at a more vertical angle than its left counterpart. The bronchi join with the lung, becoming the lobar bronchi, and further branch into subsequently smaller bronchi, eventually being called the bronchioles.

The bronchi serve primarily to transport air between the trachea and the lungs. They bring freshly oxygenated air into the lungs from the outside environment and transport old, carbon dioxide-filled air out of the lungs.

Disorders and Diseases

The bronchi are susceptible to a variety of diseases and dysfunctions, the most common being bronchitis. Bronchitis is an inflammation of the bronchi and can be secondary to various mechanisms. Acute bronchitis is usually infectious and is most common during the winter season. The symptoms are nonspecific and can include fever, cough, nasal congestion, and wheezing. Acute bronchitis can be caused by viruses such as influenza and bacteria such as *Mycoplasma pneumoniae* and *Chlamydia pneumoniae*. It can also be caused by various noninfectious outdoor or household irritants. Treatment consists of antibiotics for bacterial causes, bronchodilator inhalers, over-the-counter fever reducers and cough suppressants, fluids, and rest. Chronic bronchitis is a separate disorder of inflammation of the bronchi that is common in smokers. A cough productive of sputum for three months and occurring for at least two years in a row is required for formal diagnosis. Symptoms are similar to those of acute bronchitis. There is no cure for chronic bronchitis, but treatment aimed at symptom control often involves bronchodilator inhalers, steroids, and smoking cessation.

Asthma involves chronic inflammation of the lungs with consequent narrowing of the bronchi and airway obstruction, leading to episodes of coughing, wheezing, and difficulty breathing. Treatment involves bronchodilators such as albuterol, steroids, and leukotriene modifiers.

Additionally, the precipitous downward angle of the right mainstem bronchus lends itself to foreign body impaction, especially in children. It also makes it easier for liquids to enter the right lung, causing an aspiration pneumonia.

—*Jennifer Birkhauser, M.S., M.D.*

See also: Asthma; Bronchiolitis; Bronchitis; Chest; Coughing; Emphysema; Influenza; Lung cancer; Lung surgery; Lungs; Pneumonia; Pulmonary diseases; Pulmonary medicine; Pulmonary medicine, pediatric; Respiration; Respiratory distress syndrome; Smoking; Wheezing.

For Further Information:

American Lung Association. "How Lungs Work." *American Lung Association*, 2013.

Balch, Phyllis. "Bronchitis." In *Prescription for Nutritional Healing*, edited by Phyllis Balch. New York: Avery, 2006.

Lazaroff, Michael. "What Goes In Must Come Out." In *The Complete Idiot's Guide to Anatomy and Physiology*, edited by Jennifer Chisholm. New York: Alpha Books, 2004.

MedlinePlus. "Bronchial Disorders." *MedlinePlus*, June 26, 2013.

National Heart, Lung, and Blood Institute. "The Respiratory System." *National Institutes of Health*, July 17, 2012.

Orenstein, David. "The Respiratory System." In *Cystic Fibrosis: A Guide for Patient and Family*, edited by David Orenstein. New York: Lippincott Williams & Wilkins, 2003.

Bronchiolitis

Disease/Disorder

Anatomy or system affected: Chest, lungs, respiratory system

Specialties and related fields: Family medicine, internal medicine, pediatrics, pulmonary medicine

Definition: An inflammation of the bronchioles that affects breathing and the transfer of oxygen to the bloodstream.

Causes and Symptoms

Bronchiolitis is caused by an infection that inflames and narrows the bronchioles, the smallest branches in the respiratory system, which carry air from the large bronchial tubes to microscopic air sacs in the lungs. The infection is most often viral, though it can also be bacterial or a combination of the two. It usually affects children under two, sometimes after a cold, and is contagious and may become epidemic. Symptoms include sudden breathing difficulty characterized by rapid, shallow breathing, wheezing, fever, dehydration, and retractions of the chest and abdomen. In severe cases, the skin or nails may turn blue.

Information on Bronchiolitis

Causes: Viral or bacterial infection

Symptoms: Sudden breathing difficulty (rapid, shallow breathing), wheezing, fever, dehydration, retractions of chest and abdomen

Duration: Temporary, sometimes chronic

Treatments: Moist air, antibiotics, antiviral medications, bronchodilators

Treatment and Therapy

The general treatment of bronchiolitis involves keeping the patient's room as humid as possible with a cool-mist humidifier or by running cold or hot water in the shower with the windows and doors closed. In the case of bacterial infections, a doctor can prescribe antibiotics, and antiviral medications may be helpful in severe cases of viral infection. In addition, bronchodilators, drugs that widen the airways in the lungs, may prove helpful. The patient should frequently drink clear fluids, such as water, carbonated drinks, lemonade, weak bouillon, diluted fruit juice, or gelatin, to help thin mucus secretions and avoid dehydration. Diagnostic measures include parental observation of symptoms, physical examination by a doctor, laboratory blood studies, and x-rays of the lungs. With proper treatment, the disorder is typically curable within seven days.

Perspective and Prospects

Bronchiolitis is usually a disease of early infancy, with almost 90 percent of the patients being less than one year of age. It is important that bronchiolitis be diagnosed and treated properly because it can lead to chronic bronchitis, collapse of a small portion of a lung, repeated bouts of pneumonia, and, in some cases, chronic obstructive pulmonary disease. Studies also indicate that infants who have two or more episodes of bronchiolitis prior to age two are more prone to developing allergies and asthma.

—*Alvin K. Benson, Ph.D.*

See also: Antibiotics; Bacterial infections; Bronchi; Bronchitis; Childhood infectious diseases; Common cold; Lungs; Pneumonia; Pulmonary medicine, pediatric; Respiration; Viral infections; Wheezing.

For Further Information:

"Bronchiolitis." *MayoClinic.com*, Sept. 25, 2010.

Kaneshiro, Neil K., and David Zieve. "Bronchiolitis." *MedlinePlus*, Aug. 2, 2011.

Mason, Robert J., et al., eds. *Murray and Nadel's Textbook of Respiratory Medicine*. 5th ed. Philadelphia: Elsevier/Saunders, 2010.

Myers, Adam K. *Respiratory System*. Philadelphia: Elsevier/Mosby, 2006.

Niederman, Michael S., George A. Sarosi, and Jeffrey Glassroth. *Respiratory Infections*. 2d ed. Philadelphia: Lippincott Williams & Wilkins, 2001.

Pennington, James E. *Respiratory Infections: Diagnosis and Management*. 3d ed. Hoboken, N.J.: Raven Press, 1994.

West, John B. *Pulmonary Pathophysiology: The Essentials*. 8th ed. Philadelphia: Lippincott Williams & Wilkins, 2013.

Bronchitis

Disease/Disorder

Anatomy or system affected: Chest, lungs, respiratory system

Specialties and related fields: Family medicine, internal medicine, pulmonary medicine

Definition: An inflammation of the bronchial tree of the lungs.

Causes and Symptoms

The inflammation associated with bronchitis may be localized or diffuse, acute or chronic, and it is usually caused by infections or physical agents. In its infectious form, acute bronchitis is part of a general, acute upper respiratory infection, sometimes brought on by the common cold. It

Information on Bronchitis

Causes: Upper respiratory infection, chronic pulmonary disease, physical and chemical irritants

Symptoms: Swollen mucous membranes, bronchial spasms, shortness of breath

Duration: Acute

Treatments: Antibiotics, bed rest, exposure to warm, moist air

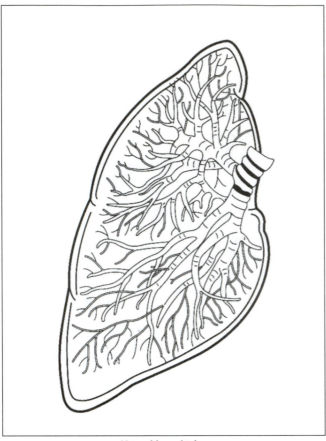

Normal bronchioles.

can also develop from a viral infection of the nasopharynx, throat, or tracheobronchial tree. Acute bronchitis is most prevalent in winter. Factors contributing to the onset of the disease include exposure, chilling, malnutrition, fatigue, or rickets. The inflammation may be serious in debilitated patients and those with chronic pulmonary disease, and the real danger rests in the development of pneumonia. Certain physical and chemical irritants can bring on acute bronchitis. Such agents as mineral and vegetable dusts, strong acid fumes, volatile organic compounds, and tobacco smoke can trigger an attack.

The disease causes thickening of the bronchi and a loss of elasticity in the bronchial tree. Changes in the mucous membranes occur, leukocytes infiltrate the submucosa, and a sticky, mucopurulent exudate is formed. The normally sterile bronchi are invaded by bacteria and cellular debris. A barking cough is often present, and this serves as an essential mechanism for eliminating bronchial secretions.

Chronic bronchitis is characterized by swollen mucous membranes, tenacious exudate, and spasms in the bronchiolar muscles. The result is dyspnea, the ventilatory insufficiency known as shortness of breath.

Treatment and Therapy

Acute bronchitis is treated with bed rest and medication to counteract the symptoms of inflammation. The room air should be kept warm and humid. Steam inhalation and cough syrup sometimes give relief from the severe, painful cough.

All surveys have demonstrated a high incidence of bronchitis in cigarette smokers when compared with nonsmokers, thus providing a good reason for the cessation of smoking.

—*Jane A. Slezak, Ph.D.*

See also: Asbestos exposure; Chronic obstructive pulmonary disease (COPD); Coughing; Inflammation; Lungs; Oxygen therapy; Pneumonia; Pulmonary diseases; Pulmonary medicine; Pulmonary medicine, pediatric; Respiration; Wheezing.

For Further Information:
American Lung Association. *American Lung Association*, 2013.
Center for Disease Control and Prevention. "Bronchitis (Chest Cold). *CDC*, May 1, 2012.
Goldman, Lee, and Dennis Ausiello, eds. *Cecil Textbook of Medicine*. 23d ed. Philadelphia: Saunders, 2007.
Niederman, Michael S., George A. Sarosi, and Jeffrey Glassroth. *Respiratory Infections*. 2d ed. Philadelphia: Lippincott, 2001.
Shuman, Jill. "Bronchitis (Acute Bronchitis; Lower Respiratory Tract Infection)." *HealthLibrary*, Mar. 29, 2013.
Shayevitz, Myra, and Berton R. Shayevitz. *Living Well with Chronic Asthma, Bronchitis, and Emphysema*. Yonkers, N.Y.: Consumer Reports Books, 1991.
Smolley, Laurence A., and Debra Fulghum Bruce. *Breathe Right Now: A Comprehensive Guide to Understanding and Treating the Most Common Breathing Disorders*. New York: Norton, 1998.
West, John B. *Pulmonary Pathophysiology: The Essentials*. 7th ed. Philadelphia: Lippincott, 2008.

Brucellosis

Disease/Disorder

Also known as: Malta fever, undulant fever

Anatomy or system affected: Brain, heart, joints, liver, musculoskeletal system, nervous system, reproductive system, spine, spleen

Specialties and related fields: Bacteriology, cardiology, epidemiology, microbiology, neurology, occupational health, preventive medicine, public health, rheumatology

Definition: A bacterial infection transmitted to humans from infected livestock and wildlife that is usually acquired from unpasteurized dairy products.

Key terms:

antibiotics: drugs that inhibit or kill bacteria and are used to treat bacterial infections

chronic: a disease of long duration, typically several weeks, months, or years

pasteurization: a method first described by the French scientist Louis Pasteur for killing bacteria in food and beverages

relapse: the recurrence of signs and symptoms after they have subsided or ceased

vaccine: a substance, usually injected, that stimulates the immune system to protect the body against a specific infectious disease

zoonotic: an infection of animals that can be transmitted to humans

Causes and Symptoms

Brucellosis is a zoonotic disease, an infection that humans acquire from infected animals. Brucellosis is caused by

Brucella bacteria transmitted to humans from cattle, sheep, goats, elk, bison, caribou (reindeer), and wild pigs. The bacteria have been found in porpoises, harbor seals, some types of whales, and dogs. Most human cases are acquired by consuming unpasteurized milk, cheese, and other dairy products. People working in microbiology labs, slaughterhouses, and meat-packing plants get brucellosis by inhaling airborne droplets contaminated with the bacteria. The bacteria also enter the body through contact with wounds and mucous membranes (eyes, nose, and mouth). Veterinarians and hunters are exposed to brucellosis in this way. Person-to-person transmission is rare, as is transmission by breast milk, transplant, and transfusion (blood donation). Transmission by sexual contact has not been documented.

After ingestion, inhalation, or contact, the bacteria move into the blood. *Brucella* do not remain in the blood for long; they invade a variety of human cells, which protects the bacteria from the immune system. Once in the blood, the bacteria enter white blood cells called neutrophils. The neutrophils normally seek out, ingest, and destroy bacteria. However, *Brucella* enter neutrophils and remain alive because the bacteria produce substances that inhibit the immune functions of neutrophils. The infected neutrophils enter the lymphatic system, a network of vessels that filters tissue fluids (called lymph when inside the vessels) and returns it to the circulatory system. In this way, *Brucella* spread throughout the body and invade cells of nearly every organ system. The bacteria infect the liver, spleen, kidneys, joints, breasts, and central nervous system. Reproduction of the bacteria in these organs causes tissue damage, and triggers the characteristic signs and symptoms of brucellosis.

Symptoms arise days to months following exposure to *Brucella*. The first symptoms resemble a severe flu-like illness, and include fever, headache, fatigue, malaise (a feeling of ill health), anorexia (loss of appetite), and pain in muscles, back, and joints. These symptoms are caused by the immune system's response to the infection. However, the immune response to these bacteria is ineffective because most of the bacteria reside inside the body's cells. Fever and symptoms often decline during infection. However, bacterial reproduction kills cells, which release the bacteria, inducing another wave of fever and symptoms. Brucellosis has been called undulant fever for these returning fevers. If untreated, the disease progresses and becomes chronic. A chronic infection lasts many weeks or months, perhaps years.

Chronic infection is characterized by recurrent fevers and relapses. A relapse is the return of signs and symptoms. Chronic brucellosis is associated with arthritis, inflammation of joints, and spondylitis, inflammation of the joints between bones of the spinal column. Arthritis and spondylitis are painful and disabling. Endocarditis, inflammation of the inner lining of the heart, is a particularly dangerous aspect of chronic brucellosis. In addition, brucellosis affects the nervous system, causing encephalitis, inflammation of the brain, and meningitis, inflammation of membranes surrounding the brain and spinal cord.

Information on Brucellosis

Causes: Bacterial infection; consumption of unpasteurized dairy products from infected animals; contact with infected livestock or wildlife
Symptoms: Recurrent fever, headache, muscle, back, and joint pain, arthritis, fatigue
Duration: Several weeks or chronic
Treatments: Antibiotics

Encephalitis and meningitis are serious complications of brucellosis. The bacteria cause swelling in other organs, including the liver, spleen, testes, epididymis (tubes that carry sperm from the testes), and scrotum. Some patients experience chronic fatigue and depression. Brucellosis is rarely fatal, resulting in death in probably less than 2 percent of cases in the United States. Most fatalities are related to endocarditis or severe neurologic disease (meningitis or encephalitis).

Infected animals exhibit no external signs of disease. Infected livestock such as cattle, goats, sheep, and domestic bison may abort spontaneously or produce weak offspring. Reduced milk production is associated with infection, but can be caused by other diseases and disorders. Fortunately, brucellosis has been nearly eradicated from domestic livestock in the United States.

Treatment and Therapy

Most cases of brucellosis turn out well. However, early diagnosis and treatment are important for making full recovery and preventing serious, disabling complications associated with chronic, relapsing disease. Diagnosis is based on the symptoms, laboratory tests, and a history of recent activities, such as travel abroad, that may have resulted in exposure to brucellosis. Brucellosis is well-controlled in U.S. livestock and outbreaks of brucellosis among humans are unexpected. Most brucellosis cases in the United States are acquired abroad through consumption of unpasteurized dairy products, particularly cheese from goats and sheep in countries where brucellosis is not well controlled. An outbreak in the United States is so unlikely that any brucellosis outbreak is investigated as a possible bioterrorist event. Thus, given a history of exposure, and symptoms consistent with brucellosis, laboratory tests confirm the presence of an ongoing infection.

Blood tests permit detection of antibodies to the bacteria. Antibodies are substances produced by white blood cells in response to infectious agents such as viruses and bacteria. The body produces antibodies that are specific for each type of infectious agent. Thus, the presence of antibodies for *Brucella* is a reliable sign of brucellosis. If the bacteria are present in the blood, the blood may be cultured in a microbiology lab. A blood culture applies a sample of blood to nutrients that promote the growth of bacteria. Once the bacteria grow they can be identified as *Brucella*. Because *Brucella* travel widely through the body, other body fluids and bone marrow can also be cultured. To determine if meningitis or encephalitis is related to brucellosis, cerebrospinal fluid is sampled and studied in the laboratory. Cerebrospinal fluid surrounds and protects the brain and spinal cord. The fluid is obtained by lumbar puncture, a procedure in which a needle is inserted between the vertebrae of the lower back to draw fluid into a syringe. Healthy cerebrospinal fluid contains no bacteria. An echocardiogram, an image of the heart's internal structure, detects signs of endocarditis.

Antibiotics are drugs that kill bacteria and these drugs are an effective treatment for brucellosis. Six weeks to several months of antibiotic therapy are required, depending on the severity of the infection. In many cases, people take a combination of two different antibiotics. Arthritis and spondylitis are treated with analgesics, medications that reduce pain. Meningitis and encephalitis are treated with drugs that suppress inflammation.

Brucellosis can be prevented by reducing the risk of exposure. Unpasteurized dairy products, including milk and cheese, should not be consumed, especially when traveling abroad. So-called "village cheeses," usually made from goat and sheep milk are known to carry brucellosis. Meat should always be fully cooked before serving. Workers in meat-packing and slaughterhouse facilities should follow their employer's and OSHA (Occupational Safety Health Administration) standards regarding safe handling of meat. These procedures may include the use of personal protective gear such as gloves and eye protection (to prevent splashes with contaminated fluids). Microbiology laboratory workers who study material contaminated with brucellosis bacteria should also follow similar precautions established by the laboratory employer and OSHA. Hunters should wear gloves to protect their hands when dressing game, especially elk, moose, and wild pigs. Game meat should be stored properly and cooked thoroughly before serving.

Perspective and Prospects

A Scottish physician, Sir David Bruce, first described the *Brucella* bacteria in 1887. Bruce made important discoveries about the disease among goats on the Mediterranean island of Malta, which is the source of this disease's former name, Malta fever.

Brucellosis once caused enormous losses in the U.S. livestock industry. In 1952, reduced milk production and livestock losses cost the industry $400 million. Infected cattle and other livestock drove a relatively high rate of human brucellosis in the United States. As of 2013 brucellosis is uncommon in the United States, affecting about 100 people each year. The infection has become uncommon because of the Cooperative State Federal Brucellosis Eradication Program, begun in 1934. This program has nearly eradicated brucellosis among domestic livestock. In 1934 11.5 percent of cattle herds in the United States tested positive for brucellosis. As of 2000, only six herds tested positive, and they had a low infection rate of less than 0.25 percent.

Continued prevention of human infections depends on effective control of animal brucellosis. The disease is in-

curable in animals. Thus, control has relied on vaccination and herd screening, followed by removal and killing of infected animals. The vaccine is effective at preventing infection in cattle. However, it is less effective at preventing disease in domestic bison. Scientists are seeking an improved vaccine because bison can transmit the infection to cattle. Wildlife such as elk and bison in the Yellowstone area carry and can transmit brucellosis to domestic livestock. Control of brucellosis in wild elk and bison has proven to be difficult because these animals migrate and gather in large numbers near food during winter. Congregating elk and bison are more likely to spread the infection within a herd. More important, wild elk and bison can enter ranchland and expose domestic cattle and bison to infection. To prevent congregation of wild herds of elk and bison, the United States Animal Health Association recommends that wildlife managers stop the practice of feeding wild herds during the winter. However, most human cases of brucellosis in the United States do not occur in the states of Yellowstone (Montana, Wyoming, and Idaho). Over half of human infections occur in California, Texas, Arizona, and Florida.

Worldwide, brucellosis is not well controlled in domestic and wild animals, which results in enormous economic losses and about 500,000 human infections each year. Brucellosis is most common in countries with underdeveloped public health or domestic animal health programs, and where pasteurization and animal vaccination is not systematically practiced. Most cases of brucellosis occur in countries around the Mediterranean Sea, Eastern Europe, Africa, Middle East, India, Latin America, and the Caribbean.Considerable effort has been focused on developing more effective vaccines to control the infection in domestic livestock.

Vaccines have been effective in the United States, even though several species of *Brucella* are known. Only a few species cause disease in humans. These include *Brucella melitensis, B. suis, B. abortus,* and *B. canis.* Of these, *B. melitensis* causes the most serious disease in humans. It is transmitted by sheep and goats and has been eradicated in the United States, although it continues to cause disease worldwide. *B. suis* infects wild pigs and occasionally infects hunters. *B. abortus* has been nearly eradicated in the United States, although it persists in wild elk and wild bison. *B. canis* infects dogs and is an uncommon cause of infection in veterinarians and dog breeders. *B. ceti* infects porpoises and whales, and *B. pinnipediae* infects harbor seals. These rarely cause disease in humans.

—*Mark Zelman, Ph.D.*

See also: Antibodies; Bacteriology; Cardiology; Environmental health; Fatigue; Immunology; Immunopathology; Microbiology; Neurology; Rheumatology; Vascular medicine

For Further Information:
Biddle, Wayne. *Field Guide to Germs.* New York: Random House, 2002. All major infectious diseases are discussed in an engaging style for nonspecialists. It includes the historical significance of each infectious disease.

Corbel, Michael J., and Nick J. Beeching. "Brucellosis." *Harrison's Principles of Internal Medicine,* edited by Antony S. Fauci, et al., 16th ed. New York: McGraw-Hill, 2004. This excellent chapter on brucellosis is aimed at specialists, clinicians, and researchers.

Franco, Maria Pia, Maximilian Mulder, Robert H. Gilman, and Henk L. Smits. "Human Brucellosis." *Lancet Infectious Diseases* 7 (2007): 775-786. This review article summarizes current knowledge about the advances and challenges regarding the treatment and prevention of brucellosis.

Mackay, Katurah. "Bison Plan Called 'Absurd.'" *National Parks* 72, nos. 7-8 (November-December, 1998): 14-15. This article reports the difficulties ranchers and wildlife biologists face when planning brucellosis control measures in the western Unites States, where brucellosis persists in wild bison and wild elk.?

Pommerville, Jeffrey C. *Alcamo's Fundamentals of Microbiology.* 9th ed. Sudbury, MA: Jones and Bartlett, 2011. An excellent, comprehensive college level text on the principles and practice of microbiology. It includes a discussion of the fundamentals of many infectious diseases.

Professional Guide to Diseases. 10th ed. Springhouse, PA: Lippincott Williams & Wilkins, 2013. This book describes the cause, signs and symptoms, diagnosis, treatment, and prevention for human diseases.

Radostits, Otto M., Clive C. Gay, Douglas C. Blood, and Ken W. Hinchcliff. *Veterinary Medicine: A Textbook of the Diseases of Cattle, Sheep, Pigs, Goats and Horses.* London: Harcourt Publishers Limited, 2000. This comprehensive specialist text summarizes the diagnosis, treatment, and prevention of most diseases in these animals. The text is aimed at doctors of veterinary medicine and researchers.

Bruises

Disease/Disorder

Also known as: Ecchymoses, contusions, hematomas

Anatomy or system affected: Blood vessels, lymphatic system, skin

Specialties and related fields: Emergency medicine, family medicine, hematology, pediatrics, vascular medicine

Definition: A bruise is an area of skin that has become discolored, usually as a result of trauma (a fall or hit to the affected area).

Causes and Symptoms

A bruise is a usually benign condition that happens when an individual has some type of injury. It may be a fall or a direct blow to any part of the body. As a result of the trauma, the affected body part undergoes various changes. A bruise can also occur spontaneously (a more serious illness or disease state) or from an allergic reaction. In most cases, bruises are not serious and resolve without any medical treatment.

Bruises occur when small blood vessels that are just beneath the skin are broken. They then begin to leak their contents (blood) into the surrounding soft tissue underneath the skin, which produces the characteristic black-and-blue discoloration. There are three types of bruises: subcutaneous (just beneath the skin), intramuscular (in the underlying muscle), and periosteal (in the bone). Bruises can last from several days to months. The typical black-and-blue mark begins to fade as the blood that leaked into the surrounding tissue is reabsorbed. The discoloration turns to a light yellowish-green and then fades completely.

Information on Bruises

Causes: Bleeding under the skin following injury; sometimes an allergic reaction or clotting disorder

Symptoms: Black-and-blue skin discoloration, pain, swelling

Duration: Acute

Treatments: Ice, analgesics, sometimes heat

Treatment and Therapy

The initial treatment of bruises should include decreasing the bleeding, minimizing any swelling, and controlling the pain. Ice is very effective and should be applied to the affected area for thirty to sixty minutes at a time. This can be done several times a day for two to three days. The ice should be in a container and covered by a towel to prevent damage to the skin. If possible, the affected area should be elevated above heart level. This helps in minimizing the swelling, which also helps decrease pain. If there is still discomfort after this period, then heat can be applied for twenty minutes at a time. The application of heat will help the blood to be reabsorbed into the tissue. The last component of the treatment regimen should include pain control. Pain can be easily controlled by using acetaminophen (Tylenol) or ibuprofen (Advil or Motrin).

Medical care should be sought if there is increased pain, a decrease in function (the affected part can no longer be used), headache, dizziness, fever (101 degrees Fahrenheit or more), or a noticeable change in vision, or if the symptoms continue.

Perspective and Prospects

Bruises are benign conditions that usually resolve without treatment. Simple self-care therapies will generally decrease discomfort and aid in a complete return to normal. Bruises are significant, however, in an individual experiencing bruising without any clear reason for the occurrence. In this case, bruises can be indicative of something more serious, such as clotting disorders or other diseases.

—*Rosslynn S. Byous, D.P.A., PA-C*

See also: Accidents; Bleeding; Blood and blood disorders; Dermatology; Dermatology, pediatric; Emergency medicine; Emergency medicine, pediatric; Hematology; Hematology, pediatric; Safety issues for children; Safety issues for the elderly; Skin; Skin disorders.

For Further Information:

"Bruise." *Medline Plus*, May 1, 2011.

"Bruises, First Aid." *Logical Images*, December 22, 2008.

"Bruising and Bleeding." *Merck Manual Home Health Handbook*, May 2012.

Gottlieb, William. *Alternative Cures: More than One Thousand of the Most Effective Natural Home Remedies*. Emmaus, Pa.: Rodale, 2008.

Griffith, H. Winter. *Complete Guide to Sports Injuries: How to Treat Fractures, Bruises, Sprains, Strains, Dislocations, Head Injuries*. 3d ed. New York: Body Press/Perigee, 2004.

The Doctors Book of Home Remedies. Rev. ed. New York: Bantam Books, 2009.

Bulimia

Disease/Disorder
Also known as: Bulimia nervosa
Anatomy or system affected: Blood, brain, gastrointestinal system, gums, heart, intestines, musculoskeletal system, nerves, psychic-emotional system, teeth
Specialties and related fields: Biochemistry, family medicine, gastroenterology, nutrition, psychiatry, psychology
Definition: An eating disorder that is characterized by repeated, uncontrollable episodes of overeating followed by induced vomiting or laxative abuse to eliminate the undigested food.

Information on Bulimia

Causes: Emotional and psychological disorders pertaining to body image
Symptoms: Intense preoccupation with food and weight, eating binges followed by self-induced vomiting or ingestion of laxatives, depression, suicidal feelings, nutritional deficiencies, dehydration, hormonal changes, gastrointestinal problems, heart disorders, persistent sore throat, tooth and gum damage
Duration: Chronic
Treatments: Psychotherapy, nutritional counseling, medication

---

Causes and Symptoms

Bulimia is typically regarded as a psychologically based disorder caused by childhood experiences, family influences, and social pressures, particularly on young women to be thinner than natural. Many people who develop bulimia have been overweight in the past and suffer from poor self-image and depression. Body weight is often within normal limits, but persons with bulimia perceive themselves as fat and are often obsessed with their body image. Others may have a history of sexual or physical abuse or of alcohol or drug abuse. Medical research suggests that bulimia may be partially caused by impaired secretion of cholecystokinin (CKK), a hormone that normally induces a feeling of fullness after a meal, or by depletion of the chemical serotonin in the brain, which contributes to a craving for carbohydrates.

Intense preoccupation with food and weight are invariably present, and eating binges are followed with self-induced vomiting or the ingestion of laxatives to rid the body of the consumed food. Depression and suicidal feelings sometimes accompany bulimia. The disorder can cause nutritional deficiencies, dehydration, hormonal changes, gastrointestinal problems, changes in metabolism and blood chemistry, heart disorders, persistent sore throat, and teeth and gum damage as a result of the acidic nature of regurgitated food.

Treatment and Therapy

Treatment of bulimia requires a combination of nutritional counseling, medication, and psychotherapy. Psychotherapists try to get to the root of any underlying psychological problems and resolve them. Various modes of group and cognitive behavioral therapy have proven effective.

Cognitive therapy usually includes confronting people with bulimia about their inaccurate perceptions of body weight and making contracts with them to shift their focus to nutrition rather than weight gain in exchange for rewards. Group therapy has helped many bulimics stop their binge eating, while treatment with antidepressant drugs, especially fluoxetine (Prozac), has helped many bulimic patients gain partial or full relief from their symptoms. Hospitalization is common treatment and is virtually always necessary if body weight is more than 30 percent below ideal.

Perspective and Prospects

Bulimia was classified as a distinct disorder by the American Psychiatric Association in 1980; the name was officially changed to bulimia nervosa in 1987. The disorder occurs mostly in adolescent and young adult females, with only about 10 percent of cases in males. Many cases of bulimia end after a few weeks or months but may reoccur. Other cases last for years without interruption.

In 2006, researchers developed a new test that analyzes carbon and nitrogen in hair, which is suggestive of eating disorders. This technique is beneficial because eating disorders are difficult to diagnose, in part because sufferers sometimes do not know that they have an eating disorder or do not want to be honest. By analyzing just five strands of hair, researchers were able to diagnose anorexia and bulimia accurately 80 percent of the time. This test may hasten treatment and prove an effective and objective method of monitoring recovery.

—Alvin K. Benson, Ph.D.;
updated by LeAnna DeAngelo, Ph.D.

See also: Anorexia nervosa; Eating disorders; Hyperadiposis; Malnutrition; Nausea and vomiting; Nutrition; Obesity; Phobias; Psychiatric disorders; Psychiatry, child and adolescent; Puberty and adolescence; Weight loss and gain; Weight loss medications; Women's health.

For Further Information:
Fairburn, Christopher G., and Kelley D. Brownell, eds. *Eating Disorders and Obesity: A Comprehensive Handbook*. 2d ed. New York: Guilford, 2005.
Maj, Mario, et al., eds. *Eating Disorders*. New York: Wiley, 2003.
National Association of Anorexia Nervosa and Associated Disorders. *ANAD*, 2013.
National Eating Disorders Association. *NEDA*, n. d.
Parker, James M., and Philip M. Parker, eds. *The 2002 Official Patient's Sourcebook on Binge Eating Disorder*. San Diego, Calif.: Icon Health, 2002.
Reindl, Shiela M. *Sensing the Self: Women's Recovery from Bulimia*. Cambridge, Mass.: Harvard UP, 2001.
Swain, Pamela I., ed. *Anorexia Nervosa and Bulimia Nervosa: New Research*. New York: Nova Science, 2006.
Vorvick, Linda J. "Bulimia." *MedlinePlus*, Feb. 13, 2012.
Wood, Debra. "Bulimia Nervosa (Bulimia)." *Health Library*, Sept. 10, 2012.

Bunions

Disease/Disorder
Anatomy or system affected: Bones, feet

Specialties and related fields: Family medicine, general surgery, orthopedics, podiatry

Definition: An enlargement that develops on the joint of the big toe, producing deformity, pain, and discomfort.

Causes and Symptoms

A bunion, or hallux valgus, is a swelling on the foot, usually at the joint of the big toe, that is caused by a misaligned bone in the joint. Bunions often develop with aging as a result of widening of the feet, arthritic conditions, or the wearing of improperly fitted shoes. Typically, the misaligned bone protrudes outward at the joint of the big toe, giving the bunion its bulging appearance. The bursa, a fluid-filled sac in the joint, becomes inflamed and swells, often twisting the big toe toward the second toe. Since the big toe supports most of the body's weight every time an individual pushes off the ground, a bunion can cause severe pain and discomfort. In addition, because bunions can change the shape of the feet, it becomes much harder for an aging sufferer to find shoes that fit properly.

While bunions themselves cannot be inherited, an individual can inherit the tendency to develop bunions by being born with extra bone near a toe joint. The risk of developing bunions can be reduced by exercising daily to keep the muscles of the feet and legs in good condition and by wearing wide-toed shoes that fit well. Women tend to develop bunions more than men do, possibly because many women wear shoes that are too small or narrow. Symptoms of bunions include pain, redness, stiffness, swelling, thickness of the skin over the bunion, fluid accumulation under the thickened skin, and the eventual development of osteoarthritis that impairs the joint's flexibility.

Treatment and Therapy

If a bunion is not severe, greater comfort can come from simply wearing a different style of shoe, including those that have been stretched in the big toe area, that are made of soft leather, or that have cushioned insoles. Sandals with

---

Information on Bunions

Causes: Misaligned bone joint from aging, arthritic conditions, improperly fitting shoes

Symptoms: Toe deformity, pain, discomfort, redness, stiffness

Duration: Acute to chronic

Treatments: Well-fitting shoes, bunion pads, moist heating pad or ice pack, anti-inflammatory medication, outpatient surgery

---

cross straps and athletic shoes are best for providing maximum comfort for people with bunions. Other ways to relieve the pain include using shoe inserts called bunion pads, using a moist heating pad on the bunion at night, applying an ice pack to reduce swelling, and taking an over-the-counter anti-inflammatory medication such as aspirin or ibuprofen (Advil or Motrin). Aging persons with medical conditions should read product labels carefully and consult their doctor or a pharmacist before taking pain-relieving medications. If home care measures do not provide relief, a podiatrist (foot doctor) may prescribe a special shoe insert known as an orthotic device.

For severe bunions, outpatient surgery may be required. The most common surgery reduces the angle between the big and second toes. Bones in the big toe are realigned, and the bunion is shaved away. Ligaments and tendons on the outside of the toe may be tightened to hold the joint properly, while any tight tendons on the inside of the toe are released. Bunion surgery can reduce pain and improve the appearance of the feet. Recovery involves the use of crutches to keep weight off the foot, and the majority of healing typically occurs within a few weeks. After surgery, pain will gradually subside and deformity of the foot will improve. However, tight shoes must still be avoided.

—*Alvin K. Benson, Ph.D.*

See also: Bones and the skeleton; Fallen arches; Feet; Foot disorders; Hammertoe correction; Hammertoes; Orthopedic surgery; Orthopedics; Podiatry.

For Further Information:

Bentley, George, and Robert B. Greer, eds. *Orthopaedics*. 4th ed. Oxford, England: Linacre House, 1993.

"Bunion Removal." *Medline Plus*, March 1, 2012.

"Bunions." *Medline Plus*, February 27, 2012.

Copeland, Glenn, and Stan Solomon. *The Foot Doctor: Lifetime Relief for Your Aching Feet*. Rev. ed. Toronto, Ont.: Macmillan Canada, 1996.

Frowen, Paul, et al., eds. *Neale's Disorders of the Foot*. 8th ed. New York: Churchill Livingstone/Elsevier, 2010.

Lippert, Frederick G., and Sigvard T. Hansen. *Foot and Ankle Disorders: Tricks of the Trade*. New York: Thieme, 2003.

Rose, Jonathan D. *The Foot Book: A Complete Guide to Healthy Feet*. Baltimore: John Hopkins University Press, 2011.

"What to Ask Your Foot and Ankle Surgeon about Bunion Surgery." *American College of Foot and Ankle Surgeons*, December 15, 2009.

A bunion, a bony overgrowth of the big toe, can be removed surgically by cutting off the excess segment of bone, thus reshaping the foot.

Burkitt's lymphoma

Disease/Disorder

Anatomy or system affected: All, especially lymphatic system

Specialties and related fields: Family medicine, hematology, internal medicine, oncology, pediatrics

Definition: A highly aggressive lymphoma often presenting in extranodal sites or as an acute leukemia.

Causes and Symptoms

The three different clinical variants of Burkitt lymphoma-endemic, sporadic, and immunodeficiency-associated-have varying clinical manifestations and epidemiologies. Endemic Burkitt lymphoma occurs in equatorial Africa and Papua, New Guinea, most commonly in children. In this form, the jaws and other facial bones are the site of manifestation in about half of the cases. Other extranodal sites may be involved, such as the distal ileum, cecum, omentum, ovaries, kidneys, and breasts, as well as the central nervous system. Sporadic Burkitt lymphoma occurs throughout the world and mainly in children and young adults. In this form, jaw tumors are less frequent, and the majority of these cases manifest as abdominal masses. Immunodeficiency-associated Burkitt lymphoma is seen primarily in association with human immunodeficiency virus (HIV) infection.

Epstein-Barr virus (EBV) plays an important role in endemic Burkitt lymphoma, and the EBV genome is present in the majority of the neoplastic cells of these patients. In sporadic Burkitt lymphoma, however, the frequency of EBV association is much lower (less than 30 percent of cases). In immunodeficiency-associated Burkitt lymphoma, EBV is identified in only 25 to 40 percent of cases. While the exact relationship of EBV to the pathogenesis of Burkitt lymphoma is not understood, it is known that genetic abnormalities involving chromosome 8 play an essential role in Burkitt lymphoma.

Treatment and Therapy

In endemic and sporadic Burkitt lymphoma, the tumor is highly aggressive but potentially curable. Endemic Burkitt lymphoma is highly sensitive to intensive combination chemotherapy and results in high cure rates (up to 90 percent) in patients with low-stage disease and significant cure rates (60 to 80 percent) in patients with advanced disease. Bone marrow and central nervous system involvement are associated with a poor prognosis, especially in sporadic Burkitt lymphoma. If Burkitt disease manifests as an acute leukemia, the treatment consists of very intensive chemotherapy of relatively short duration, which differs substantially from the current treatment of acute lymphoblastic leukemia.

Perspective and Prospects

Burkitt lymphoma is one of the first human cancers in which characteristic chromosomal translocations have been shown to be related to the development of the malignancy. This finding may be an important clue to the basic mechanism of the development of this cancer and hopefully will result in the prevention and complete cure of the disease.

—*Cherie H. Dunphy, M.D.*

See also: Cancer; Chemotherapy; Epstein-Barr virus; Human immunodeficiency virus (HIV); Leukemia; Lymphadenopathy and lymphoma; Lymphatic system; Malignancy and metastasis; Oncology; Radiation therapy.

For Further Information:

Dugdale III, David C., and David Zieve. "Burkitt Lymphoma." *MedlinePlus*, June 5, 2012.

Dugdale III, David C., and David Zieve. "Non-Hodgkin's Lymphoma." *MedlinePlus*, Mar. 4, 2012.

Gorczyca, Wojciech, with James Weisberger and Foxwell N. Emmons. *Atlas of Differential Diagnosis in Neoplastic Hematopathology.* 2d ed. New York: Taylor & Francis, 2008.

Jaffe, Elaine S., et al., eds. *Pathology and Genetics of Tumours of Haematopoietic and Lymphoid Tissues.* New York: Oxford University Press, 2001.

Knowles, Daniel M., ed. *Neoplastic Hematopathology.* 2d ed. Philadelphia: Lippincott Williams & Wilkins, 2001.

McCoy, Krisha, Rebecca J. Stahl, and Kari Kassir. "Non-Hodgkin's Lymphoma-Child." *Health Library*, Jan. 30, 2013.

"Non-Hodgkin Lymphoma in Children Overview." *American Cancer Society*, Oct. 30, 2012.

Burns and scalds

Disease/Disorder

Anatomy or system affected: Skin, other tissues in severe cases

Specialties and related fields: Critical care, dermatology, emergency medicine, physical therapy, plastic surgery

Definition: Injury to skin and other tissues caused by contact with dry heat (fire), moist heat (steam or hot liquid), chemicals, electricity, lightning, or radiation.

Key terms:

burn: an injury to tissues caused by contact with dry heat (fire), moist heat (steam or a hot liquid), chemicals, electricity, lightning, or radiation

burndegrees: system of classification for burns based on the depth of damage to the skin

major (or severe) burn: a burn covering more than 20 percent of the body and any deep burn of the hands, face, feet, or perineum

minor burn: a superficial burn of less than 5 percent of the body that can be treated without hospitalization

moderate burn: a burn that requires hospitalization but not specialized care

rule of nines: a system used to designate areas of the body, represented by various body parts; used in determining the extent of a burn

skin graft: a surgical graft of skin from one part of the body to another or from one individual to another

---

Information on Burkitt's Lymphoma

Causes: Unknown; may be related to chromosomal abnormalities, infection with HIV or Epstein-Barr virus

Symptoms: Jaw and facial tumors, abdominal masses, acute leukemia, bone marrow and central nervous system involvement

Duration: Chronic or acute

Treatments: Chemotherapy

Causes and Symptoms

Burns are injuries to tissues caused by contact with dry heat (fire), moist heat (steam or a hot liquid, also called scalds), chemicals, electricity, lightning, or radiation. The word "burn" comes from the Middle English *brinnen* or *brennen* (to burn) and from the Old English *byrnan* (to be on fire) combined with *baernan* (to set afire). Each year in the United States, more than two million people are burned or scalded badly enough to need medical treatment, and about seventy thousand require admission to a hospital. Globally, an estimated 265,000 deaths occur annually due to fires; fire-related deaths alone rank among the fifteen leading causes of death among individuals aged five to twenty-nine years (these figures do not include burns from scalding, electricity, chemicals, or radiation). Burns are most common in children and older people and in low-income countries; many burns are caused by accidents in the home that are preventable.

The severity of the burn is classified by how much of the surface area of the body is involved as well as the depth of the burn. Classification of burns are described as superficial-thickness wounds, partial-thickness wounds, full-thickness wounds, and deep full-thickness wounds.

Superficial-thickness burns involve damage only to the epidermis of the skin, and may be caused by a sunburn or exposure to high-intensity heat. There is redness with mild swelling, pain, and increased sensitivity to heat as a result of the burn. These types of burns heal quickly in 3 to 6 days without scarring.

Partial-thickness burns involve loss of tissue to the entire epidermal layer of the skin and some layers of the dermis. Depending on the depth, these wounds are further divided into superficial partial-thickness burns and deep partial-thickness burns. Superficial partial-thickness burns injure the upper third of the dermis, are pink and moist, and blanch when pressure is applied. Blisters are common and these wounds are painful due to exposed nerve endings. These burns heal within 10 to 21 days without scarring. Deep partial-thickness wounds involve deeper layers of the dermis. Typically there are no blisters. The wound is red and dry with white areas and it may or may not blanch. Pain is less than with superficial burns because more of the nerve endings have been destroyed. These wounds heal in 2 to 6 weeks and do scar.

Full-thickness burns destroy the entire epidermis and dermis. It has a hard, dry, leathery appearance of destroyed skin called eschar, which must be removed in order for healing to occur. It takes weeks to months to heal these wounds.

Deep full-thickness burns involve the skin and damage muscle, bone, and tendons. The wound is blackened and sensation is destroyed. Skin grafting is needed for healing.

Burns are also classified by the amount of total body surface area (TBSA) burned. Partial-thickness burns less than 10% TBSA or full-thickness burns less than 2% TBSA are classified as minor burns. Partial-thickness burns of 15-25% TBSA or full-thickness burns of 2-10% TBSA are classified as moderate burns. Partial-thickness burns

> ## Information on Burns and Scalds
>
> **Causes:** Fire, steam or hot liquid, chemicals, electricity, lightning, radiation
> **Symptoms:** Swelling, blisters, low blood pressure, very low urine output, infection, shock
> **Duration:** Temporary and acute; may be followed by long-term rehabilitation
> **Treatments:** Varies widely; ranges from cooling agents and antiseptic medication, to antibiotics and pain relief, to skin grafts, fluid and electrolyte maintenance, and high-protein diet

greater than 25% TBSA or full-thickness burns greater than 10% TBSA; any burn involving the eyes, ears, face, hands, feet, perineum; electrical injury; or inhalation injury is classified as a major burn.

The depth of the injury is proportional to the intensity of the heat of the causative agent and the duration of exposure. Burns can be classified according to the agent causing the damage. Some examples of burns according to this classification are brush burns, caused by friction of a rapidly moving object against the skin or ground into the skin; chemical burns, caused by exposure to a caustic chemical; flash burns, caused by very brief exposure to intense radiant heat (the typical burn of an atomic explosion); radiation burns, caused by exposure to radium, x-rays, or atomic energy; and respiratory burns, caused by inhalation of steam or explosive gases. Burns can also be classified as major or severe (involving more than 20 percent of the body and any deep burn of the hands, face, feet, or perineum), moderate (a burn that requires hospitalization but not specialized care, as with burns covering 5 to 20 percent of the body but without deep burns of hands, face, feet, or perineum), or minor (a superficial burn involving less than 5 percent of the body that can be treated without hospitalization).

While many domestic burns are minor and insignificant, more severe burns and scalds can prove to be dangerous. The main danger for a burn patient is the shock that arises as a result of loss of fluid from the circulating blood at the site of the burn. This loss of fluid leads to a fall in the volume of the circulating blood in the area. The maintenance of an adequate blood volume is essential to life, and the body attempts to compensate for this temporary loss by withdrawing fluid from the uninjured areas of the body into the circulation. In the first forty-eight hours after a severe burn is received, fluid from the blood vessels, salt, and protein pass into the burned area, causing swelling, blisters, low blood pressure, and very low urine output. The body loses fluids, proteins, and salt, and the potassium level is raised. Such low fluid levels are followed by a shift of fluid in the opposite direction, resulting in excess urine, high blood volume, and low concentration of blood electrolytes. If carried too far, this condition begins to affect the viability of the body cells. As a result, essential body cells such as those of the liver and kidneys begin to suffer, eventually causing the liver and kidneys to cease proper function. Liver and renal failure are revealed by the development of

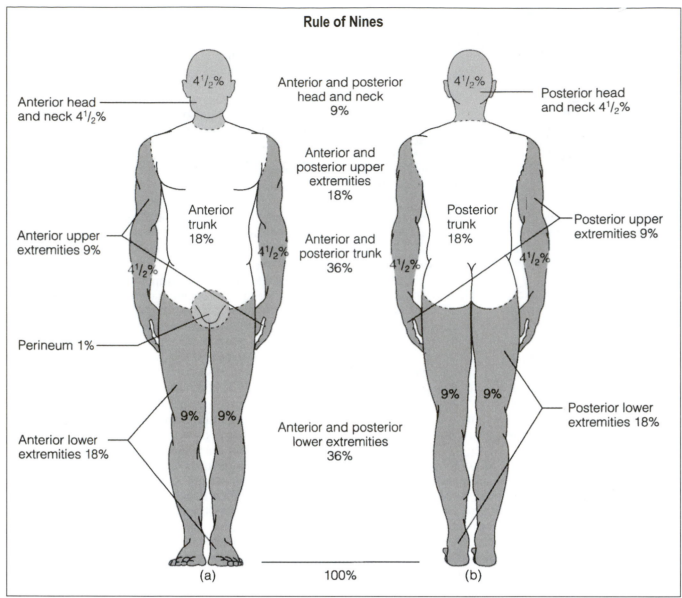

Rule of Nines

Anterior and posterior head and neck 9%

Anterior head and neck 4½%

Posterior head and neck 4½%

Anterior and posterior upper extremities 18%

Anterior trunk 18%

Posterior trunk 18%

Posterior upper extremities 9%

Anterior upper extremities 9%

Anterior and posterior trunk 36%

Perineum 1%

Posterior lower extremities 18%

Anterior lower extremities 18%

Anterior and posterior lower extremities 36%

(a)   100%   (b)

The "rule of nines" specifies the extent and hence seriousness of a burn in relation to the body's surface area.

jaundice and the appearance of albumin in the urine. In addition, the circulation begins to fail, with a resultant lack of oxygen in the tissues. The victim becomes cyanosed, restless, and collapsed, and in some cases death ensues. Other possible problems related to burns include collapse of the circulatory system, shutdown of the digestive and excretory systems, shock, pneumonia, and stress ulcers.

In addition, particularly with severe burns, there is a strong risk of infection. Severe burns can leave a large area of raw skin surface exposed and extremely vulnerable to any microorganisms. The infection of extensive burns may cause fatal complications if effective antibiotic treatment is not given. The combination of shock and infection can often be life-threatening unless expert treatment is immediately available.

The immediate outcome of a burn is more determined by its extent (amount of body area affected) than by its depth (layers of skin affected). The "rule of nines" is used to as-

sess the extent of a burn in relation to the surface of a body. The head and each of the arms cover 9 percent of the body surface; the front of the body, the back, and each leg cover 18 percent; and the crotch accounts for the remaining 1 percent. The greater the extent of a burn, the more seriously ill the victim will become from loss of fluid. The depth of the burn (unless it is very great) is mainly of importance when the question arises as to how much surgical treatment, including skin grafting, will be required. An improvement over the rule of nines in the evaluation of the seriousness of burns is the Berkow formula, which takes into account the age of the patient.

A burn caused by chemicals differs from a burn caused by fire only in that the outcome of the chemical burn is usually more favorable, since the chemical destroys the bacteria on the affected part and reduces the chance of infection. Severe burns can also be caused by contact with electric wires. As current meets the resistance in the skin, high tem-

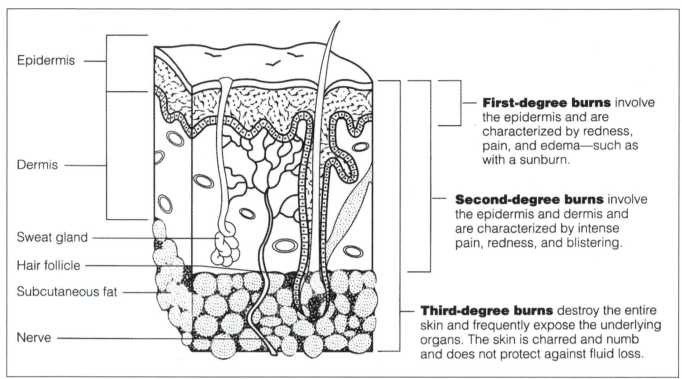

Epidermis

Dermis

Sweat gland

Hair follicle

Subcutaneous fat

Nerve

First-degree burns involve the epidermis and are characterized by redness, pain, and edema—such as with a sunburn.

Second-degree burns involve the epidermis and dermis and are characterized by intense pain, redness, and blistering.

Third-degree burns destroy the entire skin and frequently expose the underlying organs. The skin is charred and numb and does not protect against fluid loss.

Burns are measured by the layer(s) of skin affected.

peratures are reached and burning of the victim takes place. Exposure to 220 volts burns only the skin, but higher voltage can cause severe underlying damage to any tissue in its path. Electrical burns normally cause minimal external skin damage, but they can cause serious heart damage and require evaluation by a physician. Explosions and the action of acids and other chemicals also cause burns. Severe and extensive fire burns are most frequently produced by the clothes catching fire.

Treatment and Therapy

General treatment of a burn injury includes pain relief, the control of infection, the maintenance of the balance of fluids and electrolytes in the system, and a good diet. A high-protein diet with supplemental vitamins is prescribed to aid in the repair of damaged tissue. The specific treatment depends on the severity of the burn. Major burns should be treated in a specialized treatment facility, while minor burns can be treated without hospitalization. A moderate burn normally requires hospitalization but not specialized care.

In the case of minor burns or scalds, all that may be necessary is to hold the body part in cool water until the pain is relieved, as cooling is one of the most effective ways of relieving the pain of a burn. However, the application of ice to a burn may cause more harm to the skin, as ice will restrict blood flow to the affected area and slow the healing process. If the burn involves the distal part of a limb-for example, the hand and forearm-one of the most effective ways of relieving the pain is to immerse the burned part in lukewarm water and add cold water until the pain disappears. If the pain does not return when the water warms up,

the burn can be dressed in the usual way (a piece of sterile gauze covered by cotton with a bandage on top). The part should be kept at rest and the dressing dry and clean until healing takes place. Blisters can be pierced with a sterile needle, but the skin should not be cut away. No ointment or oil should be applied, and an antiseptic is not always necessary. Even minor burns can be serious if it covers as much as two-thirds of the body area. On a child, such burns are dangerous on an even smaller area of the skin, and special attention should be given to the patient. In the case of moderate burns or scalds, it is advisable to use antiseptics (such as chlorhexidine, bacitracin, and neomycin), and the patient should be taken to a doctor. Treatment may consist of applying a dressing with a suitable antibiotic or an antiseptic or pain-relieving cream and covering the burn with a dressing sealed at the end. This dressing is left on for four to five days and removed if there is evidence of infection or if pain occurs.

For severe burns and scalds, the patient must go to the hospital. Unless there is a need for resuscitation, or attention to other injuries, nothing should be done on the spot except to make sure that the patient is comfortable and to cover the burn with a sterile cloth. Clothing should be removed from the burned area only if this does not traumatize the skin further. Burned clothing should be sent to the burn center, as it may help determine the chemicals and other substances that either caused or entered the wound. Once the victim is in the hospital, the first thing to check is the extent of the burn and whether a transfusion is necessary. If the burn covers more than 9 percent of the body surface, a transfusion is required. It is essential to prevent infection or to bring it under control. A high-protein diet with ample fluids is needed to compensate for the protein that has been lost along with the fluid from the circulation. The process of healing is slow and tedious, including careful nursing, physiotherapy, and occupational therapy. The length of hospital stay can vary from a few days in some cases to many weeks in the case of severe and extensive burns.

In some cases, depending on the extent of the burn, it will be necessary to consider skin grafting, in which a graft of skin from one part of the body (or from another individual) is implanted over another part. Skin grafting is done soon after the initial injury. The donor skin is best taken from the patient, but when this is not possible, the skin of a matched donor can be used. Prior to grafting, or in some cases as a substitute for it, the burn may be covered with either cadaver or pig skin to keep it moist and free from exogenous bacterial infection. Newly developed artificial skin holds great promise for treating severe burns.

In the case of chemical burns, treatment can be specific and depends on the chemical causing the burn. For example, phenol or lysol can be washed off promptly, while acid or alkali burns should be neutralized by washing with sodium bicarbonate or acetic acid, respectively, or with a buffer solution for either one. In many cases, flushing with water to remove the chemical is the first method of action. Victims who have inhaled smoke may develop swelling and inflammation of the lungs, and they may need special care for burns of the eyes. People who have suffered an electrical burn may suffer from shock and may require artificial respiration, which should begin as soon as contact with the current has been broken.

Perspective and Prospects

Burns have been traditionally classified according to degree. The French surgeon Guillaume Dupuytren divided burns into six degrees, according to their depth. A first-degree burn is one in which there is simply redness; it may be painful for a day or two. This level of burn is normally seen in cases of extended exposure to sunlight or x-rays. A second-degree burn affects the first and second layers of skin. There is great redness, and the surface is raised up in blisters accompanied by much pain. Healing normally occurs without a scar. A third-degree burn affects all skin layers. The epidermis is entirely peeled off, and the true skin below is destroyed in part, so as to expose the endings of the sensory nerves. This is a very painful form of burn, and a scar follows on healing. With a fourth-degree burn, the entire skin of an area is destroyed with its nerves, so that there is less pain than with a third-degree burn. A scar forms and later contracts, and it may produce great deformity in the affected area. A fifth-degree burn will burn the muscles as well, and still greater deformity follows. In a sixth-degree burn, a whole limb is charred, and it separates as in gangrene.

In current practice, burns are referred to as superficial (or partial thickness), in which there is sufficient skin tissue left to ensure regrowth of skin over the burned site, and deep (or full thickness), in which the skin is totally destroyed and grafting will be necessary. It is difficult to de-

---

In the News: Treating Burns with Artificial Skin

Since the end of the twentieth century, surgeons have been using biosynthetic skin substitutes (sometimes called artificial skin or cellularwound dressings) to manage extensive or deep burns . Integra and TransCyte, approved by the Food and Drug Administration (FDA) in 1996 and 1997, respectively, are common substitutes. Both are layered products composed of synthetic silicone and a biologically active, collagen-based composite that promotes healing. TransCyte also has a nylon mesh between the two layers. Integra is produced by Integra LifeSciences Corporation in Plainsboro, New Jersey; TransCyte is produced by Advanced Tissue Sciences in La Jolla, California. TransCyte is a temporary skin substitute for partial thickness or less serious burns; it is removed after the wound heals or in preparation for a skin graft . Integra is a permanent skin substitute for full thickness or deep burns; however, after the patient's dermal layer regenerates, the silicone layer is replaced with a thin skin graft . A "one-step" skin substitute does not yet exist for deep burn wounds .

In the past, surgeons relied exclusively on biological skin to cover burn wounds or to promote wound closure. Typically, surgeons used xenografts from other species, such as pigs; allografts, human skin from cadavers; or autografts, from the patient's own skin.

Biosynthetic substitutes were developed to meet the needs both of increasing numbers of serious burn survivors and of survivors of extensive burns where fewer donor sites for autografts exist. Biosynthetic substitutes adhere to cleaned wounds, serve as a protective barrier, and minimize pain as well as length of hospital stay. For deep burns, substitutes promote regeneration of the survivor's own dermis and minimize scarring . Ideally, a skin substitute should look and feel like the patient's healthy skin. In reality, artificial skin may not match the patient's skin color and texture. Also, biosynthetic substitutes may transmit disease via the biological component or may seal in deep infection at the wound site. Although the development of biosynthetic skin substitutes is an important medical advance, bioengineering of skin tissue in the first decade of the twenty-first century is a relatively new science.

—*Tanja Bekhuis, PhD;*
updated by Geraldine Marrocco

---

termine the depth of a wound at first glance, but any burn involving more than 15 percent of the body surface is considered serious. As far as the ultimate outcome is concerned, the main factor is the extent of the burn-the greater the extent, the worse the outlook.

Unfortunately, burns are most common in children and older people, those for whom the outcome is usually the worst. Many burns are caused by accidents in the home, which are usually preventable. In fact, among the primary causes of deaths by burns, house fires account for 75 percent of the incidents. Safety measures in the home and on the job are extremely important in the prevention of burns. Severe and extensive burns most frequently occur when the clothes catch fire. This rule applies especially to cotton garments, which burn quickly. Particular care should always be exercised with electric fires and kettles or pots of boiling water in houses where small children or elderly people are present. In the United States, most severely burned patients are given emergency care in a local hospital and are then transferred to a large burn center for intensive long-term care.

The kind of environment provided in special burn units in large medical centers varies, but all have as their main objective avoiding contamination of the wound, as the major cause of death in burn victims is infection. Some special units use isolation techniques and elaborate laminar airflow systems to maintain an environment that is as free of microorganisms as possible.

The patient who has suffered some disfigurement from burns will have additional emotional problems in adjusting to a new body image. Burn therapy can be long and tedious for the patient and for family members. They will need emotional and psychological support as they work their way through the many problems created by the physical and emotional trauma of a major wound.

—Maria Pacheco, PhD;
updated by Mary Dietmann, EdD, APRN, CNS

See also: Blisters; Critical care; Critical care, pediatric; Dermatology; Electrical shock; Emergency medicine; First aid; Grafts and grafting; Healing; Heat exhaustion*and heatstroke; Intensive care unit(ICU); Radiationsickness; Shock; Skin; Wounds.*

For Further Information:

"Burns." *Health Library*, September 30, 2012. "Burns: First Aid." *Mayo Clinic*, February 1, 2012. "Fire Deaths and Injuries: Fact Sheet." *Centers for Disease Control and Prevention*, October 11, 2011.

Glanze,Walter D., Kenneth N. Anderson, and Lois E. Anderson, eds. *The Signet Mosby Medical Encyclopedia*. New York: Signet, 1996.

Jeschke, Marc G. *BurnCare and Treatment: A Practical Guide*. Medford: Springer, 2013.

Landau, Sidney I., ed. *International Dictionary of Medicine and Biology*. New York: John Wiley & Sons, 1986.

Leikin, Jerrold B., and Martin S. Lipsky, eds. *American Medical AssociationComplete Medical Encyclopedia*. New York: Random House Reference, 2003.

Marcovitch, Harvey, ed. *Black's Medical Dictionary*. 42d ed. Lanham, Md.: Scarecrow Press, 2010.

Miller, Benjamin F., Claire Brackman Keane, and Marie T. O'Toole. *Miller-Keane Encyclopedia and Dictionary of Medicine, Nursing, and Allied Health*. Rev. 7th ed. Philadelphia: Saunders/ Elsevier, 2005.

Sheridan, Robert Leo. *Burns: A Practical Approach to Immediate Treatment and Long-Term Care*. London: Manson Publishing, 2012.

Bursitis

Disease/Disorder

Anatomy or system affected: Hands, joints, knees, legs
Specialties and related fields: Internal medicine, rheumatology
Definition: An inflammation of a bursa, one of the membranes that surround joints.

Causes and Symptoms

Bursas are flattened, fibrous sacs that minimize friction on adjacent structures during activity involving a joint. The most well known bursas are around the knees, elbows, and shoulders. These protective joint sacs are lined with a fluid-producing membrane called the synovial membrane.

Information on Bursitis

Causes: Inappropriate or excessive joint use, pressure, friction, infections, injury
Symptoms: Warm, painful, swollen joints
Duration: Temporary to chronic
Treatments: Rest, avoidance of pain-inducing activity, ice packs, anti-inflammatory medications, antibiotics, surgery, physical therapy

---

Bursas are common in sites where ligaments, muscles, skin, or tendons overlie and may rub against bone. Most bursas are present at birth, but false bursas may develop at any site where there is excessive motion.

Bursitis is inflammation of a bursa, causing it to become warm, painful, and often swollen. Bursitis is usually caused by the inappropriate or excessive use of a joint. For example, pressure, friction, infections, or injury to a joint and surrounding tissues can cause membranes of the bursa to become inflamed.

Bursitis of the kneecap (prepatellar bursitis, or "housemaid's knee") is commonly caused by prolonged kneeling on a hard surface such as the floor. Similarly, olecranon bursitis ("student's elbow") is caused by pressure of the elbow against a table or desk. Perhaps the most common type of bursitis is of the shoulder joint, called subdeltoid bursitis.

Treatment and Therapy

The treatment for bursitis caused by overuse is usually rest and avoidance of the activity that resulted in the condition. Several days of rest is typically all that is needed for the swelling to subside. Ice packs may help relieve some of the minor pain and inflammation. If the inflammation does not subside after a few days, a physician may prescribe anti-inflammatory drugs such as ibuprofen or naproxen to reduce the inflammation and pain. Occasionally, a doctor will inject the inflamed bursa with a corticosteroid such as triamcinolone. In rare cases, where the symptoms are recurrent, a physician may remove the bursa (bursectomy). If the bursitis is caused by an infection, the most appropriate treatment is antibiotic therapy. During and after medical or surgical treatment, physical therapy may be recommended to improve the strength and mobility of the joint.

—Matthew Berria, Ph.D.

See also: Arthritis; Gout; Inflammation; Joints; Osteoarthritis; Rheumatoid arthritis; Rheumatology.

For Further Information:

Leach, Robert E. "Bursitis." *Health Library*, Nov. 26, 2012.

Leikin, Jerrold B., and Martin S. Lipsky, eds. *American Medical Association Complete Medical Encyclopedia*. New York: Random, 2003.

Marieb, Elaine N., and Katja Hoehn. *Human Anatomy and Physiology*. 9th ed. San Francisco: Pearson, 2010.

MedlinePlus. "Bursitis." *MedlinePlus*, Apr. 24, 2013.

Parker, James N., and Philip M. Parker, eds. *The Official Patient's Sourcebook on Shoulder Bursitis*. San Diego, Calif.: Icon, 2002.

Bypass surgery

Procedure

Anatomy or system affected: Abdomen, blood vessels, chest, circulatory system, gastrointestinal system, heart, intestines, legs

Specialties and related fields: Cardiology, gastroenterology, general surgery

Definition: Surgical provision of an additional or alternative channel to divert blood or the contents of the digestive system around an obstruction or narrowing.

Key terms:

angina: severe chest pains caused by insufficient blood supply to the heart

angiography: the injection of radiopaque dye into the arteries to make narrowing and blockages visible in X rays

angioplasty: the insertion of an inflatable probe into an artery, followed by inflation of a balloon to clear obstructions to blood flow

ischemia: a decrease in the blood supply to a body organ caused by a constriction or obstruction of blood vessels

laparoscope: a fiber-optic tube that can be used to examine internal organs

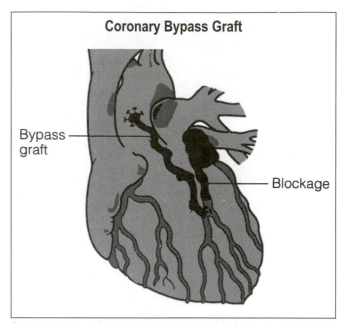

Coronary Bypass Graft

Bypass graft

Blockage

Bypass surgery can be performed in any part of the body where a blood vessel has become blocked; a common location for such a procedure is the heart, where from one to four arteries may require the placement of bypass grafts.

Indications and Procedures

Coronary artery bypass surgery is needed when angiography reveals a narrowing or blockage in heart arteries causing angina that cannot be controlled by medication or relieved by angioplasty. The traditional method of open chest bypass surgery, which first became popular in the 1970s, requires that the patient be fully anesthetized. The surgeon cuts open the patient's chest, saws through the breastbone, and spreads the halves of the ribcage to expose the heart. The heart is stopped and cooled, and the major heart vessels are attached to a heart-lung machine, which oxygenates and circulates the blood. At the same time, another surgeon removes a leg vein and prepares grafts to be sewn around blockages in the heart arteries. Mammary arteries are also employed to redirect blood flow around obstructed arteries. After the bypasses are satisfactorily implanted, the heart-lung machine is disconnected and the heart resumes pumping on its own. The two halves of the breastbone are reattached with stainless steel wire, and the incision is sewn closed. Patients are taken to a cardiac intensive care unit overnight and are normally discharged from the hospital within a week. They recover fully in one to three months.

An obstruction in the intestines can be treated surgically by removing the blocked region and sewing together the healthy portions of the gut. Severe problems may require creating an opening for the digestive tract through the abdominal wall, called a stoma, through which its contents can empty into a removable plastic bag. The procedure may be permanent or temporary, to allow the affected gut to heal. After successful healing, the bypass and bag are removed and the intestine segments are reattached.

Removal of part of the stomach or small intestine is sometimes used to treat cases of extreme obesity. The operation improves the patient's quality of life and may also extend its duration.

Uses and Complications

Traditional coronary artery bypass surgery is profoundly invasive. The heart-lung machine can create problems, even though newer machines are less stressful than the original models. The action of the pump is more powerful than that of a normal heart and can generate turbulence that damages blood cells and other organs. The machines have been blamed for blood clot formation, causing strokes and heart attacks during an operation. Patients, especially the elderly, often experience memory loss and confusion following surgery; though usually temporary, the problem can last for years. Surgeons, therefore, have been seeking less stressful and invasive methods of treating coronary artery disease.

Neither peripheral artery surgery nor intestinal bypass surgery involves using heart-lung machines, but the large incisions commonly used in such operations can also lead to complications by exposing extensive body areas to possible infection. Although traditional surgery is highly successful, innovators continue to seek the development of less invasive procedures.

Perspective and Prospects

The goal of research is minimally invasive surgery. Intestinal surgeons led the way with the development of laparoscopic gallbladder and kidney stone surgery in the 1980s. Only small circular incisions are needed to insert a fiber-optic instrument that transmits enlarged images of the surgical site to a screen. Laparoscopic tools are introduced though several additional small incisions. Segments of bowel can then be removed though tubes and their ends joined without opening the abdomen. The use of laparoscopic techniques reduces the tissue damage caused by traditional surgery. The patient feels less pain after the operation, experiences a shorter hospitalization, returns to normal activity sooner, and develops a smaller scar.

To make coronary artery surgery less invasive heart surgeons have used angioplasty. Using a catheter, a balloon is inserted into the blocked artery and inflated. This procedure pushes the deposits which cause the blockage against the artery walls making the opening larger. Although this is not a by-pass technique it is a better option for many patients.

To avoid use of the heart-lung machine, and its medical complications, cardiac surgeons have experimented with open chest surgery on a beating heart. This very delicate operation involves temporarily immobilizing the area of the heart where the surgeon intends to attach a graft, slowing the heartbeat with drugs, and stitching the bypass into place between heartbeats. Only the most skilled surgeons succeed in mastering this difficult technique.

In the 1990s, cardiac surgeons, following intestinal surgeons, adopted the use of fiber-optic tubes that permit so called keyhole surgery. Incisions of 3.0 inches in the chest and holes 0.5 inch in diameter under the armpit are sufficient to gain entry to the heart, thereby eliminating any need to open the chest cavity. Immobilizing segments of the heart and sewing grafts to the rhythm of the heartbeat, however, is considerably more difficult when done through a tube while viewing a television screen. In the twenty-first century, surgeons have begun using computer-controlled robots to carry out the intricate maneuvers needed to repair ailing hearts.

—*Bradley R.A. Wilson, PhD*

See also: Angina; Angioplasty; Arteriosclerosis; Bariatric surgery; Cardiac surgery; Cardiology; Cardiology, pediatric; Circulation; Coronary artery bypass graft; Gastrectomy; Gastroenterology; Gastrointestinal system; Gastrostomy; Heart; Heart disease; Heart valve replacement; Ileostomy and colostomy; Intestines; Obesity; Vascular medicine; Vascular system.

For Further Information:

Coppenrath, Larry. *Fixing A Damaged Heart: My Personal Experience with Coronary Artery Bypass Graph Surgery*. Kindle Edition, 2017.

Coronary Artery Bypass Grafting. *Health Library*, September 26, 2012.

Douglas, Eric L. *Heart Survivor: Recovery After Heart Surgery*. The Whole Picture Press, 2017.

Montgomery, Eugene (Ed.). *GastricBypass Surgery: Procedures, Benefits and Health Risks (Surgery - Procedures, Complications, and Results)*. Hauppauge NY: Nova Science Publishers, Inc., 2016.

Otto, Ru, *My Roux-en Y GastricBypass Surgery: A Personal Journey*. Kindle Edition, 2017.

Smith, Orleatha. *Weight Loss Surgery Success: Secrets You Must Know About GastricBypass*. CreateSpace Independent Publishing Platform, 2015.

Caffeine

Biology

Anatomy or system affected: Central and peripheral nervous system.

Specialties and related fields: Biochemistry, pharmacology, neurology.

Definition: A compound having the chemical formula $C_8H_{10}N_4O_2$ that acts, among other ways, to stimulate the central and peripheral nervous system.

Structure and Functions

Caffeine, known as 1,3,7-trimethylpurine-2,6-dione, was first isolated by the German chemist Ferdinand Runge, who published his discovery in 1820. Caffeine is found naturally in a variety of plants, where it acts as an insecticide, protecting the plant from insect predators. Caffeine is also present in various drinks, such as coffee and tea, energy drinks, soft drinks, frozen desserts, chocolate and other candies, and weight loss supplements.

Caffeine is one of the most extensively used psychoactive substances in the world. It causes a variety of behavioral and physiological effects. Most notably, caffeine acts as a stimulant, and temporarily improves mood, and increases endurance, concentration, reaction time, alertness, wakefulness and perceived feelings of energy. Caffeine causes many of its effects by indirectly affecting the release of various neurotransmitters. Neurotransmitters are chemical messengers which allow communication between nerve cells. Neurotransmitters regulate the majority of systems in the human body, including breathing, brain activity, movement, and heart rate. Neurotransmitters typically exert their influence by binding to receptor proteins at the end of nerve cells, which causes a cascade of cellular events.

Neurotransmitters may be divided into two broad categories: excitatory and inhibitory. Excitatory neurotransmitters lead to stimulation whereas inhibitory neurotransmitters prevent stimulation. Caffeine indirectly affects the release of various neurotransmitters due to its structural similarity to adenosine, a chemical that has many functions in the human body, including acting as an inhibitory neurotransmitter in the brain. Caffeine binds to cellular adenosine receptors, thus preventing adenosine from binding and exerting its inhibitory effects. In the process, excitatory neurotransmitters are released which contribute to the observed stimulatory effects of caffeine.

Caffeine intake also leads to the release of adrenaline, a stress hormone, from the adrenal glands. Adrenaline is called a stress hormone as it is one of the substances released into the bloodstream in the "fight or flight" response to prepare one for a stressful event. Release of adrenaline causes, among other things, blood pressure and heart rate to increase, expansion of the lung air passages, enlarged pupils and blood to be directed to the muscles.

Disorders and Diseases

Although caffeine is only clinically indicated for the treatment of headaches and infant apnea (reduction and stopping of breathing during sleep), it may have a role in preventing and treating Parkinson's disease and Alzheimer's disease, and may relieve constipation due to its ability to stimulate smooth muscles. Caffeine also has the ability to increase metabolic rate and energy expenditure, and has therefore been included in weight loss supplements, either alone or in combination with other substances.

Coffee and tea are the two beverages that contain the highest amount of naturally occurring caffeine. For this reason, many studies have utilized such beverages to examine the effect of caffeine intake on risks of developing various diseases. For example, coffee intake has been associated with a decreased risk of gastrointestinal cancer (oropharyngeal and hepatic) and prostate cancer, while no effect on such intake has been found with respect to ovarian cancer. A weak protective effect on endometrial cancer has been shown with coffee, but not with tea. The effect of coffee and caffeine intake on breast cancer is unclear, with some studies suggesting a protective effect and others that indicate no protective effect. Although a study found a 20% increase in urinary tract cancer with coffee drinkers, but not with tea drinkers, a causative relationship was not definitively shown. Finally, although an increase in lung cancer has been found with coffee, it is not clear whether caffeine, or other factors, was responsible. Moreover, care must be used in interpreting studies where caffeine is provided in the form of coffee and/or tea, as other substances are present in these beverages that could give rise to the protective and/or deleterious effects reported.

Although there is no current evidence that intake of small to moderate amounts of caffeine (i.e., the amount of caffeine found in less than or equal to about six cups of coffee) increases the risk of cardiovascular disease, caffeine has been found under certain circumstances to have negative effects on the cardiovascular system. For example, administration of caffeine has been shown to increase blood pressure (by no more than about 10 mm Hg) in both habitual and non-habitual caffeine users, although only non-habitual users experienced an increase in blood pressure in response to coffee consumption. Moreover, caffeine increases arterial stiffness, which affects coronary blood flow, the mechanical integrity of arteries, and is considered a marker of, and predictor of, cardiovascular disease. Although the relation between caffeine intake and sudden cardiac arrest has not been extensively studied, an increased association has been shown in patients with coronary artery disease only with intake of ten cups or more of coffee per day.

Caffeine, depending on the dosage, can cause, nausea, tremors, increased urination, vomiting, restlessness, insomnia, headaches, dizziness, anxiety, irritability, and lightheadedness. Caffeine intake has been associated with decreased bone density, which could lead to osteoporosis, and can prevent the absorption of calcium. Habitual use of caffeine can lead to physical dependence, and requires more caffeine to obtain similar, desired effects. Withdrawal symptoms from abruptly stopping caffeine intake primarily include drowsiness and headaches, but the following symptoms have been reported at a lower frequency: irritability, feelings of apathy, listlessness, inability to concentrate, tremors, nausea and vomiting.

—*Jason J. Schwartz, PhD, Esq.*

See also: Addiction; Brain; Ergogenic aids; Headaches; Neurology; Osteoporosis; Cancer; Weight loss medications; Dementias; Parkinson's Disease.

For Further Information:

Bordeaux, B. and H. R. Lieberman. "Benefits and risks of caffeine and caffeinated beverages." In Lipman, T.O. and Sullivan, D.J. (Eds.), *UpToDate*. Retrieved from http://www.uptodate.com/contents/benefits-and-risks-of-caffeine-and-caffeinated-beverages?source=search_result&search=caffeine&selectedTitle=1%7E150.

Giardina, E.G. "Cardiovascular effects of caffeine and caffeinated beverages." In Gersch, B.J., Libman, H. and Saperia, G.M. (Eds), *UpToDate*. Retrieved from http://www.uptodate.com/contents/cardiovascular-effects-of-caffeine-and-caffeinated-beverages.

National Institutes of Health, U.S. National Library of Medicine, Medline Plus. Caffeine. Retrieved from https://medlineplus.gov/caffeine.html.

Temple, J.L., C. Bernard, S.E. Lipshultz, J.D. Czachor, J.A. Westphal, and MA Mestre. "The Safety of Ingested Caffeine: A Comprehensive Review." *Front. Psychiatry*, 8:80, 2017. Published online at https://doi.org/10.3389/fpsyt.2017.00080

Wikoff, D., B.T. Welsh, R. Henderson, G.P. Brorby, J. Britt, E. Myers, and C. Doepker, (2017). Systematic review of the potential adverse effects of caffeine consumption in healthy adults, pregnant women, adolescents and children. *Food Chem. Toxicol (2017).* Advance Online Publication. https://doi.org/10.1016/j.fct.2017.04.002

Campylobacter infections

Disease/Disorder

Also known as: Campylobacteriosis, food poisoning

Anatomy or system affected: Abdomen, gastrointestinal system, intestines, stomach

Specialties and related fields: Bacteriology, gastroenterology, internal medicine, microbiology

Definition: An acute disease, often spontaneously resolving, caused by bacterial infection; sometimes called food poisoning.

Key terms:

bacteremia: a bacterial infection in the blood

hepatitis: infection of the liver

pancreatitis: infection of the pancreas

spontaneously resolve: to get better without any treatment

Causes and Symptoms

Campylobacter refers to a class of bacteria of which there are sixteen species and six subspecies. The most common types related to human disease are *Campylobacter jejuni*, *Campylobacter coli*, *Campylobacter laridis*, and *Campylobacter upsaliensis*.

Infection with *Campylobacter* bacteria is one of the most common causes of gastrointestinal problems. It usually results from contact with contaminated food or water, though the bacteria may be transmitted through fecal matter, such as from changing diapers for an infected child. These bacteria exist in the digestive system of many animals, and domestic animals or pets can transmit the bacteria through feces. Usually, babies (under one year of age), teens, and young adults are affected.

These bacteria attack the lining of the intestines, and infection causes symptoms such as diarrhea, cramps, fever, headache, or vomiting. In rare cases, the bacteria can enter the bloodstream and cause bacteremia, which needs to be treated with antibiotics. Untreated *Campylobacter* infections may also cause hepatitis, pancreatitis, or miscarriage in pregnant women. These bacteria have also been linked to arthritis and Guillain-Barré syndrome, a rare autoimmune disorder. To make a definitive diagnosis, a doctor may send a stool sample to a laboratory for analysis.

Treatment and Therapy

Often, *Campylobacter* infection will spontaneously resolve. If the patient is a young child or someone who is immunocompromised, or if the symptoms are severe and do not go away, then antibiotics may be prescribed. If the symptoms are relatively mild, then treatment involves drinking plenty of fluids and monitoring the patient for signs of dehydration. Good handwashing hygiene and the careful handling of raw foods (particularly poultry), drinking water, and nonhomogenized milk can help prevent future bouts with this bacterial infection.

Perspective and Prospects

For unknown reasons, cases of *Campylobacter* infections have been increasing, both in the developed and in the developing world. These infections are a major cause of death in children under age two in developing countries.

—*Marianne M. Madsen, M.S.*

See also Antibiotics; Arthritis; Bacterial infections; Bacteriology; Botulism; Childhood infectious diseases; Diarrhea and dysentery; *E. coli* infection; Enterocolitis; Food poisoning; Gastroenterology; Gastroenterology, pediatric; Gastrointestinal disorders; Guillain-Barré syndrome; Hepatitis; Infection; Microbiology; Nausea and vomiting; Pancreatitis; Salmonella infection; Staphylococcal infections; Strep throat; Streptococcal infections; Zoonoses.

For Further Information:

Bell, Chris, and Alec Kyriakides. *Campylobacter: A Practical Approach to the Organism and Its Control in Foods.* Malden, Mass.: Wiley-Blackwell, 2009.

"*Campylobacter.*" *National Center for Emerging and Zoonotic Infectious Diseases*. Centers for Disease Control and Prevention, Apr. 18, 2013.

"Campylobacter Infections." *MedlinePlus*, Mar. 4, 2013.

Carson-DeWitt, Rosalyn, and Daus Mahnke. "Food Poisoning." *Health Library*, Mar. 22, 2013.

Information on *Campylobacter* Infections

Causes: Contaminated food or water, contact with infected feces

Symptoms: Cramps, diarrhea, fever, headache, vomiting

Duration: Symptoms last two to five days; full recovery within a week to ten days

Treatments: Often resolves on its own; may be treated with antibiotics

Nachamkin, Irving, Christine M. Szymanski, and Martin J. Blaser, eds. *Campylobacter*. 3d ed. Washington, D.C.: ASM Press, 2008.

Newell, Diane G., Julian M. Ketley, and Roger A. Feldman, eds. *Campylobacters, Helicobacters, and Related Organisms*. New York: Springer, 1997.

Cancer

Disease/Disorder

Anatomy or system affected: All

Specialties and related fields: Cytology, histology, immunology, oncology, orthopedics, radiology

Definition: Inappropriate and uncontrollable cell growth within one of the specialized tissues of the body, threatening normal cell and organ function and in serious cases traveling via the bloodstream to other areas of the body.

Key terms:

carcinogen: a cancer-causing substance; usually a chemical that causes mutations

cell: the basic functional unit of the body, each of which contains a set of genes and all the other materials necessary for carrying out the processes of life

cell cycle: a step-by-step process whereby one cell duplicates itself to form two cells; it is the way in which most growth occurs, and the cycle leads to cancer if it becomes defective

gene: a master molecule that encodes the information needed for the body to carry out one specific function; many thousands of genes working together are needed to sustain normal human life

immortalized: the state of a cancer cell that allows it to divide an unlimited number of times

initiation: the first abnormal change that starts a cell along the pathway to cancer

messenger RNA: The messenger ribonucleic acid molecule is encoded from DNA in a process called transcription; this molecule is then translated into protein

metastasis: the process whereby tumor cells spread from one part of the body to another

mutation: damage to a gene that changes how it works

oncogene: a gene that functions normally to allow cells to progress through the cell cycle; when mutated, such genes can cause cancer

promotion: the second step in tumor development, which causes initiated cells to begin growing into tumors

telomerase: the enzyme that synthesizes the repeated sequences called telomeres at the ends of chromosomes

telomere: the repeated sequences at the end of chromosomes

transformation: genetic change in cancer cells which results in loss of growth control and often immortalization

tumorsuppressor genes: genes that normally keep cell division in check, orderly, and properly timed; when mutated, they can cause cancer

Causes and Symptoms

Cancer is a disease of abnormal cellular growth. Growth is a feature of all living things, but it must be precisely regulated for development to occur properly. All growing cells pass through a strictly regulated series of events called the cell cycle, where most cellular structures are duplicated. At the end of the cycle, one cell is separated into two "daughter cells," each receiving one copy of the duplicated structures. The most important structures to be duplicated are the genes, which govern all cellular activities.

Human life begins as a fertilized egg which divides again and again; the adult human body is composed of a trillion cells, each with a specific job to perform. At adulthood, most cells stop duplicating. Some cells, however, must continue dividing to replace worn-out cells in places like the blood, skin, and intestine. Such growth is accurately controlled so excess cells are not produced. Sometimes, however, a mutation arises in one or more genes, resulting in needless cell duplication and ultimately loss of growth control: a malignant transformation. This is the start of cancer.

At first, these cells resemble their neighbors. For example, newly altered blood cells look like normal blood cells, and in most respects are. However, cancer cells differ in a number of ways from "normal" cells. First, cancer cells grow uncontrollably. They may or may not grow faster than normal cells, but cancer cells do not cease growth. If placed in a laboratory cell culture dish, cancer cells will pile upon one another in a manner analogous to the formation of a tumor. By contrast, normal cells grow in a single layer

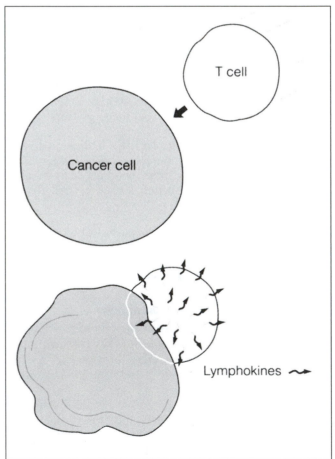

Cancer cells are fast-growing, irregular cells; normally, the body releases killer T cells that interact with antigens on the surface of the cancer cell, releasing lymphokines that are toxic to the cancer cell.

(monolayer) and stop replicating when they reach the edges of their dish when cellular signals instruct them to halt. Second, cancer cells often grow independently of hormones and growth factors, like insulin, required by other cells. They become "growth factor independent." Third, cancer cells are immortal. Normal cells are able to replicate themselves a regulated number of times, usually approximately fifty divisions, while cancer cells have no such limit. For example, HeLa cells, originally obtained from a woman with cervical cancer in the mid-1950s, have been cultured in laboratories for more than fifty years. Fourth, cancer cells in later stages change shape and size compared to normal cells. They may look very different. Oncologists (cancer specialists) use this information to identify cancer types and make prognoses.

The first event triggering cancer is initiation, precipitated by a mutation in one of the genes controlling some feature of the cell cycle. There are several hundred such genes regulating different aspects of the cell cycle and cellular growth. These genes have mundane jobs governing the life of the cell until they become damaged. When there is a mutation in a controlling gene, it functions improperly. It does not govern the cell cycle correctly, and the cell cycle proceeds when it should be halted. Such cancer-causing genes are called oncogenes.

After initiation, additional mutations and defects begin to accumulate, and the defective cells become increasingly abnormal. Tumor suppressor genes, normally functioning to keep cell division from becoming disorganized, are the site of these second-stage mutations. Those cells whose division and growth genes have mutated (oncogenes) and whose division and growth inhibitor genes (tumor suppressor genes) have also mutated will become cancer cells. Typically, a further change, "promotion," must take place before cancer cells begin growing freely. Promotion allows cells to escape the monitoring activity of the body. For example, various hormones instruct cells how to behave; a change of the promotion type may allow a cell to ignore such instructions. Both initiation and promotion occur randomly. Many initiated cells fail to grow into tumors. It is only those few cells that happen to acquire both defects that cause a problem. Fortunately, few cells have both their oncogenes turned "on" and their tumor suppressor genes turned "off."

At this point in the process, the new cancer cell is dividing and producing larger numbers. These cells grow into a mass called a tumor-except in blood and lymph tissues, where cancer cells circulate individually. Nevertheless, these cells look normal at this early stage and are relatively easy to control with surgery. The excess cells may not cause much harm. Warts, for example, result from underlying skin cells exhibiting abnormal growth control. Such harmless tumors are called benign.

Unfortunately, as cells continue to replicate uncontrollably, more mutations develop. The most harmful changes result in complete loss of growth control. Cancer cells spread, resulting in damage to other parts of the body. For example, cancer cells may acquire the ability to digest their way

---

Information on Cancer

Causes: Genetic, environmental, or lifestyle factors; viruses

Symptoms: Varies widely; may include tumor growth, headaches, lethargy, fever, bloating, pain, swelling

Duration: Chronic, possibly recurrent

Treatments: Surgery, chemotherapy, radiation

---

through nearby tissues, a process called invasion. Eventually, the functioning of organs containing such cells becomes impaired. Other cancer cells may break loose from the tumor and travel to other parts of the body in the circulatory or lymphatic systems. This process is called metastasis. In advanced stages, a cancer patient may actually have dozens or hundreds of tumors, all of which developed from a single tumor cell. Cells that can invade or metastasize are called malignant. It becomes increasingly difficult to eradicate cancer cells as they become more malignant. Because each event leading to tumor development is rare, it may take years for the several acquired mistakes to aggregate in a single cell, resulting in a malignant tumor.

Cancer-causing mutations occur when outside forces cause oncogenes and tumor suppressor genes to function abnormally. For example, genes may be chemically damaged by a number of highly active and dangerous chemicals known as carcinogens. Additionally, several kinds of radiation can damage genes: ultraviolet radiation, gamma radiation, nuclear radiation, and possibly electromagnetic field radiation. Finally, several kinds of viruses, including certain strains of the human papillomavirus or human herpesviruses, can cause oncogenes to function improperly. In most cancers, however, the origin of the disease is unknown and may result simply from a genetic mistake that takes place during gene duplication.

Treatment and Therapy

The most common cancer treatments fall into three categories: surgery, chemotherapy, and radiotherapy. The oldest treatment, going back several hundred years, is the surgical removal of tumors. If performed at an early stage, before metastasis, this method can be highly successful. Even so, surgery is much easier and less dangerous for some cancers (like that of the skin) than others (like that of the brain, which can be difficult to reach and remove). Surgery is not an option for blood and lymph cancers that are widely distributed.

The second most common type of cancer treatment for tumors is radiotherapy. The radiation of choice is X-rays, which can penetrate the body to reach a tumor in very high dosages using modern equipment. X-rays can be focused on a specific small area or be administered over the whole body in the case of metastasized cancer. Therapeutic radiation damages genes to such an extent that they become physically fragmented and nonfunctional, ending the life of the target cell.

Radiotherapy has major drawbacks. The most serious problem is that normal cells in the path of the radiation will also be killed. Bone marrow, the source of blood cells, is destroyed with whole-body cancer treatments. This problem can be overcome after radiotherapy by transplanting new bone marrow into the patient, so that a treated patient can begin to manufacture new blood cells. Ironically, radiation designed to kill cancer cells can also cause malignant mutations in normal cells. Recent innovations in radiotherapy include instrumentation such as the gamma knife, a method to direct radiation precisely into the center of a tumor. In this manner, damage to surrounding cells may be minimized.

If a patient has metastasized tumor cells, radiation and surgery are not the treatments of choice. Neither of these therapies acts systemically. The most common systemic treatment used that can reach everywhere in the body is chemotherapy. Patients are treated with chemicals that prevent cells from duplicating or slow the process. Such drugs reach all parts of the body much more effectively than surgery when cancer has reached a later stage of distribution. Different kinds of chemicals work in different ways to achieve this result.

The most common and difficult problem with the chemotherapeutic approach to cancer management is that normal cells are also affected by the same drugs that halt the growth of cancer cells. This reaction causes many difficulties for patients. Probably the most serious problems are with the immune system. Growth of the white blood cells that make antibodies is necessary to fight an infectious disease. Chemotherapy often depresses the immune system so it functions inefficiently; therefore patients in chemotherapy are more vulnerable to bacterial and viral illnesses. Red blood cells may also diminish during chemotherapy, making patients breathless and "sickly." Skin often becomes pale and unhealthy looking. The digestive tract cells stop dividing, causing weight loss and digestive problems. Finally, certain chemotherapy drugs cause hair loss, since hair follicles are also prevented from growing.

Fortunately, newer drugs and treatments are being developed to attack cancer in different ways. Targeted therapies are drugs or other substances that precisely identify cancer cells while preventing damage to normal cells. Targeted therapies focus on how the cancer cell is different from the normal cell; then works to either block or turn off chemical signals, change proteins within the cell, stop making new blood vessels for the cancer cell, trigger the immune system, or carry toxins to the cancer cells. This results in cancer death while sparing the death of normal cells. While some people do not experience many side effects from targeted therapies, others may experience skin changes, high blood pressure, swelling, and other drug specific side effects. (ACS, 2017)

Using the body's own immune system to identify cancer

In the News:
Drugs Targeting Cancer Stem Cells

An important change in strategy is occurring in the development of drugs to treat cancer. This shift is highlighted in two studies—published in the August, 2009, issue of *Cell* by Piyush B. Gupta and colleagues at the Massachusetts Institute of Technology and the October, 2009, issue of *Cancer Research* by Heather A. Hirsch and colleagues at Harvard Medical School.

Historically, cancer treatment has focused on triggering the self-destruction (apoptosis) of cells that are multiplying rapidly, a prominent feature of cancer. It has long been suspected, however, that these cells may not be the ones that initiate and spread the cancer to new locations (metastasis). Nevertheless, only in the last decade has the existence of a unique cell type responsible for metastasis been demonstrated. These cells turn out to be very similar to stem cells; in fact, some appear to be stem cells gone wild (stem cells are like seeds that can grow into organs, tissues, and replacement cells). Most tissues maintain an extremely limited reserve of stem cells scattered among their other cells, which makes stem cells exceedingly difficult to identify and isolate. Cancer stem cells are equally rare, and targeting them is like trying to find the proverbial needle in a haystack. Also like normal stem cells, cancer stem cells do not replicate very often, which makes them highly resistant to chemotherapy.

In the studies noted above, researchers reported great news—some well-known drugs already available can selectively kill stem cells causing breast cancer. Two such drugs were metformin (normally used to treat type 2 diabetes) and salinomycin (fed to farm animals as an antibiotic). The hope is that these chemicals in combination with traditional therapies will deliver a one-two punch that knocks out the cancer permanently. However, much research still needs to be done. Cancer is not a single disease but more than a hundred different diseases; so far, fewer then 10 percent have been attributed to stem cells. Cancer stem cells also differ for each type of cancer, suggesting that no single compound will treat all cancers. Clearly, the battle is not over, and clinical trials are only just beginning, but drugs that target cancer stem cells reflect a major conceptual advance in the war against cancer.

—*Brad Rikke, Ph.D.*

---

and destroy it is another growing area of research called immunotherapy. Stimulation of the immune system to work harder and smarter is one form of immunotherapy and administering synthetic proteins to boost the immune system is another. Immunotherapy can be very general or specific, depending on the type of treatment that is being used. It works better for some types of cancers than others, and some people respond better to immune therapy than others. This is an area that is under a great deal of research and has great promise for the future of cancer treatment. (ACS, 2017)

Perspective and Prospects

Expanding research in the area of immunotherapy and cancer treatment continues. Currently there are four types of immunotherapy being used. The first type are monoclonal antibodies which are proteins designed to attack specific parts of the cancer cell. Antibodies are proteins that attach to antigens (the cancer cell). Once the antibody attaches to the antigen it kills it. In order to make a monoclonal antibody, the researcher must identify the antigen (the cancer cell). An example of a frequently used monoclonal antibody is trastuzumab (Herceptin), used for women with breast cancer with the Her2 protein. The second type of immune therapy, the immune checkpoint inhibitor, helps the immune system recognize and attack the cancer cell by "taking the brake off" of the immune system. The immune system uses checkpoints that allow an immune response to be activated. Cancer cells find ways to avoid these checkpoints so these drugs are able to target the cancer at the checkpoint. PD-1 is a checkpoint protein that is found on certain types of cells in the immune system called T cells. The function of PD-1 is to keep T cells from attacking other cells in the body, including cancer cells which contain PD-L1. When a PD-1 Inhibitor such as pembrolizumab (Keytruda) is given to a person with cancer, it blocks or "inhibits" the binding of the PD-1 to the T cell so that the T cell is free to kill the cancer cells. Cancer vaccines, a third type of immunotherapy, inject substances into the body to prevent the development of cancer. There are viruses that cause cancer and can be prevented by the administration of a vaccine. Two examples are the human papilloma virus (HPV) which is linked to cervical, anal, and throat cancers and the hepatitis B virus (HBV), which places individuals at higher risk for liver cancer. Nonspecific immune therapies are general treatments that boost the immune system and attack cancer cells. Examples of nonspecific therapies are the interferons and interleukins. (ACS, 2017)

Early detection and treatment have significantly improved the prognosis for people diagnosed with cancer. Nevertheless, there are millions of cancer cases diagnosed each year, many of them fatal. In 2017, according to the American Cancer Society, 1,688,780 new cases of cancer will be diagnosed worldwide and 600,920 cancer deaths will occur in the U.S. alone.

—Howard L. Hosick, PhD, Connie Rizzo, MD, PhD, and
James J. Campanella, PhD;
updated by Richard Adler, PhD, Mary Dietmann EdD,
APRN, CNS, and Geraldine Marrocco

See also: Anal cancer; Antioxidants; Biopsy; Bladder*cancer; Bladderremoval; Bone cancer; Bone marrowtransplantation; Brain tumors; Breastbiopsy; Breastcancer; Burkitt's lymphoma; Carcinogens; Carcinoma; Cells; Cervical, ovarian, and uterine cancers; Chemotherapy; Colonoscopyand sigmoidoscopy; Colorectal cancer; Colorectal polypremoval; Colorectal surgery; Cytology; Cytopathology; Dermatopathology; Endometrial biopsy; Epstein-Barr virus; Gallbladdercancer; Gastrectomy; Genomics; Hodgkin's disease; Hysterectomy; Imagingand radiology; Immunology; Immunopathology; Kaposi's sarcoma; Kidneycancer; Laryngectomy; Leukemia; Livercancer; Lung cancer; Lung surgery; Lymphadenopathyand lymphoma; Malignancyand metastasis; Mammography; Mastectomyand lumpectomy; Melanoma; Mouthand throatcancer; National CancerInstitute(NCI); National Institutes of Health(NIH); Oncology; Plastic surgery; Polyps; Prostatecancer; Prostateglandremoval; Radiationtherapy; Sarcoma; Screening; Skin cancer; Skin lesionremoval; Stem cells; Stomach, intestinal, and pancreatic cancers; Terminally ill: Extended care; Testicular cancer; Tumorremoval; Tumors.*

For Further Information:
American CancerSociety (ACS), 2017.
Bognar, David, et al. *Cancer: Increasing Your Odds for Survival-AResource Guide for Integrating Mainstream, Alternative, and Complementary Therapies.* Alameda, Calif.: Hunter House, 1998.
Cairns, John. *Matters of Life and Death: Perspectives on Public Health, Molecular Biology, Cancer, and the Prospects for the Human Race.* Princeton, N.J.: Princeton University Press, 1998.
"Cancer." *MedlinePlus,* May 2, 2013.
"Cancer." *World Health Organization,* Jan. 2013.
CancerCare, 2013.
"CancerStatistics."*WorldCancerResearchFund International,* 2008.
Dollinger, Malin, et al. *Everyone's Guide to CancerTherapy.* Rev. 5th ed. Kansas City, Mo.: Andrews McMeel, 2008.
Greaves, M. F. *Cancer: The Evolutionary Legacy.* NewYork: Oxford University Press, 2002.
McKinnell, Robert Gilmore, ed. *The Biological Basis of Cancer.* 2d ed. New York: Cambridge University Press, 2006.
"Understanding Cancer Series: Cancer." *National CancerInstitute,* Sept. 30, 2009.
Weinberg, Robert. *The Biology of Cancer.* 2d ed. New York: Garland Science, 2013.

Candidiasis

Disease/Disorder

Anatomy or system affected: Abdomen, bladder, blood, gastrointestinal system, genitals, immune system, mouth, reproductive system, skin, urinary system

Specialties and related fields: Epidemiology, family medicine, immunology, internal medicine

Definition: An acute or chronic fungal infection of humans and animals that can be superficial or deep-seated, caused by a species of the fungus *Candida.*

Key terms:

acquired immunodeficiency syndrome (AIDS): a severe and usually fatal disease caused by infection with the human immunodeficiency virus (HIV); infection results in progressive impairment of the immune system

antifungal agents: drugs that can result in the inhibition of growth or killing of fungi; these drugs may be topical or systemic in application

cell-mediated immunity: protection mediated by thymus-derived lymphocytes; this type of immunity is particularly important for certain types of pathogenic organisms such as *Candida*

chlamydoconidia (chlamydospores): budding organisms that form directly from vegetative mycelia (molds); they differ from true spores, which are the result of sexual reproduction

culture: the propagation of organisms, such as fungi, on artificial media; *Candida* organisms grow in many kinds of media in both the yeast and mold forms

dimorphism: the ability of a fungus to exist in two forms, yeasts and molds; yeasts are unicellular round, oval, or cylindrical cells, and molds are branching tubular structures called hyphae

germ tube test: an initial laboratory test used to identify unknown yeasts and performed by microscopically examining a colony of yeast inoculated into rabbit or human plasma

histopathology: the study of the appearance and structure of abnormal or diseased tissue under the microscope

phagocytosis: the progress of ingestion and digestion by cells that are part of the immune system; this process is one of the ways that mammals use to defend themselves against infectious invaders, including *Candida* organisms

Causes and Symptoms

Candida is a genus of dimorphic fungi found widely in nature. This fungus may be found in soil, inanimate objects, plants, and most important, as a harmless parasite of humans and other mammals. It can exist in two forms: as a yeast and as a mold. In the yeast phase, this fungus exists as a normal inhabitant in and on human bodies. Nearly all infections are of such endogenous origin, but human-to-human transmission may occasionally occur from mother to newborn or between sexual partners. The yeasts reproduce asexually by budding, and a sexual stage has been recognized only in a few species. Pseudohyphae develop when yeasts and their progeny adhere to one another, forming chains. Hyphae, the branching tubular structures of molds, are formed in tissue invaded by the fungus.

Identification of *Candida* as the causative agent in clinical infections depends largely on the microscopic examination of infected tissue or secretions and on a culture of *Candida* prepared from infected material. Histopathological examination may reveal yeast forms and/or hyphal or pseudohyphal forms. The microscopic appearance of these organisms is similar to those of some other fungi, and a culture is necessary to confirm this fungus as the responsible pathogen. *Candida* will grow on many types of artificial microbiologic media and can usually be grown on the same media used to grow bacteria. With some types of infection, however, the use of special media or techniques may lead to a higher yield from cultures. After an unknown yeast is grown on artificial media, tests must be performed to determine its identity. Most laboratories initially use the germ tube test, in which yeast is introduced into rabbit or human plasma at 35 degrees Celsius for one to two hours. In this test, a structure called a germ tube is observed if the yeast is *Candida albicans*, *Candida stelloidea*, or rare strains of *Candida tropicalis*. If this test is positive (a germ tube is produced), then most laboratories assume that the microorganism is *C. albicans*-it is by far the most common species causing disease-and conduct no further, and usually more expensive, tests. Simple cultural tests may also be used to identify *C. albicans*, including the formation of spiderlike colonies on eosin methylene blue agar or the production of chlamydoconidia on cornmeal agar. The identification of *Candida* antigens in the serum of patients with widespread or disseminated infection is sometimes used to assist in the diagnosis of candidiasis, but this test is neither sensitive nor specific.

The bodies of humans and other mammals possess multiple defense mechanisms against candidiasis. The skin and mucous membranes provide a protective wall, but breaks in the mucocutaneous barrier may occur in many ways, including trauma, surgery, and disease. A balanced microbial flora in the gastrointestinal tract prevents the overgrowth of *Candida* organisms, which can lead to penetration of this fungus into the lining of the gastrointestinal tract and its entrance into the bloodstream. When invasion occurs, phagocytic cells (including monocytes, neutrophils, and eosinophils) further protect the body by ingesting and killing *Candida* organisms. Phagocytosis is assisted by serum

> ### Information on Candidiasis
> **Causes:** Fungal infection
> **Symptoms:** Dependent on region; may include white patches on tongue, difficult or painful swallowing, endocarditis, vaginal discharge, intense itching, diaper rash, urinary tract infection
> **Duration:** Temporary or chronic
> **Treatments:** Antifungal drugs, removal of foreign material or infected tissue

proteins called opsonins. Lymphocytes are also important defenders against this fungus and are part of the cell-mediated immune system. Candidiasis may result when cell-mediated immunity is defective, as is the case with the hereditary condition of chronic mucocutaneous candidia- sis or with acquired immunodeficiency syndrome (AIDS). Approximately 80 percent of healthy people exhibit delayed hypersensitivity reactions to *Candida* antigens, indicating the presence of a previously induced cell-mediated immunity directed against such an infection.

Candidiasis may be divided into superficial mucocutaneous and deep-seated, tissue-invasive types. There are more than one hundred fifty species of this fungus, but only ten are recognized as human pathogens, and *C. albicans* is the most important. Oral candidiasis, or thrush, is a common infection characterized by white patches on the tongue and oral mucosal surfaces (oropharyngeal infection). Scrapings taken from these patches contain masses of yeasts, pseudohyphae, and hyphae. Culturing is not as useful as clinical appearance and microscopic examination, since *Candida* organisms can be grown from normal mouths. Thrush is particularly common when the immune system is impaired, as in patients with cancer or AIDS or in asthmatics treated with inhaled steroids. Infection of other parts of the gastrointestinal tract, especially the esophagus, may occur in patients with a variety of underlying conditions, including an impaired immune system, gastrointestinal surgery, and antibiotic treatment. Esophageal involvement often results in difficult or painful swallowing. Only about half of patients with esophageal candidiasis will also have the more easily diagnosed oropharyngeal infection. Some patients with gastrointestinal candidiasis will develop systemic or disseminated infection.

Vaginal candidiasis, the most common type of vaginitis, is a common form of the infection associated with an overgrowth of *Candida* organisms in the vagina followed by mucocutaneous invasion. The patient will have a thick, curdlike vaginal discharge and itching of the surrounding skin areas. Antibiotic therapy, pregnancy, birth control pills, diabetes, and AIDS all predispose women to this form of infection. Recurrent or chronic infection can occur and may be associated with tissue invasion or impaired response of lymphocytes to the infection in some patients.

Cutaneous infection is common with candidiasis. This fungus is often the cause of diaper rash in infants; the condition often results from infection of skin under wet diapers by *Candida* organisms from the gastrointestinal tract. Intertrigo is another skin condition produced by candidiasis in the warm, moist area of skin folds, and similar environments result in perianal or scrotal infections that cause intense itching (pruritus). A widespread eruption of infection involving the trunk, thorax, and extremities is occasionally seen in both children and adults. Disseminated candidiasis, usually in association with persistent candidemia (the presence of the fungus in the bloodstream), may be associated with widely distributed, nodular skin lesions. Candidiasis of the skin, mucous membranes, hair, and nails beginning early in life and associated with defective cell-mediated immunity has been called chronic mucocutaneous candidiasis. This disease is often associated with a variety of endocrine diseases, including diabetes mellitus and decreased function of the parathyroid, thyroid, and adrenal glands.

Deep-organ involvement with candidiasis is serious and often life-threatening. The placement in the body of foreign material used for medical therapy may provide the initial breeding ground for the infection. Examples of these devices are vascular catheters, artificial heart valves, artificial vascular grafts, and artificial joints and other orthopedic implants. The environment created by these foreign materials makes it impossible for the normal defense mechanisms of the body to function.

Urinary tract infection with *Candida* organisms is seen in association with urinary catheters, especially when usage is chronic. Colonization of the urine with *Candida* organisms may also occur following a course of antibiotics or in diabetic patients. Infection of the kidney can result if the candidiasis spreads upward from the bladder through the ureter or via the bloodstream. Renal involvement has been reported in up to 80 percent of patients with disseminated candidiasis. In disseminated disease, infection is spread to the kidney through the bloodstream, with the formation of renal abscesses. Primary renal infection occurs when the kidney is invaded directly without concomitant invasion through the blood. Such direct infection may occur in association with urinary catheters or following surgical procedures involving the genital and urinary tracts. A particularly severe form of ascending renal infection, more frequent in diabetic patients, causes necrosis of the renal papillae and renal failure.

Ocular candidiasis (endophthalmitis) may occur when the eye is infected with *Candida* organisms either by direct invasion or through the bloodstream. Virtually any portion or structure of the eye may be involved. Examination of the retina using an ophthalmoscope can reveal white spots, resembling cotton balls, indicating *Candida* organisms in the blood vessels of the eye. This finding may also be a clue to infection elsewhere in the body that has spread through the bloodstream to the eye.

Endocarditis (inflammation of the lining of the heart) occurs when a native or artificial heart valve becomes infected. Candidiasis is an increasingly frequent cause of endocarditis of the native valves of intravenous drug abusers and artificial valves of all varieties. Such endocarditis is presumptively diagnosed when the organism is grown from blood specimens in the presence of a heart murmur. Abnormal growth on the heart valves, called vegetation, can usually be demonstrated using echocardiography. Fragments of vegetation may break off and circulate in the bloodstream, leading to the obstruction of vessels in many organs of the body, including the brain, eyes, lungs, spleen, and kidneys. Without treatment, this disease is uniformly fatal.

Disseminated candidiasis is seen in the most susceptible patients, including those with cancer, prolonged postoperative illness, and extensive burns. In these patients, further risk is associated with the use of central venous or arterial catheters, broad-spectrum antibiotic therapy, artificial feeding, or abdominal surgery. Dysfunction of neutrophils, or neutropenia, may increase the susceptibility of the patient to widespread infection with *Candida* organisms and can also be seen with AIDS. The kidney, brain, heart, and eye are the most common organs to be involved. Despite severe and extensive disease, specific diagnosis of disseminated candidiasis is difficult during life and is often only made at the time of postmortem examination.

Treatment and Therapy

Candidiasis may be prevented by avoiding or ameliorating the underlying predisposing factor or disease state and by decreasing or halting growth of the fungi. Dry or cracked skin can be treated with dermatologic lubricants. Invasive devices used for medical treatment should be placed in the body under the most sterile conditions and only employed when absolutely necessary. Care of these devices, including urinary catheters, intravascular lines, and peritoneal renal dialysis catheters, must be performed by skilled personnel using the most sterile approach possible. If antibacterial therapy is used excessively, fungal overgrowth may occur; *Candida* organisms can grow with ease in the gastrointestinal tract and vagina when bacteria are inhibited or killed by antibiotics, and overgrowth can lead not only to local infection but also to bloodstream invasion and secondary infection elsewhere in the body. Moreover, the treatment of underlying disease states such as diabetes mellitus, neoplasia, and AIDS will lessen the detrimental effects of candidiasis on the immune system.

Growth of *Candida* organisms can be decreased by altering the local conditions that favor their proliferation. For example, changing a baby's diaper frequently and applying a drying powder can avoid the wet and warm conditions that can result in diaper rash. Obese patients can lose weight, which will minimize skin fold infections. Wearing nonocclusive clothing, especially cotton fabrics, is often helpful in discouraging candidiasis.

Antifungal agents are often used to prevent candidiasis. Hospitalized patients recovering from surgery who have received antibacterial agents are given nystatin, an oral, nonabsorbed antifungal, to prevent the overgrowth of *Candida* organisms in the gastrointestinal tract. For cancer patients receiving chemotherapy, systemic antifungal drugs are often employed during the period when the cancer chemotherapy has had the most deleterious effects on the immune system.

Antifungals are employed by the topical, oral, parenteral (through a blood vessel or muscle), or irrigation routes for treatment of candidiasis. Among the many antifungal agents, nystatin, flucytosine, amphotericin B, and a variety of imidazole agents are the most commonly used. Antifungals utilize a number of different mechanisms that impede the metabolic activities of the organism or disrupt the integrity of the cell membrane on the outer surface of the fungus. Amphotericin B and fluconazole are useful in the treatment of systemic or deep-organ disease. Amphotericin B is produced by the fungus *Streptomyces nodosus* and is administered intravenously for systemic and deep-organ disease and by bladder irrigation for lower urinary tract infection (cystitis). When administered intravenously, amphotericin B has serious side effects, including fever, chills, kidney failure, liver abnormalities, and bone marrow suppression.

Fluconazole has fewer adverse effects and can be administered by the oral or intravenous routes; for these reasons, it is now commonly used as the initial therapy for candidiasis. Amphotericin B remains the treatment of choice for serious or life-threatening infection or when a *Candida* species isolated from a patient has been demonstrated by laboratory testing to be resistant to other antifungal agents.

In addition to antifungals, removal of foreign material or infected tissue is often necessary to treat severe candidiasis. Catheters, vascular grafts, artificial heart valves, artificial joints, and other devices must be removed and then replaced, if necessary, while the patient is receiving antifungal therapy or after the infection is cured. In some cases, such as with endocarditis, the infected tissue must be surgically removed to ensure a cure.

As with prevention, treatment of the underlying disease state greatly assists other measures directed against candidiasis. Gaining control of hyperglycemia in diabetes mellitus patients, viral infection in AIDS patients, and bone marrow suppression in cancer patients will aid in the treatment of candidiasis when it is present.

Perspective and Prospects

More than two thousand years ago, the Greek physicians Hippocrates and Galen described oral lesions that were probably thrush, but it was not until 1839 that fungi were found in such lesions. Deep-seated infection was first described in 1861, and endocarditis was identified in 1940. Candidiasis was recognized as an indicator disease in the 1987 surveillance definition for AIDS by the Centers for Disease Control in the United States. *Candida* ranks among the most common pathogens in hospital-acquired infections.

Candidiasis is on the increase largely because of increasingly sophisticated medical therapies and the worldwide epidemic of AIDS. Medical devices, immunosuppressive medical therapies, and organ transplantation are all becoming more common, and it is anticipated that candidiasis will increase in a corresponding manner. Likewise, as patients infected with human immunodeficiency virus (HIV) progress to clinical illness, the cases of candidiasis are expected to rise dramatically.

More effective preventive and therapeutic measures will be necessary to combat such an increase in cases of candidiasis. New antifungal agents will need to be developed to treat resistant strains of *Candida*. Laboratory testing to determine whether various antifungal agents can kill or inhibit the growth of *Candida* species isolated from patients will need to be more widely available and more frequently performed if organisms resistant to antifungals are to be identified. Early identification of resistant organisms will benefit patients by providing more effective antifungal therapy early in the course of treatment. Testing procedures will need to employ better methodology that is standardized to enable laboratories in different locations to compare results and determine regional or national trends in antifungal resistance.

—*H. Bradford Hawley, M.D.*

See also Acquired immunodeficiency syndrome (AIDS); Endocarditis; Fungal infections; Opportunistic infections; Rashes; Women's health.

For Further Information:
Betts, Robert F., Stanley W. Chapman, and Robert L. Penn, eds. *Reese and Betts' A Practical Approach to Infectious Diseases*. 5th ed. Philadelphia: Lippincott Williams & Wilkins, 2003.
Biddle, Wayne. *A Field Guide to Germs*. 3d ed. New York: Anchor Books, 2010.
Calvagna, Mary, and Andrea Chisholm. "Vaginal Yeast Infection." *Health Library*, Sept. 10, 2012.
"Candidiasis." *Centers for Disease Control and Prevention*, Mar. 15, 2012.
Hellwig, Jennifer, and Kari Kassir. "Thrush." *Health Library*, Sept. 10, 2012.
"Invasive Candidiasis." *Centers for Disease Control and Prevention*, May 6, 2013.
Kwon-Chung, K. J., and John E. Bennett. *Medical Mycology*. Philadelphia: Lea & Febiger, 1992.
Mandell, Gerald L., John E. Bennett, and Raphael Dolin, eds. *Mandell, Douglas, and Bennett's Principles and Practice of Infectious Diseases*. 7th ed. New York: Churchill Livingstone/Elsevier, 2010.
Martin, Jeanne Marie. *Complete Candida Yeast Guidebook: Everything You Need to Know About Prevention, Treatment, and Diet*. Rev. 2d ed. New York: Three Rivers Press, 2000.
Parker, James N., and Philip M. Parker, eds. *The Official Patient's Sourcebook on Genital Candidiasis*. San Diego, Calif.: Icon Health, 2002.
Winn, Washington C., Jr., et al. *Koneman's Color Atlas and Textbook of Diagnostic Microbiology*. 6th ed. Philadelphia: Lippincott Wiliams & Wilkins, 2006.
"Yeast Infections." *MedlinePlus*, Apr. 25, 2013.

Canker sores

Disease/Disorder
Also known as: Aphthous ulcers, ulcerative stomatitis
Anatomy or system affected: Mouth, skin
Specialties and related fields: Dentistry, family medicine
Definition: Small, round ulcers of the mucous membranes that line the mouth.

Causes and Symptoms

Aphthous ulcers are the most common lesions of the mucous membranes that line the mouth. The exact cause of this easily recognized problem is unknown; however, some evidence points to infection with the human herpesvirus 6, one of a family of viruses that cause a variety of diseases, including cold sores, genital herpes, and shingles. Possible triggers may include mouth injury, stress, vitamin deficiency, hormonal changes, and food allergies.

In most cases, a canker sore is a painful, small, round ulcer on a red base with a yellowish center. The redness also surrounds the lesion like a halo. Sores are usually about one to two millimeters in diameter but may be as large as one to two centimeters. They may occur as either single or multiple lesions and are found on the mucous membranes lining the mouth and tongue. These lesions tend to recur; the recurrences may be associated with stress or illness. The associated pain usually lasts for a week to ten days, and the ulcers heal completely within three weeks. Major aphthous ulcers, another variety, start out as nodules under the mucous membranes, which then break down and form craterlike ulcers that may last more than a month.

Aphthous ulcers may occur on their own, but they may also be associated with some diseases and disorders of the collagen, gastrointestinal problems such as Crohn's disease, bacterial infections, and Behçet's disease. This last condition is a syndrome that involves painful ulcers of the tongue and oral mucous membranes, in addition to a variety of eye, skin, joint, gastrointestinal, and central nervous system problems.

Treatment and Therapy

The treatment of canker sores is geared toward relieving the associated pain rather than curing the lesion. Treatments include a steroid-containing gel or paste applied directly to the ulcer, an anesthetic spray, or a mouthwash that the patient "swishes and spits." Oral antibiotic rinses may be prescribed; however, an oral infection known as "candidiasis" or "thrush" may develop as a result. In severe cases, oral steroids tapered over one week may provide relief.

Perspective and Prospects

In patients with human immunodeficiency virus (HIV) infection, aphthous ulcers may be extremely painful or extensive. If the ulcers do not respond to conventional treatment, then the drug thalidomide may be useful. However, it must be used with extreme caution, as this drug is known to cause severe birth defects if taken during pregnancy.

—*Rebecca Lovell Scott, Ph.D., PA-C*

See also Cold sores; Dental diseases; Dentistry; Dentistry, pediatric; Herpes; Lesions; Shingles; Skin; Skin disorders; Stress; Ulcers; Viral infections.

For Further Information:
A.D.A.M. Medical Encyclopedia. "Canker Sore." *MedlinePlus*, February 17, 2011.
AAOM Web Writing Group. "Canker Sores." *American Academy of Oral Medicine*, December 31, 2007.
Komaroff, Anthony, ed. *Harvard Medical School Family Health Guide*. New York: Free Press, 2005.
National Institute of Dental Research. *Fever Blisters and Canker Sores*. Rev. ed. Bethesda, Md.: National Institutes of Health, 1992.
National Institute of Dental and Craniofacial Research. "Mouth Problems and HIV." *National Institutes of Health*, March 25, 2011.
Norwood, Diane, and Michael Woods. "Aphthous Ulcers." *Health Library*, November 26, 2012.
Porter, Robert S., et al., eds. *The Merck Manual Home Health Handbook*. Whitehouse Station, N.J.: Merck Research Laboratories, 2009.
Sutton, Amy L., ed. *Dental Care and Oral Health Sourcebook*. 3d ed. Detroit, Mich.: Omnigraphics, 2008.

Capgras syndrome

Disease/Disorder
Also known as: Capgras delusion
Anatomy or system affected: The pathway connecting the ventral stream to the limbic system; the patient's belief evaluation system
Specialties and related fields: Neuropsychiatry, neurology, psychology
Definition: The delusional belief that at least one family member or friend or significant other has been replaced by an impostor
Key terms:

circumscribed: not impacting on the patient's other beliefs, meaning that these other beliefs are not adjusted

delusional misidentification: a delusional belief about the identity of an individual or thing such that the individual or thing is misidentified (e.g., that different people are the same person in disguise [Frégoli delusion] or that one's wife is an impostor)

monothematic: restricted to one type of belief or theme, rather than expanding to include multiple themes

skin conductance response (also galvanic skin response): a change in the skin's ability to conduct electricity owing to increased/decreased sweating brought on by changes in autonomic arousal

Causes and Symptoms

The Capgras delusion represents one of several rare psychiatric disorders that share a common theme: that of delusional misidentification. A typical claim made by the Capgras patient involves the replacement of one or more close relatives and/or friends or some "significant other" by exact doubles. The fact that the significant other has been "replaced" indicates that the patient does not perceive both individuals simultaneously. The real person is always absent, leaving just a single, yet identical impostor. The Capgras delusion is universal. Similar delusional beliefs occur in individuals from all cultures. It affects both sexes and strikes at all ages from adolescence upwards.

Within the Capgras patient there appears to exist a conflict of recognition: a seeming paradox in which the object of perception (the significant other) is and yet is not recognized by the patient. Physically, including all mannerisms and voice patterns, the impostor is said to be just like the real person but is not recognized as being that person.

The disorder is not the result of some global perceptual problem, nor is the "impostor belief" ubiquitous: the patient correctly identifies and believes in the authenticity of the vast majority of other people. Instead, the delusion is specific; it is directed towards persons of significance only; it is monothematic and circumscribed.

Over the years, more and more evidence has been amassed implicating some form of organic disturbance in the etiology of the Capgras delusion. Yet it has remained difficult to understand how organic disease, cerebral lesion, or head trauma could account for the high degree of selectivity evident in the delusional content. Why is this person, specifically, an impostor? To illustrate, image that a lesion to Broca's areas (which causes a disruption in language production) prevented a patient from communicating with his wife or son only, whereas with everyone else he was able to speak normally.

More recently, explanations of the Capgras delusion have tended to have at their base a neurological disturbance within the face recognition system. According to an established account of normal facial recognition, when presented with a familiar face, the face recognition unit (FRU) triggers information stored in person identity nodes (PINs). In simple terms, this enables overt or conscious identification of the face. In addition, there exists a separate pathway connecting the ventral stream to the limbic system and, in particular, the amygdala. In the presence of familiar faces heightened arousal occurs, the index of which is increased skin conductance response (SCRs). This is often interpreted as a measure of covert recognition. The mirror-image model proposes that Capgras patients have an intact overt recognition system but a dysfunctional covert system. In the presence of a familiar face, there is no heightened autonomic arousal (no increased SCR). As an aside, prosopagnosic patients (who are unable to consciously recognize familiar faces) show increased SCR when in the presence of familiar faces. They are believed to have a dysfunctional overt pathway and a functioning covert pathway, the mirror-reverse of the Capgras patient: hence, the mirror-image model.

Contemporary accounts of the Capgras delusion tend to involve either one or two explanatory stages. One-stage models hold that the neurological disturbance, in the otherwise rational individual, results in an anomalous experience. In the presence of his wife (for example), something feels wrong to the patient. The oddness he feels is explained by forming the "impostor" belief. Two-stage models, in contrast, maintain that the anomalous experience is not sufficient to form the delusional belief. In addition, there is a disruption in the patient's belief evaluation system (or some other form of cognitive disruption: e.g., attribution bias). It is the culmination of first-stage neurological disturbance and second-stage cognitive disruption that produces the impostor belief.

Treatment and Therapy

There is no single recognized treatment for the Capgras delusion. Treatment and therapy is often determined on an individual case-by-case basis. Case study reports indicate the successful use of antipsychotic drugs (such as olanzapine, pimozode, and prophylaxis) or antidepressants (mirtazapine). Cognitive techniques such as reality testing may also prove successful. The Capgras delusion can also prove resistant to treatment.

Perspective and Prospects

Prior to the aforementioned one- and two-stage accounts and the mirror-image model, the psychoanalytic approach sought to explain the Capgras delusion in terms of splitting the significant other into real and false personas. The patient's act of splitting was said to be symptomatic of their ambivalence towards the significant other. The Capgras delusion was therefore seen as a way of resolving the love-hate conflict underlying this ambivalence. The son can direct hostile feelings towards his mother, for example, if he believes that she is really an impostor. He is thus free to express his aggression without experiencing any guilt.

The Capgras delusion has thus been transformed from a psychoanalytic disorder of function, stemming from an unconscious conflict and a means of resolving it, to a neurocognitive disorder. The most recent discussion on the delusional state has centered on the extent to which those processes that bring about the delusional belief occur subpersonally (below conscious awareness) and so do not involve (require, even) anomalous patient experience.

—*Garry Young, Ph.D.*

See also Psychoanalysis; Psychiatric disorders

For Further Information:
Coltheart, Max, and Martin Davies. *Pathologies of Belief.* Oxford: Blackwell, 2000.
Davies, Martin, and Andy Egan. "Delusion: Cognitive Approaches Bayesian Inference and Compartmentalisation." *The Oxford Handbook of Philosophy and Psychiatry,* edited by K.W.M. Fulford, et al. Oxford: Oxford University Press, 2013.
Ellis, Hadyn D., and Michael B. Lewis. "Capgras Delusion: A Window on Face Recognition." *Trends in Cognitive Science* 5, no. 4 (2001): 149-156.
Young, Garry. "Capgras Delusion: An Interactionist Model." *Consciousness and Cognition,* 17, no. 3 (2008): 863-876.

Carbohydrates

Biology
Also known as: Sugars, saccharides
Anatomy or system affected: Blood, brain, endocrine system, gastrointestinal system, intestines, kidneys, muscles, pancreas

Specialties and related fields: Biochemistry, endocrinology, nutrition

Definition: Organic compounds consisting of carbon, hydrogen, and oxygen, in which hydrogen and oxygen are in a 2:1 ratio. The simplest carbohydrates (monosaccharides) contain an aldehyde or a ketone functional group and usually one hydroxyl group per carbon atom.

Digestion and Absorption

Dietary carbohydrates include monosaccharides, such as glucose, fructose, and lactose; disaccharides (two monosaccharides linked together), such as sucrose and lactose; and polysaccharides (many monosaccharides linked together in polymers), such as starches and fiber.

Starches are first broken down in the mouth by salivary alpha-amylase and then in the small intestine by alpha-amylases of both salivary and pancreatic origin. The resulting simpler sugars are further digested by enzymes linked to the inner lining of the small intestine: maltase, sucrase, and trehalase, which yield absorbable monosaccharides. These sugars cross the cells lining the small intestine via specialized molecular transport mechanisms and then diffuse into the intestinal capillaries and reach the bloodstream.

Metabolism

In the body, the main role of carbohydrates is energy production and storage. Carbohydrates can also be joined to proteins (glycoproteins, for cell-cell interactions) or fatty acids (glycolipids, which provide energy and can be markers for cellular recognition).

The body converts most digestible carbohydrates into glucose, which is a universal energy source for cells. Excess glucose is stored as glycogen (glycogenesis), which can then be broken down (glycogenolysis) when energy is needed. Glucose is maintained at a constant level in the blood by the interplay of insulin, gulcagon, and other hormones.

Carbohydrate-related diseases are often genetic in nature, linked to inborn errors in enzymes or cellular transporters. Examples are galactosemia, glycogen storage diseases, and lactose intolerance. Diabetes mellitus is a metabolic disorder characterized by excessive blood glucose. Type 1 diabetes is caused by insulin deficiency; type 2 can be the result of insulin resistance, impaired insulin secretion, and increased glucose production.

According to current recommendations, carbohydrates, preferably starches and natural sugars, should represent 40 to 60 percent of total calorie intake. Refined simple sugars provide calories but very little nutrition, and their intake should therefore be limited.

Perspective and Prospects

Food availability in developed countries has reached unprecedented levels, and the per capita consumption of carbohydrates, particularly in the form of refined sugars, increased dramatically in the late twentieth and early twenty-first centuries. Since the 1990s, the incidence of obesity has been climbing steadily, and so has the incidence of diabetes and related health problems. Current research in nutrition and carbohydrate metabolism is addressing the problem, which has reached epidemic proportions. Great progress is being made in dietary manipulations and drug development.

—*Donatella M. Casirola, Ph.D.*

See also Celiac sprue; Diabetes mellitus; Dietary reference intakes (DRIs); Digestion; Eating disorders; Enzymes; Fiber; Food biochemistry; Food Guide Pyramid; Gluten intolerance; Glycogen storage diseases; Insulin resistance syndrome; Lipids; Metabolic disorders; Metabolism; Nutrition; Obesity; Obesity, childhood; Protein.

For Further Information:

A.D.A.M. Medical Encyclopedia. "Carbohydrates." *MedlinePlus*, May 16, 2012.

Centers for Disease Control and Prevention. "Carbohydrates." *Centers for Disease Control and Prevention*, December 11, 2012.

Mayo Clinic. "Carbohydrates: How Carbs Fit into a Healthy Diet." *Mayo Foundation for Medical Education and Research*, February 8, 2011.

McGraw-Hill Encyclopedia of Science and Technology. 10th ed. 20 vols. New York: McGraw-Hill, 2007.

Sherwood, Lauralee. "The Digestive System." In *Human Physiology: From Cells to Systems.* 7th ed. Pacific Grove, Calif.: Brooks, 2010.

Stanhope, K. L., and P. J. Havel. "Fructose Consumption: Considerations for Future Research on Its Effects on Adipose Distribution, Lipid Metabolism, and Insulin Sensitivity in Humans." *Journal of Nutrition* 139, no. 6 (June, 2009): 1236S-41S.

Carcinogens

Disease/Disorder

Anatomy or system affected: All

Specialties and related fields: All

Definition: A substance or agent that causes or precipitates cancer.

Types and Effects

Carcinogens include chemicals, radiation, or viruses that can alter the DNA (deoxyribonucleic acid) in a normal human cell and eventually mutate it into a cancer cell. Some carcinogens change DNA structure directly, while others make DNA more susceptible to damage from other sources or increase the possibility of DNA changes by causing cells to divide faster than normal. This means that the mechanism for how to regulate their growth stops working properly. This is known as the inhibiting of cell regulation division.

Susceptibility to different carcinogens varies widely from person to person and is highly dependent upon genetic makeup, physiology, exposure time, dose of the carcinogen, and nutrition available to the cells affected.

The Report on Carcinogens (RoC) released by the U.S. government in 2011 identifies over 50 known carcinogens. The government also made available a list, last updated in 2010, that identifies reasonably suspected carcinogens, which have not yet been proven to be carcinogenic (cancer-causing). There are currently known viral carcinogens present on the list, including hepatitis B virus (HBV), hepatitis C virus (HVC), and human papillomaviruses (HPVs). Lately, vaccines have been used to prevent infection and subsequent cancer formation from such etiologies. A list of carcinogens is also published by the International Agency for Research on Cancer (IARC).

Classification and Reducing Risk

Identification and classification of carcinogens is made from human observation and from laboratory studies that include animal experimentation and cell cultures. The RoC data include information about the ability of each substance to cause cancer, its ability to damage genes, and the biological changes that it can produce in the body. It reports the potential for human exposure to the listed substances and the federal regulations that are imposed to limit exposure. The RoC also gives updates on current efforts to investigate potential public health concerns. For example, they explain a current effort by the National Toxicology Program to investigate any potential health hazards from exposure to cell phone radiation.

A number of important measures can lower the risk of exposure to carcinogens. Avoiding cigarette smoking, excessive alcohol consumption, and abnormal exposure to ultraviolet (UV) radiation from sunlight reduces the risk of many cancers. Another way to protect against exposure to carcinogens is to be informed about the carcinogenic (cancer-causing) substances that may be present at home or in the workplace. Exercising the necessary precautions can be beneficial in avoiding exposure and risk. It is very important to follow the directions on any chemical containers.

Perspective and Prospects

The identification of cancer-causing agents, or carcinogens, dates back to the 1930s when dozens of substances, including industrial pollution and tobacco smoke, were classified as carcinogens. U.S. federal law requires that the secretary of Health and Human Services publish the RoC through the National Toxicology Program (NTP) every two years. In addition to listing carcinogens, the IARC report also lists substances that have been studied and determined not to be carcinogens.

But even potential carcinogens can be a cause of concern. For example, RoC and IARC reports indicated that acrylamide, a chemical in French fries and potato chips, is a possible carcinogen, as well as the charred residue on barbecued meats. The Food and Drug Administration (FDA) reported that in a test of 124 cosmetics, over half of them contained the carcinogens triethanolamine (TEA) and diethanolamine (DEA). To complicate matters even more, beneficial drugs can also have carcinogenic side effects. Perhaps the best example is the drug tamoxifen, which, while used effectively in the treatment of breast cancer, increases the risk of some types of uterine cancer.

—*Alvin K. Benson, Ph.D.;*
updated by Joshua Lampert, MS-III

See also Asbestos exposure; Cancer; Environmental diseases; Environmental health; Hepatitis; Human papillomaviruses (HPV); Mutation; Smoking.

For Further Information:
Adami, Hans-Olov, David Hunter, and Dimitrios Trichopoulos. *Textbook of Cancer Epidemiology.* 2nd ed. New York: Oxford University Press, 2008.
Benigni, Romualdo, ed. *Quantitative Structure-Activity Relationship (QSAR) Models of Mutagens and Carcinogens.* Boca Raton, FL: CRC Press, 2003.
McKinnell, Robert Gilmore, ed. *The Biological Basis of Cancer.* 2nd ed. New York: Cambridge University Press, 2006.
Milman, Harry A., and Elizabeth K. Weisburger, eds. *Handbook of Carcinogen Testing.* 2nd ed. Park Ridge, NJ: Noyes, 2001.
Pohanish, Richard P., ed. *Sittig's Handbook of Toxic and Hazardous Chemicals and Carcinogens.* Vols. 1 and 2. 5th ed. Norwich, NY: William Andrew, 2008.
Weinberg, Robert. *The Biology of Cancer.* New York: Garland Science, 2007.

Carcinoma

Disease/Disorder
Anatomy or system affected: All
Specialties and related fields: Cytology, dermatology, histology, immunology, oncology
Definition: A malignant neoplasm or tumor that arises in epithelial cells.

Causes and Symptoms

The term "carcinoma" is often used as a synonym for cancer. A carcinoma is a malignant neoplasm or tumor that arises in the epithelial cells of tissues that line the surface layer of skin or that cover the internal organs. The most common carcinomas develop in the lungs, breasts, colon, small intestine, prostate (in men), and cervix (in women). In contrast, a sarcoma is a malignant neoplasm that affects mesenchymal tissue, the precursor to bone, muscle, and fat. Carcinomas are spread in the body through lymphatic fluid, most frequently to nearby lymph nodes, while sarcomas are spread in the body through the blood.

In general, carcinomas appear to be caused by a disturbance in the delicate balance of cell growth and death regulation. The immune system normally detects and stops dysfunctional cell growth, but an abnormality in this system can cause cell growth regulators to malfunction, leading to an eventual development of cancerous cells. Other potential causes of carcinoma include genetics, certain viruses, radiation, toxins, and environmental and social factors such as tobacco, pollution, sunlight, and diet. It is important to understand, however, that the causes of most cancers are still not completely known. Therefore, the best preventive measure against cancer is the avoidance and cessation of products and actions that are definitely known to be cancer-causing. Tobacco has been clearly linked to lung cancer, and excessive sunlight exposure has been linked to skin cancer. A healthy diet, exercise, and regular medical examinations are some of the preventive steps recommended by the American Cancer Society to lessen the risks of developing most cancers.

Symptoms of carcinoma depend on the type and location of the tumor, or neoplasm. For example, skin cancer may appear as a mole that changes in color and texture in a short period of time or an open sore that does not heal properly, while lung cancer may manifest itself as a serious and pain-

Information on Carcinoma

Causes: Tumor in epithelial cells of skin or internal organs; related to genetics, certain viruses, radiation, toxins, environmental and social factors (tobacco, pollution, sunlight, diet)

Symptoms: Dependent on type and location of tumor (e.g., mole or open sore for skin cancer; painful cough, hoarseness, and chest pain for lung cancer); in general, headaches, chills, fever, fatigue, unusual bleeding, unintentional weight loss, vomiting

Duration: Chronic, sometimes recurrent

Treatments: Surgery, chemotherapy, radiation

ful cough accompanied by hoarseness and chest pain. Though some cancers may not have a specific symptomology, certain symptoms are common to most, including headaches, chills, fever, fatigue, unusual bleeding, unintentional weight loss, and vomiting.

Treatment and Therapy

The goal of most cancer treatments is to eliminate the carcinoma. The course of treatment taken depends entirely on the location and type of cancer. Three kinds of cancer treatment are most frequently used: surgery, chemotherapy, and radiation. In cases where the carcinoma is confined to a specific organ or lymphatic nodule, surgery may be the prescribed course of treatment. When the carcinoma has spread throughout the body, radiation and chemotherapy may be the best viable options. Some cancers require a combination of all three modes of treatment.

Prognosis depends entirely on the carcinoma and the stage of the cancer when first diagnosed. Some carcinomas are successfully treated with little chance of recurrence, while others prove to be nonresponsive and eventually lead to death.

—Nicholas Lanzieri

See also Anal cancer; Bladder cancer; Brain tumors; Breast cancer; Cancer; Cervical, ovarian, and uterine cancers; Chemotherapy; Colorectal cancer; Epstein-Barr virus; Gallbladder cancer; Hodgkin's disease; Kidney cancer; Leukemia; Liver cancer; Lung cancer; Lymphadenopathy and lymphoma; Malignancy and metastasis; Mouth and throat cancer; National Cancer Institute (NCI); Oncology; Prostate cancer; Radiation therapy; Sarcoma; Screening; Skin cancer; Stomach, intestinal, and pancreatic cancers; Testicular cancer; Tumor removal; Tumors.

For Further Information:
American Cancer Society (ACS), 2013.
"Cancer." *MedlinePlus*, May 2, 2013.
Cancer Care, 2013.
Cooper, Geoffrey M. *Elements of Human Cancer*. Boston: Jones and Bartlett, 1992.
Dollinger, Malin, et al. *Everyone's Guide to Cancer Therapy*. 5th ed. Kansas City, Mo.: Andrews McMeel, 2008.
Holleb, Arthur I., ed. *The American Cancer Society Cancer Book: Prevention, Detection, Diagnosis, Treatment, Rehabilitation, Cure*. Garden City, N.Y.: Doubleday, 1986.
McKinnell, Robert Gilmore, ed. *The Biological Basis of Cancer*. 2d ed. New York: Cambridge University Press, 2006.
"Understanding Cancer Series: Cancer." *National Cancer Institute*, Sept. 30, 2009.
Weinberg, Robert. *The Biology of Cancer*. 2d ed. New York: Garland Science, 2013.

Cardiac arrest

Disease/Disorder

Anatomy or system affected: Circulatory system, heart

Specialties and related fields: Cardiology, emergency medicine

Definition: A complete cessation of the mechanical and/or electrical activity of the heart.

Causes and Symptoms

Many conditions, such as drug overdoses, drowning, poisoning, and electrocution, can result in cardiac arrest, but the major cause is insufficient oxygen supply to the heart as a result of a heart attack. When a major coronary artery becomes blocked, blood cannot flow to the heart muscle cells to deliver oxygen. Without sufficient oxygen, the heart is unable to pump blood to the rest of the body. Within seconds, the blood flow to the brain is inadequate and the individual loses consciousness and stops breathing. If blood flow is not resumed within several minutes, permanent brain damage will occur, frequently followed by death.

The major symptoms of cardiac arrest are lack of a pulse and lack of normal breathing. Medical personnel can also use an electrocardiogram (ECG or EKG) to identify specific problems with the heart, including too rapid of a heart rate to pump blood, quivering of the heart muscle, the complete absence of electrical activity, or the absence of contractions with normal electrical activity. Any of these cases is a medical emergency and treatment is required.

Treatment and Therapy

Cardiopulmonary resuscitation (CPR) is the initial treatment for cardiac arrest. The sooner the blood flow to the brain is restored, the better is the prognosis. Breathing into the victim's mouth and externally compressing the chest over the heart can circulate oxygenated blood throughout the body. However, emergency medical treatment is generally required to get the heart beating on its own. Cardioversion, the use of an external defibrillator to shock the heart, is administered to restore the heart's normal cardiac rhythm. Additionally, medical personnel will administer specific medications such as atropine, epinephrine, and lidocaine. In some extreme cases, emergency surgery is required.

Perspective and Prospects

One of the best strategies to save the lives of those who suffer cardiac arrest is to decrease the time that it takes to restore blood flow and get the heart beating on its own again.

CPR was first promoted to the general public as a tool to save lives in the 1970s. By teaching many individuals how to respond to this emergency situation, the likelihood of receiving CPR quickly increases. Unfortunately CPR cannot save everyone. In recent years, automatic external defibrillators (AEDs) have been placed in public areas and worksites to improve survival. AEDs can be administered

Information on Cardiac Arrest

Causes: Usually a heart attack; also, drug overdose, drowning, poisoning, electrocution

Symptoms: Lack of pulse, loss of consciousness, and cessation of breathing; if blood flow is not resumed quickly, permanent brain damage and sometimes death

Duration: Acute

Treatments: Cardiopulmonary resuscitation (CPR), defibrillation, medications (atropine, epinephrine, lidocaine), sometimes surgery

by nonmedical personnel who have been trained how to use them, thus greatly decreasing the time that it takes to restart a normal cardiac rhythm.

—Bradley R. A. Wilson, Ph.D.

See also Brain damage; Cardiac rehabilitation; Cardiology; Cardiology, pediatric; Cardiopulmonary resuscitation (CPR); Circulation; Defibrillation; Drowning; Electrical shock; Electrocardiography (ECG or EKG); Emergency medicine; Emergency medicine, pediatric; Emergency rooms; First aid; Heart; Heart attack; Infarction; Pacemaker implantation; Palpitations; Poisoning; Resuscitation; Shock; Vascular medicine; Vascular system.

For Further Information:

American Medical Association. *American Medical Association Family Medical Guide.* 4th rev. ed. Hoboken, N.J.: John Wiley & Sons, 2004.

Berra, Kathleen, et al. *Heart Attack! Advice for Patients by Patients.* New Haven, Conn.: Yale University Press, 2002.

"Cardiac Arrest." *American Heart Association,* 2013.

"Cardiac Arrest." *MedlinePlus,* May 13, 2013.

Klag, Michael J., et al., eds. *Johns Hopkins Family Health Book.* New York: HarperCollins, 1999.

Komaroff, Anthony, ed. *Harvard Medical School Family Health Guide.* New York: Free Press, 2005.

Sherwood, Lauralee. *Human Physiology: From Cells to Systems.* 8th ed. Pacific Grove, Calif.: Brooks/Cole/Cengage Learning, 2013.

Wood, Debra, and Michael J. Fucci. "Cardiac Arrest." *Health Library,* Sept. 10, 2012.

Cardiac rehabilitation

Treatment

Anatomy or system affected: Chest, circulatory system, heart

Specialties and related fields: Cardiology, exercise physiology, nursing, nutrition, occupational health, physical therapy, psychology

Definition: The activities that ensure the physical, mental, and social conditions necessary for returning cardiac patients to good health.

Key terms:

aerobic exercise: exercise that requires oxygen for energy production and that can be sustained for prolonged periods of time; involves large muscle groups, increases the heart rate and breathing rate, and is rhythmic and continuous

atherosclerosis: a buildup of fatty deposits or plaques that effectively reduces the inner diameter of the arteries, thus obstructing the normal flow of blood

cardiovascular disease: any of a group of diseases that affect the circulatory system, including coronary artery disease, hypertension, congestive heart failure, congenital heart defects, and valvular heart disease

coronary artery bypass graft(CABG): a surgical procedure in which a blocked coronary artery is bypassed using a vein or artery; this intervention provides a blood supply to areas beyond the distal attachment of the graft

coronary artery disease(CAD): a disease that results in a narrowing of the coronary arteries and a concomitant reduction of blood flow

electrocardiogram(EKG or ECG): a mechanical representation of the electrical activity generated by the heart and recorded on paper or displayed on a cathode-ray tube

invasive testing: techniques involving the puncture or incision of the skin or the insertion of an instrument or foreign material into the body

MET: a measure of human energy expenditure; 1 MET is equal to the amount of energy expended at rest (approximately 3.5 milliliters of oxygen per kilogram of body weight per minute)

myocardial infarction: irreversible damage to heart muscle tissue caused by insufficient oxygen supply to that tissue

percutaneous transluminal coronary angioplasty(PTCA): a procedure undertaken to increase the internal diameter of a coronary artery by inflating a small balloon-like device at the site or sites where the artery has narrowed because of plaque buildup

risk factors: those habits or conditions that increase the likelihood of developing a disease or disorder

target heart raterange: a heart rate range that is to be maintained during exercise training

Indications and Procedures

Cardiovascular disease (CVD), or heart disease, is the leading cause of death and disability in most of the industrialized nations of the world. For those persons who survive a cardiac event, discharge from a hospital or medical setting without further assistance may lead to financial, physical, and mental incapacity.

Just as interventional procedures and medical care are important for the initial treatment of acute cardiac events, such as a myocardial infarction (heart attack) or angina (chest pain), cardiac rehabilitation influences long-term morbidity and mortality. Such preventive cardiology assists persons with CVD in three main areas: education, behavior modification, and patient and family support. The two primary goals of the rehabilitation program are to help increase the patient's functional capacity (the ability to perform activities of daily living) and to counteract or arrest the patient's disease process using a multidisciplinary educational approach. To provide direction in prevention and rehabilitation, research studies have clearly defined several modifiable risk factors for heart disease, which are presented to patients. Among the most significant are smoking, high serum cholesterol, hypertension, physical inactivity, overweight, diabetes, and depression. Assistance with education about and modification of these risk factors, through risk factor counseling and participation in physical activity, is provided in modern cardiac rehabilitation programs.

Methods for providing education on risk factor modification can vary greatly from program to program but may include such means as didactic lecturing, slide presentations, printed material for patients to read, demonstrations (such as cooking and stress reduction techniques), providing loaner books, and one-on-one counseling.

The exercise portion of the cardiac rehabilitation is most often the time-consuming element of the program. It involves controlling and monitoring four major variables: mode (type of activity, such as bicycling, walking, or stair-stepping), duration (length of time the patient exercises), frequency (number of times per week that exercise is performed), and intensity (exertion level of the patient, usually assessed by the heart rate response).

To become involved in the cardiac rehabilitation program, a patient is initially screened by a physician, nurse practitioner, or other clinical specialist and directed to the appropriate level (or phase) of intervention. There are three to four clinical phases involved with cardiac rehabilitation, as various groups categorize them differently. Phase 1 occurs while the patient is still in the hospital. It begins when the patient's condition is stabilized, sometimes as soon as forty-eight hours after the coronary event or procedure. This phase can begin in the coronary care unit (CCU) or the intensive care unit (ICU). Phase 1 incorporates several disciplines, including physical therapy, nursing, psychiatry, dietetics, occupational therapy, and exercise science. It is designed to prevent the deleterious physiological effects of bed rest.

The physical components of this phase include maintaining a range of motion and gradually returning to activities of daily living. Patients gradually advance through stages until they are able to walk up to 200 or 400 feet. Before discharge, patients are encouraged to walk up and down one flight of stairs. Stair climbing is done while accompanied by a physical therapist or other clinician who monitors heart rate and blood pressure. The level of exertion during the early portion of this phase is normally 1 to 2 metabolic equivalents (METs). Thus, in phase 1, the mode of exercise focuses on motion (sitting, standing, and finally walking), the frequency is seven days per week, the duration of exercise is usually five to ten minutes at a time, and the intensity of activity should not cause the heart rate to exceed twenty beats above the resting rate while standing.

For coronary artery bypass graft (CABG) patients who have not experienced a myocardial infarction, progress during this phase is usually faster than for heart attack patients. Percutaneous transluminal coronary angioplasty (PTCA) patients may receive only a few days of rehabilitation, as they are usually discharged from the hospital sooner than heart attack or CABG patients.

The mental components of phase 1 include risk factor modification education and an introduction to rehabilitation concepts. Risk factor education at this point provides a good foundation for the basic concepts that will be explained during the education program in phase 2. For those patients who are appropriate candidates for a phase 2 program, information on that phase is then provided.

Phase 2 customarily begins within three weeks of discharge from the hospital and lasts for four to twelve weeks. During phase 2, patients are exposed to a level of exertion commensurate with several criteria: the patient's clinical status (stable or unstable, depending on whether the patient is experiencing problems related to the disease); the patient's functional capacity, or fitness level; orthopedic limitations, such as muscle or joint problems; the goals for functional capacity (which tasks the patient wants to be able to perform); and any other special circumstances or situations. In a given phase 2 program, there are a variety of patients, all with varying levels of physical fitness. Through variations in the mode, duration, frequency, or intensity of exercise, these differing levels of fitness can be accommodated. A variety of exercise modes are presented in the phase 2 program, including walking, stationary cycling, stationary rowing, simulated stair-climbing, water aerobics, swimming, and upper body ergometry. The exercise frequency for this phase is three to five days per week, the duration consists of twenty to forty-five minutes of continuous aerobic activity, and the intensity should produce a heart rate that is 60 to 85 percent of the symptom-limited maximal heart rate. Muscle-strengthening and flexibility exercises may also be recommended. Exercises are monitored by an exercise specialist or other sports medicine clinician and a cardiovascular fitness nurse. Exercise intensity is determined in most cases by heart rate and may be monitored by electrocardiogram (EKG or ECG) telemetry on a number of patients simultaneously. One of the interesting psychological components to phase 2 cardiac rehabilitation is that most programs are arranged so that new participants are coming into the program as participants who have been in the program for several sessions are leaving. Newer participants are able to identify with those already in the program as a result of similarities in cardiac experiences. It has been suggested that this identification decreases the anxiety level of a patient who is just becoming involved in the program.

Patients move into phase 3 of cardiac rehabilitation, a community- based outpatient program, when cardiovascular and physiological responses to exercise have been stabilized and the patient has achieved the goals initially set. Phase 3 is generally considered to be an extended, supervised program that usually lasts from four to six months but can continue indefinitely. Participants in phase 3 programs become more involved in and responsible for their own exercises. Typically, these programs do not include EKG monitoring. Individuals are given more responsibility with respect to maintaining their own heart rates in their training heart rate range. Usually, an exercise specialist, nurse, or physician is available to oversee the exercises. The mode, frequency, duration, and intensity of exercise in this phase is similar to that of phase 2. Phase 4 is a maintenance program. Although many rehabilitation settings label this part of the phase 3 program, the phase 4 program is considered the longest-term, ongoing phase and is of indefinite length. Many phase 2 cardiac rehabilitation program graduates remain in phase 3 or phase 4 programs for years. The mode,

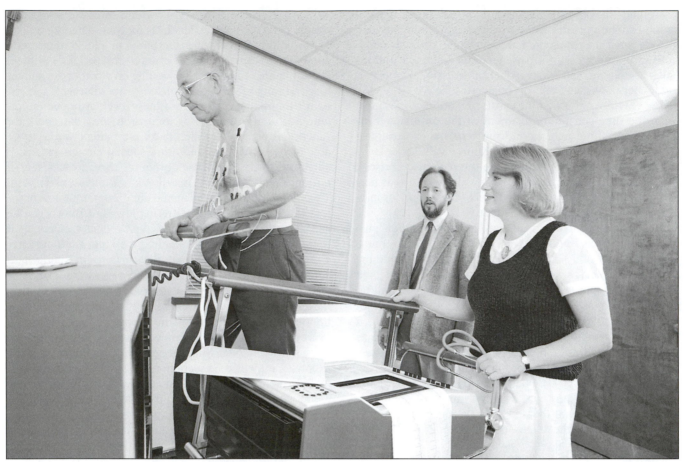

An elderly patient undergoes a cardiac stress test to evaluate heart function. (Digital Stock)

frequency, duration, and intensity of the exercise program for phase 4 are also similar to those of phase 2.

Uses and Complications

Traditionally, cardiac rehabilitation has been recommended for individuals convalescing from myocardial infarctions or heart surgery (CABG, PTCA, or valve replacement). More recently, the eligibility for cardiac rehabilitation has been extended to include heart transplant recipients and others with cardiac-related illnesses.

Improvement of work capacity is one of the goals of cardiac rehabilitation. The mechanisms involved in increasing work capacity (aerobic capacity and maximal oxygen consumption) normally include increases in both central (cardiac output, stroke volume, and heart rate) and peripheral (muscle changes, atrioventricular oxygen difference) adaptations. Nevertheless, this does not preclude patients with reduced left ventricular (LV) function from participation in a medically supervised exercise program. For the reduced LV function patient, improvement in exercise tolerance can occur; this improvement may be attributable mainly to peripheral adaptations.

For the low-risk patient, cardiac rehabilitation may seem unnecessary since unsupervised exercise programs have been demonstrated to be safe and effective and to improve exercise capacity. For healthy lifestyle modification to take place, however, the educational component of cardiac rehabilitation may provide the patient with invaluable knowledge. To reduce the chance of recurrence or severity of a myocardial infarction in an effective manner, a healthy lifestyle is encouraged. Additional potential benefits of participation include improved self-esteem, positive mental attitude, and decreased anxiety and depression.

Low-risk patients, who account for about one-third to one-half of heart attack patients and about three-quarters of CABG patients, have a first-year mortality of less than 2 percent. Moderate-risk patients have a first-year mortality rate of between 10 percent and 25 percent. High-risk patients' mortality rates are greater than 25 percent. While cardiac rehabilitation is not effective in all circumstances, proper assessment of an individual's clinical situation and competent administration of the program can optimize the outcome for participants. Increasing numbers of cardiac rehabilitation programs are accepting unconventional patient populations. These patients now include heart transplant recipients, congestive heart failure patients, individuals suffering from ischemic heart disease, and those with dysrhythmias and/or pacemakers.

Although most of the prescribed exercise regimens for these patients parallel those for the conventional cardiac patient, there are subtle differences. In the heart transplant population, for example, heart rate response differs from non-transplant patients. The adjustment of heart rate to various workloads lags in acute heart transplant recipients; that is, the heart rate does not increase as rapidly as it does for normal people. To accommodate this difference, researchers have suggested that, in place of heart rate response, clinicians use a "rating of perceived exertion" scale to monitor the patients' responses to exercise.

Even patients who have orthopedic limitations, such as arthritis or chronic injuries, may be accommodated in the exercise portion of the cardiac rehabilitation program. Exercises can be adjusted to allow participants to derive cardiovascular benefits without causing them unnecessary discomfort. Although cardiac rehabilitation is safe in general, several factors may emerge during graded exercise testing (a screening for entry into a cardiac rehabilitation program) that can identify those patients who may be at increased risk. These factors include a significant depression or elevation of the ST wave segment from a resting ECG, angina, extensive left ventricular dysfunction and severe myocardial infarction, ventricular dysrhythmias, inappropriate blood pressure response to exercise, achieving a peak heart rate of fewer than 120 beats per minute (if not taking a negative chronotropic medication, which slows down the heart rate), and a functional exercise capacity of fewer than 4 to 5 METs. Inclusion in one of these categories does not preclude participation in a cardiac rehabilitation program, but it may warrant specific exercise guidelines and close monitoring. Among the criteria for exclusion from a cardiac rehabilitation program are unstable angina, acute systemic illness, uncontrolled dysrhythmias, uncontrolled resting heart rate of greater than 120 beats per minute, uncontrolled diabetes, symptomatic congestive heart failure, a resting systolic blood pressure over 180 millimeters of mercury (mm Hg) or a resting diastolic blood pressure over 110 mm Hg, third-degree heart block without a pacemaker, and significant aortic stenosis.

For those who meet the criteria for inclusion in a cardiac rehabilitation program, risk stratification (lowest, moderate, or highest risk) may be employed. This allows an appropriate amount of supervision to be in place based on each patient's goals and condition. Clinical observations and tests allow each patient to be assessed individually. Within each phase, levels of risk may be established. Various proposals have been made for risk stratification prior to entry into a cardiac rehabilitation program, including stratification based on several factors: the degree of left ventricular dysfunction, presence or absence of myocardial ischemia, extent of myocardial injury, and presence of ventricular dysrhythmias.

Some of the most widely examined noninvasive assessment tools include the extent of QRS wave abnormalities on a resting EKG and the results of exercise stress testing, twenty-four hour ambulatory EKG monitoring, radionuclide ventriculography, and echocardiography. A combination of these test results may be used to determine the course of action provided to an individual.

As with any effective therapy, exercise as a form of cardiac rehabilitation is neither without hazard nor always beneficial. If appropriate clinical guidelines are utilized, however, the benefit-risk ratio can be very favorable. The low incidence of cardiac-related adverse events during participation in outpatient cardiac rehabilitation programs is probably attributable to improved risk stratification, the use of appropriate medical and surgical therapies, and improved exercise guidelines. On the rare occasions when cardiac events occur, reports have indicated that up to 90 percent of all patients with exercise-related cardiac arrest are successfully resuscitated when the patient experiences the event in a properly equipped and supervised program.

Perspective and Prospects

Until the 1940s, patients recovering from acute myocardial infarctions met with restriction of physical activity, bed rest, and psychological apprehension about exertion. Over the next two decades, the deleterious physiological effects of prolonged bed rest began to be described. During this time, a few investigators were beginning to encourage early treatment of the patient who has experienced an acute heart attack, including armchair work and walking within four weeks of the acute event.

In the 1950s, British physician Jeremy Morris and his colleagues conducted research that initiated interest in the relationship between coronary artery disease (CAD) and a sedentary lifestyle. In this study, he found that London bus drivers had twice the risk of developing CAD than their more physically active bus conductor counterparts. In addition, among those drivers and conductors who had experienced a heart attack, the drivers were twice as likely as the conductors to die either during or within two months of their heart attack. During the 1960s, the beginnings of what are now considered cardiac rehabilitation programs incorporated exercise training on a somewhat limited basis. Restricted exercise regimens began a few weeks after cardiac events and increased in intensity on a very gradual basis. Generally, the patient population considered appropriate for such programs consisted of those individuals who had experienced uncomplicated myocardial infarctions. Some risk factor modification education was initiated, but not on a large scale primarily because data supporting improved patient outcomes were not proven.

Soon afterward, the On Ward program, designed to begin on the tenth day following a heart attack, was introduced based on work by William P. Blocker Jr. and colleagues. In 1971, J. M. Kaufman suggested that rehabilitation of uncomplicated myocardial infarction patients could begin as early as two days after the heart attack. At this time, many hospitals had some form of cardiac rehabilitation program; most of them, however, consisted almost exclusively of exercise training. This approach addressed the physiological changes necessary for improving the functional capacity of the patients but did not address long-term behavior modification and education.

In 1986, Ralph S. Paffenbarger Jr. published a prominent exercise and heart disease study. In his study using 16,936 Harvard University alumni from thirty-five to seventy-four years of age, he validated the concept that physical inactivity is independently related to CAD. In the next seven years, various research on a total of more than 32,000 people was done confirming that hypothesis.

Also in 1986, another group of physicians and researchers described some of the deleterious effects of bed rest, including decreased physical work capacity, decreased cardiac output, skeletal muscle wasting, orthostatic hypotension (abnormally low blood pressure upon standing), decreased blood volume, loss of muscular strength, and reduced pulmonary function. Exercise was shown to be beneficial in reducing some of these effects.

Based on the information outlined above, a multifactorial approach to cardiac rehabilitation has been undertaken in order to provide patients with the information and skills necessary to alter their lifestyles. This approach includes education, in the form of lectures, handouts, videos, and informal discussions; behavior modification, by way of regularly scheduled, supervised aerobic exercise programs and nutritional counseling; and support, by means of cardiac rehabilitation classroom meetings and support groups. With this increased scope of care for the cardiac patient, some institutions are providing cardiac patients with access to a broader base of clinicians. This group may include physicians, nurses, exercise specialists or physiologists, dietitians, physical therapists, social workers, psychologists, and occupational therapists. Even with all these components in place, however, exercise training remains the focal point of most contemporary cardiac rehabilitation programs. Recent studies using meta-analysis have substantiated the hypothesis that exercise-based cardiac rehabilitation programs that include risk factor/behavior modification significantly decrease mortality. Decreasing the number and/or magnitude of the known risk factors for heart disease has been shown to affect a significant improvement in the cardiovascular risk profile for these patients. Research has demonstrated the fact that, although various degrees of CAD may remain after participation in a cardiac rehabilitation program, patients can achieve a sense of well-being. For some patients, this benefit alone may improve health and reduce the financial burden often associated with post-infarction convalescence.

—Bradley R.A. Wilson, PhD

See also: Angina; Arrhythmias; Bypass surgery; Cardiac arrest; Cardiac surgery; Cardiology; Cardiology, pediatric; Cardiopulmonary resuscitation (CPR); Circulation; Congenital heart disease; Coronary artery bypass graft; Echocardiography; Electrocardiography (ECG or EKG); Exercise physiology; Heart; Heart attack; Heart disease; Heart transplantation; Heart valve replacement; Infarction; Ischemia; Pacemaker implantation; Physical rehabilitation; Preventive medicine; Stress reduction.

For Further Information:

American Association of Cardiovascular and Pulmonary Rehabilitation. *Guidelines for Cardiac Rehabilitationand Secondary Prevention Programs*. 5th ed. Champaign, Ill.: Human Kinetics, 2013.
American College of Sports Medicine. *ACSM's Guidelines for ExerciseTesting and Prescription*. 10th ed. Philadelphia, PA: Wolters Kluwer Health, 2018.
"Cardiac Rehabilitation." Mayo Foundation for Medical Education and Research, August 9, 2017.
"Cardiac Rehab and Your Heart." WebMD, January 14, 2017.
McConnell, Larry. *Cardiac Champs: How To Live A Healthy, Vigorous, Happy Life After A Heart Attack*. CreateSpace Independent Publishing, 2014.
National Heart, Lung, and Blood Institute. "Explore Cardiac Rehabilitation." *National Institutes of Health, US Department of Health and Human Services*, December 9, 2016.
Niebauer, Josef (Ed.). *Cardiac RehabilitationManual*. Cham, Switzerland: Springer International Publishing, 2017.
Singleton, Susan S Rose and Eleanor Branch. *Advances in Cardiac and PulmonaryRehabilitation*. New York: Routledge, 2017.
Smith, William, Keith Burns, and Christopher Volgraf. *Exercises for Cardiac Recovery: The Strong Heart FitnessProgram for Life After Heart Attack & Heart Surgery*. Hobart, NY: Hatherleigh Press, 2017.
"What Is Cardiac Rehabilitation?" *American Heart Association*, July 2016.

Cardiac surgery

Specialty

Anatomy or system affected: Circulatory system, heart

Specialties and related fields: Cardiology, internal medicine, preventive medicine, vascular medicine

Definition: Medical specialization focusing on surgical procedures of the heart and vascular system.

Key terms:

aneurysm: a weakening in the wall of the heart or blood vessel

atrial fibrillation: a condition in which the atria contract too rapidly to pump blood effectively

cardiac catheterization: insertion of a flexible tube into a blood vessel that is manipulated into the heart in order to perform a procedure

coronary artery disease: formation of fatty deposits or plaque on the blood vessel walls

heart failure: a condition in which the heart cannot pump enough blood to meet the body's needs

Science and Profession

Cardiac surgeons are part of the broader field of thoracic surgery that includes all physicians who perform surgery on organs in the chest. Thoracic surgeons specialize in surgery of the chest that includes the lungs, the area between the lungs, the esophagus, and the chest wall. Surgery on the heart and the large vessels near the heart are performed by cardiac surgeons.

Cardiologists are also physicians who specialize in heart disorders. However, cardiologists do not perform open-heart surgeries. They diagnose and treat heart ailments using medications and cardiac catheterization procedures, in which a thin, flexible tube is inserted into a major blood vessel in the arm, upper thigh, or neck and threaded to the heart. If major surgery is needed, then a cardiologist refers the patient to a cardiac surgeon.

One of the major diseases treated by cardiac surgeons is coronary artery disease, in which the arteries that supply blood to the heart muscle become blocked with fatty deposits. Failure to treat coronary artery disease adequately can result in a heart attack. Heart valve problems are also surgically repaired by cardiac surgeons. If a heart valve allows blood to leak back in the wrong direction or is blocked, then the valve can be repaired and normal blood flow can be restored. Heart failure in its early stages is managed by a cardiologist. In its later and more severe stages, heart failure is treated by cardiac surgeons, who can either put in a ventricular assist device that helps to pump the blood or perform a heart transplant. These procedures will help the heart pump the amount of blood necessary to keep the patient alive and improve quality of life.

Another condition treated by cardiac surgeons is atrial fibrillation, in which the upper chambers (atria) of the heart contract so fast and chaotically that they fail to pump extra blood into the lower chambers (ventricles). In its early stages, atrial fibrillation is managed by cardiologists. Prior to the refinement of cardiac catheterization techniques, cardiac surgeons would perform the Maze procedure, in which the conducting pathways of the atria are interrupted by intentionally damaging the tissue to form scar tissue that can interrupt unwanted electrical impulses. Cardiologists can now perform this procedure using catheterization, but when other procedures that require open-heart surgery are needed, the Maze procedure can be done at the same time by the cardiac surgeon.

An aneurysm is a weakening in the wall of the heart or a blood vessel. A major concern is the rupture of the aneurysm and the subsequent loss of blood through the opening. One common location where aneurysms are found is in the aorta, the major artery that carries blood from the left ventricle of the heart. If the aneurysm gets too large, then a cardiac surgeon can repair it. As with other heart ailments, a cardiologist generally manages the treatment until the condition becomes severe and then surgery is performed by a cardiac surgeon.

Becoming a cardiac surgeon requires extensive education and training. Typically, there is four years of undergraduate education followed by four years of medical school. In the last year of medical school, students apply for a general surgery residency program. During this five-year program, residents complete rotations in various surgical specialties, including cardiothoracic surgery. In the fourth year of the general surgery residency, the student must apply for another residency in cardiothoracic surgery, which will last another two to three years. Upon completion of the residency program, the newly trained surgeon must pass the American Board of Thoracic Surgery exams. To specialize in cardiac surgery, an additional fellowship of one to two years is required. The actual years of training at the various levels may be slightly different in the many training programs available.

Diagnostic and Treatment Techniques

Most diagnostic testing for heart conditions is performed by cardiologists. Cardiac surgeons deal primarily with the surgical treatment of heart ailments. A major intervention performed by cardiac surgeons is coronary artery bypass graft surgery. The purpose of this procedure is to restore adequate blood flow through coronary arteries that have blockages from coronary artery disease. The surgeon will open up the chest by sawing through the bones of the rib cage and then stop the heart. Blood is pumped by a heart-lung machine during the surgery. A blood vessel is removed from another part of the body, usually the upper leg. The coronary artery is cut above the blockage, and the transplanted vessel is sutured at the incision. The coronary artery is then cut below the blockage, and the other end of the transplanted vessel is sutured to the coronary artery. The result is a bypass around the blockage and through the grafted vessel, restoring normal blood flow to the heart muscle. The heart is restarted, and the incision is closed. If there are multiple blockages, then multiple bypass grafts can be performed in one surgery.

Another common surgery performed by cardiac surgeons is valve repair or replacement. The procedure begins like coronary artery bypass surgery by opening the chest and stopping the heart. If the valve can be repaired, then the surgeon may sew a ring around the valve opening to strengthen it. Sometimes the surgeon modifies the valve to make it function better by cutting and separating tissue. In more severe cases, the valve can be replaced with a biological or mechanical valve. Biological valves come from pigs, cows, or human donors. Mechanical valves are made from synthetic materials. Mechanical valves last longer than biological valves but require blood-thinning medication for life so that blood clots do not form. After the damaged valve is removed and the new valve is sutured in place, the heart is restarted and the chest is closed.

Aortic aneurysms that have a risk of bursting can be repaired by a cardiac surgeon. Usually the surgeon will open the chest. The location of the incision is dependent upon the location of the aneurysm. When the aneurysm is exposed, the surgeon replaces the affected area with a synthetic graft. The material of the graft is stronger than the damaged aorta, thus eliminating the bulge.

Sometimes cardiac surgeons perform the Maze procedure, usually in conjunction with other open-heart surgeries. Maze surgery begins by gaining access to the atria of the heart. When performed by cardiac surgeons the chest is opened and the patient is placed on a heart-lung machine. Some patients are able to have the surgery without a heart-lung machine. This is called off-pump surgery and is performed while the heart is beating. In either case, the surgeon makes small incisions in the left and right atria. These lesions will interrupt unwanted electrical impulses through the atria. After the procedure is completed, the chest is closed.

When the heart muscle is damaged, often due to a heart attack, it becomes weaker and begins to lose its shape. Cardiac surgeons can reform the ventricle with a surgical procedure called ventricular remodeling. The surgeon first opens the chest and stops the heart. A heart-lung machine pumps and oxygenates the blood. The correct size and shape of the ventricle is calculated, and a balloon of the appropriate size is inserted. A patch and circular sutures are used to bring the ventricle back to its preferred shape. A mesh stent may also be inserted to help the vessel remain open. The balloon is removed, and the heart maintains the new, optimal configuration. Then the heart is restarted and the chest is sutured shut.

If the damage to the heart is extensive, then ventricular remodeling may not be possible. In severe cases, patients may need a ventricular assist device or a heart transplant. Candidates for a heart transplant must go on a waiting list for a donor match. When a match is found, the surgery is scheduled. The cardiac surgeon opens the chest and connects the great vessels to the heart-lung machine. Then the patient's heart is removed. The donor heart is sutured to the patient's great vessels and then started. The heart-lung machine is removed and the chest is closed. If a donor is not available, then a ventricular assist device can be implanted. This device weighs one to two pounds and is placed in the chest. The pump is connected to the major vessels. Generally a tube is passed through the skin to connect it to batteries and controls. Sometimes the pump is placed outside the body with the controls and batteries. The ventricular assist device may be temporary until a donor is found or can be permanent.

Some traditional open-heart surgeries can be performed using minimal-access cardiac surgery. Cardiac surgeons, instead of opening the chest, use scopes to reach the heart through smaller openings in the chest cavity. This technique can be used for bypass surgery on one or two vessels, some valve repairs and replacements, Maze surgery, and some types of aortic aneurysms. If minimal-access procedures can be used, then there is generally a quicker recovery and less time in the hospital for the patient.

Perspective and Prospects

Surgeries on the heart date back to the late 1890s. They were generally to repair penetration wounds to the heart. Open-heart surgery has been performed since 1960, when an effective heart-lung machine was developed. The heart-lung machine made many heart procedures possible. Heart surgeries increased in numbers and types through the late twentieth century and into the twenty-first century because of this machine. In the 1990s, off-pump heart surgeries were developed, so that the heart continues to beat during surgery. Techniques to stabilize the moving heart made this advance possible, but not all patients are candidates for this surgery.

Minimally invasive heart surgery techniques have been developed as well. These surgeries can be performed with three small incisions. The instrument used is a robot controlled by the cardiac surgeon with three scopes that are inserted through the holes. Minimally invasive techniques are expensive, but the recovery time for patients is much less.

Another technique that is reducing the need for open-heart surgery is cardiac catheterization. Cardiac catheterization was first used on humans in the 1930s. Over the years, more applications to heart surgeries have been discovered. New catheterization techniques continue to be developed to replace open-heart surgeries because they are less expensive, have fewer risks, and require shorter recovery times. In the future, open-heart surgeries will continue

to be replaced by minimally invasive and catheterization procedures.

The techniques used by cardiac surgeons continue to evolve, and as the population ages, more people will likely need heart surgeries. Cardiac surgeons will continue to have patients in need of surgery and better surgical techniques to correct the various heart conditions.

—*Bradley R. A. Wilson, Ph.D.*

See also Angiography; Angioplasty; Arrhythmias; Arteriosclerosis; Bypass surgery; Cardiac arrest; Cardiac rehabilitation; Cardiology; Cardiology, pediatric; Congenital heart disease; Coronary artery bypass graft; Electrocardiography (ECG or EKG); Heart; Heart attack; Heart disease; Heart transplantation; Heart valve replacement; Pacemaker implantation; Thoracic surgery; Transplantation; Vascular medicine; Vascular system.

For Further Information:

Bhimji, Shabir, and David Zieve. "Open Heart Surgery." *Medline Plus*, May 6, 2011.

Bojar, Robert M. *Manual of Perioperative Care in Adult Cardiac Surgery.* 5th ed. Hoboken: Wiley-Blackwell, 2011.

"Cardiac Procedures and Surgeries." *American Heart Association*, March 22, 2013.

Kouchoukos, Nicholas T., Eugene H. Blackstone, Frank L. Hanley, and James K. Kirklin. *Kirklin/Barratt-Boyes Cardiac Surgery.* 4th ed. Philadelphia: Elsevier-Saunders, 2013.

Morris, Charles R. *The Surgeons: Life and Death in a Top Heart Hospital.* New York: W. W. Norton, 2007.

Stoney, William S. *Pioneers of Cardiac Surgery.* Nashville, Tenn.: Vanderbilt University Press, 2008.

Weisse, Allen B. *Heart to Heart: The Twentieth Century Battle Against Cardiac Disease: An Oral History.* Piscataway, N.J.: Rutgers University Press, 2002.

Cardiology

Specialty

Anatomy or system affected: Chest, circulatory system, heart

Specialties and related fields: Emergency medicine, preventive medicine, vascular medicine

Definition: The branch of medicine concerned with the diagnosis and treatment of diseases of the heart and the coronary arteries, including arteriosclerosis, hypertension, and congenital defects.

Key terms:

acute: referring to the onset of a disease process

chronic: referring to a lingering disease process

coronary arteries: the two arteries that surround the heart and supply the heart muscle with oxygen and nutrients

heart attack: the common term for a myocardial infarction

heart failure: a condition in which the heart pumps inefficiently, allowing fluid to back up into the lungs or body tissue

sudden cardiac death: a situation in which the heart stops beating or beats irregularly, stopping blood flow

Science and Profession

Cardiology is the study of the heart and its various diseases: inflammation of the heart muscle, diseases of the heart valves, atherosclerosis and arteriosclerosis (*athero* meaning "deposits of soft material," *arterio* meaning "pertaining to the arteries," and *sclerosis* meaning "hardening"), and congenital defects. This field also concerns related diseases, such as hypertension (high blood pressure) and certain renal, endocrine, and lung disorders.

The heart contains four chambers, the right and left atria on top and the right and left ventricles below. The walls of the heart are three layers of tissue: the outer layer, the epicardium; the middle layer, the myocardium; and an inner layer, the endocardium, which includes the heart valves. The heart is contained in a protective sac, called the pericardium.

The pumping of the heart is a coordinated contraction. The right atrium receives blood from the veins and contracts, pumping blood through the tricuspid valve into the right ventricle. The right ventricle then contracts, pumping blood through the pulmonary valve into the lungs, where it gives up carbon dioxide and receives oxygen. Blood then enters the left atrium and travels through the mitral valve to the left ventricle. The blood then enters the venous system, first into the venules (tiny veins that lead to larger veins) and finally to one of the two branches of the vena cava: the superior vena cava from the upper part of the body, and the inferior vena cava from the lower. They connect outside the heart and bring blood back into the right atrium.

The heartbeat, the rhythmic contraction of the heart muscle, is controlled by the conduction system. Electrochemical impulses cause muscle fibers to contract, pumping blood through the chambers, and relax, letting the chambers fill again. The contractions are initiated by specialized "pacemaker" tissues in the sinoatrial (S-A) or sinus node, in the junction of the superior vena cava and the right atrium. The pacemaker signal travels to the atrioventricular (A-V) node, near the tricuspid valve. The impulse crosses the A-V node and travels to the bundle of His, specialized fibers that carry it to the ventricles.

Virtually every part of the heart is subject to disease: each layer of the heart muscle, each valve, each chamber, and the coronary arteries. The coronary arteries are quite small and are subject to the accumulation of plaque on their inner walls, a condition known as atherosclerosis. This plaque can be cholesterol, scar tissue, clotted blood, or calcium. As the plaque accumulates, the artery narrows, reducing the flow of blood into the heart muscle. The reduction in blood flow reduces the heart's supply of oxygen, causing myocardial ischemia (lack of blood). There is usually a signal of pain called angina pectoris (*angina* meaning "choking pain" and *pectoris* meaning "of the chest"). Often, the patient feels tightening in the chest with sharp pain behind the sternum. The pain can radiate into either arm or the jaw. It is usually caused by overexertion, exposure to cold, stress, or overeating.

As a rule, an attack of angina pectoris lasts only a few minutes and is relieved by rest, but it can signal the beginning of a heart attack. In addition, coronary arteries contain muscle fibers that can go into spasm and tighten, reducing blood flow into the heart. This condition, too, can cause anginal pain, heart attack, and death. Some patients who have myocardial ischemia do not have anginal pain. This is known as silent ischemia, and it is usually discovered only with an electrocardiogram (ECG) or exercise stress test.

There are four major classes of angina pectoris: stable angina, in which pain begins when the heart's need for oxygen exceeds the amount that it receives; unstable angina, which is significantly more serious than stable angina; variant angina, which is characterized by chest pain at rest and may be caused by spasm of the coronary arteries; and postinfarction angina, unstable angina that appears after acute myocardial infarction.

When atherosclerotic plaque builds up in the coronary arteries, the inner lining of the vessel becomes rough. As a result, a blood clot (thrombus) can form on the plaque, making the vessel even narrower or clogging it completely (coronary thrombosis). When this occurs, blood flow to parts of the heart is stopped, and heart cells die from lack of oxygen. This condition is medically known as myocardial infarction (from *infarct*, meaning "an area of dead cells") and commonly known as a heart attack.

The prognosis for patients who survive a heart attack is variable. In two-thirds of patients, spontaneous thrombolysis (the dissolution of the blood clot) starts to occur within twenty-four hours. About half of heart attack patients, however, will go on to develop postinfarction angina, which usually indicates severe, multivessel coronary artery disease.

Diseases of the conduction system can result in arrhythmias, or disturbances in the regularity of the heartbeat. Arrhythmias can be relatively benign or can severely restrict the patient's physical activity. They can also cause sudden cardiac death. The most common arrhythmias are bradycardia, slowing of the heartbeat, and tachycardia, quickening of the heartbeat.

Normally, the chambers beat in synchronization with each other. In some arrhythmias, the chambers of the heart beat out of synchronization. These arrhythmias include atrial fibrillation, paroxysmal atrial tachycardia, ventricular tachycardia, and ventricular fibrillation. In atrial fibrillation, the atria beat very rapidly (three hundred beats per minute), out of synchronization with the ventricles. When the condition is prolonged, blood clots may form in the atria and may be carried to the cerebral vessels, where they cause a stroke, or the stoppage of blood flow in a blood vessel. With paroxysmal atrial tachycardia, a disturbance in the conduction of the A-V node causes the heart to beat up to two hundred fifty times a minute. The condition is usually not serious, but if it persists, fainting or heart failure could develop. Ventricular tachycardia exists when ectopic, or irregular, beats develop in the ventricular muscle; if they go on, blood pressure falls. In ventricular fibrillation, which is the leading cause of sudden cardiac death, ventricular contractions are weak, ineffective, and uncoordinated. Blood flow stops, and the patient faints. If the condition is not corrected, the patient can die in minutes.

Heart block can be another consequence of conduction disease. If, for various reasons, all the impulses from the sinus node do not pass through the A-V node and the bundle of His, the result is one of three degrees of heart block. First-degree heart block, which is not apparent to the patient, appears on the ECG as a delay in the impulse from the atria to the ventricles. Second-degree heart block occurs when some of the impulses from the atria fail to reach the ventricles. Often, the result is an irregular pulse. This condition can be attributable to a certain heart drug and may disappear when the drug is discontinued. In third-degree heart block, impulses from the pacemaker tissues fail to reach the ventricles. A lower pacemaker assumes the function of stimulating contractions of the ventricles in an "escape rhythm." When this occurs in third-degree heart block, the heart rate often slows down so precipitously that blood flow to the brain and other organs is severely restricted. Dizziness and loss of consciousness may follow. Heart block can also result from a congenital defect, inflammation, myocardial infarction, or other causes.

Disorders in the valves of the heart are most often caused by congenital defects or the effects of rheumatic fever. Rheumatic fever is caused by streptococcal bacteria and usually begins with a throat infection. If this "strep throat" is not treated, rheumatic fever may develop. Acute rheumatic fever is associated with mitral or aortic valve insufficiency (leakage). Chronic rheumatic heart disease can include mitral or aortic stenosis (narrowing). Valves are scarred with fibrous tissue and/or calcific (calcium-containing) deposits that cause the valve openings to become narrower.

Mitral stenosis usually develops slowly. Ten to twenty years after rheumatic fever, the valve narrows so much that blood flow from the atrium into the ventricle is impeded. As blood accumulates in the left atrium, pressure within the atrium increases, and the chamber becomes enlarged. Blood is forced back into the lungs, resulting in pulmonary edema (fluid in the lungs). Blood vessels in the lungs become engorged; the increased pressure forces fluid into the air sacs. Symptoms of mitral stenosis include shortness of breath, fatigue, feelings of suffocation, wheezing, agitation, and anxiety. In severe cases, fluid may also accumulate in the lower extremities. Mitral stenosis can also cause atrial fibrillation, which in turn can generate potentially lethal blood clots.

Mitral "regurgitation" (or insufficiency), another mitral valve disorder, can be due to rheumatic fever or other causes. The valve fails to close completely during left ventricle contraction. Blood leaks back into the left atrium, and blood flow into the aorta is reduced. The heart has to work harder to pump blood into the body. Mitral regurgitation may lead to enlargement of the left atrium and left ventricle. Pulmonary edema, shortness of breath, fatigue, and palpitations are late symptoms of severe disease.

Still another disorder is mitral valve prolapse, which can also result in mitral regurgitation. The mitral valve consists of two leaflets of tissue that fall apart to open and come together to close. Prolapse occurs when either or both of these leaflets bulge into the left atrium, as occurs in a significant percentage of the population whose valves consist of "floppy" (myxomatous) tissue. The condition is usually of little clinical significance, but some patients experience palpitations and chest pain, and some have a heart murmur.

In rare cases, significant valve leakage occurs, requiring surgery.

The aortic valve consists of three leaflets or "cusps" that can become fused, calcified, or otherwise compromised because of rheumatic fever or a congenital heart defect. The opening narrows, and blood flow into the aorta is reduced. Pressure increases inside the left ventricle, causing it to pump harder. The wall of the left ventricle thickens, a condition called ventricular hypertrophy. Aortic stenosis may not be evident until it is quite advanced. Symptoms include heart murmur, weakness, fatigue, anginal pain, breathlessness, and fainting.

Tricuspid stenosis and regurgitation are relatively rare, as is pulmonary regurgitation. Pulmonary or pulmonic valve stenosis, however, is a common congenital heart defect. There is a characteristic heart murmur produced by turbulence of blood through the narrow pulmonary valve. Pressure increases in the right ventricle. Fainting and heart failure are possible in severe cases.

In congestive heart failure, the heart pumps inefficiently, failing to deliver blood to the body and allowing blood to back up into the veins. It may occur on the left or the right side, or both. If the left side of the heart is pumping inefficiently, blood flows back into the lungs, causing pulmonary edema. If the right side of the heart is inefficient, blood seeps back into the legs, resulting in edema of the extremities. Blood can also back up into the liver and the kidneys, resulting in engorgement and reduced arterial flow that prevent these organs from getting the nutrition and oxygen they need to function. The most common cause of heart failure is ischemic cardiomyopathy due to coronary artery disease, other cardiomyopathies, and valvular disease.

Cardiomyopathy refers to diseases of the myocardium. There are many possible causes, including "end-stage" coronary artery disease; infectious agents such as fungi, viruses, and parasites; overconsumption of alcohol; or genetic defects. The three main classes of cardiomyopathy are dilated congestive cardiomyopathy, hypertrophic cardiomyopathy, and restrictive cardiomyopathy. In dilated congestive cardiomyopathy, either all of the heart chambers are involved (diffuse) or some but not all chambers are involved (nondiffuse). The cause of this class of cardiomyopathy is usually ischemia, but viral infection (myocarditis), drugs, alcohol, and nonviral diseases may be responsible. The heart pumps inefficiently, causing fatigue, breathlessness, and edema in the lower extremities. The heart chambers may enlarge, and blood clots may form. With hypertrophic cardiomyopathy, the myocardium thickens and reduces the cavity of the left ventricle so that blood flow into the aorta is reduced. The condition is usually chronic, with fainting, fatigue, and breathlessness as symptoms. Restrictive cardiomyopathy is rare. With this condition, the heart muscle loses elasticity and cannot expand to fill with blood between contractions. Symptoms include edema, breathlessness, and atrial and ventricular arrhythmias.

The endocardium and the pericardium can become inflamed because of infection or injury, resulting in endocarditis or pericarditis. Bacterial endocarditis usually affects abnormal valves and heart structures that have been damaged by rheumatic fever or congenital defects. Fulminant (sudden and severe) infections can destroy normal heart valves, especially with intravenous drug abuse. The symptoms of bacterial endocarditis are fever, weight loss, malaise, night sweats, fatigue, and heart murmurs. The condition can be fatal if the invading organism is not eradicated. Nonbacterial thrombotic endocarditis or noninfective endocarditis arises from the formation of thrombi on cardiac valves and endocardium caused by trauma, immune complexes, or vascular disease. Pericarditis often occurs concomitantly with, or as a result of, viral respiratory infection. The inflamed pericardium rubs against the epicardium, causing acute pain. Large amounts of fluid may develop and press on the heart in "cardiac tamponade." This condition can impede heart action and blood flow and can be life-threatening. In constrictive pericarditis, the pericardium becomes thicker and contracts. This action prevents the heart chambers from filling, decreasing the amount of blood drawn into the heart and pumped out to the body.

Primary cardiac tumors, those originating in the heart, are rare. While usually benign, they can have fatal complications. Malignant tumors also occur, and metastasis (movement of cancer cells throughout the body) may bring malignancies to the heart.

Congenital heart defects occur in approximately eight in every 1,000 live births. Ventricular septal defect, a hole in the wall between the ventricles, is the most common. It is detected by a loud murmur. Atrial septal defect is common but rarely leads to symptoms until the third decade of life.

Diagnostic and Treatment Techniques

The stethoscope, ECGs, and the x-ray are basic tools that the cardiologist uses for the diagnosis of heart conditions. By listening to heart sounds through the stethoscope, the physician can learn much about the status of heart function, particularly heart rhythm, congenital defects, and valve dysfunction.

ECG patterns of electrical impulses help the physician discover chamber enlargement and other cardiac abnormalities. In a stress test, the ECG is attached to a patient who is running on a treadmill or riding an apparatus similar to a bicycle. The test assesses the exercise tolerance of patients with coronary artery disease and other conditions.

The chest x-ray provides a picture of the size and configuration of the heart, the aorta, the pulmonary arteries, and related structures. It can detect enlarged chambers and vessels and other disorders. In some cases, radioactive isotopes are injected into the patient, and the patterns that they form in the heart and surrounding arteries are read by a scanner to help the physician make a diagnosis. The echocardiogram uses ultrasound to outline heart chambers and detect abnormalities within them and in the myocardium. It is also used to analyze patterns of blood flow.

More sophisticated instruments the cardiologist uses in-clude fast-computed tomography, called cine-CT because it gives the physician a visualization of heart activity. Magnetic resonance imaging (MRI), MR spectroscopy, and positron emission tomography (PET) scanning help the cardiologist investigate heart function and anatomy.

These techniques and procedures are conducted outside the body. Sometimes it is necessary, however, to go into the body. One such technique is diagnostic catheterization with angiography. A thin flexible tube (catheter) is inserted into a blood vessel in the groin or arm and threaded into a coronary artery or the heart. Pressures and blood oxygen are measured in the heart chambers. A radiopaque dye is then injected through the catheter. The inside of the artery or the heart becomes visible to the x-ray and is recorded on film (a process sometimes called cineangiography). Angiography can also be used with radioactive isotopes. The radiation detected by a scanner can help the physician discover abnormalities in the coronary arteries and the heart.

Diagnosis of angina pectoris is usually based upon the patient's complaint of chest pain. An ECG can help confirm the diagnosis. Yet many patients with coronary artery disease have normal ECGs at rest, so stress testing with the ECG is considered more reliable. Patients may be given pharmacologic stress tests if they are unable to do physical exercise.

Drug therapy for coronary artery disease and angina pectoris is directed at keeping the coronary arteries open and avoiding myocardial ischemia. Primary among the drugs used is nitroglycerin, taken under the tongue or in a transdermal (through-the-skin) patch-or, in emergencies, intravenously. There are many nitrate compounds that fulfill similar functions. Beta-adrenergic blocking agents, or beta-blockers, decrease heart rate and blood pressure, reducing the heart's oxygen requirement and workload, thus reducing the incidence of angina. Some serious arrhythmias are also suppressed. Calcium-channel blockers dilate coronary arteries and maintain coronary blood flow while decreasing blood pressure, reducing heart work, and stabilizing heart rhythm. Angiotensin-converting enzyme (ACE) inhibitors help to relax the blood vessels, thereby reducing blood pressure. Cholesterol-lowering medications help to reduce the amount of cholesterol in the blood, thereby reducing plaque deposits and helping to prevent atherosclerosis, and low-dose aspirin and other blood thinners can also help to reduce to the risk of obstruction of the coronary arteries by blood clots.

If coronary artery disease progresses to the point where there is risk of myocardial infarction, various catheter and surgical procedures may be considered. Coronary angioplasty is used to open a clogged artery mechanically. The cardiologist threads a catheter with a tiny balloon into the clogged artery and inflates the balloon at the site of the blockage. This procedure is repeated until the vessel is open. A stent may be inserted into the artery to help prevent future blockages. Another procedure used when coronary arteries are blocked is coronary artery bypass surgery. The surgeon takes sections of vein or artery from another part of the body and implants them between the aorta and the heart, creating new coronary arteries and bypassing those that are clogged.

When clogged coronary arteries cause a myocardial infarction, the patient should be treated in a special medical facility, preferably in a coronary care unit (CCU). Heart attacks rarely begin in the hospital, however, so the medical team must keep the patient alive on the way to the CCU. Primary ventricular fibrillation is the greatest danger, and it must be corrected immediately by medication or electrical defibrillation. Sometimes heart block and profound bradycardia occur, which could cause a drop in blood pressure that could in turn cause cardiac arrest.

The aims of emergency myocardial infarction treatment are to ease discomfort, minimize the mass of infarcted myocardial tissue, reduce heart work, stabilize heart rhythm, and maintain oxygen perfusion throughout the body by regulating blood pressure. Treatment and medications used in the CCU include continuous ECG monitoring (both during and after the heart attack), oxygen, nitroglycerin, antiarrhythmia agents, analgesics for pain, thrombolytic agents to dissolve clots, diuretics, agents to treat shock, and sedatives. Beta-blockers, calcium-channel blockers, anticoagulants, and antianxiety drugs may also be used.

About 60 percent of patients who have suffered from myocardial infarction develop congestive heart failure. In treating congestive heart failure from heart attacks or other causes, the cardiologist uses both dietary instruction and medication. Salt restriction is recommended to reduce edema. The three most commonly prescribed drugs are diuretics to reduce edema, digitalis (digoxin or digitoxin) to increase the force of the heart's contraction, and vasodilators to reduce the resistance of blood vessel walls, to facilitate blood flow, and to reduce heart work. Intractable congestive heart failure may be a reason for a heart transplant.

The main goals of therapy for cardiac arrhythmias are to improve heart function and to prevent sudden cardiac death. Drug therapy must be individualized to correct the particular arrhythmia. Digitalis, procainamide, tocainamide, and atropine are often used. Beta-blockers and calcium-channel blockers are also helpful in stabilizing heart rhythm. If heart block becomes severe, an artificial pacemaker is implanted in the chest to regulate the heartbeat.

Disorders of the heart valves are not usually treated with drugs. While awaiting surgery, it may be necessary to treat heart failure, or the effects of valve disease in other parts of the body. For example, diuretics may be required to reduce edema, an antiarrhythmia agent may be needed to control atrial fibrillation, or anticoagulants may be used to prevent blood clots. Some stenotic valves can be opened using a modification of the balloon catheter technique, or surgical reconstruction may be possible. Often, it is necessary to replace the valve with a new one made of human or porcine tissue, or with a mechanical valve.

Pulmonary edema is a severe form of heart failure and is life-threatening. In emergencies, oxygen is given, in severe cases by inserting a breathing tube into the patient's trachea. Medications are given to relieve pulmonary congestion, and if the pumping action of the heart is compromised, digitalis or another medication can strengthen the contractility of the heart.

In treating dilated cardiomyopathy, the cardiologist uses appropriate medications that may include diuretics, vasodilators, antiarrhythmia agents, and digitalis. Alcohol restriction is required.

If bacteria or other microorganisms are involved, appropriate antibiotic therapy must be instituted to eradicate the cause. Patients with congenital or valvular heart disease are high risks for cardiac and valve infection. They are given preventive antibiotic therapy before undergoing surgical or dental procedures.

In acute pericarditis, if excessive fluid builds up, a procedure called pericardiocentesis may be performed to drain the fluid between the pericardium and the heart wall. In cardiac tamponade, pericardiocentesis may be life-saving. In chronic constrictive pericarditis, an operation may be necessary to remove tissue that has stiffened and strangled the heart.

Perspective and Prospects

Cardiology is a major medical specialty because heart disease is the leading cause of death worldwide. Today's cardiologist turns increasingly to preventive medicine as a means of reducing morbidity (the relative incidence of a disease) and mortality. These measures include programs against smoking and programs advocating cholesterol reduction, stress reduction, increased exercise, and other measures that have been found useful in preventing heart disease.

Ongoing studies continue to accumulate data on increasingly large populations in more and more countries. Links between behavior, habits, nutrition, and ecology may be found that will give a clearer picture of how to prevent and treat heart disease. Increased knowledge will improve diagnosis and treatment, improving patient care and the quality of life for sufferers of heart disease.

—*C. Richard Falcon*

See also Aneurysmectomy; Aneurysms; Angina; Angiography; Angioplasty; Arrhythmias; Arteriosclerosis; Biofeedback; Blue baby syndrome; Bypass surgery; Cardiac arrest; Cardiac rehabilitation; Cardiac surgery; Cardiology, pediatric; Cardiopulmonary resuscitation (CPR); Chest; Cholesterol; Circulation; Congenital heart disease; Coronary artery bypass graft; Cyanosis; Echocardiography; Electrocardiography (ECG or EKG); Endocarditis; Exercise physiology; Heart; Heart attack; Heart disease; Heart failure; Heart transplantation; Heart valve replacement; Hypercholesterolemia; Hypertension; Infarction; Ischemia; Kawasaki disease; Mitral valve prolapse; Pacemaker implantation; Palpitations; Rheumatic fever; Sports medicine; Thoracic surgery; Thrombolytic therapy and TPA; Thrombosis and thrombus; Transplantation; Vascular medicine; Vascular system.

For Further Information:

Baum, Seth J. *The Total Guide to a Healthy Heart: Integrative Strategies for Preventing and Reversing Heart Disease*. New York: Kensington, 2000.

Bonow, Robert O., et al., eds. *Braunwald's Heart Disease: A Textbook of Cardiovascular Medicine*. 9th ed. Philadelphia: Elsevier-Saunders, 2011.

"Coronary Artery Disease - Coronary Heart Disease." *American Heart Association*, July 17, 2013.

Crawford, Michael H., ed. *Current Diagnosis and Treatment-Cardiology*. 4th ed. New York: McGraw-Hill Medical, 2013.

Eagle, Kim A., and Ragavendra R. Baliga, eds. *Practical Cardiology: Evaluation and Treatment of Common Cardiovascular Disorders*. 2d ed. Philadelphia: Lippincott Williams & Wilkins, 2008.

"Heart Surgery Overview." *Texas Heart Institute*, August 2012.

Litin, Scott C., ed. *Mayo Clinic Family Health Book*. 4th ed. New York: HarperResource, 2009.

Murphy, Jospeh G., and Margaret A. Lloyd. *Mayo Clinic Cardiology: Concise Textbook*. 4th ed. Rochester: Mayo Clinic Scientific Press, 2012.

Piscatella, Joseph, and Barry Franklin. *Prevent, Halt & Reverse Heart Disease: 109 Things You Can Do*. Rev. ed. New York: Workman, 2011.

Swanton, R. H. *Cardiology*. 6th ed. Malden, Mass.: Blackwell Science, 2008.

"Your Guide to Living Well with Heart Disease." *National Heart, Lung, and Blood Institute*, January 2006.

Zaret, Barry L., Marvin Moser, and Lawrence S. Cohen, eds. *Yale University School of Medicine Heart Book*. New York: William Morrow, 1992.

Cardiopulmonary resuscitation (CPR)

Procedure

Anatomy or system affected: Circulatory system, heart, lungs, respiratory system

Specialties and related fields: Cardiology, emergency medicine

Definition: A procedure that combines chest compressions and artificial breathing for a person whose breathing and heart contractions have stopped.

Key terms:

automated external defibrillator: a computerized unit that can be used to defibrillate the heart by trained nonmedical personnel

chest compression: pressure applied to the bottom half of the breastbone to pump blood from a heart in cardiac arrest

defibrillation: the sending of an electric shock through the chest to enable the heart to resume normal contractions

mouth-to-mouth breathing: the expiration of air from a rescuer's mouth into a victim's mouth to send oxygen into the victim's lungs

sudden cardiac arrest: the cessation of heart contractions or insufficient contractions to pump blood to the brain and other vital organs

Indications and Procedures

Cardiopulmonary resuscitation (CPR) is generally performed on a person who is in cardiac arrest. In the United States, someone dies from sudden cardiac arrest (SCA) every two minutes. Cardiac arrest occurs when a person has no heartbeats or insufficient heartbeats to pump blood to the brain and other vital organs. Without sufficient blood flow, these organs do not receive enough oxygen to function normally; after about four minutes, they begin to die. This life-threatening situation requires immediate attention to keep the person alive. If medical personnel are not immediately available, then emergency medical services (EMS) should be called and CPR should be initiated.

Cardiac arrest can have many causes. The most common is a severe heart attack. Many heart attacks do not require CPR, but if a person is unconscious with no pulse, then CPR should begin as soon as possible. Other causes of cardiac arrest that may require CPR are drowning, suffocation, drug overdose, electrocution, stroke, and other types of brain damage. In each of these situations, the heart is not contracting and pumping blood.

CPR includes two distinct operations, breathing air into the person's lungs and compressing the chest. In mouth-to-mouth breathing, sometimes called artificial respiration, the rescuer breathes air into the person's lungs, causing the chest to rise and fall with each breath. The rescuer's expired air is 16 percent oxygen, as compared with 21 percent oxygen in room air. This expired air has enough oxygen to maintain life. It is recommended that an individual providing mouth-to-mouth breathing use a protective device, such as a CPR mask or shield, to avoid transmission of potentially infectious body fluids. The mask or shield devices can be purchased for a small cost online or from uniform stores or university medical bookstores.

Chest compressions involve the application of pressure to the lower half of the breastbone. The external pressure increases the pressure in the chest, pushing blood to the brain and the rest of the body. Although this procedure circulates only 25 to 33 percent of normal blood flow, it is sufficient to keep the person alive when used in conjunction with mouth-to-mouth breathing.

In an emergency situation, CPR can be administered by one or two people. One person can alternate mouth-to-

Firefighters practice CPR using an automatic external defibrillator during a first responder training class. (AP/Wide World Photos)

mouth breathing and chest compressions. Performing CPR for several minutes, however, can be exhausting. If two certified rescuers are present, one can do the mouth-to-mouth breathing while the other performs chest compressions. Two people can do the procedure more efficiently and for longer periods of time.

Uses and Complications

Cardiopulmonary resuscitation should be used only if a person is suffering from cardiac arrest. There are no other applications. Even when CPR is correctly performed by experienced, certified medical personnel, injury can occur to the individual receiving CPR. These injuries may include broken ribs, bruising of the heart, and tearing of the liver and/or the spleen. However, these injuries should not deter an individual from performing CPR. Cardiopulmonary resuscitation is only performed when a person is clinically dead, without a pulse or respiration. Individuals should take a course and become certified to learn the most effective and safest techniques.

Effective CPR sends oxygen to the vital organs to prevent permanent tissue death, but it cannot alter abnormal electrical energy that may be occurring in the heart muscle. This abnormal electrical energy does not allow the heart to pump blood adequately throughout the body. Medical attention is generally needed to restart the heart contractions, and CPR must be continued until EMS personnel arrive. Emergency medical personnel will defibrillate the heart by sending an electric shock through the chest in an attempt to correct the abnormal electrical energy in the heart so that it can resume normal contractions.

Almost anyone can become certified in CPR. The American Heart Association and the American Red Cross offer classes with certification. These organizations are also involved in campaigns to have as many people certified as possible because CPR doubles a victim's chances of sudden cardiac arrest survival. Therefore, the more people that are certified, the more likely it is that someone can perform CPR in an emergency and the more likely it is the victim will survive.

Another program to reduce deaths from sudden cardiac arrest includes the use of automated external defibrillators (AEDs). These units are computerized and allow a person with minimal training to defibrillate a heart. An AED unit has simple steps to follow with voice and print instructions. The machine has built-in safety features to prevent a person from receiving defibrillation that is not needed. AED units have been placed in work sites, stadiums, airports, and other places where large numbers of people are found. Designated people in these areas are trained to use the AEDs. If the first defibrillation shock is administered within six minutes, then the victim has an approximately 45 percent chance of survival.

Perspective and Prospects

Mouth-to-mouth breathing dates to biblical times, when it was used by midwives to resuscitate newborns. However, it fell out of practice until the 1950s, when it was rediscovered by James Elam and Peter Safer. In 1960, other physicians found that chest compressions could attain sufficient circulation, and these compressions were combined with mouth-to-mouth breathing to create a CPR procedure similar to what is used today.

—Bradley R. A. Wilson, Ph.D.;
updated by Amy Webb Bull, D.S.N., A.P.N.

See also Arrhythmias; Cardiac arrest; Cardiac rehabilitation; Cardiology; Cardiology, pediatric; Circulation; Defibrillation; Echocardiography; Electrocardiography (ECG or EKG); Emergency medicine; Emergency medicine, pediatric; Emergency rooms; First aid; Heart; Heart attack; Pacemaker implantation; Paramedics; Respiration; Resuscitation.

For Further Information:

American Academy of Orthopaedic Surgeons and Alton L. Thygerson. *First Aid, CPR, and AED.* 6th ed. Sudbury, Mass.: Jones and Bartlett, 2011.

American Heart Association. "2005 AHA Guidelines for CPR and ECC." http://www.americanheart.org, 2013.

American Red Cross.*American Red Cross First Aid: Responding to Emergencies.* 4th rev. ed. Yardley, Pa.: StayWell, 2007.

Bergeron, David J., et al. *First Responder.* 8th ed. Upper Saddle River, N.J.: Pearson/Prentice Hall, 2009.

"CPR: Are We Doing It Wrong?" *Harvard Health Letter*30, no. 7 (May, 2005): 1-3.

Finucane, Brendan T., and Albert H. Santora. *Principles of Airway Management.* 4th ed. New York: Springer, 2011.

Kohnle, Diana. "Cardiopulmonary Resuscitation for Children Age 1 to Early Teens." *Health Library,* March 15, 2013.

Kohnle, Diana. "Cardiopulmonary Resuscitation for Infants." *Health Library,* March 15, 2013.

Kohnle, Diana. "Cardiopulmonary Resuscitation for Teens and Adults." *Health Library,* March 15, 2013.

MedlinePlus. "CPR." *MedlinePlus,* May 22, 2013.

Carotid arteries

Anatomy

Also known as: Carotid pulse

Anatomy or system affected: Blood vessels, brain, circulatory system, heart, neck

Specialties and related fields: Cardiology, critical care, emergency medicine, exercise physiology, family medicine, internal medicine, neurology, nursing, vascular medicine

Definition: The two major arteries supplying blood to the head and neck. Each divides into an external common carotid and an internal common carotid branch.

Structure and Functions

The internal and external carotid arteries branch from the common carotid arteries at about the level of the thyroid cartilage. The left common carotid artery stems directly from the aortic arch, but the right common carotid artery is derived from the brachiocephalic artery. The external carotid arteries supply blood to the face, thyroid, tongue, and pharynx. A branch from the external carotid arteries, the middle meningeal artery, supplies the deep structures of the face and sends a large branch to the dura mater in the brain. A slight dilation in the internal carotid arteries just past the bifurcation is called the carotid sinus. Specialized nerve endings within the carotid sinuses respond to changes in arterial blood pressure to maintain blood supply to the brain and body. The anterior cerebral arteries provide blood supply to structures such as the frontal and parietal lobes of the brain. An occlusion (obstruction) in the main trunk of an anterior cerebral artery results in a contralateral hemiplegia (paralysis) that is greater in the leg than in the arm. Bilateral paralysis and sensory impairment result when there is total occlusion of both anterior cerebral arteries. The middle cerebral arteries supply arterial blood to portions of the temporal, parietal, and frontal lobes of the cerebral cortex. Occlusion of the middle cerebral artery results in severe aphasia (loss of speech) when the language hemisphere is involved, loss of position sense and touch discrimination, and a severe hemiplegia in the upper extremities and the face.

Disorders and Diseases

Major clinical features associated with arterial insufficiency to the brain may cause a cerebral vascular accident, or stroke. Strokes are associated with signs and symptoms such as weakness in one to four extremities; increased tendon reflexes; ataxia; bilateral Babinski sign; dysphagia; dysarthria; syncope, stupor, coma, dizziness, or memory disturbances; visual disturbances (diplopia, nystagmus, ptosis, paralysis of single eye movements); numbness of the face; confusion; dementia; coma; hemiparesis; visual aphasia or word blindness; occasional blindness; disturbance of all functions involving speech and communication; and dysphasia.

A thorough history and physical examination should be done on all patients with cerebrovascular disease. An inadequate history is probably the most frequent cause of diagnostic error. Often neither the patient nor the family can recall when initial symptoms started. Two significant phenomena that are characteristic of all varieties of stroke are the suddenness of occurrence and the findings of some degree of improvement following stabilization. Hemiplegia is the classic sign of stroke and is found in lesions involving the cerebral hemispheres or brain stem.

—*Jane C. Norman, Ph.D., R.N., C.N.E.*

See also Aneurysmectomy; Aneurysms; Blood vessels; Brain; Brain damage; Brain disorders; Circulation; Embolism; Head and neck disorders; Hemiplegia; Paralysis; Strokes; Thrombosis and thrombus; Transient ischemic attacks (TIAs); Vascular medicine; Vascular system.

For Further Information:

A.D.A.M. Medical Encyclopedia. "Carotid Artery Disease." *MedlinePlus*, July 31, 2011.

A.D.A.M. Medical Encyclopedia. "Carotid Artery Surgery." *MedlinePlus*, June 4, 2012.

Guyton, Arthur C., and John C. Hall. *Guyton and Hall Textbook of Medical Physiology*. 12th ed. Philadelphia: Elsevier/Saunders, 2011.

Moore, Keith L. *Clinically Oriented Anatomy*. Philadelphia: Lippincott Williams & Wilkins, 2009.

National Heart, Lung, and Blood Institute. "What Is Carotid Artery Disease?" *National Institutes of Health*, November 1, 2010.

Naylor, A. Ross. *Carotid Artery Surgery: A Problem-Based Approach*. New York: Elsevier Health Sciences, 2000.

Rohen, Johannes W. *Color Atlas of Anatomy: A Photographic Study of the Human Body*. Philadelphia: Lippincott Williams & Wilkins, 2006.

Rosenberg, Norman. *Handbook of Carotid Artery Surgery*. New York: Taylor & Francis, 1994.

Carpal tunnel syndrome

Disease/Disorder

Anatomy or system affected: Arms, hands, joints, nerves, tendons

Specialties and related fields: Neurology, occupational health

Definition: A common disorder that causes discomfort and decreased hand dexterity via excessive pressure on the median nerve at the wrist, often caused by repetitive wrist and hand movements.

Key terms:

carpal tunnel: a narrow tunnel formed by a U-shaped cluster of eight bones called carpals at the base of the palm and the inelastic transverse carpal ligament that lies across the arch

median nerve: a nerve running through the carpal tunnel that carries sensory impulses from the thumb, index and middle fingers, and half of the ring finger to the central nervous system; it has a motor branch that supplies the thenar muscles on the thumb side of the hand

Causes and Symptoms

The carpal tunnel is a narrow passage of ligament and bones that contains the median nerve and tendons. Carpal tunnel syndrome, also known as median nerve palsy, is caused by the transverse carpal ligament compressing the median nerve. This nerve passes through the carpal tunnel alongside nine tendons attached to the muscles that enable the hand to close and the wrist to flex. The tendons have a lubricating lining called the synovium, which normally allows the tendons to glide back and forth smoothly through the tunnel during wrist and hand movements. The median nerve is the softest component within the tunnel and becomes compressed when the tendons are stressed and become swollen. Median nerve compression most often results when the synovium becomes thick and sticky as a result of the wear and tear of aging or repeatedly performing stressful motions with the hands while holding them in the same position for extended periods. The carpal tunnel is smaller in some people than in others, predisposing them to carpal tunnel syndrome. Entrapment of the median nerve is less commonly caused by rheumatoid arthritis, diabetes mellitus, poor thyroid gland or pituitary function, excessive fluid retention during pregnancy or menopause, medications, vitamin B_6 or B_{12} deficiency, or bone protruding in the tunnel from previous dislocations or fractures of the wrist.

Initial symptoms of carpal tunnel syndrome include tingling and numbness in the hands, often beginning in the thumb and index and middle fingers, that causes the hand to feel as though it were asleep and shooting pain from the thenar region radiating as far up as the neck. Later symptoms include burning pain from the wrist to the fingers, changes in touch or temperature sensation, clumsiness in the hands, and muscle weakness creating an inability to grasp, pinch, and perform other thumb functions. Swelling of the hands and forearms and changes in sweat gland func-

Information on Carpal Tunnel Syndrome

Causes: Repetitive movement of hands and wrists
Symptoms: Discomfort, decreased hand dexterity, numbness, tingling, shooting or burning pain, changes in touch or temperature sensation, clumsiness in the hands
Duration: Temporary or chronic
Treatments: Splinting of wrist, changes in hand movement and problem-causing activity, anti-inflammatory drugs, surgery

tioning in the hands may also be noted. Symptoms can be intermittent or constant and often progress to the point of regularly awakening the patient at night. Temporary relief is sometimes available by elevating, massaging, and shaking the hand. Although very treatable if diagnosed early, carpal tunnel syndrome can escalate into persistent pain, which can become so crippling that workplace duties and such simple tasks as holding a cup, writing, and buttoning a shirt are compromised. Carpal tunnel syndrome usually occurs in adults and is more common in women than in men.

A clinical examination for confirmation of median nerve impingement includes wrist examination, an X-ray for previous injury and arthritis, and assessment of swelling and sensitivity to touch or pinpricks. Tapping of the median nerve (Tinel's test) will cause tingling or shocklike sensations in the fingers. Holding the wrist in a flexed position for several minutes with the heel of the hands touching for several minutes (Phalen's test) will result in tingling or numbness in the hands. Nerve conduction tests, which measure nerve transmission speed by electrodes placed on the skin, and electromyogram evaluation, which notes muscle function abnormalities, may also assist in a diagnosis. Ultrasound identifies whether motion of the median nerve is impeded.

Treatment and Therapy

Early diagnosis and the taking of appropriate preventive measures, such as ergonomic modifications in the way that upper extremity movements are performed, often reduce the risk of developing advanced carpal tunnel syndrome. The need to compensate for weak muscles with an inappropriate wrist position can be reduced by maintaining a neutral (straight) wrist position instead of a flexed, extended, or twisted wrist position; utilizing the entire hand and all the fingers to grasp and lift objects, instead of gripping solely with the thumb and index finger; minimizing repetitive movements; allowing the upper extremities regular rest periods; using power tools, instead of hand tools; alternating work activities; switching hands; reducing movement speed; and stretching and using strengthening exercises for the hand, wrist, and arm. Keeping the hands warm to maintain good blood circulation and avoiding smoke-filled environments, which reduce peripheral blood flow, are also recommended.

Treatment generally begins with splinting of the wrist and medication, but surgery may be required if symptoms do not subside within six months. Both nocturnal splints and job-specific occupational splints can effectively keep the wrist in a neutral position, thus avoiding the extreme wrist flexion or extension that narrows the carpal tunnel. Wrist supports lying on the desk in front of a computer keyboard are often helpful, but the benefit of strapping on wrist splints while typing is controversial because disuse atrophy may result, potentially creating a muscle imbalance. Aspirin and other oral nonsteroidal anti-inflammatory drugs (NSAIDs) may reduce swelling and inflammation, relieving some nerve pressure. Corticosteroids and cortisone-like medications injected directly into the carpal tunnel can help confirm diagnosis if the symptoms are relieved. Diuretics and vitamin supplementation may also be benefi-

Carpal Tunnel Syndrome

Median nerve

Superficial branch of the nerve supplies the palm

Median nerve

Muscles at base of the thumb

Tough membrane roofing the carpal tunnel

Tendons

Carpal bones

(Cross section of the left wrist)

Repetitive wrist motion such as typing may put excessive pressure on the median nerves and cause numbness and tingling in the hands, a condition known as carpal tunnel syndrome. If rest, wrist splints, and painkillers do not alleviate the problem, surgery may be needed to relieve the pressure.

Though most patients who have carpal tunnel surgery recover completely, recovery can take months.

Perspective and Prospects

The historic roots of carpal tunnel syndrome can be traced back to the 1860s, when meatpackers complained of pain and loss of hand function, which physicians initially attributed to reduced circulation. Modern occupations that require repetitive motions for extended periods-such as typing on a computer keyboard, construction and assembly-line work, and jackhammer operation-have caused a dramatic rise in cumulative trauma disorders such as carpal tunnel syndrome, while other workplace injuries have leveled off.

—*Daniel G. Graetzer, Ph.D.;*
updated by Sharon W. Stark, R.N., A.P.R.N., D.N.Sc.

See also Nervous system; Neuralgia, neuritis, and neuropathy; Neurology; Neurosurgery; Occupational health; Pain management; Upper extremities.

For Further Information:

Biundo, Joseph J., and Perry J. Rush. "Carpal Tunnel Syndrome." *American College of Rheumatology*, Sept. 2012.

"Carpal Tunnel Syndrome." *MedlinePlus*, Apr. 19, 2013.

Johansson, Philip. *Carpal Tunnel Syndrome and Other Repetitive Strain Injuries*. Berkeley Heights, N.J.: Enslow, 1999.

McCabe, Steven J. *101 Questions and Answers About Carpal Tunnel Syndrome: What It Is, How to Prevent It, and Where to Turn for Treatment*. New York: McGraw-Hill, 2002.

National Institute of Neurological Disorders and Stroke (NINDS). "Carpal Tunnel Syndrome Fact Sheet." *National Institutes of Health*, May 1, 2013.

Rosenbaum, Richard B., and José L. Ochoa. *Carpal Tunnel Syndrome and Other Disorders of the Median Nerve*. 2d ed. Boston: Butterworth-Heinemann, 2002.

Smoots, Elizabeth, and John C. Keel. "Carpal Tunnel Syndrome." *Health Library*, Oct. 31, 2012.

Zaidat, Osama A., and Alan J. Lerner. *The Little Black Book of Neurology*. 5th ed. Philadelphia: Mosby/Elsevier, 2008.

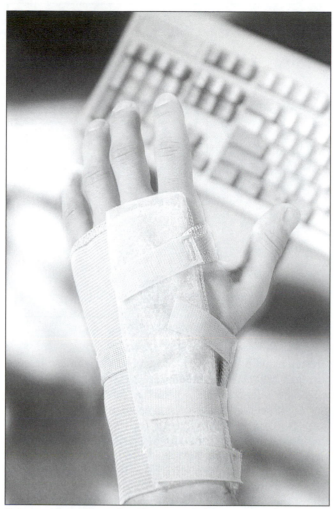

Patients with carpal tunnel syndrome may find that wearing a brace relieves pressure on the nerve in the wrist. (Adobe)

cial. Vitamin B_6 has shown promise in reducing the symptoms of carpal tunnel syndrome. Exercises can be performed, under the guidance of a physical or occupational therapist, to stretch and strengthen the wrists. Acupuncture and chiropractic may benefit some who suffer from carpal tunnel syndrome; however, their effectiveness has not been supported. Pain reduction and improved grip strength have been documented among patients who practice yoga.

If initial symptoms do not subside, pain increases, or the risk of permanent nerve and muscle damage exists, then surgery may be necessary, with subsequent rehabilitation and ergonomic counseling with a physical or occupational therapist. Carpal tunnel release is one of the most common surgical procedures in the United States. It is often recommended for individuals who experience carpal tunnel symptoms for more than six months. This outpatient surgical procedure involves dividing the transverse ligament to open the carpal tunnel to relieve pressure and remove thickened synovial tissue. Endoscopic surgery using a fiber-optic camera allows the surgeon to visualize and cut the carpal ligament. This procedure results in faster recovery and minimizes postoperative discomfort and scarring.

Carticel®

Procedure/Treatment

Anatomy or system affected: Knee joint and cartilage
Specialties and related fields: Orthopedic surgery.
Definition: autologous cultured chondrocytes, initially isolated from a patient's knee cartilage, cultured in the laboratory, and subsequently implanted into the same individual to repair knee cartilage defects

Key terms:

aminoglycosides: antibiotics such as gentamicin, streptomycin, and others that inhibit protein synthesis in bacteria and are used to treat or prevent bacterial infections

arthrofibrosis: scar tissue in a joint that develops after surgery, implant, or joint replacement

arthroscopy: a procedure where a surgeon uses an instrument called an arthroscope to look inside a joint

arthrotomy: a procedure where a surgeon opens or cuts into a joint

articulating: where a joint or juncture between bones or cartilages is present for motion

autologous cultured chondrocytes: cells obtained from an individual's own cartilage

bovine: related to cattle, buffalo

Carticel®: an FDA-approved cellular product obtained from an individual's own knee cartilage cells (chondrocytes), which are processed to multiply cell growth and then used as an implant to treat knee cartilage defects

chondromalacia: deterioration or softening of cartilage under the knee cap

chondrosis: the formation of cartilage

gentamicin: an aminoglycoside antibiotic

graftdelamination: a splitting of tissue layers after implant

graft: in medical terms, any tissue or organ for implantation or transplant

implant: insertion of tissue, cells or prosthetic into a person's body at a specific location in the body

marrow stimulation technique: marrow stimulation involves an orthopedic surgeon making tiny incisions, called microfractures, with an instrument in the underlying bone. These microfractures allow blood and bone marrow to percolate to the surface and form a super clot that contains stem cells and growth factors, which produce healthy cartilage

kneecartilagedefects: an area of damaged cartilage in the knee

periosteal flap: an orthopedic surgeon makes a flap in the periosteum, specialized connective tissue covering all bones of the body and possessing bone-forming potential. Periosteum also serves as a point of attachment for certain muscles

stem cells: human cells with the ability to grow into any one of the body's more than 200 cell types. Stem cells contribute to the body's ability to renew and repair its tissues

Indications and Procedures

Cartilage is a thick, but slippery and movable tissue that provides cushioning for the knee joint as well as other joints in the body. Carticel® is used to repair damage to knee cartilage caused by repeated knee trauma, or in individuals who have had prior, unsuccessful arthroscopic surgery or cleaning of the defective cartilage. Carticel® implants are not recommended in patients with cartilage damage from osteoarthritis or who have had all their cartilage previously removed unless there has been cartilage reconstruction prior to implant.

The use of Carticel® in individuals over age 65 or in children has not been studied. Also, individuals with a known history of allergies to gentamicin, other aminoglycoside antibiotics, or materials of bovine origin are not eligible for Carticel® implant.

Potential Carticel® candidates should check with their health insurance company to inquire about coverage for Carticel® implantation.

Procedure

The initial stage of Carticel® implantation begins with an orthopedic surgeon taking a biopsy of cartilage cells (chondrocytes) from the individual's non-weight bearing area (a non-articulating surface) of the knee. Only

Courtesy of meganscacicarticelsurgery.blogspot.com

physicians who complete a surgical training program specific to Carticel® administration can perform this procedure. The cells are sent to a special lab (Vericel®) where they are processed and grown in a specific cell culture system. It usually takes three to five weeks for the chondrocytes to proliferate to the point where they are numerous enough for implantation into the patient's knee.

The newly-grown chondrocyte cells are then implanted into the damaged knee by the surgeon by means of an arthrotomy. A periosteal flap is created by the surgeon prior to the implant in order to secure and stabilize the implant of chondrocyte graft. The surgeon then slowly injects the chondrocyte cells through a catheter.

After the implant, the patient needs to gradually increase activity, at first limiting weight bearing on the affected knee using crutches, etc. It can take six to eight weeks to resume normal physical activity, and the activity level is based on the physician's recommended rehabilitation activity plan and how the individual is recovering. Ice packs are usually needed to reduce swelling. The patient should watch for any sharp pain, locking, or increased swelling of the knee and should report these symptoms to their surgeon.

Uses and Complications

The safety of implanted autologous chondrocytes is derived from primarily four main research studies and post-marketing reporting. The primary studies are: Study of the Treatment of Articular Repair (STAR); the Registry Based Study (RBS); the Cartilage Repair Registry (CRR); the Swedish Series; and post-marketing adverse event reporting.

The most common serious complications overall (greater than 5%) reported in the STAR study included arthrofibrosis/joint adhesion, implant graft overgrowth, chondromalacia or chondrosis, cartilage injury, graft complication, cartilage lesion development, and graft delamination.

Also in the STAR study, the most common complications reported were joint adhesions (16%) in the first six months after Carticel® implant, and after six months, the need for a subsequent surgical procedure to remove excess cartilage growth (15%).

Data from the RBS study for Carticel-treated individuals, showed that 39% (38/97) of patients needed another surgical procedure within three years for removal of excess knee cartilage growth. After the procedure, it was reported that the subsequent procedure relieved patients' symptoms. In the RBS, 67% (16/24) of patients who required arthroscopy after Carticel® had a good clinical benefit in terms of improved function and relief of symptoms.

Of 153 patients treated with autologous cultured chondrocyte implantation in the Swedish Series, 22% (34/153) of patients experienced complications. About 1% of patients developed severe adhesions resulting in "frozen knee" and significant swelling of the joint, pain with postoperative fever, and pooling of blood in the surgical area following arthroscopy. In this study, arthroscopy was scheduled for chondrocyte implantation patients at 18 months of follow-up, regardless of patient symptoms. Of the patients who had arthroscopy, 43% (37/86) had excess cartilage growth that needed trimming.

As of July 31, 2006, approximately 12,500 patients were implanted with Carticel, and 559 reported serious adverse reactions after treatment. The most frequently identified serious complications reported, in descending order of frequency, were graft overgrowth, graft delamination (partial or complete), arthrofibrosis, joint adhesions, meniscus lesion or tear, graft complications, chondromalacia, loose body in knee joint, and joint malalignment.

Many surgical procedures have been used to promote repair of knee cartilage, and a few studies have evaluated the composition of cartilage cells and function resulting from these interventions. Procedures such as marrow stimulation techniques (MST) have been shown to produce fibrocartilage or hybrid mixtures of fibrocartilage and hyaline cartilage. However, the long-term success of marrow stimulation is limited, especially in older patients with large cartilage defects. Published data show that autologous chondrocyte implantation (ACI) such as Carticel, is more likely than MST to result in hyaline-like cartilage at the repair site. However, because of differences in study design, variation in lesion size and associated patient conditions, there is not sufficient data to draw conclusions about the long-term correlation of histology and clinical outcomes.

The adverse reaction rates as well as the rate and type of subsequent surgical procedures from Carticel® studies of different designs have not been directly compared with each other. However, the reports from these studies regarding complications provide a basis for identifying adverse reactions that may be related to Carticel® use and for estimating their frequency.

As individuals grow older, joint issues—especially knee joints—can be challenging. In addition to the use of Carticel, other new procedures are being studied to restore or replace damaged knee cartilage. Among them are the use of stem cells to promote cartilage growth, novel anti-inflammatory pharmaceuticals to stifle the inflammation in osteoarthritis, and growth factors for cartilage regrowth.

—*Joanne R. Gambosi, BSN, MA*

See also: Aging; Knee surgery; Cartilage repair; Meniscus repair; Torn cartilage

For Further Information:

Brittberg M, Lindahl A, Nilsson A, et al. "Treatment of deep cartilage defects in the knee with autologous chondrocyte transplantation." *New England Journal of Medicine* 1994; 331: 889-895.

Eustice C. "Treatments for Osteoarthritis of the Knee: 18 Alternative to Knee Replacement Surgery." *Very Well*. September 21, 2017.

Ingraham P. "A review of the science of Carticel® (autologous chondrocyte implantation, or ACI): Implanting your own cartilage cells to repair knee joint surfaces." *Pain Science*. July, 2016.

Peterson L, Brittberg M, Kiviranta I, et al. "Autologous chondrocyte transplantation. Biomechanics and long-term durability." *American Journal of Sports Medicine* 2002; 30:2-12.

Zaslav K, Cole B, Brewster R, et al. "A prospective study of autologous chondrocyte implantation in patients with failed prior treatment for articular cartilage defect of the knee: results of the Study of the Treatment of Articular Repair (STAR) clinical trial." *American Journal of Sports Medicine* 2009; 37(1):42-55.

Cartilage

Biology

Anatomy or system affected: Musculoskeletal, respiratory

Specialties and related fields: Geriatrics, orthopedics, otolaryngology, radiology, rheumatology

Definition: Versatile connective tissue with several functions, most prominently strength and flexibility, found in many structures throughout the body

Key terms:

chondrocyte: the cell type responsible for secreting the collagen and elastin components of the cartilage matrix

proteoglycan: a compound found in connective tissue, and other places in the body, composed of a protein to which chains of sugar-based groups are attached

Structure and Function

Cartilage represents a vital tissue component of the human body and is responsible for numerous functions ranging from structural support to shock absorption. It is a subtype of the broader category of connective tissues and thus embodies many of the features of this class. Notably, as a connective tissue, cartilage does not receive any innervation from neurons or nerve cells, nor does it receive a blood supply like muscle or epithelial tissue. In addition, connective tissue is composed of an extracellular matrix—a conglomeration of fibers that provides the structural backbone and ground substance, which helps the tissue retain water. In the case of cartilage, these components are collagen fibers, a triple helix of protein fibrils that helps provide strength against resistance, and various types of proteoglycans.

Chondrocytes are the cells primarily responsible for production of the cartilage matrix and are diverse in their function of maintaining the flexible yet resilient nature of cartilage. During development, chondrocytes develop from the line of embryonic stem cells, specifically the subsequent mesenchymal cells that hold the ability to become fibroblasts or the precursors to bone. Chondrocytes secrete two primary elements of cartilage: collagen, which is a protein building block that provides strength, and elastin, which allows for flexibility. Unlike other similar tissues made of an extracellular matrix, cartilaginous cells themselves make up only about 10% of the overall structure of cartilage, a much lower percent than other connective tissues. One hypothesis for the low cellular population is that cartilage relies heavily on diffusion for its nutrition, given that it does not have its own blood or immunologic supply.

Three types of cartilage exist: hyaline, elastic, and fibrous. Each one has its own histologic structure and unique function. Hyaline cartilage is the most abundant type and includes articular cartilage, which is the cartilage found in joint surfaces. Its major role is to help reduce friction and maintain the composition of joints, since these surfaces are under constant motion throughout the day. As such, hyaline cartilage is located in the throat, larynx, nose, and at the costal cartilages that attach the ribs to the sternum. This allows ribs to bounce back to their original position with respiration. Structurally, hyaline cartilage is about 5-10% chondrocytes. Approximately 70% of the remaining mass of cartilage is made up of water. The remaining 20-25% of cartilage is made up of various proteins and extracellular components, such as type 2 collagen and proteoglycans.

The remaining 90-95% is composed of various proteins such as type 2 collagen and proteoglycans, i.e. proteins with sugar groups, which help to retain the approximately 70% water component.

On the other hand, fibrous cartilage, which is located in the disks that sit between vertebrae and in the structure that fuses the two pubic bones, functions primarily to provide rigidity and resist compressive forces. In the spine, the fibrous cartilage helps resist and cushion the continuous downward compressive forces from walking and gravity. In the pubic symphysis, which fuses the pubic bones, it maintains structure against the turning forces from the two halves of the pelvis that articulate with the legs. The structure of fibrous cartilage is distinct from hyaline in that the chondrocytes, while similar in quantity, secrete much thicker collagen fibers, which thus resist compression.

Elastic cartilage, the third type, is even more distinct from hyaline cartilage. It is located in the ears and epiglottis and helps to spring the tongue back into its resting position with each swallow. This type of cartilage contains a much larger cell population than either hyaline or fibrous cartilage, and the chondrocytes here produce many more elastic fibers, providing the necessary flexibility.

Disorders and Diseases

Diseases associated with cartilage can arise in a number of different forms, including degeneration, congenital problems, and inflammatory conditions. In general, the theme involves disruptions in the balance of cartilage production and maintenance. Because of the vast number of structures in the body reliant on cartilage, these effects can potentially be devastating. While the list can be extensive, the most common disorders affecting cartilage include osteoarthritis, costochondritis, spinal disc herniation, and disc degeneration.

Osteoarthritis is a widespread disease, affecting as many as 3 million people worldwide. Osteoarthritis has been linked to local inflammatory changes that can occur with increases in body fat and the metabolic changes of aging. Such changes alter the fine balance between the cartilage-producing chondrocytes and various catabolic or destructive elements, such as oxygen atoms with unpaired electrons. Because articular cartilage in weight-bearing joints, such as the knees and hips, is particularly affected in OA, individuals with this condition report joint discomfort that is worse at the end of the day. Radiologic findings include narrowing of the joint space from loss of the cartilage, sclerosis or stiffening of the joint capsule, and bony cyst formation. Treatment involves a combination of medications targeted to reduce this inflammation, including non-steroidal anti-inflammatory drugs, or NSAIDs, like naproxen or ibuprofen, and steroid injections directly into the joint space. Rheumatoid arthritis, a close cousin of osteoarthritis, likewise involves degradation of the cartilage's extracellular matrix, but is associated with an autoimmune phenomenon in which the body develops a reaction to its own cartilage, leading to cellular destruction.

Costochondritis is a contributing cause of extra-cardiac chest pain, and due primarily to inflammation of the hyaline cartilage that exists at the costochondral junctions. Like osteoarthritis, costochondritis is primarily controlled by NSAIDs and possible steroid injections.

Spinal disc herniation occurs when the nucleus pulposus, or the central component of a vertebral disc, begins to herniate or leak into the surrounding annulus fibrosus and cause swelling that irritates nearby nerves. On a similar note, disc degeneration involves weakening of both layers, starting from the hyaline-type pulposus and extending to the fibrous annulus. Studies have shown early loss of the proteoglycan component within both layers to be a contributing factor.

Perspective and Prospects

Cartilage damaged by degenerative, inflammatory, and traumatic etiologies has shown a limited ability to regenerate, thus afflicting millions of people. As such, the future of managing such conditions will be reliant on restorative and regenerative technologies to restore or reduce the damage on cartilage. Current research has ranged from implementing template-like devices to laying down a foundation for various proteins. Some research has also considered carbohydrate polymer gels that mimic the extracellular matrix. Other tools include injection of growth factors to stimulate proliferation of chondrocytes and even injection of mesenchymal stem cells to increase the chondrocyte population.

Of these research techniques, the field of cartilage tissue

engineering has advanced significantly over the last 5-10 years. Despite the proliferation of technologies, significant challenges persist, as none of these methods have been proven to fully replicate the structure and function of original cartilage. In addition, various obstacles exist, including regulatory concerns and ethical liabilities associated with the use of embryonic stem cell-based products.

—*Derek T. Nhan, BS and Walter Klyce, BA*

For Further Information:

Firestein, Gary S., et al., eds. *Kelley's Textbook of Rheumatology*. 8th ed. Philadelphia: Elsevier, 2008.

Grassel, Susanne, and Attila Aszodi, eds. *Cartilage: Volume 2: Pathophysiology*. New York, NY: Springer, 2017

Pham, Phuc Van, ed. *Bone and CartilageRegeneration*. New York, NY: Springer, 2016

Casts and splints

Treatment

Anatomy or system affected: Arms, bones, hands, joints, knees, legs, ligaments, musculoskeletal system, neck, nose, skin, tendons

Specialties and related fields: Emergency medicine, family medicine, general surgery, internal medicine, nursing, orthopedics, pediatrics, physical therapy, sports medicine

Definition: Casts are solid, firm dressings formed with plaster of Paris or similar material around a limb or other body part to provide immobilization for healing. Splints are orthopedic devices made from rigid metal or plaster or from flexible felt or leather that support, immobilize, or restrain any part of the body during the healing process.

Key terms:

callus: a bony deposit formed between and around the broken ends of a fractured bone during healing

hematoma: a swelling that contains blood

ischemia: lack of blood supply resulting in tissue damage

Indications and Procedures

The general objectives of fracture management are to realign the bone fragments, to maintain the alignment by immobilization, and to restore function to the limb or part. Closed reduction is the manipulation of the bone fragments until the bone is realigned. Manual traction and rotation of the limb may be necessary. This type of reduction is done with a general anesthetic or sedation. The realigned bone is then immobilized by application of a cast or splint. Immobilization is essential after the fracture is realigned. If the bone fragments are not immobilized, then the necessary hematoma and callus formation will be disrupted and the bone will heal slowly, in poor alignment, or fail to heal. Restoration of function is accomplished by preventing complications during immobility and by rehabilitation methods that prepare the patient for mobility and maintain muscle strength, tone, and range of motion.

Uses and Complications

Complications of fractures include infection (osteomyelitis), problems of bone union, compartment syndrome, nerve damage, and cast syndrome. Delayed union of the fracture occurs when the bone does not unite in the usual amount of time. The delay may have various causes, including infection, poor circulation to the bone, and inadequate reduction. Nonunion is the failure of healing so that firm union does not take place. Malunion is a complication in which union occurs in a deformed or angulated position. Compartment syndrome occurs when swelling develops within a confined space. Tight splints and casts may cause pressure from outside the compartment, or inflammation and resulting edema or hemorrhage may cause pressure from within, compromising circulation in the extremity. Ischemia of the muscle occurs if enough pressure builds and leads to nerve damage. The first symptom of compartment syndrome is pain that increases in severity and is unrelieved by narcotics. Other symptoms and signs include paralysis, paresthesias, and decreased or absent pulses. Irreversible damage begins in the muscles and nerves after six hours of ischemia, and the extremity becomes useless after twenty-four to forty-eight hours with loss of motor and sensory function. Nerve damage can result from the original injury itself or from the casting. Cast syndrome, a complication of body casts, is caused by compression of part of the duodenum by the superior mesenteric artery, resulting in gastric or intestinal obstruction. The condition can become fatal if allowed to progress. Treatment includes gastrointestinal decompression, no intake of food or fluid by mouth, fluid and electrolyte intravenous replacement, and removal of the cast.

Nursing management of fracture patients involves efficient care of the cast. Analgesics are administered prior to cast application, if needed. The skin under the area of the cast will be inspected for redness, abrasions, open lesions, or bruising. These areas will need careful evaluation through a cast window to determine that the skin is not breaking down. The skin will be cleaned and dried thoroughly. A tubular stockinette long enough to extend beyond both edges of the cast will be applied to the limb. Rolls of a feltlike material are wrapped around the limb. Bony prominences are wrapped sufficiently to prevent friction and pressure from the cast when applied. The plaster cast is applied over the protective coverings. An X ray should be taken to ensure proper bone alignment following cast application. The nurse will teach the patient to avoid allowing any objects or crumbs to fall under the cast, as such objects would become pressure points and could cause skin breakdown. The patient should be taught not to scratch under the cast with any object. If itching occurs, then the cool air of a hair dryer may be directed through the open end of the cast to alleviate the sensation. The nurse will monitor the casted limb for odors indicating infection. Hot spots along the cast may also be an indication of infection of the skin underneath. Drainage through the cast is a sign of infection or bleeding. A patient who believes that bleeding has occurred should circle the drainage area with ink and label the date and time on the cast. The nurse should remember to check the undersurface of the cast, as drainage flows downward. The creation of a cast window to expose the area of skin that requires care may be necessary.

Neurovascular assessment should be made frequently for the first twenty-four hours following application of a cast. If neurovascular impairment is not recognized early, then irreversible damage can result with loss of function or even loss of the extremity. These assessments include evaluating the circulatory status-color, temperature, capillary refill, edema, and pulses. Neurologic status includes sensation, mobility, presence of numbness and tingling, or pain. Patients should be taught to self-monitor and self-evaluate their casted extremity.

When the fracture is healed, the cast is split with an electric cast remover that vibrates rather than cuts. The patient will feel only pressure, vibration, and heat. When the cast is removed, the extremity will appear thin and flabby, and the skin will be scaly and may be foul smelling. The nurse should prepare the patient for the appearance of the limb, explaining that when the part begins to be used once again, the muscle will return to its former size. The weakened limb will need support when moved; it may be painful. The limb can swell if held in a dependent position, Patients will be instructed to continue to elevate the extremity and should be reassured that with activity and exercise the tendency for swelling will subside.

Perspective and Prospects

Humans have had to contend with broken or malformed bones since prehistory. Ancient Egyptian hieroglyphics depict injured limbs wrapped and braced to heal normally. The earliest methods of holding a reduced fracture involved using splints. These are rigid strips laid parallel to each other alongside the bone. The Egyptians used wooden splints made of bark wrapped in linen. Plaster of Paris bandages were introduced in different forms by a surgeon in the Dutch army in 1851. The bandages hardened rapidly and provided an exact fit.

—*Jane C. Norman, Ph.D., R.N., C.N.E.*

See also Bone disorders; Bone grafting; Bones and the skeleton; Fracture and dislocation; Fracture repair; Healing; Hip fracture repair; Orthopedic surgery; Orthopedics; Orthopedics, pediatric; Physical rehabilitation; Wounds.

For Further Information:

"Care of Casts and Splints." *OrthoInfo*, April 2011.

"Elbow Fractures in Children." *OrthoInfo*. November 2011.

Farrell, Jane. *Illustrated Guide to Orthopedic Nursing*. Philadelphia: Lippincott Williams & Wilkins, 1986.

"Forearm Fractures in Children." *OrthoInfo*, January 2010.

Maher, Ann Butler. *Orthopaedic Nursing*. New York: Elsevier Health Sciences, 1994.

Schoen, Delores Christina. *Adult Orthopaedic Nursing*. Philadelphia: Lippincott Williams & Wilkins, 2000.

CAT scans. *See* Computed tomography (CT) scanning.

Cataract surgery
Procedure
Anatomy or system affected: Eyes

Specialties and related fields: Ophthalmology, optometry
Definition: The surgical management of cataracts.
Key terms:

cornea: the transparent, curved front surface of the eye

phacoemulsification: the insertion of an ultrasound device through a small incision in the eye to break a cataract into small fragments, which are then aspirated with the same device

retina: a thin membrane at the back of the eyeball where light is converted into nerve impulses that travel to the brain

ultrasound: high-frequency sound waves

Indications and Procedures

Cataract surgery refers to the surgical removal of the lens from the eye, generally because of a decrease in vision or other visual complaints, such as difficulty with night vision, glare, or loss of contrast. The decision to undergo cataract surgery, however, depends most often on the individual's subjective threshold for what constitutes unacceptable vision.

Every eye contains a lens that allows images to be focused on the retina, much like a camera focuses light. Over time, most people develop some degree of opacity in their lens, which can only be remedied by surgically removing the lens and replacing it with an artificial one. The artificial lens can be made from a variety of materials, such as silicone, acrylic, or other biocompatible synthetic substances.

Because of the refinement in instrumentation and technique, general anesthesia is rarely indicated in cataract surgery, and the procedure is often performed on an outpatient basis. Anesthesia is generally administered by injection of the anesthetic solution around the eye or by placing anesthetic drops on the eye. The surgical approach to lens extraction depends to some extent on the nature of the cataract and the surgeon's preference. The majority of surgeons use

The presence of a cataract, cloudiness of the eye lens that obscures vision, often requires the removal of the entire lens and its replacement with an artificial lens (shown here), which is held in place with loops.

an ultrasound device to break the cataract into small fragments, which are then aspirated with the same device (phacoemulsification). This procedure is often performed through a very small incision, which may be left to close by itself or be closed with one small suture. Under certain circumstances, the ophthalmologist may elect to remove the entire lens in a single piece (extracapsular surgery), in which case a larger opening is needed into the eye to gain access to the cataract.

Once the cataract is removed, a clear artificial intraocular lens (IOL) is often placed in its position to allow the eye to continue to focus light properly. The IOL may be single focus (focusing at only one distance) or multifocal (focusing at both near and far distances). In general, cataract surgery is performed on one eye at a time, since a resulting infection in both eyes, albeit rare, can be quite devastating. The length of the procedure is often significantly less than one hour, provided there are no complications or special needs.

In most cases, the patient returns home the same day and may wear a patch over the eye until the next postoperative day, when he or she is seen on follow-up. The patient is then asked to start using a combination of antibiotic and anti-inflammatory agents to prevent infection and reduce inflammation. Alternatively, some surgeons recommend starting drops immediately following surgery in order to hasten recovery. Some ophthalmologists also suggest using these drops prior to surgery in order to minimize the risk of infection and inflammation even further. Visual recovery varies greatly among individuals and may be as short as a day or as long as several months.

Uses and Complications

Although cataracts are mostly a condition affecting the elderly, they can occur at any age and even in newborns. Cataracts may have various causes, although the most common is related to simple aging and does not necessarily reflect a significant disease of the eye or the body. The presence of cataracts in young children or young adults is never normal, however, and must be promptly addressed, especially in newborns. Potentially more serious conditions may mask themselves as cataracts in the young child. Therefore, unlike the adult cataract, the progression of which can be carefully followed over time, the cataract in the newborn must be quickly referred to an ophthalmologist for surgical care.

With the many refinements in technique and technology, the overall morbidity of this procedure has significantly diminished, and the majority of patients who undergo cataract surgery find it to be a positive life-altering experience. As with most surgical procedures, infection and bleeding can occur during cataract surgery. Although rare, a resulting eye infection, known as "endophthalmitis," can have devastating consequences and must be addressed immediately. The signs and symptoms of endophthalmitis include decreased vision, pain, and redness. A more common complication of surgery is swelling of the retina (macular edema). This condition may lead to suboptimal vision fol-

---

Information on Cataracts

Causes: Aging, diabetes, injury, exposure to X rays or nuclear radiation, congenital defect
Symptoms: Loss of clear vision, typically one eye at a time
Duration: Chronic
Treatments: Surgery

---

lowing surgery but can generally be treated with anti-inflammatory drops. Finally, one or more fragments of the lens may become dislodged in the eye as a result of a rupture of the capsule surrounding the cataract. If the surgeon deems it unsafe to proceed further, then the eye may be closed and approached at a later time with the help of a retinal surgeon, who can then safely remove any remaining fragments from the eye. It is not uncommon for a secondary cataract to form on the implanted IOL; this is treated using a laser technique called "posterior capsulotomy." Other rare but potential complications include the loss of the clarity of the cornea, retinal detachment, glaucoma, or long-standing inflammation.

Perspective and Prospects

The word "cataract" is derived from a Greek and Latin word meaning "waterfall," referring to the visible veil that forms in the pupil. Cataracts constitute the most common cause of preventive blindness throughout the world. In 2010, close to twenty million people around the world were blind as a result of cataracts. No medicinal treatments are currently available for cataracts. There is some evidence that a healthy lifestyle with proper precaution against ultraviolet (UV) light can slow the formation or progression of cataracts.

Future trends in the management of cataracts point to less invasive surgical approaches, with smaller incisions and devices that produce less collateral heat. Laser devices for cataract surgery continue to improve and may one day equal or surpass ultrasound devices in their ability to address most cataracts safely.

Significant progress continues to be made in the realm of artificial intraocular lenses. Many IOLs can now be folded or injected into the eye through very small incisions. Some progress has been made to manufacture lenses that provide true accommodation, much like a young individual's eyes, thus obviating the need for reading glasses. Finally, with the advent of better antibiotic solutions, the potential risk of infection is significantly reduced.

—*Ebrahim Elahi, M.D.*

See also Aging; Aging: Extended care; Astigmatism; Blindness; Blurred vision; Cataracts; Corneal transplantation; Eye infections and disorders; Eye surgery; Eyes; Glaucoma; Laser use in surgery; Macular degeneration; Microscopy, slitlamp; Ophthalmology; Optometry; Optometry, pediatric; Vision; Vision disorders.

For Further Information:
A.D.A.M. Medical Encyclopedia. "Cataract Removal." *MedlinePlus*, September 14, 2011.

Albert, Daniel M. *Ophthalmic Surgery: Principles and Techniques*. 2 vols. Malden, Mass.: Blackwell Science, 1999.

Buettner, Helmut, ed. *Mayo Clinic on Vision and Eye Health: Practical Answers on Glaucoma, Cataracts, Macular Degeneration, and Other Conditions*. Rochester, Minn.: Mayo Foundation for Medical Education and Research, 2002.

Cheyer, Christopher, ed. "Cataract Removal." *Health Library*, February 28, 2012.

Eye Smart. "Cataract Surgery." *American Academy of Ophthalmology*, 2013.

Gottsch, John D., Walter J. Stark, and Morton F. Goldberg, eds. *Ophthalmic Surgery*. 5th ed. New York: Oxford University Press, 1999.

Houseman, William. "The Day the Light Returned." *New Choices for Retirement Living* 32 (April, 1992): 54-58.

Parker, James N., and Philip M. Parker, eds. *The Official Patient's Sourcebook on Cataract Surgery*. Rev. and updated ed. San Diego, Calif.: Icon Health, 2005.

"Prevention of Blindness and Visual Impairment: Priority Eye Diseases-Cataract." *World Health Organization*, 2013.

Shulman, Julius. *Cataracts-From Diagnosis to Recovery: The Complete Guide for Patients and Families*. Rev. ed. New York: St. Martin's Griffin, 1995.

Spaeth, George L., ed. *Ophthalmic Surgery: Principles and Practice*. 4th ed. Philadelphia: W. B. Saunders, 2012.

Sutton, Amy L., ed. *Eye Care Sourcebook: Basic Consumer Health Information About Eye Care and Eye Disorders*. 3d ed. Detroit, Mich.: Omnigraphics, 2008.

Cataracts

Disease/Disorder
Anatomy or system affected: Eyes
Specialties and related fields: Geriatrics and gerontology, ophthalmology, optometry
Definition: Dark regions in the lens of the eye that cause gradual loss of vision.
Key terms:

artificial lens implant: a plastic lens inserted permanently into the eye to replace a defective natural lens that has been removed

cornea: the transparent front surface of the eye; its curvature produces about 60 percent of the focusing power needed to produce an image on the retina

extracapsular cataract extraction: a procedure in which the lens is emulsified (broken up) with an ultrasonic probe and the pieces are suctioned out

intracapsular cataract extraction: a procedure in which the faulty lens is removed in one piece while still inside its capsule

iris: the colored portion of the eye that regulates the amount of light entering the pupil at its center

laser: an intense light beam, used in eye surgery to reattach a detached retina or to open a secondary cataract

microsurgery: surgery performed with the aid of a microscope

retina: the dark membrane on the inside rear surface of the eye, where light is converted into nerve signals sent to the brain

Causes and Symptoms

Cataracts are imperfections in the clarity of the eye lens that reduce its ability to transmit light. They are a very common medical problem. There are many misconceptions about cataracts. Cataracts are not an infection, a growth, a disease, or a film on the surface of the lens. They do not cause pain, redness, tears, or other discomforts of the eye. The initial symptom is a gradual deterioration of vision, usually in one eye at a time. There is no known treatment other than to remove the lens surgically. After surgery, neither the lens nor the cataracts can grow back. The formation of cataracts is a normal part of aging, like gray hair or hardening of the arteries. All people would develop cataracts eventually if they lived long enough.

In a discussion of cataracts, it is helpful to review the structure of the human eye. The eye is often compared to a camera lens. The camera lens, however, can be moved back and forth slightly to focus on objects at different distances, whereas the eye lens is squeezed into a thicker shape by muscular action to change its focus. Both camera and eye have a variable-size diaphragm to regulate the amount of light that is admitted.

When light enters the eye, it first encounters a transparent, tough outer skin called the "cornea." There are no blood vessels in the cornea, but many nerve cells make it sensitive to touch or other irritation. Immediately behind the cornea is the clear aqueous fluid that carries oxygen and nutrients for cell metabolism. Next comes the colored portion, the iris of the eye, with a variable-size opening at its center called the "pupil." The pupil has no color but rather looks black, like the opening of a cave. A person looking at his or her own eye in a mirror and then shining a flashlight on it can see the black pupil quickly shrink in size.

Next comes the lens of the eye, surrounded by an elastic membrane called the "capsule." The lens is suspended by ligaments, or short strands, which are attached to a sphincter muscle. When the muscle contracts, the lens becomes thicker in the middle, thus increasing its focusing strength. The transparent lens has no blood vessels, so its metabolism is provided by the aqueous fluid. Behind the lens is the vitreous fluid, which fills about two-thirds of the eyeball and maintains its oval shape. At the back of the eye is the retina, where special visual cells convert light into electrical signals that travel to the brain via nerve fibers.

The lens of the eye is not simply a homogeneous fluid, but has a unique, internal structure and growth pattern. It continues to grow larger throughout the life of the individual. New cells originate at the front surface of the lens, just inside the capsule enclosure. These cells divide and grow into fibers that migrate toward the nucleus, or middle, of the lens. The whole structure has been compared to the layers of an onion, with the oldest cells at the center. The protein molecules in the nucleus are less soluble and more rigid than those in the outer part of the lens. By the age of forty, in most people, the firm nucleus has enlarged until the lens has lost much of its elasticity. Even with considerable muscular strain, the curvature of the lens surface will no longer bulge enough to focus on nearby objects. The eye loses its power of accommodation, and reading glasses will be needed.

The mechanism by which cataracts form in the lens is not yet clearly understood. Like the loss of accommodation, however, it is a normal part of the aging process. One pro-

Cataracts are dark regions in the eye lens that lead gradually to obscured vision and blindness.

posed biochemical explanation is the Maillard reaction, in which glucose and protein molecules combine when heated to form a brown product. The Maillard reaction is responsible for the browning of bread or cookies during baking. The same process is thought to occur even at body temperature, though very slowly over a period of years. Some scientists have theorized that wrinkled skin, hardening of the arteries, and other normal features of aging may be caused by this reaction. The biochemistry of aging is an active area of research, in which the deterioration of the eye lens is only one example.

The most common symptom of cataracts is a loss of clear vision that cannot be corrected with eyeglasses; among the indicators of cataract-related vision loss are reduced night vision, loss of color contrast and intensity, inability to focus, double vision, and increased sensitivity to glare. Brighter lighting can partially help to overcome the blockage of light transmission. However, there is one paradoxical situation reported by some patients, whose vision becomes worse in bright light. The explanation for this problem is that brightness causes the pupil to become smaller. If the cataract is centered right in the middle of the lens, it will block a larger fraction of the incoming light. In dimmer light, the pupil opening is larger, so light can pass through the clear periphery of the lens.

By far the most common cataracts are those attributable to normal aging, called "senile cataracts." (This has nothing to do with the common use of the term "senility" to describe declining mental ability.) "Secondary cataracts" can also develop in special circumstances. For example, exposure to x-rays or nuclear radiation will increase the probability of cataracts, and the eye lens seems to be particularly sensitive to the effects of ionizing radiation. Certain medications such as cortisone, which is used in arthritis treatment, increase the risk of cataracts. A diet deficient in protein, especially in developing countries, has been associated with cataract formation. A blow to the eye from a sports injury or an accident can lead to a cataract. Diabetics are more likely to develop cataracts than the general public. Some studies have suggested that electric shock, ultraviolet rays, or certain environmental pollutants may be other causes.

Some babies are born with cataracts. These congenital cataracts are frequently associated with the mother having had German measles (rubella) during the first three months of pregnancy; they are also commonly found with a number of birth defects, such as Down syndrome and trisomy 13. Congenital cataracts are characterized by an infant having cloudy pupils, moving the eye rapidly, and/or appearing unable to see. For moderate and severe cases, surgery on the infant's eye must be done with little delay to prevent permanent blindness.

Cataracts are much more prevalent in developing nations as compared to industrialized countries. It is not clear yet what roles race, diet, and life habits may play in cataract formation. Some ophthalmologists believe that cataracts run in families, suggesting a genetic influence. The evidence is not conclusive, and further studies are needed. What causes cataracts is much less understood than how to treat them surgically.

Treatment and Therapy

When cataracts begin to form in the eye lens, no medication can remove them and they will not get better on their own. The patient's vision will continue to deteriorate as the cataracts mature, although the process may be quite slow. Fortunately, modern techniques of surgery for cataract removal have a success rate of better than 95 percent.

When a patient's eye examination reveals the onset of senile cataracts (as a result of aging), he or she is referred to an ophthalmologist, who assesses the need for surgery. If surgery is not needed immediately, the ophthalmologist may recommend more frequent, semiannual checkups. Reading or other eye-straining activities will not accelerate cataract growth, but brighter lighting and better eyeglasses will help the patient to see more clearly. Over the course of several years, the cataracts slowly darken and increase in size. Eventually, distance vision may deteriorate markedly in one or both eyes, and the ability of the patient to drive a car or perform other normal activities becomes seriously impaired, even with corrective lenses. Surgery is then indicated. Operating on one eye while the other one is still fairly clear is recommended.

Once the decision has been made to go ahead with surgery, it is necessary for the patient to have a thorough physical examination. The doctor checks for possible health problems that could complicate cataract surgery. Among these are diabetes, high blood pressure, kidney disease, anemia, and glaucoma (excess pressure in the eye). Normally, extracting the cataractous lens and implanting an artificial, plastic one are done at the same time. Before proceeding with surgery, the ophthalmologist must determine what the proper strength of the implant lens should be, so that light will focus properly on the retina. An accurate measurement is made by reflecting a beam of high-frequency sound waves (ultrasound) from the back of the eye. Measuring the time for an echo to return gives the needed data for calculating the strength of the implant lens.

On the day of the surgery, an injection is given to make the patient drowsy, and eye drops are administered to dilate the patient's pupil. Gradually, more eye drops are administered to produce a large dilation, so that access to the lens is easier. In the operating room, local anesthetic is injected to keep the eyelids from closing and to deaden the normally very sensitive surface of the cornea. To prepare for surgery, a microscope is moved into place above the eye. Making an incision in the cornea, removing the defective lens, inserting and fastening the artificial lens, and finally closing the incision with a very fine needle and thread are all performed by the surgeon while looking through the microscope. Its magnification and focus controls are operated using foot pedals, so that both of the surgeon's hands are free.

There are three basic types of cataract extraction. Each method has its advantages and disadvantages. The first method is called "intracapsular extraction." The capsule is the membrane that surrounds the lens. "Intracapsular" means that the lens and capsule are removed together-that is, with the lens still inside its capsule. The advantage of this method is that no part of the lens is left behind to cause possible problems with infection or swelling later. The disadvantage is that the incision at the edge of the cornea must be fairly large to allow the lens and capsule to be pulled out together. Five to ten stitches are needed to close the incision. The patient must avoid strenuous activity for about a month to permit thorough healing. Before 1962, forceps were used to bring the lens and capsule out of the eye. Then Charles D. Kelman introduced the cryoprobe, which uses a freezing process. When the rather slippery lens is touched by the cold cryoprobe, it freezes to the probe and can be pulled out in one piece. Most eye surgeons have adopted the cryoprobe for intracapsular extraction.

A second method of cataract surgery is called "extracapsular extraction," in which the lens is removed while the capsule is left in the eye. The advantage is that the unbroken back surface of the capsule can prevent leakage of fluid from the rear of the eye and therefore can decrease the chances for damage to the retina. A disadvantage is that small fragments of the lens may remain behind, causing infection or irritation. The size of the incision and the recuperation period are about the same as for the intracapsular method.

The third method of cataract surgery is an improvement of extracapsular extraction, first developed by Kelman in 1967. An ultrasonic probe is used to emulsify, or break up, the lens. The small pieces are then suctioned out of the capsule while fluid is washed into the opening. The main advantage of emulsification is that the incision can be very small, because the lens is brought out in fragments, not as a whole. The incision may be only three millimeters long, and a single suture to close it would heal rapidly. This method requires very specialized training, however, because surgeons must learn to operate the microscope, the ultrasonic generator, and the suction apparatus with their feet while manipulating the probe with their hands.

After the eye lens has been extracted, an artificial intraocular lens (IOL) is inserted in its place. The implant is made of clear plastic, about the size of an aspirin tablet. Two spring loops embedded in the plastic are used to center the implant and to keep it there permanently. A variety of different spring loop attachments have been designed by ophthalmologists. (Contact lenses may be used on infant patients instead of IOLs).

To complete the surgery, the incision in the cornea is closed. During the recuperation period, the patient is instructed to avoid strenuous exercise and to protect the eye from any hard contact. Normally, there is little pain, although some eye irritation should be expected during the healing process. An IOL has a fixed focal length, with no power of accommodation for different distances. It is like a box camera that gives a good picture at a set distance, while near and far objects are somewhat blurry. After the eye has healed thoroughly, the patient is fitted with prescription glasses for reading and for distance vision, respectively.

A number of minor complications can develop after cataract surgery. Between 10 and 50 percent of the patients develop a "secondary cataract," which is a clouding of the capsule membrane just behind the implant. This condition is easily corrected with a laser beam to open the membrane, requiring no surgery. Another potential complication is astigmatism. The eye is squeezed and flattened slightly, and the curvature of the surface will differ between the flattened and the more rounded regions. During surgery, the symmetry of the corneal surface can be distorted if some sutures are tighter than others. Astigmatism is relatively easy to correct with prescription glasses. For infants who undergo cataract removal surgery, infection, inflammation, and bleeding pose slight risks.

All operations have some risks, and a small percentage of cataract surgeries can lead to serious complications. Among these are a detached retina, glaucoma caused by scar tissue, and hemorrhage into the vitreous fluid in front of the retina. Fortunately, such problems are rare, and the percentage of successful eye surgeries continues to improve.

Perspective and Prospects

In the history of medicine, surgery for cataracts has been traced back to Roman times. The method was called "couching." The physician would insert a needle through the white of the eye into the lens and try to push the lens down out of the line of vision, leaving it in the eyeball. The procedure must have been painful, with a high chance for infection. The complete extraction of a lens from the eye was done for the first time in 1745. A French ophthalmologist named Jacques Daviel was performing a couching operation but was unable to push the lens out of the line of sight. On the spur of the moment, he decided to make a small cut in the cornea, through which he was able to extract the lens. The operation was successful. During the following ten years, he repeated his procedure more than four hundred times with only fifty failures, a much better result than with couching.

A major advance in eye surgery was the discovery of local anesthesia by Carl Koller in 1884. Together with the famous psychiatrist Sigmund Freud, Koller had been investigating the psychological effects of cocaine. He noticed that his tongue became numb from the drug and wondered if a drop of cocaine solution locally applied to the eyes might work as an anesthetic. He tried it first on a frog's eye and then on himself, and the cocaine made his eye numb. He published a short article, and the news spread to other physicians. Synthetic substitutes such as novocaine were developed and came into common use, thereafter making eye surgery virtually painless.

When the lens of the eye is surgically removed, it be-

comes impossible to focus light on the retina. A strong replacement lens is needed. For example, the French painter Claude Monet had cataract surgery in the 1920s, and photographs show him with the typical thick cataract glasses of that time. Today, contact lenses or artificial lens implants are much better alternatives to restore good vision.

The recovery period after cataract surgery used to be several weeks of bed rest, with the head kept absolutely still, because the cut in the cornea had to heal itself without any stitches. The development of microsurgery made it possible for the surgeon to see the extremely fine thread and needle that can be used for closing the cut. With stitches in place, the patient can usually carry on normal activities within a day after surgery.

In the 1960s, the cryoprobe and the ultrasound probe were developed to replace forceps for removing an eye lens. The size of the required incision was smaller and the healing time correspondingly shorter. In the 1980s, reliable lens implants became available, making near-normal vision possible again. In the future, perhaps drugs can be found that will prevent or delay the onset of cataracts, so that surgery will not be necessary. Further research is needed to obtain a better understanding of biochemical changes in the eye lens that occur with aging.

—*Hans G. Graetzer, Ph.D.*

See also Aging; Blindness; Cataract surgery; Eye infections and disorders; Eye surgery; Eyes; Ophthalmology; Optometry; Vision; Vision disorders.

For Further Information:

A.D.A.M. Medical Encyclopedia. "Cataract." *MedlinePlus*, September 16, 2011.

A.D.A.M. Medical Encyclopedia. "Congenital Cataract." *MedlinePlus*, September 14, 2011.

Buettner, Helmut, ed. *Mayo Clinic on Vision and Eye Health: Practical Answers on Glaucoma, Cataracts, Macular Degeneration, and Other Conditions*. Rochester, Minn.: Mayo Foundation for Medical Education and Research, 2002.

Eballé, André Omgbwa, et al. "Secondary Cataract: An Epidemiologic and Clinical Survey at the Yaounde Gynaeco-obstetric and Paediatric Hospital." *Clinical Ophthalmology*, June 22, 2011.

Eden, John. *The Physician's Guide to Cataracts, Glaucoma, and Other Eye Problems*. Yonkers, N.Y.: Consumer Reports Books, 1992.

Houseman, William. "The Day the Light Returned." *New Choices for Retirement Living* 32 (April, 1992): 54-58.

Oliff, Heather, and Christopher Cheyer. "Cataract." *Health Library*, September 1, 2011.

Parker, James N., and Philip M. Parker, eds. *The Official Patient's Sourcebook on Cataracts*. San Diego, Calif.: Icon Health, 2002.

Sardegna, Jill, et al. *The Encyclopedia of Blindness and Vision Impairment*. 2d ed. New York: Facts On File, 2002.

Shulman, Julius. *Cataracts-From Diagnosis to Recovery: The Complete Guide for Patients and Families*. Rev. ed. New York: St. Martin's Griffin, 1995.

Sutton, Amy L., ed. *Eye Care Sourcebook: Basic Consumer Health Information About Eye Care and Eye Disorders*. 3d ed. Detroit, Mich.: Omnigraphics, 2008.

Taylor, Allen, ed. *Nutritional and Environmental Influences on the Eye*. Boca Raton, Fla.: CRC Press, 1999.

Catheterization

Procedure

Anatomy or system affected: Bladder, blood vessels, circulatory system, genitals, heart, reproductive system, throat, urinary system

Specialties and related fields: Anesthesiology, cardiology, critical care, emergency medicine, general surgery, pulmonary medicine, radiology, urology

Definition: The insertion of a tube into a cavity of the body to withdraw fluids from or to introduce fluids into that cavity.

Key terms:

bladder: the organ that stores urine until it is discharged from the body

urethra: the tube that transfers urine from the bladder to outside the body

Indications and Procedures

Many different types of catheters exist, and they can be used for many different purposes. What they all have in common is the placement of a tube (catheter) into a body cavity. The tube is used to draw a gas or liquid from the cavity or to inject a gas or liquid into the cavity. The most common uses of catheterization are the opening of an airway for breathing, the withdrawal of urine from the bladder, and the injection of dye or other substances such as an intravenous (IV) drip into blood vessels.

Catheterization can be used to assist in the breathing process. This procedure may be necessary when the patient's airway is blocked, the patient is unconscious and unable to breathe, or the patient needs help to breathe. The tube or catheter is placed into the mouth, nose, throat, or lungs. Oxygen passes through the tube and into the lungs, where it can be absorbed by the blood. Catheters can also be used to remove secretions from these same areas to open the airway and improve breathing. They are also necessary in many emergency situations to open and maintain breathing. At times, a catheter must be introduced directly into the lungs through an incision in the neck, near the Adam's apple; this procedure is known as a tracheostomy. A catheter may also be introduced into the patient's nose to transport oxygen into the lungs. Catheterization is important for maintaining breathing during surgery under general anesthesia, when the body's breathing mechanisms are shut down.

Another common catheterization procedure involves the introduction of a urethral catheter. This type of catheter is inserted into the urethra to drain urine from the bladder. Such a procedure may be necessary to empty the bladder when the urethra is blocked, or it may be used to collect urine when the person is unable to control his or her own bladder.

An area where catheters are being used more frequently is heart diagnosis and surgery. In cardiac catheterization, a catheter is inserted into a large blood vessel (a vein or artery) in the upper arm or groin area. The physician then maneuvers the catheter into the heart and uses it to inject a dye directly into the organ. An X ray can show the distribution of the dye within the heart, allowing the physician to see if and where any coronary arteries are blocked. In addition, cardiac catheters can be used to determine blood pressures within the heart, the amount of oxygen in the blood in the heart, and how the valves are functioning. More recently, cardiac catheters have been developed to perform some types of surgery. A good example is balloon angioplasty. Using similar procedures to insert the catheter, the cardiologist guides a specialized catheter into the coronary artery to the area of the blockage. A small balloon on the end of the catheter is inflated, pushing the fatty material blocking the artery against the blood vessel wall and opening the artery to allow for the normal flow of blood.

Uses and Complications

Catheterization has been used safely and successfully for many years. When people are unable to breathe on their own, airway catheters have been instrumental in saving lives and making such patients more comfortable. Such procedures have been widely used on a daily basis, with few complications.

Likewise, urethral catheters are routinely employed to control the flow of urine from the bladder. This type of catheterization can be seen in many clinical settings. Although caution must be used to prevent the introduction of bacteria into the bladder and subsequent infection, this procedure is considered to be safe and effective.

The overall success rate of cardiac catheterization has been good, with few deaths resulting from the procedure. It is a valuable tool for the diagnosis of heart diseases and disorders because a major incision in the chest is avoided. This procedure is performed many times each day in all cardiac care units. Angioplasty has also been successful, but it is useful for only some types of blockages. A major risk of angioplasty is rupture of the artery if the balloon is inflated too much. When this happens, open heart surgery is necessary to prevent death. The death rate from angioplasty is less than 1 percent, however, and the success rate exceeds 90 percent. Another problem with balloon angioplasty is that in 33 percent of the cases, the blockages re-form within six months. Nevertheless, this procedure offers a good alternative to coronary artery bypass surgery.

Perspective and Prospects

The use of catheterization for airway management was first tried in 1871 by Friedrich Trendelenburg. Through the years, such procedures have been improved. Catheters will continue to be instrumental for airway management.

The cardiac catheterization of a living human being was done by Werner Forssmann in the 1920s: He performed the procedure on himself. His techniques were further developed by André Frédéric Cournand in the 1940s, for which he won the Nobel Prize in Physiology or Medicine in 1956. Continued advances in the procedure and improved technology have increased the applications of cardiac catheterization. New and better procedures, which will continue to replace some types of open heart surgery, are expected in the future.

—Bradley R. A. Wilson, Ph.D.

See also Amniocentesis; Anesthesia; Anesthesiology; Angiography; Angioplasty; Biopsy; Blood testing; Cardiology; Circulation; Heart; Intensive care unit (ICU); Intravenous (IV) therapy; Lumbar puncture; Pharmacology; Phlebotomy; Radiopharmaceuticals; Respiration; Resuscitation; Surgical procedures; Tracheostomy; Transfusion; Urinary system; Urology; Vascular medicine; Vascular system.

For Further Information:

Askari, Arman. T, and Medhi H. Shishehbor, eds. *Introductory Guide to Cardiac Catheterization*. Lippincott, Williams, & Wilkins, 2010.

Finucane, Brendan T., and Albert H. Santora. *Principles of Airway Management*. 3d ed. New York: Springer, 2003.

Karch, Amy Morrison. *Cardiac Care: A Guide for Patient Education*. New York: Appleton-Century-Crofts, 1981.

Kern, Morton J., ed. *Cardiac Catheterization Handbook*. 3d. Philadelphia: Saunders, 2012.

Nordlicht, Scott M., Alan N. Weiss, and Philip A. Ludbrook. *Why Me? Approaching Coronary Heart Disease, Cardiac Catheterization, and Treatment Options from a Position of Strength*. St. Louis, Mo.: Northern Lights, 1999.

"What Is Cardiac Catheterization?" *nhlbi.nih.org*, January 30, 2012.

Cavities

Disease/Disorder
Also known as: Dental caries
Anatomy or system affected: Gums, teeth
Specialties and related fields: Dentistry
Definition: Cavities are erosions of the surface of teeth that can excavate the tooth surface and damage tooth structure.

Causes and Symptoms

The oral cavity is filled with a variety of bacteria, some of which can ferment foods, especially complex and simple sugars, into organic acids. A mixture of oral bacteria, organic acids, food debris, and saliva combine to form a sticky, creamy-colored substance called plaque. Plaque forms on all teeth, but some are more susceptible to plaque buildup than others. A failure to remove plaque causes it to mineralize into tartar. The combination of plaque and tartar irritates the gums, which results in gingivitis and can ultimately cause an infection of the ligaments and bones that support the teeth (periodontitis). The acids in plaque also dissolve the enamel surface of the tooth, generating a hole that is known as a cavity.

Untreated, tooth decay can hollow out a tooth and destroy the nerves and blood vessels inside, resulting in a tooth abscess.

The earliest sign of a cavity is a chalky, white spot on the surface of a tooth, which indicates demineralization of the tooth enamel. At this point, the process is reversible, but the white spot can turn brown and develop into a breach in the enamel. Once the cavity forms, the affected tooth structure cannot be regenerated. Large cavities can cause toothache, particularly after consuming cold, hot, or sweet foods or drinks, but most cavities are typically painless until they grow large enough to affect the nerves. Dental X-rays can detect cavities even before they are visible to the naked eye, and cavities usually cause soft spots that are sticky when the tooth is pressed with a probe.

Treatment and Therapy

Treatment of dental cavities requires drilling the tooth to remove the enamel and dentin eroded by the invasion of acid-producing bacteria. Once the affected hard tissues have been removed, a dental filling made from dental amalgam, composite resin, porcelain, or gold is placed into the tooth to restore its structural integrity. For large cavities that have eroded so much of the tooth structure that restorative material cannot be placed within it, a cap called a crown, made of gold, porcelain, or porcelain fused to metal, is fitted over what remains of the tooth. Sometimes, the

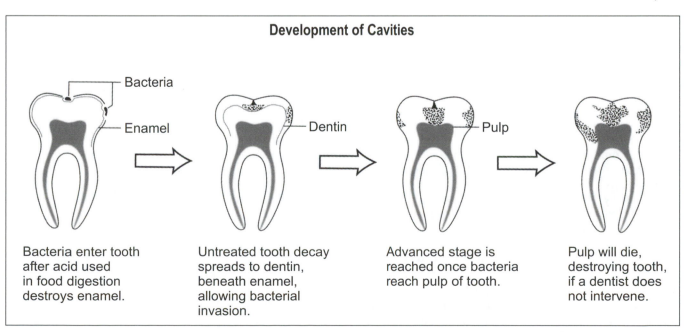

Development of Cavities

Bacteria — Enamel — Dentin — Pulp

Bacteria enter tooth after acid used in food digestion destroys enamel.

Untreated tooth decay spreads to dentin, beneath enamel, allowing bacterial invasion.

Advanced stage is reached once bacteria reach pulp of tooth.

Pulp will die, destroying tooth, if a dentist does not intervene.

damage is great enough to continually stress the nerve in the tooth, leading the nerve to die and decay. Endodontic therapy is then employed. An endodontic file hollows the center of the tooth, forming a "root canal," and removes the nerve tissue. The tissue often appears as thin wispy fibers. Endodontic therapy also involves filling the canal with gutta percha, a rubber-like substance. If the decay is too great for the tooth to be treated and saved, the tooth must be extracted.

Conscientious personal dental hygiene consists of daily brushing and flossing, regular dental examinations at least twice a year, and diet modification that reduces the intake of simple sugars. This personal dental hygiene can reduce the risk of cavities and keep teeth and gums healthy.

—*Michael A. Buratovich, Ph.D.*

See also Dental diseases; Dentistry; Dentistry, pediatric; Endodontic disease; Gingivitis; Gum disease; Periodontal surgery; Periodontitis; Plaque, dental; Root canal treatment; Teeth; Tooth extraction; Toothache.

For Further Information:
Alan, Rick. "Tooth Decay." *Health Library*, Oct. 31, 2012.
Fotek, Paul. "Dental Cavities." *MedlinePlus*, Feb. 22, 2012.
Frost, Helen. *Food for Healthy Teeth*. Mankato, Minn.: Capstone, 2006.
Sutton, Amy L, ed. *Dental Care and Oral Health Sourcebook*. 3d ed. Detroit, Mich.: Omnigraphics, 2008.
Taintor, Jerry F., and Mary Jane Taintor. *The Complete Guide to Better Dental Care*. New York: Checkmark, 1999.
UConn Health Center. "Your Dental Health: A Guide for Patients and Families." *Healthnet: Connecticut Consumer Health Information Network*, Nov. 27, 2012.

Celiac sprue

Disease/Disorder

Also known as: Nontropical sprue, gluten-sensitive enteropathy

Anatomy or system affected: Intestines, joints

Specialties and related fields: Gastroenterology, internal medicine, nutrition, pediatrics

Definition: Inflammation of the small intestine resulting from an abnormal response to gluten in the diet.

Causes and Symptoms

The most common symptoms of celiac sprue are diarrhea and weight loss. Patients develop an inflammatory reaction to gluten, a protein found in wheat, rye, oats, and barley.

This inflammation causes flattening of the fingerlike projections in the small intestine known as "villi," thereby decreasing the surface area available for nutrient and fluid absorption. Thus, patients often have anemia (from malabsorption of iron and folic acid) and bone disease (from malabsorption of calcium and vitamin D). Other symptoms of celiac sprue can include muscle weakness, infertility, epilepsy, and psychiatric illnesses, although the mechanisms underlying these manifestations are less clear. Some patients develop a blistering, itchingrash on the skin known as "dermatitis herpetiformis." Most patients come to medical attention at two years of age, after wheat is introduced into the diet. A small number of people develop the disease as adults. Research suggests that stress can trigger celiac sprue reactions, including extreme emotional stress, pregnancy, surgery, and infections.

Treatment and Therapy

The mainstay of therapy is elimination of gluten from the diet, which calms the inflammation and eventually allows the flattened villi to grow back. Symptoms usually improve within two weeks. Lack of improvement is most often the result of incomplete elimination of gluten. Alternative diagnoses-including infection, food allergies, inflammatory bowel disease, and lymphoma of the intestines-must also be considered.

The avoidance of gluten sounds straightforward, but it often requires significant dietary changes that must be rigorously followed throughout life. Most breads, pastas, and pastries must be avoided. Patients often benefit from counseling with a dietitian, since many processed foods contain gluten. Patients may also need to be screened for vitamin and mineral deficiencies. Folic acid supplementation is especially important for women of childbearing age. An x-ray to determine bone mineral density is sometimes helpful in patients with suspected vitamin D deficiency.

Perspective and Prospects

Celiac sprue is a genetic disease. It is known to be caused by a mutation on chromosome 6, and attempts to identify the specific gene further are ongoing. Testing to determine whether one has celiac sprue includes blood tests for antibodies against gliadin, the offensive component of gluten. About 1 percent of the global population suffers from celiac sprue. People at higher risk for celiac sprue include those who have diabetes mellitus, an autoimmune disease, Down syndrome, or anemia and those with a family member who has celiac sprue.

—Ahmad Kamal, M.D.;
updated by LeAnna DeAngelo, Ph.D.

See also Allergies; Anemia; Diarrhea and dysentery; Gastroenterology; Gastroenterology, pediatric; Gastrointestinal system; Gluten intolerance; Intestinal disorders; Intestines; Malabsorption; Malnutrition; Nutrition; Vitamins and minerals; Weight loss and gain.

For Further Information:

A.D.A.M. Medical Encyclopedia. "Celiac Disease." *MedlinePlus*, January 20, 2010.

Green, Peter H. R., and Rory Jones. *Celiac Disease: A Hidden Epidemic*. Rev. ed. New York: William R. Morrow, 2010.

Holmes, Geoffrey, C. Catassi, and Alessio Fasano. *Celiac Disease*. Abingdon, England: Health Press, 2009.

Korn, Danna. *Kids with Celiac Disease: A Family Guide to Raising Happy, Healthy, Gluten-Free Children*. Bethesda, Md.: Woodbine House, 2001.

Mahadov, Srihari, and Peter H. R. Green. "Celiac Disease: A Challenge for All Physicians." *Gastroenterology & Hepatology* 7, no. 8 (August, 2011): 554-556.

Parker, James N., and Philip M. Parker, eds. *The Official Patient's Sourcebook on Celiac Disease*. San Diego, Calif.: Icon Health, 2002.

Shepard, Jules E. Dowler. *The First Year: Celiac Disease and Living Gluten-Free-An Essential Guide for the Newly Diagnosed*. Cambridge, Mass.: Da Capo Lifelong, 2009.

Tessmer, Kimberly A. *Gluten-Free for a Healthy Life: Nutritional Advice and Recipes for Those Suffering from Celiac Disease and Other Gluten-Related Disorders*. Franklin Lakes, N.J.: New Page Books, 2003.

Wood, Debra, and Daus Mahnke." Celiac Disease." *Health Library*, January 28, 2013.

Cells

Biology

Anatomy or system affected: Bones, immune system, musculoskeletal system, nerves, nervous system, skin

Specialties and related fields: Bacteriology, cytology, histology

Definition: The fundamental structural and functional units of all living organisms.

Key terms:

chromosome: one DNA molecule of the cell nucleus, in combination with chromosomal proteins

cytoskeleton: a network of filaments (including microtubules, microfilaments, and intermediate filaments) that supports the cytoplasm and extensions of the cell surface

endoplasmic reticulum: a system of cytoplasmic membrane-bound sacs that, with attached ribosomes, synthesize proteins destined to enter membranes or to be stored or secreted

gene: a segment of DNA encoding a protein; RNA molecules such as messenger and ribosomal RNA

Golgi complex: a system of membrane sacs in which proteins are chemically modified, sorted, and routed to various cellular destinations

membrane: a thin layer of lipid and protein molecules that controls transport of molecules and ions between the cell and its exterior and between membrane-bound compartments within the cell

mitochondrion: a membrane-bound cytoplasmic organelle that constitutes the primary location of oxidative reactions providing energy for cellular activities

nucleolus: a nuclear structure formed through the activity of chromosome segments in the production of ribosomal RNA and the assembly of ribosomal subunits

peroxisome: a membrane-bound organelle that contains reaction systems linking biochemical pathways taking place elsewhere in the cell; also called a microbody

ribosome: a cytoplasmic particle assembled from ribosomal RNA and ribosomal proteins that uses messenger RNA molecules as directions for synthesizing proteins

Structure and Functions

Cells are the basic components of all living things, and the human body is made up of approximately 10 trillion cells. Cells contain complex biochemical systems that use energy sources to power cellular activities such as growth, movement, and reaction to environmental changes or external stimuli. The information required to assemble the enzymatic and structural molecules involved in these activities is stored in a cell's deoxyribonucleic acid (DNA) and is duplicated and passed on in cell division.

A cell can be divided into two major internal regions, the nucleus and cytoplasm, which reflect a fundamental division of labor. In the nucleus are the DNA molecules that store the hereditary information required for cell growth and reproduction. The nucleus also contains enzymes that are capable of copying the hereditary information into ribonucleic acid (RNA), which is used as instructions for making proteins in the cytoplasm. Enzymes within the nucleus also duplicate the DNA in preparation for cell division. The cytoplasm makes proteins according to the directions copied in the nucleus and also synthesizes most other molecules required for cellular activities. The cytoplasm carries out several additional vital functions, including motility and the conversion of fuel substances into usable forms of chemical energy.

Cells are encapsulated by membranes. These layers of lipid and protein molecules, not much more than 7 to 8 nanometers thick, form an outer boundary, called the plasma membrane, that separates the cell contents from the exterior. Several internal membrane systems divide the cell interior into specialized compartments called organelles. The lipid part of membranes consists of a double layer of molecules called a bilayer. The lipid bilayer provides the structural framework of membranes and acts as a barrier to the passage of water-soluble substances. Membrane proteins, which are suspended in the lipid bilayer or attached to its surface, carry out the specialized functions of membranes.

The plasma membrane forming the outer cell boundary has a variety of functions. The most significant is the transport of substances between the cytoplasm and the cell's exterior, which is carried out by proteins that form channels in the membrane. These channels pass specific water-soluble molecules or ions. The plasma membrane also contains proteins functioning as receptors, which recognize and

The Structure of a Cell

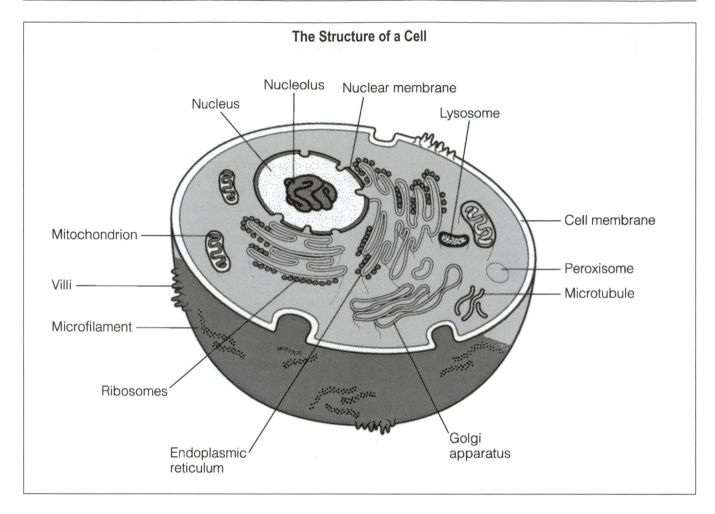

bind to specific molecules from the surrounding medium. On binding to their target molecules, which include peptide hormones, many receptors trigger internal cellular responses that coordinate the activities of cells in tissues and organs. Other plasma membrane proteins recognize and adhere to molecules on the surfaces of other cells or to extracellular structures such as collagen. These adhesive functions are critical to the development and maintenance of tissues and organs. Other plasma membrane proteins identify cells as part of the individual or as foreign intruders.

The nucleus is separated from the cytoplasm by two concentric membranes, one layered just inside the other, forming a system known as the nuclear envelope. At closely spaced intervals, the envelope is perforated by pores, about 70 to 90 nanometers in diameter, which form channels between the nuclear interior and the surrounding cytoplasm. The pores are filled by a ringlike mass of proteins that control the movement of large molecules, such as proteins and RNA, through the nuclear envelope.

Within the nucleus are chromatin fibers containing the nuclear DNA, held in association with two major types of proteins, the histone and nonhistone chromosomal proteins. The histones are primarily structural molecules that pack DNA into chromatin fibers. The nonhistones include proteins that regulate gene activity. The hereditary information of the human nucleus is subdivided among forty-six

linear DNA molecules. Each individual DNA molecule, with its associated histone and nonhistone proteins, is a chromosome of the nucleus.

Each segment of a chromosome containing the information used to make an RNA copy constitutes a gene. One type of gene encodes messenger RNA (mRNA) molecules, which contain information required to make proteins. Another type of gene encodes ribosomal RNA (rRNA) molecules. Ribosomal RNA forms part of ribosomes, complex RNA-protein particles in the cytoplasm that assemble proteins according to the directions carried in mRNA molecules. The regions of the chromosomes active in making rRNA are collected into structures called nucleoli. Within nucleoli, rRNAs are assembled with proteins into subunits of ribosomes.

The cytoplasm surrounding the nucleus is packed with ribosomes and a variety of organelles. The boundary membranes of the organelles set them off as distinct chemical and molecular environments, specialized to carry out different functions. Ribosomes may be either freely suspended in the cytoplasm or attached to the surfaces of a system of flattened, membranous sacs called the endoplasmic reticulum. Freely suspended ribosomes make proteins that enter the cytoplasmic solution as enzymes, structural supports, or motile elements. Ribosomes attached to the endoplasmic reticulum assemble proteins that become part of membranes or eventually enter small, membrane-bound sacs for storage or release to the cell exterior.

Proteins made in the rough endoplasmic reticulum-those sacs with ribosomes-are modified chemically in another system of membranous sacs, the Golgi complex or apparatus. This system usually appears as a cup-shaped stack of flattened, ribosome-free sacs. The modifications carried out in the Golgi complex may include the addition of chemical groups such as sugars, and the clipping of surplus segments from proteins. Following modification, proteins are sorted into small, membrane-bound sacs that pinch off from the Golgi membranes. These sacs may be stored in the cytoplasm or may release their contents to the cell exterior.

One type of membrane-bound sac containing stored proteins, the lysosome, is particularly important to cell function. Lysosomes contain a group of enzymes collectively capable of breaking down all major molecules of the cell. Many substances taken into cells are delivered to lysosomes, where they are digested by the lysosomal enzymes. Lysosomes may also release their enzymes into the cytoplasm or to the cell exterior. Release within the cell causes cell death, which may occur due to pathological conditions or as part of normal development.

Most of the chemical energy required for cellular activities is produced by reactions taking place in another cytoplasmic organelle, the mitochondrion. Mitochondria are surrounded by two separate membranes, one enclosed within the other. Within mitochondria occur most of the oxidative reactions that release energy for cellular activities. Fuel for these reactions is provided by the breakdown products of all major cellular molecules, including carbohydrates, fats, proteins, and nucleic acids.

The oxidative functions of mitochondria are supplemented by the activities of peroxisomes (also called microbodies). These structures, which consist simply of a boundary membrane surrounding a solution of enzymes, carry out reactions that link major oxidative pathways occurring elsewhere in the cytoplasm. Microbodies are particularly important to the oxidation of fatty acids.

Almost all cell movements are generated by one of two cytoplasmic structures, microtubules or microfilaments. Microtubules form the motile elements of sperm tails; microfilaments are responsible for the movements of skeletal, cardiac, and smooth muscle. Microtubules are fine, hollow cylinders about 25 nanometers in diameter, assembled from subunits of a protein known as tubulin. Microfilaments are thin, solid fibers 5 to 7 nanometers in diameter, assembled from subunits of a different protein, actin. Both structures produce motion through protein cross-bridges that work as transducers converting chemical energy to mechanical energy. One end of a cross-bridge attaches to the surface of a microtubule or microfilament; the opposite, reactive end attaches to another microtubule or microfilament or to other cell structures. The cross-bridge produces motion by making an attachment at its reactive end, forcefully swiveling a short distance, and then releasing. Distinct proteins form the swiveling cross-bridges for the two motile elements.

In addition to their functions in cell motility, both microtubules and microfilaments form supportive networks inside cells collectively called the cytoskeleton. Another group of supportive fibers with diameters averaging about 100 nanometers, the intermediate filaments, also forms parts of the cytoskeleton. Intermediate filaments assemble from a large family of related proteins that is distinct from the tubulins and actins forming microtubules and microfilaments.

Disorders and Diseases

Because cell structure and function underlie the totality of bodily functions, all aspects of health and disease reflect normal and abnormal cellular activities. Perhaps the most critical and important of these activities to contemporary medical science is the conversion of normal cellular activity to abnormal activity, which is responsible for cancer. Cancer occurs when cells grow and divide uncontrollably, break free from their normal cell contacts, and migrate to other regions of the body.

The cell transformations occurring in the development of cancer involve changes at several levels. Most of these changes reflect an alteration of one or more genes in the cell nucleus from normal to aberrant forms called oncogenes. Most oncogenes encode proteins involved in a relatively small number of activities. These include nonhistone proteins regulating gene activity, growth hormones, receptors in the plasma membrane for peptide hormones, and proteins taking part in internal cellular response systems triggered by receptors. Directly or indirectly, the altered proteins encoded in oncogenes induce internal changes that lead to uncontrolled cell division and loss of normal adhesions to neighboring cells.

For example, the oncogene *src* encodes a protein that adds phosphate groups to other proteins as a cellular control measure. In many types of cancer cells, the *src* gene or its product is hyperactive. One of the targets of the enzyme encoded in the gene is a receptor protein of the plasma membrane. In some cancer cells, uncontrolled addition of phosphate groups to the receptor causes it to lose its attachment to extracellular structures that hold the cells in place. This loss contributes to the tendency of tumor cells to break loose and migrate to other parts of the body.

In some cases, movement of DNA segments from one chromosome to another is involved in the transformation of cells from normal to cancerous types, including several types of leukemia. For example, in some types of leukemia, breaks occur in chromosomes 8 and 14 in cell lines producing leukocytes, and segments are exchanged between the chromosomes. The exchange moves the gene *myc* from its normal location in chromosome 8 to a region of chromosome 14 that encodes a major segment of antibody proteins. In its normal location, the *myc* gene encodes a chromosomal regulatory protein that controls genes involved in cell division. When translocated to chromosome 14, *myc* comes under the influence of DNA sequences that promote the high activity of the antibody gene. As a result, *myc* becomes hyperactive in triggering cell division and contributes to the uncontrolled division of white blood cells characteristic of leukemias.

Alterations in cytoplasmic organelles are also directly responsible for some human diseases. The enzymes contained in lysosomes are abnormally secreted in many human diseases. The degenerative changes of arthritis, for example, are suspected to be caused in part by the abnormal release of enzymes from the lysosomes of bone or lymph cells into the fluids that lubricate joints. Some of the damage to lung tissues caused by the inhalation of silica fibers in silicosis is also related to lysosomal function. Microscopic silica fibers are taken in by macrophages and other cells in the lungs; these fibers are delivered to lysosomes for breakdown, as are many other substances. The fibers accumulate in the lysosomes, causing lysosomal enlargement and eventually breakage, causing the destructive release of lysosomal enzymes into the cytoplasm. Other human diseases related to lysosomes are caused by inherited mutations that destroy the activity of lysosomal enzymes. For example, an inherited deficiency in one lysosomal enzyme, hexosaminidase, interferes with reactions clipping carbohydrate segments from molecules removed from the cell surface. As a result, the subparts of these molecules accumulate in lysosomes and cannot be recycled. Their concentration on cell surfaces is diminished; loss of these molecules from nerve cells, particularly a group called gangliosides, can lead to seizures, blindness, loss of intellect, and early death.

Human disease has also been linked to inherited changes in mitochondria. The mutations interfere with the oxidative reactions inside the organelle or have detrimental effects on the transport of substances through the mitochondrial membranes. The mutations cause the most severe problems in locations where the energy supplied by mitochondria is highly critical, particularly in the central nervous system and skeletal and cardiac muscle. Mitochondrial deficiencies in these locations are typically responsible for symptoms such as muscular weakness, irregularities in the heartbeat, and epilepsy.

Deficiencies in motile systems based on microtubules and microfilaments are also associated with human disease. For example, a group of inherited defects known as the immotile cilia or Kartagener's syndrome is characterized by acute bronchitis, sinusitis, chronic headache, male sterility, and reversal of the position of the heart from the left to the right side of the body. In individuals with the disease, the cyclic cross-bridges driving microtubule-based motion are missing. Male sterility results from loss of motility by sperm tails; other deficiencies result from the immotility of cilia on cells lining the respiratory system and the cavities of the brain. (Cilia are microtubule-based cellular appendages that beat like sperm tails to maintain the flow of fluids over cell surfaces.) In the respiratory system, loss of ciliary beating stops the flow of mucus that normally removes irritating and infectious matter from the lungs and respiratory tract. This deficiency explains the sinusitis and bronchitis. Presumably, an insufficient flow of fluids in the ventricles of the brain, normally maintained by ciliated cells lining these cavities, produces the headaches. The reversed position taken by the heart remains unexplained.

Even the cytoskeleton has been associated with human disease. For example, deficiencies in intermediate filaments of the cytoskeleton have been implicated in the hereditary disease epidermolysis bullosa. In this disease, skin cells are fragile, and slight abrasions that would cause little or no problem in normal individuals lead to severe blistering, ulceration, and scarring.

Perspective and Prospects

Knowledge of cell structure and function developed gradually from the first morphological descriptions of cells in the seventeenth century. By the 1830s, enough information had accumulated for Theodor Schwann and Matthias Schleiden to propose that all living organisms are composed of one or more cells and that cells are the minimum functional units of living organisms. Their conclusions were supplemented in 1855 by a third postulate by Rudolf Virchow: that all cells arise only from preexisting cells by a process of division. Further work established that the cell nucleus contains hereditary information and that the essential feature of cell division is transmission of this information from parent to daughter cells.

The study of cell chemistry and physiology began in the late eighteenth and early nineteenth centuries. By the end of the nineteenth century, investigators had isolated, identified, and synthesized many organic substances found in cells and worked out the structural components of proteins and nucleic acids. This chemical work was complemented by biochemical studies leading to the discovery of enzymes. The gradual integration of cell structure, physiology, and biochemistry continued; by the 1930s, the field had shifted from morphological observations to biochemical and molecular studies of cell function. Crucial to this shift was the research of George Beadle and Edward Tatum, who concluded from their studies that mutant genes encode a faulty form of an enzyme necessary to produce a substance needed for normal growth. On this basis, they proposed that each gene codes for a single enzyme-the famous "one gene-one enzyme" hypothesis.

Further biochemical work revealed the oxidative reactions providing chemical energy for cell activities. This research was integrated with structural studies of cytoplasmic organelles by Albert Claude, who developed a technique for isolating and purifying cell parts by cell fractionation and centrifugation. Claude and his associates successfully isolated ribosomes, endoplasmic reticulum, Golgi complexes, lysosomes, microbodies, and mitochondria by these methods, which allowed biochemical analysis of the fractions. This work was facilitated by development of the electron microscope, allowing elucidation of the ultrastructure of many of the organelles studied biochemically in cell fractions.

Experiments in the 1940s implicating DNA as the hereditary molecule sparked an intensive effort to work out the three-dimensional structure of this molecule, culminating in the discovery of DNA's double-helix structure in 1953 by James D. Watson and Francis Crick. Their discovery led to an effort to determine the molecular structure of genes and their modes of action, which was greatly facilitated by the development of rapid methods for nucleic acid sequencing. Using these methods, many genes have been completely sequenced; the sequences, in turn, allowed deduction of the amino acid sequences of many proteins. The comparisons of gene and protein sequences and structure in normal and mutant forms made possible by these developments provided fundamental insights into the mechanisms controlling and regulating genes and the molecular functions of proteins, revolutionizing biology and medicine.

—Stephen L. Wolfe, Ph.D.

See also Amniocentesis; Antibiotics; Bacteriology; Biopsy; Cancer; Cholesterol; Chorionic villus sampling; Cloning; Cytology; Cytopathology; DNA and RNA; Enzymes; Gene therapy; Genetic engineering; Genetics and inheritance; Glycolysis; Gram staining; Immunology; Immunopathology; Karyotyping; Laboratory tests; Microbiology; Microscopy; Mutation; Oncology; Pathology; Proteomics; Stem cell research.

For Further Information:

Alberts, Bruce, et al. *Molecular Biology of the Cell*. 5th ed. New York: Garland, 2008.

Reece, Jane B., et al. *Campbell Biology: Concepts and Connections*. 7th ed. San Francisco: Pearson/Benjamin Cummings, 2011.

Karp, Gerald. *Cell and Molecular Biology: Concepts and Experiments*. 7th ed. Hoboken: Wiley, 2013.

Kindt, Thomas J., Richard A. Goldsby, and Barbara A. Osborne. *Kuby Immunology*. 7th ed. New York: W. H. Freeman, 2013.

Lewin, Benjamin. *Genes IX*. 9th rev. ed. Sudbury, Mass.: Jones and Bartlett, 2008.

Lodish, Harvey, et al. *Molecular Cell Biology*. 7th ed. New York: W. H. Freeman, 2012.

Rasmussen, Nicolas. *Picture Control: The Microscope and the Transformation of Biology in America, 1940-1960*. Stanford, Calif.: Stanford University Press, 1997.

Stipp, David. "Quiet Little Traitors." *Scientific American* 307.2 (2012): 68-73.

Wolfe, Stephen L. *Molecular and Cellular Biology*. Belmont, Calif.: Wadsworth, 1993.

Centers for Disease Control and Prevention (CDC)

Organization

Definition: One of the divisions of the U.S. Department of Health and Human Services; the CDC is the highest level governmental health organization in the United States.

Key terms:

Department of Health and Human Services: a federal organization, headed by a member of the U.S. president's cabinet, concerned with the health of the nation's citizens

health organizations: organizations that help to shape people's ability to respond effectively to health-related issues by protecting and promoting good health

Role in the United States

The Centers for Disease Control and Prevention (CDC) is located in DeKalb County, Georgia, near Atlanta. The mission of the CDC is to promote health and improve quality of life by preventing and controlling disease, injury, and disability. The organization is charged with protecting the public health of the United States by providing leadership and direction in the prevention and control of disease and other preventable conditions and by responding to public health emergencies.

The CDC is responsible for maintaining, recording, and analyzing disease trends of all types of diseases, including communicable diseases and diseases resulting from lifestyle, occupational, and environmental causes. The CDC also publishes reports on all these diseases, including the *Morbidity and Mortality Weekly Report* (MMWR), which reports updated incidence and prevalence statistics for a number of reportable diseases. The MMWR also provides a means of disseminating and describing new regularity changes or health information pertinent to public health and safety. As a federal government health agency, the CDC supports state and local health departments and cooperates with similar national health organizations of other countries. The CDC also provides guidelines for disease prevention. The structure of the CDC is formed by centers, institutes, and officers, which carry out the diverse functions of disease prevention and control. Its various divisions are responsible for specific aspects of public health.

The mission of the National Center for Environmental Health (NCEH) is to provide national leadership through science in order to promote health and improve quality of life by preventing or controlling disease, birth defects, disabilities, or deaths that result from interactions between people and their environment, such as from exposure to toxins. NCEH especially is committed to safeguarding the health of populations that are particularly vulnerable to certain environmental hazards, including children, the elderly, and people with disabilities.

NCEH conducts research in the laboratory and in the field to investigate the effects of the environment on health. NCEH tracks and evaluates environment-related health problems through surveillance systems. NCEH also helps domestic and international agencies and organizations prepare for and respond to natural, technologic, humanitarian, and terrorism-related environmental emergencies. The scope of NCEH work also includes educating various audiences about environmental health, developing new standards and guidelines in this field, helping to formulate public policy, and providing training and technical assistance to officials of state and local health agencies in preventing and responding to public health challenges.

The National Center for Health Statistics (NCHS) is the US government's principal vital and health statistics agency. The mission of NCHS is to provide statistical information that will guide policies to improve the health of the American people. Since 1960, when the National Office of Vital Statistics and the National Health Survey merged to form NCHS, the agency has provided a wide variety of data to monitor national health. NCHS data systems include data on vital events, such as birth and death, as well as information on health status, lifestyle, exposure to unhealthy influences, the onset and diagnosis of illness and disability, and the uses of health care. These data are used by governmental policy makers, by medical researchers, and by others in the health community.

The National Vital Statistics System in NCHS includes birth data, mortality data, fetal death data, and linked births/infant deaths. Some of the important NCHS health data systems include the National Health Interview Survey, National Health Interview Survey on Disability, National Health and Nutrition Examination Survey, National Health Care Survey, Ambulatory Health Care Data, National Hospital Discharge Surgery Data, National Home and Hospice Care Survey, National Nursing Home Survey, National Employer Health Insurance Survey, National Survey of Family Growth, National Maternal and Infant Health Survey, and National Immunization Survey.

Prevention and Health Promotion

The mission of the National Center for Chronic Disease Prevention and Health Promotion is to prevent death and disability from chronic diseases; to promote maternal, infant, and adolescent health; to promote healthy personal behaviors; and to accomplish these goals in partnership with health and education agencies, major voluntary associations, the private sector, and other federal agencies.

Chronic diseases are health conditions that last longer than three months. In the United States, the leading causes of death are chronic diseases, such as heart disease, cancer, stroke, and diabetes, which often stem from an unhealthy lifestyle. Within the center, there are divisions of cancer prevention and control, diabetes, arthritis, epilepsy, genomics, smoking and health, nutrition and physical activity, reproductive health, oral health, adolescent and school health, and adult and community health.

Within this center there are several divisions: the Division of HIV/AIDS Prevention Research, the Division of Sexually Transmitted Diseases Prevention, and the Division of Tuberculosis Elimination. As the name implies, the mission of the Division of HIV/AIDS Prevention Research is to prevent HIV infection and reduce illness and death related to HIV/AIDS. In collaboration with community, state, national, and international partners, the Division of HIV/AIDS Prevention Research conducts research on behavioral intervention, program evaluation, and epidemiology of HIV/AIDS. It also provides community assistance, technical information, training, and prevention services related to HIV/AIDS.

The Division of Sexually Transmitted Diseases Prevention provides national leadership through research, policy development, and support of effective services to prevent sexually transmitted diseases (STDs) and their complications, such as infertility, adverse outcomes of pregnancy, and reproductive tract cancer. The Division of STD Prevention assists health departments, health care providers, and nongovernmental organizations through the development of goals and policies; synthesis, translation, and dissemination of timely science-based information; and the development and support of science-based programs that meet the needs of communities. The Division of STD Prevention also conducts surveillance; epidemiological, be-

havioral, and operational research; and program evaluation related to STDs, including syphilis, gonorrhea, chlamydia, human papillomavirus, genital herpes, and hepatitis B.

The Division of Tuberculosis Elimination works to provide leadership in preventing, controlling, and eventually eliminating tuberculosis (TB). The activities that are carried out in the Division of Tuberculosis Elimination include developing and advocating effective and appropriate TB prevention and control policies; supporting a nationwide framework for monitoring TB morbidity and mortality; detecting and investigating TB outbreaks; conducting clinical, epidemiological, behavioral, and operational research to enhance TB prevention and control efforts; evaluating prevention effectiveness; providing funding and technical assistance to state and local health departments; and providing training, education, and technical services to state and local health departments.

The mission of the National Center for Infectious Diseases (NCID) is to prevent illness, disability, and death caused by infectious disease in the United States and around the world. Infectious diseases are diseases that are caused by bacteria, viruses, or other microorganisms and can be transmitted from one person to another. With widespread immunization and effective antibiotics, the public health threat of infectious diseases has been lessened in industrialized countries. However, infectious diseases are the leading cause of death worldwide. Deaths from infectious disease in the United States have been increasing recently because new diseases emerge, old diseases rebound, inappropriate use of antibiotics results in drug-resistant germs, and falling rates of childhood immunization due to the unfounded fear that vaccines are linked to autism. To meet this challenge, NCID conducts surveillance, epidemic investigations, epidemiological and laboratory research, training, and public education programs. NCID also develops, evaluates, and promotes prevention and control strategies for infectious diseases.

As the lead federal agency for injury prevention, the National Center for Injury Prevention and Control (NCIPC) works closely with other federal agencies; national, state, and local organizations; state and local health departments; and research institutes to prevent and reduce injury, disability, death, and costs associated with injuries outside the workplace. Injury is the leading cause of death and disability among children and young adults. Injury is a serious public health problem because of its impact on the health of the United States, including premature death, disability, and the burden on the health care system. Common sources of unintentional injuries are falls, fires, drownings, poisonings, motor vehicle accidents, recreational activities accidents, and playground and day care accidents. Intentional injuries are related to suicide, youth violence, family and intimate partner violence, and homicide. Injury prevention strategies focus primarily on environmental design (such as road construction that permits optimum visibility), product design, human behavior and education, and legislative and regulatory requirements that support environmental and behavioral change.

Vaccination and Immunization

The National Vaccine Program Office is designated to provide leadership and coordination among federal agencies and to oversee that they work together to carry out the goals of the National Vaccine Plan. The National Vaccine Plan provides a framework, including goals, objectives, and strategies, for pursuing the prevention of infectious diseases through immunizations. This office develops and implements strategies for achieving the highest possible level of prevention of human diseases through immunization and the highest possible level of prevention of adverse reactions to vaccines.

The National Immunization Program (NIP) is a disease prevention program that provides leadership for the planning, coordination, and conduct of immunization activities nationwide. NIP provides consultation, training, and statistical, educational, epidemiological, and technical services to assist health departments in planning, developing, and implementing immunization programs. NIP assists health departments in developing vaccine information management systems to facilitate identification of children who need vaccinations, to help parents and providers to ensure that all children are immunized at the appropriate age, to assess vaccination levels in state and local areas, and to monitor the safety and efficiency of vaccines by linking vaccine administration information to adverse event reporting and disease outbreak patterns. NIP also administers research and operational programs for the prevention and control of vaccine-preventable diseases.

Other Agencies and Offices

As a federal agency, the National Institute for Occupational Safety and Health (NIOSH) is responsible for conducting research into the full scope of occupational disease and injury and making recommendations for the prevention of work-related disease, injury, and disability. The occupational diseases range from lung disease in miners to carpal tunnel syndrome in computer users. Each day in the United States, an average of nine thousand workers sustain disabling injuries on the job, seventeen workers die from an injury sustained at work, and 137 workers die from work-related diseases. The economic burden of occupational health problems is high. NIOSH is a diverse organization made up of professionals representing a wide range of disciplines including industrial hygiene, nursing, epidemiology, engineering, medicine, and statistics. NIOSH investigates potentially hazardous working conditions when requested by employers or employees and provides training to occupational safety and health professionals.

The public health of the United States depends on the health status of its minority populations. The major minority groups in the United States include African Americans, Asian and Pacific Islander Americans, Native Americans, and Hispanic Americans. Compared to the United States as a whole, minority populations, particularly African Americans, suffer higher rates of morbidity and mortality. Native Americans and Hispanic Americans also have worse health outcomes than the total population. Although Asian American and Pacific Islanders overall have reasonably good health indicators, some subgroups have very poor health status. By providing health promotion and communication strategies, policy recommendations, research, and program development, the Office of Minority Health is committed to developing cooperative and interagency agreements among various federal, state, local, and private agencies and organizations concerned with minority health.

Because of the globalization of the world economy, health problems associated with global movements of people and commerce are increasing. One country's health problems today can become another country's health problems tomorrow. Diseases are losing their boundaries, and global health efforts are necessary. The mission of the Office of Global Health is to improve health worldwide by providing leadership, coordination, and support for the CDC's global health activities in collaboration with the CDC's health partners worldwide. This office provides leadership in the development of cross-cutting policies, plans, and programs related to the CDC's global health interests; assists the CDC's divisions, other federal agencies, or nongovernmental agencies in the implementation of appropriate policies, plans, and programs for which they have responsibilities; and enhances global health partnerships by serving as the entry point for external organizations with an interest in the CDC's global health activities.

Advances in human genetics have demonstrated the potential public health impact of effectively applying genetics to disease prevention. Several CDC programs have been heavily involved with genetics for many years. The Office of Public Health Genomics works to integrate advances in human genetics into public health research, policy, and program development and evaluation and to provide a coordinated focus for the CDC's genetics efforts with particular emphasis on communication and training.

Perspective and Prospects

The CDC had its origin in the US antimalaria program of World War II and was recognized as the Communicable Disease Center in 1946, when the main health problems were infectious diseases. It became the Center for Disease Control in 1970, then the Centers for Disease Control in 1980, and the words "and Prevention" were added in 1992, though Congress requested that "CDC" remain the agency's initials. Currently, the CDC conducts research into the origin and occurrence of communicable diseases as well as noncom- municable diseases and develops methods for their control and prevention. The CDC is a powerful leader in the public health in the United States and worldwide.

—Kimberly Y. Z. Forrest, Ph.D.

See also Accidents; Acquired immunodeficiency syndrome (AIDS); Bacterial infections; Bacteriology; Childhood infectious diseases; Department of Health and Human Services; Ebola virus; Environmental diseases; Environmental health; Epidemics and pandemics; Epidemiology; Immunization and vaccination; Microbiology; National Institutes of Health (NIH); Occupational health; Preventive medicine; Safety issues for children; Safety issues for the elderly; Tuberculosis; Viral infections; World Health Organization.

For Further Information:

Brunette, Gary W., ed. *The Yellow Book: CDC Health Information for International Travel 2014*. Oxford: Oxford University Press, 2013.

"Diseases & Conditions." *Centers for Disease Control and Prevention*, February 8, 2013.

Etheridge, Elizabeth W. *Sentinel for Health: A History of the Centers for Disease Control*. Berkeley: University of California Press, 1992.

Kramer, Alexander, Mirjam Kretzschmar, and Klaus Krickeberg. *Modern Infectious Disease Epidemiology: Concepts, Methods, Mathematical Models, and Public Health*. Berlin: Springer, 2009.

McCormick, Joseph B., Susan Fisher-Hoch, and Leslie Alan Horvitz. *Level 4: Virus Hunters of the CDC*. Rev. ed. New York: Barnes & Noble, 1999.

Mintzer, Richard. *The National Institutes of Health*. Philadelphia: Chelsea House, 2002.

Potter, Polyxeni. *Art in Science: Selections from Emerging Infectious Diseases*. Oxford: Oxford University Press, 2013.

Regis, Edward. *Virus Ground Zero: Stalking the Killer Viruses with the Centers for Disease Control*. New York: Pocket Books, 1996.

Rom, Mark Carl. *Fatal Extraction: Kimberly Bergalis, the Centers for Disease Control, Health Care Workers, and HIV*. San Francisco: Jossey-Bass, 1997.

Cerebral palsy

Disease/Disorder

Also known as: Little's disease

Anatomy or system affected: Brain

Specialties and related fields: Dentistry, epidemiology, family medicine, neurology, obstetrics, orthopedics, pediatrics, physical therapy, podiatry, preventive medicine, psychology, public health, speech pathology

Definition: A motor disability evident early in life (often by one year of age and certainly by age two) that is caused by a brain abnormality present by the end of the newborn period (one month of age) and unchanged after that time.

Key terms:

athetosis: involuntary movements that are slow and writhing

chorea: rapid involuntary movements

in utero: occurring in the womb

intraventricular: within the brain spaces called the lateral ventricles

Moro reflex: an involuntary movement in which both arms go outward and upward

motor disability: difficulty in carrying out voluntary movements

posterior rhizotomy: a surgical procedure done on the lower back in which some of the sensory (posterior) nerve roots to the leg muscles are cut

premature infant: an infant born before thirty-seven weeks of pregnancy

prevalence: the number of persons with a disorder divided by the number of persons in the population

primitive reflexes: reflexes present in infants but gone by one year of age

term infant: an infant born after thirty-seven weeks of pregnancy

white matter: the brain fibers that connect neurons

Causes and Symptoms

Cerebral palsy is not a single disorder. Rather, it is a group of disorders that affect the brain at some time before a child is one month old, resulting in a lack of normal control of movements. While problems with making normal movements may be apparent at birth, this symptom is often not noticeable until the child is nine or ten months of age; on occasion, it may not be apparent before eighteen or twenty-four months of age because the areas of the brain that control movement are immature and not very effective early in life. Until the child reaches an age at which these areas are functional, a lack of function may go unrecognized. For example, problems using the legs may not be evident until the child is old enough to try to walk. Sometimes, a child is so severely affected that the motor problems-noticeable as either decreased or increased motor tone, or tension on the tendons-may be apparent in the first days or months of life.

Abnormal motor function can have both negative and positive symptoms. Negative symptoms can include the inability to do normal motor activities such as reach for a toy, pick up a raisin with the fingers, or walk. Positive symptoms can consist of abnormal movements such as the involuntary flexion of the foot when trying to walk, resulting in toe walking, or the persistence of primitive reflexes (such as the Moro reflex), which impede voluntary movements. These positive manifestations can result in unusual arm or leg postures that make some of these children easily recognizable. On the other hand, many children with cerebral palsy do not have these symptoms and are normal in appearance. Others have motor problems so mild that they are never diagnosed but are simply considered clumsy or maladroit.

By definition, any brain abnormality that causes cerebral palsy is not progressive, which means that the brain does not deteriorate. Actually, most children with cerebral palsy show improved motor coordination as they become older. A child with mild cerebral palsy at one year of age may be able to move normally by the second grade. Children correctly diagnosed with cerebral palsy early in life may no longer suffer from the disorder later in life. Therefore, the number of children with cerebral palsy decreases with age. The rate in developed countries is approximately two per one thousand school-age children. The vast majority of children with cerebral palsy reach adulthood, with most having a full life span. As a group, those who are never able to walk are more likely to die younger.

There is no single cause of cerebral palsy. Any abnormality of the brain that can develop either in utero or before the infant is one month old can cause cerebral palsy. Cerebral palsy is more common among children born prematurely; they account for approximately one-third of all children with cerebral palsy. One theory holds that these children develop a brain abnormality while in the womb which causes the child both to be born prematurely and to have cerebral palsy. Alternatively, especially among very low birth weight infants, their difficult first weeks of life may cause intraventricular hemorrhage and brain injury, most commonly of the white matter adjacent to the lateral ventricles. The pattern referred to as diplegia, in which the legs are more severely affected than the arms, is characteristic in premature infants with cerebral palsy.

Approximately 78 percent of term infants who develop cerebral palsy are healthy at birth. Only later, when they reach the appropriate developmental stage, does their condition become apparent. It is widely believed that these children have a brain abnormality that occurred while the brain was developing in the womb. The underlying cause of such abnormalities is unclear. About 22 percent of term infants with cerebral palsy are unwell at birth. These children have had various physiological insults-including stroke, infection, or lack of oxygen-either in the womb or at the time of birth. Children who suffer a lack of oxygen or hypotension (low blood pressure) during the birth process account for about 10 percent of infants who develop cerebral palsy. Sometimes, maternal hemorrhage or placental abnormalities deprive the infant of oxygen. Errors committed by the delivering doctor or midwife are an uncommon cause of cerebral palsy. Enhanced fetal monitoring during labor and delivery using electronic devices and delivery by cesarean section have not lowered the rate of cerebral palsy.

Since cerebral palsy is a motor disorder, it is classified by motor patterns. Children with cerebral palsy are generally divided into two major groups: those with increased tone (also called spasticity) and those with decreased tone. This is a somewhat artificial distinction since some children have decreased tone in infancy and increased tone later in life, while others may have decreased tone when lying down but increased tone when sitting or standing. A major advantage of this division is the recognition that persistent and severe decrease in motor tone makes walking more difficult, while increased tone makes the development of contractures (shortened tendons) more likely. In addition, children are classified by pattern of limb involvement. The common pattern in children born prematurely is diplegia, in which the legs are more severely affected than the arms. About 50 percent of children affected with diplegia are able to walk. Another common pattern is hemiplegia, in which the arm and leg on one side are affected and the other side is normal. The arm is more severely involved than the leg, and the prognosis for walking is good, with almost all these children able to walk if they do not have any other motor problem. When all four limbs are involved, the condition is called quadriplegia (or double hemiparesis or tetraplegia). These youngsters have the least likelihood of being able to walk and are most likely to have associated problems such as mental retardation. The pattern wherein the limbs produce markedly abnormal movements whenever the child attempts voluntary movements is uncommon. These abnormal movements can be sharp and sudden in nature (called chorea) or slower and more writhing (called athetosis), although often the movements are a combination of the two patterns and thus not easily classified. In the past, this motor pattern was caused by severe hyperbilirubinemia (a very high accumulation of bilirubin) shortly after birth. Today, modern therapies such as exchange transfusion and light therapy usually prevent the bilirubin level from rising to dangerous levels.

Information on Cerebral Palsy

Causes: Unknown; likely a brain abnormality that develops in utero
Symptoms: Lack of normal control of movements, unusual arm or leg postures, weak muscle tone, facial distortion, labored speech
Duration: Chronic
Treatments: None

The motor impairment can affect more than the child's limbs. Speech, chewing, drinking, and swallowing can be abnormal when the motor disability affects the face, tongue, and lips. This is most commonly seen in children with quadriplegia. It is widely noted that many of these children have weak face muscles and tend to keep their mouths open and to drool. When speech is affected, the patient often speaks slowly, has a nasal quality to the voice, and has poor enunciation. When this disability is severe, patients may find it impossible to speak any intelligible words even when their understanding of speech is not affected. Children with this type of motor problem may have difficulty with the fine lip and tongue movements necessary for chewing and may be able to eat only soft foods. Some of these children also have difficulty handling liquids such as water and may choke on clear liquids; they may prefer thickened soft foods. The motor disability can be severe enough that the swallowing movements of the esophagus and stomach are disturbed. Normally, there is a well-organized progression of such movements that propel food down the esophagus and through the stomach into the intestines. When this normal motor progression does not occur, children may regurgitate their food, since the food is inadvertently propelled up and out instead of down and into the intestines. This is referred to as reflux. When present to a minor degree, reflux can be merely a cosmetic problem, and the child may need to wear a bib much of the day. When present to a more severe degree, reflux can interfere with normal nutrition. Having food returning into the mouth in a child who has difficulty coordinating swallowing can lead to aspiration, the inadvertent passage of food down the windpipe and into the lungs, which can cause frequent bouts of pneumonia.

The brain abnormalities that cause cerebral palsy can produce other brain-related disabilities. In a survey of children with cerebral palsy in Atlanta, 75 percent had another disability, 65 percent had mental retardation, 46 percent had epilepsy, and 15 percent had sensory loss. Many of the children had more than one additional disability. Children with quadriplegia are the most likely to have other disabilities.

Treatment and Therapy

Only in unusual circumstances is there any direct treatment available for the brain abnormality that causes the motor disability of cerebral palsy. On the other hand, a variety of resources are available for helping the child cope with motor problems. Physical aids such as wheelchairs, walkers, and crutches have long been available. Modern ones are extremely adjustable and made of lightweight and durable materials. Lightweight plastic can be custom molded and fitted to supplement or replace the more traditional leg braces. Physical therapy helps interfere with involuntary and primitive reflex patterns that hinder voluntary movements. Therapy can also facilitate normal patterns of arm and leg use. Occupational therapy focuses on developing fine motor skills and improving the ability to dress, eat, write, and perform other daily activities. To be successful, all these therapies must be done every day. As a practical matter, this means performing the activities at home with parental assistance under the periodic supervision of a therapist. Orthopedic surgery, when used judiciously, can improve muscle aalance, release contractures, and correct scoliosis. The surgeon must consider carefully how the child's growth in height and weight in the years following the surgery might affect the outcome either favorably or adversely.

Abnormal tone is difficult to alter. No medicines exist that can increase tone, while several medications such as diazepam, dantrolene, and baclofen can sometimes decrease tone for children who have spasticity. Side effects such as sleepiness greatly limit the use of such medications. In addition, many children have both weakness and increased tone. The tone often helps them do activities such as standing, since the tone stiffens their legs. The loss of tone can actually make the child less able to stand. A surgical procedure called posterior rhizotomy can decrease the tone for children with diplegia who have mild gait abnormalities. These youngsters can walk with minimal assistance, usually walking up on their toes, and they have no problem with truncal balance. In this surgical procedure performed on the lower back, some of the sensory (posterior) innervating nerves to the leg muscles are severed. The procedure can produce some postoperative sensory loss, which usually disappears. Long-term adverse effects include weakness and scoliosis. It is generally believed that to be effective, the procedure should be accompanied by an aggressive program of physical therapy.

School programs have become increasingly sophisticated in assisting pupils with motor disabilities. Techniques include the use of computers for written work as well as computers with voice simulators for youngsters who cannot speak adequately to participate in the classroom. All schools in the United States are required to be physically accessible to motor-disabled students and to structure gym and recess programs so that all students can participate.

Medications are available that can help control muscle spasms and seizures. Spasticity may be treated with botulinum toxin, baclofen, diazepam, or tizanidine. Glycopyrrolate can be prescribed to help ease drooling. Pamidronate can be given to help treat related osteoporosis.

Perspective and Prospects

The Centers for Disease Control and Prevention reported in September 2012 that cerebral palsy is the most common motor disability to occur during childhood, with an estimated global incident rate of 1.5 to more than four cases per thousand live births or children in a defined age group. The brightest hope lies in research to understand better the abnormalities of fetal development that lead to cerebral palsy, in the expectation of finding preventive measures. In addition, since premature infants are disproportionately represented among those with cerebral palsy, the prevention of prematurity and improvements in the management of children born prematurely also provide hope for decreasing the occurrence of the disorder. Newer medicines such as gabapentin that hold the potential for decreasing the adverse effects of increased tone with fewer side effects are also appearing. Finally, the potential of computers and computer-assisted physical devices to help motor-impaired persons is being actively explored.

—*Robert J. Baumann, M.D.*

See also Birth defects; Motor skill development; Muscle sprains, spasms, and disorders; Muscles; Nervous system; Neurology; Neurology, pediatric; Palsy; Reflexes, primitive; Seizures.

For Further Information:

Centers for Disease Control and Prevention. "Facts about Cerebral Palsy." *CDC*, May 18, 2012.

Centers for Disease Control and Prevent. "Data & Statistics for Cerebral Palsy." *CDC*, Sept. 7, 2012.

Geralis, Elaine, ed. *Children with Cerebral Palsy: A Parent's Guide.* 2d ed. Bethesda, Md.: Woodbine House, 1998.

Grether, Judith K., and Karin B. Nelson. "Maternal Infection and Cerebral Palsy in Infants of Normal Birth Weight." *Journal of the American Medical Association* 278, no. 3 (July 16, 1997): 207-11.

Hutton, J. L., T. Cooke, and P. O. Pharoah. "Life Expectancy in Children with Cerebral Palsy." *British Medical Journal* 309, no. 6952 (August 13, 1994): 431-35.

Kramer, Laura Shapiro. *Uncommon Voyage: Parenting a Special Needs Child.* 2d ed. Berkeley, Calif.: North Atlantic, 2001.

MedlinePlus. "Cerbral Palsy." *MedlinePlus*, Mar. 25, 2013.

Pimm, Paul. *Living with Cerebral Palsy.* Austin, Tex.: Raintree, 1999.

Stanton, Marion. *The Cerebral Palsy Handbook.* London: Vermilion, 2002.

Swaiman, Kenneth F., Stephen Ashwal, and Donna M. Ferriero, eds. *Pediatric Neurology: Principles and Practice.* 4th ed. Philadelphia: Mosby, 2006.

United Cerebral Palsy. *UCP*, 2013.

Wood, Debra. "Cerebral Palsy." *Health Library*, Feb. 1, 2013.

Cervical, ovarian, and uterine cancers

Disease/Disorder

Anatomy or system affected: Genitals, lymphatic system, reproductive system, uterus

Specialties and related fields: Gynecology, immunology, obstetrics, oncology

Definition: Primary cancers of the female reproductive system.

Key terms:

benign: refers to a non-malignant tumor made up of a mass of cells that do not metastasize (leave the site where they develop)

cancer: diseases in which abnormal cells divide uncontrollably and may enter nearby tissues or migrate to other parts of the body; malignant growth or tumor

cervix: the narrowest part of the uterus, which opens into

the vagina

endometrium: the inner lining of the uterus, which normally thickens before being sloughed off during each menstrual cycle; estrogens cause its growth and development, and progesterone prepares it for possible pregnancy

fallopian tubes: slender tubes of tissue that connects the ovary to the uterus and allows eggs to pass from an ovary to the uterus; normally there is one ovary and one fallopian tube on each side connected to the uterus

malignant: refers to a tumor which can lose cells that can travel via blood or lymph fluid to other sites

metastasis: the process by which malignant tumors invade other tissues either locally or distally

ovary: the female gonad located in the pelvic cavity, where egg production occurs; the principal organ that produces the hormones estrogen and progesterone

tumor: a mass of cells characterized by uncontrolled growth; can be either benign or malignant

uterus: the female organ in which the embryo develops; it is in the pelvic cavity and is connected to the ovaries by the fallopian tubes

Causes and Symptoms

Although people commonly talk about cancer as a single disease, it is a category that includes more than one hundred different diseases that do appear to have a commonality. All cancer cells divide without obeying the normal control mechanisms. These abnormal cells have altered deoxyribonucleic acid (DNA) that causes them to divide and form other abnormal cells, which again divide and eventually form a neoplasm, or tumor. Cancers may arise in the tissues or blood-forming organs.

If the neoplasm has the potential to leave its original site and invade other tissues, it is called malignant. If the tumor stays in one place, it is benign. One major difference between these tumors is that malignant cells seem to have lost the cellular glue that holds them to one another, allowing them to metastasize, leaving the tumor and infiltrating nearby tissues. Metastatic cells can also travel to distant sites via the blood or lymph systems.

Medical scientists do not know exactly what causes a cell to become cancerous. It is likely that several different factors in varying combinations cause cancer. Genetic, viral, hormonal, immunological, toxic, environmental and physical factors may all play a role. Whatever the cause, cancer is a common disease and causes one out of four deaths in the United States. Tumors of the reproductive tract occur in relatively high rates in women. Cervical cancer accounts for 6 percent, ovarian cancer 3 percent, and cancer of the lining of the uterus (endometrial cancer) 7 percent of all cancers in women.

Cervical cancer was once one of the most common cancers in women but now ranks 14th. The situation has been improved primarily by increased screening and, more recently, vaccines. Cervical cancer is most frequently found in women over the age of 30. The Human Papilloma Virus (HPV), a sexually transmitted virus, is the most common cause of cervical cancer. Several factors may be involved in

Information on Cervical, Ovarian, and Uterine Cancers

Causes: Genetic, viral, hormonal, immunological, toxic, and/or physical factors
Symptoms: Abdominal pain and swelling, gastrointestinal disorders (changes in bowel habits), bloating, abnormal vaginal bleeding
Duration: Chronic, possibly recurrent
Treatments: Surgical removal of affected organ, hormonal therapy, chemotherapy, radiation

the development of this cancer: young age at first intercourse; number of sexual partners (as well as the number of the partner's partners); infection with sexually transmitted diseases such as herpes simplex type 2 and human papillomavirus; the presence of HIV; long-term use of birth control; having three or more children; and cigarette smoking

Since most patients do not experience noticeable symptoms, regular checkups are necessary. The Pap (Papanicolaou) test performed in a physician's office will detect the presence of cervical cancer. It is generally recommended that Pap Tests begin when a woman is 21, but the decision should be made between the patient and her doctor. In this procedure, the physician obtains a sample of the cervix by swabbing the area and placing the cells on a microscope slide for examination.

Ovarian cancer accounts for more deaths than any other cancer of the female reproductive system. It is the 8th most common cancer in women, and the 5th most common cause of death from cancer. While the cause of ovarian cancer is unknown, there are several factors that increase a woman's

Tubal carcinoma
Endometrial carcinoma
Cervical carcinoma
Vaginal carcinoma
Vulval carcinoma

Common sites of cancer in the female reproductive system.

risk of developing the disease. According to the Centers for Disease Control, having close relatives on either the mother's or father's side with ovarian cancer; being older; prior patient history of colorectal, breast or uterine cancer; an Ashkenazi or Eastern European Jewish background; never having children; trouble getting pregnant; or having endometriosis, a condition in which the tissue escapes the uterus and grows elsewhere in the body, all increase risk. Researchers recently discovered that the genes *BRCA1* and *BRCA2*, usually associated with hereditary forms of breast cancer, are also connected to an increased rate of ovarian cancer. About 5 to 10 percent of ovarian cancers appear to have a strong hereditary association, particularly in patients who develop the cancer at a young age. Its incidence is slightly decreased in women who use oral contraceptives for many years. Ninety percent of ovarian tumors occur after the age of 40 with the majority after the age of 60.

There are two major types of ovarian cancer: epithelial and germ cell neoplasms. About 90 percent of ovarian cancers are epithelial and develop on the surface of the ovary. These tumors are often bulky and involve both ovaries. Germ cell tumors are derived from the eggs within the ovary and, if malignant, tend to be highly aggressive. Malignant germ cell neoplasms tend to occur in women under the age of thirty.

Ovarian cancer is generally considered a silent disease, as the signs and symptoms are vague and often ignored. Abdominal pain or pressure in the pelvic region is the most obvious symptom, followed by abdominal swelling. Bloating, a sensation of feeling full after eating small amounts, and back pain may also occur. Some patients also report changes in bowel habits involving more frequent urination or constipation. Abnormal vaginal bleeding, including after menopause, or vaginal discharge may occur, but like other symptoms this is not unique to this disease. Diagnosis is made using imaging techniques such as ultrasound, computed tomography (CT) scanning, and magnetic resonance imaging (MRI). The presence and identification of the BRCA1 and BRCA2 genes also allows a woman to aggressively monitor her health, even though her predisposition for ovarian cancer cannot be changed.

Uterine cancer refers to cancers that develop in the uterus. Endometrial cancer is the most common type of uterine cancer and forms in the lining or endometrium of the uterus. It is the 4th most common cancer in women and the most commonly diagnosed gynecologic cancer. It most frequently affects women after the age of 50. Symptoms are very similar to ovarian cancer and careful diagnosis is indicated using endometrial biopsy and transvaginal ultrasound. Like most cancers, the cause of endometrial cancer is not clear but risk factors may include age, obesity, estrogen replacement therapy without progesterone during menopause, the use of Tamoxifen for breast cancer, and family history

Treatment and Therapy

Specialists have achieved a measure of success in prevention of cervical cancer with the use of HPV vaccines that will prevent the disease in many individuals. Gardasil®, Gardasil 9®, and Cervarix® have been approved by the government to treat HPV infection, the cause of about 70% of cervical cancers in women. Gardisil and Gardisil 9 are approved for females 9-26. Cervarix is approved for females 9-25. Gardisil is approved for males 9-26 and Gardisil 9 is approved for males 9-15 for prevention of anal cancer caused by HPV, anal lesions, and genital warts. None of the vaccines protect against all HPV infections so even vaccinated females need to continue cervical cancer screening. The remaining 30% of women whose cervical cancer is not caused by HPV will need routine screening and treatment.

A variety of treatments are available for patients with cancers of the reproductive tract: surgical removal of the organ, hormonal therapy, chemotherapy, or radiation therapy. The treatment of cervical cancer depends on the size and location of the tumor, how early the disease is diagnosed and whether the cells are benign or malignant. If the patient is no longer capable of or interested in childbearing, then she may choose to have her uterus, including the cervix, removed in a procedure known as a hysterectomy. The

---

In the News:
Cervical Cancer Vaccines; Chemotherapy Pumped into Abdomen for Ovarian Cancer

In June, 2006, the Food and Drug Administration (FDA) approved the first vaccine for cervical cancer and made it available for females between the ages of nine and twenty-six. Manufactured by Merck and known as Gardasil, the vaccine protects against the two main strains of human papillomavirus (HPV) that cause nearly 70 percent of all cervical cancer cases. In October, 2009, the FDA approved a second vaccine for cervical cancer, Cervarix, manufactured by GlaxoSmithKline. Like Gardasil, Cervarix protects against the two main strains of HPV. Although the two vaccines do not protect against existing HPV infections or against other HPV types that can produce cervical cancer, they will protect an individual against future infections of the two main viruses that cause cervical cancer. No serious side effects were reported from the vaccines, which are administered as a series of three shots in six months. Eventually, Pap samplings may not be needed.

Medical research results published in early 2006 report that pumping chemotherapy drugs into a patient's abdomen, known as intraperitoneal therapy, can extend the lives of ovarian cancer victims by an additional year or more. The downside is serious side effects that include stomach pain, numbness to the extremities, and possible infection, resulting in a lower quality of life for these patients compared to those taking only an intravenous (IV) regimen. One year after termination of treatment, patients who received IV or intraperitoneal therapy experienced the same quality of life. In January, 2006, the National Cancer Institute recommended an individualized combination of IV and intraperitoneal therapy for ovarian cancer patients.

—*Alvin K. Benson, Ph.D.*

physician may also use a laser, cryotherapy (use of a cold instrument), or electrocautery (use of a hot instrument) to destroy the tumor without removing the uterus. Malignant tumors may require a total hysterectomy and removal of associated lymph nodes, which can contain metastatic cells. This surgery may be followed by radiation and/or chemotherapy if there is a possibility that all cancer cells have not been removed.

Cervical cancer diagnosed in a pregnant patient can complicate the treatment, but fortunately, only about 1 percent of cervical cancers are found in pregnant women. If the cancer is restricted to the cervix (that is, it has not metastasized), treatment is usually delayed until after childbirth. It is interesting to note that a normal vaginal delivery may occur without harming the mother or the infant. Malignant cervical cancer must be treated in a similar way as in non-pregnant women. If the cancer is found in the first trimester, a hysterectomy or radiation therapy or both is used to help eradicate the malignancy. Obviously, these approaches terminate the pregnancy. During the second trimester, the uterus must be emptied of the fetus and placenta, followed by radiation therapy or removal of the affected reproductive organs. In the third trimester, the physician will typically try to delay treatment until he or she believes that the fetus has developed sufficiently to stay alive when delivered by cesarean section. A vaginal delivery is not recommended, as it has been shown to lower the cure rate of malignant cervical cancer. Treatment after delivery consists of surgery, radiation therapy, and chemotherapy. The prognosis in patients who have elected surgical removal of the tumor is a five-year survival rate of up to 90 percent. Cure rates for patients undergoing radiation therapy are between 75 and 90 percent. Chemotherapeutic agents have not had as much effect, as they significantly reduce only 25 percent of tumors. It is important to note that the best outcomes are achieved with early diagnosis.

Ovarian cancers are treated with a similar approach. Surgery may involve the removal of the ovaries, fallopian tubes, and uterus, as well as associated lymph nodes depending upon the extent of malignancy. Radiation and chemotherapy are usually employed but may be less effective. The most commonly used chemotherapies are platinum based regimens such as carboplatin (Paraplatin®) or cisplatin with a taxane such as paclitaxel (Taxol®) or docetaxel (Taxotere®). Chemotherapy may be administered intravenously (into a vein, IV) or directly into the abdominal cavity using a small tube. Avastin, a newer drug, is showing promise in treating ovarian cancer and works by cutting off blood vessel growth to the tumor, which cuts off the tumor's nutrients.

In the News: Ovarian Cancer Test OvaSure

OvaSure is a blood test to detect ovarian cancer. A screening test developed at Yale University, the test provides a probability of ovarian cancer being present by measuring the levels of six proteins and putting those into a predictive algorithm.

A validation study of the test's performance was published in the journal *Clinical Cancer Research* in February, 2008, and the test became clinically available through LabCorp in June, 2008. While the test did not have Food and Drug Administration (FDA) approval, LabCorp claimed that the test was developed and marketed by a single company, and thereby met an FDA exemption.

The main concern of the FDA, shared by the Society of Gynecologic Oncologists, was that the test was being implemented before having adequate clinical validation. Specifically, it was questioned if the research participants included in the initial publication were comparable to the broader population of women.

Controversy ensued as to the use of OvaSure, as well as to the appropriate regulatory agency to provide oversight. However, the product was discontinued in October, 2008. As of 2010, no similar test was available. Further, the FDA continues to send warning letters to laboratories and companies offering the test, requiring them to stop.

While ovarian cancer is not a common cancer, a screening test to find it at early stages is greatly needed. The vast majority of ovarian cancers are diagnosed at later stages, when treatment options are more limited and five-year survival might be only 30 percent. With any screening test, however, positive results might lead women to have surgical removal of their ovaries. False positive screening results might thereby result in women having normal ovaries unnecessarily removed, leading to the consequences of menopause. Thus, the accuracy of any screening test for detecting ovarian cancer is paramount.

OvaSure is not an available test, but a test like it is greatly needed. While the sometimes difficult balance continues between making new tests clinically available with protecting the public health, additional studies are needed to determine if this particular test becomes available in the future.

—*Judy Mouchawar, M.D., M.S.P.H.*

Ovarian cancer typically has a more negative outcome than cervical or endometrial cancers, since the disease is usually in an advanced stage by the time it is diagnosed. The overall survival rate without evidence of recurrence in patients with ovarian cancers depends on how early the disease is found and is referred to as Stage at Diagnosis on a scale of I to IV

The overall survival rate is 45 percent but if caught early (Stage I or Stage II out of the four stages) it may be as high as 95 percent. The more uncommon germ cell ovarian cancers have a much more variable prognosis. With early diagnosis, aggressive surgery, and the use of newer chemotherapeutic agents, the long-term survival rate for all ovarian cancer patients is expected to increase as newer drugs and interventions are employed.

Surgery is often the treatment of choice for uterine/endometrial cancer, which usually occurs in women 55 and older. As with cervical cancer, treatment depends upon the extent of the disease and the patient's wishes relative to reproductive capabilities and family planning. A hysterectomy, or removal of the fallopian tubes, ovaries, and surrounding lymph nodes, is usually indicated. Chemotherapy and radiation therapy are occasionally utilized as adjunctive therapy, as is progesterone. Chemotherapies may include paclitaxel (Taxol®), carboplatin, doxorubicin (Adriamycin®), liposomal doxorubicin (Doxil®) or cisplatin in varying combinations. Progesterone (medroxyprogesterone or hydroxyprogesterone) may benefit patients with advanced disease, as it seems to cause a decrease in tumor size and regression of metastases. Progesterone therapy in patients with advanced or recurrent endometrial cancer leads to regression in about 40 percent of cases. Progesterone therapy also has produced regression in tumors that have metastasized to the lungs, vagina, and chest cavity.

The outcome of endometrial cancer is influenced by the aggressiveness of the tumor, the age of the woman (older women tend to have a poorer prognosis), and the stage at which the cancer was detected. Almost two-thirds of all patients live without evidence of disease for five or more years after treatment. Unfortunately, 28 percent die within five years. For cancer identified and treated early, almost 90 percent of patients are alive five years after treatment.

Perspective and Prospects

Even though medical science has advanced the ability to detect and treat cancers in much earlier stages, many lives are still lost to cancer each year. According to the American Cancer Society 2017, projections estimate diagnosis of cervical cancer in 12,820 women with 4,210 dying from the disease. 22,400 are expected to be diagnosed with ovarian cancer with 14,080 dying from the disease. There are 61,380 expected cases of uterine cancers with 10,920 deaths in 2017. According to the World Health Organization, cervical cancer was the second most common cancer in women in developing countries in 2012, accounting for 270,000 deaths. Therefore, as with most diseases, prevention may be a significant way to reduce a patient's chances of getting cancer or to reduce the effects of cancer itself.

The National Institute of Health and the American Cancer Society have made several suggestions for reducing the risk of cancer. The dietary guidelines include reducing fat intake to less than 30 percent of total calories, eating more high-fiber foods, such as whole-grain breads and cereals, and eating more fruits and vegetables, especially those high in vitamins A, C, and E. Scheduling regular checkups with a health care provider may increase the likelihood of detecting cervical, ovarian, and uterine cancers early, even if no symptoms are present. Pelvic examinations should be performed every three years for women under the age of forty and yearly thereafter. Pap testing for cervical cancer should be undertaken yearly from the time that a woman becomes sexually active. Some physicians will take an endometrial tissue biopsy from women at high risk and at the time of the menopause.

Some data suggest that modifying lifestyle may help reduce the incidence of cervical cancer. The cervix is exposed to a variety of factors during intercourse, including infections and physical trauma. Having multiple sexual partners increases the risk of sexually transmitted diseases which may predispose the cervix to cancer. This factor is compounded by the fact that infectious agents and other carcinogens can be transmitted from one individual to another. Therefore, the cervix can theoretically be exposed to carcinogens from a partner's sexual partners. Regular intercourse begun in the early teens also predisposes one to cervical cancer, as the tissue of the cervix may be more vulnerable at puberty. Barrier methods of contraception, especially condoms, reduce the risk of developing cervical cancer by reducing the exposure of the cervix to potential carcinogens. Smoking increases the risk of cervical cancer, perhaps because carcinogens in tobacco enter the blood, which in turn has access to the cervix. Thus, practicing lifestyle changes such as safer sexual practices, quitting smoking, and dietary changes would be beneficial to someone wanting to reduce the chance of having cervical cancer.

Women who are twenty or more pounds over ideal body weight are twice as likely to develop endometrial cancer, and the risk increases with increased body fat. Some estrogens are produced in fat tissue, and this additional estrogen may play a role in the development of endometrial cancer. Therefore, reduction of excess body fat through diet and exercise may be important for a woman who wishes to reduce her chances of developing uterine cancer.

In May 2013, investigators from the Cancer Genome Atlas Research Network reported the results of their comprehensive genomic analysis of close to four hundred endometrial tumors. Their findings, published in the journal *Nature*, suggest that molecular characteristics can help determine and differentiate types of endometrial cancer and possibly yield insights into effective treatment strategies. The investigators also found four new tumor subtypes and identified similarities between endometrial cancer and other types of cancers. Also in 2013, Dr. Devansu Tewari of Southern California Permanente Medical Group presented the results of a long-term study he authored on the effectiveness of using intraperitoneal chemotherapy to treat ovarian cancer. The study demonstrated that intraperitoneal chemotherapy, in which the patient's stomach area is bathed in chemotherapeutic agents, significantly increased survival rates for patients with advanced ovarian cancer. Patients who received intraperitoneal treatment were 17 percent more likely to survive longer than patients who received conventional intravenous therapy.

—*Matthew Berria, PhD;*
updated by Patricia Stanfill Edens, PhD, RN, LFACHE

See also: Biopsy; Cancer; Cervical procedures; Chemotherapy; Cryosurgery; Endometrial biopsy; Genital disorders, female; Gynecology; Human papillomavirus (HPV); Hysterectomy; Malignancy and metastasis; National Cancer Institute (NCI); Ovaries; Pap test; Radiation therapy; Reproductive system; Screening; Uterus; Women's health.

For Further Information:
American Cancer Society (ACS). *ACS*, 2013.
Badash, Michelle. "Uterine Cancer." *Health Library*, Mar. 14, 2013.
Cancer Facts and Figures 2017. *American CancerSociety*. Downloaded on August 24, 2017 from https://www.cancer.org/content/dam/cancer-org/research/cancer-facts-and-statistics/annual-cancer-facts-and-figures/2017/cancer-facts-and-figures-2017.pdf
Centers for Disease Control and Prevention. "Gynecological Cancers: Cervical Cancer." *CDC*, August 24, 2017.

Centers for Disease Control and Prevention. "Gynecological Cancers: Ovarian Cancer." *CDC*, August 24, 2017.

Centers for Disease Control and Prevention. "Gynecological Cancers: Uterine Cancer." *CDC*, August 24, 2017.

Links to Gynecologic Cancer Information . *Gynecologic OncologyGroup*. 2017 Information available at http://www.gog.org/gyneco logiccancerinformation.html.

HealthNews."HealthDay: Abdominal 'Chemo Bath' May Extend Survival in Ovarian Cancer Patients." *MedlinePlus*, Mar. 11, 2013.

Kerr, Shelly K., and Robin M. Mathy. *Preventive Health Measures for Lesbianand BisexualWomen*. New York: Haworth, 2006.

LaRusso, Laurie. "Cervical Cancer." *Health Library*, Feb. 1, 2013.

LaRusso, Laurie. "Ovarian Cancer." *Health Library*, Sept. 27, 2012.

McGinn, Kerry Anne, and Pamela J. Haylock. *Women's Cancers: How to Prevent Them, How to Treat Them, How to Beat Them*. Alameda, Calif.: Hunter, 2003.

MedlinePlus. "Cervical Cancer." *MedlinePlus*, May 1, 2013.

National Cancer Center Dictionaries, Downloaded August 24, 2017 from https://www.cancer.gov/publications/dictionaries.

National Cervical Cancer Coalition. *NCCC*, 2017 Information available at http://www.nccc-online.org/.

National Institutes of Health. "Study Establishes Basis for Genomic Classification of Endometrial Cancers." *NIH*, May 1, 2013.

World Health Organization. "Media Centre: Cancer." *WHO*, Downloaded August 24, 2017 from www.who.org.

Cervical procedures

Procedure

Anatomy or system affected: Genitals, reproductive system, uterus

Specialties and related fields: Gynecology

Definition: Such procedures as biopsy, conization, cryosurgery, and electrocauterization, which are performed to analyze cervical tissue for abnormal cell development and/or to remove abnormal or cancerous tissue from the cervix.

Indications and Procedures

Surgical procedures performed on the cervix (the opening of the uterus into the vagina) such as biopsy, conization, cryosurgery, and electrocauterization are used to diagnose and treat cervical abnormalities. The first indication of a potential problem is usually a routine gynecological examination that reveals inflammation of the cervix or an abnormal Pap test. In Pap testing, a cell sample is scraped from the surface of the cervix and analyzed microscopically. Abnormal results range from slightly abnormal cell growth (dysplasia) to invasive cancer. If the Pap testing results indicate a condition more serious than dysplasia, further tests are conducted.

The first step in the diagnosis of a cervical abnormality is colposcopy and cervical biopsy. The colposcope is a lighted magnifying instrument similar to a pair of binoculars. When placed at the vaginal opening, it permits detailed viewing of the cervix. The cervix is treated with vinegar to produce an aceto-whitening reaction, abnormal areas are visualized, and small tissue samples of cervical cell layers are punched out for further analysis. Cervical biopsy is performed in an outpatient setting by physicians and, in some cases, by nurse practitioners and certified nurse midwives, and anesthesia is not required, though a local anesthetic may be applied.

In cases of severe dysplasia or cancer localized to the cervix, a cone biopsy may be performed. Conization is conducted in an outpatient setting with local anesthesia or in a hospital under general anesthesia. A circular incision is made around the cervical opening with a knife or laser and is extended up at an angle to obtain a cone of tissue, including some from the cervical canal. The edges of the incision are sutured or cauterized. Examination of the cone can determine the severity and extent of cancer. In some cases, excision of the cone may have eliminated all the cancerous cells from the cervix.

Cryosurgery, also known as "cryotherapy," freezes and destroys abnormal tissue with liquid nitrogen. This procedure can be done in an outpatient setting and takes only a few minutes to perform. It can be used successfully to treat dysplasia, localized cancer cells, and reddened areas that sometime develop around the cervical opening, called "cervical erosions."

Dysplasia, cancer, and cervical erosions are also treated with electrocauterization, in which an electrically heated instrument is used to destroy abnormal cells. This procedure is performed in a doctor's office, without anesthesia, just after a woman's menstrual period. A speculum is used to open the vagina, and the tip of the electrocautery device is applied to the abnormal tissue. A scab forms and allows new healthy tissue to grow. Healing is complete in seven to eight weeks.

Pregnant women who have a history of miscarriage during the second trimester of pregnancy due to cervical incompetence may undergo a cervical cerclage, a procedure used to temporarily stitch the cervix closed. A cervical cerclage will help keep the cervix closed as the baby grows. The stitches are generally removed at the thirty-seventh week of pregnancy, allowing for a normal delivery. The procedure successfully prevents miscarriage or premature delivery due to cervical incompetence in 85 to 90 percent of cases.

Uses and Complications

Mild dysplasias typically revert to a normal state spontaneously and are merely monitored for possible slow progression to a more serious state. When Pap testing, punch biopsies, or both indicate more serious development of abnormal cells, cryotherapy or electrocauterization is used to destroy the suspicious tissue. While colposcopy is nearly painless, a punch biopsy may cause some cramping. Side effects of electrocauterization include cervical swelling, discharge for up to three weeks, and, rarely, infection or infertility caused by the removal of too many cervical mucous glands. Scarring may occur, making future Pap tests difficult to interpret. Cryotherapy causes much less damage to the cervical opening than electrocauterization does, but it may produce a temporary watery discharge and changes in cervical mucus.

If repeated colposcopies or Pap tests confirm severe dysplasia or localized cancer, and if the abnormal tissue extends into the cervical canal, a cone biopsy is performed. If analysis of the cone reveals that the abnormal tissue extends beyond the borders of the biopsied tissue, a second, larger conization may be performed. This conization is major surgery performed under general anesthesia, and bleeding and infection are common complications. Removal of too many cervical mucous glands may lead to infertility. Removal of cervical muscle may lead to an incompetent cervix, an inability of the cervix to maintain a pregnancy to term. There are surgical interventions, however, that can eliminate this problem.

If tests indicate that the cancer has become invasive and has spread beyond the borders of the cervix, a hysterectomy and possible removal of the lymph nodes is performed. This serious surgery renders the woman infertile and carries the same risks as any major surgery.

Perspective and Prospects

In the 1940s, George Papanicolaou discovered that premalignant as well as malignant changes caused the cervix to shed cells that could be analyzed microscopically. Simultaneously, the colposcope was developed. Together, the Pap test and colposcopies caused a revolution in the early detection and prevention of cervical cancer.

Cervical cancer has become a more preventable and easily monitored disorder as a result of advances in the classification of abnormalities from mild to severe and the discovery that human papilloma viruses (HPV), genital herpes virus, multiple sexual partners or mates with a history of multiple partners, smoking, and environmental toxins can all contribute to the development of cervical malignancies. The HPV vaccine is now recommended for female patients aged nine to twenty-six, as well as boys and young men, in order to reduce the transmission of HPV infection and incidence of cervical cancer, among other genital malignancies. Public education may also lead to a decrease in the incidence of this disease.

New surgical techniques have improved the efficiency of abnormal tissue destruction, with fewer side effects. The loop electrosurgical excision procedure (LEEP) uses a low-voltage electrical current that runs through a thin wire loop to scoop out abnormal tissue from the cervix in a matter of seconds. Carbon dioxide laser treatment uses a laser beam to destroy cells in a small area, without damaging healthy tissue. Little bleeding occurs, and healing is rapid. Future advances in deoxyribonucleic acid (DNA) analysis may help to identify those who may be at risk for developing cervical cancer so that they may take preventive action and be closely monitored for early, successful treatment.

—*Karen E. Kalumuck, Ph.D.*

See also Biopsy; Cervical, ovarian, and uterine cancers; Cryosurgery; Electrocauterization; Genital disorders, female; Gynecology; Hysterectomy; Infertility, female; Oncology; Pap test; Uterus; Women's health.

For Further Information:

A.D.A.M. Medical Encyclopedia. "Cold Knife Cone Biopsy." *MedlinePlus*, February 26, 2012.

A.D.A.M. Medical Encyclopedia. "Colposcopy-Directed Biopsy." *MedlinePlus*, February 26, 2012.

Boston Women's Health Collective. *Our Bodies, Ourselves: A New Edition for a New Era*. 35th anniversary ed. New York: Simon & Schuster, 2005.

Carlson, Karen J., Stephanie A. Eisenstat, and Terra Ziporyn. *The New Harvard Guide to Women's Health*. Cambridge, Mass.: Harvard University Press, 2004.

"Human Papillomavirus (HPV) Vaccines." *National Cancer Institute, National Institutes of Health*, December 29, 2011.

"Cervical Cryotherapy." *American Society for Colposcopy and Cervical Pathology*, April, 2010.

"Loop Electrosurgical Excision Procedure." *American College of Obstetricians and Gynecologists*, February, 2013.

McGinn, Kerry Anne, and Pamela J. Haylock. *Women's Cancers: How to Prevent Them, How to Treat Them, How to Beat Them*. Alameda, Calif.: Hunter House, 2003.

Rushing, Lynda, and Nancy Joste. *Abnormal Pap Smears: What Every Woman Needs to Know*. Rev. ed. Amherst, N.Y.: Prometheus Books, 2008.

Stewart, Susan Cobb, and the American Medical Women's Association. *The Women's Complete Healthbook*. New York: Dell Books, 1996.

Cesarean section

Procedure

Anatomy or system affected: Abdomen, reproductive system, uterus

Specialties and related fields: Anesthesiology, emergency medicine, general surgery, gynecology, neonatology, obstetrics, perinatology

Definition: The surgical procedure used to remove a fetus by incisions into the mother's abdominal and uterine walls.

Key terms:

amniotic fluid: the liquid that surrounds the fetus to protect it from injury and to help maintain a stable temperature

breech: a commonly encountered abnormal fetal presentation in which any part other than the head presents first

cervix: the lower part of the uterus, which is continuous with the vaginal canal; it must enlarge significantly prior to vaginal delivery

incision: a cut made with a scalpel during a surgical procedure

labor: the physiological process by which the fetus and placenta are expelled from the uterus; labor involves strong uterine contractions

placenta: the spongy organ containing blood vessels that provides the fetus with nutrients and oxygen from the mother via the umbilicus

umbilicus: the cord that contains the blood vessels connecting the fetus to the placenta

Indications and Procedures

Cesarean section was initially intended to be performed when it is impossible or dangerous to deliver a baby vaginally. For example, the operation is necessary if the fetus is unable to fit through the mother's pelvis or if it shows signs of fetal distress. Fetal distress is detected by abnormal changes in the fetal heart rate, which may indicate that the fetus is not receiving adequate oxygen from the placenta. Other reasons for the procedure include a placenta that is lying over the cervix, which blocks the opening to the birth canal (placenta previa); scarring of the uterus from other

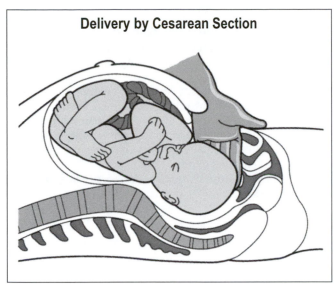

Delivery by Cesarean Section

Several conditions may necessitate the delivery of a baby through an incision in the lower abdomen instead of through the birth canal, including fetal distress or the inability of the baby's head to fit through the mother's pelvis.

surgical procedures (or previous cesarean section), which reduces the ability of the uterus to contract; unsuccessful induction of labor with oxytocin (Pitocin); breech presentation, in which any part other than the head presents first; and postmaturity, in which gestation and fetal development indicate that labor should have begun yet is delayed.

These medically necessary indications for a cesarean section have been largely overshadowed by a tremendous increase in cesareans because of patient choice and/or by an overuse of the practice by physicians for a variety of reasons, including over-medicalization of birth, support of often misinformed patient choice, or convenience. In 2010, more than 32 percent of live births were delivered by cesarean. One major reason for this increase is that after a woman has a cesarean, vaginal delivery in subsequent births becomes less likely.

A cesarean section allows the delivery of a baby through a horizontal or vertical incision through the mother's abdominal and uterine walls. Prior to surgery, an anesthesiologist gives the mother an epidural or spinal anesthetic so that she can remain conscious but free of pain during the procedure. Occasionally, under certain emergency conditions such as severe fetal distress, a general anesthetic is given. The use of epidural anesthesia, however, is preferred in the majority of deliveries. The anesthesiologist administers epidural anesthesia by injecting a locally acting anesthetic into the space that surrounds the spinal cord. This space is known as the epidural space, and when it is filled with anesthetic agents, the nerves to the abdominal and pelvic cavities are blocked.

A catheter is inserted into the urinary bladder to empty it prior to making an incision into the abdomen. Typically, a horizontal incision is made just above the pubic bone, as this type of cut heals more readily and is more cosmetically acceptable. Once the pregnant uterus is exposed, a second transverse incision is made in the lower region of the

uterus. The amniotic fluid is drained off by suction, and the baby is delivered. Once the infant's head is exposed, its mouth and nose are cleared of any fluid that may hinder respiration. After completely removing the baby from the uterine cavity, the physician clamps the umbilical cord, cuts and ties it, and hands the baby to the parents or a member of the surgical team. Vertical incisions are more likely to be made in emergency situations, since they allow for quicker delivery; however, they result in poorer healing of the uterine muscle. After the placenta is delivered, the physician sutures the uterine and abdominal walls and provides postoperative care to the patient. A drug known as ergonovine can be used after delivery of the infant to stimulate uterine contractions and to aid in preventing postpartum bleeding. A patient in pain or discomfort may be given analgesics such as meperidine or morphine as needed. The medical staff closely monitors the patient's vital signs, such as her heart rate, blood pressure, and urine flow, as well as the status of the uterus, including abnormal bleeding.

Uses and Complications

The major adverse effects to women undergoing cesarean section have been complications caused by anesthesia, infection, hemorrhaging, and blood-clotting disorders, such as thromboembolic episodes in which a blood clot breaks loose from a vessel and causes a stroke, heart attack, or pulmonary embolism. One of the most frequent complications from cesarean section is postoperative fever. Physicians can reduce the incidence of fever, however, by administering antibiotics prophylactically. Some women also experience damage to internal organs during the surgery, especially the bowel and bladder. Risks to the fetus include entrapment of a fetal head or limb in the uterine incision, which may result in injury to the head or spine and in limb fractures, and wounding of the fetus when the incision is made in the uterine wall.

Patients and their health care providers must weigh these potential adverse effects against the benefits of cesarean sections. Cesarean section is often performed when a normal vaginal delivery is possible, and women may not be fully aware of the risks involved. For most patients who are failing to progress in labor or whose baby is in the breech position or in distress, a cesarean is indicated. It is not always necessary, however, for a cesarean to be performed on a patient who has had a previous cesarean. Research supports the use of attempted vaginal births after cesarean (VBACs) for women who are appropriately selected, counseled, and managed.

Perspective and Prospects

Cesarean section was first performed in ancient Rome when the law required physicians to examine the fetus in the event of a mother's death. Some medical historians have proposed that Julius Caesar was delivered in this way; the term for the procedure is derived from his name. Whether this story is truth or legend, however, is still a matter of debate. In the eighteenth century, many women attempted to perform the procedure as a method of abortion. These self-surgeries usually resulted in the mother's death.

The rate for delivery by cesarean section has increased in the United States since the 1960s. In 1965, 4.5 percent of babies were born via cesarean. By 2010, more than 32 percent of all children born in the United States were delivered by cesarean. The cesarean delivery rate declined during the late 1980s through the mid-1990s but has been on the rise since 1996. Because fetal monitoring during labor is much more sophisticated than it was in the past, problems with the fetus are more easily detected, leading to an increased number of cesareans; still, far too many cesareans are being performed for reasons other than medical necessity. There is a great deal of controversy currently about the practice of cesarean delivery on maternal request (CDMR), and about whether women are adequately informed of the risks of the procedure.

—Clair Kaplan, A.P.R.N./M.S.N.; additional material by Matthew Berria, Ph.D., and Douglas Reinhart, M.D.; Robin Kamienny Montvilo, R.N., Ph.D.

See also Childbirth; Childbirth complications; Emergency medicine; Obstetrics; Reproductive system; Uterus; Women's health.

For Further Information:

Crombleholme, William R. "Obstetrics." In *Current Medical Diagnosis and Treatment 2006*, edited by Lawrence M. Tierney, Jr., Stephen J. McPhee, and Maxine A. Papadakis. New York: McGraw-Hill Medical, 2006.

"Cesarean Birth." *acog.org*, June 18, 2013.

Cesarean Section: Understanding and Celebrating Your Baby's Birth. Baltimore: Johns Hopkins University Press, 2003.

Cunningham, F. Gary, et al., eds. *Williams Obstetrics*. 23d ed. New York: McGraw-Hill, 2010.

Greene, R. A., C. Fitzpatrick, and M. J. Turner. "What Are the Maternal Implications of a Classical Caesarian Section?" *Journal of Obstetrics and Gynaecology* 18, no. 4 (July, 1998): 345-347.

Menacker, F., E. Declercq, and M. F. Macdorman. "Cesarean Delivery: Background, Trends, and Epidemiology." *Seminars in Perinatology* 30, no. 5 (2006): 235-241.

Menaker, F. "Neonatal Mortality Risk for RepeatÂ CesareanÂ Compared to VaginalÂ BirthÂ afterCesareanÂ (VBAC) Deliveries in the United States, 1998-2002Â BirthÂ Cohorts." Maternal & Child Health Journal. 14,2. (March 2000): 147-154.

Murphy, Magnus. *Choosing Cesarean: A Natural Birth Plan*. Amherst, New York: Prometheus Books, 2012.

Tower, Clare L., B. K. Strachan, and P. N. Baker. "Long-Term Implications of Caesarean Section." *Journal of Obstetrics and Gynaecology* 20, no. 4 (July, 2000): 365.

Chagas' disease
Disease/Disorder

Anatomy or system affected: Immune system, nervous system, skin

Specialties and related fields: Family medicine, public health

Definition: An acute disease that is most common in children and caused by the protozoan *Trypanosoma cruzi*.

Causes and Symptoms

Chagas disease, also known as American trypanosomiasis or South American trypanosomiasis, is a parasitic disease that affects millions of persons in both North and South

---

Information on Chagas' Disease

Causes: Protozoan transmitted by conenose bug (also called reduviid, assassin, or kissing bug) through bite or feces

Symptoms: Acute phase includes anemia, loss of strength, nervous disorders, chills, muscle and bone pain, heart failure, sometimes death; chronic phase also includes central and peripheral nervous system dysfunction eventually leading to heart failure

Duration: Acute and chronic

Treatments: Nifurtimox and benznidazole for acute infections

America. More than 15 million persons are infected-most from Mexico south throughout South America-and about 50,000 die from the disease each year. More than 100 million are at risk of contracting the disease.

The protozoan *Trypanosoma cruzi* that causes Chagas disease is transmitted by the conenose bug (order Hemiptera, family Reduviidae, subfamily Triatominae), also known as the reduviid, assassin, or kissing bug. The feces of the bugs contain the parasites, which enter a human host through broken skin or mucous membranes. Entry of the parasites into cells in the subcutaneous tissue triggers an acute local inflammatory reaction. Within one to two weeks of infection, the trypanosomes spread to the regional lymph nodes and begin to multiply in the cells that phagocytose (digest) them. Chagas disease also can be transmitted by blood transfusion; by organ transplantation, especially heart; and by triatomine bugs.

Chagas disease is manifested in acute and chronic phases. Symptoms of the acute phase (most common in children) include anemia, loss of strength, nervous disorders, chills, muscle and bone pain, and varying degrees of heart failure. Death may ensue three to four weeks after infection. Symptoms of the chronic phase (most common in adults) include those of the acute phase, plus central and peripheral nervous dysfunction, which may last for many years and eventually lead to heart failure.

Treatment and Therapy

Unlike many other trypanosomes of humans, *T. cruzi* does not respond well to chemotherapy. The most effective drugs kill only the extracellular protozoa, but the intracellular forms defy the best efforts at eradication. The reproductive stages, which occur inside living host cells, seem to be shielded from the drugs. Nifurtimox and benznidazole have been shown to be somewhat effective in curing acute infections, but they require long treatment durations and have significant side effects.

Perspective and Prospects

In 1910, Carlos Chagas dissected a number of assassin bugs and found their hindguts swarming with trypanosomes some twenty years before they were known to cause disease. A century later, progress in controlling this harmful disease has been slow.

The 2005 report of the Scientific Working Group on Chagas Disease calls for, among other things, pediatric formulations of the two main drugs used to treat the disease, better diagnostic tools, better ways to screen donated blood to prevent transmission by transfusion, and improvements in control of the insects involved in transmission of the disease.

—Jason A. Hubbart, M.S.;
updated by David M. Lawrence

See also Bites and stings; Insect-borne diseases; Leishmaniasis; Parasitic diseases; Protozoan diseases; Sleeping sickness; Tropical medicine; Zoonoses.

For Further Information:

Dorn, Patricia L., et. al. "Autochthonous Transmission of *Trypanosoma cruzi*, Louisiana." *Emerging Infectious Diseases* 13, no. 2 (April, 2007).

Mascola, L., et. al. "Chagas Disease After Organ Transplantation-Los Angeles, California, 2006." *Morbidity and Mortality Weekly Report (MMWR)* 55, no. 29 (July 28, 2006): 798-800.

MedlinePlus. "Chagas Disease." *MedlinePlus*, Jan. 14, 2013.

Perleth, Matthias. *Historical Aspects of American Trypanosomiasis (Chagas Disease)*. Frankfurt, Germany: Lang, 1997.

Tarleton, Rick L. "Pathology of American Trypanosomiasis." *Immunology and Molecular Biology of Parasitic Infections*, edited by Kenneth S. Warren. 3d ed. Boston: Blackwell, 1993.

World Health Organization. *Control of Chagas Disease: Second Report of the WHO Expert Committee on Chagas Disease*. Geneva, Switzerland: Author, 2002.

Charcot-Marie-Tooth disease

Disease/Disorder

Also known as: Charcot-Marie-Tooth neuropathy, hereditary motor and sensory neuropathy, peroneal muscular atrophy

Anatomy or system affected: Arms, ears, feet, hands, joints, legs, muscles, musculoskeletal system, nervous system, spine

Specialties and related fields: Audiology, genetics, neurology, occupational health, orthopedics, pediatrics, physical therapy

Definition: A group of inherited neurological disorders that damage peripheral nerves.

Key terms:

axon: a typically long, single extension of a neuron that conducts nerve impulses away from the cell body

myelin sheath: a layer of protein and fatty substances that surround and insulate the axons of particular nerves in the brain, spinal cord and peripheral nervous system and increase the speed of nerve impulse transmission

neuron: impulse conducting cells in the brain, spinal cord, and peripheral nervous system that consist of a nucleated cell body, dendrites, and an axon

osteotomy: a surgical procedure that cuts a bone to shorten, lengthen, or change its alignment

peripheral nervous system: the part of the nervous system that lies outside the brain and spinal cord

Wallerian degeneration: axon degeneration after injury to a neuron that degrades the axon from the point of injury to its tip while leaving the rest of the neuron intact

---

Information on Charcot-Marie-Tooth Disease

Causes: Inherited mutations that deactivate proteins involved in axon and Schwann cell function and cause myelin sheath abnormalities and neuron dysfunction

Symptoms: Weakness and loss of muscle mass in legs, ankles, and feet; high foot arches; hammertoes; foot drop; abnormal gait; frequent tripping or falling; decreased sensation in legs and feet; neuropathic pain; eventual spreading of symptoms to hands

Duration: Symptoms begin within the first two decades of life and become progressively worse throughout life

Treatments: Physical and occupational therapy, orthopedic devices and surgery, medications for neuropathic pain

---

Causes and Symptoms

Charcot-Marie-Tooth disease (CMT) is one of the most common inherited neurological disorders. In the United States, it affects approximately 1 in 2,500 people. Mutations that affect the structural integrity of the myelin sheath that surrounds particular peripheral nerves or the survival of the nerves themselves cause CMT. In the peripheral nervous system, Schwann cells make the myelin sheath by wrapping around the nerve axon much like a cinnamon roll. Abnormalities of the myelin sheath or the Schwann cells make it disrupt nerve function and eventually lead to nerve degeneration.

There are several different types of CMT. Many are inherited in a dominant fashion, which means that individuals only need to inherit one copy of the mutation in order to acquire CMT. Those types of CMT that affect the myelin sheath are called demyelinating neuropathies. CMT1A, the most common form of CMT, results from the duplication of a gene located on chromosome 17 that encodes Peripheral Myelin Protein-22 (PMP-22). Overproduction of PMP22 disrupts the structure and function of the myelin sheath. CMT1B results from loss-of-function mutations in the MPZ gene, which encodes Myelin Protein Zero (P0). Hereditary neuropathy with predisposition to pressure palsy, or HNPP, is caused by deletion mutations in the PMP22 gene. CMT1X, the second-most frequent form of CMT, results from mutations in the GJB1 gene, which is located on the X chromosome and encodes a protein called Connexin 32. Schwann cells make Connexin 32 and without it, they cannot properly communicate with neurons to make the myelin sheath. There are also other rare types of CMT1 caused by mutations in other genes. CMT3 or Dejerine-Sottas disease, a very severe form of CMT, results from loss-of-function mutations in the MPZ, PMP22, PRX, or EGR2 genes.

Those types of CMT that disrupt the nerve and cause neuronal death are called axonal neuropathies. CMT2 consists of a group of dominantly-inherited axonal neuropathies. Mutations in the MFN2 gene that encodes the Mitofusin 2 protein, a protein associated with the fusion of mitochondria (the energy-making structure of the cell),

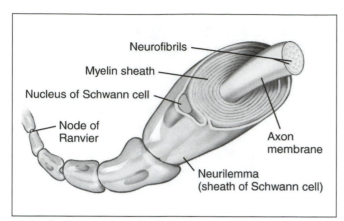

Neurofibrils

Myelin sheath

Nucleus of Schwann cell

Node of Ranvier

Axon membrane

Neurilemma (sheath of Schwann cell)

Myelin sheath. (Mosby's Medical Dictionary, 8th edition. © 2009, Elsevier.)

cause CMT2A. Other rare types of CMT2 caused by mutations in other genes also exist.

Recessive forms of CMT also exist, which means that individuals must inherit two copies of the mutations in particular genes to acquire CMT. CMT4, which consists of recessively-inherited demyelinating neuropathies, results from mutations in several different genes, all of which encode proteins that play integral roles in axonal and Schwann cell biology.

The time of onset of symptoms and their severity varies, but symptoms usually begin between mid-childhood and early adulthood. For example, individuals with CMT1A first show symptoms in their legs during the first two decades of life, but those with Dejerine-Sottas disease initially show symptoms as infants. Symptoms include foot deformities such as feet that have high arches and do not flatten when bearing weight (pes cavus) and foot drop (an inability to hold the foot horizontal), loss of lower leg muscle mass that gives the patient a kind of "inverted bottle" appearance, numbness in the foot or leg, weakness in the hips, legs, or feet, and an abnormal gait (manner of walking or moving on foot). Later, similar symptoms may also appear in the arms and hands, leading to a claw-like hand.

Unfortunately, even though the motor and sensory nerves degenerate in CMT patients, the nerves that conduct pain impulses are completely normal. Therefore, if CMT patients continue to use the affected extremity, they might develop pain, cramps, numbness, and spasms in that limb. Other conditions, such as pregnancy, emotional stress, or depression can exacerbate CMT.

CMT patients have also shown changes in touch, vision, and hearing, scoliosis, malformation of the hip sockets, and atrophy of the vocal cords. Tremors, difficulty eating and swallowing, and limited mobility are other possible symptoms. Rarely, CMT patients may have difficulty breathing.

Treatment and Therapy

CMT diagnosis is initially made based on the clinical presentation and family medical history. If CMT is suspected, then other tests, including electromyography, nerve conduction velocity, nerve biopsy, and genetic testing, are conducted to confirm the diagnosis.

Electromyography (EMG) measures the electrical activity produced by muscles. A small needle electrode is inserted into a muscle, after which the patient contracts her muscle, and the electrode detects the electrochemical activity produced by the muscle. Nerve conduction velocity (NCV) tests are usually done at the same time as EMGs. NCV tests measure the time it takes for nerve impulses to run between two inserted electrodes. For demyelinating types of CMT (CMT1, CMTX) conduction velocities are decreased 60 to 80 percent (normal nerve conduction rates range from 50 to 60 meters per second) with values below 38 meters per second. Such slowing can also be found in individuals who show no symptoms. For this reason, family members of the patient are often tested to aid in the diagnosis, including those who have no signs of weakness.

Nerve biopsies can be helpful in equivocal cases. Patients with CMT1 show nerve demyelination and multiple layers of remyelination (onion bulbing). CMT2 patients have axon loss with Wallerian degeneration. More importantly, nerve biopsies show a complete absence of inflammatory infiltrates that indicate an autoimmune demyelinating process, as in multiple sclerosis.

Genetic testing for CMT Type 1A is now commercially available and this provides a definitive diagnosis, even in asymptomatic individuals. However, only 50 to 60 percent of cases are positive.

Presently no treatments exist to reverse or slow the progression of CMT. Patients often are evaluated and treated symptomatically by a team that includes a neurologist, physiatrist, orthopedic surgeon, physical therapist, and occupational therapist. Orthopedic equipment (braces or orthopedic shoes) or surgery might make it easier to walk, and physical and occupational therapy may help maintain muscle and improve independent functioning.

Severe pes cavus, scoliosis, and other joint deformities require orthopedic surgery. The age of the patient and severity of deformity determine the treatment. There are three types of surgical procedures used to treat severe CMT deformities: soft tissue, osteotomy, and joint stabilization. Surgical procedures are usually staged, starting with soft tissue surgeries (tendon releases or tendon transfers), followed by osteotomies, and then joint stabilization (arthrodesis).

Acetaminophen (Tylenol) or nonsteroidal anti-inflammatory drugs alleviate neuropathic pain in some CMT patients. Tricyclic antidepressants or antiepileptic drugs such as carbamazepine or gabapentin may also provide relief from chronic pain in some CMT patients. CMT patients should avoid drugs known to damage nerves (e.g., nitrofurantoin, isoniazid, vincristine).

Perspective and Prospects

CMT is named for the three physicians who first identified it in 1886: Jean Martin Charcot and Pierre Marie from Paris, France, and Howard Henry Tooth from Cambridge, England. All three reported the main clinical features of CMT, including inheritance, skeletal deformities, and progressive distal muscle weakness and wasting. Tooth was the first to correctly attribute the symptoms of CMT to peripheral nerve degeneration (neuropathy) rather than degeneration of the spinal cord (myelopathy). Less than a decade later (1893), Joseph Jules Dejerine and Jules Sottas reported a case involving two siblings who had a more severe neuropathy with much earlier onset.

In 1957, R.W. Gilliat and P.K. Thomas and later, in 1968, P.J. Dyck and E.H. Lambert used electrophysiological studies to show that CMT patients showed markedly slower rates of nerve conduction. The combination of electrophysiological studies, inheritance patterns, and clinical descriptions were used by Thomas and A.E. Harding to construct a rational classification of the different types of CMT.

Several laboratories have successfully regenerated the myelin sheath in laboratory animals by using cultured Schwann cells, differentiated pluripotent stem cells, and other cell types. Small human trials examining the safety and efficacy of stem cell-based treatments are presently in progress, and larger trails might commence in the near future.

—*Michael A. Buratovich, Ph.D.*

See also Audiology; Fatigue; Genetic counseling; Neurology; Occupational health; Ophthalmology; Orthopedics; Pain; Paralysis; Pathology; Physical rehabilitation

For Further Information:

Li, Jun. "Inherited Neuropathies." *Seminars in Neurology* 32, no. 3 (July, 2012): 204-214.

Li, Jun, Brett Parker, Colin Martyn, Chandramohan Natarajan, and Jiasong Guo. "The PMP22 Gene and Its Related Diseases." *Molecular Neurobiology* 47 (2013): 673-698.

Patzko, Agnes, and Michael A. Shy. "Update on Charcot-Marie-Tooth Disease." *Current Neurology and Neuroscience Reports* 11, no. 1 (February, 2011): 78-88.

Pareyson, Davide, and Chiara Marchesi. "Diagnosis, Natural History, and Management of Charcot-Marie-Tooth Disease." *Lancet Neurology* 8. no. 7 (July, 2009): 654-667.

Parker, James N., and Philip M. Parker, eds. *The Official Patient's Sourcebook on Charcot-Marie-Tooth Disorder: A Revised and Updated Directory for the Internet Age.* San Diego, CA: Icon Health Publications, 2002.

Chemotherapy

Treatment

Anatomy or system affected: All

Specialties and related fields: Alternative medicine, genetics, microbiology, nuclear medicine, oncology, pharmacology, preventive medicine, toxicology

Definition: The use of chemical compounds to treat diseases, especially infectious diseases and cancer.

Key terms:

adjuvant chemotherapy: the use of combinations of drugs or treatments in addressing metastatic cancer

antibiotics: substances produced by groups of microorganisms that are cytotoxic to other groups of microorganisms

cancer stem cells: the small proportion of cells in cancers that have the potential for long-term replication and metastasis

cytotoxic: referring to the cell-killing properties of a drug

selective toxicity: the properties of a drug that make it selectively destructive to an infectious agent or diseased cell, without harming normal cells of the body

Indications and Procedures

Chemotherapy refers to the concept of using chemicals in a therapeutic manner. Although chemotherapy is commonly associated with cancer, its concept and history encompass the use of medicinal approaches to treat many different types of human disease, such as bacterial and viral infections. In the early part of the twentieth century, Paul Ehrlich coined the term "chemotherapy" and defined it descriptively as a "chemical knife." The work of Ehrlich established the principle that chemical substances could be used effectively in the treatment of human diseases. The success of chemotherapy is based on the simple principle of selective toxicity, which can be defined as the capacity of a drug to recognize and destroy an infectious agent or diseased cell without seriously harming the human body. The chemical knife envisioned by Ehrlich must be a selective one, or both the host and the pathogen will die.

In antibiotics, this targeting is achieved largely because of the vast structural differences between bacterial cells and human cells. For example, penicillin, discovered by British scientist Alexander Fleming as a product of the mold *Penicillium notatum*, targets a unique compound found only in bacterial cells. When antibiotics such as penicillin target the bacterial cell wall, the bacterial cell lyses, or falls apart and dies. Human cells lack cell walls and peptidoglycan; therefore, the cells of the body are not affected by the antibiotic. Most antibiotics follow this principle of selective cytotoxicity by targeting bacterial structures or metabolic processes unique to bacterial cells, thereby permitting the human host, which is designed differently, to survive the attack.

Many of the same principles have been applied to the development of chemical approaches to cancer treatment; however, the target in cancer therapy is significantly different from that of bacterial antibiotics. One of the most challenging and intractable problems in the treatment of cancer involves the fact that cancer cells are derived from host cells within the body and share many similarities to the cells and tissues of origin, thereby complicating treatment approaches. Unlike bacteria, which differ profoundly from human cells in both form and function, cancer cells evolve within the host and share many if not most cytologic and immunologic properties.

How, then, can the principle of selective cytotoxicity be utilized in the treatment of cancer? Traditional approaches have targeted the abnormal functions of tumor cells, which are largely associated with abnormalities of cell proliferation. For this reason, chemicals that interfere with processes associated with cell reproduction were the major therapeutic approach in the treatment of cancer in the second half of the twentieth century. This theoretical approach targets quantitative differences, such as the rates of deoxyribonucleic acid (DNA) synthesis and/or cell division, rather than qualitative differences, such as structural or biochemical differences, as the basis or rationale for selective

Two young girls with acute lymphoblastic leukemia (ALL) receive chemotherapy. (Bill Branson/National Cancer Institute)

targeting treatment approaches. These treatment approaches have largely involved the use of drugs that target DNA synthesis or that block mitosis (cell division), since these are the principal pathways that are quantitatively dysregulated in malignant tumor cells.

This mode of selective toxicity, however, is less precise than the chemical knife of antibiotic therapies, which are based on qualitative rather than quantitative differences between the target and host. This lack of precision is attributable to the fact that the processes of DNA synthesis and mitosis are not restricted only to cancer cells but occur in many other tissues of the body. Many of the side effects of chemotherapy-including anemia, immunosuppression, nausea and vomiting, mouth ulcers, and hair loss-are the result of the effects of these chemicals on normally dividing cells of the body. These side effects are largely temporary, and normal tissue functions are restored once chemotherapy treatments are completed. Chemotherapy may also produce cumulative and long-term effects on organ systems of the body such as the heart, kidneys, and nervous system, depending on the drug regimen, the time course, and the total accumulated dose received by the patient.

Thus, the similarities between cancer cells and normally dividing cells of the body make it much more difficult to design chemotherapy in a way that selectively targets the tumor while sparing the normally dividing cells of the body. Any selective targeting that is achieved depends on the increased rate of cell division in the tumor cells as compared to normal cells. The observed selective toxicity of a chemotherapeutic drug for a tumor is referred to as its therapeutic index, which refers to the ratio between its cytotoxicity for the tumor cells versus normally dividing cells of the body. The higher the therapeutic index, the more selective and presumably effective is the chemotherapeutic drug for a given tumor type. The intrinsic similarities between cancer cells and their normal tissue counterparts, however, ultimately limit the maximum tolerable doses of chemotherapeutic drugs and their clinical effectiveness.

An important concept related to therapeutic index is that of growth fraction, which is defined as the percentage of cells in a normal tissue or tumor that is actively proliferating. Since most chemotherapeutic drugs target cells that are engaged in DNA synthesis or mitosis, malignancies with a higher growth fraction (such as leukemias) will be more sensitive to these drugs than are tumors with a low growth fraction (such as many solid tumors). Most standard chemotherapeutic drugs affect cycling cells, that is, cells that are in the active cell division cycle. These drugs are classified as phase-specific since they are active against tumor cells only in certain phases of the cell cycle. Because they are phase-specific, they are much more cytotoxic to rapidly dividing cells than to nondividing cells.

Another important principle of chemotherapy involves

the observation that most conventional chemotherapeutic drugs kill cancer cells with first-order kinetics, which means that the drug induces death in a constant percentage of cells over time rather than a constant number of cells. Therefore, even if the drug is 99.9 percent effective, 0.1 percent of the total number of cancer cells will remain even after drug treatment is completed. This small remaining base of tumor cells may eventually produce tumor recurrence. This problem of tumor recurrence as a result of the mechanism of cell destruction may be countered in part by a combined chemotherapy approach, utilizing multiple drugs, in which each targets a different abnormal component of the cancer cell.

Combined therapy is also designed to address the problem of drug resistance, which has shadowed oncologists and their patients since the earliest treatments for leukemia were developed in the 1950s. In fact, the early therapy protocols involving the use of 6-mercaptopurine and methotrexate in the treatment of childhood acute lymphoblastic leukemia (ALL) immediately exposed some of the fundamental difficulties associated with the use of chemotherapy. Initially, many children with ALL died immediately after treatment, since it was not realized that the therapeutic index of these drugs was so low that overdoses readily occurred. When the dosing regimen was finally adjusted, many children treated with these new drugs recovered rapidly, displaying dramatic drops in white cell counts and restored health. Sadly, some of these children subsequently suffered relapses of disease that no longer responded to chemotherapy. From these early clinical studies, the problem of drug resistance was first identified, and it remains one of the main reasons that chemotherapy treatments may ultimately fail.

More than half a century has passed since the early clinical trials with 6-mercaptopurine in childhood ALL, and oncologists still do not completely understand the phenomenon of drug resistance, although many studies have suggested that it is linked to abnormal gene function and the genetic instability of tumor cells. Most important, more recent research studies have provided significant evidence that, regardless of the mechanism of action, chemotherapeutic drugs ultimately trigger cell death "suicide" pathways that are regulated by the damaged cell. Activation of these internally regulated cell death pathways involves a complex process called apoptosis. A key finding that has emerged from these studies is that, as a result of defects in genes such as the tumor suppressor *p53*, cancer cells may be less able to enter the death pathway and commit "suicide" in response to chemotherapy than are normal cells whose death pathways are intact.

Uses and Complications

Conventional chemotherapeutic drugs are divided into separate groups depending on their chemical properties and mechanism of cell destruction. Most clinical treatment protocols involve combination chemotherapy using several drugs with different cell targets. This approach is designed to employ multifaceted targeting as a way of achieving maximum cell destruction in a single round of treatment and, in conjunction with high-dose or "dose dense" approaches, is thought to produce maximum effects with the least likelihood of triggering the new growth of drug-resistant tumors. All treatment protocols are designed and implemented only after rigorous preclinical trials are conducted to ascertain their effectiveness against a particular type of cancer. The important classes of standard anticancer drugs are summarized below.

Alkylating agents block the synthesis of DNA by chemically modifying its structure. The nitrogen mustards were the first chemical drugs to be used in the treatment of cancer. Today, cyclophosphamide is commonly used in combined treatment approaches in patients with leukemia and lymphoma. The nitrosoureas, a second group of alkylating agents, interact with DNA by forming chemical cross-links that result in DNA strand breakage. They can enter the cerebrospinal fluid and are therefore used to treat brain tumors. Examples include carmustine and busulfan.

The antimetabolites share structural similarities to DNA precursor components. There are three general groups of antimetabolites: folate antagonists (methotrexate), purine analogues (6-mercaptopurine), and pyrimidine analogues (5-flurouracil). Each of these antimetabolites blocks a normal pathway required for DNA synthesis in the tumor cell, thereby blocking its reproduction.

The anticancer antibiotics are the natural products of microorganisms that display toxic effects toward cancer cells. In general, they interfere with the processes of DNA synthesis or messenger ribonucleic acid (RNA) production. Doxorubicin (Adriamycin) inserts itself between the base pairs of DNA in a process called intercalation, which greatly disrupts DNA structure and function. This drug is effective for many types of cancer; however, its use is limited by its cumulative cytotoxic effects on the heart, which restrict the maximum lifetime dosage that a patient can receive.

Hormonal therapy may be effective against cancers arising in tissues whose growth is hormonally sensitive, such as cancers of the breast and prostate gland. Tamoxifen is a competitive estrogen receptor (ER) antagonist, which means that it binds to estrogen receptors in competition with estrogen. Tamoxifen use has significantly decreased the recurrence of breast cancer in patients with estrogen-sensitive tumors, by 60 percent. Studies with a different class of antiestrogens called aromatase inhibitors, which block estrogen synthesis directly, have also shown very promising results.

A number of naturally occurring products have been found to display anticancer properties. Important members of this group are the vinca alkaloids, which are the natural products of periwinkle plants. Vincristine and vinblastine, the best-known chemical agents of this group, both work by blocking the process of mitosis. These drugs are commonly used in combined therapies with other chemotherapeutic drugs to treat leukemias and lymphomas. Another naturally occurring product is etoposide, a toxic plant alkaloid found in the mandrake (mayapple) plant. It induces a cell cycle arrest that blocks cell proliferation and is used to treat several types of cancer.

A recently discovered drug is paclitaxel, better known as Taxol. This drug, originally isolated from the bark of the rare Pacific yew tree, was found to disrupt the process of mitosis by binding to the filaments called microtubules that pull the chromosomes apart during the process of cell division. Taxol freezes these structures, thereby paralyzing the cell division machinery. In synthetic form, it is used to treat ovarian and breast cancer.

Most recently, there has been a renewed interest in some of the naturally occurring components of herbal medicines and plants that have been used for centuries in the treatment of myriad ailments and diseases. One of the most dramatic examples is the traditional Chinese medicine used to treat patients in rural China with a rare form of leukemia called acute promyelocytic leukemia (APL). The results convinced a team of European and American oncologists to visit rural China and study the properties of this curative herbal extract. After the many components of this complex herbal medicine were purified, it was found that the active anticancer component was arsenic. Indeed, further studies showed that very low dose arsenic by itself was capable of eliciting complete remission in patients with formerly incurable APL. Many other plants and flowers produce anti-inflammatory substances with documented anticancer properties. Perhaps the best known is aspirin. Its chemical name is acetylsalicylic acid, and it occurs naturally in the bark of the willow tree. For centuries, it was used as an anti-inflammatory agent, and over the past few years it has been shown to have chemopreventive effects against colon cancer. The chemically synthesized cyclo-oxygenase-2 (COX-2) inhibitors may also have anticancer effects, further strengthening the suggested link between abnormal inflammatory pathway activities within the cell and responses to chemotherapy.

Beginning in the late twentieth century, the understanding of the molecular basis of cancer increased dramatically, and oncologists have been extremely eager to apply this knowledge to the development of newer targeted treatment approaches that would selectively destroy cancer cells and spare the normal cells of the body. One of the greatest successes in this area of research to date has been in the treatment of a form of leukemia called chronic myeloid leukemia (CML) with a drug called Gleevec, produced by Novartis Pharmaceutical Company, that selectively targets the primary gene product that is abnormal in this type of leukemia. CML patient responses to Gleevec were so dramatic that the drug was quickly approved by the Food and Drug Administration (FDA). Because of its greater selective toxicity as a result of a gene-targeted mechanism of action, Gleevec causes few side effects, unlike traditional chemotherapeutic drugs.

Perspective and Prospects

The idea of chemotherapy is not a new one; it dates back to the days of antiquity. Approximately 2,500 years ago, ancient Egyptian writings about cancer first appeared, along

---

In the News: PARP Inhibitors

PARP inhibitors are a promising new class of anticancer drugs. In mid-2009, results from phase 1 and 2 clinical trials with two PARP-1 inhibitors, BSI-201 from BiPar (Sanofi-Aventis) and olaparib from AstraZeneca, were reported. The drugs showed increased patient survival and tumor shrinkage, to the extent that BSI-201 has advanced to stage 3 clinical trials.

PARP is short for poly (ADP-ribose) polymerase, an enzyme participating in deoxyribonucleic acid (DNA) damage repair in the cell. The double-stranded cellular DNA can suffer single strand breaks and double-strand breaks, among other forms of DNA damage. PARP-1 has a role in repairing single-strand breaks, or "nicks." The BRCA (BReast CAncer) proteins 1 and 2 are involved in repairing double-strand breaks. Mutations of the *BRCA* genes which render their respective protein products inactive are associated with increased risk of several cancers, in particular breast cancer.

Two studies published in the journal *Nature* in 2005 paved the way to the development of PARP inhibitors-based chemotherapy. In these studies, cells containing inactive BRCA protein did not survive PARP inhibition. This finding suggested that at least one of the DNA repair pathways, fixing single- or double-strand DNA breaks, has to function for cells to survive. When both pathways are inactive, cellular death follows. Indeed, as expected from these studies, the PARP-1 inhibitor olaparib is effective against BRCA-deficient cancers. Moreover, normal cells which have an active BRCA protein are not expected to respond to PARP-inhibitors. PARP inhibitors thus have the potential for targeting mainly cancerous cells while minimally affecting normal cells, which are often indiscriminately targeted by many current chemotherapy drugs.

—*Nadja Rozovsky, Ph.D.*

---

with treatment recommendations such as the use of barley, castor beans, and pig ears to treat cancers of the stomach and uterus. After the ancient Egyptians, among the earliest recorded chemotherapies involved the use of mercury to treat outbreaks of syphilis in Europe in the late fifteenth century. In North America, early American Indians chewed the bark of the cinchona tree to ward off malaria, and by 1630 it was recognized by Europeans that this medicinal bark contained an antimalarial substance called quinine, which eventually became a widely used treatment for malarial infections.

One of the most significant advances in the development of modern chemotherapy was the pioneering work of Paul Ehrlich in the early part of the twentieth century. His efforts to find a "magic bullet" to selectively destroy infectious disease agents culminated in the isolation of a synthetic arsenic compound called salvarsan, which was used in the treatment of syphilis.

In 1929, Alexander Fleming made the monumental discovery that penicillin, an extract from a common mold, could kill infectious bacterial pathogens. He made this astonishing finding upon examining a set of moldy, contaminated culture dishes that he was preparing to discard when he noticed that no bacterial colonies grew in the vicinity of the mold. Thus the modern age of antibiotics was born. In

1935, Gerhard Domagk, a scientist at Bayer Pharmaceutical Company, isolated a chemical substance whose active component, sulfanilamide, was capable of killing several types of infectious bacteria and was later used to save his own daughter from a near-fatal streptococcal infection. This was the first sulfonamide, and it led to the chemical synthesis of a class of related drugs with antimicrobial activity called sulfa drugs. Selman Waksman, another pioneer of this time, isolated the antibiotic streptomycin from the soil microbe *Streptomyces griseus*. It was Waksman who first proposed the term "antibiotic" to define a chemical substance made by one microorganism that kills other microorganisms at low concentrations. Since those early days of drug discovery, many antibiotics and synthetic drugs have been developed. These discoveries transformed the world of medicine and have saved countless lives worldwide.

During the second half of the twentieth century, the term "chemotherapy" became increasingly associated with the treatment of cancer. Several important discoveries of this time were largely responsible for this transition in modern thinking. The earliest discovery occurred in the 1930s as scientists were studying the aftermath of World War I and the effects of sulfur mustard on soldiers exposed to this toxic gas. These findings and later studies on nitrogen mustard showed that among the side effects of exposure to these poisonous gases were decreases in white blood cell (lymphocyte) production by the bone marrow. Ultimately, this led to the notion that low doses of these toxic chemicals might be used as a medicinal approach in the treatment of leukemias and lymphomas resulting from the abnormal production of lymphocytes in the bone marrow. Nitrogen mustard was used for the first time to treat lymphoma in the 1940s. Early promising results quickly established the principle that toxic chemicals could be used to destroy cancer cells within the body. In 1951, landmark research by Gertrude Elion and George Hitchings led to the synthesis of a chemical called 6-mercaptopurine, which was found to block DNA synthesis in rapidly dividing leukemia cells. 6-mercaptopurine was used successfully to treat the most common form of childhood leukemia, ALL. Before this treatment was developed, the average survival time for children diagnosed with ALL was only three to four months. Upon introduction of this new chemotherapeutic treatment, approximately 80 percent of children diagnosed with ALL improved or recovered from this disease.

Since those early days of cancer chemotherapy, more than fifty chemotherapeutic drugs have been used successfully in the treatment of cancer. The greatest successes have been observed for childhood leukemia, Hodgkin's disease, some adult leukemias and lymphomas, and some other rare childhood tumors. The mixed results and lower success rates obtained for many adult epithelial carcinomas have prompted continued research into the development of novel therapeutic approaches to the treatment of cancer.

The twenty-first century promises to be the beginning of a new era in the history of chemotherapy. As the molecular basis of disease is increasingly well understood, the scope of potential targets for therapy and prevention steadily increases. Some of these developments have resulted from the discovery that some cancers express unusual proteins on their surface, unique to the tumor, which may serve as targets for new forms of treatments. For example, certain types of cancers, including breast cancer and some leukemias, may develop from what have been called cancer stem cells. These represent the small minority of cells that are capable of growing or metastasizing; most of the other cells which constitute the cancer do not metastasize and have limited tumorigenic potential. It was found these stem cells often have unique markers on their surface, markers which differentiate them from either normal cells or other cancer cells which have limited survival potential. The development of methods of chemotherapy which target only these stem cells may provide another mechanism to target certain cells.

Another form of treatment has been called adjuvant chemotherapy, the use of combination of drugs. By using these drugs sequentially, it is sometimes possible to reduce their concentrations, thereby reducing the extent of side effects while at the same time providing effective therapy. Adjuvant chemotherapy has shown some evidence of success in treating metastatic cancers such as those associated with breast or lung cancer. In April 2013, the *Journal of the American Medical Association* published a study reporting that the drug duloxetine (known commercially as Cymbalta) is potentially helpful for paitents suffering from the side effects of chemotherapy.

—*Sarah Crawford, Ph.D.;*
updated by Richard Adler, Ph.D.

See also Antibiotics; Bacterial infections; Bacteriology; Cancer; Carcinoma; Cells; Drug resistance; Immune system; Immunology; Leukemia; Lymphadenopathy and lymphoma; Malignancy and metastasis; Microbiology; Oncology; Pharmacology; Radiation therapy; Sarcoma; Tumor removal; Tumors.

For Further Information:
"Antidepressant Lessens Chemo-Related Pain." *Medline*, April 2, 2013.
Bruning, Nancy. *Coping with Chemotherapy*. Rev. ed. New York: Ballantine Books, 1993.
Brunton, Laurence L., et al., eds. *Goodman and Gilman's "The Pharmacological Basis of Therapeutics."* 11th ed. New York: McGraw-Hill, 2006.
"Chemotherapy." *Mayo Clinc*, June 24, 2013.
Clarke, Michael, et al. "Stem Cells: The Real Culprit in Cancer?" *Scientific American* 295, no. 1 (July, 2006): 52-59.
Fischer, David S. *The Cancer Chemotherapy Handbook*. 6th ed. St. Louis, Mo.: Mosby, 2003.
Quillin, Patrick. *Beating Cancer with Nutrition*. Rev. ed. Tulsa, Okla.: Nutrition Times Press, 2005.
Simon, Stacy. "Study Shows Duloxetine Reduces Pain from Chemotherapy." *cancer.org*, April 3, 2013.

Chest

Anatomy

Anatomy or system affected: Circulatory system, lungs, muscles, musculoskeletal system, respiratory system

Specialties and related fields: Cardiology, pulmonary medicine

Definition: The region of the body from the diaphragm to the neck, both within the rib cage (heart and lungs) and in front of it (breasts and muscles).

Key terms:

breast: the mammary gland, along with the nipple in front of it and the surrounding fatty tissue

diaphragm: a curved muscular sheet that separates the chest cavity from the abdominal cavity

heart: a muscular pump that propels the blood through the circulatory system

lungs: the air sacs that are the principal respiratory organs; located in the chest

ribs: the bones that support the chest and define its outline

thoracic: pertaining to the chest

thorax: another name for the chest region

Structure and Functions

The chest, or thorax, consists of those parts of the body lying between the diaphragm and the neck. Included here are the rib cage, diaphragm, heart, lungs, chest muscles, and breasts.

The skeletal support of the chest consists of the thoracic vertebrae and rib cage. In humans, there are usually twelve pairs of ribs and twelve thoracic vertebrae. Each thoracic vertebra consists of a cylindrical portion, the centrum or body, and a neural arch attached to the dorsal side of the centrum. The neural arch surrounds and protects the spinal column. A spinous process extends dorsally from the neu-

ral arch of each thoracic vertebra and serves as a site for muscle attachment. Near the base of each neural arch are two pairs of articular processes (zygapophyses). The superior pair of one vertebra face toward each other and articulate with the inferior articular processes of the adjacent vertebrae.

Attached to each thoracic vertebra is a rib. There are usually twelve pairs of ribs, but this number occasionally varies. Each rib consists of a bony portion and a cartilaginous extension, the costal cartilage. At its vertebral end, each rib has two articulating processes, the head (capitulum) and the tubercle (tuberculum). The costal cartilages of the first seven ribs (the number occasionally varies) extend all the way to the sternum. The next two or three ribs have costal cartilages that attach to the costal cartilage above them. The remaining ribs have costal cartilages that are "floating" and have no attachments. Together, the ribs make up a cagelike structure called the rib cage, which shapes the chest and protects the heart and lungs from injury.

The sternum, or breastbone, runs along the front of the chest in the midline of the body. It consists of a flattened top portion called the manubrium; a long, extended body (corpus); and an extension called the xiphoid process, which is made mostly of cartilage. The manubrium has notches for the attachment of the clavicle and the first rib on either side. The attachment for the second rib lies between the manubrium and corpus and is shared by both bones. The

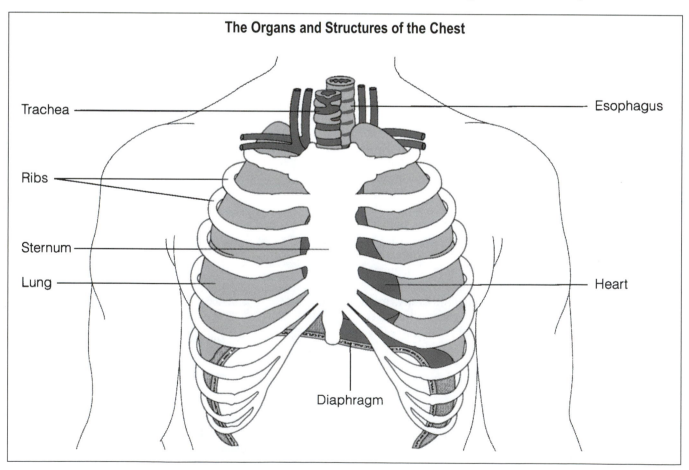

The Organs and Structures of the Chest

Trachea

Esophagus

Ribs

Sternum

Lung

Heart

Diaphragm

corpus of the sternum is formed by the fusion of five individual parts called sternebrae. The costal cartilages of the second through seventh ribs articulate with the corpus of the sternum and mark the boundaries between the individual sternebrae. Beyond the notch for the attachment of the seventh costal cartilage, the xiphoid process extends downward along the midline.

A muscular diaphragm marks the boundary between the chest cavity and the abdominal cavity. Although it is located at the lower end of the chest cavity, it originates in the neck region and derives its nerve supply, the phrenic nerve, from within the neck. The diaphragm is the principal muscle used in breathing. Normally dome-shaped and bowed upward, the diaphragm flattens when its muscles contract, expanding the chest cavity and resulting in the inhalation of air. Relaxation of the diaphragm returns the curvature of the dome upward, compressing the chest cavity and resulting in the exhalation of air. The diaphragm has openings for the passage of the esophagus and the major blood vessels, especially the descending aorta and inferior vena cava.

The heart and major blood vessels lie within the chest cavity and are protected by the rib cage. The heart is a muscular pump that has four chambers (two atria and two ventricles). The right atrium receives oxygen-poor blood from the body's organs via the superior vena cava (from the head and upper extremities) and the inferior vena cava (from the abdominal region, pelvic region, and lower extremities). Blood from the right atrium passes through the tricuspid valve to the right ventricle, from which it is pumped into the pulmonary artery. The pulmonary artery then divides in two branches that run separately to each lung. Oxygen-rich blood from the lungs returns to the heart by means of the pulmonary veins, which empty into the left atrium. Blood from the left atrium passes through the bicuspid valve and empties into the left ventricle, which has an extremely thick, muscular wall. Contraction of the left ventricle propels the blood out of the aorta and through the body via the arteries.

Contractions of the heart originate in a location known as the sinoatrial node, located on the surface of the right atrium. From this point, contractions spread to the atrioventricular node, located at the point where all four chambers meet. The wave of contraction then spreads rapidly down the septum between the two ventricles and up the side walls of each ventricle. A specialized bundle of cardiac muscle called the bundle of His, composed of modified muscle fibers (Purkinje fibers), is responsible for this rapid conduction.

Except for the pulmonary arteries, the arteries of the chest region are all branches of the aorta, the major artery that flows out from the left ventricle of the heart in an upward direction. The aorta can be subdivided into an initial portion (the ascending aorta), an aortic arch, and a longer descending aorta which extends from the thoracic region into the pelvis. The coronary arteries are small but important branches that arise from the ascending aorta as it leaves the heart. These arteries supply blood to the muscular wall of the heart itself. From the arch of the aorta, the most common pattern of branching is that of a brachiocephalic trunk, which then splits into a right common carotid and right subclavian artery, followed by a left common carotid artery and then a left subclavian artery. There is considerable variation, however, in this pattern of branchings. The carotid arteries run up the sides of the neck to supply blood to the head and neck.

The subclavian arteries of either side run first upward and then laterally through the chest cavity, continuing toward the upper extremity as the axillary artery. Along its course, each subclavian artery gives off the following branches: vertebral artery, thyrocervical trunk, internal thoracic artery, costocervical artery, and descending scapular artery. The vertebral artery, the largest branch, supplies blood to the vertebrae of the neck region and ultimately to the base of the brain. The short thyrocervical trunk divides almost immediately into three branches: an inferior thyroid artery to the larynx, trachea, esophagus, and surrounding muscles; a suprascapular artery to the subclavius and sternocleidomastoid muscles and to the overlying skin; and a transverse cervical artery to the muscles of the shoulder region.

The right and left internal thoracic arteries (also called internal mammary arteries) run along the ventral side of the chest, just beneath the costal cartilages and just to either side of the sternum. Each internal thoracic artery gives off branches to the diaphragm, the pleura, the pericardium, the thymus, the transverse thoracic muscle, the ribs and intercostal muscles, the pectoral muscles, and the mammary glands. Beyond the sixth rib, each internal thoracic artery divides into a musculophrenic branch to the last six ribs and the diaphragm and a superior epigastric artery, which descends along the abdominal surface, supplying the muscles of this region before meeting the inferior epigastric artery that ascends from the pelvic region.

The veins of the chest region include the external and internal jugular veins, draining the head and neck, and the subclavian veins, draining the upper extremities. These veins come together to form the right and left brachiocephalic veins, which then drain into the superior vena cava. The superior vena cava also receives several smaller tributaries, including the azygos vein, the paired internal thoracic and inferior thyroid veins, the highest intercostal vein, and several smaller veins of the vertebral column. The azygos vein (on the right) and the hemizygous vein (on the left) run parallel to each other on either side of the vertebral column along the dorsal or rear wall of the chest cavity, draining blood from the muscles of the back, the bronchi, the ribs, and the mediastinum. The right and left internal thoracic veins receive tributaries from the ribs and intercostal muscles as well as the diaphragm, pericardium, and mediastinum. The highest intercostal veins drain the first two or three intercostal spaces on either side, also receiving smaller tributaries from the bronchi and the upper portion of the diaphragm. The inferior thyroid veins drain the thyroid gland, esophagus, trachea, and larynx. In addition to the veins listed above, the veins of the heart muscle all drain into a coronary sinus, which runs between the left atrium and ventricle, then drains directly into the right atrium near the inferior vena cava.

The lungs, the principal organs of respiration, consist of several lobes. The right lung has superior, medial, and inferior lobes; the left lung has superior and inferior lobes only. Inhalation of air, or inspiration, is brought about by the lowering (contraction) of the diaphragm and by the raising and outward expansion of the rib cage. Exhalation of air, or expiration, is brought about by the raising (relaxation) of the diaphragm and by the relaxation of the intercostal muscles, lowering and contracting the rib cage. Under most conditions, inspiration is an active process requiring muscular contraction, while expiration takes place passively as the muscles relax.

Together, the heart, the lungs, and the thoracic portion of the esophagus occupy the thoracic cavity, or chest cavity. Each of these organs is surrounded by a thin membrane, the visceral pleura. This membrane is continuous with the parietal pleura, another thin membrane that lines the outer walls of the chest cavity. The right and left visceral pleura come together to form a septum called the mediastinum, which separates the bulk of the thoracic cavity into right and left pleural cavities, each containing one of the lungs. The pericardial cavity, containing the heart, is inserted between the layers of the mediastinum. Also occupying part of the thoracic cavity is a large mass of lymphoid tissue, the thymus body. The thymus is irregular in shape and occupies the highest portion of the thoracic cavity above the heart.

Muscles of the chest region may be divided into those associated developmentally with the upper extremity and those that are associated with the trunk of the body. One muscle, the trapezius, is a modified gill muscle that belongs developmentally to neither group. Fibers of the trapezius muscle originate from the cervical and thoracic vertebrae, including the adjoining ligaments and the adjacent part of the skull. These fibers converge onto the spine and acromion of the scapula and onto the clavicle. The muscles associated with the trunk of the body are called axial muscles. Of those in the chest or thoracic region, four are responsible primarily for movements of the shoulder blade (scapula), twelve for movements of the rib cage, and another eleven for movements of the vertebral column.

The levator scapula runs from the transverse processes of the first four cervical vertebrae to the vertebral border of the scapula; by contracting, it raises and rotates the scapula. The two rhomboid muscles run from the vertebral column to the vertebral border of the scapula. The rhomboideus minor originates from the spinous processes of the seventh cervical and the first thoracic vertebra and from the nuchal ligament that runs from these spinous processes to the skull. The rhomboideus major originates from the spinous processes of the second through fifth thoracic vertebrae. Both rhomboideus muscles run diagonally from the vertebral column to the vertebral border of the scapula, including the base of the scapular spine. The serratus anterior, also called serratus ventralis, is a sheetlike muscle that lies between the scapula and the rib cage. Its fibers originate from the ribs as a series of strips that converge slightly; they

all insert onto the vertebral border of the scapula. The attachments of this muscle to the ribs resemble a series of angular sawteeth (serrations) that give the muscle its name. The four preceding muscles all share a common embryological origin, and all have a common nerve supply from the dorsal scapular nerve.

The axial muscles associated with movements of the rib cage include the scalenus anterior, scalenus medius, scalenus posterior, intercostals, subcostals, levatores costarum, transversus thoracis, serratus posterior superior, serratus posterior inferior, rectus abdominis, and diaphragm. The three scalene muscles, as their name implies, are all shaped like elongated scalene triangles (with three sides of different lengths). The scalenus anterior arises from the transverse processes of the third through sixth cervical vertebrae and inserts (attaches) onto the first rib. The largest of the scalene muscles is the scalenus medius, which runs from the transverse processes of the last six cervical vertebrae to an insertion on the first rib. The scalenus posterior arises from the transverse processes of the last two or three cervical vertebrae and inserts onto the second rib.

The intercostal muscles run between the ribs in two sets of fibers. The external intercostals run from each rib to the next in a diagonal direction; the upper end of each fiber is situated closer to the vertebral column than is the lower end. The internal intercostals also run diagonally from each rib to the next, but deep to the fibers of the external intercostals and perpendicular to them, so that the lower end of each fiber is closer to the vertebral end of each rib than is the upper end. Both sets of intercostals are broad, extending nearly along the entire extent of each rib, but the fibers are in each case short, extending only from one rib to the next. The subcostals are similar in position and orientation to the internal intercostals, except they are usually confined to the last few ribs and they span two or three intercostal spaces at a time. The levatores costarum are a continuation of the external intercostals onto the transverse processes of the vertebrae, from the last cervical vertebra to the eleventh thoracic vertebra. Each levator costarum is a triangular slip located in the angle between one of the ribs and the vertebra in front of it, running from the transverse process of the vertebra onto the rib.

The transversus thoracis is a flat muscle that covers part of the inside of the rib cage. Its fibers originate from the corpus and xiphoid process of the sternum; these fibers radiate both horizontally and diagonally upward to insert on the deep surfaces of the second through sixth ribs. The serratus posterior superior arises from the spinous processes of the first few thoracic vertebrae and the seventh cervical vertebra, as well as from the ligaments connecting these spinous processes with one another and with the skull. The fibers converge only slightly and are inserted in four separate slips onto the superior margins of the second through fifth ribs. The serratus posterior inferior is a similar but broader muscle located farther down the spine. It arises from the spinous processes of the last two thoracic and first few lumbar vertebrae, runs diagonally upward, and divides into four separate slips that insert onto the inferior margins of the last four ribs. The rectus abdominis, obliquus externus, obliquus internus, and transversus abdominis are abdominal muscles that pull down on the chest and particularly on the rib cage. The rectus abdominis consists of a strip of muscle fibers running vertically along the ventral midline. The other abdominal muscles are sheetlike and cover the majority of the abdominal surface. Contractions of these muscles generally pull downward on the ribs and oppose the expansion of the rib cage.

The diaphragm is also an axial muscle of the chest cavity. Its muscle fibers originate from the inside of the xiphoid process of the sternum (the sternal portion), from the inner surfaces of the last six ribs and their costal cartilages (the costal portion), and from two muscular arches and two tendinous crura that make up the lumbar portion. The medial lumbocostal arch forms a passage for the greater psoas muscle, while the lateral lumbocostal arch forms a passage for the lumbar quadrate muscle. The right and left crura arise from the ventral surfaces of the first few lumbar vertebrae. Together, the sternal, costal, and lumbar portions of the diaphragm converge upon a sheetlike central tendon, which is divided into large left and right leaflets and a small middle leaflet.

The axial muscles concerned with movements of the thoracic vertebrae include the longus and splenius muscles and the muscles of the erector spinae complex. The longus colli arises from the centra of the last few cervical and first few thoracic vertebrae along their ventral surfaces; it runs upward to insert onto the bodies of the first four cervical vertebrae and the transverse processes of the fifth and sixth cervical vertebrae. The splenius capitis originates from the spinous processes of the last cervical and the first three or four thoracic vertebrae and from the ligaments connecting these processes to one another and to the back of the skull. The muscle inserts onto the occipital and temporal bones on the back of the skull, including the mastoid process. The splenius cervicis arises from the spinous processes of the third through sixth thoracic vertebrae and runs to an insertion on the transverse processes of the first few cervical vertebrae. The muscles of the erector spinae complex include the iliocostalis, longissimus, spinalis, semispinalis, multifidius, rotatores, and intertransversarii. Collectively, these muscles are responsible for dorsal movements (extension) of the vertebral column throughout the lumbar, thoracic, and cervical regions.

The muscles associated developmentally with the extremities are called appendicular muscles. Appendicular muscles of the chest region include the pectoralis, latissimus dorsi, and subclavius. The pectoralis major is triangular in shape; it originates from the sternum, costal cartilages, and a portion of the clavicle, from which its fibers converge toward an insertion onto the greater tuberosity of the humerus. The pectoralis minor originates from the third through fifth ribs and inserts onto the coracoid process of the scapula. The latissimus dorsi is a broad, flat muscle that originates from the lower half of the vertebral column (and part of the ilium) by way of a tough tendinous sheet (the lumbar aponeurosis); it inserts high on the humerus. The

subclavius muscle runs from the bottom surface of the clavicle diagonally onto the first rib. Upon contraction, this muscle helps pull the shoulder inward and the rib cage upward.

Each of the paired breasts consists of a mammary gland, nipple (papilla), areola, and surrounding fat tissue. The breasts are small in children and remain small in most adult men, but they become larger during puberty in women and enlarge even more during late pregnancy and throughout lactation. Toward the end of pregnancy, the gland begins to secrete milk, a white, nutritive fluid containing lactose (milk sugar), proteins, and some fats (more sugar and less fat than in cow's milk). The secretion of milk is known as lactation. During lactation, the mammary gland continues to secrete milk as long as the baby continues nursing. When the child is weaned, the mammary gland undergoes a process of involution (shrinkage). The smaller ducts of the mammary gland collect into larger ducts, each draining a wedge-shaped section of the breast. These larger ducts converge toward a raised nipple (papilla) from which the milk exudes. The nipple is surrounded by a circular area, the areola, characterized by thin skin which is a bit more heavily pigmented (usually redder) than the remainder of the breast.

Disorders and Diseases

A wide variety of medical problems can occur in the chest region, including a number of diseases and traumatic injuries. Because of the presence of the heart and lungs, injuries and diseases of the chest region are often life-threatening and may be fatal. These include diseases of the heart and major vessels, diseases of the lungs and bronchi, and cancer of the breast. Common heart disorders include myocardial infarction, coronary artery disease, and chest pain (angina pectoralis); less serious disorders include arrhythmias and heart murmurs. Disorders of the lungs and bronchi include lung cancer, pulmonary emphysema, and such infectious diseases as tuberculosis, lobar pneumonia, and bronchial pneumonia.

Thoracic specialists include heart specialists (cardiologists), respiratory specialists (pulmonologists), cancer specialists (oncologists), and neuromuscular specialists. Thoracic surgeons specialize in the surgery of the chest. Thoracotomy is a cutting into the thoracic cavity, usually for the repair of the heart, the lungs, or both. Thoracotomy is the first step in open heart surgery, coronary bypass surgery, pacemaker implantation, and heart or lung transplants.

Disorders of the breast are so distinctive that many different specialists are involved. The most fatal of these diseases is breast cancer, often treated by surgical removal of the tumor or of the entire breast. Other breast disorders include mastitis, an inflammation of the breast in women. Rare conditions include the presence of extra (supernumerary) breasts in either sex. Also rare are the hormonal or reproductive disorders that result in the premature enlargement of the female breast or in its failure to develop during adolescence. Enlargement of the breast in males is a condition known as gynecomastia; it often results from abnormal levels of steroid hormones associated with aging and chronic liver disease, but it may arise from other causes. Usually only the fat tissue enlarges in this condition; the mammary gland, nipple, and areola remain underdeveloped. Much less common is a condition called Klinefelter syndrome, in which a tall, thin male develops breasts comparable in size to those of a thirteen-year-old girl. This condition is controlled by a chromosomal defect (XXY). The opposite chromosomal defect (XO) results in Turner syndrome, in which a short female has breasts that enlarge only slightly and that never develop fully. Both Klinefelter and Turner syndromes result in a degree of intellectual disability and in sterility.

Breast surgery may be performed by several types of surgeons, including general surgeons, thoracic surgeons, cancer surgeons, and plastic surgeons. Common surgical operations include the removal of a breast tumor (lumpectomy) or of the entire affected breast (mastectomy) in cases of breast cancer. In addition, plastic surgeons may perform such cosmetic operations as breast augmentation or reduction.

Perspective and Prospects

The heart, lungs, breasts, and major muscles and bones of the chest region were studied by the ancients. The Latin names that are used today are derived in large measure from the writings of Galen, or Caius Galenus, physician to the Roman army in the second century. Renaissance artists such as Leonardo da Vinci (1452-1519) and Michelangelo (1475-1564) dissected human corpses illegally in order to gain further knowledge of these anatomical structures. These studies were followed by the well-illustrated anatomical texts of Andreas Vesalius (1514-1564), who corrected many of Galen's errors.

Good medical understanding of the circulatory system began with the studies of the Renaissance physician William Harvey (1578-1657), who examined the veins in the arms of many patients. It was Harvey who discovered the valves in the veins and who proved that the blood circulates outward from the heart and then back. Anatomists who have described the finer details of the structure of the heart include Jan Evangelista Purkinje (1787-1869) and Wilhelm His Jr. (1863-1934).

—*Eli C. Minkoff, Ph.D.*

See also Anatomy; Aspergillosis; Asthma; Avian influenza; Bones and the skeleton; Breasts, female; Bronchitis; Bypass surgery; Cardiac rehabilitation; Cardiac surgery; Cardiology; Cardiology, pediatric; Cartilage; Choking; Chronic obstructive pulmonary disease (COPD); Common cold; Congenital heart disease; Coronary artery bypass graft; Coughing; Croup; Cystic fibrosis; Electrocardiography (ECG or EKG); Embolism; Emphysema; Heart; Heart transplantation; Heart valve replacement; Heartburn; Hyperbaric oxygen therapy; Interstitial pulmonary fibrosis (IPF); Legionnaires' disease; Lung cancer; Lungs; Pacemaker implantation; Pleurisy; Pneumonia; Pneumothorax; Pulmonary diseases; Pulmonary medicine; Pulmonary medicine, pediatric; Respiration; Respiratory distress syndrome; Resuscitation; Thoracic surgery; Tuberculosis; Wheezing; Whooping cough.

For Further Information:

Agur, Anne M. R., and Arthur F. Dalley. *Grant's Atlas of Anatomy.* 13th ed. Philadelphia: Wolters Kluwer Health/Lippincott Williams & Wilkins, 2012.
"Chest Pain: First Aid." *Mayo Clinic*, February 3, 2012.
Crouch, James E. *Functional Human Anatomy.* 4th ed. Philadelphia: Lea & Febiger, 1985.
Marieb, Elaine N. *Essentials of Human Anatomy and Physiology.* 10th ed. San Francisco: Pearson/Benjamin Cummings, 2011.
Rosse, Cornelius, and Penelope Gaddum-Rosse. *Hollinshead's Textbook of Anatomy.* 5th ed. Philadelphia: Lippincott-Raven, 1997.
Standring, Susan, et al., eds. *Gray's Anatomy.* 40th ed. New York: Churchill Livingstone/Elsevier, 2008.

Chest pain. *See* Angina; Heart attack; Pain.

Chiari malformations

Disease/Disorder
Also known as: Arnold-Chiari malformation
Anatomy or system affected: Brain, muscles, neck, nervous system, spine
Specialties and related fields: Neurology, neurosurgery
Definition: A group of disorders where the cerebellum extends below the opening of the spinal canal (the foramen magnum). Chiari malformations are classified according to severity and how much of the brain extends into the spinal canal: Type I is the most common and may be asymptomatic, type II is considered the classic Chiari malformation, and types III and IV are rare and the most serious.

Key terms:
cerebellum: the part of the brain in the lower rear of the head located just above the brain stem; it controls balance, coordination, and motion
decompression surgery: removal of tissue or bone pressing against the spinal cord or a nerve to make more space and relieve the pressure
dura: a sac that surrounds the brain and spinal cord
foramen magnum: an opening at the bottom of the skull where the nerves from the brain pass through and connect with the spinal cord
herniation: a bulge or protrusion of a body organ beyond the space where it is usually contained
spina bifida: an incomplete closure in the spinal column in which the spinal cord and the membrane around it may stick out through an opening in the back
spinal canal: a tube or tunnel that runs down the spine and contains the spinal cord, which carry the nerves from the brain to the body
syringomyelia: a cyst filled with cerebrospinal fluid that forms in the spinal canal, expands the spinal cord, and stretches the nerve tissue

Causes and Symptoms

Primary or congenital Chiari malformations are a result of structural flaws during fetal development of the brain of spinal canal. The classification of Chiari malformations into four types is based on the extent of the structural flaws. Chiari malformations may also occur after surgery of the head and neck area or after an injury; they are considered secondary or acquired Chiari malformations.

Information on Chiari Malformations

Causes: Structural flaws in the brain and spinal cord during fetal development; for Type I Chiari malformation, sometimes injury or surgery later in life

Symptoms: May be asymptomatic; headaches that are worse with coughing and straining, neck pain, difficulty swallowing, occasionally difficulty speaking, problems with balance and motion, feeling of numbness in arms and legs

Duration: Chronic

Treatments: Pain medication, surgery

Some individuals with type I do not have any symptoms and may not even know they have a Chiari malformation. This type is considered the adult form of the disorder because often symptoms first appear in adolescence or adulthood. Headaches, neck pain, balance problems, dizziness, hearing and vision problems, and numbness in the arms and legs are the symptoms that result from the pressure on nerves caused by the herniation of the cerebellum into the foramen magnum; the symptoms may come and go. A secondary condition called a syringomyelia may develop in some cases, and it can cause permanent nerve damage.

Type II, also known as an Arnold-Chiari malformation, is considered the classic Chiari malformation. In this type, both the cerebellum and part of the brain stem are pushed into the foramen magnum. Type II is a pediatric disorder, and it almost always involves a form of spina bifida.

Types III and IV, also pediatric disorders, are the most serious forms of Chiari malformations and involve significant brain and neurologic defect. Children with these types do not usually live past two years of age.

Treatment and Therapy

Treatment is not necessary for those individuals who do not have symptoms. Otherwise, treatment is based on the severity of the disorder. Pain medications or nonsteroidal anti-inflammatory drugs (NSAIDs), or both, are used to reduce the pain.

Surgery, specifically some type of decompression surgery, is used to alleviate the pressure on the spinal cord and nerves. Various surgical procedures may be performed to reduce pressure by making more room. One frequently used procedure is a posterior fossa decompression, in which a small piece of the skull at the back of the head is taken out; sometimes a piece of synthetic tissue, called a dura patch, is used to enlarge the area for the brain. Another surgical procedure that is used to relieve pressure and make more room is a laminectomy, in which some of the bony border of the spinal canal is removed.

Other surgical procedures, such as insertion of a shunt for drainage of a syringomyelia or surgical closure of the spinal column in spina bifida, may be necessary. Some surgeries for treatment of the pediatric forms of the disorder are done before birth.

Surgery does not cure Chiari malformations, and it cannot undo the nerve damage that has already occurred. Nevertheless, the various surgical procedures can reduce the pressure and relieve the symptoms. Surgery is not always effective, however, and it is possible that a more severe Chiari malformation may result after surgery.

—*Vicki J. Miskovsky*

See also Brain; Brain damage; Brain disorders; Craniotomy; Dizziness and fainting; Head and neck disorders; Headaches; Nervous system; Neuralgia, neuritis, and neuropathy; Neuroimaging; Neurology; Neurology, pediatric; Neurosurgery; Numbness and tingling; Spina bifida; Spinal cord disorders; Spine, vertebrae, and disks.

For Further Information:

McCoy, Krisha. "Arnold-Chiari Syndrome." *Health Library*, Sept. 30, 2012.

National Institute of Neurological Disorders and Stroke. "Chiari Malformation Fact Sheet." *NINDS*, Apr. 18, 2013.

Novegno, F., M. Calderelli, A. Massa, et al. "The Natural History of Chiari Type I Anomaly." *Journal of Neurosurgery Pediatrics* 2, no. 3 (September, 2008): 179-87.

Oakes, W. Jerry, and R. Shane Tubbs. "Management of the Chiari Malformation and Spinal Dysraphism." In *Clinical Neurosurgery*, edited by Guy M. McKhann. Denver: Lippincott Williams and Wilkins, 2004.

Parker, James N. *The Official Parent's Sourcebook on Chiari Malformations*. San Diego, Calif.: Icon Health, 2003.

Chickenpox

Disease/Disorder

Also known as: Varicella

Anatomy or system affected: Mouth, nose, skin

Specialties and related fields: Dermatology, epidemiology, family medicine, immunology, pediatrics, public health, virology

Definition: A highly infectious viral disease occurring primarily in children. Chickenpox is characterized by weakness, fever, and a generalized body rash.

Key terms:

antihistamine: a medicine used to treat allergic reactions

encephalitis: inflammation of the brain

malaise: a feeling of weakness or discomfort

pruritus: itching

vesicles: small, fluid-filled bumps

Causes and Symptoms

Chickenpox is an acute, highly infectious viral disease occurring primarily, but not exclusively, in children. Each year, between three and four million cases are reported in the United States, with the highest incidence occurring during the late winter and early spring. About ten to thirteen thousand of those affected became so ill that they require hospitalization; since the introduction of the varicella-zoster virus vaccine, the number of cases and the number of hospitalizations have dropped significantly.

The varicella-zoster virus (VZV) is responsible for chickenpox infection. Physical contact with an infected individual is not required, as the virus is transmitted from person to person via an airborne route.

Symptoms begin to appear about eleven to fifteen days after exposure. At first, they may resemble those of the common cold: sore throat, runny nose, malaise, and fever. Soon, red spots appear on the body, usually beginning on the trunk and scalp and spreading outward. Occasionally, the mucous membranes are affected as well, with spots appearing in the mouth and nasal passages. The spots develop into vesicles-raised bumps with clear, teardrop-shaped blisters that turn rapidly to crusty lesions within six to eight hours. The rash occurs in waves, with new spots developing as old ones heal and disappear. By the fifth or sixth day, no new lesions will develop, and the crusts will be gone in less than twenty days.

Chickenpox causes intense itchiness. The impulse to scratch can be overwhelming and can lead to one of the most common complications: bacterial skin infections. Scratching the lesions can also lead to ugly pox scarring. Other possible complications of chickenpox include viral pneumonia and viral encephalitis.

The diagnosis of chickenpox is almost always done on the basis of its symptoms, most notably its characteristic rash accompanied by fever. In the event that confirmation of the disease is necessary, the fluid in the lesions can be cultured, although by the time results are obtained (five to ten days), the disease is usually on its way to resolution.

Treatment and Therapy

In children, chickenpox, uncomfortable although it may be, is not considered a serious illness. The vast majority of

A child with chickenpox. (AP/Wide World Photos)

Information on Chickenpox
Causes: Infection with varicella-zoster virus
Symptoms: Generalized body rash, intense itching, malaise, weakness, fever, sore throat, runny nose
Duration: Two to three weeks
Treatments: None; alleviation of symptoms

cases are uncomplicated and resolve themselves within two to three weeks. Treatment is therefore primarily symptomatic, with an emphasis on controlling itching and reducing fever.

Oral antihistamines such as Benadryl (diphenhydramine) and Atarax (hydroxyzine) are effective in managing pruritus. Topical treatments, such as calamine lotion, and wet compresses may offer almost immediate relief. Fever is treated with acetaminophen. Aspirin is not an option because of its link to Reye's syndrome, a potentially fatal condition characterized by vomiting, disorientation, and eventual coma. Ibuprofen should also be avoided, as it may be linked to secondary infections.

Some parents trim short the fingernails of infected children to keep them from scratching away the crusts of chickenpox lesions. This is one way of reducing the risk of secondary bacterial infections. Frequent bathing is also helpful in preventing this complication.

Although there is no cure for chickenpox, the oral antiviral drugs acyclovir, valacyclovir, and famciclovir have been shown to be effective in decreasing the intensity of itching, hastening the healing of skin lesions, and generally shortening the duration of the disease. To be effective, treatment must begin within twenty-four hours of the appearance of the rash.

The use of acyclovir is not recommended for most children because of the relatively benign nature of the disease in this age group. However, for some high-risk children, such as premature infants, therapy should be started within twenty-four hours of the onset of illness. In adolescents older than age thirteen, adults, and immunocompromised individuals, however, chickenpox may have severe complications, and this increased risk may be lessened with acyclovir therapy.

Affected newborns and immunocompromised persons may receive gammaglobulin intravenously or oral acyclovir immediately following exposure to the virus.

Perspective and Prospects

Chickenpox has been around for so long that there are conflicting accounts about how it got its name. One theory has it that when chickenpox was first described, it was noted that its lesions looked as if they were placed upon the skin rather than arising from the skin itself. They were compared to chickpeas-hence the name. Another idea is that the term "chickenpox" was intended to distinguish this weaker pox illness from the more life-threatening smallpox-the term "chicken" being used, as in "chickenhearted," to mean weak or timid.

Chickenpox was not considered a distinct rash disease

until 1553, when the Italian physician Filippo Ingrassia differentiated it from scarlet fever. In 1785, the English physician William Heberden gave the earliest clear description of varicella, having distinguished it from smallpox in 1768. In 1924, T. M. Rivers and W. S. Tillett reported the isolation of the chickenpox virus.

Throughout history, the treatment of chickenpox has been symptomatic. In the 1970s, however, a vaccine became available for persons in high-risk categories. In 1995, a vaccine called Varivax was approved by the US Federal Food and Drug Administration for use in children over the age of one; other brands of the vaccine are available in Canada, the United Kingdom, and Australia. Varivax is 70 to 90 percent effective in preventing chickenpox over the short term. Vaccinated individuals who still develop chickenpox get a milder form of the disease. Immunity from the vaccine may wane over time, so booster shots may be needed. The vaccine's ability to provide long-term protection from chickenpox is still unknown.

—Robert T. Klose, Ph.D.

See also Childhood infectious diseases; Herpes; Immunization and vaccination; Itching; Lesions; Rashes; Shingles; Skin disorders; Viral infections.

For Further Information:

A.D.A.M. Medical Encyclopedia. "Chickenpox." *MedlinePlus*, August 2, 2011.

Alan, Rick, and Michael Woods. "Chickenpox (Varicella)." *Health Library*, October 11, 2012.

Behrman, Richard E., et al. *Nelson Textbook of Pediatrics*. 19th ed. Philadelphia: Saunders/Elsevier, 2011.

Kiple, Kenneth F., ed. *The Cambridge World History of Human Disease*. New York: Cambridge University Press, 2008.

Kump, Theresa. "Chicken-Pox Survival Guide." *Parents* 69, no. 5 (May, 1994): 29-31.

Marquis, Julie. "Chickenpox Vaccine Is Swaying Skeptics." *Los Angeles Times*, June 21, 2000, p. 1.

National Center for Immunization and Respiratory Diseases, Division of Viral Diseases. "Monitoring the Impact of Varicella Vaccination."*Centers for Disease Control and Prevention*, August 30, 2012.

Sadovsky, Richard. "Safety and Effectiveness of Varicella Vaccine." *American Family Physician* 61, no. 7 (April 1, 2000): 2209.

"Varicella (Chickenpox)." In *Conn's Current Therapy*, edited by Rick D. Kellerman et al. Philadelphia: Saunders/Elsevier, 2012.

Whitley, Richard J. "Varicella-Zoster Virus." In *Mandell, Douglas, and Bennett's Principles and Practice of Infectious Diseases*, edited by Gerald L. Mandell, John F. Bennett, and Raphael Dolin. 7th ed. New York: Churchill Livingstone/Elsevier, 2010.

Childbirth

Biology

Anatomy or system affected: Reproductive system, uterus

Specialties and related fields: Gynecology, neonatology, obstetrics, perinatology

Definition: The process whereby a fetus moves from the uterus to outside the mother's body-a natural event that normally requires no, or minimal, medical intervention.

Key terms:

birth canal: the passageway from the uterus to the outside of the mother's body formed by the fully opened cervix in continuity with the vagina

cervix: a ring of tissue at the lowest and narrowest part of the uterus forming a canal that opens into the vagina

contraction: a squeezing action of the uterus that results in birth

dilation: the opening of the cervix to allow passage of the fetus through the birth canal

hormone: a chemical carried in the blood that acts as a messenger between two or more body parts

labor: the period in the birth process in which forceful and rhythmic uterine contractions are present

placenta: a structure located inside the uterus during pregnancy that provides oxygen to the fetus, removes fetal wastes, and produces hormones; also known as the afterbirth

prostaglandins: chemical messengers that are not carried in the blood and that function only locally

uterus: the organ in the female pelvis that supports the fetus during pregnancy and expels it during birth; also known as the womb

vagina: the stretchy tubular structure that leads from the uterus to the outside of the mother's body; part of the birth canal

Process and Effects

In humans, pregnancy lasts an average of forty weeks, counting from the first day of the woman's last menstrual cycle. Actually, ovulation, and therefore conception and the start of pregnancy, does not normally occur until about two weeks after the beginning of the last menstrual period, but because there is no good external indicator of the time of ovulation, obstetricians and other health care providers typically count the weeks of pregnancy using the easily observed last period of menstrual bleeding as a reference point. Because of the uncertainty about the actual time of ovulation and conception, the calculated due date for an infant's birth may be inaccurate by as much as two weeks in either direction.

There is incomplete understanding of the processes that determine the timing and initiation of childbirth. Near the end of pregnancy, the uterus undergoes changes that prepare it for the birth process: The cervix softens and becomes stretchy, the cells in the uterus acquire characteristics that enable them to contract in a coordinated fashion, and the uterus becomes more responsive to hormones that cause contractions.

A number of substances are involved in the preparation of the uterus for birth, including the hormones estrogen and progesterone (produced within the placenta), the hormone relaxin (from the maternal ovary and/or uterus), and prostaglandins (produced within the uterus). The fetus participates in this preparation, since it provides precursors necessary for the uterine synthesis of estrogens. In addition, the amnion and chorion (the placenta and umbilical cord), two membranes surrounding the fetus, are capable of producing prostaglandins that assist in the preparation of the uterus.

Once labor begins, the hormone oxytocin (from the maternal pituitary gland) and uterine prostaglandins cause uterine contractions. It is not known what triggers the onset of labor or how the preparatory hormones and prostaglandins work together. However, a 2009 study indicated that labor may be triggered by elevated levels of placental corticotrophin-release hormone (CRH), which promotes the production of a steroid hormone called DHEAS by the fetal adrenal gland. The placenta is then thought to convert the steroid hormone into estriol, and the increasing imbalance between estriol and estradiol (both estrogens) may be responsible for inducing labor. Typically, estradiol blocks estriol's actions, but as the imbalance between these two estrogens increases, estriol is able to activate proteins in the uterine muscles, which then produce prostaglandins that promote muscle cell contraction.

In humans, the onset of labor is indicated by one or more of three signs: the beginning of regular, rhythmic uterine contractions; the rupture of the amniotic membrane, a painless event that is usually accompanied by the leakage of clear fluid from the vagina; and the expulsion of a slightly bloody mucus plug from the cervix, which is an indication that the cervix is beginning to dilate. These signs may appear in any order, or occasionally one sign may be absent or unnoticed. For example, the amniotic membrane may fail to rupture spontaneously; in this case, the attendant will usually pierce the membrane to facilitate the birth.

Uterine contractions are the most prominent indication of labor, which is divided into three stages. In the first stage of labor, the contractions have the effect of dilating the cervix from its initial size of only a few millimeters to full dilation of 10 centimeters, large enough to permit the passage of the fetus. When the first stage of labor starts, the contractions may be up to twenty minutes apart, with each contraction of relatively short duration. As the first stage progresses, the contractions become longer and closer together, so that by the end of the first stage there may be only a minute between contractions. There is no downward movement of the fetus during the first stage of labor, but the contractions do force the fetus against the cervix, and this

Stages of Childbirth

Stage one

Symphysis pubis
Urinary bladder
Urethra
Vagina
Cervix
Rectum

Ruptured amniotic sac

Placenta

Placenta
Uterus
Umbilical cord

Ties

Stage two

Stage three

force is important in causing cervical dilation. This first stage lasts for an average of eleven hours in women giving birth for the first time, but up to twenty hours is considered normal. The average length of the first stage of labor in women who have previously delivered is reduced to seven hours, with a norm of up to fourteen hours.

In the second stage of labor, the fetus moves downward through the fully dilated cervix and then into the vagina as a result of the force exerted by the continuing uterine contractions. Voluntary contractions of the abdominal muscles by the mother can help shorten this stage of labor by applying additional force, but in the absence of voluntary contractions (as with an anesthetized mother), the uterine contractions are usually sufficient to cause delivery. In approximately 96 percent of human births, the fetus is situated so that the head is downward and thus is first to pass through the birth canal. Because the vagina does not lie in the same line as the cervix and uterus, the head of the fetus must flex and rotate as the fetus progresses downward past the mother's pelvic bones. The final barrier to the birth of the fetus is the soft tissue surrounding the vaginal opening; once the head of the fetus passes through and stretches this opening, the rest of the body usually slips out readily. The average duration of this second stage of labor in women delivering for the first time is slightly more than one hour; the average duration is shortened to twenty-four minutes in women who have previously delivered. Most women agree that the actual birth of the child during the second stage is less uncomfortable than the strong uterine contractions that occur at the very end of the first stage of labor, when the cervix is dilating the last centimeter or so.

Most infants begin to take regular, deep breaths immediately upon delivery. These breaths serve to inflate the lungs with air for the first time. The infant now becomes dependent on breathing to supply oxygen to the blood, whereas oxygen had been supplied to the fetal blood by circulation through the placenta.

Following delivery of the infant, the mother enters the third stage of labor, during which continued uterine contractions serve to reduce the size of the uterus and expel the placenta. The placenta usually separates from the uterus and is expelled five to fifteen minutes after the birth of the infant.

Uterine contractions do not end with the delivery of the placenta; they continue, with decreasing frequency and intensity, for as long as six weeks following childbirth. These later contractions, known as afterpains, serve to reduce bleeding from the site of placental attachment and to return the uterus and cervix to their prepregnancy condition.

Another significant process that occurs in the mother's body following delivery is the onset of milk production. During pregnancy, the breasts are prepared for later milk production by a number of hormones, but actual milk production does not begin until about the second day after delivery. It appears that the decrease in progesterone levels caused by the removal of the placenta at birth allows milk production to commence.

Most obstetrical attendants agree that the ideal childbirth situation is a labor and delivery with a minimum of medical intervention. If all goes well, the role of the attendant will be primarily that of a support person. Most women are admitted to a hospital or birthing center during the first stage of labor. The mother's blood pressure and temperature will be checked frequently. In addition, the strength and timing of contractions will be assessed either by a hand placed lightly on the abdomen or by an electronic monitor that detects uterine activity through a sensor belt placed around the abdomen. The fetal heart rate will be measured with a stethoscope or by this same electronic monitor placed on the mother's abdomen. Fetal well-being may also be monitored by an electrode placed on the scalp of the fetus through the cervix. This scalp pH probe indicates whether the fetus is tolerating labor well or is in distress. Cervical dilation can be assessed by a vaginal examination: The attendant will insert one or more fingers into the cervix to determine its state of dilation. It is also important that the attendant provide emotional support and reassurance to the mother throughout the delivery.

During the second stage of labor, the attendant will monitor the progress of the fetus through the birth canal. By inserting a hand into the vagina and feeling for the fetal skull bones, the attendant can determine the exact placement of the fetus within the birth canal. As the infant's head appears at the vaginal opening, an incision called an episiotomy is usually performed to prevent accidental tearing of these tissues. Many physicians believe that episiotomy should be done to prevent possible vaginal tearing, since a planned incision is easier to repair than an accidental tear. Another advantage of episiotomy is that it tends to speed the expulsion of the infant, which may be an advantage to both the mother and the child at this stage. The episiotomy incision is made after the injection of a local anesthetic to numb the area, and the incision is stitched closed following the delivery of the placenta.

Once the infant's head has emerged from the vagina, the attendant uses a suction device to clear the infant's nose and mouth of fluid. As the rest of the infant emerges, the attendant supports the body; a quick examination is conducted at this time to determine whether the infant has any major health problems. The umbilical cord that joins the infant to the placenta is usually cut within a few minutes after birth. When the placenta is delivered, the attendant will examine it for completeness and then will perform a thorough examination of the mother and child to ensure that all is well.

Complications and Disorders

If the labor and delivery do not progress normally, the attendant has available a number of medical interventions that will promote the safety of both the mother and the baby. For example, labor may be induced by administration of oxytocin through an intravenous catheter. Such induction is performed if the amniotic membrane ruptures without the spontaneous onset of uterine contractions, if the pregnancy progresses well beyond the due date, or in response to maternal indicators such as hypertension. The induction of labor has been found to be safe, but careful monitoring of the progress of labor is required.

Another fairly common procedure is the use of forceps to assist delivery. These tonglike instruments have two large loops that are placed on the sides of the fetal head when the head is in the birth canal. Forceps are not used to pull the fetus from the birth canal; instead, they are used to guide the fetus through the birth canal and to assist in the downward movement of the fetus during contractions. The use of forceps can help to speed the second stage of labor, and injury to the fetus or the mother is minimal when the forceps are not applied until the fetal head is well within the birth canal, as is the convention. Some type of anesthesia is always used with a forceps delivery. In some areas, vacuum extraction of the fetus is preferred. As the name implies, vacuum extraction makes use of a suction cup on the end of a vacuum hose; the suction cup is affixed to the fetal scalp.

Many women require some type of pain relief during labor, although this need can be reduced by thorough education and preparedness during the pregnancy. A wide range of pain-reducing drugs (analgesics), sedatives, and tranquilizers is available for use during the first stage of labor. These are typically administered by injection; they work at the level of the brain to alter the perception of pain and to promote relaxation. The goal is to use the minimum drug dose that allows the woman to be comfortable. The main danger is that these drugs reach the fetus through the placental circulation; side effects in the infant, which can persist for many hours after delivery, may include depressed respiration, irregular heart rhythm or rate, and sleepiness accompanied by poor suckling response.

Anesthetics that numb pain-carrying nerves in the mother may also be used during the first and second stages of labor. Two routes of delivery are in common use: epidural and spinal, both of which involve the injection of anesthetic drugs into or near the membranes around the mother's spinal cord. The epidural route of injection places the anesthetic in a space that lies outside the spinal cord membranes; with spinal anesthesia, the injection is made slightly deeper into the membranous layers. An advantage of both methods is that the mother remains awake during the delivery and can assist by pushing during the second stage.

Although the disadvantages of both anesthetics, and especially of epidurals, have been downplayed, these procedures do impose restrictions on the mother. Once an epidural has been given, for example, a woman must stay in bed because it will be difficult for her to move her legs; some hospitals do offer "mobile epidurals," which use a type of drug that blocks the pain while still allowing the woman to walk around, but these are the exception. Because walking helps to stimulate labor, the use of epidurals can be counterproductive. The use of epidurals is also associated with a prolongation of the second stage of labor and with increased need for forceps to assist delivery. Headaches, backaches, low blood pressure, nausea, and other side effects may result in the mother following the use of anesthetics. Moreover, contrary to past evidence, recent studies have suggested that the drugs in epidurals do cross the placenta to the baby, causing health risks.

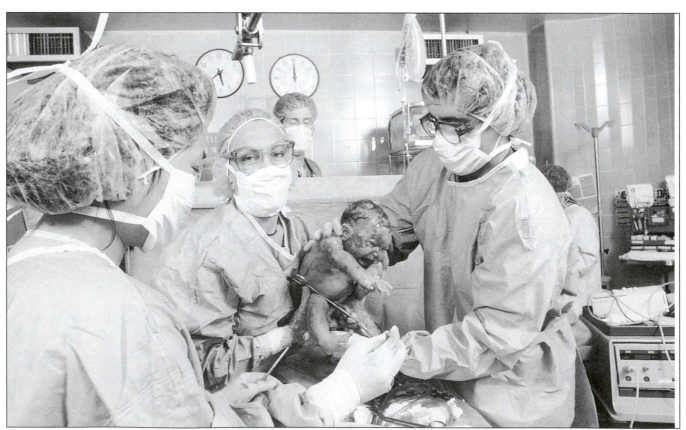

A newborn is delivered by cesarean section. (PhotoDisc)

General anesthesia refers to the use of drugs that induce sleep; they may be administered by inhalation or by injection. Because of profound side effects in both the mother and child, most physicians use general anesthesia only in an emergency situation requiring an immediate cesarean section.

Cesarean section refers to the delivery of the fetus through an incision made in the mother's abdominal and uterine walls. (The name derives from an unsubstantiated legend that Julius Caesar was delivered in this way.) Cesarean deliveries may be planned in advance, as when a physician notes that the fetus is in a difficult-to-deliver position, such as breech (buttocks downward) or transverse (sideways). Multiple fetuses may also be delivered by cesarean section in order to spare the mother and her infants excessive stress. Alternatively, cesarean delivery may be performed as an emergency measure, perhaps after labor has started. As fetal monitoring techniques have improved, problems are noted more quickly and with greater frequency, leading to a larger number of cesarean sections. One indication of the need for emergency cesarean delivery is fetal distress, a condition characterized by an abnormal fetal heart rate and rhythm. Fetal distress is thought to be an indication of reduced blood flow to the placenta, which may be life-threatening to the fetus. Cesarean section may be performed using spinal or epidural anesthesia, as well as general anesthesia. A woman who delivers one child by cesarean section does not necessarily require a cesarean for later deliveries; each pregnancy is evaluated separately. Attempted vaginal births after cesareans (AVBACs) are still being done but are decreasing in frequency due to increased likelihood of problems.

Perspective and Prospects

Prior to 1800, most women were attended during childbirth by female midwives. In some areas, a midwife was provided a salary by the town or region; her contract might stipulate that she provide services to all women regardless of financial or social status. In other areas, midwives worked for fees paid by the clients. Midwives of this time had little, if any, formal training and learned about birth practices from other women. Because birth was considered a natural event requiring little intervention on the part of the attendant, the midwife's medical role was limited and the few doctors available were consulted only in difficult cases. Although birth statistics were not kept at the time, anecdotal accounts from the diaries of midwives and doctors suggest that the births were most often successful, with rare cases of maternal or infant deaths.

The nineteenth century saw a gradual shift away from the use of midwives to a preference for formally trained male doctors. This shift was made possible by the establishment of medical schools that provided scientific training in obstetrics. Because these schools were generally closed to women, only men received this training and had access to the instruments and anesthesia that were coming into use.

Maternity hospitals came into being during the nineteenth century but were at first used primarily by poor or unmarried women. Women of higher social status still preferred to deliver their children in the privacy of their homes. Indeed, home birth was safer than hospital birth, since the building of hospitals had outpaced the knowledge of how to sanitize them. Rates of infection and maternal and infant death were higher in hospitals than in homes.

By the 1930s, the situation had reversed: Hospital births had become safer than home births, because sanitation and surgical procedures had improved. There followed an increasing trend for women to enter hospitals for delivery, so that the percentage of women giving birth in hospitals increased from about 25 percent in 1930 to almost 100 percent by 1960. In the same period, maternal and infant mortality showed a dramatic reduction. The shift to hospital birth had coincided with an interventionist philosophy: Most women were anesthetized during delivery, and forceps deliveries and episiotomy became more common.

By the 1960s, the older idea of "natural" childbirth-that is, a birth that encourages active labor and the use of drug-free types of pain relief with as little medical intervention as possible-had regained popularity. This change in attitude was brought about in part by recognition that analgesic and anesthetic drugs often had profound effects on the infant and often prevented strong mother-infant bonding in the immediate hours after delivery.

It was also brought about by the Lamaze method of childbirth, conceived by French doctor Fernand Lamaze and introduced to the United States with Marjorie Karmel's book *Thank You, Dr. Lamaze* (1959). In this method, women learn controlled breathing techniques to relax and to cope with contractions during labor. A labor coach, who is often the baby's father, helps to initiate and facilitate these techniques. Because natural childbirth must be learned, usually through childbirth classes offered in hospitals during the last trimester of pregnancy, it is also called prepared childbirth. As an extension of natural childbirth, the LeBoyer method has been proposed, allowing for delivery to take place underwater, so that the fetus is expelled from the fluid-filled amniotic sac into a warm, peaceful, fluid-filled environment, allowing for an easier transition to extrauterine life.

By the latter part of the twentieth century, a compromise between the more radical approaches of the past seemed to have been reached, with common practice in obstetrics being to allow the birth to proceed naturally when possible, but with the advantage of having refined drugs, diagnostics, and surgical techniques available if needed. The midwife has been reinstated as a specially trained advanced practice nurse (certified nurse midwife) who provides comprehensive health care to pregnant and nonpregnant women, and who conducts deliveries under a variety of settings, collaborating with physician colleagues as necessary for medically complicated labor and birth.

—Marcia Watson-Whitmyre, Ph.D. and
Cassandra Kircher, Ph.D.;
updated by Robin Kamienny Montvilo, R.N., Ph.D.

See also Amniocentesis; Assisted reproductive technologies; Birth defects; Breast-feeding; Cesarean section; Childbirth complications; Chorionic villus sampling; Conception; Ectopic pregnancy; Embryology; Episiotomy; Fetal alcohol syndrome; Gynecology; In vitro fertilization; Miscarriage; Multiple births; Neonatology; Obstetrics; Perinatology; Placenta; Postpartum depression; Pregnancy and gestation; Premature birth; Reproductive system; Stillbirth; Ultrasonography; Umbilical cord; Uterus; Women's health.

For Further Information:

Ammer, Christine. *The New A to Z of Women's Health: A Concise Encyclopedia*. 6th ed. New York: Checkmark Books, 2009.

Beckmann, Charles R. B., et al., eds. Obstetrics and Gynecology. 7th ed. Baltimore: Lippincott Williams & Wilkins, 2013.

Creasy, Robert K., et al., eds. *Creasy & Resnik's Maternal-Fetal Medicine: Principles and Practice*. 6th ed. Philadelphia: W. B. Saunders, 2008.

Cunningham, F. Gary, et al., eds. *Williams Obstetrics*. 23d ed. New York: McGraw-Hill, 2010.

DeCherney, Alan, et al., eds. Current Diagnosis & Treatment: Obstetrics & Gynecology. 11th ed. New York: McGraw Hill, 2012.

Klaus, Marshall H., John H. Kennell, and Phyllis H. Klaus. *Doula Book: How a Trained Labor Companion Can Help You Have a Shorter, Easier, and Healthier Birth*. 2d ed. Reading, Mass.: Perseus, 2002.

Klein, M. C., et al. "Why Do Women Go Along with This Stuff?" *Birth* 33, no. 3 (September, 2006): 245-250.

"Labor and Birth." *US Department of Health and Human Services Office on Women's Health*, September 27, 2010.

Lees, Christoph, and Grainne McCarten. *Pregnancy and Birth: Your Questions Answered*. Rev. ed. New York: DK, 2012.

Quilligan, Edward J., and Frederick P. Zuspan, eds. *Current Therapy in Obstetrics and Gynecology*. 5th ed. Philadelphia: W. B. Saunders, 2000.

Simkin, Penny, et al. *Pregnancy, Childbirth, and the Newborn: The Complete Guide*. 4th ed. Minnetonka, Minn.: Meadowbrook Press, 2010.

Childbirth complications

Disease/Disorder

Anatomy or system affected: Reproductive system, uterus

Specialties and related fields: Gynecology, neonatology, obstetrics

Definition: The difficulties that can occur during childbirth, either for the mother or for the baby.

With medical monitoring and diagnostic tests, about 5 to 10 percent of pregnant women can be diagnosed as having high-risk pregnancies, and appropriate precautions and preparations for possible complications can be made prior to labor. Yet up to 60 percent of complications of labor, childbirth, and the postpartum period (immediately after birth) occur in women with no prior indications of possible complications. Difficulties in childbirth can be placed into two general categories-problems with labor and problems with the child-and encompass a wide range of causes and possible treatments.

Complications of labor. Cesarean birth (also called cesarean section, C-section, or a section) is the surgical removal of the baby from the mother. An increasing number of infants are delivered by cesarean birth. In this procedure, one incision is made through the mother's abdomen and a second through her uterus. The baby is physically removed from the mother's uterus, and the incisions are closed. This type of surgery is very safe but carries with it the general risks of any major surgery and requires approximately five days of hospitalization. In some cases, diagnosed preexist-

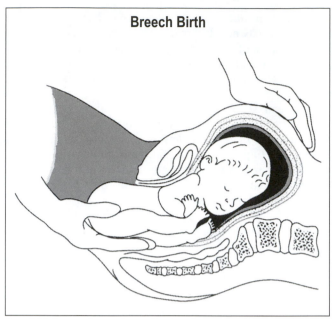

Breech Birth

Breech birth, one of several complications that may occur during childbirth, is the emergence of the infant buttocks-first rather than head-first; such a birth is risky for the child, and often birth is accomplished by cesarean section, a surgical procedure to eliminate that risk.

ing conditions suggest that a cesarean birth is necessary and can be planned; in the majority of cases, unexpected difficulties during labor dictate that an emergency cesarean section be performed.

Some conditions leave no question about the necessity of a cesarean section. These absolute indications include a variety of physical abnormalities. Placenta previa is a condition in which the placenta has implanted in the lower part of the uterus instead of in the normal upper portion, thereby totally or partially blocking the cervix. The baby would not be able to pass down the birth canal without dislodging or tearing the placenta, thereby interrupting the baby's blood and oxygen supply. Placenta previa is frequently the cause of painless bleeding after the twentieth week of pregnancy, and it can be definitively diagnosed by ultrasound. Sometimes a low-lying placenta will migrate to a higher uterine position, but this condition requires careful monitoring. Bed rest may be ordered, and a cesarean section may be performed before the onset of labor.

Placental separation, also known as placenta abruptio, is the result of the placenta partially or completely separating from the uterus prior to birth. This condition results in painful bleeding, with either mild or extreme blood loss depending on the severity of the separation. If severe, up to four pints of blood may be lost, increasing risks related to maternal hemorrhage, including disseminated intravascular coagulation (DIC). Transfusions may be ordered, along with emergency cesarean section.

Occasionally, as the baby begins traveling down the birth canal, the umbilical cord slips and lies ahead of the baby. This condition, called prolapsed cord, is very serious because the pressure of the baby against the cord during a vaginal delivery would compress the cord to the extent that the baby's blood and oxygen supply would be cut off. This condition necessitates an emergency cesarean section.

Some conditions that occur during labor are judged for their potential for causing harm to either the mother or the baby. The physician's decision to proceed with vaginal delivery will be based on the severity of the complication and consideration of the best option for the mother and baby. A few of the more common indicators for possible cesarean section which occur during labor include a fetal head size that is too large for the mother's birth canal; fetal distress, evidenced by insufficient oxygen supply reaching the baby; rupturing of the membranes without labor commencing or prolonged labor after membranes burst (usually twenty-four hours); and inelasticity of the pelvis in first-time mothers over forty years of age.

Other maternal conditions are diagnosed prior to the onset of labor, and the physician or midwife may or may not recommend a cesarean birth based on the severity of the complication. These include postmaturity, in which the onset of labor is at least two weeks overdue and degeneration of the placenta may compromise the health of the baby; maternal diseases, such as diabetes mellitus and eclampsia, in which the stress of labor would be highly risky to the mother; and previous cesarean section.

Complications with the baby. Premature labor can occur between twenty and thirty-six weeks gestation, and a premature infant is considered to be any infant born before thirty-seven weeks of gestational age. Certain maternal illnesses or abnormalities of the placenta can lead to premature birth, but in 60 percent of the cases there is no identifiable cause. If labor begins six weeks or more before the due date, the best chance of infant survival occurs when the baby is delivered and cared for at a hospital with a perinatal center and specialized intensive care for premature infants. The survival rate of premature infants increases with age, weight, and body system maturity.

In about 4 percent of births, the baby is in the breech position-buttocks first or other body part preceding the head-rather than in the normal head-down position. Delivery in this position is complicated because the cervix will not dilate properly and the head may not be able to pass through the cervix. Other complications of breech position are prolapse or compression of the umbilical cord and trauma to the baby if delivered vaginally. Manual techniques may be used to rotate the baby into the correct position. Vaginal delivery may be attempted, frequently aided by gentle forceps removal of the baby. Breech babies are frequently born by cesarean section.

Cephalopelvic disproportion is a condition in which the baby's head is larger than the pelvic opening of the mother. This can be determined only after labor has begun, because the mother's muscles and joints expand to accommodate the baby's head. If at some point during labor it is determined that the baby will not fit through the mother's pelvic opening, a cesarean section will be performed.

—*Clair Kaplan, A.P.R.N./M.S.N.;
additional material by Karen E. Kalumuck, Ph.D.*

See also Birth defects; Cesarean section; Childbirth; Diabetes mellitus; Episiotomy; Gestational diabetes; Multiple births; Obstetrics; Placenta; Postpartum depression; Preeclampsia and eclampsia; Pregnancy and gestation; Premature birth; Reproductive system; Stillbirth; Toxemia; Umbilical cord; Uterus; Women's health.

For Further Information:
Campos, Bonnie C., and Jennifer Brown. *Protect Your Pregnancy.* New York: McGraw, 2004.

Carlson, Karen J., Stephanie A. Eisenstat, and Terra Ziporyn. *The New Harvard Guide to Women's Health.* Cambridge, Mass.: Harvard UP, 2004.

Gonik, Bernard, and Renee A. Bobrowski. *Medical Complications in Labor and Delivery.* Cambridge, Mass.: Blackwell, 1996.

Hotchner, Tracie. *Pregnancy and Childbirth.* Rev. ed. New York: Quill, 2003.

MedlinePlus. "Childbirth Problems." *MedlinePlus*, May 6, 2013.

Mishell, Daniel R., et al. *Management of Common Problems in Obstetrics and Gynecology.* 4th ed. Hoboken, N.J.: Wiley, 2010.

Moore, Keith L., and T. V. N. Persaud. *The Developing Human.* 8th ed. Philadelphia: Saunders, 2008.

Sears, William, and Martha Sears. *The Birth Book: Everything You Need to Know to Have a Safe and Satisfying Birth.* Boston: Little, 1994.

Stoppard, Miriam. *Conception, Pregnancy, and Birth.* Rev. ed. New York: DK, 2005.

Childhood infectious diseases
Disease/Disorder

Anatomy or system affected: Gastrointestinal system, immune system, lungs, muscles, musculoskeletal system, nose, respiratory system

Specialties and related fields: Bacteriology, epidemiology, family medicine, immunology, internal medicine, pediatrics, public health, virology

Definition: A group of diseases including diphtheria, tetanus, measles, polio, rubella (German measles), mumps, varicella (chickenpox), hepatitis, and pertussis (whooping cough).

Key terms:

anorexia: diminished appetite or aversion to food

conjunctivitis: inflammation of the conjunctiva, which lines the back of the eyelid, extends into the space between the lid and the globe of the eye, and goes over the globe to the transparent tissue covering the pupil

erythematous: related to or marked by reddening

malaise: a general feeling of discomfort, of being "out of sorts"

nuchal rigidity: stiffening of the back of the neck

oophoritis: inflammation of the ovary

orchitis: inflammation of the testis

photophobia: dread or avoidance of light

prodrome: a forewarning symptom of a disease

rhinitis: inflammation of the nasal mucous membrane

salivary glands: the glands that produce saliva

Causes and Symptoms

Acute communicable diseases occur primarily in childhood because most adults have become immune to such diseases, either by having acquired them as children or by having been inoculated against them. For example, prior to the use of vaccine for measles-a highly contagious disease found in most of the world-the peak incidence of the disease was in five- to ten-year-olds. Most adults were immune. Before a vaccine was developed and used against measles, epidemics occurred at two- to four-year intervals in large cities. Today, most cases are found in nonimmunized preschool children or in teenagers or young adults who have received only one dose of the vaccine.

Measles, a highly contagious virus, is a leading cause of fatalities among children worldwide. A person infected with red measles (also known as rubeola) becomes contagious about ten days after exposure to the disease virus, at which time the prodromal stage begins. Typically, the infected person experiences three days of slight to moderate fever, a runny nose, increasing cough, and conjunctivitis. During the prodromal stage, Koplik's spots appear inside the cheeks opposite the lower molars. These lesions-grayish white dots about the size of sand particles with a slightly reddish halo surrounding them that are occasionally hemorrhagic-are important in the diagnosis of measles.

After the prodrome, a rash appears, usually accompanied by an abrupt increase in temperature (sometimes as high as 104 or 105 degrees Fahrenheit). It begins in the form of small, faintly red spots and progresses to large, dusky red confluent areas, often slightly hemorrhagic. The rash frequently begins behind the ears but spreads rapidly over the entire face, neck, upper arms, and upper part of the chest within the first twenty-four hours. During the next twenty-four hours, it spreads over the back, abdomen, entire arms, and thighs. When it finally reaches the feet after the second or third day of the rash, it is already fading from the face. At this point, the fever is usually disappearing as well.

The chief complications of measles are middle-ear infections, pneumonia, and encephalitis (a severe infection of the brain). There is no correlation between the severity of the case of measles and the development of encephalitis, but the incidence of the infection of the brain runs to only one or two per every thousand cases. Measles can also exacerbate tuberculosis.

The incubation period for rubella (German measles) lasts between fourteen and twenty-one days, and the disease occurs primarily in children between the ages of two and ten. Like the initial rash of measles, the initial rash of rubella usually starts behind the ears, but children with rubella normally have no symptoms save for the rash and a low-grade fever for one day. Adolescents may have a three-day prodromal period of malaise, runny nose, and mild conjunctivitis; adolescent girls may have arthritis in several joints that lasts for weeks. The red spots begin behind the ears and then spread to the face, neck, trunk, and extremities. This rash may coalesce and last up to five days. Temperature may be normal or slightly elevated. Complications from rubella are relatively uncommon, but if pregnant women are not immune to the disease and are exposed to the rubella virus during early pregnancy, severe congenital anomalies may result. Because similar symptoms and rashes develop in many viral diseases, rubella is difficult to diagnose clinically. Except in known epidemics, laboratory confirmation is often necessary.

The patient with mumps is likely to have fever, malaise, headache, and anorexia-all usually mild-but "neck swelling," a painful enlargement of the parotid gland near the ear, is the sign that often brings the child to a doctor. Maximum swelling peaks after one to three days and begins in one or both parotid glands, but it may involve other salivary glands. The swelling pushes the earlobe upward and outward and obscures the angle of the mandible. Drinking sour liquids such as lemon juice may increase the pain. The opening of the duct inside the cheek from the affected parotid gland may appear red and swollen.

The painful swelling usually dissipates by seven days. Abdominal pain may be caused by pancreatitis, a common complication but one that is usually mild. The most feared complication, sterility, is not as common as most believe. Orchitis rarely occurs in prepubertal boys and occurs in only 20 to 30 percent of older males. In 35 percent of patients with orchitis, both testes are involved, and a similar percentage of affected testes will atrophy. Surprisingly, impairment of fertility in males is only about 13 percent; absolute infertility is rare. Ovary involvement in women, with pelvic pain and tenderness, occurs in only about 7 percent of postpubertal women and with no evidence of impaired fertility. Mumps during early pregnancy may cause miscarriage, but this is a rare complication for females who have been immunized.

Hemophilus influenzae type B is the most common cause of serious bacterial infection in the young child. It is the leading cause of bacterial meningitis in children between the ages of one month and four years, and it is the cause of many other serious, life-threatening bacterial infections in the young child. Bacterial meningitis, especially from *Hemophilus influenzae* and pneumococcus, is the major cause of acquired hearing impairment in childhood.

Poliomyelitis (polio), an acute viral infection, has a wide range of manifestations. The minor illness pattern accounts for 80 to 90 percent of clinical infections in children. Symptoms, usually mild in this form, include slight fever, malaise, headache, sore throat, and vomiting but do not involve the central nervous system. Major illness occurs primarily in older children and adults. It may begin with fever, severe headache, stiff neck and back, deep muscle pain, and abnormal sensations, such as of burning, prickling, tickling, or tingling. These symptoms of aseptic meningitis may go no further or may progress to the loss of tendon reflexes and asymmetric weakness or paralysis of muscle groups. Fewer than 25 percent of paralytic polio patients suffer permanent disability. Most return in muscle function occurs within six months, but improvement may continue for two years. Twenty-five percent of paralytic patients have mild residual symptoms, and 50 percent recover completely. A long-term study of adults who suffered the disease has documented slowly progressive muscle weakness, especially in patients who experienced severe disabilities initially.

Tetanus is a bacterial disease which, once established in a wound of a patient without significant immunity, will build a substance that acts at the neuromuscular junction, the spinal cord, and the brain. Clinically, the patient experiences "lockjaw," a tetanic spasm causing the spine and extremities to bend with convexity forward; spasms of the facial muscles cause the famous "sardonic smile." Minimal stimulation of any muscle group may cause painful spasms.

Diphtheria is another bacterial disease that produces a virulent substance, but this one attacks heart muscle and nervous tissue. There is a severe mucopurulent discharge from the nose and an exudative pharyngitis (a sore throat accompanied by phlegm) with the formation of a pseudomembrane. Swelling just below the back of the throat may lead to stridor (noisy, high-pitched breathing) and to the dark bluish or purplish coloration of the skin and mucous membranes because of decreased oxygenation of the blood. The result may be heart failure and damaged nerves; respiratory insufficiency may be caused by diaphragmatic paralysis.

Clinically, pertussis (whooping cough) can be divided into three stages, each lasting about two weeks. Initial symptoms resembling the common cold are followed by the characteristic paroxysmal cough and then convalescence. In the middle stage, multiple, rapid coughs, which may last more than a minute, will be followed by a sudden inspiration of air and a characteristic "whoop." In the final stage, vomiting commonly follows coughing attacks. Almost any stimulus precipitates an attack. Seizures may occur as a result of hypoxia (inadequate oxygen supply) or brain damage. Pneumonia can develop, and even death may occur when the illness is severe.

Varicella (chickenpox) produces a generalized itchy, blister-like rash with low-grade fever and few other symptoms. Minor complications, such as ear infections, occasionally occur, as does pneumonia, but serious complications such as infection in the brain are rare. It is a very inconvenient disease, however, requiring the infected person to be quarantined for about nine days or until the skin lesions have dried up completely. Varicella, a herpes family virus, may lie dormant in nerve linings for years and suddenly emerge in the linear-grouped skin lesions identified as herpes zoster. These painful skin lesions follow the distribution of the affected nerve. Herpes zoster is commonly known as shingles.

Hepatitis type B is much more common in adults than in children, except in certain immigrant populations in which hepatitis B viral infections are endemic. High carrier rates appear in certain Asian and Pacific Islander groups and among some Inuits in Alaska, in whom perinatal transmission is the most common means of perpetuating the disease. Having this disease in childhood can cause problems later in life. An estimated five thousand deaths in the United States per year from cirrhosis or liver cancer occur as a result of hepatitis B. Carrier rates of between 5 and 10 percent result from disease acquired after the age of five, but between 80 and 90 percent will be carriers if they are infected at birth. The serious problems of hepatitis B occur most often in chronic carriers. For example, approximately, 15 to 40 percent of carriers will ultimately develop liver cancer. The virus is fifty to one hundred times more infectious than human immunodeficiency virus (HIV), the virus that causes acquired immunodeficiency syndrome (AIDS). Health care workers are at high risk of contracting hepatitis B, but virtually everyone is at risk for contracting this disease because it is so contagious.

Hepatitis type A is a virus that causes jaundice, fatigue, abdominal pain, nausea, diarrhea, and fever. Approximately 15 percent of those who have the disease will have relapsing symptoms for six to nine months. Hepatitis A is usually spread through fecal contamination, and during epidemic years over 35,000 cases are diagnosed in the United States.

Treatment and Therapy

The Centers for Disease Control and Prevention (CDC) and the US Department of Health and Human Services recommend immunizing all infants soon after birth and again at age one to two months, with a final dose after the age of twenty-four weeks. The Committee on Infectious Diseases of the American Academy of Pediatrics recommends extending hepatitis B immunization to all adolescents, if possible. Based on field trials, the hepatitis B vaccine appears to be between 80 and 90 percent effective. The plasma-derived vaccine is protective against chronic hepatitis B infection for at least nine years. Newer, yeast-derived vaccines appear to be safe for administration to all, including pregnant women and infants: Both the vaccine and a placebo evoke the same incidence of adverse reactions. These yeast-derived vaccines will be monitored to see if a booster dose is needed.

The incidence of infection with hepatitis B increases rapidly in adolescence, but teenagers are less likely to comply with immunization than are infants. Asking adolescents to participate in a three-dose immunization program over a six-month period is likely to result in high dropout rates. Therefore, the American Academy of Pediatrics has recommended combining vaccination at birth with vaccination of teenagers. Two states, Alaska and Hawaii, have implemented universal immunization of infants with hepatitis B vaccine, and so have twenty nations. Thirty-four states require vaccination for students before entry to middle school. Hepatitis A vaccine is recommended by the CDC for all children between twelve and twenty-three months of age. Two doses of the vaccine should be given, at least six months apart.

Primary vaccination with DTaP (diphtheria, tetanus, and acellular pertussis) vaccine is recommended at two months, four months, and six months of age, followed by boosters at fifteen to eighteen months and upon entry into school (at four to six years of age).

Once a child reaches fifteen months of age, only one dose of the Hemophilus influenzae type B vaccine is necessary, but vaccination should begin at two months of age. Three vaccines are licensed for use in infants. Depending upon which vaccine is used, shots are given at ages two, four, and six months, with a booster between twelve and fifteen months. These vaccines are safe and at least 90 percent effective in preventing serious illness, such as sepsis and meningitis, from influenza B.

At two and four months of age, infants should receive an inactivated poliovirus vaccination, with boosters between six and eighteen months and upon entry into school (four to six years of age).

MMR (measles, mumps, rubella) vaccination should take place at twelve and fifteen months and at four to six years of age. If the infant lives in a high-risk area, the first dose should occur at twelve months of age. While women who are pregnant or plan to become pregnant in the next three months should not receive MMR vaccination, children may receive the vaccine even if the mother is pregnant, since the viruses are not shed by immunized individuals. Children who have not received the second dose should be vaccinated at eleven to twelve years.

In the 1990s, researchers announced that they had developed a vaccine to prevent chickenpox. According to the CDC, the first dose of varicella vaccine should be given to children between twelve and fifteen months of age who have not had chickenpox. The second dose is given between ages four and six, but may be given as soon as three months after the first dose. Individuals age thirteen and older who have never had chickenpox or the vaccine should get two doses given at least twenty-eight days apart. The chickenpox vaccine is contraindicated for those who have had life-threatening allergic reactions to a prior dose of the vaccine, gelatin, or neomycin; children who are taking aspirin or other salicylates should not be given the vaccine. Those who are ill at the scheduled vaccination time and pregnant women should wait before being vaccinated. Those who have immune system diseases, are taking drugs that affect the immune system, have cancer, are receiving cancer treatments, or have had a recent blood transfusion or other blood products should check with their health care provider before receiving the vaccine.

The CDC states that a combination vaccine called MMRV containing both chickenpox and MMR vaccines can be given instead of the two individual vaccines to children twelve and under. The combination vaccine is associated with rash and higher rates of fever than the two vaccines administered separately; seizures caused by a fever are also more frequently reported with the combination vaccine.

Influenza vaccine, containing two strains of type A and one strain of type B, is now recommended to be administered to all children to prevent infection with seasonal influenza viruses. Annual vaccination is necessary as influenza viruses continually mutate, resulting in new strains not present in previous vaccines. Sometimes, special strains of influenza, such as H1N1 (swine) influenza, may necessitate adding a separate influenza vaccine. Vaccination is particularly important for children with chronic heart and lung disease, diabetes, HIV, sickle cell disease, and other chronic conditions that place them at greater risk for severe influenza.

Pneumococcal vaccine is now routinely given to children aged two to twenty-three months and to certain children aged twenty-four to fifty-nine months who are at risk of overwhelming pneumococcal infections. For example, children without spleens and children with sickle cell disease should be considered for vaccination against pneumococcal disease.

Meningococcal vaccine, which protects against bacteremia and meningitis caused by some strains of meningococci, should be given to children with certain immune deficiency states, including the absence of a functioning spleen. The vaccine may also be given if there is an outbreak of meningococcal disease caused by a strain included in the vaccine, or if the child is traveling to a part of the world where the disease is common.

Some parents refuse to have their children vaccinated against pertussis because of concerns about the vaccine's safety. Media focus on the safety of pertussis vaccines, as well as lawsuits, has frightened many physicians as well, the result being that they may be overly cautious in interpreting vaccine contraindications. Yet primary care physicians have also been sued for failing to give timely immunizations, which may result in complications from preventable disease. The Tennessee Medicaid Pertussis Vaccine Data should reassure them of the vaccine's safety. Other pertussis vaccine safety information is also available, including reports from the American Academy of Pediatrics Task Force on Pertussis and Pertussis Immunization. Some parents have feared that there is a link between vaccinations and neurological disorders such as autism, but studies have found no connection.

The means exist to prevent many serious illnesses from infectious diseases in childhood, but both parents and health care professionals must make the effort to vaccinate all children at the appropriate times in their lives.

Perspective and Prospects

Some vaccines are more protective than others; effectiveness may hinge on a number of factors. In 1989, for example, 40 percent of people who developed measles had been vaccinated correctly under the old guidelines of one dose. Recommendations were therefore revised to include a booster dose. In the case of the hepatitis B vaccine, initial recommendations for administration of the vaccine established no injection site (only intramuscular), but studies revealed that there were fewer vaccine failures in recipients who were vaccinated in the deltoid region of the arm as opposed to the buttocks. The recommendation for injection site was therefore revised.

In the United States, vaccine coverage increased by the late 1990s after having been woefully inadequate during the 1980s. One state's department of health, in a 1987 study, discovered that only 64 percent of children who were two years old were adequately vaccinated with DTaP, oral polio, and MMR vaccines. Although by 2000, rates were closer to 80 percent, in 2011, the rates had only moved to 82 percent. Undoubtedly, multiple and interacting factors have inhibited full vaccine coverage for all American children, including physicians' attitudes and practice behaviors. For parents, the cost of vaccination, lack of health insurance, and other barriers to health care frustrate their efforts to get their children immunized. Some parents, for ideological or other reasons, may even be disinterested in or opposed to vaccination. In today's highly mobile society, however, all persons should keep a standard personal

immunization record to facilitate immunization coverage.
—*Wayne R. McKinny, M.D.;*
updated by Lenela Glass-Godwin, M.W.S.

See also Bacterial infections; Bacteriology; Bronchiolitis; Chickenpox; Common cold; Epidemics and pandemics; Epidemiology; Epiglottitis; Family medicine; Fifth disease; Giardiasis; Hand-foot-and-mouth disease; Hemolytic uremic syndrome; Hepatitis; Herpes; H1N1 influenza; Immunization and vaccination; Impetigo; Infection; Influenza; Kawasaki disease; Measles; Microbiology; Mononucleosis; Mumps; Noroviruses; Parasitic diseases; Pediatrics; Pinworms; Poliomyelitis; Rabies; Rheumatic fever; Roseola; Rotavirus; Roundworms; Rubella; Scarlet fever; Smallpox; Strep throat; Tapeworms; Tetanus; Tonsillitis; Tuberculosis; Viral infections; Whooping cough; Worms.

For Further Information:

Beers, Mark H., et al., eds. *The Merck Manual of Diagnosis and Therapy.* 18th ed. Whitehouse Station, N.J.: Merck Research Laboratories, 2006.

Behrman, Richard E., Robert M. Kliegman, and Hal B. Jenson, eds. *Nelson Textbook of Pediatrics.* 18th ed. Philadelphia: Saunders, 2007.

Biddle, Wayne. *A Field Guide to Germs.* 2d ed. New York: Anchor, 2002.

Centers for Disease Control and Prevention. "Chickenpox Vaccine: What You Need to Know." *CDC*, Mar. 13, 2008.

Centers for Disease Control and Prevention. "Immunization Schedules." *CDC*, Jan. 29, 2013.

Child Trends. "Immunization." *Child Trends Data Bank*, Sept. 2012.

Kimball, Chad T. *Childhood Diseases and Disorders Sourcebook: Basic Consumer Health Information About Medical Problems Often Encountered in Pre-adolescent Children.* Detroit, Mich.: Omnigraphics, 2003.

Kumar, Vinay, Abul K. Abbas, and Nelson Fausto, eds. *Robbins and Cotran Pathologic Basis of Disease.* 8th ed. Philadelphia: Saunders, 2010.

MedlinePlus. "MMR Vaccine (Measles, Mumps, and Rubella." *MedlinePlus*, July 18, 2012.

Preidt, Robert. "HealthDay: Measles Can Spread Further Than Thought on Airplanes: Study." *MedlinePlus*, Mar. 20, 2013.

Woolf, Alan D., et al., eds. *The Children's Hospital Guide to Your Child's Health and Development.* Cambridge, Mass.: Perseus, 2002.

Zieve, David. "DTaP Immunization (Vaccine)." *MedlinePlus*, Feb. 1, 2012.

Chiropractic

Specialty

Anatomy or system affected: Back, bones, hips, musculoskeletal system, nervous system, spine

Specialties and related fields: Neurology, orthopedics, preventive medicine

Definition: The art and science of adjusting the spine and other bony articulations of the body to restore and maintain normal structure and function in the nervous system.

Key terms:

adjustment: a thrust delivered into the spine or its articulations with the purpose of reestablishing normal joint and nerve function

nerve interference/pressure: chiropractic term that refers to a disturbance of normal nerve impulse transmission, usually via compression, stretch, or chronic irritation

neuromusculoskeletal: pertaining to the interrelationship between the nerves, muscles, and skeletal aspects of the body

palpation: the act of feeling with the hand; the application of the fingers with light pressure to the surface of the body for the purpose of determining the consistency of the parts beneath for physical diagnosis

subluxation: an incomplete or partial dislocation of a joint, which creates abnormal neurological and physiological symptoms in neuromusculoskeletal structures and/or other body systems via interference with nerve impulse transmission

Science and Profession

The major premise of the field of chiropractic states that vertebrae of the spine can, and frequently do, become misaligned, causing interference in normal conduction of nerve impulses from the brain to the organs and tissues of the body. Although most spinal misalignments are corrected naturally through normal body movement, some become fixated. As a result, normal nerve transmission is impaired for long periods of time, and the health of the patient suffers as a result. Chiropractors perform adjustments aimed at correcting alignment problems in order to ease pain and improve bodily function.

What distinguishes doctors of chiropractic from other health care professionals is that they work primarily to identify, analyze, and adjust the vertebrae and pelvis to their correct positions. Treatment is directed at restoring and maintaining normal structure and mechanical function of the spine in order to reduce irritation of the spinal cord and spinal nerves. These irritations lead to pain and distress of the muscles and joints of the body. Less acknowledged and still in want of corroborating research is the relationship between the subluxation (partial dislocation), the neuromusculoskeletal system, and internal organ dysfunction.

Doctors of chiropractic may examine, diagnose, analyze, and use x-rays for diagnostic purposes according to generally recognized procedures taught in accredited chiropractic colleges. Clinical practice generally encompasses consultation and taking the medical history of the patient; physical, neurological, orthopedic, and chiropractic examinations; x-ray analysis of the spine and articulating structures; the administration of adjustments; physiotherapy; nutritional support; and the use of orthopedic supports. In most countries, chiropractic practice does not include the prescription or administration of medicine or drugs, performance of surgery, administration of radiation therapy, treatment of infectious or sexually transmitted diseases, performance of internal exams, reduction of fractures, or administration of anesthetics. Historically, chiropractic physicians practiced either solo or in a group setting with other chiropractors and did not have hospital privileges. This is changing as some chiropractic physicians are entering into group practice settings with other health care specialists and gaining admittance to hospitals in a limited capacity.

Chiropractic history dates back to ancient medical writings dating from 2700 BCE. Chiropractic was popularized in the United States in 1895, when D. D. Palmer experimented with a spinal adjustment on Harvey Lillard; Lillard, a janitor, had experienced a "popping sensation" in his up-

A chiropractor performs a manipulation on the neck of a young patient. (PhotoDisc)

per spine caused by heavy lifting and subsequently suffered a loss of hearing. After treatment, Lillard's hearing improved and Palmer formulated the early chiropractic scientific premise and philosophy: that illness is essentially functional in nature and becomes organic only as an end process. His son, B. J. Palmer, is credited with refining and promoting the work of his father. The early educational program organized by D. D. Palmer was admittedly crude, abbreviated, and inadequate. As the profession grew and matured, however, so did the educational standards, to the current level. Chiropractic has emerged as a viable alternative health care system.

In the United States, chiropractic colleges are accredited by the Council on Chiropractic Education, which is in turn approved by the US Office of Education. The chiropractic curriculum is designed to prepare the chiropractic student to evaluate and manage conditions from a holistic point of view, in which the various factors that affect a person's health are taken into consideration, including diet, nutritional supplementation, exercise, stress, and lifestyle.

Chiropractors have a full medical curriculum enabling them to make diagnoses. The education of a chiropractor begins with two years of preprofessional college study, with concentration in the human sciences. Although this prerequisite of two years is all that is required, the majority of students entering chiropractic college possess at least a bachelor's degree. The student then begins the doctor of chiropractic (DC) course of study at an accredited chiropractic college. The DC program is composed of four academic years of study. The initial phase of study is much like any curriculum in the medical, dental, or veterinary schools, consisting of courses in the basic sciences: organic chemistry, biochemistry, anatomy of the musculoskeletal system (including limbs, trunk, and head), anatomy of the internal structures of the body (including all the organs, blood vessels, and internal systems), neuroanatomy (the anatomy of the brain, spinal cord, and entire nervous system), physiology (the study of how these systems function), neurophysiology, pathology (the study of disease), bacteriology, histology (the microscopic study of body tissues), and microbiology. The remainder of the courses are concentrated on the clinical sciences: x-ray physics, positioning, and interpretation; laboratory diagnosis (blood and urine studies); physical examination and diagnosis; neurology; orthopedics; cardiology; pediatrics; geriatrics; dermatology; gastrointestinal and genitourinary systems; physical therapy nutrition; and chiropractic adjustment techniques.

During the later part of the student chiropractor's matriculation, he or she will see patients in a college-affiliated clinic as an "extern," which prepares the future doctor for patient care and management. In addition to the basic chiropractic curriculum, there are residencies available in both radiology and orthopedics. A chiropractic graduate may apply to study an additional three years in order to become either a chiropractic radiologist or a chiropractic orthopedist. The training received in these programs is highly specialized, and both of these chiropractic specialists are the equal of their medical counterparts in terms of diagnostic abilities. In addition, comprehensive 360-hour programs of study in orthopedics, neurology, radiology, and sports medicine exist; doctors completing such programs are eligible to sit for an examination to be awarded diplomate status by chiropractic boards in the corresponding specialties. Postgraduate education for the practicing chiropractor includes seminars and workshops in soft tissue injuries, disc syndromes, lower back pain, and other common and difficult conditions. Interdisciplinary seminars and conferences in nutrition, fitness, biochemical imbalances, and numerous other areas of common interest allow physicians from every discipline the opportunity to exchange views and perspectives. The licensing procedure for the graduate chiropractic doctor varies from state to state and country to country.

Diagnostic and Treatment Techniques

To understand fully how chiropractic health care works, it is necessary to understand the spine and the role that it plays in overall body function. The nervous system-consisting of the brain, cranial nerves (nerves that originate in the head), the spinal cord, and thirty-one pairs of spinal nerves that branch out much as the limbs of a tree do-generates and regulates all activities in the body. Signals, or impulses, travel along the nerve fibers conveying information between the brain and the rest of the body. Since every tissue and organ of the body is connected to and controlled by nerves from the spinal cord and brain, removal of nerve interference can bring dramatic results. Interference with the transmission of these impulses results in alteration of normal body function. The cranium (skull) and spinal column, composed of twenty-four bones called vertebrae, house the brain and spinal cord. In addition to protecting the spinal cord, the spine is the core of the skeletal framework that supports upright posture, provides for organ and muscle attachment, and allows for the dynamics of human movement. Given this monumental job, the spine and its connecting framework are subject to much activity and abuse.

For the mechanics of body motion to occur properly, there must be full, free, and harmonious movement in every one of the spinal joints. The working unit of the spine is referred to as the motor unit. The motor unit is composed of two vertebrae joined by cartilage cushions called discs and four posterior joints called facet joints, two located to attach the superior vertebra and two to attach the inferior vertebra. The discs separate the vertebrae while allowing flexibility and shock absorption for the spine. They also maintain openings between the vertebrae that are necessary for the passage of the spinal nerves. The facet joints provide additional movement and are limited in their range of motion by ligaments. Restriction in any of them can be compensated for only by the other joints and adjoining structures (such as ribs, muscles, or tendons), thus producing strain in the compensating structures.

It is at the location of the facet joints of the spine where subluxation occurs-an alteration of the alignment and proper movement of the spinal joint resulting in irritation of the exiting spinal nerve via compression, stretch, or chronic (constant) irritation-and leads to alteration of normal body functions. Subluxations can result from various factors, including trauma, toxic irritation, muscular imbalance caused by disuse or repetitive tasks, ligamental weakening, organic dysfunction, and stress. The altered nerve impulse transmission, left uncorrected, results in accumulative dysfunction in the tissue cells of the body.

Spinal biomechanics, the basis of the chiropractor's evaluation, refers to the manner in which the spine works in movement. Restoration of spinal motion is the primary treatment on which chiropractors depend to alleviate patients' symptoms. The single most distinguishing element of chiropractic procedures is the spinal adjustment. This chiropractic adjustment is a technique of physically moving the spine by hand or by instrument with the objective of mobilizing a fixated joint. It is a gentle but dynamic thrust applied to a specific joint in a way that generates joint movement in a specific direction. Basically, it is a way to "coax" a restricted joint into moving. Applied repeatedly over a period of time, spinal adjustments are capable of restoring mobility to even the most chronic spinal subluxations. Deep-rooted subluxations that have existed for several years typically require months of care. Fixations of

lesser duration and severity respond in less time, often the mildest in one treatment. The procedure works because the restoration of the proper mechanics of spinal motion via the spinal adjustment improves joint function, corrects specific joint problems, and helps prevent injury through increased spinal strength brought about by spinal joints that function properly.

Chiropractic health care can be useful for the detection and correction of existing health problems and for preventive purposes. Chiropractors look for the reason that a patient's symptom developed, including such contributing factors as environmental conditions, lifestyle, systemic stress, and malfunction. For example, instead of giving medication to stop the pain of headache, the chiropractor analyzes possible irritating factors, including subluxation, that may be causing the headache and addresses that factor first. Thus, in many cases, the prescription of medication can be avoided.

Perspective and Prospects

Chiropractic history dates back to 2700 BCE. Modern chiropractic originated in the second half of the nineteenth century during a time when many theories of healing were being promulgated. Chiropractic and osteopathy shared their early beginnings amid the emergence of several alternatives to the regular school of healing (medicine), including the Thomsonian system (the use of botanicals), the Hygienic movement (the use of fresh fruits and vegetables, fresh air, exercise, and better food preparation), and homeopathy. Daniel David Palmer, born in 1845 in Canada, was involved in making and losing several small mercantile fortunes when he made his way to Iowa in 1886 to become a magnetic healer. Over the next decade, he would attract patients from throughout the Midwest until one day in September 1895, a janitor named Harvey Lillard came into his office, received an "adjustment," and regained his lost hearing. Soon afterward, the term "chiropractic" (Greek meaning "done by hand") was coined by Samuel Weed, a Palmer patient. D. D. Palmer began giving instruction at Dr. Palmer's School and Cure, later becoming Palmer Institute and Chiropractic Infirmary and finally Palmer Chiropractic College.

Brian Inglis, a distinguished British historian, commentator, and author of the two-volume work *The History of Medicine* (1965), has declared: "The rise of chiropractic... has been one of the most remarkable social phenomena in American history... yet it has gone virtually unexplored." In spite of its humble origins and formulative years, chiropractic has had a decided impact on the evolution of health care attitudes. For more than a century, it fought for its very survival, overcoming a strong medical lobby in 1977 when the American Medical Association (AMA) reversed its long-standing policy against professional interrelationships between medical doctors and chiropractors. In March 1977, the AMA's Judicial Council announced:

A physician may refer a patient for diagnostic or therapeutic services to another physician, a limited practitioner, or any other provider of health care services permitted by law to fur-

nish such services, whenever he believes that this may benefit the patient. As in the case of referrals to physician-specialists, referrals to limited practitioners should be based on their individual competence and ability to perform the services needed by the patient.

Despite the AMA's policy change toward chiropractic, however, complete acceptance by the medical profession has not occurred. This reluctance has not been attributable solely to the attitudes of the medical profession. Rather, it is the result of a combination of the continued opposition of the medical profession and the resistance of chiropractors to subordinate themselves to medical prescription, as with physical therapists who practice under medical supervision. Chiropractors have been independent practitioners for too long, functioning at a high level in the diagnosis and treatment of illness, for them to be willing to regress in status.

It is likely that the chiropractic profession will continue on its present course of becoming a health profession with parallels to general medicine. Emphasizing the uniqueness of chiropractic treatment and the contrasting philosophical approaches of health maintenance and therapy, chiropractic has not only survived but also flourished. Whether used as a preventive means to ensure good health or as a way to help the body cure itself of disease, chiropractic has sometimes succeeded where other health care measures have failed.

—Cindy Nesci, D.C.

See also Alternative medicine; Anxiety; Bone disorders; Bones and the skeleton; Massage; Muscle sprains, spasms, and disorders; Muscles; Pain; Pain management; Physical rehabilitation; Spinal cord disorders; Spine, vertebrae, and disks; Stress; Stress reduction.

For Further Information:

Bergmann, Thomas F., and David H. Peterson. *Chiropractic Technique: Principles and Procedures*. 3d ed. St. Louis, Mo.: Mosby/Elsevier, 2010.

"Chiropractic Adjustment." *Mayo Clinic*, October 10, 2012.

"Chiropractic: An Introduction" *National Center for Complementary and Alternative Medicine*, February 2012.

"Chiropractic: A Safe Treatment Option." *American Chiropractic Association*, 2009.

Coulter, Ian Douglass. *Chiropractic: A Philosophy for Alternative Health Care*. Boston: Butterworth-Heinemann, 1999.

Haldeman, Scott, ed. *Principles and Practice of Chiropractic*. 3d ed. New York: McGraw-Hill, 2005.

Lenarz, Michael, and Victoria St. George. *The Chiropractic Way*. New York: Bantam, 2003.

"Spinal Manipulation for Low-Back Pain." *National Center for Complementary and Alternative Medicine*, April 2013.

Tousley, Dirk, and David M. Lees. *The Chiropractic Handbook for Patients*. 3d ed. Independence, Mo.: White Dove, 1985.

Chlamydia

Disease/Disorder

Anatomy or system affected: Eyes, genitals, lungs, lymphatic system, reproductive system, urinary system

Specialties and related fields: Gynecology, microbiology

Definition: The most common sexually transmitted bacterial disease in the United States, which primarily infects the reproductive tract and is caused by the bacterium *Chlamydia trachomatis*.

Key terms:

contact tracing: also known as partner referral; a process that consists of identifying sexual partners of infected patients, informing the partners of their exposure to disease, and offering resources for counseling and treatment

screening procedures: tests that are carried out in populations which are usually asymptomatic and at high risk for a disease in order to identify those in need of treatment

sexually transmitted disease: an infection caused by organisms transferred through sexual contact (genital-genital, orogenital, or anogenital); transmission of infection occurs through exposure to lesions or secretions which contain the organisms

Causes and Symptoms

Chlamydia is one of the most common sexually transmitted bacterial diseases , with a prevalence of about 2 to 12 percent in sexually active men and women worldwide. Chlamydia is caused by a bacterium, *Chlamydia trachomatis*, that infects cells on mucosal surfaces, such as the genital tract, urinary tract, anorectal tract, eyes, and throat. These infections cause inflammation of the cervix, urethra, prostate, or epididymis. In women, symptoms may include urinary discomfort, lower abdominal pain, and abnormal vaginal discharge. Women are commonly asymptomatic in the early stages of the disease. In men, symptoms may involve urinary discomfort and unusual discharge from the urethra. Men may also be asymptomatic in early stages of the disease.

Most cases of chlamydia are asymptomatic, and many patients are diagnosed based on screening procedures. Nevertheless, asymptomatic patients are able to infect others and can suffer serious consequences of chlamydia infection, such as pelvic inflammatory disease (PID) and infertility. PID occurs when chlamydia infection ascends the female reproductive tract to involve the uterus, Fallopian tubes, and pelvic cavity. This infection of the upper reproductive tract can lead to scarring of these organs and puts the patient at increased risk of infertility and ectopic pregnancy.

In rare cases, chlamydia can travel to regional lymph nodes and cause abscesses, a condition termed lymphogranuloma venereum. This condition is commonly accom-

---

Information on Chlamydia

Causes: Bacterial infection of mucosa (genital tract, urinary tract, anorectal tract, eyes, throat) through sexual transmission or childbirth

Symptoms: Often none, but may include urinary discomfort, lower abdominal pain, abnormal discharge from vagina or urethra, complications such as pelvic inflammatory disease (PID) and infertility; in infants, eye infection, visual impairment, blindness, respiratory tract infection

Duration: Chronic until treated

Treatments: Antibiotics (doxycycline, azithromycin, erythromycin, ofloxacin)

panied by systemic symptoms such as fever, chills, and muscle and joint aches.

An infant may contract chlamydia as it passes through the birth canal of an infected mother. The disease can lead to eye infection that results in visual impairment and blindness, as well as infection of the respiratory tract.

Treatment and Therapy

A patient receives antibiotic therapy if laboratory tests indicate infection with *C. trachomatis*. Uncomplicated chlamydia infection can be treated effectively with antibiotics such as doxycycline, azithromycin, erythromycin, or ofloxacin. A patient with risk factors for sexually transmitted diseases (STDs) or symptoms of the disease may be treated presumptively with antibiotic therapy, even before the results of laboratory tests for chlamydia return.

Because chlamydia is associated with other STDs, such as gonorrhea, human immunodeficiency virus (HIV), syphilis, and hepatitis B and C, the patient should be advised to undergo testing for these diseases as well. Approximately 35 to 50 percent of patients with gonorrhea also have chlamydia, so an antibiotic against chlamydia is given along with an antibiotic for gonorrhea, unless laboratory tests have declared the patient free of chlamydia. If chlamydia and gonorrhea are treated early, complications such as PID or infertility can be avoided.

In addition to antibiotics, a key component of chlamydia treatment involves counseling in the prevention of STDs. To minimize future exposure to chlamydia and other STDs, patients are encouraged to use barrier methods such as condoms during intercourse and to avoid high-risk sexual behaviors.

Another key component to the treatment of chlamydia and other STDs is contact tracing, which occurs once the infection is confirmed with laboratory testing. With the cooperation of the patient, all sexual partners of the patient are notified regarding their exposure to disease. Partners are encouraged to seek medical attention, even if they have no symptoms themselves, in order to prevent reinfection of the patient during subsequent sexual encounters or further spread of the disease to other sexual partners.

In the United States, erythromycin eyedrops are given prophylactically to all newborns to prevent eye infections with chlamydia that could lead to visual impairment.

Perspective and Prospects

Diseases caused by *C. trachomatis* have been described as early as ancient Egyptian times. It was not until 1907, however, that the bacterium was actually identified, and there was some controversy about whether it was a true bacterium because it requires host cells to live (obligate intracellular parasite). The organism favors cells that are more available on the cervix of young (versus older) women, which is partly why rates of chlamydia are so much higher in the young. In the 1960s, a clinically useful diagnostic test was developed that allowed screening of a large number of specimens within a few days. The development of a relatively easy test for chlamydia enabled clinicians to screen a large number of asymptomatic but at-risk patients (such as those under age twenty-five or those with multiple sexual partners).

A promising area of research is the search for a vaccine to *C. trachomatis*. This research focuses on identifying antigens on the bacterium that are important for its function, such as proteins responsible for bacterial attachment to or uptake into cells. The premise is to use these proteins to generate an immune response in patients so that when patients are exposed to chlamydia, their immune systems are prepared to respond against it.

—*Clair Kaplan, A.P.R.N./M.S.N.;
additional material by Anne Lynn S. Chang, M.D.*

See also Acquired immunodeficiency syndrome (AIDS); Antibiotics; Bacterial infections; Blindness; Conjunctivitis; Epidemiology; Genital disorders, female; Genital disorders, male; Gonorrhea; Gynecology; Hepatitis; Herpes; Human immunodeficiency virus (HIV); Infertility, female; Men's health; Pelvic inflammatory disease (PID); Reproductive system; Screening; Sexually transmitted diseases (STDs); Syphilis; Trachoma; Women's health.

For Further Information:

Badash, Michelle. "Chlamydia." *Health Library*, October 11, 2012.

Centers for Disease Control and Prevention. "Chlamydia-CDC Fact Sheet." *Centers for Disease Control and Prevention*, December 2012.

Centers for Disease Control and Prevention. "Sexually Transmitted Diseases Treatment Guidelines, 2010." Morbidity and Mortality Weekly Report 59, no. RR-12 (2010).

Holmes, King K., et al., eds. *Sexually Transmitted Diseases*. 4th ed. New York: McGraw-Hill Medical, 2008.

Longo, Dan, et al., eds. *Harrison's Principles of Internal Medicine*. 18th ed. New York: McGraw-Hill, 2011.

Ryan, Kenneth J., et al., eds. *Sherris Medical Microbiology: An Introduction to Infectious Diseases*. 5th ed. New York: McGraw-Hill, 2010.

Choking

Disease/Disorder

Anatomy or system affected: Chest, lungs, neck, respiratory system, throat

Specialties and related fields: Emergency medicine

Definition: A condition in which the breathing passage (windpipe) is obstructed.

Causes and Symptoms

A person who is choking may cough, turn red in the face, clutch his or her throat, or any combination of the above. If the choking person is coughing, it is probably best to do nothing; the coughing should naturally clear the airway. The true choking emergency occurs when a bit of food or other foreign object completely obstructs the breathing passage. In this case, there is little or no coughing-the person cannot make much sound. This silent choking calls for immediate action.

Treatment and Therapy

An individual witnessing a choking emergency should first call for emergency help and then perform the Heimlich maneuver. The choking person should never be slapped on the back. The Heimlich maneuver is best performed while the

Information on Choking

Causes: Blockage of airway, injury
Symptoms: Coughing, red face, grabbing at throat
Duration: Acute
Treatments: Heimlich maneuver, emergency care

choking victim is standing or seated. If possible, the person performing the Heimlich maneuver should ask the victim to nod if he or she wishes the Heimlich maneuver to be performed. If the airway is totally blocked, the victim will not be able to speak and may even be unconscious.

The individual performing the Heimlich maneuver positions himself or herself behind the choking victim and places his or her arms around the victim's waist. Making a fist with one hand and grasping that fist with the other hand, the rescuer positions the thumb side of the fist toward the stomach of the victim-just above the navel and below the ribs. The person performing the maneuver pulls his or her fist upward into the abdomen of the victim with several quick thrusts. This action should expel the foreign object from the victim's throat, and he or she should begin coughing or return to normal breathing.

The Heimlich maneuver is not effective in dislodging fish bones and certain other obstructions. If the airway is still blocked after several Heimlich thrusts, a finger sweep should be tried to remove the obstruction. First, the mouth of the victim must be opened: The chin is grasped, and the mouth is pulled open with one hand. With the index finger of the other hand, the rescuer sweeps through the victim's throat, pulling out any foreign material. One sweep should be made from left to right, and a second sweep from right to left. The Heimlich maneuver may then be repeated if necessary.

—*Steven A. Schonefeld, Ph.D.*

See also Asphyxiation; Coughing; Cyanosis; First aid; Heimlich maneuver; Hyperventilation; Respiration; Resuscitation; Unconsciousness.

For Further Information:
"Acute Upper Airway Obstruction." *Medline Plus*, July 16, 2011.
American College of Emergency Physicians. *Pocket First Aid*. New York: DK, 2003.
Castleman, Michael. "Life Saving Moves from EMS Experts." *Family Circle* 107, no. 4 (March 15, 1994): 37.
"Choking First Aid." *Mayo Clinic*, October 13, 2011.
"Choking Prevention." *American Academy of Pediatricians*, May 11, 2013.
"Infant Choking: How to Keep Your Infant Safe." *Mayo Clinic*, June 6, 2013.
Stern, Loraine. "Mom, I Can't Breathe!" *Woman's Day* 57, no. 6 (March 15, 1994): 18.

Cholecystectomy

Procedure
Anatomy or system affected: Abdomen, gallbladder, gastrointestinal system
Specialties and related fields: General surgery
Definition: The surgical removal of a diseased gallbladder.

Indications and Procedures

Cholecystectomy is indicated when the patient exhibits nausea, vomiting, and abdominal pain and examination reveals gallstones. Gallstones, which consist mostly of crystallized cholesterol and bile, form in the gallbladder and may lodge in the bile duct. The stones can be dissolved with medication or broken up with ultrasound and passed from the body. They can (and often do) form again, however, with renewed symptoms. Removal of the gallbladder is the method of choice to prevent the recurrence of symptoms. Surgery is performed under general anesthesia.

In open surgery, the abdomen is cleaned and a 7.5- to 15-centimeter (3- to 6-inch) incision made with a scalpel through the skin and abdominal tissues. The gallbladder is isolated from the liver. A duct and artery are tied off with surgical staples or sutures, and they are cut in order to free the gallbladder. The organ is removed, and the tissues are closed with sutures or staples.

In laparoscopic surgery, the surface is cleaned and the surgeon makes four small holes. A 1.3-centimeter (0.5-inch) cut is made at or near the navel and another just below the breastbone, as well as two small punctures to the right of the incisions. The laparoscope, with a video camera and light, is inserted into the navel incision. Long, thin dissecting instruments are passed through the three punctures, and the gallbladder is cut free as in open surgery. The organ is removed through the navel incision, which is then closed with sutures or staples. The punctures are closed with small adhesive bandages.

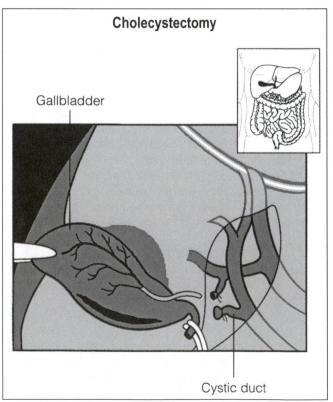

Cholecystectomy

Gallbladder

Cystic duct

The removal of the gallbladder may be indicated with severe infection of the organs or with repeated attacks of biliary colic caused by the presence of gallstones; the inset shows the location of the gallbladder.

Uses and Complications

Open surgery for cholecystectomy requires a hospital stay of five to eight days and a recovery time of four to six weeks. Complications occur in 1.0 to 9.4 percent of the surgeries and range from postoperative bleeding and diarrhea to intestinal obstruction. Rare but major complications include severing the common bile duct that connects the liver and small intestine, or puncturing a major blood vessel. Overall, the mortality rate is low: 0.2 to 0.6 percent.

Laparoscopic surgery may require an overnight stay and a recovery period of five to seven days. The complication rate is lower than the rate in open surgery, but this may be a reflection of the fact that sicker patients with more complex diseases and, therefore, greater risk factors are generally referred for open surgery; not all patients are good candidates for the limited approach afforded by laparoscopy.

—Albert C. Jensen, M.S.

See also Cholecystitis; Gallbladder; Gallbladder cancer; Gallbladder diseases; Gastroenterology; Gastrointestinal system; Laparoscopy; Stone removal; Stones.

For Further Information:

American College of Surgeons. "Cholecystectomy: Surgical Removal of the Gallbladder." *FACS*, n.d..

Carson-DeWitt, Rosalyn. "Cholecystectomy-Laparoscopic Surgery." *Health Library*, May 28, 2013.

Carson-DeWitt, Rosalyn. "Cholecystectomy-Open Surgery." *Health Library*, May 28, 2013.

Chellappa, M. *Laparoscopic Cholecystectomy*. Teaneck, N.J.: World Scientific, 1994.

Dunn, David C., and Christopher J. E. Watson. *Laparoscopic Cholecystectomy: Problems and Solutions*. Cambridge, Mass.: Blackwell Science, 1992.

Parker, James N., and Philip M. Parker, eds. *The Official Patient's Sourcebook on Gallstones*. [N. p.]: ICON Group, 2007.

Porter, Robert S., et al., eds. *The Merck Manual Home Health Handbook*. Whitehouse Station, N.J.: Merck Research Laboratories, 2009.

Valverde, A., and H. Mosnier. "Laparascopic Cholecystectomy." *Journal of Visceral Surgery* 148, no. 5 (October, 2011):353-360.

Cholecystitis

Disease/Disorder

Anatomy or system affected: Abdomen, gallbladder, gastrointestinal system, liver, pancreas

Specialties and related fields: Emergency medicine, family medicine, gastroenterology, internal medicine, pathology

Definition: An inflammation of the gallbladder.

Causes and Symptoms

There are basically two types of cholecystitis, calculous and acalculous, both of which could present as acute or chronic inflammation of the gallbladder. The calculous type is seen in 90 percent of cases and is caused by an obstruction of the neck of the gallbladder by gallstones, which are usually composed of cholesterol. The cholesterol stones may block the gallbladder neck and cause an acute attack of cholecystitis, or they may act as chemical irritants and result in chronic inflammation. About 10 percent of cases of cholecystitis are not the result of gallstones and are

---

Information on Cholecystitis

Causes: Usually obstruction of gallbladder by gallstones; sometimes sepsis, severe trauma, severe burns

Symptoms: Severe, progressive upper-right abdominal pain, with nausea, vomiting, fever, sometimes jaundice

Duration: Often chronic, with acute episodes lasting one to three days

Treatments: None (spontaneous resolution), sometimes gallbladder removal

---

hence called acalculous. A variety of factors may precipitate an acute attack, such as sepsis, severe trauma, severe burns, and even the postpartum state. Approximately 75 percent of patients with acute cholecystitis are women.

Acute cholecystitis may first come to a medical attention in the emergency room, with the patient complaining of severe, progressive upper-right quadrant pain (biliary colic), which may be associated with nausea, vomiting, and fever and could radiate to the back. Jaundice (yellowish skin) may or may not be present, depending on the degree of obstruction of the gallbladder neck. The attack usually follows a large, fatty meal and can last one to three days. Chronic cholecystitis is usually more insidious in onset and may be relatively asymptomatic; it also may be associated with a vague sensation of indigestion, which eventually progresses to mild, right-upper abdominal distress or long-standing pain.

Diagnosis is usually made with an ultrasound of the abdomen that demonstrates calcified gallstones. Obstruction of the gallbladder neck cannot be visualized, however, and thus requires another imaging test called a hepatobiliary iminodiacetic acid (HIDA) scan. An elevated white blood cell count is also seen in most cases.

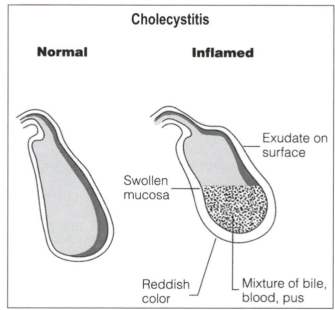

A normal gallbladder and one inflamed by cholecystitis.

Treatment and Therapy

Most acute attacks of cholecystitis may resolve spontaneously, but they should always be considered for surgery, as removal of the gallbladder (cholecystectomy) is the only definitive therapy for the disease. The gallbladder is usually removed using laparoscopic surgery, wherein small incisions are made in the abdomen through which surgical instruments and a fiber-optic camera are passed. In some cases, particularly if the gallbladder is highly inflamed, an open procedure is necessary. In acute attacks, it may also be necessary to maintain adequate nutrition and fluid replacement. A low-fat diet is usually recommended for these patients.

In those patients who decide against surgery, there is a risk of recurrent infections, pain, and even perforation of the gallbladder; the perforation of the gallbladder has a 15 percent mortality rate. Perforation of the gallbladder occurs in less than 3 percent of cases of acute cholescystitis.

—*Rashmi Ramasubbaiah, M.D. and*
Venkat Raghavan Tirumala, M.D., M.H.A.

See also Cholecystectomy; Gallbladder; Gallbladder diseases; Gastroenterology; Internal medicine; Stone removal; Stones.

For Further Information:

American Medical Association. *American Medical Association Family Medical Guide.* 4th ed. Hoboken, N.J.: John Wiley & Sons, 2004.

Frazier, Margaret Schell, and Jeanette Wist Drzymkowski. *Essentials of Human Diseases and Conditions.* 5th ed. St. Louis, Mo.: Saunders/Elsevier, 2012.

Longo, Dan, et al., eds. *Harrison's Principles of Internal Medicine.* 18th ed. New York: McGraw-Hill, 2011.

Longstreth, George F. "Chronic Cholecystitis." *Medline Plus,* February 27, 2011.

Mayo Clinic Staff. "Cholecystitis." *Mayo Clinic,* September 1, 2011.

Porter, Robert S., et al., eds. *The Merck Manual Home Health Handbook.* 3d ed. Whitehouse Station, N.J.: Merck, 2011.

Rakel, Robert E., ed. *Textbook of Family Practice.* 6th ed. Philadelphia: W. B. Saunders, 2002.

Cholera

Disease/Disorder

Anatomy or system affected: Circulatory system, gastrointestinal system, intestines, kidneys

Specialties and related fields: Environmental health, epidemiology, gastroenterology, internal medicine, microbiology, public health

Definition: An acute bacterial disease transmitted by polluted water and contaminated food.

Key terms:

epidemic: an acute disease prevalent and spreading rapidly in a community

pandemic: a worldwide epidemic

pathogen: a disease-causing organism

rice-water stools: extremely dilute feces comprising a whitish liquid containing rice-shaped flecks of solid mucous material; a characteristic symptom of cholera

Causes and Symptoms

The comma-shaped bacterium *Vibrio cholerae* causes the life-threatening disease cholera. The organism is spread when people ingest water or raw food contaminated with fecal matter. Studies have shown that the bacterium can live in both oceanic salt water and freshwater. In the ocean, it adheres to a type of zooplankton called copepods, which are eaten by certain types of shellfish. Therefore, people who consume shellfish grown in contaminated water can ingest the cholera organism. Also, people eating crops fertilized with human feces can ingest the organism.

Cholera affects particularly underdeveloped nations with poor sewage disposal and sanitation practices. It is endemic in Africa, Southeast Asia, the Indian subcontinent, and Central and South America. Even in developed nations, however, cholera may emerge after major disasters, such as hurricanes and earthquakes. Most of those cases were caused by the ingestion of contaminated raw shellfish. In 2011 the World Health Organization (WHO) reported 589,854 cases worldwide; 32 percent of cases were in Africa while 61.2 percent were in North and South America, mostly attributed to an outbreak in Haiti that began after the 2010 earthquake there. The WHO's reports do not include an additional estimate 500,000-700,000 unreported or misdiagnosed cases.

After a person ingests contaminated food or water, between twenty-four and seventy-two hours elapse before the symptoms of cholera develop. Normally, between ten million to a billion *V. cholerae* bacteria must be present to cause infection, due to the large number that die in stomach acid. If an individual has taken antacids to neutralize stomach acid, however, then only about one thousand organisms are necessary to cause infection. Fewer organisms are also required if they enter the body via food, because the food protects some of the bacteria from the stomach acid.

The organisms that survive travel to the small intestine, attach to the epithelial cells there, and produce a toxin that causes a tremendous loss of water and electrolytes though extreme diarrhea and sometimes vomiting. Patients can lose more than twenty quarts of fluid per day. The extremely dilute feces are primarily a whitish liquid containing flecks of solid mucous material resembling rice grains, and hence are commonly called rice-water stools. The tremendous loss of fluids and electrolytes can lead to hypotension (low blood pressure), an increase in both pulse and respiratory rates, cardiac arrhythmia, kidney failure, and the appearance of sunken eyes and cheeks. Shock, resulting from changes in blood acidity and extremely low blood volume, can lead to death within a few hours, especially in children.

Some strains of *V. cholerae* may produce almost no symptoms or only mild diarrhea in some individuals, but the majority of infected people experience very severe disease. Left untreated, approximately 60 percent of patients die; however, immediate rehydration therapy normally saves all but about 1 percent of patients. Nonfatal cases spontaneously resolve themselves after a few days, since both the organisms and the toxin that they produce are ejected from the patient's body in the diarrhea.

Treatment and Therapy

The best method for controlling cholera is prevention. Societies with adequate sanitation and sewage treatment are normally protected, except for contaminated seafood. Underdeveloped nations should be encouraged to improve their sanitation and sewage treatment practices and to cease using human feces as crop fertilizer. Also, especially in infected areas, raw foods and unpurified water should be avoided.

Although different vaccines have been developed, the immunity that they produce appears to be short-lived and not effective against all strains. Prophylactic antibiotic treatment for travelers entering affected areas has not been shown to be effective. Given the large number of bacteria needed for the disease to occur, however, proper hygienic practices alone should provide sufficient protection.

Treatment for cholera patients is primarily supportive, with rehydration and restoration of the electrolyte balance being paramount. Secondary treatment with antibiotics may reduce the presence of organisms and their production of toxin, thus ameliorating the symptoms. Because of the high volume of watery diarrhea, the antibiotic tends to be released from the body very rapidly. Doxycycline is usually the preferred drug, but trimethoprim-sulfamethoxazole or tetracycline have also been used. Unfortunately, certain strains of *V. cholerae* have been discovered to be resistant to the latter two antibiotics. Using antibiotics to more effectively eliminate the organism may be important, since it has been estimated that up to 20 percent of patients continue to carry *V. cholerae* asymptomatically for a time after recovery from the disease.

Perspective and Prospects

Historically, cholera has been a very important epidemic pathogen credited with causing seven different pandemics. These pandemics have affected various areas, including Asia, the Middle East, and Africa. Between 1832 and 1836, two pandemics (the second and fourth) affected the North American continent, resulting in two hundred thousand American deaths. While studying and trying to limit the effects of the 1854 cholera epidemic in London, physician John Snow founded the science of epidemiology and introduced techniques that are still in use today. The seventh pandemic occurred in 1961, starting in Indonesia and spreading to South Asia, the Middle East, and portions of both Europe and Africa.

In 1991, Peru suddenly reported new cases after being free of cholera for more than a century. Contaminated bilge water discharged from a freighter into the Peru harbor has been hypothesized as being responsible for the disease's reappearance. The water supply in the capital city of Lima was not chlorinated, and the organism rapidly multiplied and infected the inhabitants. In two years, more than 700,000 cases and 6,323 deaths were recorded in South and Central America, and spread of this cholera strain continues today.

The 1961 pandemic strain caused over five million cases of cholera and more than 250,000 deaths. In 1992, a genetic

---

Information on Cholera

Causes: Bacterial infection via contaminated food or water

Symptoms: Diarrhea, vomiting

Duration: Several days

Treatments: Fluid and electrolyte replacement, antibiotics

---

variant of this strain appeared in Bangladesh, causing an epidemic and spreading to neighboring countries. In January 2010 an earthquake hit Haiti and devastated much of the country's capital and the surrounding areas. The first case of cholera was confirmed in October 2010 and the disease quickly spread; by January 2013 the epidemic had killed more than eight thousand people and affected more than six hundred thousand more.

—*Steven A. Kuhl, Ph.D.*

See also Bacterial infections; Bacteriology; Diarrhea and dysentery; Environmental health; Epidemics and pandemics.

For Further Information:

Badash, Michelle. "Cholera." *Health Library*, November 26, 2012.

"Cholera." *MedlinePlus*, May 30, 2012.

"Cholera - *Vibrio cholerae* Infection." *Centers for Disease Control and Prevention*, February 24, 2011.

Ezzell, Carol. "It Came from the Deep." *Scientific American* 280 (June, 1999): 22-24.

Pennisi, Elizabeth. "Infectious Disease: Cholera Strengthened by Trip Through Gut." *Science* 296 (June, 2002): 1783-1784.

Reidl, Joachim, et al. "*Vibrio cholerae* and Cholera: Out of the Water and into the Host." *FEMS Microbiological Reviews* 26 (June, 2002): 125-139.

Wachsmuth, Kaye, et al. *"Vibrio cholerae" and Cholera: Molecular to Global Perspectives.* Washington, D.C.: American Society for Microbiology, 1994.

Zimmer, Carl. "Infectious Diseases: Taming Pathogens-An Elegant Idea, but Does It Work?" *Science* 300 (May, 2003): 1362-1364.

Cholesterol
Biology

Anatomy or system affected: Blood vessels, cells, circulatory system, gastrointestinal system

Specialties and related fields: Biochemistry, cytology, family medicine, internal medicine, nutrition, preventive medicine, vascular medicine

Definition: A lipid substance that is a structural component of cell membranes and that makes up the surface of lipoproteins.

Key terms:

cholesterol: a lipid substance that is a component of cell membranes and the surface of circulating lipoproteins

cholesteryl ester: cholesterol linked to a fatty acid; it is stored in lipid droplets in the cytoplasm of cells and circulates in the core of lipoproteins

lipids: substances that are poorly soluble in water; in animal tissues, the principal lipids are triglycerides (fat), phospholipids, cholesterol, and cholesteryl esters

lipoproteins: lipid aggregates that transport fat and cholesteryl esters in the circulation; associated apolipoproteins determine how rapidly they are taken up by the liver or other tissues

sterols: a class of chemically related lipids; cholesterol is the principal sterol in vertebrates, but in plants its functions are served by related substances

Structure and Functions

Living cells are bounded by a cell membrane composed of a double layer of phospholipid, which is traversed by proteins that have catalytic, transportation, and signaling functions. Variable amounts of sterol are interspersed among the molecules of phospholipid in each membrane layer. Sterols are essential components in the membranes of fungal, plant, and animal cells (but not in bacteria). In vertebrates, the predominant sterol is cholesterol. There is little or no cholesterol in plant cell membranes; its place is taken by chemically related substances, chiefly sitosterol. This fact is of nutritional significance; only animal products add cholesterol to the diet.

In mammals, cholesterol is the precursor of steroid hormones, which are essential for mineral balance, adjustment of the body to stress, and normal reproductive function. It is also the precursor of bile acids, which are required for the absorption of dietary lipids. Bile acids play a role in cholesterol balance; the body can dissolve excess cholesterol in bile so that it may be expelled as waste, or the body may convert cholesterol to produce more bile acid.

Cholesterol itself is required for normal functioning of the mammalian cell membrane. Cholesterol alters the membrane's fluidity-the ease with which proteins embedded in the membrane can move about and interact with one another-and also affects the activity of enzymes and transport proteins embedded in the membrane. Cultured cells that are prevented from making their own cholesterol will not grow unless it is provided in the medium.

Cholesterol may either be free or esterified (cholesterol becomes esterified when an ester bond binds a fatty acid to the hydroxyl group of cholesterol). Free cholesterol is confined to cellular membranes. Cholesterol content is highest (about one molecule of cholesterol for every one or two molecules of phospholipid) in the outer cell membrane that forms the boundary between a cell and its environment. It is much lower in intracellular membranes. Although cholesterol synthesis is completed within the endoplasmic reticulum, the ratio of cholesterol to phospholipid in this membrane is less than one to twenty. In a typical cell, it is estimated that between 80 and 90 percent of the total free cholesterol is located in the outer cell membrane.

Cholesterol in excess of normal proportions is coupled (esterified) to long-chain fatty acids. The resulting cholesteryl ester accumulates, along with triglyceride, in lipid droplets in the cytoplasm. The activity of the enzyme catalyzing this esterification is increased when cholesterol is imported into the cell in excess of its needs. The ability to esterify and sequester cholesterol defends the cell against excessive membrane concentration of the free sterol.

Free cholesterol and cholesteryl ester are carried in plasma in lipoproteins. Lipoproteins are aggregates of several thousand molecules of lipid and one or more molecules of specific proteins (apolipoproteins). Each lipoprotein particle consists of a core of triglyceride and cholesteryl ester surrounded by a single layer of phospholipid and free cholesterol. The apolipoproteins are embedded in the surface of the particle. Lipoproteins differ in size and relative lipid composition. In humans, about two-thirds of circulating cholesterol is contained in low-density lipoprotein (LDL), a core of cholesteryl ester with a single molecule of apolipoprotein B on the surface. LDL transports cholesterol from the liver to peripheral tissues. Most of the remaining circulating cholesterol is carried in high-density lipoprotein (HDL), which transports cholesterol from peripheral tissues back to the liver for disposal. Under normal conditions, LDL is the principal source of exogenous cholesterol available to a cell.

Uptake of LDL is mediated by a specific protein on the cell's surface, the LDL receptor, which is concentrated in pockets in the cell membrane termed coated pits. LDL receptors bind apolipoprotein B and particles such as LDL that contain this protein. Coated pits continually pinch off to form sealed vesicles (endosomes) inside the cell. At the same time, new coated pits form on the cell surface. When a coated pit pinches off, it carries with it LDL receptors and associated LDL. The fluid within the endosome is acidified, which causes LDL to dissociate from its receptor and float free. The LDL is transferred to lysosomes, where cholesteryl ester is cleaved to liberate cholesterol; along with the free cholesterol that formed part of the LDL surface, this liberated cholesterol is now available for use within the cell. The LDL receptor is returned to the cell surface, where it can again become associated with a coated pit and participate in a new round of LDL uptake.

The rate at which LDL is removed from the circulation depends on the concentration of LDL receptors in cells of the liver and other tissues. (Although there are other mechanisms for removing LDL, these are less efficient than uptake via the LDL receptor.) This process is subject to feedback regulation. When a cell contains an adequate supply of cholesterol, the synthesis of new LDL receptors is inhibited. This inhibition occurs at the transcriptional level: The rate at which the gene for the LDL receptor is copied into messenger ribonucleic acid (mRNA) is reduced. With less mRNA for this protein reaching the cytoplasm, the rate at which new copies of the protein are made also falls. Following normal turnover of existing receptors, the concentration of LDL receptors at the cell surface declines and the uptake of cholesterol is accordingly reduced.

The gene for the LDL receptor contains short stretches of deoxyribonucleic acid (DNA), termed sterol response elements (SREs), that make transcription sensitive to cholesterol-induced "down-regulation." These can be spliced out and inserted into another gene that codes for a bacterial protein. The foreign gene can be inserted into a mammalian cell, which will then begin to produce the corresponding protein. If the foreign gene does not contain an SRE, the rate of synthesis of the coded protein is unaffected by the cholesterol content of the recipient cell. When an SRE has been inserted into the gene in an appropriate location, however, excess cholesterol down-regulates transcription of the foreign gene just as it does that for the LDL receptor.

The signal that causes down-regulation of the cholesterol receptor has not been clearly identified, although some researchers have suggested it may be mediated by excess lipoprotein cholesterol. It is also possible that an internal regulatory pool of cholesterol-such as the cholesterol content of certain internal membranes or the concentration of individual cholesterol molecules bound to some cytoplasmic protein carrier-is responsible. Some evidence points to oxysterol analogues of cholesterol, rather than to cholesterol itself, as mediators of down-regulation. These analogues arise as minor metabolites of cholesterol and as intermediates and by-products of cholesterol synthesis. They are much more potent than cholesterol itself in inhibiting the synthesis of LDL receptors. A cytoplasmic oxysterol-binding protein has been identified whose affinity for different oxysterols parallels their relative potency in down-regulating the transcription of LDL receptor genes.

Mammalian cells also have the capacity to synthesize their own cholesterol. The enzymes catalyzing the successive reactions along this pathway are located in the cytoplasm and in the membranes of the endoplasmic reticulum. The starting material from which cholesterol is made is acetic acid in the form of acetyl coenzyme A (acetyl CoA). This material is generated in mitochondria as an intermediate in the oxidation of glucose and of fatty acids. To be utilized for synthesis of cholesterol, it must first be transported from the mitochondria to the cytoplasm; a specific shuttle exists for this purpose. The synthesis of fatty acids from acetyl CoA also takes place in the cytoplasm, and more of the translocated precursor is used for this purpose than to make cholesterol.

An early step on the pathway to cholesterol is the reduction of hydroxymethylglutaryl coenzyme A (HMG CoA) to mevalonic acid, catalyzed by HMG CoA reductase. The enzymatic capacity to catalyze this reaction is substantially lower than that for other steps on the pathway, so that the overall rate of cholesterol synthesis is largely determined by the activity of this enzyme. Both amount and activity are regulated to match the rates of cholesterol synthesis to the needs of the cell. When the cell has adequate supplies of cholesterol, HMG CoA reductase activity is low and, simultaneously, uptake via the LDL receptor is reduced. Conversely, when more cholesterol is needed, HMG CoA reductase activity and overall cholesterol synthesis are increased, as are expression of the LDL receptor and the uptake of cholesterol.

HMG CoA reductase activity is regulated at several points, including transcription of the gene, efficiency with which its mRNA is translated into protein, turnover of the enzyme protein, and inactivation by chemical modification. Regulation of the transcription of the HMG CoA reductase gene and regulation of the LDL receptor gene appear to have the same fundamental mechanism. The gene for HMG CoA reductase contains an SRE similar in sequence to those in the gene for the LDL receptor.

Oxysterols that repress transcription of the LDL receptor exert the same effect on transcription of the gene for HMG CoA reductase, and with the same relative potency. Mutant cells that have lost the capacity to respond to oxysterols by repressing the synthesis of LDL receptors also fail to respond by repressing the synthesis of HMG CoA reductase.

Excess cholesterol also increases the rate at which HMG CoA reductase is broken down. This might be a response to changes in cholesterol concentration in the internal membranes in which HMG CoA reductase is embedded. When the gene for HMG CoA reductase is altered to remove the sequences that anchor it to the membrane and the altered gene is inserted into a recipient cell, the mutant protein is located unattached in the cytoplasm. In contrast to the native enzyme, the rate of turnover of the altered gene product is not affected by the cholesterol content of the recipient cell.

Phosphorylation (attachment of a phosphate to specific amino acid residues) of HMG CoA reductase is a third mechanism by which the synthesis of cholesterol is altered. This is best documented in the liver (which is also the principal site within the body for the synthesis of cholesterol). Liver cells contain an enzyme that phosphorylates and inactivates HMG CoA reductase; the same enzyme also phosphorylates and inactivates the enzyme catalyzing the rate-determining step in the synthesis of fatty acids, acetyl CoA carboxylase. The phosphorylation of both enzymes is promoted, and the synthesis of fatty acids and cholesterol is correspondingly inhibited, under fasting conditions. In the fed state, the reverse is true. These changes appear to be a response to circulating levels of the hormone insulin.

Most of the mevalonic acid that is produced by HMG CoA reductase activity is converted to cholesterol. Since its formation is the rate-determining step on the pathway, the addition of mevalonic acid itself to the cell results in much higher rates of cholesterol synthesis than can be achieved with acetyl CoA as starting material. Moreover, the synthesis of cholesterol from mevalonic acid is not controlled by feedback inhibition. Under these circumstances, expression of HMG CoA reductase and expression of the LDL receptor are maximally repressed.

Mevalonic acid is also the precursor of other substances needed by the cell. These include dolichol (a coenzyme needed for the addition of carbohydrate residues to proteins), ubiquinone (a participant in electron transport reactions in mitochondria), and isoprenyl side chains that are attached to specific proteins. Although their synthesis consumes only a minor portion of the mevalonic acid produced by HMG CoA reductase, these substances are essential to normal cell function. When HMG CoA reductase is inhibited by lovastatin, a drug that competes with the substrate HMG CoA for binding to the enzyme, cell growth is inhibited even when supplies of cholesterol in the medium are adequate. Resumption of cell growth requires the addition of small amounts of mevalonic acid as well as cholesterol. Mutant cell lines have been obtained that, even without lovastatin, are unable to grow unless mevalonic acid is present. The requirements of these cells can be met with a large amount of mevalonic acid in the medium or with a small amount of mevalonic acid plus a large amount of cholesterol.

The multiple roles of mevalonic acid are also reflected in the way that HMG CoA reductase activity is regulated. Although transcription of the HMG CoA reductase gene is reduced when cholesterol levels in the cell are high, some transcription continues to allow enough mevalonic acid to be produced to meet other needs of the cell. Adding small amounts of mevalonic acid further decreases the synthesis of HMG CoA reductase by decreasing the rate at which its mRNA is translated into protein. In contrast, expression of the LDL receptor is not under dual regulation; maximal suppression can be obtained with cholesterol alone.

Disorders and Diseases

Excessive levels of LDL cholesterol are associated with an increased risk of coronary heart disease and stroke. Efforts to reduce LDL cholesterol through changes in diet or through drugs take advantage of what is known about cholesterol balance in individual cells and in the body as a whole. The latter is determined by three factors: the dietary intake of cholesterol, the rate of cholesterol synthesis within the body (principally by the liver), and the rate of cholesterol disposal (also principally by the liver, through secretion of free sterol into the bile and by the conversion of cholesterol to bile acids). Accordingly, levels of LDL cholesterol can be diminished by limiting the intake and synthesis of new cholesterol, reducing cholesterol secretion by the liver (in the form of an LDL precursor particle), promoting LDL uptake by the liver (mediated by the LDL receptor), and increasing the formation and secretion of bile acids and free cholesterol.

The body can meet its need for cholesterol through synthesis; there is no dietary requirement. Cholesterol deficiency does not arise in humans even on a purely vegetarian (cholesterol-free) diet. The average Western diet, rich in meat and dairy products, contains between 250 and 400 milligrams of cholesterol per day. Small amounts of cholesterol in the diet are fairly well absorbed, but efficiency declines with larger quantities; on average, about half of the cholesterol consumed per day is assimilated. Absorption of cholesterol and other lipids in the small intestine requires the presence of bile acids. These mix with cholesterol and partially degraded dietary triglyceride to form small droplets that facilitate the absorption of lipids by the cells lining the small intestine. In the process, most of the bile acid (as well as cholesterol secreted in the bile) is reabsorbed and returned to the liver. The absorbed cholesterol is esterified and secreted into the lymph, along with triglyceride, in the core of chylomicrons. These large lipoproteins are reduced in size by removal of triglyceride in capillary beds, and the remnants, containing all the original cholesteryl ester, are taken up by the liver. Thus, the cholesterol absorbed in the intestine passes initially to the liver.

The liver is the most important site for cholesterol synthesis within the body. As explained above, hepatic synthesis of cholesterol is under feedback control. HMG CoA reductase activity and cholesterol synthesis are suppressed when large amounts of dietary cholesterol reach the liver and are augmented when the diet is cholesterol-free. Drugs such as lovastatin that inhibit HMG CoA reductase are useful in reducing cholesterol levels in the circulation, since they limit the ability of the liver to respond by making more cholesterol when the dietary intake is reduced.

Cholesterol within the liver may be incorporated into very low-density lipoprotein (VLDL) and secreted into the circulation. VLDL is secreted primarily to transport triglyceride to other tissues for use as a metabolic fuel or for storage. After serving this function, most of the VLDL remnants return to the liver. Those that escape hepatic reabsorption are transformed in the circulation into LDL. LDL is also taken up by the liver (and elsewhere), but at a much slower rate than VLDL remnant particles, so that this lipoprotein accumulates in the circulation. It is deposition of LDL in the lining of blood vessels that initiates the formation of atherosclerotic plaques-the beginning of atherosclerotic disease. Since cholesterol is required for the secretion of VLDL, HMG CoA reductase inhibitors that cause a partial depletion of cholesterol in liver cells reduce the rate at which it enters the bloodstream. By the same means, they also increase expression of LDL receptors in liver cells, which results in a more rapid removal of LDL from the circulation. Both mechanisms reduce circulating levels of LDL cholesterol.

Cholesterol in the liver may also be converted to bile acids and secreted in the bile. Although most of the secreted bile acid comes back to the liver, some escapes reabsorption in the small intestine. The bile acid that is lost must be replaced by the metabolization of more cholesterol. Bile acid sequestrants such as cholestyramine are also used to reduce circulating cholesterol. They act by forming complexes with bile acids in the small intestine and interfere with their reabsorption. A larger fraction of the secreted bile acid is thus lost by excretion, and the rate of conversion of cholesterol to bile acid in the liver is correspondingly increased.

The liver secretes a large amount of free cholesterol into the bile. Most of this biliary cholesterol is reabsorbed and returned to the liver. Since bile acids are required for the intestinal uptake of cholesterol, a second beneficial action of bile acid sequestrants is to increase the fraction of biliary cholesterol that escapes reabsorption and is excreted. The combination of bile acid sequestrant and HMG CoA reductase inhibitor is especially effective in lowering blood levels of LDL cholesterol by limiting the uptake of cholesterol from the diet, limiting the synthesis of cholesterol in the liver, increasing the clearance of cholesterol from the blood by the liver, and increasing the conversion of hepatic cholesterol to bile acids.

Other drugs used to reduce circulating LDL cholesterol levels include nicotinic acid, fibiric acid derivatives, and probucol. Nicotinic acid (niacin) is also a vitamin, but the amounts required to affect plasma cholesterol levels are far in excess of the daily requirement for this compound as an essential nutrient. At these pharmacologic doses, side effects such as itching, facial flushing, and gastric distress are common. Nicotinic acid decreases the formation of VLDL triglyceride in the liver and therefore reduces the formation of LDL; it also promotes the uptake of LDL through LDL receptors and increases the concentration of HDL cholesterol (cholesterol being returned to the liver for disposal). The underlying mechanisms for these actions have not been determined. Fibric acid derivatives, such as gemfibrazole, also reduce VLDL secretion and promote LDL uptake by the liver; again the mechanism of drug action is uncertain. Probucol acts primarily to prevent chemical modification of LDL in the circulation that makes it more likely to be deposited in the walls of blood vessels.

Although high circulating levels of LDL cholesterol call for drug intervention, the risk of atherosclerotic disease can be reduced in most adults by attention to the dietary factors that affect cholesterol balance. Dietary studies have had a controversial history because of frequently contradictory findings. A few principles are, however, well supported by the data. First, eliminating cholesterol from the diet, with no other intervention, produces a significant drop in the levels of cholesterol in circulating LDL. Second, intake of calories beyond actual energy needs raises serum cholesterol. Excess fuel is stored as triglycerides, which to a large extent are formed in the liver and exported in VLDL. Since VLDL contains cholesterol, and since it is the precursor of LDL, high rates of triglyceride formation in the liver promote the accumulation of cholesterol in plasma LDL, which is especially likely to occur if the calories are ingested in the form of triglyceride. Not only does this increase the requirement for the liver to secrete VLDL, but the fatty acids derived from triglyceride also stimulate cholesterol synthesis. Third, saturated fatty acids have the strongest tendency to elevate plasma cholesterol levels. This is the case even when these fatty acids are consumed as vegetable oils (such as palm oil and coconut oil) unaccompanied by cholesterol. The basis for this effect is not well understood but appears to result from decreased expression of LDL receptors in the liver. The American Heart Association recommends that not more than 300 milligrams per day of cholesterol be consumed in a diet which is matched to caloric need and in which not more than 25 to 30 percent of calories are consumed as fat (and not more than 7 percent as saturated fat and not more than 1 percent trans fat). Individuals with heart disease or with LDL cholesterol levels greater than 100 milligrams per deciliter should limit their cholesterol intake to less than 200 milligrams each day.

Perspective and Prospects

The average adult body contains about 150 grams of cholesterol. Less than 5 percent of this cholesterol is in circulating lipoproteins or trapped in atherosclerotic lesions. The remainder performs essential functions as a structural component of membranes and as the precursor of other vital substances. Although researchers have learned much about the subcellular distribution, the pathway for biosynthesis, and the mechanisms for transport of cholesterol, important questions remain. It is not clearly understood how cholesterol is transported within the cell or what determines its relative distribution among different cellular membranes. It is not known what signals suppress the synthesis of HMG CoA reductase and LDL receptors or how the message is transmitted to the nucleus to diminish transcription of these genes. Some product of mevalonic acid metabolism other than cholesterol also regulates the

---

In the News:
Cholesterol-Lowering Drugs

Since high cholesterol level contributes to major health problems including hypertension, heart disease, and stroke, it is essential that cholesterol levels be kept in check. While lifestyle changes including diet and exercise may help to lower cholesterol, most individuals with elevated cholesterol levels are placed on medication. These cholesterol-lowering medications fall into several different categories. Patients may be placed on one drug or on a combination of drugs. The major categories of cholesterol-lowering drugs are statins, selective cholesterol absorption inhibitors, bile acid sequestrants (resins), fibric acid derivatives (or fibrates), and nicotinic acid (niacin). The most commonly used of these medications are statins. These drugs work in the liver to inhibit the production of HMG CoA reductase, which controls the production of cholesterol. Statins have been found to decrease cholesterol levels between 20 and 60 percent by slowing the production of cholesterol, while increasing the ability of the liver to remove low-density lipoproteins (LDL) from the blood, and increasing high-density lipoproteins (HDL). This class of drugs includes Lipitor (atorvastatin), Crestor (rosuvastatin), Zocor (simvastatin), and Pravachol (pravastatin). Statins are contraindicated in people who are preganant or nursing, have liver damage, or have high alcohol intakes. A second category of cholesterol-lowering drugs are selective cholesterol absorption inhibitors. Drugs in this category interfere with the absorption of cholesterol in the intestines, allowing the body to eliminate more cholesterol, especially LDLs. Zetia (ezetimibe) is the most commonly used drug in this class. Resins also work in the intestines, although in a different manner. Resins bind to bile, so that it is eliminated and cannot be used in digestion, causing more bile to be produced. Cholesterol is used by the liver to produce bile, leaving less cholesterol in the bloodstream. Drugs in this category include Questran (cholestyramine) and WelChol (colesevelam Hcl). Fibrates are used to lower triglycerides, rather than LDLs, and may be used in combination with the statins. This category of drugs includes Lopid (gemffibrozil) and Tricor (fenofibrate). The final category of drug used to lower cholesterol is niacin, a nutritional supplement that is available over the counter and in prescription form. It acts in the liver to decrease cholesterol production. In prescription form, niacin can lower both LDL and triglycerides. Thus, physicians can use any of these medications, individually or in combination, to lower their patients' cholesterol.

—*Robin Kamienny Montvilo, R.N., Ph.D.*

expression of HMG CoA reductase, but this factor has not yet been identified. It is not known why cholesterol is an absolute requirement for functioning of mammalian cell membranes. It is not known what determines the fraction of dietary cholesterol that is absorbed across the intestinal lining. Finally, there is much to learn about factors that regulate the secretion and reuptake of lipoproteins by the liver and that control the return to the liver of cholesterol in HDL.

These questions are of practical as well as academic interest. Ischaemic heart disease and other complications of atherosclerosis are the leading causes of death, causing about 12.8 percent of deaths worldwide, according to data from the World Health Organization. Controlling and reversing this process is a serious medical challenge. While other factors such as hypertension, smoking, and diabetes mellitus contribute to the risk of atherosclerosis, reducing the level of cholesterol that circulates as a component of LDL and increasing the level transported in HDL have been shown to provide significant protection. Knowledge of how cholesterol is normally produced and assimilated has contributed to the design of drugs that reduce circulating levels by interfering with the absorption and synthesis of cholesterol and promoting its metabolism and excretion. This field of investigation continues to be a major concern of both basic and pharmaceutical scientists.

—*Lauren M. Cagen, Ph.D.*

See also Arteriosclerosis; Blood and blood disorders; Blood testing; Cells; Digestion; Food biochemistry; Heart disease; Hypercholesterolemia; Hyperlipidemia; Metabolism; Nutrition; Plaque, arterial; Preventive medicine; Strokes.

For Further Information:

Dietschy, John M. "Physiology in Medicine: LDL Cholesterol-Its Regulation and Manipulation." *Hospital Practice* 25 (June 15, 1990): 67-78.

Freeman, Mason W., with Christine Junge. *The Harvard Medical School Guide to Lowering Your Cholesterol*. New York: McGraw-Hill, 2005.

Grundy, Scott M. *Cholesterol and Atherosclerosis*. Philadelphia: J. P. Lippincott, 1990.

Hirsch, Anita. *Good Cholesterol, Bad Cholesterol: An Indispensable Guide to the Facts About Cholesterol*. New York: Avalon, 2002.

Hosomi, Ryota. "Fish Protein Decreases Serum Cholesterol in Rats by Inhibition of Cholesterol and Bile Acid Absorption." *Journal of Food Science* 76.4 (2011): H116-H121.

Jayoung Kim, et al. "The Response of the Prostate to Circulating Cholesterol: Activating Transcription Factor 3 (ATF3) as a Prominent Node in a Cholesterol-Sensing Network." *PLoS ONE* 7.7 (2012): 1-14.

Leaf, David A. *Cholesterol Treatment: A Guide to Lipid Disorder Management*. 4th ed. Durant, Okla.: EMIS, 2000.

McGowan, Mary P., and Jo McGowan Chopra. *Fifty Ways to Lower Cholesterol*. New York: McGraw-Hill, 2002.

Nesto, N. W., and Lisa Christenson. *Cholesterol-Lowering Drugs: Everything You and Your Family Need to Know*. New York: William Morrow, 2000.

Wang, Helen H., et al. "Prevention of Cholesterol Gallstones by Inhibiting Hepatic Biosynthesis and Intestinal Absorption of Cholesterol." *European Journal of Clinical Investigation* 43.4 (2013): 413-426.

Chorionic villus sampling

Procedure

Anatomy or system affected: Reproductive system, uterus

Specialties and related fields: Embryology, genetics, obstetrics, perinatology

Definition: The collection of a small sample of chorionic villi tissue from the fingerlike projections of the placenta at the point of attachment to the uterine wall. These cells are examined for genetic and chromosomal abnormalities by means of karyotyping.

Indications and Procedures

Chorionic villus sampling can be performed between the ninth and thirteenth weeks of pregnancy to detect genetic and chromosomal abnormalities. The procedure is recommended when there is increased risk of genetic disorders in the fetus such as Down syndrome, sickle cell disease, and muscular dystrophy.

Chorionic villus sampling involves collecting a small sample of the chorionic villi, the finger-like projections on the developing placenta, which delivers food and oxygen to the fetus. A sample of chorionic villi can be obtained from the point at which the placenta attaches to the uterine wall, either by inserting a needle through the abdomen or by entering the cervix with a small flexible catheter through the vagina. The choice of approach depends on the position of the placenta. An antiseptic cleansing solution is applied to the area prior to sampling, and ultrasound is used to locate the fetus and the placenta and its villi.

A 10- to 25-milligram sample is collected using a syringe, which is then purified and sometimes cultured. Since the chorionic villi originate from the same cell as the fetus, they normally have the same genetics. Results are available within one to two weeks.

Uses and Complications

Along with exposing genetic and chromosomal disorders, chorionic villus sampling can be used to determine the sex of the embryo but should never be used for this purpose alone because of the risks involved. Testing can be done early in the pregnancy. Therefore, should the woman choose to terminate her pregnancy, an easier first-trimester abortion can be performed. If the results from the test are favorable, the parents have early peace of mind.

Possible complications from chorionic villus sampling include vaginal bleeding, cramping, and uterine infection. More serious risks involve Rh incompatibility between maternal and fetal blood, spontaneous abortion (miscarriage), and even possible fetal injury. A 2003 intervention review published in the *Cochrane Database of Systematic Review* found that the rate of miscarriage is significantly higher with chorionic villus sampling than with amniocentesis, performed after sixteen weeks and yielding the same information.

Some studies suggest that chorionic villus sampling itself may cause some birth defects; others do not. Also, the procedure can be inaccurate. Abnormalities may occur in some placental cells but not in the fetus. This might lead to

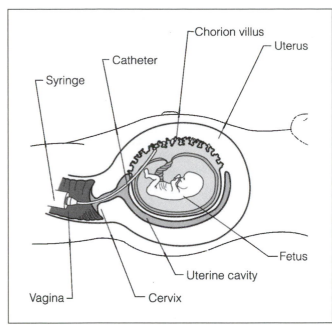

Chorionic villus sampling is one method of obtaining embryonic cells from a pregnant woman; examination of these cells helps physicians determine fetal irregularities or defects, which allows time to assess the problem and make recommendations for treatment.

aborting a healthy fetus. With the guidance of a physician, the risks and benefits should be compared with other available procedures.

—Paul R. Boehlke, Ph.D., and Pavel Svilenov; updated by Robin Kamienny Montvilo, R.N., Ph.D.

See also Abortion; Amniocentesis; Birth defects; Down syndrome; Embryology; Fetal surgery; Genetic counseling; Genetic diseases; Karyotyping; Miscarriage; Muscular dystrophy; Obstetrics; Perinatology; Pregnancy and gestation; Reproductive system; Sickle cell disease; Ultrasonography; Women's health.

For Further Information:

A.D.A..M. Medical Encyclopedia. "Chorionic Villus Sampling." *MedlinePlus*, August 7, 2012.

Caughey, Aaron B., Linda M. Hopkins, and Mary E. Norton. "Chorionic Villus Sampling Compared with Amniocentesis and the Difference in the Rate of Pregnancy Loss." *Obstetrics and Gynecology* 108, no. 3 (September, 2006): 612-616.

"Chorionic Villus Sampling." *Mayo Foundation for Medical Education and Research*, October 10, 2012.

Ettorre, Elizabeth, ed. *Before Birth: Understanding Prenatal Screening*. Brookfield, Vt.: Ashgate, 2001.

Filkins, Karen, and Joseph F. Russo, eds. *Human Prenatal Diagnosis*. 2d rev. ed. New York: Marcel Dekker, 1990.

Harper, Peter S. *Practical Genetic Counselling*. 6th ed. New York: Oxford University Press, 2004.

Lichtman, Ronnie, Lynn Louise Simpson, and Allan Rosenfield. *Dr. Guttmacher's Pregnancy, Birth, and Family Planning*. Rev. ed. New York: New American Library, 2003.

Montemayor-Quellenberg, Marjorie, and Andrea Chisholm. "Chorionic Villus Sampling-Transabdominal." *Health Library*, March 15, 2013.

Montemayor-Quellenberg, Marjorie, and Andrea Chisholm. "Chorionic Villus Sampling-Transcervical." *Health Library*, March 15, 2013.

Moore, Keith L., and T. V. N. Persaud. *The Developing Human: Clinically Oriented Embryology*. 9th ed. Philadelphia: Saunders/ Elsevier, 2013.

Pierce, Benjamin A. *The Family Genetic Sourcebook*. New York: John Wiley & Sons, 1990.

Chromosomal abnormalities. *See* Birth defects; Genetic diseases.

Chronic fatigue syndrome
Disease/Disorder
Also known as: Chronic fatigue and immune dysfunction syndrome
Anatomy or system affected: Immune system, muscles, musculoskeletal system, psychic-emotional system
Specialties and related fields: Family medicine, hematology, immunology, internal medicine, psychiatry
Definition: Chronic fatigue syndrome is a multifaceted disease state characterized by debilitating fatigue.
Key terms:
adenopathy: the enlargement of any gland (often the lymph gland)
cell-mediated immune response: an immune response that involves cells rather than antibodies, particularly T lymphocytes rather than B lymphocytes
cytokines: proteins secreted by immune cells which contribute to immune responses and inflammation
fibromyalgia: a condition of generalized chronic pain that shares many symptoms with chronic fatigue syndrome
infectious mononucleosis: acute self-limiting infection of lymphocytes by the Epstein-Barr virus
interleukin-2: a protein messenger that regulates T cell activity and differentiation during the immune response
lymphocytes: agranular leukocytes that differentiate into B lymphocytes and T lymphocytes and play a fundamental role in the immune response
polymerase chain reaction: a laboratory method used to increase the amount of DNA found in small quantities
suppressor T cell: a type of T lymphocyte that is believed to modulate the immune response

Causes and Symptoms

Chronic fatigue syndrome is a heterogeneous disease state that has been difficult to define, diagnose, and treat because of poorly understood cause-and-effect relationships. The disease can be best described in terms of long-lasting and debilitating fatigue, the etiology of which has been linked to such external factors as microbial agents, stress, and lifestyle as well as such internal factors as genetic makeup and the body's immune response. The physical disease also has psychological components, which has caused confusion in the medical community as to the exact cause of the syndrome.

Among the many names that have been used for the disease, two that demonstrate the many factors that contribute to chronic fatigue syndrome are chronic Epstein-Barr virus syndrome and chronic fatigue immune dysfunction syndrome. Because of the marked immunological aspects of the disease and the fact that different viruses have been found in patients with chronic fatigue, the disease is often referred to as chronic fatigue immune dysfunction syndrome. The US Centers for Disease Control and Prevention (CDC) continues to refer to it as chronic fatigue syndrome (CFS).

Although the disease is not specific by race, gender, or age group, it affects significantly more women than men. It is estimated by the CDC that between 20 and 40 of every 10,000 people in the United States have CFS.

CFS can manifest itself in acute and chronic phases, although some patients do not remember an acute phase presentation. Acute phase symptoms are general and flulike, with a low-grade fever, sore throat, headache, muscle pain, painful lymph nodes, and overall fatigue. Unlike with a bout of influenza, the symptoms do not subside with time, instead intensifying into a chronic phase. The fatigue can become disabling, with severe muscle and joint pain, swollen and painful lymph nodes, and the inability to develop proper sleep patterns. The similarity of CFS to fibromyalgia, diffuse muscular pain throughout the body, has resulted in cross diagnosis by many physicians of the two syndromes. Some researchers blame psychological and emotional stress, with a viral infection having triggered the initial acute phase. Although the psychological description does not fit all cases, problems of concentration, attention, and depression have been implicated to the point that researchers recognize both psychological and physical components. The working definition from both a research and a clinical perspective requires that the fatigue cause at least 50 percent incapacitation and last at least six months. The ineffectiveness of treatment, compounded by the inability to provide a concrete diagnosis, further complicates the psychological aspects of the disease for the patient.

Although the environment provides an array of agents that could trigger the physical condition of CFS, the hypothesis for a viral cause is supported by the flulike symptoms, occasional clustering of cases, and presence of antiviral antibodies in the patient's serum. The involvement of the Epstein-Barr virus in some forms of CFS seems likely because of its role as the etiological agent of mononucleosis and Burkitt's lymphoma, which are similar diseases. In both of these diseases, the Epstein-Barr virus has a unique and harmful effect on the immune system because it directly invades B lymphocytes, the antibody-producing cells of the body, using them to grow new virus particles while disrupting the proper functioning of the immune system. Like CFS, mononucleosis is characterized by flulike symptoms and fatigue, but the disease is self-limiting and the patient eventually recovers.

Despite this seeming difference in outcome, the Epstein-Barr virus can cause a chronic condition. The viruses that infect humans can become dormant within the cells that they infect. The nucleic acid of a virus can become incorporated into the deoxyribonucleic acid (DNA) of its host cell, and the body no longer shows physical signs of its presence. A virus can become active at times of physical or emotional stress and can once again trigger the physical symptoms of disease. For example, herpes simplex virus 1 remains dormant in its host cell but periodically, in response to environmental factors, causes a cold sore lesion.

Immunological dysfunction has been observed in CFS patients because they demonstrate increased allergic sensitivity to skin tests when compared to individuals without CFS. Cells and cellular chemicals directly involved with protective immunity and the regulation of the immune response have been found in these patients in abnormal concentrations. For example, they have abnormal numbers of the natural killer cells and suppressor T cells that are essential to cell-mediated immunity. A variety of cytokines, such as gamma interferon, and various interleukins that regulate the activities of the cells in the cell-mediated and humoral immune responses are seen in abnormal concentrations in some CFS patients. Some of these cytokines are already known to mediate the immune response to viral infections. Infectious agents such as bacteria, viruses, yeast, intracellular parasites, and even cancer cells are eliminated from the body when humoral and cell-mediated immune systems are operating properly. The presence of abnormally high concentrations of these cytokines may contribute to inflammatory processes sometimes found in patients with CFS. When the immune system is not working properly, however, not only is the body more susceptible to a variety of infectious agents, but the immune system can begin to damage or destroy normal tissues as well. Such disease states are referred to as autoimmune diseases. Inflammation and allergic reactions are other examples of uncontrolled immune responses.

The psychological and emotional aspects of CFS are also in question. Some studies indicate that the brain is physically affected by inflammation and hormonal changes. Other studies demonstrate that some of the known viral infective agents can have neurological effects. Psychiatric studies give ample evidence that depression, memory loss, and concentration are significant problems for some CFS patients. The extent to which stress is a factor in the disease is unknown.

Treatment and Therapy

Defining and treating chronic fatigue syndrome has been difficult because it manifests itself as a systemic disease with confusing cause-and-effect relationships involving external factors such as infectious viruses, internal factors such as the immune response, and a psychological component that is difficult to assess. The symptoms, provided by patient histories, physical examinations, and laboratory findings, involve neuromuscular, psychoneurological, and immunological changes that vary between patients. The variety of factors to consider has caused difficulty in establishing diagnostic criteria for primary care in a clinical setting or further definition of the disease and treatments in a research setting.

In 1988, the CDC established diagnostic criteria that are divided into two major criteria, eleven minor symptom criteria, and three minor physical criteria. The first major criterion defines chronic fatigue as lasting at least six months and causing debilitation to 50 percent of the patient's normal activity. The second major criterion requires that all other disease conditions that could fit the patient history, physical examination, and appropriate laboratory tests be ruled out. The categories of disease that might be similar to CFS are cancers, chronic degenerative disease, autoimmune disorders, microbial and parasitic disease, and chronic psychiatric disease. Combinations of some minor criteria that would fit a general flulike condition must be demonstrated.

In 1993, a meeting at the CDC attempted to evaluate what had been learned over the previous five-year period and to make recommendations regarding a case definition. It was suggested that the case definition format involve inclusion and exclusion criteria that would increase the number and range of cases being studied because of the heterogeneous nature of the disease. The cases should also be subcategorized to provide a homogeneity that would allow for subgroup identification and comparison. The inclusion evidence should be simple, with a descriptive interpretation of the fatigue being essential and having objective criteria to define a 50 percent reduction of physical activity. Symptoms that are specific to unexplained fatigue should be used, while the physical exam information should not be included. It was also suggested that exclusion of any cases should involve an in-depth history (both medical and psychiatric), a physical examination, and standardized testing that would involve medical, laboratory, and psychiatric information.

Because it appears that CFS overlaps with many other medical and psychiatric conditions that can be identified and treated, there is debate as to how to interpret CFS as it relates to patient care and research. Some believe that an in-depth history is fundamental to the understanding of CFS and that CFS could be caused by a variety of biological and psychosocial factors.

The minor criteria used to define CFS involve both symptom and physical criteria that have not been proved adequate to validate or define the condition. In fact, the conflicting data have only served to emphasize further the clinical heterogeneity of the disease and suggest a heterogeneity of cause. Suggestions have been made to drop the concept of minor criteria, use symptoms that are specific to the unexplained fatigue, and drop all physical examination criteria. The argument for eliminating physical criteria is that more specific criteria exist for a case definition. Because physical symptoms are inconsistent or periodic, it is believed that a documented patient history would provide more case-specific information.

Although symptom criteria have widespread support in the case definition of CFS, symptoms with the greatest sensitivity and specificity are also being debated. Night sweats, cough, gastrointestinal problems, and new and worsening allergies are not presently considered and are believed by some to be more specific than fever or chills and sore throat. Others have proposed that symptoms should be reduced to chills and fever, sore throat, neck or axilla adenopathy, and sudden onset of a main symptom complex. The most prevalent symptoms are believed to be muscle weakness and pain, problems in concentration, and sleep disturbance.

The importance of the psychiatric component in CFS continues to be a problem in case definition. Some believe that the neurological component is a major criterion in case definition and that behavioral symptoms, including stress and psychiatric illness, must be emphasized in clinical diagnosis as well as in treatment. It has been recommended that objective neuropsychological testing be used to determine cognitive dysfunction and depression. There is a general agreement that CFS patients have impaired concentration and attention, but forgetfulness and memory problems are questioned. There is also evidence that the duration and severity of myalgia are closely associated with psychological distress and that psychotherapy improves physical symptoms. Finally, it has been argued that the psychiatric component of the case definition is essential because there is evidence that the disease directly affects the brain and that CFS can cause both isolation and limitation of the patient's normal lifestyle.

Proper patient care necessitates extensive evaluation in order to identify the biological or psychological reasons for the problem. Proper CFS patient care demands the elimination of other serious disease possibilities that may appear superficially similar. Primary care physicians may find it difficult to make a diagnosis without a team of specialists in the areas of hematology, immunology, and psychiatry. Numerous laboratory tests must be made available. Although there are no specific recommended tests, those that must be performed should be tailored to specific patients.

The possibility of infectious disease, either as part of CFS (as in the case of certain viral agents) or as an autonomous infection having no relation to CFS, requires a variety of antibody tests to detect such viruses as Epstein-Barr or HIV. Skin tests such as the purified protein derivative (PPD) test for tuberculosis are used. Polymerase chain reaction and tissue culture for cytopathic effects have been developed to detect certain retroviruses for use in diagnosis.

The immune system is so intimately interactive with the entire body that most disease conditions are affected by and affect its function. Carefully monitoring the components of the immune system can provide clues to the identity of the disease that is operating because they indicate whether normal protection activity or immune dysfunction (or a combination) is occurring in the patient.

The components of the immune system can be measured

in numerous ways, from methodologies used in standard clinical laboratory procedures to research protocols used to study immune function and disease treatment. Tests are available that can measure total antibody concentration and the various subgroups IgG, IgM, IgA, IgE, and IgD; cytokines such as interleukin-2 and gamma interferon; cellular components such as T cells and their subtypes (such as suppressor T cells and natural killer cells); and B cells.

Autoimmune diseases and allergies are immune dysfunction diseases in their own right. Because there is an immune dysfunction component to CFS, tests for these conditions are important considerations. An antinuclear antibody (ANA) test determines the presence of antibodies that attack the tissues of the patient, as in systemic lupus erythematosus. The type and extent of allergic reactions can be measured using the radioimmunosorbent (RIST) tests for total IgE concentration and radioallergosorbent (RAST) tests for IgE concentration for particular antigens.

Systemic disease states, including CFS, often involve generalized inflammation that is considered part of the body's protective response. While inflammation is important to the elimination of various infective agents, it is also involved in neurological and muscle tissue damage. C-reactive protein (CRP) and the erythrocyte sedimentation rate (ESR) tests measure the intensity of the inflammatory response. A variety of other tests provide information that indicates the extent of muscle, liver, thyroid, and other vital organ damage.

Although a diagnosis can be made for CFS, there is no standard treatment. Clinical treatment essentially takes the form of alleviating the symptoms. Antidepressants such as doxepin (Sinequan) are useful in the treatment of depression and are also used to control muscle pain, lethargy, and sleeping problems. Nonsteroidal anti-inflammatory drugs (NSAIDs) provide relief for headache and muscle pain. Two drugs that have demonstrated antiviral activities are acyclovir and ampligen; ampligen can also modulate the immune response. Psychological counseling is also recommended for CFS patients in order to help them identify alternatives to work around some of the limitations that CFS creates. Physical therapy and graded exercise have also been shown to ease some of the symptoms of CFS, although patients should be careful not to overexert themselves, which could lead to a worsening of symptoms.

Because of the systemic nature of the disease, including its psychoneurological component, consideration must be given to holistic medical treatment. Any treatment protocol must be able to address the interactive factors of CFS that are still being defined in terms of cause and effect. Some researchers believe that therapeutic treatment should comprise diet, exercise, vitamins, and homeopathic medicine.

Perspective and Prospects

The vague, often "flulike" symptoms used to define chronic fatigue syndrome have historically been associated with numerous infectious agents, such as *Brucella* (brucellosis), *Coxsiella*, Epstein-Barr virus infections (infectious mononucleosis), and other chronic viral diseases.

In most cases, a specific etiological agent was discovered. Association with a specific agent allowed for treatment in many cases, or at the least a means to define the illness.

Continued technological advances and research into both the immune system and the nature of viral infection will provide new insights into more effective treatment protocols for CFS, including the role played by immune responses to the triggering agent. The neuropsychological components of the disease, as well as evidence demonstrating ties between these components and the immune system, require an active approach by the patient to achieve a healthy state. CFS provides a challenge to the patient to adapt a personal lifestyle that is conducive to a healthy mind and body.

Medical treatment and diagnostic testing can be costly as well as useless, particularly as the health care community continues to refine its understanding of the condition. Patients must remain vigilant regarding phony or trendy treatments that have no correlation to acceptable research findings; such treatments not only can be expensive but also could lead to deteriorating health.

—*Patrick J. DeLuca, Ph.D.;*
updated by Richard Adler, Ph.D.

See also Autoimmune disorders; Epstein-Barr virus; Fatigue; Fibromyalgia; Immune system; Immunology; Mononucleosis; Multiple chemical sensitivity syndrome; Stress.

For Further Information:
Afari, Niloofar, and Dedra Buchwald. "Chronic Fatigue Syndrome: A Review." *American Journal of Psychiatry* 160 (February, 2003): 221-236.
Berne, Katrina. *Chronic Fatigue Syndrome, Fibromyalgia, and Other Invisible Illnesses: The Comprehensive Guide.* 3d ed. Alameda, Calif.: Hunter House, 2002.
Bested, Alison, and Alan Logan. *Chronic Fatigue Syndrome and Fibromyalgia.* Nashville: Cumberland House, 2006.
"Chronic Fatigue Syndrome." *Medline Plus*, March 22, 2013.
Englebienne, Patrick, and Kenny DeMeirleir, eds. *Chronic Fatigue Syndrome: A Biological Approach.* Boca Raton, Fla.: CRC Press, 2002.
Friedberg, Fred. *Fibromyalgia and Chronic Fatigue Syndrome: Seven Proven Steps to Less Pain and More Energy.* Oakland, Calif.: New Harbinger, 2006.
Jason, Leonard A., and Molly M. Brown. "Subtyping Daily Fatigue Progression in Chronic Fatigue Syndrome." *Journal of Mental Health* 22, no. 1 (February, 2013): 4-11.
Mayo Clinic Staff. "Chronic Fatigue Syndrome." *Mayo Clinic*, June 18, 2011.
Patarca-Montero, Roberto. *Chronic Fatigue Syndrome and the Body's Immune Defense System.* New York: Haworth Medical Press, 2002.
Sticherling, Michael, and Enno Christophers, eds. *Treatment of Autoimmune Disorders.* New York: Springer, 2003.

Chronic granulomatous disease

Disease/Disorder

Also known as: Bridges-Good syndrome, chronic granulo- matous disorder, and Quie syndrome

Anatomy or system affected: All

Specialties and related fields: Bacteriology, critical care, dermatology, emergency medicine, family practice, gastroenterology, general surgery, genetics, immunology, internal medicine, microbiology, nephrology, pathology, pediatrics, pharmacology, proctology, pulmonary medicine, radiology, serology, urology

Definition: An inherited immune system disorder that prevents particular white blood cells (phagocytes) from effectively killing micro-organisms and leads to recurrent infections.

Key terms:

granulomas: inflammatory response in which the cell infiltrate is a collection mainly of macrophages

macrophages: a type of white blood cell within tissues and circulating blood that ingests foreign material and is produced by the division and maturation of monocytes

phagocytes: types of white blood cells capable of ingesting and absorbing micro-organisms and other small cells and particles

reactive oxygen species: oxygen-containing molecules that possess unpaired valence electrons, and as a consequence are highly reactive

Causes and Symptoms

Chronic granulomatous disease (CGD) is an inherited disorder that prevents particular white blood cells known as phagocytes from producing reactive oxygen species. Because phagocytes use reactive oxygen species to kill invading micro-organisms, white cells from CGD patients cannot stem the influx or proliferation of incoming micro-organisms.

When phagocytes encounter invading microorganisms, they extend their cell membranes around the micro-organism and fuse them in order to move the micro-organism into an intracellular compartment known as a phagosome. This process, known as phagocytosis, stimulates oxygen consumption in phagocytes. Increased oxygen consumption by phagocytes drives the production of reactive oxygen species (ROS), which are used by phagocytes to kill phagocytosed micro-organisms.

Phagocytes make ROS by means of an enzyme complex known as the phagocytic NADPH (nicotinamide adenine dinucleotide phosphate) oxidase or phox system, which consists of a five-protein complex. Inside phagocytes, the phox system lies within the membrane of a vesicle known as the lysosome. After phagocytosis, the phagosome fuses with lysosomes to form a new compartment known as the phagolysosome. Within the phagolysosome membrane, the phox system catalyzes the following reaction: $NADPH + 2O_2 \leftrightarrow NADP^+ + 2O_2^- + H^+$. The superoxide radicals, or O_2^- molecules produced by this reaction, can damage subcellular structures, but they can also react with other molecules to produce even more damaging ROS, including hydroxyl radials (OH^-), hydrogen peroxide (H_2O_2), peroxynitrite anions ($ONOO^-$), and oxyhalides ($HOCl^-$). Phagocyte production of these various ROS effectively kills phagocytosed micro-organisms.

Mutations in the genes that encode components of the phox system abrogate ROS production and prevent phagocytes from being able to kill phagocytosed micro-organisms. The five subunits of the phox system include gp91 (glycoprotein 91), p22, p47, p67, and p40. The CYBB gene encodes gp91 and is on the X chromosome. Mutations in CYBB constitute 50 to 75 percent of cases of CGD. The NCF1 gene encodes p47, and NCF1 mutations account for 20 to 40 percent of CGD cases; the NCF2 gene encodes p67, and NCF2 mutations account for less than 10 percent of all cases of CGD. The incidence of CGD in the United States ranges from 1 in 200,000 / 250,000. Internationally, CGD rates range from 1 case in 220,000 / 500,000.

CGD patients usually present symptoms in their first five years of life. The most common infections in CGD patients include skin infections, pneumonia, lung abscesses, lymphatic vessel infections (suppurative lymphangitis), gastrointestinal infections with diarrhea, abscesses around the anus and rectum, and liver and spleen abscesses. Other infections include bone infections (osteomyelitis), colonization of the bloodstream by micro-organisms (septicemia), and fungal infections.

A second feature of CGD patients is the development of granulomas in the skin, and in the gastrointestinal, reproductive, and urinary tracts, which can obstruct them.

Treatment and Therapy

Genetic tests can establish the diagnosis of CGD. Also the nitroblue tetrazolium (NBT) test can confirm a functional phox complex. Phagocytes isolated from blood convert the colorless NBT to a blue compound called formazan. Phagocytes from the blood of CGD patients cannot convert NBT to formazan.

To prevent infections, CGD patients are given trimethoprimn-sulfamethoxaxole (Bactrim). Patients with sulfa allergies are treated with trimethoprim alone and a cephalosporin. Staphylococcal infections are treated with Ciprofloxacin (Cipro). Fungal infections are treated with newer antifungals, including voriconazole (VFEND), posaconazole (Noxafil), and intraconazole (Sporanox and Onmel). Interferon-gamma improves phagocyte activity against invading micro-organisms and, therefore, is used to prevent infections in CGD. Steroid drugs such as prednisone are the agents of choice to reduce the incidence and severity of granulomas. Abscesses may require surgical drainage and resection.

Bone marrow transplantations from a compatible donor can cure CGD. Gene therapy trials in 2006 successfully inserted the CYBB gene into the bone marrow stem cells of

---

Information on Chronic Granulomatous Disease

Causes: Mutations in the CYBB, NCF1, NCF2, or CYBA genes

Symptoms: Severe recurrent bacterial and fungal infections, granulomas

Duration: Symptoms first appear by 5 years and are sustained unless a bone marrow transplant cures the patient

Treatments: Antibiotics and antifungals for frequent infections, interferon-gamma to stimulate the immune system, steroids for granulomas, surgery for abscesses, bone marrow transplants to cure the disease two different patients. Both patients showed significant phox activity and were effectively cured by gene therapy.

Perspective and Prospects

The first description of CGD comes from Janeway and his colleagues at a meeting of the Society for Pediatric Research in 1954 in which they reported the cases of five children who suffered from recurrent infections. In 1957 and 1959, Bridges, Good, and Berendes published the clinical and laboratory features of a "fatal granulomatous disease of children." In 1967, Nathan and Baeher documented the inability of phagocytes from CGD patients to reduce NBT, a test still in use to this day. Louis Kunkel's laboratory published the cloning of the CYBB gene in 1986.

Successful gene therapy trials in 2006 established the possibly of gene therapy to cure CGD. In this trial, however, the bone marrow stem cells from the CGD patients were infected with genetically engineered retroviruses. While this procedure increased gp41 levels in the patient's phagocytes, retroviral gene vectors are potentially dangerous because they randomly insert their viral genomes into the chromosomes of the host cells, which can produce mutations. Further work using nonmutagenic vectors that permanently introduce genes into bone marrow stem cells is underway to make gene therapy a viable option as a cure for CGD patients.

—*Michael A. Buratovich Ph.D.*

See also Bacterial infections; Bacteriology; Bronchitis; Candidiasis; Dermatology; Fever; Hematology; Immunology; Immunopathology; Lungs; Mastitis; Pediatrics; Pulmonary medicine

For Further Information:

Åhlin, Anders, et al. "Chronic Granulomatous Disease-Haematopoietic Stem Cell Transplantation Versus Conventional Treatment." *Acta Paediatrica doi*: 10.1111/apa.12384 (August 2013).

Murphy, Kenneth. *Janeway's Immunobiology.* 8th ed. London: Garland Science, 2011.

Sompayrac, Lauren M. *How the Immune System Works.* 4th ed. Hoboken, NJ: Wiley-Blackwell, 2012.

Chronic obstructive pulmonary disease (COPD)

Disease/Disorder

Anatomy or system affected: Lungs, respiratory system

Specialties and related fields: Geriatrics and gerontology, public health, pulmonary medicine

Definition: A progressive, irreversible disease of the lungs that causes expiratory airflow obstruction. The most common form of COPD is a combination of chronic bronchitis and emphysema.

Key terms:

alpha 1 antitrypsin: a protein that protects the lungs

alveoli: air sacs in the lungs that exchange oxygen and carbon dioxide

barrel chest: a rounded chest in which the anterior and posterior diameter is increased

bronchial tubes: branches in the airways in the lungs that allow for the exchange of oxygen and carbon dioxide

chronic bronchitis: a condition involving the inflammation and eventual scarring of the lining of the bronchial tubes and the production of excess mucus in the lungs

emphysema: airway disease involving permanent distension of distal airspaces and damage to alveolar walls of the lungs

exacerbation: worsening or intensifying

expiratory phase: exhalation, or breathing out

hypoxic: having low oxygen levels

pursed lip breathing: slow expirations from the abdomen against pursed lips

tachypnea: rapid breathing greater than twenty breaths per minute

Causes and Symptoms

Patients suffering from chronic obstructive pulmonary disease (COPD), a combination of chronic bronchitis and emphysema, have a chronic cough and shortness of breath that progressively limits their tolerance for physical activity. A physical examination may appear normal in the early stages of COPD, but as the disease progresses, tachypnea and wheezing occur. Over time, the occasional cough becomes more frequent, and greater effort is exerted to breathe. In later stages of COPD, the heart may be affected because the lungs can no longer supply an adequate amount of oxygen to the body. Other signs of advanced COPD are a barrel chest, pursed lip breathing, and a prolonged expiratory phase of respirations. Coughing produces phlegm that becomes increasingly difficult to expel as it thickens. Persons with advanced COPD cannot lie flat to sleep and may need to sit in an semiupright position in order to breathe.

The major risk factor for COPD is cigarette smoking. Other risk factors are air pollution (including exposure to mining), manufacturing (such as steel and cement), a history of childhood respiratory infections, and low socioeconomic status. In chronic bronchitis, the lining of the bronchial tubes become irritated, inflamed, and filled with mucus that blocks the airways, making it difficult to breathe. In emphysema, the alveoli become irritated, stiffen, and cannot transfer oxygen and carbon dioxide in the blood. Thus far, a deficiency of the enzyme alpha-1 antitrypsin is the only identified genetic cause of COPD.

COPD is an insidious disease that presents few symptoms until it is well developed in the lungs. It is usually not identified until the patient is fifty to sixty years old, although COPD caused by a deficiency of alpha-1 antitrypsin may be identified by thirty to forty years of age.

Confirmation of the diagnosis of COPD is made by pulmonary function tests (PFTs). PFTs are helpful in diagnosing COPD in its early stages and may be helpful in convincing patients to stop smoking, if necessary, to slow the progression of COPD. Spirometry measures the amount of air exhaled in one second, or forced expiratory volume (FEV1). The total amount of air exhaled, or forced vital capacity (FVC), is compared to the FEV1 to determine the extent of airway obstruction. A peak flow meter can show the severity of breathing impairment; after a deep breath, the patient blows into the instrument as forcefully and for as long as possible. Arterial blood gas tests measure the level

Information on Chronic Obstructive Pulmonary Disease (COPD)

Causes: Unknown; risk factors include smoking, air pollution, textile manufacturing, childhood respiratory infections
Symptoms: Chronic cough, shortness of breath, wheezing, limited physical activity
Duration: Chronic and progressive
Treatments: None; alleviation of symptoms (bronchodilators, antibiotics, steroids, oxygen therapy, vaccination against pneumonia and influenza, smoking cessation, pulmonary rehabilitation)

of oxygen and carbon dioxide in the blood. Serum alpha-1-antitrypsin levels are measured by blood samples. Finally, chest X-rays, pulmonary ventilation-perfusion scans, and chest magnetic resonance imaging (MRI) scans may all help to identify the degree of lung damage caused by COPD.

Treatment and Therapy

Because no cure exists for COPD, treatment focuses on decreasing symptoms and reducing complications. Bronchodilator medications, antibiotics, steroids, oxygen, and vaccination against pneumonia and influenza are used to treat or prevent symptoms, slow the progression of the disease, and manage any complications. Smoking cessation is vitally important for slowing the progress of COPD. Nicotine replacement therapy, antidepressant therapy, and counseling are some of the methods used to assist in smoking cessation.

Patients with COPD who are hypoxic require long-term oxygen therapy to improve their functional status and rate of survival. The purpose of oxygen therapy is to maintain adequate oxygen levels to prevent respiratory difficulties.

Pulmonary rehabilitation can help reduce hospitalizations and increase the quality of life for those with COPD, improving their overall functional status. Pulmonary rehabilitation includes therapies to enhance breathing, physical training to improve muscle strength and stamina, and the pacing of activities to avoid overexertion. Pursed lip breathing helps to relieve abnormal breathing (dyspnea) and to slow respirations.

Lung transplantation and lung reduction surgery may be options for people who suffer from severe emphysema. Lung reduction surgery, which is still in the experimental stages, is the partial removal of the most damaged areas of the lungs in order to allow for better lung expansion of the normal areas of the lung. Gene therapy and alpha-1-antitrypsin replacement therapy are presently under evaluation as treatments for alpha-1-antitrypsin deficiency, but the long-term effects of these treatments are unknown.

Perspective and Prospects

Between 80 and 90 percent of all cases of COPD are caused by cigarette smoking. According to the World Health Organization, COPD is the fourth leading cause of death in the world. The incidence of this disease is increasing every year. Those with COPD are prone to recurrent respiratory infections, and their quality of life gradually declines as the disease worsens. Smoking cessation is the single most important prevention method.

—*Sharon W. Stark, R.N., A.P.R.N., D.N.Sc.*

See also Asbestos exposure; Aspergillosis; Bronchi; Bronchitis; Chest; Cyanosis; Emphysema; Environmental diseases; Environmental health; Geriatrics and gerontology; Influenza; Lungs; Nicotine; Occupational health; Oxygen therapy; Pneumonia; Pulmonary diseases; Pulmonary medicine; Respiration; Smoking; Wheezing.

For Further Information:
Barnett, Margaret. *Chronic Obstructive Pulmonary Disease in Primary Care*. New York: Wiley, 2006.
Calverley, Peter M. A., et al., eds. *Chronic Obstructive Pulmonary Disease*. 2d ed. London: Hodder Arnold, 2003.
Haas, François, and Sheila Sperber Haas. *The Chronic Bronchitis and Emphysema Handbook*. Rev. ed. New York: John Wiley & Sons, 2000.
Jenkins, Mark. *Chronic Obstructive Pulmonary Disease: Practical, Medical, and Spiritual Guidelines for Daily Living with Emphysema, Chronic Bronchitis, and Combination Diagnosis*. Center City, Minn.: Hazelden Information Education, 1999.
Kaufman, Gerri. "Chronic Obstructive Pulmonary Disease: Diagnosis and Management." *Nursing Standard* 27, no. 21 (January, 2013): 53-62.
Parker, James N., and Philip M. Parker, eds. *The 2002 Official Patient's Sourcebook on Chronic Obstructive Pulmonary Disease*. San Diego, Calif.: Icon Health, 2002.
"What Is COPD?" *National Heart, Lung, and Blood Institute*, June 8, 2012.
Wood, Debra. "Chronic Obstructive Pulmonary Disease." *Health Library*, October 11, 2012.

Chronic wasting disease (CWD)
Disease/Disorder
Anatomy or system affected: Brain, nervous system
Specialties and related fields: Neurology
Definition: A neurological disease of deer and elk caused by an infectious protein particle called a prion.

Causes and Symptoms

Chronic wasting disease (CWD) is an invariably fatal neurological disease that affects deer, elk, and moose in North America. The disease was first described in the late 1960s in captive animals in Colorado. As of 2006, CWD-infected animals-from either wild or captive populations-had been found in Colorado, Illinois, Kansas, Montana, Nebraska, New Mexico, New York, Oklahoma, South Dakota, Utah, West Virginia, Wisconsin, and Wyoming in the United States and in the provinces of Alberta and Saskatchewan in Canada. In the late stages of the disease, infected animals show progressive weight loss, listlessness, increased salivation and urination, increased water consumption, depression, and death.

The brains of dead animals show characteristic vacuoles, or holes, that give the brain the appearance of a sponge. This pathology is characteristic of all the transmissible spongiform encephalopathies (TSEs), including bovine spongiform encephalopathy (BSE) of cows (so-called mad cow disease), scrapie of sheep, and Creutzfeldt-Jakob disease (CJD) of humans. Although CWD is similar to these other diseases, it is not identical to them. These diseases appear to be caused by the misfolding of a small protein (prion) normally located in the membranes of neurons and other cells. The normal function of this protein is unknown, but when misfolded, it accumulates in the brain, resulting in the death of neurons. The misfolded, pathogenic prion appears to be able to direct the misfolding of any normal prion present in a cell, thus replicating its aberrant structure.

Prion diseases can be either inherited or transmitted. Humans can inherit CJD or contract it from contaminated blood or brain tissue. Evidence suggests that variant CJD in humans can result from consuming beef contaminated with the BSE prion. There is concern about whether the CWD prion in deer and elk can also "jump" the species barrier to humans in a manner similar to that of BSE. Research using monkeys suggests that there is a species barrier to humans, making it unlikely that CWD will be transmitted to humans despite contact with contaminated blood or tissues.

CWD is believed to be transmitted from animal to animal through contact with body fluids or feces. Research published in 2006 indicated that the disease is most easily transmitted via saliva and blood, although other modes of transmission have not been ruled out. Two recent studies found no strong clinical or epidemiological evidence that the disease can be transmitted to humans via the consumption of contaminated meat. Laboratory studies indicate that such transmission is possible, however. Because of the long incubation period for the disease, however, it is difficult to prove or disprove transmission from deer, elk, or moose to humans.

Perspective and Prospects

Many states where CWD is prevalent have banned the baiting of deer and are thinning the deer population. Deer and elk in crowded populations, particularly captive herds, appear to be more susceptible to CWD.

Research efforts are focused on developing a sensitive field diagnostic test. Definitive diagnosis is made by autopsy, but tests based on tonsil biopsy and antibodies to detect prions in body fluids are also being developed. Transgenic mouse models of each of the known TSEs are also being created in order to learn more about transmission and pathology.

—*Michele Arduengo, Ph.D.;*
updated by David M. Lawrence

See also Brain; Brain disorders; Creutzfeldt-Jakob disease (CJD); Food poisoning; Nervous system; Neurology; Prion diseases.

For Further Information:

Bartz, Jason C., Samuel E. Saunders, and Shannon L. Barelt-Hunt. "Occurrence, Transmission, and Zoonotic Potential of Chronic Wasting Disease." *Emerging Infectious Diseases* 18, no. 3 (March, 2012): 369-376.

Brown, David R., ed. *Neurodegeneration and Prion Disease.* New York: Springer, 2005.

Harris, David A., ed. *Prions: Molecular and Cellular Biology.* Portland, Oreg.: Horizon Scientific Press, 1999.

> ### Information on
> ### Chronic Wasting Disease (CWD)
>
> **Causes:** Prion disease in deer and elk
> **Symptoms:** In animals, progressive weight loss, listlessness, increased salivation and urination, increased water consumption, depression, death; possible transmission to humans through infected game
> **Duration:** Chronic and progressive
> **Treatments:** None

Potapov, Alex, et al. "Chronic Wasting Disease: Possible Transmission Mechanisms in Deer." *Ecological Modelling* 250 (February, 2013): 244-257.

"Prion Diseases." *National Institute of Allergy and Infectious Diseases,* July 5, 2011.

Prusiner, Stanley B., ed. *Prion Biology and Diseases.* 2d ed. Cold Spring Harbor, N.Y.: Cold Spring Harbor Laboratory Press, 2004.

Race, Brent, et al. "Susceptibilities of Nonhuman Primates to Chronic Wasting Disease." *Emerging Infectious Diseases* 15, no. 9 (2009): 1366-1376.

US Geological Survey. "Chronic Wasting Disease (CWD)." *National Wildlife Health Center,* June 5, 2012.

Chyme

Biology

Also known as: Chymus
Anatomy or system affected: Gallbladder, gastrointestinal system, intestines, liver, pancreas, stomach
Specialties and related fields: Gastroenterology, internal medicine
Definition: The slurry-like mixture of food and digestive juices produced in the digestive tract.

Structure and Functions

Chewing and swallowing produces a bolus of food that descends through the esophagus into the stomach. There, the stomach walls secrete hydrochloric acid while waves of muscular contraction called peristalsis mix the stomach contents. The gastric juices break the bolus into small food particles, producing a thick fluid called chyme. Peristalsis causes the chyme to collect in the antrum, the lowest section of the stomach. The pyloric sphincter passes small portions of chyme into the duodenum at regular intervals.

Chyme is highly acidic because of the stomach acid. To protect the membrane lining the duodenum, the pancreas releases bicarbonate to neutralize the acid. In the duodenum, digestion continues. Bile produced in the liver is added to the chyme to emulsify fats into small globules. The pancreas contributes enzymes that break down fats, proteins, and carbohydrates so that nutrients, minerals, and salts can be absorbed through the membrane of the small intestine and into the bloodstream.

Over a period of three to five hours, peristalsis pushes the chyme through the small intestine and into the colon. There, bacteria convert some ingredients of the chyme into vitamin K and vitamin B, which the colon extracts along with excess water. Bacteria also produce various gases. These gases are mixed with the remaining waste matter, or feces.

Disorders and Diseases

Most disorders relating to chyme come from excessive food or water intake. When too much is eaten, the stomach distends and presses on the diaphragm. Peristalsis and the sheer bulk of the chyme can make breathing difficult and uncomfortable. When food contains a high proportion of fat, spices, or fibers and is eaten too quickly, the stomach can be overburdened. The churning of peristalsis may force some of the chyme back up the esophagus, causing a burning sensation there known as acid reflux or heartburn. This indigestion of the chyme, or dyspepsia, can make the stomach feel sour and achy and can lead to stomach ulcers. The stomach also may react to psychological stress by producing too much acid.

When the pancreas fails to produce enough bicarbonate to neutralize the acid in chyme after it enters the duodenum, the acid may burn through the mucosa in its wall and into tissue, producing a duodenal ulcer. Too much bile added to the chyme, if not reabsorbed in the distal small intestine, can lead to diarrhea, whereas too little bile can contribute to malabsorption of nutrients. Similarly, excessive water intake may leach sodium from the body or cause the intestine to process the chyme too quickly for all the nutrients to be removed from it.

—*Roger Smith, Ph.D.*

See also Acid-base chemistry; Acid reflux disease; Bile; Diarrhea and dysentery; Digestion; Enzymes; Food biochemistry; Gastroenterology; Gastroenterology, pediatric; Gastrointestinal disorders; Gastrointestinal system; Heartburn; Indigestion; Intestines; Malabsorption; Metabolism; Nutrition; Peristalsis; Ulcers; Vitamins and minerals.

For Further Information:
Corcoran, Mary K., and Jef Czekaj. *The Quest to Digest.* Watertown, Mass.: Charlesbridge, 2006.

Lipski, Elizabeth. Digestive Wellness. 4th ed. New York: McGraw-Hill, 2012.

Parker, Steve. *The Human Body Book.* New York: DK Adult, 2001.

Seymour, Simon. *Guts: Our Digestive System.* New York: HarperCollins, 2005.

Circulation

Biology

Anatomy or system affected: Blood, blood vessels, circulatory system, liver

Specialties and related fields: Cardiology, hematology, vascular medicine

Definition: The flow of blood throughout the body; the circulatory system consists of the heart, lungs, arteries, and veins.

Key terms:

aneurysm: a localized enlargement of a vessel, usually an artery

atherosclerosis: accumulation of plaque within the arteries

calcification: the deposit of lime salts in organic tissue, leading to calcium in the arterial wall

capillaries: hairlike vessels that connect the ends of the smallest arteries to the beginnings of the smallest veins

claudication: muscle cramps that occur when arterial blood flow does not meet the muscles' demand for oxygen

diastole: the period of relaxation in the cardiac cycle

hypertension: a blood pressure higher than what is considered to be normal

lumen: the space within an artery, vein, or other tube

stenosis: the constriction or narrowing of a passage

systole: the period of contraction in the cardiac cycle

thrombus: a blood clot that, commonly, obstructs a vein but may also occur in an artery or the heart

vasoconstriction: a decrease in the diameter of a blood vessel

vasodilation: an increase in the diameter of a blood vessel

Structure and Functions

The cardiovascular system is made up of the heart, arteries, veins, capillaries, and lungs. The heart serves as a pump to deliver blood to the arteries for distribution throughout the body. The veins bring the blood back to the heart, and the lungs oxygenate the blood before returning it to the arterial system.

Contraction of the heart muscle forces blood out of the heart. This period of contraction is known as systole. The heart muscle relaxes after each contraction, which allows blood flow into the heart. This period of relaxation is known as diastole. A typical blood pressure taken at the upper arm provides a pressure reading during two phases of the cardiac cycle. The first number is known as the systolic pressure and represents the pressure of the heart during peak contraction. The second number is known as the diastolic pressure and represents the pressure while the heart is at rest. A typical pressure reading for a young adult would be 120/80. When blood pressure is abnormally elevated, it is commonly referred to as high blood pressure, or hypertension.

The heart is separated into two halves by a wall of muscle known as the septum. The two halves are known as the left and right heart. The left side of the heart is responsible for high-pressure arterial distribution and is larger and stronger than the right side. The right side of the heart is responsible for accepting low-pressure venous return and redirecting it to the lungs.

Because of these pressure differences from one side of the heart to the other, the vessel wall constructions of the arteries and the veins differ. Strong construction of the arterial wall allows tolerance of significant pressure elevations from the left heart. The arterial wall is made up of three major tissue layers, known as tunics. Secondary layers of tissue that provide strength and elasticity to the artery are known as elastic and connective tissues. As with the artery, the wall of the vein is made up of three distinct tissue layers. Compared to that of an artery, the wall of a vein is thinner and less elastic, which allows the wall to be easily compressed by surrounding muscle during contraction.

While the heart is at rest, between contractions, newly oxygenated arterial blood passes from the lungs and enters the left heart. Each time the heart contracts, blood is forced from the left heart into a major artery known as the aorta. From the aorta, blood is distributed throughout the body. Once depleted of nutrients and oxygen, arterial blood passes through an extensive array of minute vessels known as capillaries. A significant pressure drop occurs as blood is dispersed throughout the immense network of capillaries. The capillaries empty into the venous system, which carries the blood back to the heart.

The primary responsibility of the venous system is to return deoxygenated blood to the lungs and heart. Much more energy is required from the body to move venous flow compared to arterial flow. Unlike the artery, the vein does not depend on the heart or gravity for energy to move blood. The venous system has a unique means of blood transportation known as the "venous pump," which moves blood toward the heart.

The components making up the venous pump include muscle contraction against the venous wall, intra-abdominal pressure changes, and one-way venous valves. Compression against the walls of a vein induces movement of blood. Muscle contraction against a vein wall occurs throughout the body during periods of activity. Activity includes every movement, from breathing to running. Variations in respiration cause fluctuations in the pressure within the abdomen, which produces a siphonlike effect on the veins, pulling venous blood upward. Valves are located within the veins of the extremities and pelvis. A venous valve has two leaflets, which protrude inward from opposite sides of the vein wall and meet one another in the center. Valves are necessary to prevent blood from flowing backward, away from the heart.

The venous system is divided into two groups known as the deep and superficial veins. The deep veins are located parallel to the arteries, while the superficial veins are located just beneath the skin surface and are often visible through the skin.

Disorders and Diseases

Numerous variables may affect the flow of blood. The autonomic nervous system is connected to muscle within the wall of the artery by way of neurological pathways known as sympathetic branches. Various drugs and/or conditions can trigger responses in the sympathetic branches and produce constriction of the smooth muscle in the arterial wall (vasoconstriction) or relaxation of the arterial wall (vasodilation). Alcohol consumption and a hot bath are examples of conditions that produce vasodilation. Exposure to cold and cigarette smoking are examples of conditions that produce vasoconstriction. Various drugs used in the medical environment are capable of producing similar effects. The diameter of the lumen of an artery influences the pressure and the flow of blood through it.

Another condition that alters the arterial diameter is atherosclerosis, a disease primarily of the large arteries, which allows the formation of fat (lipid) deposits to build on the inner layer of the artery. Lipid deposits are more commonly known as atherosclerotic plaque. Plaque accumulation reduces the diameter of the arterial lumen, causing various degrees of flow restriction. Plaque is similar to rust accumulation within a pipe that restricts the flow of water. A restriction of flow is referred to as a stenosis. The majority of stenotic lesions occur at the places where arteries divide into branches, also known as bifurcations. In advanced

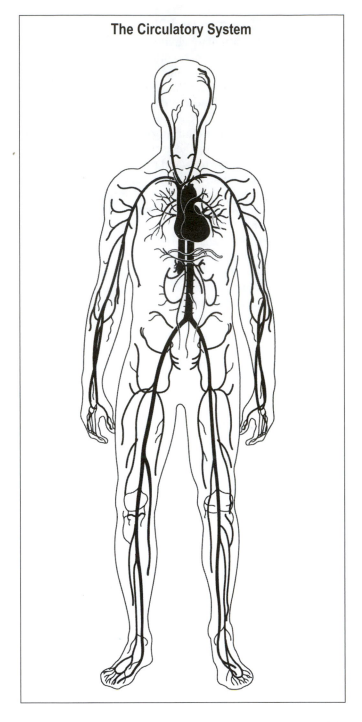

The Circulatory System

stages of plaque development, plaque may become calcified. Calcified plaque is hard and may become irregular, ulcerate, or hemorrhage, providing an environment for new clot formation and/or release of small pieces of plaque debris downstream. When pieces of plaque break off, they may move downstream into smaller blood vessels, causing a blockage and restricting the flow of oxygenated blood; this can cause tissue death, stroke, and heart attack.

An arterial wall may become very hard and rigid, a condition commonly known as hardening of the arteries. Hardened arteries may eventually become twisted, kinked, or dilated as a result of the hardening process of the arterial wall. A hardened artery which has become dilated is known as an aneurysm.

Normal arterial flow is undisturbed. When blood cells travel freely, they move together at a similar speed with very little variance. This is known as laminar flow. Nonlaminar (turbulent) flow is seen when irregular plaque or kinks in the arterial wall disrupt the smooth flow of cells. Plaque with an irregular surface may produce mild turbulence, while a narrow stenosis produces significant turbulence immediately downstream from the stenosis.

Many moderate or severe stenoses can be heard with the use of a standard stethoscope over the vessel of interest. A high-pitched sound can be heard consequent to the increased velocity of the blood cells moving through a narrow space. (A similar effect is produced when a standard garden hose is kinked to create a spray and a hissing sound is heard.) Medically, this sound is often referred to as a bruit. *Bruit* (pronounced "broo-ee") is a French word meaning noise.

Patients with significant lower extremity arterial disease will consistently experience calf pain and occasionally experience thigh discomfort with exercise. The discomfort is relieved when the patient stands still for a few moments. This is known as vascular claudication and occurs from a pressure drop as a consequence of a severely stenotic (reduced in diameter by greater than 75 percent) or occluded artery. If the muscle cannot get enough oxygen as a result of reduced blood flow, it will cramp, forcing the patient to stop and rest until blood supply has caught up to muscle demand. Alternate pathways around an obstruction prevent pain at rest, when muscle demand is low. Alternate pathways are also referred to as collateral pathways. Small, otherwise insignificant branches from a main artery become important vessels when the body uses them as collateral pathways around an obstruction. Time and exercise help to collateralize arterial branches into larger, more prominent arterial pathways. If collateral pathways do not provide enough flow to prevent the patient from experiencing painful muscle cramps while performing a daily exercise routine or to heal a wound on the foot, it may be necessary to perform either a surgical bypass around the obstruction or another interventional procedure such as angioplasty, atherectomy, or laser surgery.

Claudication may also occur in the heart. The main coronary arteries lie on the surface of the heart and distribute blood to the heart muscle. Patients suffering from coronary artery disease (CAD) may experience tightness, heaviness, or pain in the chest subsequent to flow restriction to the heart muscle as a result of atherosclerotic plaque within the coronary arteries. These symptoms are known as angina pectoris, or simply angina, usually occurring with exercise and relieved by rest. Intensity of the symptoms is relative to the extent of disease. A myocardial infarction (heart attack) is the result of a coronary artery occlusion.

Unlike the arteries, the venous system is not affected by atherosclerosis. The primary diseases of the veins include blood clot formation and varicose veins. A varicose vein is an enlarged and meandering vein with poorly functioning valves. A varicosity typically involves the veins near the skin surface, the superficial veins, and is often visualized as an irregular and/or raised segment through the skin surface. Varicosities are most common in the lower legs.

Valve leaflets are common sites for development of a thrombus. Thrombosis is the formation of a clot within a vein, which occurs when blood flow is delayed or obstructed for many hours. Several conditions that may induce venous clotting include prolonged bed rest (postoperative patients), prolonged sitting (long airplane or automobile rides), and the use of oral contraceptives. Cancer patients are at high risk of clot formation secondary to a metabolic disorder that affects the natural blood-thinning process.

Because numerous tributaries are connected to the superficial system, it is easy for the body to compensate for a clot in this system by rerouting blood through other branches. The deep venous system, however, has fewer branches, which promotes the progression of a thrombus toward the heart. A thrombus in the deep venous system is more serious because the risk of pulmonary emboli, commonly known as blood clots in the lungs, is much higher than superficial vein thrombosis. The further a thrombus propagates, the higher the risk to the patient.

Lower extremity venous return must take an alternate route via the superficial venous system when the deep system is obstructed by a thrombus. This is known as compensatory flow around an obstruction.

Perspective and Prospects

Historically, the vasculature of the human body was evaluated by placing one's fingers on the skin, palpating for the presence or absence of a pulse, and making note of the patient's symptoms. Prior to the 1960s, treatment of the circulatory system was very limited or nonexistent, resulting in a high death rate and large numbers of amputations, strokes, and heart attacks. The development of arteriography (the angiogram), a procedure in which dye is injected into the vessels while x-rays are obtained, revealed more about the vasculature and the nature of disease involving it. In conjunction with arteriography came corrective bypass surgery.

This period of development was followed by vast improvements in diagnostics, treatment, and knowledge of preventive maintenance. Today, synthetic bypass grafts are commonplace and are used to reroute flow around an obstruction. In many cases, procedures such as atherectomy and angioplasty, in which plaque or a thrombus is removed through a catheter inserted into the vessel, are often performed as outpatient procedures. In cases where an artery been seriously narrowed or weakened, a stent, a small mesh tube, may be inserted into the blood vessel to keep it open and unobstructed following the angioplasty procedure.

Diagnostic imaging of the cardiovascular system and the study of hemodynamics with the use of ultrasound have been useful for patient screening, the monitoring of disease progression, and the postoperative evaluation of surgical/interventional procedures. Ultrasound is a particularly valuable diagnostic tool because, compared to x-rays or arteriography, it is less expensive; it is also quick, painless, and noninvasive (no radiation, needle, or dye is required).

In addition to technological advances, new medications have been made available to reduce the risk of graft rejection, hypertension, and clotting, and to lower blood cholesterol. Preventive measures such as a healthy diet, weight maintenance, and regular exercise, however, constitute the most effective approach to good cardiovascular health. Much new information has been made available to improve the knowledge of the general public regarding diet, exercise, and the avoidance of unhealthy habits such as cigarette smoking as the way to create and maintain a healthier cardiovascular system.

—*Bonnie L. Wolff*

See also Aneurysmectomy; Aneurysms; Angina; Angiography; Angioplasty; Arteriosclerosis; Biofeedback; Bleeding; Blood and blood disorders; Blood testing; Blood vessels; Bypass surgery; Cardiopulmonary resuscitation (CPR); Catheterization; Chest; Cholesterol; Claudication; Coronary artery bypass graft; Cyanosis; Diabetes mellitus; Dialysis; Disseminated intravascular coagulation (DIC); Echocardiography; Edema; Embolism; Endarterectomy; Exercise physiology; Heart; Heart disease; Heat exhaustion and heatstroke; Hematology; Hematology, pediatric; Hemorrhoid banding and removal; Hemorrhoids; Hormones; Hypercholesterolemia; Hypertension; Ischemia; Kidneys; Lymphatic system; Phlebitis; Phlebotomy; Preeclampsia and eclampsia; Pulmonary hypertension; Shock; Shunts; Stents; Strokes; Systems and organs; Thrombolytic therapy and TPA; Thrombosis and thrombus; Transfusion; Transient ischemic attacks (TIAs); Varicose vein removal; Varicose veins; Vascular medicine; Vascular system; Vasculitis; Venous insufficiency.

For Further Information:

Ford, Earl S. "Combined Television Viewing and Computer Use and Mortality from All-Causes and Diseases of the Circulatory System among Adults in the United States." *BMC Public Health* 12.1 (2012): 70-79.

Guyton, Arthur C., and John E. Hall. *Human Physiology and Mechanisms of Disease.* 6th ed. Philadelphia: W. B. Saunders, 1997.

Marder, Victor J., et al., eds. *Disorders of Thrombosis and Hemostasis: Basic Principles and Clinical Practice.* 6th ed. Philadelphia: Lippincott Williams & Wilkins, 2012.

Marieb, Elaine N., and Katja Hoehn. *Human Anatomy and Physiology.* 9th ed. San Francisco: Pearson/Benjamin Cummings, 2012.

Saltin, Bengt, et al., eds. *Exercise and Circulation in Health and Disease.* Champaign, Ill.: Human Kinetics, 2000.

Strandness, D. Eugene, Jr. *Duplex Scanning in Vascular Disorders.* 4th ed. London: Lippincott Williams & Wilkins, 2009.

Circumcision, female, and genital mutilation

Procedure

Anatomy or system affected: Genitals, reproductive system

Specialties and related fields: General surgery, gynecology, plastic surgery, psychiatry

Definition: The partial or complete surgical removal of the clitoris, labia minora, or labia majora (or all) for cultural reasons. Often performed without anesthesia or sterilized instruments, and often performed on young females without assent or understanding.

Key terms:

clitoridectomy: the removal of the entire clitoris, the prepuce, and adjacent labia

deinfibulation: an anterior episiotomy

episiotomy: the incision of the labia

infibulation: a clitoridectomy followed by the sewing up of the vulva

pharaonic circumcision: another term for infibulation

prepuce: the covering of the clitoris

sunna circumcision: the removal of the tip of the clitoris and/or the prepuce

Indications and Procedures

The various forms of female circumcision and female genital mutilation, although not universal to all cultures, have been practiced in numerous societies of the world for nearly two thousand years. Recorded evidence cites that female circumcision predates the advent of both Christianity and Islam and that early Christians, Muslims, and the Jewish group Falashas practiced circumcision on young girls. Historically, during the nineteenth century and until the 1940s, clitoridectomies were performed in Europe and America as a procedure to "cure" female masturbation, nervousness, and other specific types of perceived psychological dysfunction.

The 1989-1990 Demographic Health Survey of Circumcision stated that circumcision is still performed annually on an estimated 80 to 114 million women; 85 percent of these procedures involve clitoridectomy, while approximately 15 percent involve infibulation. Infibulation, or pharaonic circumcision, is the removal of the clitoris, the labia minora, and much of the labia majora; on occasion, the remaining sides of the vulva are stitched together to close up the vagina, except for a small opening maintained for the passage of blood and urine.

Certain contemporary cultures of Africa, the Middle East, and parts of Yemen, India, and Malaysia continue these practices. Contemporary Middle Eastern countries practicing female circumcision and genital mutilation are Jordan, Iraq, Yemen, Syria, and southern Algeria. In Africa, it is practiced in the majority of the countries, including Egypt, the Ivory Coast, Kenya, Mali, Mozambique, Sudan, and Upper Volta. It has been estimated that 99 percent of northern Sudanese women aged fifteen to forty-nine are circumcised. In and around Alexandria, Egypt, 99 percent of rural and lower-income urban women are circumcised. The World Health Organization estimates that as of 2013, approximately 140 million women worldwide have been circumsized during their childhood, with 101 million of these women in Africa.

Cross-culturally, there are essentially four types of female genital circumcision and female genital mutilation. Circumcision, or sunna circumcision, is removal of the prepuce or hood of the clitoris, with the body of the clitoris remaining intact. Sunna means "tradition" in Arabic. Excision circumcision, or clitoridectomy, is the removal of the entire clitoris (both prepuce and glans) and all or part of the adjacent labia majora and the labia minora. Intermediate circumcision is the removal of the clitoris, all or part of the labia minora, and sometimes part of the labia majora.

All types of female genital mutilation frequently may create severe, long-term effects, such as pelvic infections that usually lead to infertility, chronic recurrent urinary tract infections, painful intercourse, obstetrical complications, and in some cases, surgically induced scars that can cause tearing of the tissue and even hemorrhaging during childbirth. In fact, it is not unusual for women who have been infibulated to require surgical enlargement of the vagina on their wedding night or when delivering children. Unfortunately, babies born to infibulated women may frequently suffer brain damage because of oxygen deprivation (hypoxia) caused by a prolonged and obstructed delivery. Babies may die during the painful birthing process because of a damaged birth canal. Other physical and psychological difficulties for the circumcised woman may be sexual dysfunction, delayed menarche, and genital malformation.

From a cultural perspective, there are numerous reasons or justifications given for these procedures. They are often described as rites of passage and proof of adulthood, and it is often argued that the procedures raise a woman's status in her community, because of both the added purity that circumcision brings and the bravery that initiates are called upon to demonstrate. The procedure also is believed to confer maturity and inculcate positive character traits, such as the ability to endure pain and to be submissive. In some cultures, the circumcision ritual is considered to be positive because the girl is the center of attention. She receives presents and moral instruction from her elders, creating a bond between the generations, as all women in the society must undergo the procedure; they thus share an important experience.

Furthermore, it is thought that a girl who has been circumcised will not be troubled by lustful thoughts or sensations or by physical temptations such as masturbation. Therefore, there is less risk of premarital relationships that can end in the stigma and social difficulties of illegitimate birth. The bond between husband and wife may be closer because one or both of them will never have had sex with anyone else. The relationship may be motivated by love rather than lust because there will be no physical drive for the wife, only an emotional one. There is little incentive for extramarital sex for the wife; hence, the marriage may be more secure. Children may be better cared for because the husband can be more confident that he is their father. Generally, a girl who is not circumcised is considered unclean by local villagers and therefore unmarriageable. In some societies, a girl who is not circumcised is believed to be dangerous, even deadly, if her clitoris touches a man's penis.

All of these arguments for female genital mutilation and female circumcision must be weighed against the pain and terror, the lack of consent, and the subjugation of girls and women that is inherent in the practice. The practice must also be weighed against the medical risks.

Female genital circumcision and female genital mutilation surgeries are invariably conducted in unsanitary conditions in which a midwife or close female relative uses unsterile sharp instruments, such as pieces of glass, razor blades, kitchen knives, or scissors. The induction of tetanus, septicemia, hemorrhaging, and even shock are not uncommon. Human immunodeficiency virus (HIV) can be transmitted. No anesthesia is used. These procedures usually are experienced by the girl at approximately three years of age, although the actual age depends upon the customs of the particular society or village. To minimize the risk of the transmission of viruses, countries such as Egypt have made it illegal for female genital mutilation to be practiced by anyone other than trained doctors and nurses in hospitals.

Treatment and Therapy

There is no information regarding the surgical restoration of severed or damaged genitals. Because of severe cultural sanctions by the participating groups, which continue to hold tenaciously to such practices, female genital circumcision is seldom discussed with outsiders. Those who follow these customs do not report their occurrence. Consequently, there are few data concerning the frequency of female genital circumcision and female genital mutilation within the United States, despite the knowledge that some immigrant groups from Africa, the Middle East, and Asia continue to practice these surgeries. Health care workers estimate that, within the United States, approximately ten thousand girls undergo these surgical procedures each year. Usually, the procedure is conducted in the home. Those who can pay physicians to perform the surgery may do so; in these cases, local anesthesia is used and the risk of infection is less.

Perspective and Prospects

Because of the high number of female genital mutilations and the deaths that this procedure has caused, it is now prohibited in some communities in the United States, Great Britain, France, Sweden, and Switzerland, and in some countries of Africa, such as Egypt, Kenya, and Senegal. The National Organization of Circumcision Information Resource Centers (NOCIRC) is opposed to the procedures, as well as to male circumcision. The United Nations Children's Fund (UNICEF) and the World Health Organization (WHO) consider female genital mutilation to be a violation of human rights and recommend its eradication. In the United States, former representative Patricia Schroeder had introduced a bill that would outlaw female genital mutilation. The bill, called the Federal Prohibition of Female Genital Mutilation Act of 1995, was passed in 1996. The Canadian Criminal Code was enacted to protect children who are ordinarily residents in Canada from being removed from the country and subjected to female genital mutilation.

Both female genital circumcision and female genital mutilation perpetuate customs that seek to control female bodies and sexuality. It is hoped that with increasing legislation and attitude changes regarding bioethical issues, fewer girls and young women will undergo these mutilating surgical procedures. One problem in this campaign is the conflict between cultural self-determination and basic human rights. Feminists, physicians, and ethicists must work respectfully with, and not independently of, local resources for cultural self-examination and change.

—*John Alan Ross, Ph.D.*

See also Bleeding; Childbirth; Childbirth complications; Circumcision, male; Episiotomy; Ethics; Genital disorders, female; Gynecology; Infertility, female; Menstruation; Psychiatry; Reproductive system; Septicemia; Sexual dysfunction; Sexuality; Stillbirth; Women's health.

For Further Information:

Bacquet-Walsh, Caroline. "Female Genital Cutting Fact Sheet." *WomensHealth.gov*, Dec. 15, 2009.

Benedek, Wolfgang, et al., eds. *The Human Rights of Women: International Instruments and African Experiences*. London: Zed, 2002.

"Female Gential Mutilation/Cutting." *UNICEF*, May 15, 2013.

"Female Genital Mutilation." *World Health Organization*, Feb. 2013.

"Female Genital and Sexual Mutilation." *WIN News* 26, no. 2 (Spring, 2000): 51-59.

Galanti, Geri-Ann. *Caring for Patients from Different Cultures*. 4th ed. Philadelphia: University of Pennsylvania Press, 2008.

Gruenbaum, Ellen. *The Female Circumcision Controversy: An Anthropological Perspective*. Philadelphia: University of Pennsylvania Press, 2001.

James, Stanlie M., and Claire C. Robertson, eds. *Genital Cutting and Transnational Sisterhood: Disputing U.S. Polemics*. Urbana: University of Illinois Press, 2002.

Larsen, Ulla, and Sharon Yan. "Does Female Circumcision Affect Infertility and Fertility? A Study of the Central African Republic, Cote d'Ivoire, and Tanzania." *Demography* 37, no. 3 (August, 2000): 313-321.

Sarkis, Marianne. "Female Genital Cutting (FGC): An Introduction." *Female Genital Cutting Education and Networking Project*, 2003.

"Sexual Problems in Women." *MedlinePlus*, June 10, 2013.

Walker, Alice, and Pratibha Parmar. *Warrior Marks: Female Genital Mutilation and the Sexual Blinding of Women*. New York: Harcourt Brace, 1993.

Williams, Deanna Perez, William Acosta, and Herbert A. McPherson, Jr. "Female Genital Mutilation in the United States: Implications for Women's Health." *American Journal of Health Studies* 15, no. 1 (1999): 47-52.

Circumcision, male

Procedure

Anatomy or system affected: Genitals, reproductive system

Specialties and related fields: General surgery, pediatrics, urology

Definition: The removal of the foreskin (prepuce) covering the head of the penis.

Key terms:

chordee: the downward curvature of the penis, most apparent on erection, caused by the shortness of the skin on the downward side of the penile shaft

glans or *glans penis*: the head of the penis

necrosis: the death of one or more cells or a portion of a tissue or organ resulting from irreversible damage

phimosis: the narrowing of the opening of the skin covering the head of the penis sufficient to prevent retraction of the skin back over the glans

sepsis: an infection in the circulating blood

smegma: a pasty accumulation of shed skin cells and secretions of the sweat glands which collects in the moist areas of the foreskin-covered base of the glans

urinary tract infections : infections of the bladder, the kidneys, the urethra (which connects the bladder to the opening at the end of the penis), and the ureters (which connect the bladder to the kidneys); infection may be limited to one area of these organs or spread throughout the urinary tract

Indications and Procedures

Routine circumcision of the newborn male-in which the foreskin of the penis is stretched, clamped, and cut-is becoming an increasingly controversial procedure. Famed pediatrician Benjamin Spock once contended that circumcision is a good idea, especially if most of the boys in the neighborhood are circumcised; then a boy feels "regular." Yet, many wonder if that is justification for circumcision. Allowing routine circumcision of newborns as a religious and cultural rite still leaves the debate over medical necessity. The United States is the only country in the world that circumcises a majority of newborn males without a religious reason. In fact, circumcision has been termed a "cultural surgery."

True medical indications for the surgery are seldom present at birth. Such conditions as infections of the head and/or shaft of the penis may be indications for circumcision; an inability to retract the foreskin in the newborn (phimosis) is not an indication. Some argue that circumcision should be delayed until the foreskin has become retractable, making an imprecise surgical procedure presumably less traumatic. In 96 percent of infant boys, however, the foreskin is not fully retractable; it is normally so tight and adherent that it cannot be pulled back and the penis cleaned. By age three, that percentage decreases to 10 percent.

There are other definite contraindications to newborn circumcision. Circumcising infants with abnormalities of the penal head or shaft makes treatment more difficult because the foreskin may later be needed for use in reconstruction. Prematurity, instability, or a bleeding problem also preclude early circumcision. The foreskin is a natural protective membrane, representing 50 to 80 percent of the skin system of the penis, having 240 feet of nerve fibers, more than one thousand nerve endings, and three feet of veins, arteries, and capillaries. It keeps the sensitive head protected, facilitating intercourse, and prevents the surface of the glans from thickening and becoming desensitized. Also, within the inner surface of the foreskin are a series of tiny ridged bands that contribute significantly to stimulating the glans.

The two most persistent arguments for the operation, however, are the risks of infection and cancer in the uncircumcised. Without circumcision, smegma accumulates beneath the base of the covered head of the penis. This cheeselike material of dead skin cells and secretions of the sweat glands is thought to be a cause of cancer of the penis and prostate gland in uncircumcised men and cancer of the cervix in their female partners. Doctors who argue against circumcision, however, say that the presence of smegma in the uncircumcised is simply a sign of poor hygiene and that poor sexual hygiene, inadequate hygienic facilities, and sexually transmitted diseases cause an increased incidence of cancer in ethnic groups or populations that do not practice circumcision. Doctors who argue against circumcision also point out that complete circumcision is found as often in male partners of women without cancer of the cervix as in male partners of women who have cervical cancer. In Sweden, moreover-where newborn circumcision is not routinely practiced but where good hygiene is practiced-the rates of these cancers are essentially the same as those found in Israel, where ritualistic circumcision is practiced.

The increased incidence of urinary tract infections and sexually transmitted diseases (STDs) in uncircumcised males sufficiently argues for circumcision, say its proponents. They warn that the intact foreskin invites bacterial colonization, which leads to urethral infection ascending to the bladder that ultimately may spread upward to the kidneys and sometimes cause permanent kidney damage. On the other hand, no proof exists that uncircumcised male infants who sustain urinary tract infections will have future urologic problems. Furthermore, the operation is not a simple procedure and is not without peril. Penile amputation, life-threatening infections, and even death have been well documented.

Slightly increased rates of infection with sexually transmitted diseases in the uncircumcised argue the case for some proponents, but it is acquired immunodeficiency syndrome (AIDS) that they most fear. In Africa, where male circumcision is seldom practiced, the acquisition of AIDS by heterosexual men from infected women during vaginal intercourse is the most common mode of transmission.

Proponents say that infection with human immunodeficiency virus (HIV), the virus that leads to AIDS, depends on a break or an abrasion of the skin to gain entry. The intact foreskin provides a site for the transfer of infected cervical secretions. In Africa, doctors at the University of Nairobi noted a relationship of HIV infection to genital ulcers and lack of circumcision. Uncircumcised men had a history of genital ulcers more often than did the circumcised, and they were more often HIV-positive. They were also more frequently HIV-positive even if they did not have a history of genital ulcer disease.

Every evaluation of circumcision, pro or con, should reflect the confounding genetic and environmental variables, as well as the actual increased risks and benefits. All the pros and cons should be explained to parents before informed consent is obtained.

Uses and Complications

In 1989, the American Academy of Pediatrics' Task Force on Circumcision concluded that "newborn circumcision has potential medical benefits and advantages as well as disadvantages and risks. When circumcision is being considered, the benefits and risks should be explained to the parents and informed consent obtained." This neutral statement does not lessen the anxiety of parents who are trying to weigh the pros and cons of routine newborn circumcision, but examination of the evidence does allow parents to weigh the individual benefits and risks and see if the scale tips in either direction.

Worldwide studies of predominantly uncircumcised populations have shown a higher incidence of urinary tract infection in boys during the first few months of life, which is the reverse of what is found in older infants and children, where girls predominate. In 1986, Brooke Army Medical Center in Fort Sam Houston, Texas, took a closer look. The doctors found the incidence of urinary tract infection in circumcised infant males to be 0.11 percent but 1.12 percent in the uncircumcised. Even without proof that the uncircumcised male infants who get urinary tract infections will have future urologic problems, the proponents for the surgical procedure claim about a 1 percent advantage.

The evidence for an increase in sexually transmitted diseases (such as genital herpes, gonorrhea, and syphilis) among the uncircumcised is conflicting. Furthermore, apparent correlations between circumcision status and these diseases do not reflect confounding genetic and environmental variables. It is also difficult to factor in the risk from HIV infections. The studies from Africa do not look at any variables in the transmission of HIV except circumcision status and previous history of genital ulcers. The nutritional and economic status of the men was not examined, even though it is known that malnourishment suppresses the immune systems. Moreover, if everyone practiced safer sex, the argument for circumcision would be moot.

Almost all the surgical complications of circumcision can be avoided if doctors performing the procedure adhere to strict asepsis, are properly trained and experienced in the procedure, remove the appropriate and correct amount of tissue, and provide adequate hemostasis. The variety of circumstances, populations, and physicians affects the incidence of complications. In the larger, teaching hospitals, often the newest physicians with the least experience or supervision perform the operation. As a result, complications may arise. Excessive bleeding is the most frequent complication. The incidence of bleeding after circumcision ranges from 0.1 percent to as high as 35 percent in some reports. Most of the episodes are minor and can be controlled by simple measures, such as compression and suturing, but some of these efforts can lead to diminished blood supply to the head and shaft of the penis with necrosis of the affected part. Chordee can result if improper technique or bad luck intervenes, and such penile deformity begets the risk of emotional distress. The urethral opening on the end of the penis can become infected or ulcerated when the glans is no longer protected by foreskin; such infection rarely occurs in the uncircumcised. Finally, any surgical procedure runs the risk of infection. These localized infections rarely spread to the blood, but death from sepsis and its sequelae has been documented.

Overall, the surgical complication rate after circumcision runs around 0.19 percent, which could be lowered with strict protocols, meticulous technique, strict asepsis, and well-trained, experienced physicians. Strict protocols, it is hoped, would ensure that absolute contraindications to the procedure-such as anomalies of the penis, prematurity, instability, or a bleeding disorder-were honored.

Another human factor must be considered. Many insurance companies do not provide payment for newborn care, since it is considered preventive medicine. In 1997, a physician's fee for performing a circumcision ranged to approximately $400, with a nationwide average of $137. Interestingly, a growing number of circumcised men are undergoing expensive foreskin restoration procedures.

In part because of an additional cost that arises with anesthesia, the vast majority of infant circumcisions are performed without pain control. The surgery is painful, yet some physicians claim that the minute that the operation ends, the circumcised baby no longer cries and frequently falls asleep. Continuing pain, therefore, is probably not present.

Another perspective to examine is the experience of adult males, who are circumcised by their own choice. Many complain of at least a week's discomfort after the operation. The most compelling argument against adult circumcision, however, comes from their answer to "Would you do it again?" In one study of several hundred men who were circumcised as adults, they were asked five years later if they would do it again. All said no.

Perspective and Prospects

Routine newborn circumcision originated in the United States in the 1860s, ostensibly as prophylaxis against disease. Some medical historians, however, believe that nonreligious circumcision was a deliberate surgical procedure to desensitize and debilitate the penis to prevent masturbation. During this era, and for nearly one hundred years afterward, most American physicians viewed masturbation as an inevitable cause of blindness, weak character, insanity, nervousness, tuberculosis, sexually transmitted disease, and even death. One physician maintained that a painful circumcision would have a salutary effect upon the newborn's mind, so that pain would be associated with masturbation. As late as 1928, the *American Medical Journal* published an editorial that justified male circumcision as an effective means of preventing the dire effects of masturbation. During World Wars I and II, soldiers were forcibly circumcised under threat of court martial, being told that the surgery was for reasons of hygiene and the prevention of epilepsy and other diseases.

Eventually, a general change in attitude occurred, notably in Great Britain and New Zealand, which virtually have abandoned routine circumcision. Rates of circumcision have also fallen dramatically in Canada, Australia, and even the United States. As recently as the mid-1970s, approximately 90 percent of US male babies were circumcised. Not until 1971 did the American Academy of Pediatrics determine that circumcision is not medically essential. In 1999, an estimated 65 percent of US male babies were circumcised; by 2010, the incidence of newborn circumcision had declined to 55 percent.

In 1971, the American Academy of Pediatrics' Committee on the Fetus and Newborn issued an advisory that said, "There are no valid medical indications for routine circumcision in the neonatal period." In 1978, when the American

College of Obstetricians and Gynecologists affirmed this statement, the circumcision rate had already declined to an estimated 70 percent of newborn males, compared to previous rates of between 80 and 90 percent.

Undoubtedly, the future will bring improved surgical techniques. More emphasis will be placed on avoiding surgical complications by more rigid monitoring of the operation and who performs the procedure. It is unlikely that circumcision will disappear completely.

Organizations such as Doctors Opposing Circumcision and the National Organization to Halt the Abuse and Routine Mutilation of Males, however, are actively proposing an end to routine neonatal circumcision. Some nursing groups and concerned mothers have formed local groups to oppose circumcision in male neonates. They argue that subjecting a baby to this procedure may impair mother-infant bonding. Another question posed by some physicians and parents is the ethics involved in the unnecessary removal of a functioning body organ, particularly without the patient's consent. Others claim that the baby's rights are being violated, noting that it is the child who must live with the outcome of the decision to perform a circumcision. As a result of these efforts, the rates of circumcision will probably continue to fall.

—*Wayne R. McKinny, M.D.;*
updated by John Alan Ross, Ph.D.

See also Circumcision, female, and genital mutilation; Ethics; Genital disorders, male; Men's health; Neonatology; Pediatrics; Reproductive system; Urology, pediatric.

For Further Information:

Apuzzio, Joseph J., Anthony M. Vintzileos, and Leslie Iffy, eds. *Operative Obstetrics*. 3d ed. New York: Taylor & Francis, 2006.

Behrman, Richard E., Robert M. Kliegman, and Hal B. Jenson, eds. *Nelson Textbook of Pediatrics*. 19th ed. Philadelphia: Saunders/Elsevier, 2011.

Bigelow, Jim. *The Joy of Uncircumcising! Exploring Circumcision-History, Myths, Psychology, Restoration, Sexual Pleasure, and Human Rights*. Rev. ed. Aptos, Calif.: Hourglass, 1998.

"Circumcision." *HealthyChildren.org*. American Academy of Pediatrics, May 11, 2013.

"Circumcision." *MedlinePlus*, May 13, 2013.

Gollaher, David L. *Circumcision: A History of the World's Most Controversial Surgery*. New York: Basic Books, 2000.

Kerr, Sarah J., and Michael Woods. "Child Circumcision." *Health Library*, May 13, 2013.

King, Lowell R., ed. *Urologic Surgery in Neonates and Young Infants*. Philadelphia: W. B. Saunders, 1998.

"Male Circumcision." *Centers for Disease Control and Prevention*, Apr. 15, 2013.

Snyder, Howard M. "To Circumcise or Not." *Hospital Practice* 26 (January 15, 1991): 201-207.

Woods, Michael. "Newborn Circumcision." *Health Library*, Sept. 27, 2012.

Cirrhosis
Disease/Disorder
Anatomy or system affected: Liver
Specialties and related fields: Family medicine, internal medicine, psychology
Definition: The formation of scar tissue in the liver, which interferes with its normal function.

Causes and Symptoms

The liver is a large, spongy organ that lies in the upper-right abdomen. Regarded as primarily part of the digestive system because it manufactures bile, the liver has many other functions, including the synthesis of blood-clotting factors and the detoxification of such harmful substances as alcohol.

Cirrhosis describes the fibrous scar tissue (or nodules) that replaces the normally soft liver after repeated long-

> ### Information on Cirrhosis
>
> **Causes:** Buildup of scar tissue in liver from toxins (alcohol, viruses)
> **Symptoms:** May include jaundice, fatigue, weakness, appetite loss, easy bruising
> **Duration:** Chronic
> **Treatments:** None

term injury by toxins such as alcohol or viruses. The liver may form small nodules (micronodular cirrhosis), large nodules (macronodular cirrhosis), or a combination of the two types (mixed nodular cirrhosis). Cirrhosis is a frequent cause of death among middle-aged men, and increasingly among women. While alcoholism is the most common cause, chronic hepatitis and other rarer diseases can also produce the irreversible liver damage that characterizes cirrhosis. The resulting organ is shrunken and hard, unable to perform its varied duties. Because of its altered structure, the cirrhotic liver causes serious problems for surrounding organs, as blood flow becomes difficult. The barrier to normal circulation leads to two serious complications: portal hypertension (the buildup of pressure in the internal veins) and ascites (fluid leakage from blood vessels into the abdominal cavity).

Treatment and Therapy

Diagnosis is usually made from a history of alcoholism. A physical examination may reveal jaundice; a large nodular liver or a small shrunken one, depending upon the stage; or a fluid-filled abdomen (ascites). Laboratory studies may show elevated liver enzymes released from damaged cells and low levels of products that the liver normally produces (protein, clotting factors). A definitive diagnosis can be made only by biopsy, although radiographic methods such as computed tomography (CT) scanning and magnetic resonance imaging (MRI) can be quite conclusive.

The mortality rate is very high, as the damage is irreversible. Deaths from internal vein rupture and hemorrhage (the results of portal hypertension) and from kidney failure are most common. Repeated hospitalizations attempt to control the variety of complications that arise with agents that stop bleeding, bypass tubes that relieve pressure, the removal of the ascitic fluid, and nutritional support for malnutrition. Eventually, kidney failure ensues or one of these control measures fails, and death rapidly follows. Liver transplantation is considered in some cases. Cases of mild cirrhosis, where sufficient normal tissue remains, have a clearly better course.

In 2013, a study led by Dr. W. Kim Ray, of the Mayo Clinic in Rochester, Minnesota, found a link between advanced fibrosis and higher death rates in patients with nonalcoholic fatty liver disease. The incidence of nonalcoholic fatty liver disease has risen over the last twenty-five years and it is now the most frequently occurring liver disease in the United States.

—*Connie Rizzo, M.D., Ph.D.*

Cirrhosis

Micronodular (cross-section)

Macronodular (cross-section)

Mixed nodular (cross-section)

Cirrhosis appears in three forms, detectable under the micro-scope, each depending primarily on the cause of the liver damage. All are characterized by the replacement of normally soft, spongy tissue with hard, fibrous scarring. Alcohol-related cirrhosis usually produces the micronodular form.

See also Alcoholism; Endoscopic retrograde cholangiopancreatography (ERCP); Hepatitis; Jaundice; Liver; Liver cancer; Liver disorders; Liver transplantation; Nonalcoholic steatohepatitis (NASH).

For Further Information:

Dallas, Mary Elizabeth. "HealthDay: Scarring May Raise Death Risk from Fatty Liver Disease." *MedlinePlus*, Apr. 16, 2013.

Fishman, Mark, et al. *Medicine.* 5th ed. Philadelphia: Lippincott, 2004.

Goldman, Lee, and Dennis Ausiello, eds. *Cecil Textbook of Medicine.* 23d ed. Philadelphia: Saunders, 2007.

MedlinePlus. "Cirrhosis." *MedlinePlus*, Apr. 17, 2013.

Parker, James N., and Philip M. Parker, eds. *The Official Patient's Sourcebook on Primary Biliary Cirrhosis.* San Diego, Calif.: Icon Health, 2002.

Parker, James N. and Philip M. Parker. *The Official Patient's Sourcebook on Cirrhosis of the Liver: A Reference Manual for Self-Directed Patient Research.* San Diego, Calif.: Icon Health, 2004.

Wood, Debra. "Cirrhosis." *Health Library*, Oct. 11, 2012.

Zelman, Mark, et al. *Human Diseases: A Systemic Approach.* 7th ed. Upper Saddle River, N.J.: Pearson, 2010.

Claudication

Disease/Disorder

Anatomy or system affected: Blood vessels, circulatory system, legs

Specialties and related fields: Vascular medicine

Definition: Pain in the calf or thigh muscle brought on by walking and relieved by rest.

Causes and Symptoms

Claudication is pain that develops in the calf or thigh muscle during walking. The pain increases if the patient continues walking and is relieved within a few minutes after walking is terminated. The medical term for this condition is intermittent claudication. The pain is caused by a narrowing in the arteries that supply the leg with blood. This narrowing is commonly caused by atherosclerosis, in which fatty material builds up on the inside wall of the artery. At first, as the fatty material accumulates in the artery, it creates no symptoms. Only after more than 50 percent of the artery is narrowed do symptoms occur. The first symptom is mild cramping or heaviness that develops during a long walk. Over time, the narrowing increases and the distance that the individual is able to walk decreases. If not treated, the narrowing of the artery may increase further and the pain will be present all the time, signaling a more serious condition called rest pain that may lead to limb loss.

Factors that may lead to this condition include smoking, high blood pressure, heart disease, high cholesterol, and advanced age. Elderly people are more likely to develop intermittent claudication, but younger individuals with multiple risk factors for vascular disease may develop this problem at any age. Sometimes a thrombus may obstruct an artery, causing claudication symptoms to occur suddenly instead of slowly as with atherosclerosis.

The diagnosis of claudication is fairly simple. Clinically, true intermittent claudication can be differentiated from a similar but unrelated condition by noting if the symptoms happen every time that the patient walks a similar distance. True claudication will develop every time, while pain from

---

Information on Claudication

Causes: Narrowing in leg arteries from atherosclerosis; risk factors include smoking, high blood pressure, heart disease, high cholesterol, advanced age

Symptoms: Mild cramping or heaviness during long walks, progressing to leg pain at rest and sometimes amputation

Duration: Chronic, progressive without treatment

Treatments: Smoking cessation, lowering of cholesterol levels, program of long-distance walking, medications (pentoxifylline, cilostazol), surgery (angioplasty, bypass surgery, stents)

---

other conditions will occur at some times but not others.

To be more precise in diagnosing this condition, a Doppler study can be performed on an outpatient basis in a hospital or a doctor's office. The examination, called an ankle-brachial index (ABI), is simple and painless. Blood pressures are taken at the ankles and in the arms before and after exercise. If the pressure at the ankles drops with exercise and goes back to normal a few minutes later, then the diagnosis of intermittent claudication can be made. Ultrasound imaging or angiogram studies may be done to identify the exact location of the narrowing.

Treatment and Therapy

Treatment depends on the severity of the symptoms. Stopping smoking, lowering cholesterol levels, and beginning a program of long-distance walking may provide enough relief to allow some patients to return to near-normal routines. Medications such as pentoxifylline (Trental or Pentoxil) or cilostazol (Pletal) may provide limited relief from symptoms. More severe cases may require angioplasty, surgery to bypass the narrowed artery, or stenting of the diseased artery.

Perspective and Prospects

Claudication has become more common in the United States as the population ages and sedentary lifestyles become more popular. Although some treatments are effective, it is a difficult problem to manage. Education programs are available to help those at risk for this condition make necessary lifestyle changes that may lessen their chances of developing this ailment. Those changes may include getting plenty of exercise (brisk walking being the best), not smoking, lowering cholesterol, and keeping diabetes under control.

In March 2013, the US Preventive Services Task Force stated that, after reviewing available research, it did not find enough evidence to make a recommendation one way or the other about the use of ABI as a way to assess heart disease risk in patients who show no symptoms of peripheral artery disease. The task force called for more research into the matter.

—Steven R. Talbot, R.V.T.

See also Arteriosclerosis; Bypass surgery; Cholesterol; Circulation; Exercise physiology; Hypercholesterolemia; Lower extremities;

Pain management; Plaque, arterial; Stents; Thrombosis and thrombus; Vascular medicine; Vascular system; Vasculitis.

For Further Information:
Hershey, Falls B., Robert W. Barnes, and David S. Sumner, eds. *Noninvasive Diagnosis of Vascular Disease*. Pasadena, Calif.: Appleton, 1984.
Mohler, Emile R., III. "Patient Information: Peripheral Artery Disease and Claudication (Beyond the Basics)." *UpToDate*, May 2, 2013.
Preidt, Robert. "HealthDay: Experts Question Use of Ankle Blood Pressure to Gauge Heart Risks." *MedlinePlus*, Mar. 18, 2013.
Rutherford, Robert B., ed. *Vascular Surgery*. 6th ed. Philadelphia: Saunders/Elsevier, 2005.
Zwiebel, William J., and John S. Pellerito, eds. *Introduction to Vascular Ultrasonography*. 5th ed. Philadelphia: Saunders/Elsevier, 2005.

Cleft lip and palate
Disease/Disorder

Anatomy or system affected: Bones, musculoskeletal system

Specialties and related fields: Neonatology, otorhinolaryngology, pediatrics, plastic surgery, speech pathology

Definition: A fissure in the midline of the palate, resulting from the failure of the two sides to fuse during embryonic development; in some cases, the fissure may extend through both hard and soft palates into the nasal cavities.

Key terms:

alveolus: the bony ridge where teeth grow

ectrodactyly: a congenital anomaly characterized by the absence of part or all of one or more of the fingers or toes

hard palate: the bony portion of the roof of the mouth, contiguous with the soft palate

Logan's bow: a metal bar placed, for protection and tension removal, on the early postoperative cleft lip

obturator: a sheet of plastic shaped like a flattened dome which fits into the cleft and closes it well enough to permit nursing

soft palate: a structure of mucous membrane, muscle fibers, and mucous glands suspended from the posterior border of the hard palate

syndactyly: a congenital anomaly characterized by the fusion of the fingers or toes

uvula: the small, cone-shaped projection of tissue suspended in the mouth from the posterior of the soft palate

Causes and Symptoms

Cleft palate is a congenital defect characterized by a fissure along the midline of the palate. It occurs when the two sides fail to fuse during embryonic development. The gap may be complete, extending through the hard and soft palates into the nasal cavities, or may be partial or incomplete. It is often associated with cleft lip or "harelip." About one child in eight hundred live births is affected with some degree of clefting, and clefting is the most common of the craniofacial abnormalities.

Cleft palate is not generally a genetic disorder; rather, it is a result of defective cell migration. Embryonically, in the first month, the mouth and nose form one cavity destined to be separated by the hard and soft palates. In addition, there is no upper lip. Most of the upper jaw is lacking; only the part near the ears is present. In the next weeks, the upper lip and jaw are formed from structures growing in from the sides, fusing at the midline with a third portion growing downward from the nasal region. The palates develop in much the same way. The fusion of all these structures begins with the lip and moves posteriorly toward, and then includes the soft palate. The two cavities are separated by the palates by the end of the third month of gestation.

If, as embryonic development occurs, the cells that should grow together to form the lips and palate fail to move in the correct direction, the job is left unfinished. Clefting of the palate generally occurs between the thirty-fifth and thirty-seventh days of gestation. Fortunately, it is an isolated defect not usually associated with other disabilities or with developmental delays.

If the interference in normal growth and fusion begins early and lasts throughout the fusion period, the cleft that results will affect one or both sides of the top lip and may continue back through the upper jaw, the upper gum ridge, and both palates. If the disturbance lasts only part of the time that development is occurring, only the lip may be cleft, and the palate may be unaffected. If the problem begins a little into the fusion process, the lip is normally formed, but the palate is cleft. The cleft may divide only the soft palate or both the soft and the hard palate. Even the uvula may be affected; it can be split, unusually short, or even absent.

About 80 percent of cases of cleft lip are unilateral; of these, 70 percent occur on the left side. Of cleft palate cases, 25 percent are bilateral. The mildest manifestations of congenital cleft are mild scarring or notching of the upper lip. Beyond this, clefting is described by degrees. The first degree is incomplete, which is a small cleft in the uvula. The second degree is also incomplete, through the soft palate and into the hard palate. Another type of "second-degree incomplete" is a horseshoe type, in which there is a bilateral cleft proceeding almost to the front. Third-degree bilateral is a cleft through both palates but bilaterally through the gums; it results in a separate area where the teeth will erupt, and the teeth will show up in a very small segment. When the teeth appear, they may not be normally aligned. In addition to the lip, gum, and palate deviations, abnormalities of the nose may also occur.

Cleft palate may be inherited, probably as a result of the interaction of several genes. In addition, the effects of some environmental factors that affect embryonic development

---

Information on Cleft Lip and Palate

Causes: Congenital defect
Symptoms: Craniofacial abnormalities, greater susceptibility to colds, poor muscle reactivity, dental problems
Duration: Correctable, usually between seven and twelve months of age
Treatments: Surgery

may be linked to this condition. They might include mechanical disturbances such as an enlarged tongue, which prevents the fusion of the palate and lip. Other disturbances may be caused by toxins introduced by the mother (drugs such as cortisone or alcohol) and defective blood. Other associated factors include deficiencies of vitamins or minerals in the mother's diet, radiation from X-rays, and infectious diseases such as German measles. No definite cause has been identified, nor does it appear that one cause alone can be implicated. It is likely that there is an interplay between genetic and chromosomal abnormalities and environmental factors.

There are at least 150 syndromes involving oral and facial clefts. Four examples of cleft syndromes that illustrate these syndromes are EEC (ectrodactyly, ectodermal dysplasia, cleft lip/palate), popliteal pterygium syndrome, van der Woude's syndrome, and trisomy 13 syndrome. EEC and trisomy 13 both result in intellectual and developmental disabilities as well as oral clefts. Popliteal pterygium has as its most common feature skin webbing (pterygium), along with clefts and skeletal abnormalities. Van der Woude's syndrome usually shows syndactyly as well as clefting and lower-lip pitting.

Problems begin at birth for the infant born with a cleft palate. The most immediate problem is feeding the baby. If the cleft is small and the lip unaffected, nursing may proceed fairly easily. If the cleft is too large, however, the baby cannot build up enough suction to nurse efficiently. To remedy this, the hole in the nipple of the bottle can be enlarged, or a plastic obturator can be fitted to the bottle.

Babies with cleft palates are more susceptible to colds than other children. Since there is an open connection between the nose and mouth, an infection that starts in either location will easily and quickly spread to the other. Frequently, the infection will spread to the middle ear via the Eustachian tube. One end of a muscle is affixed to the Eustachian tube opening, and the other end is attached to the middle of the roof of the mouth (palate). Normal contraction opens the tube so that air can travel through the tube and equalize air pressure on both sides of the eardrum. As long as the eardrum has flexibility of movement, the basics for good hearing are in place. Children with cleft palates, however, do not have good muscle contractions; therefore, air cannot travel through the tube. If the tube remains closed after swallowing, the air that is trapped is absorbed into the middle-ear tissue, resulting in a vacuum. This pulls the eardrum inward and decreases its flexibility, and hearing loss ensues. The cavity of the middle ear then fills with fluid, which can breed bacteria, causing infection. The infection may or may not be painful; if there is no pain, the infection may go unnoticed and untreated. The accumulated fluid can cause erosion of the tiny bones, which would decrease sound transmission to the auditory nerve. This conductive hearing loss is permanent. Persistent and prolonged fluid buildup can also cause accumulation of dead matter, forming a tumorlike growth called a cholesteatoma.

Other problems associated with cleft palates are those related to dentition. In some children there may be extra teeth, while in others the cleft may prevent the formation of tooth buds so that teeth are missing. Teeth that are present may be malformed; those malformations include injury during development, fusion of teeth to form one large tooth, teeth lacking enamel, and teeth that have too little calcium in the enamel. If the teeth are misaligned,

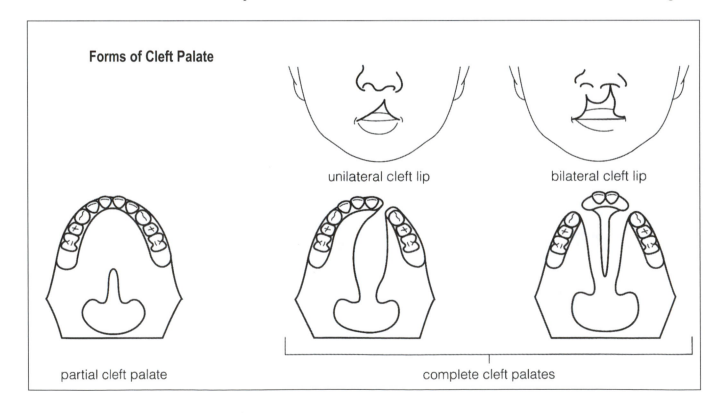

Forms of Cleft Palate

unilateral cleft lip

bilateral cleft lip

partial cleft palate

complete cleft palates

orthodontia may be undertaken. Another possible problem met by patients with a cleft palate is maxillary (upper jaw) arch collapse; this condition is also remedied with orthodontic treatment.

Treatment and Therapy

One of the first questions a parent of a child with a cleft palate will pose regards surgical repair. The purpose of surgically closing the cleft is not simply to close the hole-although that goal is important. The major purpose is to achieve a functional palate. Whether this can be accomplished depends on the size and shape of the cleft, the thickness of the available tissue, and other factors.

Cleft lip surgery is performed when the healthy baby weighs at least ten pounds; it is done under a general anesthetic. If the cleft is unilateral, one operation can accomplish the closure, but a bilateral cleft lip is often repaired in two steps at least a month apart. When the lip is repaired, normal lip pressure is restored, which may help in closing the cleft in the gum ridge. It may also reduce the gap in the hard palate, if one is present. Successive operations may be suggested when, even years after surgery, scars develop on the lip.

Surgery to close clefts of the hard and soft palate is typically done when the child is at least nine months of age, unless there is a medical reason not to do so. Different surgeons prefer different times for this surgery. The surgeon attempts to accomplish three goals in the repair procedure. The surgeon will first try to ensure that the palate is long enough to allow for function and movement (this is essential for proper speech patterns). Second, the musculature around the Eustachian tube should work properly in order to cut down the incidence of ear infections. Finally, the surgery should promote the development of the facial bones and, as much as possible, normal teeth. This goal aids in eating and appearance. All of this may be accomplished in one operation if the cleft is not too severe. For a cleft that requires more procedures, the surgeries are usually spaced at least six months apart so that complete healing can occur. This schedule decreases the potential for severe scarring.

At one time, it was thought that if surgery were performed before the child began talking, speech problems would be avoided. In reality, not only did the surgery not remedy that problem, but the early closure often resulted in a narrowing of the upper jaw and interference with facial growth as well. Thus, the trend to put off the surgery until the child was four or five years of age developed; by this age, more than 80 percent of the lateral growth of the upper jaw has occurred. However, most surgeons can perform the corrective surgery when the child is between one and two years of age without affecting facial growth.

Successful repair greatly improves speech and appearance, and the physiology of the oral and nasal cavities is also improved. Additional surgery may be necessary to improve appearance, breathing, and the function of the palate. Sometimes the palate may partially reopen, and surgery is needed to reclose it.

When the baby leaves the operating room, there are stitches in the repaired area. Sometimes a special device called a Logan's bow is taped to the baby's cheeks; this device not only protects the stitches but also relieves some of the tension on them. In addition, the baby's arms may be restrained in order to keep the baby's hands away from the affected area. (The child is fitted for elbow restraints before surgery; the elbows are encased in tubes that prevent them from bending.) A parent of a child that has just undergone cleft palate repair should not panic at the sight of bleeding from the mouth. To curb it, gauze may be packed into the repaired area and remain about five days after surgery. As mucus and other body fluids accumulate in the area, they may be suctioned out.

During the initial recovery, the child is kept in a moist, oxygen-rich environment (an oxygen tent) until respiration is normal. The patient will be observed for signs of airway obstruction or excessive bleeding. Feeding is done by syringe, eyedropper, or special nipples. Clear liquids and juices only are allowed. The child sits in a high chair to drink, when possible. After feeding, the mouth should be rinsed well with water to help keep the stitches clean. Peroxide mixed with the water may help, as well as ointment. Intake and output of fluids are measured. Hospitalization may last for about a week, or however long is dictated by speed of healing. At the end of this week, stitches are removed and the suture line covered and protected by a strip of paper tape.

An alternative to surgery is the use of an artificial palate known as an obturator. It is specially constructed by a dentist to fit into the child's mouth. The appliance, or prosthesis, is carefully constructed to fit precisely and snugly, but it must be easily removable. There must be enough space at the back so the child can breathe through the nose. While speaking, the muscles move back over this opening so that speech is relatively unaffected.

Speech problems are the most likely residual problems in the cleft palate patient. The speech of the untreated, and sometimes the treated cleft palate patient is very nasal. If the soft palate is too short, the closure of the palate may leave a space between the nose and the throat, allowing air to escape through the nose. There is little penetrating quality to the patient's voice, and it does not carry well. Some cleft palate speakers are difficult to understand because there are several faults in articulation. Certainly not all cleft lip or palate patients, however, will develop communication problems; modern surgical procedures ensure that most children will develop speech and language normally, without the help of a speech therapist.

Genetic counseling may help answer some of the family's questions about why the cleft palate occurred, whether it will happen with future children, and whether there is any way to prevent it. There are no universal answers to these questions. The answers depend on the degree and type of cleft, the presence of other problems, the family history, and the history of the pregnancy. Genetic counseling obtained at a hospital or medical clinic can determine whether the condition was heritable or a chance error and can establish the risk level for future pregnancies.

Perspective and Prospects

Oral clefts, as well as other facial clefts, have been a part of historical records for thousands of years. Perhaps the earliest recorded incidence is a Neolithic shrine with a two-headed figurine dated about 6500 BCE. The origination and causative agent of such clefts remain mysterious today.

Expectant parents are rarely alerted prior to birth that their child will be born with a cleft, so it is usually in the hospital, just after birth, that parents first learn of the birth defect. Even if it is suspected that a woman is at risk for producing a child with a cleft palate, there is no way to determine if the defect is indeed present, as neither amniocentesis nor chromosomal analysis reveals the condition. When the baby is delivered, the presence of the cleft can evoke a feeling of crisis in the delivery room.

The problems accompanying clefting may alter family morale and climate, increasing the complexity of the problem. A team of specialists usually works together to help the patient and the family cope with these problems. This team may include a pediatrician, a speech pathologist, a plastic surgeon, an orthodontist, a psychiatrist, an otologist, an audiologist, and perhaps others.

The cooperating team should monitor for the following situations: feeding problems, family and friends' reactions to the baby's appearance, how parents encourage the child to talk or how they respond to poor speech, and whether the parents are realistic about the long-term outcome for their child. The grief, guilt, and shock that the parents often feel can be positively altered by how the professional team tackles the problem and by communication with the parents. Usually the team does not begin functioning in the baby's life until he or she is older than one month. Some parents have confronted their feelings, while others are still struggling with the negative feeling that the cleft brought to bear. Therefore, the first visit that the parents have with the team is important because it establishes the foundation of a support system that should last for years.

If the cleft were only a structural defect, the solution would simply be to close the cleft. Yet, problems concerning feeding and health, facial appearance, communication, speech, dental functioning, and hearing loss, as well as the potential for psychosocial difficulties, may necessitate additional surgical, orthodontic, speech, and otolaryngological interventions. In other words, after the closure has been made, attention is focused on aesthetic, functional, and other structural deficits.

—*Iona C. Baldridge*

See also Birth defects; Cleft lip and palate repair; DiGeorge syndrome; Oral and maxillofacial surgery; Speech disorders.

For Further Information:

Berkowitz, Samuel, ed. *Cleft Lip and Palate: Diagnosis and Management.* 2d ed. New York: Springer, 2006.

"Cleft Lip and Palate" *Medline Plus*, May 4, 2012.

Clifford, Edward. *The Cleft Palate Experience.* Springfield, Ill.: Charles C. Thomas, 1987.

"Facts about Cleft Lip and Cleft Palate. *Centers for Disease Control and Prevention*, July 19, 2012.

Gruman-Trinker, Carrie T. *Your Cleft-Affected Child: The Complete Book of Information, Resources, and Hope.* Alameda, Calif.: Hunter House, 2001.

Kliegman, Robert, et al. "Cleft Lip and Palate." In *Nelson Textbook of Pediatrics*, edited by Robert Kliegman, et al. 19th ed. Philadelphia, Pa.: Elsevier, 2011.

Lorente, Christine, et al. "Tobacco and Alcohol Use During Pregnancy and Risk of Oral Clefts." *American Journal of Public Health* 90, no. 3 (March, 2000): 415-419.

Stengelhofen, Jackie, ed. *Cleft Palate.* New York: Churchill Livingstone, 1988.

Wyszynski, Diego F., ed. *Cleft Lip and Palate: From Origin to Treatment.* New York: Oxford University Press, 2002.

Cleft lip and palate repair

Procedure

Anatomy or system affected: Oral cavity, lips, muscle, bone, skin, cartilage, mucosa, and teeth

Specialties and related fields: Oral & maxillofacial surgery, plastic surgery, otolaryngology, neonatology, speech therapy, orthodontist, pediatric dentist, genetic counselor

Definition: The surgical closure of cleft lip and cleft palate, the repositioning of hard and soft tissue through multiple

The Repair of Cleft Lip

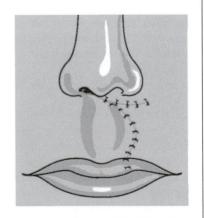

A cleft lip, a congenital deformity in which the tissues between the lip and nostril have failed to fuse, can be corrected surgically through realignment and suturing.

operations according to child development to produce a functional and cosmetic result

Indications and Procedures

Children born with clefts may have different levels of severity; cleft lip only, palate only, or cleft lip and palate. Prevalence varies according to ethnicity: Asian and American Indians are 1 in 500, Europeans are 1 in 1000, and Africans are 1 in 2500. The condition occurs more commonly in males than females and clefts are more common on the left side rather than the right.

Patients born with cleft lip and plate require a team approach for their care as they grow. The team is formed at the time they are born with the neonatologist setting the consults in motion. In the first few days of life the oral and maxillofacial surgeon, a genetic counselor, and a speech and swallow specialist are all called to consult on their care. Upon discharge from the hospital, the pediatrician becomes the leader of the team in conjunction with the surgeon's operative plan for sequencing on-going operative interventions. A pediatric dentist is consulted in the first few weeks of life to add expertise and assistance for shaping the alveolar segments. The pediatric dentist then follows them into adulthood. A speech therapist is brought into the group these children begin to learn how to speak and produce speech patterns. An orthodontist is asked to join the team when the patients are approximately 9 years old to help arrange the dental arches and to prepare these patients for bone grafting. The orthodontist continues to provide treatment until all jaw surgeries are completed.

Children afflicted with both cleft lip and palate need a minimum of five operations from infancy to adulthood. The procedures include lip closure, palate closure, alveolar bone grafting, jaw surgery, and a rhinoplasty. While there is much debate among clinicians as to what the timing and sequencing for surgical corrections for cleft lip and palate should be, the most common sequence is to repair the lip at 3 months of age, repair the palate between 12 and 16 months, perform an alveolar bone graft between 9 and 12 years, jaw surgery between 16 and 17 years, and finally, perform a rhinoplasty at 18 years of age. Surgical revisions are very common in care for these children as their course of growth and maturation is never fully known in advance. Unfortunately, there is a subgroup of these patients who have any of a variety of craniofacial syndromes and these increase dental, medical, and surgical challenges for treatment.

—Vincent Carrao, MD, DDS, FACS
and Cheryl Carrao, DO

For Further Information:

"Cleft lip and palate repair." *MedlinePlus*, June 24, 2013.
"Your child's cleft lip and palate repair." *plasticsurgery.org*, June 24, 2013.

Clinical trials

Procedure
Anatomy or system affected: All
Specialties and related fields: All

Definition: Research studies that test new drugs or treatments on human subjects to determine whether and at what dosage they are safe, effective, and better than similar products already in use.

Key terms:

blinded or *single-blind*: a study in which the patients are not told whether they are in an experimental or control group

control group: a group of patients receiving either a standard treatment or a placebo, allowing comparison with the experimental treatment

double-blind: referring to a study in which neither the patients nor the research staff knows which patients are receiving which treatment

informed consent: consent for treatment by a patient who has been educated fully about the purpose, benefits, and risks of a clinical trial

Institutional Review Board (IRB): a committee that oversees informed consent, reviews the progress of clinical trials, and safeguards participants' rights

placebo: an inactive substance resembling the experimental drug that might be given to a control group, especially when no standard treatment exists

protocol: a lengthy, technical document outlining the rules for inclusion in, scientific rationale of, and procedures for a clinical trial

randomization: assigning, by chance, patients with similar characteristics to either the experimental or the control group in a clinical trial

Indications and Procedures

Clinical trials offer the most reliable process for bringing new drugs and medical treatments into public use. The process has features that can protect human participants, avoid biases, ensure that patient improvements are due to the experimental treatment and not to other factors, and allow accurate comparison of the experimental treatment with others on the market. Clinical trials are usually initiated and managed by academic institutions (often with grant funding), pharmaceutical companies, or government research agencies, such as the National Cancer Institute.

In 1998, it was estimated that the cost of developing a new drug was, on average, $500 million, and the process could take twelve to fifteen years-from discovery and laboratory testing, through clinical trials, to Food and Drug Administration (FDA) approval, and finally getting the drug to market. By the late 1990s, a new drug might go through sixty-eight clinical trials. The average number of patients enrolled in a trial was 3,800.

Clinical trials fit into one of four types. Phase I trials, which usually involve only twenty to one hundred seriously ill patients, try to determine how to administer a new drug, the maximally tolerated dose (MTD), how the human body processes the drug, and any significant side effects. Phase II trials, which are usually randomized, treat up to several hundred patients who all have measurable rates of disease. These trials study the effectiveness of the drug. Phase III trials, which are usually randomized and blinded and which treat hundreds or thousands of patients, have more relaxed criteria for inclusion and are usually multicenter (held simultaneously at more than one site). These trials try to determine whether the new drug is better than current, standard ones. Phase IV trials, conducted once a drug is on the market, are often informal. Pharmaceutical companies may simply ask physicians to submit reports on how their patients are responding to the drug.

Uses and Complications

The 1979 Belmont Report detailed three ethical principles to guide clinical trials. They include respect for persons (abiding by their opinions and choices as autonomous agents), beneficence (doing no harm and maximizing the possible benefits while minimizing possible harm), and justice (distributing the benefits and burdens of research fairly).

Two standard features of clinical trials help ensure that ethical principles are being followed. First, all clinical trials in the United States must be approved and monitored by an Institutional Review Board (IRB), which includes both scientists and laypersons. Multicenter trials must also have a data safety and monitoring board composed of independent experts. This group monitors data from the trial regarding the treatment's effectiveness and any adverse reactions. Second, the detailed informed consent document that patients must carefully consider and sign gives a number of categories of information. Most important, anticipated physical risks and discomforts are explained, as are financial risks. Similar practices are followed in countries other than the United States as well.

Perspective and Prospects

In October, 1948, *The British Medical Journal* published an article reporting on what was probably the first study using all the methodological features of the randomized clinical trial. Since then, the randomized clinical trial has come to be regarded as perhaps the most important medical achievement of the twentieth century. It transformed biomedical research and allowed physicians to make treatment choices based on scientific evidence rather than on personal opinion and experience.

The National Cancer Institute (NCI) and other sources reported a small participation rate in clinical trials-ranging in the late 1990s from 3 to 20 percent of patients. One of many causes was that insurance companies and managed care providers frequently refused payment for experimental treatments. Their concerns were that they might be liable for adverse reactions or additional care after the trial ends and that clinical trials are more costly than conventional treatments. Because so many insurers would not cover the costs of clinical trials, researchers had trouble finding patients willing to participate, thus slowing the development of more effective drugs and treatments. Insurers gradually realized that more widespread coverage of the costs of trials might speed the development of better drugs, which could ultimately save them money. In 1998, US states began to pass laws requiring insurers to cover the routine medical costs (such as tests and office visits) of

treatment in clinical trials of drugs for life-threatening diseases.

Criticism has been leveled at clinical trials for insufficient inclusion of women, children, people of color, and the aged. When these groups are underrepresented, there is no certainty that a drug will be effective or without side effects for them.

In June 2000, the FDA added a regulation that would place a clinical hold on a phase I trial of a drug or treatment for a life-threatening disease affecting both women and men if either gender was excluded because of risk to their reproductive potential. That same month, President Bill Clinton signed an executive memorandum directing Medicare to reimburse senior citizens for routine medical costs incurred in clinical trials. A major impetus for this change came from reports that only 33 percent of cancer clinical trial participants were over sixty-five, while 63 percent of all cancer patients are over sixty-five.

—*Glenn Ellen Starr Stilling, M.A., M.L.S.*

See also Animal rights vs. research; Cancer; Clinics; Death and dying; Disease; Ethics; Food and Drug Administration (FDA); Iatrogenic disorders; Invasive tests; National Cancer Institute (NCI); Noninvasive tests; Over-the-counter medications; Pharmacology; Pharmacy; Screening; Terminally ill: Extended care.

For Further Information:

Beer, Tomasz M., and Larry Axmaker. *Cancer Clinical Trials: A Commonsense Guide to Experimental Cancer Therapies and Clinical Trials*. New York: DiaMedica, 2012.

"Clinical Trials." *MedlinePlus*, May 3, 2013.

"Clinical Trials of Medical Treatments: Why Volunteer?" *US Food and Drug Administration*, Jan. 4, 2010.

Finn, Robert. *Cancer Clinical Trials: Experimental Treatments and How They Can Help You.* Sebastopol, Calif.: O'Reilly, 1999.

Green, Stephanie, Jacqueline Benedetti, and John Crowley. *Clinical Trials in Oncology*. 3d ed. Boca Raton, Fla.: Chapman & Hall, 2012.

Harrington, David P. "The Randomized Clinical Trial." *Journal of the American Statistical Association* 95, no. 449 (March, 2000): 312-315.

"Learn about Clinical Studies." *ClinicalTrials.gov,* Aug 2012.

Malay, Marilyn. *Making the Decision: A Cancer Patient's Guide to Clinical Trials*. Sudbury, Mass.: Jones and Bartlett, 2002.

"Overview of Clinical Trials." *CenterWatch Clinical Trials Listing Service*, n.d.

Quinn, Susan. *Human Trials: Scientists, Investors, and Patients in the Quest for a Cure*. Cambridge, Mass.: Perseus, 2002.

Clinics

Health care system

Definition: Organizations that provide outpatient care to specific types of patients; they can be in-hospital or out of hospital, usually consist of a physical space with reception and examination rooms, and are staffed by doctors, nurses, and other health care professionals.

Key terms:

ambulatory surgery center: a facility providing day surgery outside a hospital setting

clinic: a site for outpatient care

hospital: an inpatient care facility that provides overnight care and in many cases intensive care, emergency care, and surgical services

inpatient care: overnight patient treatment at a hospital

outpatient care: patient treatment not requiring an overnight stay at a hospital

provider: the medical practitioner within a clinic or hospital; providers may be physicians, nurses, dentists, or other licensed health care professionals

Organization and Functions

There are three main types of patient care facilities in North America: hospitals, ambulatory surgery centers, and clinics. Hospitals care for patients who require overnight care, emergency care, or intensive care treatment. Hospital emergency rooms are not usually considered a clinic due to the highly specialized equipment needed and the fact that many patients who are treated in the emergency room are then admitted for overnight stay at a hospital. Ambulatory surgery centers provide outpatient surgery. Clinics provide outpatient nonsurgical care. In some cases, minor procedures are performed in clinics; however, a clinic does not provide outpatient surgery.

A clinic will usually consist of at least a waiting room and patient exam rooms. The number of examination rooms and size of the clinic will depend on the number of providers and the clinic type. Clinics can range in size from a solo practice with a very small office to very large multispecialty outpatient clinics such as the Mayo Clinic or Cleveland Clinic. Specialized equipment may be part of a clinic, such as in a dental clinic. Clinics may be located within a hospital, in a private building, or in a public building. Clinics can be owned and operated by a single practitioner, a group of practitioners, a private group, a public or nonprofit group, a hospital, or a government agency.

Clinics will most often have regular business hours and are not usually open overnight. Some urgent care walk-in clinics may have extended hours. Most clinics will be closed on major holidays. Some smaller solo practitioner clinics may close for one or more weeks per year when the provider is on vacation. Some clinics will have an answering service or after-hours coverage for emergency calls.

Clinic administration will depend on the ownership of the clinic. A solo private practitioner may do administration as well as provision of care. Hospital-based clinics will generally have a clinic manager who works within the administrative system of the hospital. Some clinics may be part of a publicly held company and will have an office manager who reports to a board. Most clinics will have a clinic manager and a medical director. Larger clinics will have more administrative staff, including human resource staff and marketing staff.

Each clinic serves a specific patient population that will be determined by the primary provider or providers within the clinic. For example, a solo family practice physician will serve children and adults for treatment of common illnesses and conditions. In contrast, a pediatric clinic will see only children, and some public health clinics may provide only immunization services. There are as many clinics as there are health care specialties. Some providers will work in groups, such as a multidiscipline group that may contain internal medicine, pediatrics, and dermatology.

Clinics may accept direct fee-for-service payment, insurance, or government funding such as Medicare, Veterans Administration, or Indian Health Service. In Canada, most clinics will accept fee-for-service payment, provincial health insurance payment, or both.

A large number of combinations are possible in terms of specific services offered, number of providers, payment types accepted, clinic size, and clinic location. No matter what the combination of these features, all clinics have in common the provision of nonsurgical outpatient health care services.

Staff and Services

A health care clinic will generally be staffed by a primary provider and support staff. The primary provider will often be a medical doctor but can be another type of provider such as physical therapist, chiropractor, optometrist, dentist, or naturopath. Support staff will include nurses, physician assistants, technicians, office staff, and, in some cases, specialized paraprofessionals. Providers and other specialized staff who provide direct patient care will have licensing requirements that are specific to the state or province and that will vary depending on the field. For example, physicians and dentists will have different licensing requirements.

Depending on the clinic, patients may require referral from a physician. Other clinics such as urgent care clinics will accept walk-ins without referral. Walk-in clinics may refer patients to family practice clinics or other clinics for ongoing care of chronic disease.

Services will depend on the clinic providers. For example, a family practice clinic will provide physical examination, diagnosis, and treatment recommendations for people of all ages for general nonsurgical outpatient medical care. Diagnosis might include giving a patient requisitions to have laboratory or radiology (X-ray) or other specialized tests done at a laboratory or radiology facility. Some family practice clinics may have the capacity to do some simple laboratory tests such as a dip urinalysis or electrocardiography (ECG or EKG). Treatment may include advice, prescription for medications, or treatment of minor injuries.

Another example of a clinic would be a physical therapy clinic. This type of clinic would have one or more physical therapists as providers. These providers would provide limited physical examination, usually of the musculoskeletal system. Diagnosis would be based on the physical examination. Physical therapists would not usually order specialized testing such as X rays or magnetic resonance imaging (MRI) but might comanage a patient with a physician provider if these additional diagnostic tests were needed. Treatment within a physical therapy clinic will usually consist of specialized exercises, massage therapy, heat or cold treatment, specialized physical therapy maneuvers, and, in some cases, acupuncture.

Specialized clinics will treat only specific groups of patients. For example, an obstetrics clinic will provide care only to pregnant women. Pediatrics clinics will treat only children. Ophthalmology clinics will treat both children and adults but will care only for vision and other eye-related problems. Similarly, an orthopedic clinic will be focused on musculoskeletal disorders, and sports medicine clinics will treat sports-related injuries.

Urgent care clinics are designed to treat minor illnesses and minor injuries. More significant illness or injury would be treated in a hospital emergency room. Most urgent care clinics will operate on a walk-in basis due to the nature of the clinic focus. Some hospitals have both an urgent care clinic and an emergency room to keep the emergency room available for the more seriously ill or injured.

The Mayo Clinic and the Cleveland Clinic are examples of clinics that have grown to become very large multidisciplinary clinics that provide outpatient care. These large clinics are affiliated with hospitals that provide inpatient and surgical care.

Some clinics receive public funding to serve low-income populations. This type of clinic may operate on a sliding scale for fee payment. Often this type of clinic will be located in an urban area and may serve homeless populations as well. These clinics are sometimes staffed by volunteers, including volunteer providers.

Regardless of the clinic type, the usual practice is to have the patient check in at a desk in the reception area. Patients may have to wait in the reception area until the appropriate staff is ready and until an exam or treatment room is available. Each patient will have a paper or computerized chart that will record the examinations, diagnosis, and treatment recommendations. The patient will then be taken to the exam room, where a nurse or other specialized staff will often do some preliminary testing such as blood pressure and a preliminary history to determine what services are needed. If the chart is a paper chart, then it will be taken along with the patient to the exam room. The provider will often go from one exam room to the next to examine and treat patients. The support staff will clean each exam room as it is vacated and then room the next patient. This system allows for more efficiency for the provider. Once the provider is done with examination, diagnosis, and treatment, the patient is directed back to the reception area to book additional appointments or testing, if necessary, and is then dismissed from the clinic.

A patient who comes to a clinic with a life-threatening condition or serious injury will be directed to the nearest emergency room. In some cases, an ambulance will be called to transport a patient who is in need of inpatient care, emergency treatment, or immediate surgery.

Perspective and Prospects

The word "clinic" is derived from the Greek word for bed, *kline*. Evidence exists for the use of herbs and other natural substances for the treatment of medical conditions even in prehistoric times. The provision of health care has been historically linked with religious and spiritual beliefs. In some cases, religious leaders such as shamans or monks were the providers of health care, and illness was attributed to demons or witchcraft.

Ancient Egypt has been credited with having organized houses of medicine, and Herophilos (335-280 BCE) is considered the founder of the medical school in Alexandria, Egypt. The knowledge of human anatomy was very limited, there was no understanding of sterile technique, no understanding of germ theory, and few treatment options were available; however, these early institutions served to further medical knowledge. In the Middle Ages, medical care was provided in monasteries, which in some cases had hospitals attached.

Licensing standards vary across the world, and in some places the provision of health care is still largely unregulated. There are some areas in which the only clinics in existence are provided by volunteer organizations, and in some areas these clinics are in the form of mobile trailers.

The Mayo Clinic is one of the best known multidisciplinary clinics. It was established in the aftermath of a destructive tornado in Rochester, Minnesota, in 1883. William Mayo and his sons Charles and William joined the Sisters of St. Francis to establish a hospital and clinic to care for tornado victims. It grew to be the first and largest non-profit multispecialty clinic serving more than one-half million patients annually at its three locations.

—*E. E. Anderson Penno, M.D., M.S., FRCSC*

See also Emergency care; Emergency rooms; Hospitals; Nursing; Physician assistants.

For Further Information:

Fauci, Anthony, et al. *Harrison's Principles of Internal Medicine.* 17th ed. New York: McGraw-Hill, 2008. Chapter 1, "The Practice of Medicine," outlines the standards for providing health care in the United States and discusses inpatient care, outpatient care, and different levels of care within hospitals.

Gonzalez-Crussi, F. *A Short History of Medicine.* New York: Modern Library, 2007. A compendium of medical care from ancient times to the early twenty-first century.

Kennedy, Michael. *A Brief History of Disease, Science, and Medicine from the Ice Age to the Genome Project.* Mission Viejo, Calif.: Asklepiad Press, 2004. History of medicine and disease.

Cloning

Procedure

Also known as: Nuclear transplantation

Anatomy or system affected: Cells

Specialties and related fields: Biotechnology, embryology, ethics, genetics

Definition: From a scientific perspective, the term "clone" signifies an exact genetic copy of a segment of deoxyribonucleic acid (DNA), cell, or organism. Cloning is a procedure conducted by teams of molecular biologists, geneticists, and embryologists to introduce the genetic information from one cell into another for the purpose of producing a clone.

Key terms:

blastocyst: the stage during early embryonic development, just prior to implantation in the uterus, in which the cells form a large hollow ball; at this point, the cells are undifferentiated

complementary DNA (cDNA): DNA that is made from messenger ribonucleic acid (mRNA) and thus represents the genes actively being expressed in a cell at a given time *eukaryotic*: referring to a type of cell that contains a nucleus and membrane-bound organelles; all animal cells are eukaryotic, as are those of plants and fungi

inner cell mass: a tight cluster of spherical cells inside the blastocyst-stage embryo of placental mammals that eventually give rise to the definitive structures of the later embryo and fetus

meiosis: a specific type of cell division that occurs in gamete-producing cells or germ cells, and results in four daughter cells each with half the number of chromosomes of the parent cell

parthenogenesis: the development of an adult from an unfertilized egg

pluripotent: a description for stem cells that have begun differentiation and are capable of forming limited cell types

stem cells: unspecialized cells capable of renewing themselves through cell division that can be induced, under certain conditions, to differentiate into particular types of cells

totipotent: an undifferentiated cell that still retains the ability to form any other cell type of the adult organism; cells of this type are commonly referred to as stem cells

transduction: the incorporation of a piece of DNA into the genome of a bacterium using a virus as a vector transformation: the incorporation into a cell of cell-free DNA from the environment

transgenic: referring to an organism that contains genetic material from two or more species

vector: a system that is used to carry a fragment of DNA for molecular cloning

Uses and Complications

Scientists use the word "cloning" to indicate an experimental process by which an exact genetic duplicate is made of a molecule, cell, or organism. It is frequently divided into three general categories. Molecular cloning involves copying genes, short segments of DNA, or cells (sometimes also called cellular cloning) for the purpose of producing multiple copies of a molecule or cell for further scientific study. The cloning of DNA is commonly called recombinant DNA technology or genetic engineering. Cell cloning isolates one particular cell from a large population of cells and places it in an environment where it can grow into a new homogeneous population of cells. Cloning at the organismal level, also called nuclear transplantation, has been used to create genetically identical organisms and has the potential to produce genetically identical tissues and organs from a donor.

The procedure for molecular cloning involves choosing a vector for the study of the target DNA. The choice of the vector depends on the size of the genetic information being studied and whether it is genomic DNA or complementary DNA (cDNA). Common vectors include plasmids (small circular pieces of bacterial DNA), viruses, and artificial chromosomes. For example, if the length of the DNA being studied is small, then the researcher may choose to insert it into a plasmid. By the process of transformation, the selected plasmid is moved into the bacteria (usually E. coli), and as the bacteria divide, cells are produced that are clones

for the DNA in the plasmid vector. If the researcher is unsure what area contains the gene to be cloned, then the genome is first fragmented and the individual fragments are inserted into viruses that infect bacteria, or bacteriophages. This creates a library of genetic information. Each bacteriophage vector then infects a bacterium, and the infected bacterial cells will divide to produce a colony of bacteria that contain clones of the genetic information contained within the bacteriophage vector. These colonies may then be screened using molecular techniques to isolate a colony that contains the desired section of DNA.

If the DNA fragment is larger, as is frequently the case with studies of genomic DNA, then the researcher may decide to create an artificial chromosome. The purpose is to create a small, synthetically-derived chromosome that is replicated by the host cell prior to cell division. Bacterial artificial chromosomes (BACs) and yeast artificial chromosomes (YACs) are commonly used, but human artificial chromosomes (HACs) have also been available since 1997. In all cases, the purpose is to create cells that are genetically identical, or cloned, for a specific stretch of DNA. While this is a useful technique, molecular cloning is not able to produce an entire organism that is genetically identical to the original.

In eukaryotic organisms, sexual reproduction produces offspring that contain new combinations of the parents' genomes. While this provides variability to the species, it complicates medical research since it effectively shuffles the genome every generation. Identical, or monozygotic, twins are the closest thing to clones in humans, but between even their cells small genetic differences exist. For scientific studies of development and cell biology, large numbers of cloned cells are needed.

The process of nuclear transplantation, or cloning, as it is commonly called, has the ability to create large numbers of genetically identical multicellular organisms. In theory, cloning is not a difficult process: Simply remove the DNA from the host cell, replace it with the DNA from the donor cell, and induce the new cell to divide. Procedures such as this have been performed on amphibians since the 1950s, but nuclear transplantation in mammals is slightly more complicated, since mammalian egg cells, or oocytes, are vastly smaller than those of amphibians. Fortunately technological advances in microscopy and embryology have remedied this problem. In mammalian nuclear transplantation, the embryologist uses a microscope equipped with a micropipette. The micropipette is effectively a microscopic needle that is controlled remotely by the researcher. During the procedure, the egg is held in place by a second pipette to allow for greater control. The researcher then inserts the needle from the first pipette into the oocyte through the zona pellucida (outer covering of the oocyte) and gently removes the nucleus from the cell. At this stage, the oocyte contains only the zona pellucida, cytoplasm, and the internal organelles of the cell, such as the mitochondria. The researcher then inserts a donor cell, complete with DNA, into the area between the oocyte and the zona pellucida. At this point, there are effectively two cells alongside each other-one containing nothing but cytoplasm, the other containing the donor DNA. To form a single cell, the plasma membranes of the two cells must be fused. This is done using a process called electrofusion, in which a small current is applied to the cells, temporarily disrupting the membranes and allowing the cytoplasm of the two cells (and the donor DNA) to mix. The end result is an egg cell than contains the DNA of a second cell.

However, this cell is not yet technically a clone. To produce an embryo that is genetically identical to the original donor cell, the oocyte must divide. In some species, the first cell divisions (cleavages) occur readily in response to electrofusion, but this is not always the case. Frequently, growth factors or other chemical signals need to be applied to make the cell divide. All the cells of the blastocyst are clones of one another and the DNA in the original donor cell. Once cell division ensues, the embryo eventually forms a hollow sphere with flat cells on the outside (trophectoderm) and a tight cluster of round cells on the inside (inner cell mass) known as a blastocyst.

Human oocytes begin as cells called "oogonia;" the progenitors of oocytes. During early fetal developing, oogonia divide and increase in numbers, but later in fetal development (18-22 weeks after conception), oogonia cease dividing, undergo one additional round of DNA synthesis and enter the first phase of meiosis, but become arrested in the first phase of meiosis, at which time it is known as a primary oocyte. Like all gametes (sex cells), oocytes undergo a special type of cell division known as meiosis in which the cell divides twice and reduces the number of chromosomes in the progeny cells by half. Primary oocytes remain arrested in the first stage of meiosis from fetal life through childhood until puberty, when a surge of luteinizing hormone from the anterior lobe of the pituitary gland stimulates the resumption of meiosis. This secondary oocyte, as it is now called, arrests at the metaphase stage of the second stage of meiosis and will not complete meiosis unless it is fertilized.

This introduction to the life of human oocytes explains why cloning human embryos has proven to be so technically difficult; the spindle chromosome apparatus that holds the chromosomes in place, poised to complete the second phase of meiosis, is a fragile structure that is easily disrupted by physical or chemical manipulation. Consequently, meiotic arrest in human oocytes is rather unstable and invasive manipulations tend to induce rapid, premature completion of meiosis, which disrupts normal reprogramming of the nucleus. To solve this problem, Shoukhrat Mitalipov and his colleagues at the Oregon Health & Science University treated human oocytes with caffeine to prevent premature exit from meiosis during the cloning procedure, which greatly increased cloning efficiency.

The development of improved technologies in nuclear transplantation has enabled scientists to create organisms that are genetically the same. In the media, the use of the term "clone" usually signifies an organism produced by this procedure. To create a cloned adult organism, the researcher must insert the blastocyst into the uterus of a surrogate mother, who will carry the embryo to term. To date

cloned adult sheep, cattle, goats, mules, horses, pigs, mouflons (a wild sheep), mice, rats, dogs, cats, and rabbits have been made in the laboratory. To successfully clone adult animals (reproductive cloning), scientists have adapted the techniques of in vitro fertilization (IVF). IVF retrieves eggs from the mother and fertilizes them with sperm from the father in the laboratory. Subsequently, these embryos are grown in embryo culture, and after they grow to the blastocyst stage, the embryos are transferred into the uterus of the mother. Cloning does not require the fertilization step, since the fusion of the enucleated oocyte with the adult cell takes the place of fertilization. Theoretically, once implanted, the cloned blastocyst should develop in the same manner as an embryo made by means of a natural fertilization event.

A different use of cloning, known as therapeutic cloning, uses cloned embryos (made by means of somatic cell nuclear transfer) to generate a large number of embryonic stem cells for the purpose of treating a disease. Since embryonic stem cells are pluripotent, or have the ability to produce all adult cell types, embryonic stem cells made from a cloned embryo, which are known as "nuclear transfer embryonic stem cells (NT-ESCs) should, theoretically, have the ability to take the place of damaged or diseased cells. Embryonic stem cells (ESCs) are derived from a specific group of cells within the blastocyst called the inner cell mass (ICM). ICM cells are pluripotent cells that can be harvested and grown under laboratory conditions to form an ESC line. Under specific culture conditions, ECSs can differentiate into new tissues, such as nerves, skin, bone, fat, cartilage, or pancreas.

Stem cell scientists have used NT-ESCs to treat various diseases in laboratory animals. For example, researchers from Sloan-Kettering Institute used NT-ESCs derived from cloned mouse embryos to successfully treat animals with a rodent version of Parkinson's disease. However, the use of blood-making stem cells derived from NT-ESCs to reconstitute the immune systems of mutant mice showed that cells made from NT-ESCs can still be subject to immunological rejection under certain conditions.

Another technique to make stem cells from unfertilized eggs that have been artificially activated has been utilized. Artificial activation of eggs in the absence of fertilization can cause the egg to initiate development, and this process, by which embryonic development begins in the absence of fertilization, is known as parthenogenesis. Parthenogenesis is common in amphibians and insects, but it does not occur naturally in humans. However, if a female egg cell is chemically induced to form a blastocyst without nuclear transplantation, then the resulting stem cells derived from such blastocysts could be used to generate new organs or tissues for the female. Scientists have made several parthenogenic stem cell lines from various animals and humans, and they can be differentiated into several different cell types. However, the stability of parthenogenic stem cells has been questioned by some stem cell scientists. Parthenogenesis cannot be used in males, since sperm cells lack the cytoplasmic components found in egg cells.

Indications and Procedures

By definition, the purpose of cloning is to produce genetically identical cells or individuals for scientific studies. Yet even identical (monozygotic) twins, whose cells are derived from the same fertilized egg, are not truly identical. For example, monozygotic twins do not have the same fingerprint pattern, even though they possess the same genes for ridges on the fingers. The reason for this difference is environmental. For twins, the genes establish a general pattern, but it is the touch of the fingers on the inner wall of the uterus that establishes the final pattern of fingerprints. Environment plays a significant role in the development of the embryo, and this fact has presented a challenge for scientists who wish to produce identical genetic clones. Also, the process of DNA replication, while highly efficient, is not perfect, and DNA sequence differences between monozygotic twins and cloned individuals emerge. A study by the Seoul National University compared the genomic DNA sequence of the cloned dog (Snuppy) and the donor animal, and the genomes of two identical Korean twins. Snuppy and his donor (Tai) showed approximately the same degree of DNA sequence differences as human monozygotic twins.

Therefore, Dolly, a cloned ewe, was not an exact copy of her donor, even though she possessed the same genetic information as the donor ewe. According to Ian Wimut, the scientist whose laboratory made Dolly and other cloned sheep, the cloned sheep made in his laboratory were different sizes, and had different temperaments even though they were made from cells that came from the same donor ewe. These differences stem from the fact that Dolly and her "sisters" were raised in the uterus of a surrogate mother and thus were exposed to the minor, but important, environmental variations specific to the surrogate mother. It is known that, by a process called genomic imprinting, the mother can override certain traits in the embryo and impose her own traits, regardless of the genes present in the embryo. The mother also provides all the nutrients needed for the developing embryo, and thus any metabolic problems with the surrogate mother may inhibit proper development in the cloned embryo. Also, particular random events during embryonic and fetal development can generate unique individuals who are also genetically identical.

A potential problem with nuclear transplantation is that not all the DNA in the cell is located within the nucleus. Mitochondria, the energy factories of a cell, contain small circular pieces of DNA. The genes on this DNA are inherited along with the mother's cytoplasm, so that individuals receive all mitochondrial DNA from the maternal line. During nuclear transplantation, mitochondria are not removed from the host cell, so once transplantation is complete, the new cell contains donor DNA by both host cell and donor cell mitochondria. Because mitochondrial genetic disorders exist, it is known that the genes in the mitochondria contribute to the characteristics of the organism. In fact, in the Korean study mentioned above, the cloned animals had a significantly greater number of mitochondrial mutations.

Cells age and have a finite life span. This appears to be at least partially controlled by the length of the chromosome, specifically the ends of the chromosome called the telomeres. After each cell division, the telomeres shorten like a genetic fuse, until the cell is no longer able to divide. However, work in several species has established that the telomere length of the chromosomes is reset in the cloned embryo.

One of the greatest challenges facing the process of cloning is ethical, which involves the opinion of the general public regarding the cloning of mammals and potentially, humans. Some consider the cloning of organisms to be an unnatural event, while others question the use of cloned embryos as a source of embryonic stem cells. One of the greatest concerns among the general public regarding cloning is the moral right of people to create life by artificial processes. This objection was also applied to IVF when it was introduced in 1978. Another concern is the production of human embryos solely for the purpose of destroying them. The debate over cloning shows no signs of abating and will almost certainly continue into the foreseeable future. The majority of scientists involved in cloning research are interested in either the therapeutic benefits of cell cloning or the study of embryonic development and cell differentiation, and not the creation of a cloned human.

Perspective and Prospects

While for many people the history of cloning may appear to have begun in 1996, when Ian Wilmut of the Roslin Institute in Scotland introduced the world to Dolly the cloned ewe, the reality is that the cloning of organisms had been going on for some time. The making of cloned plants had been occurring for decades and now represents a common occurrence in agriculture. If one restricts the discussion to animals, then Dolly does not really even represent the first cloned mammal, but rather the first adult animal cloned from the cells of another adult animal.

The cloning of animals by nuclear transplantation has its roots in the late nineteenth century, when early embryologists were studying cell division in the eggs of invertebrate animals. The first experiments that transferred a nucleus from one cell to another in a vertebrate animal were conducted in the early 1950s by Robert Briggs and Thomas King. Briggs and King worked with nuclear transplantation in amphibians. These researchers were not interested in the creation of a cloned frog but rather the question of nuclear programming, or whether the cells isolated from the blastocyst had the genetic ability to form a new adult frog. These experiments examined the use of embryonic cells to produce a functionally adult organism. In later experiments, researchers, including Briggs and King, set out to determine at what age of embryonic development cells differentiate to the point where they cannot be used to produce a functioning adult. In essence, they were studying the potency of the cells and beginning to distinguish between totipotent cells and pluripotent cells. For the next several decades, scientists perfected methods of nuclear transplantation in a variety of organisms, including mammals such as mice and rabbits.

In 1996, the researchers at the Roslin Institute used tissue from the mammary gland of an adult ewe in a nuclear transplantation experiment. The result was Dolly, the first mammal to be cloned from an adult cell. Although this experiment was widely reported as producing the first cloned mammal, its real importance was the demonstration that the genes of an adult cell could be expressed in an embryo to produce a living organism. For decades, scientists had debated whether adult cells were capable of being used in cloning. Adult cells are highly specialized, and many of their developmental genes are inactivated. The experiments with Dolly demonstrated that, under the right conditions, the environment within the blastocyst allows DNA from adult cells to be used. In other words, the DNA from differentiated tissue can be used to create undifferentiated stem cells. This remains a major advance in the understanding of cellular processes.

In June 2013, Masahito Tachibana in the laboratory of Shoukhrat Mitalipov at the Oregon Health & Science University reported the derivation of human embryonic stem cells from cloned human embryos. This was the first time human NT-ESCs were produced, and it represented a remarkable technical advance.

In an earlier publication, Mitalipov's laboratory showed that replacement of an oocyte nucleus by means of somatic cell nuclear transfer, followed by fertilization, can result in a normal embryo. Several scientists suggest that this procedure might allow patients who suffer from mitochondrial genetic diseases to conceive children who do not have these destructive mutations. However, until more animal studies establish the safety of this procedure, it will remain experimental.

The question may then be asked as to why scientists pursue experiments involving the cloning of organisms. Since public opinion is against the cloning of humans and no immediate need exists to clone an individual, then research in this area would appear to be at an impasse. The reality, however, is that the process of nuclear transplantation and organism cloning gives scientists the ability to answer some important questions about cellular differentiation, especially during embryonic development, and the patterns of expression of genes within cells during development.

Furthermore, while the cloning of humans may not be morally acceptable, cloning can serve society in many other ways, such as in studies using transgenic organisms and in tissue and organ transplantation. Scientific research frequently involves the use of transgenic organisms for study. In the study of human genetics and biochemistry, mice are frequently used as a model system. The ability to study the effects of a particular gene in a transgenic organism is dependent on that organism being genetically pure (homozygous) for that trait. In animals, it can take up to fifteen generations of inbreeding to develop a pure line. For organisms with long gestation periods or a small number of offspring per generation, this becomes both cost- and time-prohibitive. The cloning of new organisms that are genetically similar to the donor can facilitate research with transgenic organisms.

Organ transplantation in humans is a difficult process. Recipients of organ transplants must be carefully matched with donors for a variety of biochemical factors to ensure that the new organ is not rejected by the recipient's immune system. Even when a match is close, the use of immunosuppressant drugs increases the chances of infection in the recipient. The process of nuclear transplantation may alleviate some of these problems. Rather than being matched with a donor, a patient would contribute genetic material for nuclear transplantation. Stem cells could then be harvested and chemically induced to form the required tissue, or someday even the entire organ. Experiments are currently under way to manufacture skin for burn victims using this type of procedure. Even though the discovery of induced pluripotent stem cells have largely marginalized NT-ESCs, many scientists still think that NT-ESCs, which are probably safer than induced pluripotent stem cells, still have an important role to play in research and regenerative medicine. The applications of nuclear transplantation are almost endless, and developments in this area of research have the potential to influence directly the lives of the majority of people alive today.

—*Michael Windelspecht, Ph.D.;*
updated by Jeffrey A. Knight, Ph.D.;
further updated by Michael A. Buratovich, Ph.D.

See also Cytology; DNA and RNA; Embryology; Ethics; Gene therapy; Genetic counseling; Genetic engineering; Genomics; Gynecology; Law and medicine; Multiple births; Obstetrics; Ovaries; Premature birth; Veterinary medicine.

For Further Information:

Buratovich, Michael A. *The Stem Cell Epistles. Letters to My Students about Bioethics, Embryos, Stem Cells, and Fertility Treatments.* Eugene, OR: Cascade Books, 2013. A readable and down-to-earth assessment of stem cells, cloning, and regenerative medicine in the form of answers to letters from his students and colleagues.

Kim, Hak-Min, et al. "Whole Genome Comparison of Donor and Cloned Dogs." *Scientific Reports* 3 (October 2013): 1-4. A comparison of the genomic sequence of Snuppy, the cloned dog, and the donor dog, Tai.

Korf, Bruce R., and Mira B. Irons. *Human Genetics and Genomics.* Hoboken, NJ: Wiley-Blackwell, 2013. A textbook of human genetics that gives a solid introduction to basic Mendelian and molecular genetics and then applies it to clinical problems and medical practice.

National Institutes of Health. Department of Health and Human Services. *Regenerative Medicine* 2006. Bethesda, MD: NIH Press, 2006. A collection of articles describing advances in stem cell and cloning technologies since this resource was first published in 2001.

Nussbaum, Martha, and Cass Sunstein, eds. *Clones and Clones: Facts and Fantasies About Human Cloning.* New York: W.W. Norton, 1999. A series of contributed essays on all aspects of human cloning, including science, ethics, and legal issues.

Trounson, Alan, and Natalie D. DeWitt. "Pluripotent Stem Cells from Cloned Human Embryos: Success at Long Last." *Cell Stem Cell* 12 (June 2013): 636-638. An excellent summary of the research that led to the first successful derivation of the first human embryonic stem cell lines from cloned human embryos.

Wilmut, Ian, and Roger Highfield. *After Dolly: The Uses and Misuses of Human Cloning.* New York: W. W. Norton, 2006. The scientist who directed the laboratory that created Dolly and other cloned sheep discusses the utility of therapeutic cloning and the dangers of reproductive cloning.

Wilmut, Ian, Keith Campbell, and Colin Tudge. *The Second Creation: Dolly and the Age of Biological Control.* New York: Farrar, Straus and Giroux, 2000. Coauthored by one of the creators of Dolly, this book examines the process of cloning and the steps that led to the cloning of the first mammal. It also provides insight into the reason why Dolly was cloned.

Clostridium difficile (C. diff.)

Disease/Disorder

Also known as: c. diff, clostridium difficile-associated disease

Anatomy or system affected: gastrointestinal, immune system

Specialties and related fields: infectious disease, gastrointestinal

Definition: Clostridium difficile, often referred to as "c. diff" by health care professionals, is a spore-forming, gram-positive anaerobic bacterium. It produces exotoxins that excrete a microorganism into the environment, which is how the c. diff is spread. C. diff is usually linked to the use of broad-spectrum antibiotic use.

Key terms:

clostridium difficile: a spore-forming, gram-positive anaerobic bacterium

c. diff: the abbreviation used by health care professional for clostridium difficile

bacillus: a rod shaped bacterium

exotoxin: a toxin excreted by c. diff into the environment

pseudomembranous colitis: infection of the colon caused by c. diff

toxic megacolon: dilation of the colon accompanied by fever, bloating, and shock

colonperforation: a hole in the intestinal wall causing bowel contents to spill into the abdominal cavity

peritonitis: infection of the abdominal cavity

sepsis: a systemic infection

Causes and Symptoms

C. diff is usually linked to broad-spectrum antibiotic use but is also commonly transmitted to patients in hospitals because inactive c. diff spores can survive for months on surfaces and objects as well as the gut of healthy people. C. diff spores are shed in feces and transmitted when a person ingests the spores which become active and then produce toxins that damage intestinal cells in the colon. This ingestion leads to an inflammatory and exudative response. People who take antibiotics such as cephalosporins, fluoroquinolones, and sulfonamides, which are broad-spectrum antibiotics, are at an increased risk of developing c.diff because these antibiotics disrupt the normal intestinal flora that prevents the activation of c. diff spores.

Symptoms of c. diff are watery diarrhea, fever, loss of appetite, nausea, and abdominal pain. C. diff may lead to more serious, and life-threatening illnesses such as pseudomembranous colitis, toxic megacolon, colon perforation, sepsis, and even death. Pseudomembranous colitis signs and symptoms include watery diarrhea, abdominal pain, pus or mucus in the stool, nausea and dehydration. Toxic megacolon is a life-threatening conditioning in which the colon becomes extremely dilated and is accompanied by bloating, fever, and shock. Colon perforation is rare and results from damage to the intestine after toxic megacolon. A hole in the intestine causes bacteria to spill from the bowel into the abdominal cavity, causing a severe infection called peritonitis. This can lead to a life-threatening systemic infection called sepsis.

Individuals with unexplained diarrhea are tested for c. diff by confirmation of the c. diff toxin or toxin-producing c. diff in the individual's stool. Other tests may include a CBC to determine if the individual's white blood cell count is elevated, blood chemistry tests to evaluation hydration status, and abdominal x-rays or CT scans if toxic megacolon is suspected.

Treatment and Therapy

Once the diagnosis of c. diff is made, the individual is isolated to prevent further transmission of the disease. These individuals are placed on contact precautions, which include the use of gloves, gowns, and a single-patient room as soon as the c. diff infection is suspected. Transmission often occurs from the hands of health care providers to a patient so recommendations are for health care workers to use soap and water only when caring for individuals with c. diff. It is important to note that alcohol hand rubs do not kill c. diff spores. All visitors must use soap and water to wash their hands before and after visiting the individual with c. diff.

Initial c. diff infections are treated with metronidazole; while more severe cases of c. diff infections may require the use of vancomycin. Intravenous fluids are often administered in the hospital setting to those individuals who are dehydrated from the c. diff infection and loss of fluid through diarrhea. Antiemetics to relieve nausea may also be administered. Gastric acid suppressants are restricted for those individuals with c. diff because these drugs have been associated with the development of c. diff infections. Probiotics are encouraged as a means for prevent c. diff infection for individuals who are taking antibiotics.

Perspective and Prospects

C. diff is the most common infectious cause of healthcare-associated diarrhea in adults, accounting for 80% of healthcare-associated gastrointestinal infections. It is associated with an increase in length of hospital stay, increase in healthcare costs, and increase in morbidity and mortality. Approximately 3 million cases of diarrhea and colitis are associated with c. diff infections in the U.S. each year.

Individuals over 65 years of age, with a compromised

Information on *Clostridium Difficile* Infections

Causes: Bacterial infection

Symptoms: Fever, abdominal pain or tenderness, anorexia, nausea, watery diarrhea

Duration: Acute

Treatments: Antibiotics, sometimes IV fluids to prevent dehydration immune system, utilizing antibiotics, taking chemotherapy, and with chronic illness are most at risk for c. diff infection. Gastric acid suppressive therapy, which includes proton pump inhibitors such as omeprazole and histamine-2 blockers such as famotidine, can increase the risk of c. diff infection.

Fecal microbiota transplantation (FMT) is a procedure in which fecal matter from a healthy donor is instilled into an individual with recurrent c. diff. The transplant is done through colonoscopy, endoscopy, sigmoidoscopy, or enema. The purpose is to replace good bacteria that has been killed or suppressed. Cammarota et al., 2014 reported an 87% success rate with FMT treatment in c. diff patients.

A new, more virulent strain of c. diff, BI/NAP1/027 emerged in 2003. It is resistant to the usual treatment of metronidazole and has caused a dramatic increase in morbidity, mortality, and healthcare-associated infections.

Educate individuals that alcohol based hand sanitizers do not kill c. diff spores. Frequent handwashing with antibacterial soap is the best defense against c. diff transmission.

See also: Antibiotics; Colitis; Colon; Diarrhea*and dysenteryinfection; Infection; Intestines; Peritonitis*

—*Mary Dietmann, EdD;*
updated by Geraldine Marrocco

For Further Information:

C. difficile infection. (2016). *Mayo Clinic.* http://www.mayoclinic.org/diseases-conditions/c-difficile/home/ovc-20202264

Clostridium difficile infection information for patients. (2015). *CDCCenters for Disease Control and Prevention.* https://www.cdc.gov /hai/organisms/cdiff/cdiff-patient.html

cdifffoundation.org

Gupta, S., Allen-Vercoe, E., & Petrof, E.O. (2016). Fecal microbiota transplantation: in perspective. *TherapeuticAdvances in Gastroenterology, 9*(2), 229-239.

Smith, S., & Taylor, J. (2016). Best practices in caring for patients infected with clostridium difficile. *Critical Care Nurse, 36*(3), 71-72.

What is clostridium difficile (c. diff)? (2017) *WebMD.* http://www.webmd.com/digestive-disorders/clostridium- difficile-colitis#1

Club drugs

Disease/Disorder
Also known as: Designer drugs, psychedelics
Anatomy or system affected: All
Specialties and related fields: Alternative medicine, critical care, emergency medicine, pharmacology, preventive medicine, psychiatry, psychology, public health, toxicology
Definition: A slang term for a variety of substances of abuse that generally are used in social situations, have hallucinogenic properties, and may either excite or sedate the user.

Key terms:

amnesia: a diverse condition where there is complete or partial loss of memory for specific periods of time, for specific types of information, or both

blackout: memory loss, usually as a result of taking substances known to disrupt memory, in which the affected person may function as if aware of what is happening, despite having no memory of activities

psychedelic drugs: substances that cause alterations in perception and thinking, such as changes in awareness or sense of self and hallucinations

raves: social gatherings that are distinguished by long periods of music, dancing, and often a percentage of individuals using psychedelic drugs and other substances of abuse

synergistic effects: the combined effects of drugs interacting with one another, such that the effects of the drugs together have a compounded effect, greater than that of any one alone

Causes and Symptoms

Less expensive, easily accessible, intoxicating drugs can often be attractive to persons wanting a momentary high or psychedelic experience, when they are at a rave, dance party, or bar with friends. This desire, combined with a belief that club drugs seem safe, leads people to trying club drugs and sometimes using them regularly. Club drugs are often first used in dance clubs or with friends. The belief that such drugs are natural forms of prescription drugs or are not necessarily always illegal fuels a misconception of their safety. Because these drugs are psychedelic, the reactions that individual users have can vary quite significantly depending on the user's emotional state, concurrent use of other substances, underlying psychiatric conditions, personality, and past experience with the drug. Additionally, as they are street drugs, usually subject to some variability in their contents (such as being mixed with less expensive drugs), their quality may vary substantially. Finally, the individual situations where the substances are used can pose a variety of dangers of varying levels.

Club drugs go by many different names. They include substances such as gamma-hydroxybutyrate (GHB, Georgia Home Boy, Liquid X), ketamine hydrochloride (ketamine, special K), lysergic acid diethylamid (LSD, acid, blotter), methylenedioxymethamphetamine (MDMA, Adam, ecstasy, X), and rohypnol (roofies, roach, roche). They also include herbal ecstasy (herbal X, cloud nine, herbal bliss), which is a drug made from ephedrine or pseudoephedrine and caffeine. These substances vary in their effects but as a group cause a variety of positive reactions, including euphoria, feelings of well-being, emotional clarity, a decreased sense of personal boundaries, and feelings of empathy and closeness to others. They also can cause, however, significant negative reactions, including panic, impaired judgment, amnesia, impaired motor control, insomnia, paranoia, irrational behavior, flashbacks, hallucinations, rapid heartbeat, high blood pressure, chills, sweating, tremors, respiratory distress, convulsions, and violence. It is not uncommon for individuals to mix these drugs with alcohol, prescription drugs, and illegal drugs. Taken in combination, these substances can make these very dangerous reactions even worse.

Treatment and Therapy

The effects of club drugs vary somewhat by substance; as such, treatment also varies by substance. In general, though, club drugs may tend to be seen more in emergency care settings than in primary health care settings. This is due to the fact that some of the problems that they cause, as a group, are often of an emergency nature. For instance, overdose, strokes, allergic shock reactions, blackouts, loss of consciousness, and accidents related to these conditions may require emergency care. Similarly, dehydration and heat exhaustion can result from prolonged periods of dancing or other physical exertion, as can occur in rave situations, and result in a need for emergency care. Finally, because date rapes have been known to occur with these drugs, particularly rohypnol, injuries due to sexual assault also may need attention.

Certainly the long-term impact of problems like those described above may require some type of psychotherapy. In addition, problems related to the abuse of or dependence upon club drugs would be addressed in much the same manner as for other substances of abuse. General addiction treatment would be advised. A special area of treatment may also include exploration of what it is like to deal with blackouts, amnesia, and flashbacks, as these are features that are commonly reported with psychedelic drugs.

Perspective and Prospects

Club drugs emphasize that there is a continuing need for the social awareness of the dangers of substances that may otherwise seem harmless. Just because a substance is not listed as an illegal drug does not mean that it cannot be dangerous. Any drug, whether sold over the counter, by prescription, or any other place, can be misused and can be dangerous. Where drugs are used, how much is used, with whom they are used, and with what they are used can all make a difference.

Club drugs are also a reminder that in efforts to find ways of joining with each other, finding community, and discovering themselves and their relationships, people will sometimes resort to experimenting with substances. While the experimental use of psychedelic substances for psychotherapeutic work continues and may prove beneficial to certain groups of patients, such work is balanced by investigations into neurology, physiology, psychopharmacology, and psychology to ensure that the benefits do not outweigh the risks. Continued exploration of the neuronal, developmental, social, and other health effects of using club drugs is likely, as they pose a significant danger to public health, particularly that of younger populations.

—*Nancy A. Piotrowski, Ph.D.*

See also Addiction; Amnesia; Emergency medicine; Hallucinations; Herbal medicine; Intoxication; Marijuana; Panic attacks; Paranoia; Pharmacology; Seizures; Substance abuse; Tremors.

For Further Information:

Holland, Julie, comp. *Ecstasy: The Complete Guide-A Comprehensive Look at the Risks and Benefits of MDMA*. Rochester, Vt.: Inner Traditions International, 2001.
Jansen, Karl. *Ketamine: Dreams and Realities*. Ben Lomond, Calif.: Multidisciplinary Association for Psychedelic Studies, 2004.
Kuhn, Cynthia, et al. *Buzzed: The Straight Facts About the Most Used and Abused Drugs from Alcohol to Ecstasy*. 3d ed. New York: W. W. Norton, 2008.
O'Neill, John, and Pat O'Neill. *Concerned Intervention: When Your Loved One Won't Quit Alcohol or Drugs*. Oakland, Calif.: New Harbinger, 2003.
Stafford, Peter. *Psychedelics*. Berkeley, Calif.: Ronin, 2003.

Cluster headaches

Disease/Disorder

Anatomy or system affected: Blood vessels, brain, head, nerves, nervous system

Specialties and related fields: Neurology

Definition: The most severe headache syndrome, characterized by paroxysmal onset of one side of the head, short duration, and episodic occurrence. Cluster headaches are often confused with migraine headaches, which are a similar syndrome but with different causes, patterns, and treatments.

Key terms:

alarm clock headaches: an earlier term for cluster headaches, emphasizing the characteristic awakening of sufferers during the night

circadian rhythm: the biological clockwise regularity associated with many body processes; most sufferers of cluster headaches have attacks at the same time of day during the same season of the year

cluster period: a time period, from two weeks to four months, during which cluster headaches occur; they usually disappear, or "enter remission," after the cluster period ends

paroxysmal: having a sudden, spasmlike, and painful onset

trigeminal-autonomic reflex pathway: the nerve pathway at the base of the brain activated during cluster attacks; the trigeminal nerve, the most important facial nerve for sensations such as temperature and pain, causes the "hot-poker-in-the-eye" pain typical of cluster headaches

unilateral: occurring only on one side (for example, on one side of the head or behind one eye)

Causes and Symptoms

Cluster headache is a well-defined, rare, but often misdiagnosed syndrome characterized by excruciatingly severe unilateral headaches that last from a half hour to three hours, with an average duration of forty-five minutes. Its features include paroxysmal onset of one side of the head, a short duration, and episodic occurrence. The pain often wakes sufferers one to two hours after they fall asleep. "Cluster" refers to the original perception that the headaches emerged in groups over a period of time (called the cluster period) lasting weeks to months, followed by periods that are free of pain and attacks (called remission or interim periods). The International Headache Society divides cluster headaches into episodic cluster and chronic cluster, with chronic further subclassified into primary and secondary variants. Chronic cluster headaches do not have a cessation, or interim, period but recur for years.

The precise cause of cluster headaches is unknown, although the season of the year is the most common trigger. Because they usually begin with spring or autumn, cluster

Information on Cluster Headaches

Causes: Unknown; may be seasonal

Symptoms: Sudden headache on one side of head, with intense pain behind one eye often spreading to teeth, jaw, neck, or temple; occasionally preceded by visual aura

Duration: Recurrent, with acute episodes occurring one to six times a day and lasting a half hour to three hours each during cluster periods

Treatments: For symptom alleviation, oxygen therapy, injections of sumatriptan or dihydroergotamine, zolmitriptan tablets, intranasal lidocane, ergotamine; for prevention, verapamil, ergotamine, lithium, methysergide, prednisone, valproic acid, divalproex

headaches are often misattributed to seasonal allergies (such as hay fever) or seasonal-related stress (such as the beginning of school, final examinations, or the height of business cycles).

Positron emission tomography (PET) scanning has revealed that in cluster headaches the hypothalamus activates the trigeminal nerve, which is responsible for most of the severe pain. Located deep in the brain, the hypothalamus is also responsible for the internal biological clock that regulates the approximately twenty-four-hour sleep-wake cycle. The production and activity of the neurotransmitter serotonin, which is important in the self-regulation of these circadian rhythms, is also altered during attacks. Cluster headache is not related to the development of tumors or lesions.

Cluster headaches are rare. No more than .03 percent of the population ever experiences them. Men suffer them more than women do, although with improvements in epidemiological techniques the known ratio has been changed from 7:1 to 2:1. The age of onset is usually in the late twenties. As with migraine headaches, cluster headaches tend to run in families, with a fourteenfold increase in the chances of having them if a first-degree relative (mother, father, son, daughter, brother, or sister) suffers from the syndrome. In addition, a statistically significant incidence of migraine headaches exists in families with a cluster headache sufferer.

Cluster headache attacks, which are excruciatingly severe, debilitating, and dramatic, are almost always unilateral and occur from one to six times a day. They are most intense in, around, or behind one eye. Because the pain, commonly described as "boring" or "stabbing," often spreads into the upper teeth, jaw, neck, or temple, the headaches can be misdiagnosed as coming from dental or sinus problems. The attacks are rapid, peaking in five to ten minutes, and are occasionally, but not frequently, preceded by a visual aura. Attacks are much more likely to occur if tobacco and/or alcohol have been recently used, and they even more frequently will awaken sufferers during their first hour of napping or sleeping.

While migraine headache sufferers seek quiet, darkened places and try to remain still, cluster headache sufferers feel more pain if they try to lie down or recline in a chair. Typically, cluster headache sufferers are restless, pacing back and forth, or want to sit upright, holding their heads with their hands. A sufferer may even bang his or her head against a wall to obtain relief.

Treatment and Therapy

Treatments are oriented either toward abortive therapies or prophylactic therapies. Abortive approaches attempt to shorten the duration and/or intensity of an individual attack. Prophylactic approaches attempt to shorten or prevent the cluster periods themselves. While a fortunate characteristic of the attacks is their brevity, this feature also limits the range of abortive measures that can be undertaken; by the time that some agents are metabolized, the attack is over.

Although not always practical, a successful and safe abortive treatment is simply breathing 100 percent oxygen for ten to twenty minutes through a nonrebreathing mask. Also not always practical but effective are subcutaneous injections of sumatriptan (Imitrex) or intravenous, intramuscular, or subcutaneous injections of dihydroergotamine (Migranal). Other effective first-line therapies for acute intervention include zolmitriptan (Zomig) tablets, intranasal lidocane, or ergotamine (Cafergot).

Prophylactic, or preventive, treatments prevent attacks or at least lessen their intensity. All cluster headache sufferers should be on a prophylactic regimen (unless their cluster periods are less than two weeks, which is rarely the case). Verapamil (marketed as Calan, Covera, Isoptin, Tarka, and Verelan) is the most commonly prescribed medication because its mechanism as a calcium-channel blocker is well understood and it is usually effective. Occasionally, higher-than-typical doses must be employed. For those who do not respond well or receive sufficient relief on verapamil alone, a second medication such as ergotamine, lithium, methysergide (Sansert), or prednisone is often added. Sometimes, these second medications are effectively used alone, as are valproic acid and divalproex (Depakote).

In the event that pharmacology proves ineffective, several surgical or radiation techniques can block the trigeminal-autonomic reflex pathway. The benefits of these, or any, invasive treatments must be weighed against potential harm. For example, corneal anesthesia, needed to carry out these procedures, can put the eye at risk.

Perspective and Prospects

People have suffered from cluster headaches as long as people have suffered from headaches, although the rarity, seasonal occurrence, and symptoms of cluster headaches have made their recognition as a distinct syndrome difficult. Through PET scanning, neurovascular research has identified three areas of the brain particularly affected by cluster headaches. Because two of these areas are affected every time any sort of pain is felt, research is being concentrated on the third area, hypothalamic gray matter. Researchers expect that probes here will resolve their biggest debate: Is the vasodilation associated with cluster headache the primary problem or the result of activation of the trigeminal vascular system? Researchers do agree that cluster headaches, while distinct, belong to a family of related conditions, the cranial neuralgias.

—*Paul Moglia, Ph.D.*

See also Brain; Brain disorders; Head and neck disorders; Headaches; Migraine headaches; Pain; Pain management; Stress.

For Further Information:
Dalessio, Donald J. "Relief of Cluster Headache and Cranial Neuralgias." *Postgraduate Medicine* 109, no. 1 (January, 2001): 69-78.
Jasmin, Luc. "cluster Headache." *MedlinePlus*, Mar. 22, 2013
Kudrow, L. "Cluster Headache: Diagnosis and Management." *Headache* 19 (1979): 141-48.
Newman, Lawrence C., Peter Goadsby, and Richard B. Lipton. "Cluster and Related Headaches." In *Headache*, edited by Ninan T. Mathew. Philadelphia: Saunders, 2001.
Wood, Debra. "Cluster Headache." *Health Library*, Feb. 21, 2013.

Coccidioidomycosis

Disease/Disorder
Also known as: San Joaquin Valley fever, valley fever
Anatomy or system affected: All
Specialties and related fields: Dermatology, family medicine, general surgery, internal medicine, microbiology, pulmonary medicine
Definition: A fungal infection acquired by inhaling the spores of particular soil-based fungi. It initially attacks the lungs and often resolves without causing symptoms, but it can cause pneumonia and disseminate throughout the body.

Key terms:
arthroconidia: asexual fungal spores that are made by the segmentation of preexisting fungal hyphae
endospores: tiny, round cells produced by spherules as they divide into smaller and smaller cells that are released upon rupture
erythema nodosum: inflammation of the fatty layer of the skin that results in red, painful bumps, usually located on the front of the legs
hyphae: the long, filamentous, often branching cells of many fungi
mycelium: a body of the fungal organism that consists of a collection of hyphae
mycetoma: a progressive and chronic fungal or bacterial infection that causes overgrowth of the infected tissue and the formation of sinuses filled with the infecting organism
pulmonary nodules: small, round growths on the lung that contain either trapped microorganisms or cancer cells
spherules: a thick-walled, spherical structure that is the tissue-specific form of *Coccidioides* species

Causes and Symptoms

Coccidioidomycosis is an infection caused by the soil-based fungi *Coccidioides immitis* (*C. immitis*) and *Coccidioides posadasii* (*C. posadasii*). These fungi are found only in the Western hemisphere, and they prefer dry, alkaline soils. *C. immitis* and *C. posadasii* are endemic to the southwestern United States (south-central California, Nevada, Arizona, New Mexico, and western Texas), those regions of Mexico that border the western United States, parts of Central America (Guatemala, Honduras, and Nicaragua), and the desert regions of South America (Argentina, Paraguay, and Venezuela).

While in the soil, *Coccidioides*, like most fungi, grows as thin, branching filaments called hyphae. A collection of hyphae is called a mycelium. When it rains, the mycelium grows quite rapidly, but once the soil dries out, it forms resting cells called arthrospores. If disturbed by wind, earthquakes, or soil excavation, these arthrospores become airborne and, if inhaled, can cause coccidioidomycosis.

Once inhaled, the arthrospore transforms into a thick-walled, spherical structure called a spherule that divides itself into hundreds of small endospores. When the spherule ruptures, it releases the endospores, which grow into spherules that form more endospores.

About 60 percent of patients show no symptoms, and the disease resolves spontaneously. Those patients who show symptoms suffer from fever, sore throat, headache, cough, fatigue, painful bumps on the skin (erythema nodosum), and chest pain approximately one to three weeks after inhaling arthrospores. About 95 percent of symptomatic patients recover without further problems after several weeks. If symptoms persist beyond three months, however, then the patient has chronic progressive coccidioidal pneumonia. Between 5 and 7 percent of patients with coccidioidal pneumonia form pulmonary nodules, which are areas of the lung where the immune system has walled-off the organism from the rest of the lung. On an X-ray, these nodules can look exactly like cancerous masses in the lung. A biopsy is often necessary to distinguish between lung cancer and coccidioidal pulmonary nodules. In 5 percent of patients with coccidioidal pulmonary nodules, the nodules enlarge to form pulmonary cavities that can become infected, rupture, and bleed, causing the release of pus between the lungs and the ribs (empyema). Small cavities (less than 2.5 centimeters) can heal after one to two years, but larger cavities can persist and cause the patient to spit up blood (hemoptysis) and allow the growth of fungi throughout the cavity (mycetoma).

A minority of patients develop disseminated coccidioidomycosis, in which the organism penetrates blood vessels, invades the bloodstream, and infects any organ in the body. Disseminated coccidioidomycosis occurs weeks or months after the primary pneumonia and can even

---

Information of Coccidioidomycosis

Causes: Fungal infection
Symptoms: Chest pains, chills, cough, fever, headache, spitting up blood, loss of appetite, muscle aches and stiffness, night sweats, rash, light sensitivity, excessive sweating, weight loss, wheezing
Duration: Up to three months or more
Treatments: Antifungal drugs

develop in cases where there is no previous evidence of respiratory disease. Particular ethnic groups such as Filipinos and African Americans show increased risk of developing disseminated disease, as do pregnant women in the third trimester of their pregnancy, infants younger than one year old, diabetics, patients with acquired immunodeficiency syndrome (AIDS), or those taking drugs or suffering from diseases that suppress the immune system.

Treatment and Therapy

Asymptomatic or symptomatic infections are usually self-limited and require little more than supportive care. Patients with coccidioidal pneumonia require fluconazole or itraconazole treatment for at least twelve months and intravenous amphotericin B for stubborn cases. Pulmonary nodules are typically not treated, but they may require surgery. Pulmonary cavities are only treated with antifungal drugs if the patient shows symptoms. Surgical removal might also be warranted if the infection resists treatment. Disseminated coccidioidomycosis requires higher doses of fluconazole, and very sick patients may require amphotericin B or a combination of fluconazole and amphotericin B. Amphotericin B is preferred for pregnant women, since other drugs harm the developing fetus.

Perspective and Prospects

Coccidioidomycosis was first described in 1892 by Roberto Johann Wernicke and Alejandro Posadas in South America. The first case in the United States was reported in California in 1894. Two years later, Emmet Rixford and Thomas Caspar Gilchrist reported several clinical infections that were caused by an organism that, they thought, resembled the protozoan *Coccidia*. Therefore they named it *Coccidioides*, which means "*Coccidia*-like." In 1905, William Ophüls described the fungal life cycle and pathology of *C. immitis*. Charles E. Smith studied the epidemiology of coccidioidomycosis in the San Joaquin Valley of California and went on to develop the coccidioidin skin test and serological testing for the disease.

The Centers for Disease Control and Prevention released a study in 2013 that showed an increase in cases of coccidioidomycosis in the southwestern United States between 1998 and 2011. Cases in the states of Arizona, California, Nevada, New Mexico, and Utah increased from 2,265 reported in 1998 to 22,000 reported in 2011.

New treatments under investigation for coccidioidomycosis include posaconazole, voriconazole, caspofungin, and a new lipid-dispersal formulation of amphotericin B that reduces its kidney toxicity. Nikkomycin Z is another experimental agent that is very active against *Coccidioides* in culture and infected animals.

—Michael A. Buratovich, Ph.D.

See also Acquired immunodeficiency syndrome (AIDS); Aspergillosis; Candidiasis; Environmental diseases; Environmental health; Fungal infections; Immune system; Immunodeficiency disorders; Immunology; Immunopathology; Lungs; Microbiology; Mold and mildew; Pneumonia; Pulmonary diseases; Pulmonary medicine; Respiration.

For Further Information:

Anstead, Gregory M., and John R. Graybill. "Coccidioidomycosis." *Infectious Disease Clinics of North America* 20, no. 3 (September, 2006): 621-43.

Centers for Disease Control and Prevention. "Valley Fever Increasing in Some Southwestern States." *CDC*, Mar. 28, 2013.

Galgiani, John N. "Changing Perceptions and Creating Opportunities for Its Control." *Annals of the New York Academy of Sciences* 1111 (September, 2007): 1-18.

Kohnle, Diana. "Coccidioidomycosis." *Health Library*, Nov. 26, 2012.

Kwon-Chung, K. J., and John E. Bennett. *Medical Mycology*. Philadelphia: Lea and Febiger, 1992.

Parish, James, M., and James E. Blair. "Coccidioidomycosis." *Mayo Clinic Proceedings* 83, no. 3 (March, 2008): 343-348.

Cockayne disease

Disease/Disorder

Also known as: Weber Cockayne syndrome, Neill-Dingwall syndrome

Anatomy or system affected: All

Specialties and related fields: Audiology, dentistry, dermatology, genetics, neurology, ophthalmology, optometry, otorhinolaryngology, pediatrics

Definition: A rare, inherited genetic disease characterized by short stature and premature aging.

Key terms:

ataxia: lack of voluntary coordination of muscle movements

contractures: the replacement of normally elastic tissues by inelastic tissues that limit flexibility and prevent normal movement

microcephaly: an abnormally small head

Causes and Symptoms

Cockayne syndrome (CS) is a rare disorder that results from mutations in the ERCC8/CSA or ERCC6/CSB genes. These genes encode proteins that repair damaged DNA. Inactivating mutations in the CSA or CSB genes prevent cells from repairing their DNA, which leads to an accumulation of mutations, cell malfunction, and death. CS occurs in about 2 newborns per million live births.

There are three main types of CS, each of which differs in the age when symptoms first appear and their severity. In the case of Classical or Type I CS, symptoms usually appear after the first year of life. For the more severe, congenital Type II CS (also known as cerebro-oculo-facio-skeletal syndrome or Pena-Shokeir syndrome type II), symptoms appear at birth. Type III CS is a Cockayne Syndrome/xeroderma pigmentosum combination condition that will not be discussed further.

CS is an autosomal recessive genetic disease. Autosomal recessive diseases require that cells have two mutant copies of the gene in question in order to have the genetic disease.

CS children grow and develop at an abnormally slow rate and fail to gain weight normally (failure to thrive). In addition to microcephaly and noted mental retardation, their nervous systems deteriorate and they begin to show signs of ataxia and quick jerky movements. CS children also have skin that is highly sensitive to sun exposure (photosensitivity), thin, dry hair, hearing loss, progressive vision loss (progressive pigmentary retinopathy), and dental caries (cavities). In addition, CS children have characteristic facial features that include a pinched, narrow face with a beaked nose (bird-like face). Also, CS children who can walk have a "horse riding stance" when they stand as a result of their disproportionately long limbs, large hands and feet, and knee contractures. CS children also show accelerated aging and have an elderly look about them (progeroid appearance).

Treatment and Therapy

No cure exists for CS, but there are palliative measures that can be taken. CS patients should protect themselves from the sun at all costs; sunscreen and protective clothing are essential. Cochlear implants can minimize the effects of auditory impairment. Eye problems (optic atrophy and cataracts) require the care of an ophthalmologist. Dentists can help deal with the severe tooth decay seen in CS children. Neurological deterioration and ataxia requires consultation with a neurologist. Parents known to carry mutations in CSA or CSB should consult a geneticist for prenatal evaluation and genetic counseling.

—*Michael A. Buratovich, Ph.D.*

See also Audiology; Burns and scalds; Dentistry; Dermatology; Dermopathology; Failure to thrive; Genetic counseling; Ophthalmology; Optometry

For Further Information:

Moriwaki, Shinichi. "Hereditary Disorders with Defective Repair of UV-Induced DNA Damage." *Japanese Clinical Medicine* 4 (2013): 29-35.

Woliver, Robbie. *Alphabet Kids-From ADD to Zellweger Syndrome: A Guide to Developmental, Neurobiological and Psychological Disorders to Parents and Professionals.* London: Jessica Kingsley Publishers, 2008.

Cognitive development

Development

Anatomy or system affected: Brain, nervous system, psychic-emotional system

Specialties and related fields: Environmental health, genetics, pediatrics, psychology

Definition: The growth and age-related changes that occur over time in children's mental processes and in activities related to the faculties of attending, learning, perceiving, problem solving, thinking, and remembering.

Key terms:

adaptation: change or adjustment made to create a balance between existing thought structures and the environment

assimilation: the process of attempting to explain a new experience in terms of existing schemes

cognition: the activity of knowing and the processes through which knowledge is acquired and used

cognitive equilibrium: a term used by psychologist Jean Piaget to describe the balanced relationship between an individual's mental processes and the environment

conservation: understanding that an object's properties remain unchanged when its appearance is altered

egocentrism: seeing the world only from one's own point of view; being unable to acknowledge or recognize different perspectives

equilibration: the process of adapting or adjusting one's existing knowledge or mental structures to the new situation, thus constructing more complex and sophisticated structures

miseducation: the tendency to hurry and pressure children to perform activities and tasks for which they are not cognitively or physically ready

reflexive: referring to an automatic response to external stimuli

reversibility: the ability to negate an action by mentally reversing it or imagining its opposite

scheme: a pattern of thought constructed by the child to organize experience in a meaningful way

Physical and Psychological Factors

The mental capabilities and skills of humans develop gradually over a period of time from birth through adolescence. As a child ages, the quality of the processes by which he or she responds to and adapts thinking to particular situations and evaluates, plans, and solves problems changes over time.

In childhood, the brain develops very rapidly. At birth, the human brain already weighs about 25 percent of its adult weight. By six months of age, this figure is 50 percent. By the age of five, the child's brain has achieved 90 percent of its eventual weight. While the basic structure of the brain is genetically and biologically determined, environment and experience play a significant role in the development of cognition. Children's biological constitutions may affect the way in which they interact with and respond to their environment.

According to the Swiss psychologist Jean Piaget (1896-1980), the cognitive growth of all children follows a universal or holistic pattern of development through infancy, childhood, and adolescence. The thought processes of young children are less mature and complex than those of older children, and as children grow and experience life, their cognitive structures become more sophisticated, as well as qualitatively different from those of children in earlier or later stages of development. Cognitive structures, or "schemes" as Piaget called them, are thought patterns that children construct to explain, understand, or interpret their experiences. When children's schemes or thought processes are in harmony with their environment, they experience cognitive equilibrium. When children encounter new and puzzling events or objects, they are in a state of imbalance or disequilibrium and must achieve equilibrium via a process called equilibration. This process consists of adapting or adjusting one's existing knowledge or mental structures to the new situation, thus constructing more complex and sophisticated thought structures. Adaptation takes place through the processes of assimilation and accommodation.

Assimilation refers to the process of attempting to explain a new experience in terms of existing schemes. For example, a child who sees a pony for the first time may call it a "kitty" because a cat is the existing model of that child for four-legged animals. Noticing that there are differences between the scheme of a cat and the reality of the pony, however, the child soon attempts to modify existing mental structures to fit the new experience. This process of modification is accommodation. Through assimilation and accommodation, children organize their knowledge into schemes that better explain their observations.

Piaget's theory of cognitive development, with its emphasis on continuous and active organization and adaptation involving assimilation and accommodation, implies that children actively construct their own knowledge. This construction is based on the child's current stage of cognitive development: Piaget proposed that all children in a specific, universal cognitive stage construct similar interpretations of similar experiences.

According to Piaget, cognitive development can be divided into four major stages. The order in which these stages occur is universal, and all individuals must experience each stage. No stage can be skipped, although the rates at which children go through a stage may vary. The basis for Piaget's insistence on the unvarying sequence of cognitive stages is a concept known as epigenesis, which he used to explain the gradual development of thinking processes. Each new structure or cognitive skill is based on and develops from an earlier one. Hence, each stage, and each structure within each stage, is necessary for the development of new, more advanced structures. Piaget called this feature of development "hierarchization."

The four stages of cognitive development identified by Piaget are the sensorimotor stage (up to age two), the preoperational stage (two to seven years of age), the concrete operations stage (seven to eleven years of age), and the formal operations stage (age eleven and up).

During the sensorimotor stage, children act upon their environment and acquire knowledge of it through their senses and motor activities. In the first two years, cognition progresses from reflexive actions, such as sucking and grasping, to primitive symbolic functions or representation, such as language use and symbolic play. The sensorimotor stage can be further divided into six substages. Substage 1 lasts from birth to one month and centers on exercising basic reflexes, including eye movements, sound orientation, and vocalization, and assimilat-

ing and accommodating objects into reflexive schemes. Substage 2, from one to four months, consists of simple repetitive actions, such as thumb sucking, which are discovered by chance and acquired through repeated trials. Piaget called these actions primary circular reactions. Substage 3 appears between four and eight months of age. Piaget named this period secondary circular reactions. Infants notice stimulating events in the environment beyond their bodies-such as a noise made by squeezing a toy or a movement caused by touching an object-and attempt to re-create the events.

Between eight and twelve months of age, infants experience substage 4, or the coordination of secondary schemes. This means that infants can use two already acquired schemes to reach a simple goal. For example, they are able to remove an object to grasp a hidden toy. These early coordinations reflect intentional behavior and simple problem solving. Tertiary circular reactions are characteristic of substage 5, appearing between the ages of twelve and eighteen months. Infants display curiosity, experiment actively, and find new ways of solving problems. Their behaviors are goal-directed but are carried out through trial and error. Substage 6, from eighteen to twenty-four months, reflects inner experimentation or new mental combinations. The infant now displays symbolic functioning through language, imagery, and symbolic play. Children also begin to acquire a sense of cause and effect.

During the sensorimotor stage, children develop the ability to imitate. Piaget believed that novel actions could be imitated by infants around eight to twelve months of age and needed much practice. The ability to imitate absent models, called deferred imitation, appears between twelve and twenty-four months of age.

Another important milestone of the sensorimotor stage is the development of a sense of object permanence. Before the age of four months, objects are of interest to infants only if they can be experienced by the senses. They lose interest in objects that are hidden; such objects no longer exist for them. Between four and eight months of age, they may retain interest in partially hidden objects, and by twelve to eighteen months of age, the concept of objects is stronger. The idea that objects have permanence even when not seen appears around the age of eighteen months, when children can represent objects mentally.

The preoperational stage, the second of Piaget's stages of cognitive development, occurs between the ages of two and seven. During this stage, children increase their use of words and images to represent objects and experiences. Piaget called this stage "preoperational" because he believed that children had not yet achieved "operations," or cognitive schemes to think logically. The preoperational stage can further be divided into a preconceptual period (two to four years of age) and an intuitive period (four to seven years of age).

Characteristics of the preconceptual period include the development of symbolic representation, expressed through developing language and pretend play. Children in this stage demonstrate animism; that is, they attribute life to nonliving things. They are egocentric, seeing the world as revolving around themselves and having difficulty in understanding other points of view.

Although still egocentric during the intuitive period, children are less so than before. Piaget argued that they also display centered thinking, or the capacity to classify objects according to one feature or attribute even though several may be evident. Children in this stage find it hard to conserve, or understand that a substance or object's properties can remain unaltered even when its appearance changes. They cannot reverse actions mentally, such as realizing that water poured from a tall glass into a flat dish is the same amount of water and would look as high as before if poured back into the glass.

In the concrete operations stage, between the ages of seven and eleven, children's cognitive structures develop to include operations that help them think more competently and logically about objects and events experienced. Children are less egocentric; are able to classify, sequence, and quantify more efficiently; and display skills of conservation and reversibility. Piaget believed, however, that children are still unable to hypothesize or think about abstract concepts during this stage.

From eleven years onward, children enter the formal operations stage. They can hypothesize and reason inductively about abstract concepts such as religion, goodness, or beauty. According to Piaget, this transition from concrete to formal operations is very gradual. He also suggested that many adults reason at the formal operations level only if a problem is important or interesting to them.

Another approach to cognitive development compares individuals as information-processing systems to computers. The hardware in humans consists of physical components such as the brain, the sensory receptors, and the nervous system. The software consists of the mental processes and strategies used to store, interpret, access, and analyze information. The information-processing mechanisms of young children are elementary and immature. As children grow, as their nervous systems and brains develop, their information-processing strategies improve and become more sophisticated, like modern computers.

Humor and the appreciation of humor have also been associated with an individual's level of cognitive development. A child whose mental structures and language acquisition have developed enough to enable the child to notice incongruities or deviations from the usual and expected can perceive humor in incongruous situations. To a two-year-old, calling a bird a cat may seem hilarious or making barking sounds and pretending to be a dog may provoke much laughter. A picture of a fish in a tree will amuse a three-year-old. Seven-year-olds who can understand the double meanings inherent in language will laugh at puns and "knock-knock" jokes and can create riddles. As children's understanding of language ambiguities matures and becomes more sophisticated, they are able to appreciate more complex humor.

Sociocultural Factors

The Russian psychologist Lev Vygotsky (1896-1934) believed that cognition is sociocultural, that it is influenced by values and beliefs of cultures as well as by the specific tools that each culture uses for adaptation and problem solving. Children are born with simple mental processes such as attention, memory, perception, and sensation. These processes develop into what Vygotsky called higher mental functions, or more competent ways of using intellectual capabilities. The strategies and tools for thinking are taught to children by their culture and develop as young children interact and collaborate with capable adults or peers, who guide and model problem-solving techniques that encourage cognitive development. Vygotsky called the difference between children's level of achievement when working independently and their potential development when guided by a competent adult the zone of proximal development.

For Vygotsky, language plays an important role in cognitive growth. Adults use language to transmit the culture's ways of thinking to the child. The child uses language to plan and regulate activities and behavior and to solve problems. Language helps children organize thought and reach objectives. Younger children verbalize phrases and words aloud during this process, but older children and adults internalize speech that, although no longer uttered aloud, still organizes and guides thinking and action.

Disorders and Effects

The importance of experience on the cognitive development of children implies that when children live in intellectually impoverished environments, their cognitive development may be stunted or fail to reach its potential. Studies show the children whose parents play and interact with them in a variety of ways and provide stimulating materials to engage their interest and attention do better in school than children who lack this cognitive stimulation. Verbal interactions between parents and children, collaborative activities with competent peers, and guided activities with adults have been found to help children improve their thinking and planning abilities. Mary Ainsworth's research on mother-infant attachment showed that mothers who interacted with their infants had securely attached children who, in turn, felt confident enough to explore their environment more independently than less securely attached infants. In this way, cognitive growth was affected by social functioning. Some longitudinal studies have found that securely attached children demonstrated more cognitive competence through childhood and adolescence than children who did not have secure attachments. Parental support and responsiveness encouraged cognitive growth over time.

The effects of the curriculum within programs and schools for children can maximize or discourage cognitive development. The Cognitively Oriented Curriculum, developed at the High/Scope Institute by David Weikart and his associates, focused on active learning. It was based on Piagetian principles and involved children in planning and other cognitively oriented activities. The games that children play can also affect their thinking and can be utilized in the curriculum. Research by Constance Kamii and Rheta DeVries has shown how the use of games and play-oriented activities can help children develop numerical thinking, language competency, and other cognitive abilities, while promoting autonomy or the ability to think independently and enhancing cooperative and social skills.

As an understanding of the negative effects of poverty and lack of enriching experiences increased during the 1950s and 1960s, initiatives such as Head Start and various other compensatory early childhood programs were established in the United States to reverse the effects of early cognitive deprivation. Initial studies on the effects of such programs were extremely encouraging, and gains in intelligence quotient (IQ) scores and cognitive performance were found to be significant. It was later discovered, however, that such gains could be lost if intellectual stimulation was not maintained. The need to continue to provide stimulating educational experiences was recognized. It was found that positive attitudes toward schooling and a sense of self-esteem also occur when compensatory education and enrichment programs are provided.

The increasing evidence of brain research concerning the importance of stimulating experiences to the developmental process during the first few years of life, as well as knowledge about the growth and weight of the brain in infancy, suggests the need to provide such experiences from a very early age. Prenatal experiences and their impact on cognitive and other areas of development are also being studied.

The concept of cognitive development as a highly active process that occurs in a series of stages has certain implications for the education and well-being of children. One implication is that children in a particular stage of development should not be hurried but should be allowed to develop and mature at their own pace. Hurrying children beyond their developmental capacity can cause mental and emotional damage. David Elkind uses the term "miseducation" to refer to the tendency to hurry and pressure children to perform activities and tasks for which they are not cognitively or physically ready. He believes that miseducation is an increasingly common problem in the United States.

Another implication of the active nature of cognitive development is that children should be given numerous opportunities to explore materials and the environment, and thus acquire knowledge for themselves. Materials, equipment, and knowledge to be discovered should be appropriate to the stage of the child and should be based on the child's existing structures and schemes.

Perspective and Prospects

The cognitive and intellectual development of children was not studied seriously or scientifically until the late nineteenth century. G. Stanley Hall was the first person to develop an instrument-the questionnaire-to study the minds of children. The twentieth century saw the emergence of developmental theories such as the psychoanalytic theory of Sigmund Freud and the psychosocial theory of Erik Erikson. Behaviorism, which viewed children's learning and development as passive and therefore controllable, dominated much of the earlier part of the century. John Watson proposed that children's minds were like blank tablets on which anything could be written. In other words, children's development was thought to be shaped solely by their environment and by the people around them. This view had been held in the seventeenth century by the philosopher John Locke. Watson's theory was extended by B. F. Skinner, who evolved a learning theory based on the use of reinforcement and external stimuli to influence and control behavior. Albert Bandura's theory of social cognition departed from the earlier passive learning theories of Watson and Skinner. He believed that individuals actively process information. Bandura also emphasized the role of observational learning, or learning by observing and mimicking others and thinking about outcomes, in the process of children's development.

During the 1950s, a cognitive revolution occurred as the theory and research of Jean Piaget became known. Piaget was interested in how children think, in their "wrong" answers as indicators of their stage of cognitive development, and in their active construction of knowledge. He observed his own children's early interactions and explorations. He also utilized the clinical method, in which he interviewed children of different ages to understand the nature of their hypotheses and problem-solving strategies. The questions in this method were flexible and depended on the responses given by the child.

Piaget's theories were later criticized and were seen to underestimate children's abilities. His assumption of the heterogeneity or universality of cognitive stages was also questioned. Critics charged that Piaget did not give enough credit to the role of cultural and social factors in cognitive development. The impact of culture and social interaction on the child's thinking and use of strategies as culturally transmitted tools of thought was studied by Lev Vygotsky. In the last decades of the twentieth century, Vygotsky's ideas aroused much interest. The difference in learning styles was also studied, and it was recognized that learning styles vary across cultures as well as from individual to individual.

Many neo-Piagetian theories attempted to integrate some Piagetian assumptions with information-processing approaches. These approaches examined cognitive processes such as memory and attention and demonstrated their influence on children's cognitive development.

The influence of the environment and various activities cannot be overemphasized in its importance to cognitive development. As technologies continue to develop for use by children, ranging from toys to educational tools, it will be crucial to consider all aspects of development carefully. One example is recent research evaluating the impact on brain development of frequent video game and computer use by children. The research suggested that activities that encourage vision and movement skills, to the exclusion of other skills important to development, may be problematic. The concern is that some capacities may become overused, while others may not receive enough stimulation to encourage adequate development. More research is certainly needed to examine the potential impact of new technologies and exposure to diverse stimuli. Important lessons can be learned from history in an effort to guard against anything that impoverishes a child's learning environment.

—*Nillofur Zobairi, Ph.D.;*
updated by Nancy A. Piotrowski, Ph.D.

See also Bonding; Developmental disorders; Developmental stages; Intellectual disability; Learning disabilities; Motor skill development; Psychiatric disorders; Psychiatry, child and adolescent; Reflexes, primitive.

For Further Information:

Berk, Laura E. *Child Development*. 9th ed. Boston: Pearson/Allyn & Bacon, 2012.

Berk, Laura E., and Adam Winsler. *Scaffolding Children's Learning: Vygotsky and Early Childhood Education*. Washington, D.C.: National Association for the Education of Young Children, 1995.

Bjorklund, David F. *Children's Thinking: Developmental Function and Individual Differences*. 4th ed. Belmont, Calif.: Thomson/Wadsworth, 2005.

"Cognitive Development: One-Year-Old." *American Academy of Pediatrics*, May 11, 2013.

"Cognitive Development: Two-Year-Old." *American Academy of Pediatrics*, May 11, 2013.

Elkind, David. *Miseducation: Preschoolers at Risk*. New York: Alfred A. Knopf, 1987.

Sears, William, et al. *The Portable Pediatrician: Everything You Need to Know about Your Child's Health*. New York: Little, 2011.

Shore, Rima. *Rethinking the Brain: New Insights into Early Development*. Rev. ed. New York: Families and Work Institute, 2003.

"Zero to Three." *National Center for Infants, Toddlers, and Families*, 2012.

Cognitive enhancement

Treatment

Anatomy or system affected: Brain

Specialties and related fields: Psychiatry, neurology, cognitive psychology

Definition: An increase in one or more of the cognitive processes of the brain, including learning, memory, attention, perception, problem solving, and decision making.

Key terms:

agonist: a chemical that mimics or increases the effect of a neurotransmitter

antagonist: a chemical that inhibits or decreases the effect of a neurotransmitter

mnemonic: technique used to facilitate memory by modifying the way that information is learned

neuromodulator: a brain chemical that increases or decreases the effect of a neurotransmitter

psychostimulant: any drug that increases the overall excitability of neurons in one or more neural pathways

reaction time: the amount of time required to complete a task

transcranial direct current stimulation (tDCS): a technique that uses small electrodes placed on the surface of the scalp to excite or inhibit regions deep within the brain

Perspective and Prospects

Cognitive enhancement involves the use of a specific intervention to achieve the goal of improving one or more mental processes. The processes that may be enhanced include perception, attention, working memory, long-term memory, language, problem solving, and decision making. Some cognitive enhancers are also purported to increase intelligence.

There are many ways that people attempt to enhance cognition, including nutritional supplements, over-the-counter and prescription drugs, by modifying training paradigms, with the assistance of interactive technologies, and through the direct electrical stimulation of the brain. Although many anecdotal and popular accounts of how various substances and technologies can increase cognition exist, experimental and clinical evidence suggest that there are very few, evidence-validated methods for achieving cognitive enhancement.

The ginkgo is one of the oldest surviving species of trees. The fan-shaped leaves of the Ginkgo biloba tree have been used in traditional Chinese medicine to boost memory for centuries. Though there is evidence that ginkgo leaf extract may have some memory-restoring effects for those elderly suffering from mild dementia or Alzheimer's disease, laboratory studies have failed to find any evidence for such an effect on cognition in normal, healthy individuals. Despite the lack of research support for ginkgo as a memory enhancer, it is still a popular supplement and is touted as an ingredient in so-called "energy drinks."

Energy drinks are carbonated beverages that contain high levels of caffeine and other assorted ingredients, which are purported to affect attention and learning. Along with ginkgo, the amino acid L-taurine is a common ingredient in energy drinks. Despite claims that taurine and caffeine work together to enhance cognition, researchers have failed to find any consistent positive or negative effects of adding this substance to the diet. Indeed, when positive effects on cognition were observed, they were most often attributed to the effect of caffeine on the brain.

One of the most widely used cognitive enhancers, both today and historically, is the ubiquitous alkanoid, caffeine. Caffeine is found in varying quantities in tea, coffee, soft drinks, energy drinks, and chocolate. This drug, which is classified as a psychostimulant, requires between 20-45 minutes before the effects are experienced and has a half-life of 5-6 hours. Like most stimulants, caffeine increases the level of excitation within the brain. An antagonist of the neuromodulator adenosine, caffeine indirectly increases the release of the neurotransmitters dopamine and norepinephrine by decreasing the levels of inhibition on both.

There is general agreement that moderate levels of caffeine enhance alertness, attention, and decrease reaction time, whereas high levels of caffeine have an impairing effect on attention. What is less clear is whether caffeine has any positive effect on learning and memory. The lack of consistency in experimental studies may reflect the complex way that caffeine intake, normal patterns of use (i.e., how much does one normally ingest each day), and task difficulty and demands all interact.

Nicotine is another readily available substance that may have some mild cognitive enhancing effects. This highly addictive compound, commonly found in tobacco, is an agonist of the neurotransmitter acetylcholine. The stimulating effects of nicotine on acetylcholine networks in the brain are likely responsible for the decreases in reaction time and slight increases in working memory function that have been demonstrated.

Just like nicotine and caffeine, prescription drugs that have been reported to enhance cognition are psychostimulants. Both Ritalin (methylphenidate) and Adderall (amphetamine salts) act to increase excitation within the brain by increasing the release of dopamine. Most often prescribed to ameliorate the hyperactivity associated with attention deficit hyperactivity disorder (ADHD), these drugs have been abused by non-ADHD children and adults because of their ability to increase focus and positively impact long-term memory retention. Similarly, the anti-narcolepsy drug modafinil has gained notoriety due to its purported high level of abuse by college students and professionals striving to get ahead by working long hours. Unfortunately, there are some studies that suggest that the abuse of prescription psychostimulant medications may have adverse long-term effects on the brain and other bodily systems.

Instead of taking drugs, cognition may also be enhanced by manipulating the way that information is presented and processed. As was demonstrated by Hermann Ebbinghaus in 1885, the amount of time required to learn information may be reduced drastically if the learning trials are spread out across days rather than crammed together in one day. Similarly, mnemonics can greatly enhance the amount of information that can be learned and retrieved. Techniques such as visualizing items to be remembered, anchoring new information to existing memories, and chunking large numbers of items into meaningful units, have all been shown to enhance learning and memory in both laboratory and real-life (e.g., classroom) settings.

Despite the fact that optimal results are seen when cognitive enhancing techniques are used by individuals in face-to-face settings, some mnemonic and other cognitive enhancing techniques have been integrated into computer-based "brain training" programs. Although these programs are based on neuroscientific and cognitive psychological research findings, there are few studies that have examined the effects of computer-based training on enhancing cognition directly. What studies have shown is that though there are often moderate enhancements for the specific games that are used as training (which are designed to enhance cognition in general), there is no evidence of transfer of the computer-developed skills to novel tasks, intelligence, or other areas of cognition. In the few studies that did show transfer effects outside the computer, it should be noted that the participants were required to train on the games for extended periods (i.e., hours) each day for several weeks. Thus, such prolonged and time-consuming training regimens may be prohibitive for general use.

Rather than using computers and technology to train one's brain to become more efficient and accurate, transcranial direct current stimulation (tDCS) is being used to directly stimulate portions of the brain by modifying the local electromagnetic fields in those regions. The stimulation is facilitated by placing electrodes to the scalp and applying a small electrical current. A few studies have demonstrated that tDCS enhances attention, various forms of long-term learning and memory, and working memory. Though the technique was first developed decades ago, it has only recently begun to be used in clinical and research settings. Thus, although tDCS may hold some promise for enhancing cognition, there is more that needs to be known about the safety and efficacy of this technique. For example, studies have shown that when some cognitive processes are enhanced by tDCS, others may then be impaired.

While advances in medicine and technology continue to introduce novel ways to attempt to enhance cognition, bioethicists debate whether cognitive enhancement should be pursued in the first place. Though cognitive enhancers such as nicotine and caffeine have been present for centuries, direct stimulation of the brain and abuse of prescription drugs have prompted a reexamination of the morality concerning cognitive enhancement and, even, what it means to be human.

—*Jerome L. Rekart, Ph.D.*

See also Memory loss

For Further Information:
Buchanan, Allen. *Better Than Human: The Promises and Perils of Enhancing Ourselves.* Oxford: Oxford University Press, 2011.
Hildt, Elisabeth, and Andreas G. Franke, eds. *Cognitive Enhancement: An Interdisciplinary Perspective (Trends in Augmentation of Human Performance).* New York: Springer, 2013.
Rekart, Jerome L. *The Cognitive Classroom: Using Brain and Cognitive Science to Optimize Student Success.* Lanham, PA: Rowman & Littlefield Publishers, Education Division, 2013.
Smith, Martha J., and M. Elizabeth Smith. "Are Prescription Stimulants 'Smart Pills'? The Epidemiology and Cognitive Neuroscience of Prescription Stimulant Use by Normal Health Individuals." *Psychological Bulletin* 137, no. 5 (2011): 717-741.

Cold agglutinin disease

Disease/Disorder

Anatomy or system affected: Blood, blood vessels, chest, circulatory system, ears, feet, hands, immune system, liver, lungs, lymphatic system, nose, respiratory system, skin, spleen, urinary system

Specialties and related fields: Bacteriology, emergency medicine, hematology, histology, immunology, oncology, pathology, pediatrics, pulmonary medicine, radiology, rheumatology, serology, urology, vascular medicine, virology

Definition: A disease characterized by the production of antibodies against red blood cells that destroy them and cause anemia.

Key terms:

anemia: a deficiency of the oxygen-carrying protein hemoglobin or the red blood cells that contain hemoglobin *antibodies*: a blood protein produced by B-lymphocytes in response to the introduction of antigens into the body that binds to and neutralizes these antigens

antigens: toxins or other foreign substances introduced into the body that induce an immune response against it

complement proteins: a group of proteins in blood that initiate a biochemical cascade when an antibody is bound to a cell surface that culminates in the destruction of that cell and its clearance from the body

hemolysis: the destruction of red blood cells

plasmapheresis: a clinical procedure that removes blood from the body, separates it into liquid or plasma and cells, and then returns the cells to the body without the plasma and its components

---

Information on Cold Agglutinin Disease

Causes: Elevated blood levels of antibodies directed against red blood cells

Symptoms: Painful fingers; toes with a purplish tinge; passing dark urine, especially during exposure to cold; anemia; chronic fatigue; pallor; difficulty breathing

Duration: In children and young adults, acute hemolysis lasts 1-3 weeks and all evidence disappears within 6 months, but in older patients, the disease lasts as long as the patient is exposed to cold

Treatments: Avoiding cold, folic acid and iron supplementation, Rituximab, plasmapheresis, blood transfusions

---

Causes and Symptoms

Cold agglutinin disease (CAD) is one of a group of blood disorders known as autoimmune hemolytic anemias (AIHAs). The immune systems of patients who suffer from AIHAs attack their own red blood cells, which cause routine red blood cell destruction (hemolysis). Destruction of red blood cells faster than they can be replaced leads to anemia or an abnormally low number of red blood cells. Exposure to cold initiates symptoms in CAD patients, which sets it apart from other types of AIHA. Approximately 1 in 300,000 people suffer from CAD.

Everyone tends to have circulating antibodies against their own red blood cells. Because the concentration of these antibodies tends to be rather low, they usually do not cause any problems. However, in some people, the concentration of these anti-red blood cell antibodies increases. In the case of primary CAD, the increase in the concentration of these antibodies occurs for reasons that remain unclear. In the case of secondary CAD, though, certain types of bacterial and viral infections or particular kinds of white blood cell cancers boost the concentration of these red blood cell-specific antibodies.

At low body temperatures (usually between 28-31°C or 82-88°F), which usually prevail during the winter months, the anti-red blood cell antibodies bind to the surfaces of red blood cells. The bound antibodies cause them to aggregate and activate complement proteins. Activation of the complement pathway culminates in the boring of small holes in red blood cell membranes and hemolysis. Those red blood cells that escape destruction by complement proteins are marked by them for destruction, and are filtered out by the liver and spleen and destroyed.

The whole-scale destruction of red blood cells causes anemia and other symptoms as cell debris becomes lodged in small blood vessels and blocks blood flow. CAD symptoms include pain and a purplish tinge in the fingers and toes (Raynaud's phenomenon), pallor, trouble breathing (dyspnea), and fatigue. Upon physical examination, patients with CAD may show purplish discoloration of the ears, forehead, tip of the nose, and digits (acrocyanosis). Enlargement of the spleen (splenomegaly), jaundice, and fever are also seen in more severe CAD patients.

Treatment and Therapy

Most cases of secondary CAD result from diseases that are, themselves, self-limiting and only of short duration. For most cases of primary CAD, avoidance of the cold prevents the onset of symptoms. CAD patients should eat foods rich in folic acid (e.g., fresh fruits and vegetables) and iron (e.g., meat, egg yolks, beans, artichokes), which help build red blood cells.

For more severe cases of CAD, intravenous administration of Rituximab promptly resolves the disease. A genetically engineered antibody, Rituximab binds to the surfaces of B-lymphocytes-the cells that produce antibodies-and removes them from the body. Rituximab can provide relief

An ear affected by cold agglutinin disease. (New England Journal of Medicine)

for up to one year. Combination treatments with purine analogs (e.g., fludarabine, azathioprine, etc.) may achieve faster responses and longer remission times. Other immune-suppressing drugs that have been used to treat severe cases of CAD include cyclophosphamide, chlorambucil, prednisone, vincristine, and interferons, all with varying degrees of success.

For emergencies, plasmapheresis can reduce the concentration of those antibodies that bind red blood cells in the blood. Because it acts quickly, plasmapheresis provides time for drugs to act, or for the patient to undergo surgery. Blood transfusions with warmed, washed, carefully matched red blood cells are only used as a last resort.

CAD patients should strongly consider relocating to warmer climates and should wear protective clothing to prevent chilling the body.

Perspective and Prospects

Karl Landsteiner first described cold agglutinins in 1903. In 1918, M.C. Clough and I.R. Richter identi?ed the pathologic association between the presence of cold agglutinins and red blood cell destruction and its occurrence during respiratory infections. D.M. Horstmann and H. Tatlock reported the first case of secondary CAD in 1943 when they detected cold agglutinins in the serum of patients with pneumonia. In 1957, W.H. Christenson, J.H. Dacie and colleagues identified antibodies as the cold agglutinins, but H. Schubothe actually coined the phrase "cold agglutinin disease" in 1966.

Other types of drugs that have been developed to treat non-Hodgkin's lymphoma and multiple myeloma may also effectively treat CAD. For example, a drug called bortezomib prevents cells from degrading damaged or unwanted proteins and has been approved for the treatment of multiple myeloma. Bortezomib depletes B-cells and might be effective as a treatment for CAD. Other experimental drugs might also prove useful as future treatments for recalcitrant cases of CAD.

—*Michael A. Buratovich, Ph.D.*

See also Antibodies; Blood vessels; Hematology; Immunology; Immunopathology; Raynaud's phenomenon; Vascular medicine

For Further Information:

Jeskowiak, Antonia, and Tobias Goerge. "Images in Clinical Medicine: Cutaneous Necrosis Associated with Cold Agglutinins." *New England Journal of Medicine* 369 (July 2013): e1.

Rodak, Bernadette F., George A. Fritsma, and Elaine Keohane. *Hematology: Clinical Principles and Applications.* 4th ed. St. Louis: Elsevier, 2012.

Swiecicki, Paul L., Livia T. Hegerova, and Morie A. Gertz. "Cold Agglutinin Disease." Blood 122, no. 7 (August 2013): 1114-1121.

Cold sores

Disease/Disorder
Also known as: Fever blisters
Anatomy or system affected: Mouth, skin
Specialties and related fields: Family medicine
Definition: An infectious disease characterized by thin-walled vesicles around the mouth.

Causes and Symptoms

Cold sores are an infectious disease caused by the herpes simplex virus. Cold sores and fever blisters are two terms used for sores that develop around the mouth. They are among the most common disorders around the mouth area, causing pain and annoyance. An estimated 45 to 80 percent of adults and children in the United States have had at least one cold sore. There are two types of herpes simplex. Type 1 usually causes oral herpes, or fever blisters, while type 2 usually causes genital herpes. About 95 percent of the cold sores located on the mouth are caused by herpes simplex type 1.

Cold sores are highly contagious, more so in the first day or two of an outbreak. Once the blister has formed a dry scab, transmission is low and the herpes simplex virus usually cannot be recovered from the site. The virus can spread to others through touch; frequently, infection spreads through kissing. The chance of infection is higher if the body's defenses are weakened by stress, illness, or injury.

Once a person is infected with oral herpes, the virus remains in the nerve located near the cold sore. It may stay dormant at this site for years. People who have had fever blisters in the past can sometimes predict when an outbreak is going to occur. The appearance of cold sores may be preceded by a few hours of a tingling, burning, or itching sensation, a phenomenon called a prodrome. Typically, the sores erupt in a small cluster, with each blister about the size of a large pimple. The blisters quickly dry to form a scab. Generally, no scarring or loss in sensation occurs. Outbreaks usually last from three to ten days.

Treatment and Therapy

Treatment includes keeping the area clean and dry to prevent bacterial infection. The patient should avoid irritating the sores, as touching them may spread the virus. For example, if a person rubs the sore and then rubs an eyelid, a new sore may appear on the eyelid in a few days. When the fever blister is contagious, kissing should be avoided. People whose cold sores appear in response to stress should try to avoid stressful situations. Some investigators have suggested that adding L-lysine to the diet or eliminating certain foods (such as nuts, chocolate, and seeds) may help, although no research studies have validated these suggestions. Even sunlight has been linked as a trigger for cold sores. The National Institute of Dental and Craniofacial Research recommends the use of sunscreen on the lips to prevent sun-induced recurrences of herpes.

Antiviral therapy of mucocutaneous herpes simplex virus infection is rarely curative, but is given for treatment of severe cases and to prevent or ameliorate recurrences. Treatment can also decrease viral shedding, making transmission to other people less likely. Available antiviral compounds include nucleoside analogues, which selectively interfere with viral deoxyribonucleic acid (DNA) replication. Oral acyclovir (Avirax or Zovirax) and valacyclovir (Valtrex), antiviral drugs that keep the virus from multiplying, can be taken to prevent recurrence. Acyclovir applied locally has also been found effective, and foscarnet

Information on Cold Sores

Causes: Infection by herpes simplex virus

Symptoms: Sores around mouth that dry to form scabs; preceded by tingling, burning, or itching sensation

Duration: Chronic, with acute outbreaks lasting from three to ten days

Treatments: Keeping area clean and dry, avoidance of sore irritation or stress; prevention through antiviral compounds (acyclovir, valacyclovir, foscarnet)

(Foscavir) is useful in treating acyclovir-resistant infections. Two topical preparations, Zovirax and penciclovir (Vectavir), have been shown to influence the eruption and duration of cold sores when applied during the prodromal stage. Antibiotics may be used in treating secondary infections. An ophthalmologist should treat any eye lesions.

Some cold sore treatments that have been successful in selected people are solvents such as ether, alcohol, povidone iodine, and antiseptic mouthwash. Other patients have applied ice or toothpaste to the sores. While none of these treatments has scientific backing, eating an ice pop or applying an ice cube to the blister may relieve the discomfort.

Perspective and Prospects

Future research is aimed at determining the precise form and location of the inactive herpesvirus in nerve cells. This information might allow scientists to design antiviral drugs that can attack the virus while it lies dormant in nerves. Researchers are also trying to learn more about how sunlight, injury, and stress act as triggers so that the cycle of recurrences can be stopped.

—*Janet Mahoney, R.N., Ph.D., A.P.R.N.*

See also Blisters; Canker sores; Herpes; Lesions; Skin; Skin disorders; Stress; Stress reduction; Ulcers; Viral infections.

For Further Information:

Alan, Rick. "Cold Sores." *Health Library*, March 20, 2013.

"Cold Sore." *Mayo Clinic*, May 23, 2012.

Ignatavicius, Donna D., and M. Linda Workman, eds. *Medical-Surgical Nursing: Critical Thinking for Collaborative Care.* 7th ed. Philadelphia: Saunders/Elsevier, 2012.

Lewis, Sharon, et al., eds. *Medical-Surgical Nursing: Assessment and Management of Clinical Problems.* 8th ed. 2 vols. St. Louis, Mo.: Mosby/Elsevier, 2010.

National Institutes of Health. National Institute of Dental Research. *Fever Blisters and Canker Sores.* Rev. ed. Bethesda, Md.: Author, 1992.

Smeltzer, Suzanne C., and Brenda G. Bare, eds. *Brunner and Suddarth's Textbook of Medical-Surgical Nursing.* 12th ed. Philadelphia: Wolters Kluwer/Lippincott Williams & Wilkins, 2010.

Colic

Disease/Disorder

Anatomy or system affected: Gastrointestinal system, intestines, psychic-emotional system

Specialties and related fields: Gastroenterology, pediatrics

Definition: As a general term, a paroxysm of acute abdominal pain caused by spasm, obstruction, or twisting of a hollow abdominal organ. As a specific entity, infantile colic is a group of behaviors displayed by young infants including crying, facial grimacing, drawing-up of the legs over the abdomen, and clenching of the fists.

Key terms:

flatulence: the presence of excessive gas in the stomach and intestines, which is expelled from the body

irritability: a state of general overreaction to external stimuli

spasm: an involuntary muscle contraction; a painful spasm is called a cramp

Causes and Symptoms

As a general term, colic can arise from any site in the abdomen due to a spasm, obstruction, or twisting of an abdominal organ. For example, cramplike pain caused by a stone obstructing the bile ducts or a stone obstructing the urinary tract are known as biliary colic or renal colic, respectively. More specifically, the term "colic," when unmodified, generally refers to infantile colic. Infantile colic is a group of behaviours displayed by young infants including crying, facial grimacing, drawing-up of the legs over the abdomen, and clenching of the fists, which are not caused by a medical problem and typically resolve at three months of age.

The crying of colicky infants tends to be more prominent in the evening, although they cry more than other infants at other times of day. The "rule of threes" of infantile colic holds that infants with colic cry for more than three hours per day for more than three days per week for more than three weeks. The associated gestures suggest to some that the infant is experiencing abdominal pain and is responsible for the use of the term "colic" to describe the condition.

Several causes of infantile colic have been postulated, but conclusive evidence is lacking for any of them. This combination of behaviors has been interpreted as abdominal pain, leading to the idea that cramping somewhere in the intestine is the cause. Neurobehavioral explanations have been offered. The most common is that colic represents a state of agitation that may not require a noxious stimulus for agitation and crying to continue. Rarely is colic the result of organic disease, and the prevailing opinion is that it is a variant of normal infant behavior. Almost all babies display colicky symptoms to varying degrees. It appears to be unrelated to caregiving style or intensity. Other proposed mechanisms include difficult temperament, sleep disturbance, diarrhea, child abuse, and irritable bowel syndrome (IBS). Some theories ascribe colic to hypersensitivity to dietary protein-usually proteins derived from cow's milk, which can be secreted in breast milk-thus explaining the occurrence of colic in breast-fed infants. Mothers who are breastfeeding may want to remove dairy and caffeine from their diets to see if that helps their infant's colicky symptoms improve. Intestinal gas, either from air swallowed during feeding or crying or from fermentation of incompletely absorbed carbohydrates in the colon, has also been implicated. Parents of colicky infants frequently describe flatulence as an associated symptom.

Information on Colic

Causes: Unknown; abdominal pain suspected
Symptoms: Crying for long periods of time, facial grimacing, drawing of legs over abdomen, clenching of fists
Duration: Typically one to three months
Treatments: Switching formulas, swaddling, mimicking of in utero motion, medications

---

Treatment and Therapy

The medical treatment of the infant with colic begins with a thorough medical history and a careful physical examination. While the likelihood of finding a cause of the infant's symptoms are slight, the thoroughness of this approach provides an effective basis for reassurance and demonstrates that the parents' complaint is taken seriously.

Infantile colic virtually always resolves spontaneously, leaving the infant healthy and thriving. The essentials of therapy are demystification, reassurance, and support for the haggard and anxious parents. Demystification is the explanation of the source of the infant's distress, which alleviates the anxiety attendant on diagnostic hypotheses that occur to or are suggested to the parents. It is important for pediatricians to deal with the anxiety aroused by the infant's symptoms with reassurance, pointing out that the baby will be fine.

Quick, superficial attempts to solve the problem with formula changes or medications, particularly when not accompanied by patient demystification and reassurance, reinforce the parents' suspicion that there is something wrong with the child, ultimately increasing parental perception of the child's vulnerability. The results of studies in the medical literature investigating the usefulness of switching formulas and using agents such as simethicone to deal with intestinal gas are mixed.

More frequent, smaller feedings may help, as may increased carrying (called "walking the floor") and rocking. One theory holds that mimicking the environment in the womb is reassuring, which can be achieved through closeness to a warm person with a detectable heartbeat (sometimes called "kangaroo care"), swaddling (wrapping the baby in a blanket to restrict movement of the extremities), and rhythmic stimulation provided by background music and car or stroller rides. One commonly used method involves placing the baby in an infant seat on top of a running washer or dryer, thus exposing the infant to constant vibration. Care must be taken to stay with the baby or to secure the infant seat to prevent injury resulting from a fall off the appliance. Caretakers should experiment to see which methods best soothe their crying infant. Most colicky infants have excessive gas, and gas pains have long been suspected as being responsible for colic. Since virtually all the gas in the intestine is swallowed air, minimizing air swallowing and maximizing burping after feedings are important measures in reducing colic. The use of cereal to ease the infant's hunger and decrease the vigor with which he or she sucks on the nipple results in less air being swallowed. Unfortunately, many parents are advised to put cereal in a bottle; this increases the negative pressure required to suck the slurry of milk and cereal and increases the amount of air swallowed. Identifying and then avoiding the dietary triggers of colic and learning how to comfort the infant during crying episodes will help to soothe the infant until the symptoms of colic subside, typically at three to four months of age.

Perspective and Prospects

One theory holds that infantile colic is related to a familial prevalence of irritable bowel syndrome, also called irritable colon or spastic colon, although the evidence for this theory is limited. Diagnosis of colic is made after carefully reviewing the familial history of the infant and performing a thorough physical examination to rule out any organic causes. Although treatment is limited, most babies outgrow the symptoms of colic by three to four months of age. In the absence of an organic disease or unexplained weight loss, colic is self-limited with no long-term adverse effects on the child's development or future health.

—*Wallace A. Gleason, Jr., M.D.*

See also Bonding; Colon; Diarrhea and dysentery; Gastroenterology, pediatric; Gastrointestinal system; Irritable bowel syndrome (IBS); Lactose intolerance; Neonatology; Pediatrics.

For Further Information:
Barr, Ronald G. "Changing Our Understanding of Infant Colic." *Archives of Pediatrics and Adolescent Medicine* 156, no. 12 (December, 2002): 1172-1175.
Ben-Joseph, Elana Pearl. "Your Colicky Baby." *Nemours Foundation*, November 2011.
Brazelton, T. Berry. *Calming Your Fussy Baby: The Brazelton Way.* Cambridge, Mass.: Perseus, 2002.
"Colic." *Mayo Clinic*, July 6, 2011.
"Colic and Crying." *Medline Plus*, August 2, 2011.
Lampe, John B. "Infantile Colic: Follow-up at Four Years of Age." *Clinical Pediatrics* 29, no. 10 (October, 2000): 620.
McCormick, David P. "The Challenge of Colic." *Clinical Pediatrics* 39, no. 7 (July, 2000): 401-402.
Thompson, June. "Infantile Colic: What Is It and Are There Effective Treatments?" *Community Practitioner* 73, no. 9 (September, 2000): 767.
Thompson, June. "Low Birth Weight and Colic Linked.'" *Community Practitioner* 73, no. 8 (August, 2000): 727.
Walling, Anne D. "Diagnosing Biliary Colic and Acute Cholecystitis." *American Family Physician* 62, no. 6 (September 15, 2000): 1386.
Waltman, Alicia Brooks. "The Crying Game." *Parenting* 14, no. 3 (April, 2000): 128-132.
White, Barbara Prudhomme, et al. "Behavioral and Physiological Responsivity, Sleep, and Patterns of Daily Cortisol Production in Infants with and Without Colic." *Child Development* 71, no. 4 (July/August, 2000): 862-877.

Colitis

Disease/Disorder

Anatomy or system affected: Abdomen, gastrointestinal system, intestines, stomach

Specialties and related fields: Gastroenterology, internal medicine

Definition: A potentially fatal but manageable disease of the colon that inflames and ulcerates the bowel lining, occurring in both acute and chronic forms.

Key terms:

diarrhea: persistent liquid or mushy, shapeless stool

dysentery: bloody diarrhea caused by infectious agents affecting the colon

ileum: the last section of the small bowel, which passes food wastes to the colon through the ileocecal valve

inflammation: swelling caused by the accumulation of fluids and chemical agents

mucosa: the membrane of cells that lines the bowel; admits fluids and nutrients but also serves as the first-line protection against infectious agents and other materials foreign to the body

procedure: any medical treatment that entails physical manipulation or invasion of the body

stoma: an opening, formed by surgery, from the bowel to the exterior surface of the body

stool: the food wastes mixed with fluid, bacteria, mucus, and dead cells that exit the body upon defecation

ulcer: an area of the mucosa that has been abraded or dissolved by infection or chemicals, creating an open sore

Causes and Symptoms

The colon is the section of the lower bowel, or intestines, extending from the ileocecal valve to the rectum. It is wider in diameter than the small bowel, although shorter in length at about one meter. From behind the pelvis, the colon rises along the right side of the body (ascending colon), turns left to cross the upper abdominal cavity (transverse colon), and then turns down along the left side of the body (descending colon) until it joins the sigmoid (S-shaped) colon. The sigmoid colon empties into the rectum, a pouch that stores the waste products of digestion that are excreted through the anus. The colon absorbs most of the fluid passed to it from the small bowel, so that wastes solidify; meanwhile, bacteria in the colon break down undigested proteins and carbohydrates, creating hydrogen, carbon dioxide, and methane gases in the process.

A key structure in colonic activity is its mucosa. This thin sheet of cells lining the bowel wall permits passage of fluids and certain nutrients into the bloodstream but resists bacteria and toxins (poisonous chemical compounds). When the mucosa is torn or worn away, bacteria and toxins enter, infecting the bowel wall. The body responds to infection by rushing fluids and powerful chemicals to the endangered area to confine and kill the infecting agents. In the process, the tissues of the bowel wall swell with the fluids; this is known as "inflammation." The medical suffix denoting this response is *-itis*; when it occurs in the colon, physicians call it "colitis."

A variety of agents can cause colitis, which is divided into two major types depending on the duration of the disease: acute colitis and chronic ulcerative colitis. Acute colitis is a relatively brief, single episode of inflammation. It is often caused by bacteria or parasites. For example, *Giardia lamblia*, a bacterium in many American streams, is a common infectious agent in colitis, and the amoebas in polluted water supplies are responsible for the type of coli-

Information on Colitis
Causes: Unknown; possibly bacterial or viral infection, genetic factors, exposure to antibiotics, autoimmune reaction
Symptoms: Swelling of bowel lining, ulcers, bloody diarrhea, pain, fever, severe weight loss, anemia, lack of energy, dehydration, uncontrollable urge to defecate
Duration: Chronic, with acute episodes
Treatments: Medications (anti-inflammatory agents), surgery, dietary restrictions

tis known as "amebic dysentery." Some medicines, however, especially antibiotics, can also induce colitis. Acute colitis either disappears on its own or can be cured with drugs. Untreated, however, it may be fatal.

Chronic ulcerative colitis and Crohn's disease constitute a category of serious afflictions called inflammatory bowel disease (IBD), whose primary physical effects include swelling of the bowel lining, ulcers, and bloody diarrhea. Although some medical researchers think that these afflictions may be two aspects of the same disease, ulcerative colitis affects only the colon, whereas Crohn's disease can involve the small bowel as well as the colon. Moreover, colitis chiefly involves the colonic mucosa, but Crohn's disease delves into the full thickness of the bowel wall.

Chronic ulcerative colitis is a permanent disease that manifests itself either in recurring bouts of inflammation or in continuous inflammation that cannot be cleared up with drugs. It is commonly called "ulcerative colitis" because ulcers, open sores in the mucosa, spread throughout the colon and rectum, where the disease usually starts. Researchers have not yet discovered the causes of chronic ulcerative colitis although there are many theories, of which three are prominent. The first is bacterial or viral infection, and many agents have been proposed as the culprit. Because such a multitude of organisms commonly reside in or pass through the colon, researchers have enormous difficulty separating out a specific kind in order to show that it is always present during colitis attacks. Second is autoimmune reaction. Research in other diseases has shown that sometimes the body's police system, enforced by white blood cells, mistakes native, healthy tissue for a foreign agent and attacks that tissue in an attempt to destroy it. Yet no testing in chronic ulcerative colitis has yet proven the theory. Third is a combination of foreign infection and autoimmune response; it is as if the immune system overreacts to an infectious agent and continues its attack even after the agent has been neutralized. Many researchers have suspected that the disease is inherited, because certain families have higher rates of the disease than others. This genetic theory is not universally accepted, however, because it is just as likely that family members share infection rather than having passed on a genetic predisposition for the disease. Other theories propose food allergies as the cause; even toothpaste has been considered.

Regardless of the cause, there is no doubt that colitis is a painful, disabling, bewildering disease. When the bowel inflames, the tissues heat up and fever results. Cramps are common, and sufferers feel an urgent, frequently uncontrollable urge to defecate. When they reach the toilet (if they do so in time), they have soft, loose stool or diarrhea, which can seem to explode from the anus. They may have as many as ten to twenty bowel movements a day. Because ulcers often erode blood vessels, blood can appear in the stool, as well as mucus and pus from the bowel wall. Severe weight loss, anemia, lack of energy, dehydration, and anorexia often develop as the colitis persists. The symptoms may clear up on their own only to recur months or years later; attacks may come with increasing frequency thereafter. The first attack, if it worsens rapidly, is fatal in about 5 to 10 percent of patients, although the death rate can rise to 25 percent among first-time sufferers who are more than sixty years old.

Complications from colitis can be life threatening. These include perforation of the bowel wall, strictures, hemorrhaging, and toxic megacolon (hyperinflation of the colon, an emergency medical condition). If left untreated or if unresponsive to treatment, ulcerative colitis can led to bone loss or arthritis, rashes, inflammation of the eye, liver disease, or painful kidney stones. Furthermore, studies show that patients who have had ulcerative colitis for more than ten years have about a 20 percent chance of developing cancer in the colon or rectum.

Because colitis is a relapsing, embarrassing disease, patients often suffer psychological turmoil. In *Colitis* (1992), Michael P. Kelly reports the results of his study of forty-five British colitis patients. According to Kelly, they typically denied that early symptoms were the signs of serious illness, passing them off as the result of overeating or influenza. The denial continued until the continual, desperate urge to defecate made them despair of controlling their bowels without help. Often, they suffered embarrassment because they had to flee family gatherings or work in order to find a toilet or because they passed stool inadvertently in public. Many feared being beyond easy access to a toilet, shunned public places, and felt humiliated. Only then did some visit a physician, and even after chronic ulcerative colitis was diagnosed, a portion hoped they could still cope on their own. When they could not, they grew depressed, insomniac, angry at their fate, or antisocial. Even with treatment, the strain of enduring the disease can be debilitating.

Treatment and Therapy

Fortunately, medical science has several well-tested methods of controlling or curing colitis. In the case of acute colitis, patients usually resume normal bowel functions on their own and emerge as healthy as they were before the onset of symptoms. For chronic ulcerative colitis patients, however, the body is rarely the same again, and they must adjust to the effects of medication, surgery, or both-an adjustment that some authors claim is essentially a redefinition of the self.

After interviewing a patient and assessing the reported symptoms, the physician suspecting colitis orders a stool sample to check for blood, bacteria, parasites, and pus. If any of these are present, the physician directly examines the rectum and colon by inserting a fiber-optic endoscope into the rectum and up the colon. Early in the disease, the mucosa looks granular with scattered hemorrhages and tiny bleeding points. As the disease progresses, the mucosa turns spongy and has many ulcers that ooze blood and pus. An x-ray often helps determine the extent of inflammation, and tissue samples taken by endoscopic biopsy can establish if it is ulcerative colitis or infection, and not Crohn's disease, that is present.

There is no easy treatment for chronic ulcerative colitis. Dietary restrictions-especially the elimination of fibrous foods such as raw fruits and vegetables, of milk products, or of certain seasonings-may reduce the irritation to the inflamed colon, and symptoms then may improve if the disease is mild. Antidiarrheal drugs can firm the stool and reduce the patient's urgency to defecate, although such drugs must be used very cautiously to avoid dangerous dilation of the bowels.

Such nonspecific measures are seldom more than delaying tactics, and drugs are needed to counteract the colon's inflammation. The most common types are aminosalicylates, corticosteroids, oral immunosuppressants, and intravenous infliximab, an antitumor necrosis factor agent. Among the first class, sulfasalazine is a sulfa drug developed in the 1940s. It is an anti-inflammatory agent that is most effective in mild to moderate ulcerative colitis and helps prevent recurrence of inflammation. Aminosalicylates may be administered as pills, suppositories, or enemas. Corticosteroids behave like the hormones produced by the adrenal gland that suppress inflammation. Administered orally, intravenously, or rectally, these drugs work well in relieving the symptoms of moderate to moderately severe attacks. Immunosuppressants and infliximab may be prescribed for severe, unresponsive cases of ulcerative colitis. All of these types of drugs have serious side effects, so physicians must carefully tailor dosages for each patient and check repeatedly for reactions. In some patients, sulfasalazine induces nausea, vomiting, joint pain, headaches, rashes, dizziness, and hepatitis (liver inflammation). The effects of corticosteroids include sleeplessness, mood swings, acne, high blood pressure, diabetes, cataracts, thinning of the bones (especially the spine), and fluid retention and swelling of the face, hands, abdomen, and ankles. Women may grow facial hair, and adolescents may have delayed sexual maturation. In most cases, the side effects clear up when patients stop taking the drugs. Immunosuppressants and infliximab can lead to toxicity.

With medication, people who suffer mild or moderate chronic ulcerative colitis can control it for years, often for the rest of their lives. Severe colitis requires surgery, and sometimes patients with milder forms choose to have surgery rather than live with the disease's unpredictable recurrence or the ever-present side effects of drugs. In any case, surgery is the one known cure for chronic ulcerative colitis, although fewer than one-third of patients undergo surgical procedures. Several types of these surgeries have high success rates.

Because ulcerative colitis eventually spreads throughout the colon, complete removal of the large bowel and rectum is the surest way to eliminate the disease. This "total proctocolectomy" takes place in three steps. The surgeon first cuts through the wall of the abdomen, the incision extending from the mid-transverse colon to the rectum, and removes the colon. Next, the end of the ileum is pulled through a hole in the abdomen to form a stoma (a procedure called an ileostomy). Finally, the rectum is removed and the anus sutured shut. Thereafter the patient defecates through the stoma. Either of two arrangements prevents stool from simply spilling out unchecked. Most patients affix plastic bags around their stomas into which stool flows without their control; when full, the bag is either emptied and reattached or thrown away and replaced. To avoid external bags, some patients prefer a "continent ileostomy," so called because it allows them to control defecation. The surgeon constructs a pouch out of a portion of the ileum and attaches it right behind the stoma, a procedure called a "Kock pouch" after its inventor, Nils Kock of Sweden. When this pouch is full, the patient empties it with a catheter inserted through the stoma. Some patients can choose to have an ileoanal anastomosis. In this procedure, the surgeon forms the end of the ileum into a pouch, which is attached to the anus and collects wastes in place of the rectum. The patient continues to defecate through the anus rather than through a stoma.

None of these surgical procedures is free of problems, and all require extensive recovery in the hospital and rehabilitation. Moreover, both infections and mechanical failures can occur. If healthy portions of the colon are left intact, they often flare with colitis later, and more operations become necessary. Patients with stomas are vulnerable to bacterial inflammation of the small intestine, resulting in diarrhea, vomiting, and dehydration. Stomas and pouches sometimes leak or close up, and even after successful operations patients lose some capacity to absorb zinc, bile salts, and vitamin B_{12}, although food supplements can make up for these deficiencies.

Any major surgery is an emotional trial. One that leaves a basic function of the body permanently altered, as with proctocolectomy or ileostomy, is difficult to accept afterward, even when the surgery was an emergency measure to save the patient's life. Patients must live with a bag of stool on their abdomen or a pouch that they must empty with a plastic straw-bags and pouches that sometimes leak stool or gas and that, even when functioning smoothly, are not pleasant to handle. They must pay close attention to body functions that they rarely had to think about before the ulcerative colitis began. The changes can severely depress patients, who then may need psychiatric help and antidepressant drugs to recover their spirits. Patients with anastomoses, who continue to defecate through their anus, also find their bowel functions changed, although not so severely. For example, it takes many months before normal stool forms, and diarrhea plagues these patients.

After their operations, patients have access to considerable help in addition to physicians and surgeons. Special nurses train patients to care for their stomas, check regularly for infection or malfunction, and generally ease them into their new lives. Formal support groups and informal networks are common and provide the afflicted with information and reassurance.

Perspective and Prospects

Acute forms of colitis, especially amebic dysentery, have long been recognized as among the endemic diseases of polluted water, and until the development of antibiotics, they regularly killed significant portions of local populations, especially the young and elderly. Chronic ulcerative colitis was first described in 1859, but no effective treatment for it existed until the 1940s. At that time, Nana Svartz of Sweden noticed that when rheumatoid arthritis patients were given sulfasalazine, the bowel condition of those who had colitis improved as well. J. Arnold Bargen, an American physician, confirmed Svartz's observation in a formal clinical trial, and sulfasalazine soon was massproduced for distribution in the United States and later throughout the world. Since the 1940s, medications and surgical techniques for ulcerative colitis have proliferated, although none restores a patient's original state of health.

Because the agents causing ulcerative colitis are unknown, the historical and geographical origin of the disease likewise cannot be determined. Nevertheless, three somewhat odd social facets of the disease are recognized.

Evidence suggests that ulcerative colitis is a disease of urban industrial society. Along with Crohn's disease, colitis appears to be entrenched in Scandinavia, the United States, Western Europe, Israel, and England. It rarely occurs in rural Africa, Asia, or South America, despite the poor nutrition and sanitation in some of these areas. Yet the disease does not appear to vary solely by racial type or nationality, although Jewish people tend to fall ill with it more often than any other group. For example, African Americans, whether from families long-established in the United States or recently immigrated, show an incidence of colitis as high as residents of European descent.

Furthermore, ulcerative colitis strikes the young. It most often begins between the ages of fifteen and thirty; men and women are equally likely to come down with it. This fact, taken with the high rate of inflammatory bowel disease (IBD) sufferers who have family members also with the disease (20 to 25 percent), has led some researchers to believe that a genetic factor creates a susceptibility for IBD.

Finally, IBD patients bear some social stigma or at least believe they do. Ulcerative colitis involves bowel incontinence and often ends with surgical replacement of the anus with a stoma; in such cases, bowel movements can dominate a patient's life and become obvious to family members, coworkers, and even strangers. Because the subject of stool is taboo to many and the odor offends most people, patients can feel severe embarrassment and come to see themselves as pariahs. Even though the causes of ulcerative colitis remain obscure and the treatment is often distressing, modern medicine saves people who otherwise would die.

—*Roger Smith, Ph.D.*

See also Amebiasis; Colon; Colorectal cancer; Colorectal surgery; Crohn's disease; Diarrhea and dysentery; Diverticulosis and diverticulitis; Gastroenterology; Gastrointestinal disorders; Gastrointestinal system; Giardiasis; Intestinal disorders; Intestines; Irritable bowel syndrome (IBS); Rectum; Ulcers.

For Further Information:
Beers, Mark H., et al., eds. *The Merck Manual of Diagnosis and Therapy.* 18th ed. Whitehouse Station, N.J.: Merck Research Laboratories, 2006.

Brandt, Lawrence J., and Penny Steiner-Grossman, eds. *Treating IBD: A Patient's Guide to the Medical and Surgical Management of Inflammatory Bowel Disease.* Reprint. Philadelphia: Lippincott-Raven, 1996.

Carson-DeWitt, Rosalyn, and Daus Mahnke. "Ulcerative Colitis." *Health Library,* September 10, 2012.

Crohn's and Colitis Foundation of America. http://www.ccfa.org.

Kalibjian, Cliff. *Straight from the Gut: Living with Crohn's Disease and Ulcerative Colitis.* Cambridge, Mass.: O'Reilly, 2003.

Kelly, Michael P. *Colitis.* Reprint. New York: Taylor & Francis, 2004.

Lashner, Bret A. "Ulcerative Colitis." *Center for Continuing Education, Cleveland Clinic Foundation,* March 2013.

National Digestive Diseases Information Clearinghouse. "Ulcerative Colitis." *National Institute of Diabetes and Digestive and Kidney Diseases, National Institutes of Health,* November 15, 2011.

Parker, James N., and Philip M. Parker, eds. *The Official Patient's Sourcebook on Ulcerative Colitis.* San Diego, Calif.: Icon Health, 2005.

Saibil, Fred. *Crohn's Disease and Ulcerative Colitis: Everything You Need to Know.* 3d rev. ed. Toronto, Ont.: Firefly Books, 2011.

Sklar, Jill, Manual Sklar, and Annabel Cohen. *The First Year-Crohn's Disease and Ulcerative Colitis: An Essential Guide for the Newly Diagnosed.* 2d ed. New York: Marlowe, 2007.

Steiner-Grossman, Penny, Peter A. Banks, and Daniel H. Present, eds. *The New People, Not Patients: A Source Book for Living with Inflammatory Bowel Disease.* Rev. ed. Dubuque, Iowa: Kendall/Hunt, 1997.

Collagen

Biology

Anatomy or system affected: All, especially joints, ligaments, musculoskeletal system, skin, tendons

Specialties and related fields: Biochemistry, rheumatology

Definition: A fibrous protein that is the main component of most connective tissues; the most common protein in animals.

Structure and Functions

Collagen is a complex protein made up of three separate polypeptide chains that form a triple helix. These polypeptides are unusual because every third amino acid is a glycine and because prolines make up an additional 17 percent of the chains. There are at least twenty-eight types of collagen made up of forty-three distinct polypeptide chains, each coded for by a different gene. For example, type I collagen, the most common type, has two chains classified as alpha-1 and alpha-2. These peptides are initially produced on the rough endoplasmic reticulum (ER) and then processed in the ER lumen, where sequences at the ends are removed and hydroxyl groups are added to many of the chains' prolines and lysines. The triple helix then formed is called procollagen. Further processing, including preparation for secretion, takes place in the Golgi bodies. Once secreted, more end sequences are cleaved off to form collagen (also called tropocollagen). In the extracellular region, collagen molecules associate into collagen fibrils and eventually collagen fibers.

Collagen is a flexible but not stretchable protein that is an important component of most connective tissues. It is the primary component of tendons and ligaments, giving them the requisite strength to connect muscles to bones and bones to other bones or organs. Cartilage found at joints and in many other structures is mostly collagen. The connective tissues found in the dermal layer of the skin, the capsules surrounding internal organs, and blood vessels are also primarily made of collagen. Bones are initially formed from collagen, which then serves as a matrix for calcium phosphate deposition. (Collagen fragments have even been extracted from fossilized dinosaur bones.) During healing, excess collagen production can lead to scar tissue formation. Collagen can be heat-treated to produce gelatin or animal-based glues, and injected collagen is often used in cosmetic procedures to plump lips or smooth out wrinkles.

Disorders and Diseases

Collagen is associated with many disorders. Osteogenesis imperfecta (brittle bone disease) is caused by mutations in the gene for the alpha-1 protein in type I collagen. An inherited form of osteoporosis is caused by a defect in the same gene. Ehlers-Danlos syndrome, which results in hyperextensible joints and fragile, stretchable skin, is caused by defects in types III and V collagen. A form of early-onset osteoarthritis is caused by a lack of functional type VI collagen, and in all forms of osteoarthritis cartilage is lost from the ends of bones at joints. In rheumatoid arthritis, modification of type II collagen forms new antigens that are attacked by the immune system. Vitamin C deficiency decreases activity of the enzymes that add hydroxyl groups to proline, thus leading to lowered amounts of functional type I collagen, which causes scurvy.

—*Richard W. Cheney, Jr., Ph.D.*

See also Arthritis; Cartilage; Connective tissue; Joints; Ligaments; Osteoarthritis; Osteogenesis imperfecta; Rheumatoid arthritis; Rheumatology; Scurvy; Tendon disorders; Tendon repair; Wrinkles.

For Further Information:
Abreu-Velez, Ana Maria, and Michael S. Howard. "Collagen IV in Normal Skin and in Pathological Processes." North American Journal of Medical Sciences 4, no. 1 (2012): 1-8.

"Collagen Vascular Disease." *Medline Plus,* February 9, 2011.

Fratzl, Peter. *Collagen: Structure and Mechanics.* New York: Springer, 2008.

Myllyharju, Joahanna, and Kari Kivirkko. "Collagen and Collagen-Related Diseases." *Annals of Medicine* 33 (2001): 7-21.

"Questions and Answers about Heritable Disorders of Connective Tissue." *National Institute of Arthritis and Musculoskeletal and Skin Diseases,* October 2011.

"Types of OI." *Osteogenesis Imperfecta Foundation,* 2012.

Whitford, David. *Proteins: Structure and Function.* Hoboken, N.J.: John Wiley & Sons, 2005.

Collodion baby

Disease/Disorder

Anatomy or system affected: Hair, nails, skin

Specialties and related fields: Dermatology, neonatology, pediatrics

Definition: A baby is born encased in a tight, shiny membrane.

Key terms:

desquamation: shedding of the outer layer of skin

epidermis: the outer epithelial layer of the skin

hyperkeratosis: excessive proliferation of skin cells accompanied by accelerated sloughing

Causes and Symptoms

At birth, collodion babies are encased in a tight, translucent, shiny membrane that resembles a "collodion," or a sausage skin. This membrane sloughs (desquamates) in 10-14 days to reveal the abnormal skin underneath. Ten percent of collodion babies are "self-healing" collodion babies. In this case, normal skin underlies the collodion, and peeling of the membrane leads to healing and normal skin. The incidence of collodion baby is unknown, but occurs at an estimated rate of 1 in every 100,000 births.

The two most common diseases associated with collodion babies include lamellar ichthyosis and nonbullous congenital erythroderma. Other rarer conditions associated with collodion babies include Sjögren-Larsson syndrome, Gaucher Disease type 2, Hay-Well syndrome, Trichothyodystrophy, Comel-Netherton syndrome, ectodermal dysplasia, and neutral lipid storage disease. All of these diseases result from mutations in genes that play integral roles in establishing and maintaining the outermost layer of the skin (epidermis). Dysfunctional skin cells cause accelerated turnover and thickening of the skin (hyperkeratosis).

The sloughing of the collodion membrane reveals red, scaly skin underneath. In many cases the scaling has a plate-like appearance that resembles fish scales, but the exact nature of the scaling depends on the type of skin disease responsible for the collodion membrane. As the collodion membrane dries, it cracks. The resulting fissures compromise the barrier function of the skin, and put the baby at increased risk of infections, dehydration, and overheating or cooling. Also, the tightness of the collodion membrane physically restricts underlying tissues. These constraints

---

Information on Collodion Baby

Causes: Abnormal sloughing of the skin associated with several congenital skin disorders

Symptoms: Peeling skin that scales, dries, and cracks

Duration: Extra skin sheds in 10-14 days, but duration of skin problems depends on the nature of the underlying skin condition

Treatments: High humidity, moisturizers, pain relievers, artificial tears for eyes

---

can prevent the baby from properly suckling and feeding, restrict blood flow in the limbs, affect breathing, and turn the lower eyelids away from the eyeball (ectropion).

Treatment and Therapy

After birth, collodion babies are transferred to a neonatal intensive care unit and placed in a humidified incubator. During their time in the incubator, they are given intravenous fluids and fed through a feeding tube. The goal of treatment is to keep the skin soft and moist to reduce scaling. Emollients such as petrolatum are smeared on the skin to moisten it. A mild topical steroid treatment can reduce inflammation, and artificial tears can ameliorate severely dry eyes in the cases of severe ectropion.

—Michael A. Buratovich, Ph.D.

See also Blisters; Dehydration; Dermatology; Dermatopathology; Intensive care unit; Neonatology; Pediatrics

For Further Information:

Kinai, Miriam. *Dermatology: Ichthyosis.* Seattle: Amazon Digital Services, 2012.

Polin, Richard A., and Alan R. Spitzer. *Fetal and Neonatal Secrets.* 3rd ed. Philadelphia: Mosby, 2013.

Colon

Anatomy

Also known as: Large intestine, large bowel, large gut

Anatomy or system affected: Abdomen, gastrointestinal system, intestines, nervous system

Specialties and related fields: Alternative medicine, biochemistry, gastroenterology, general surgery, histology, internal medicine, nutrition, oncology, osteopathic medicine, pathology, pediatrics, pharmacology

Definition: The section of the gastrointestinal system where the absorption of water, sodium, and some vitamins occurs and where residual chyme is converted to semisolid feces before expulsion through the anal canal. It is connected to the small intestine through the ileo-cecal valve and is populated by commensal bacteria.

Key terms:

chyme: food in a semifluid state that reaches the large intestine after digestion in the upper gastrointestinal tract

epithelium: tissue made up of tightly adherent cells, usually lining the surfaces of the body and organs

Structure and Functions

In the average adult man, the large intestine is about 1.5 to 1.8 meters long. It is divided into the cecum; the ascending, transverse, descending, and sigmoid colon; and the rectum, ending in the anus. Its wall contains both circular and longitudinal layers of smooth muscle and innervation that controls its motility. The longitudinal musculature runs along the outside of the colon in three separate bands, called teniae coli, which converge around the sigmoid colon and the rectum. The inner layer of the large intestine consists of mucosa with sparse or no villi but with numerous invaginations (glands); it is lined with simple columnar epithelium. The glands contain goblet cells, endocrine cells, and absorptive cells. There are no digestive enzymes linked to the inner surface of the colon.

The main function of the colon is to absorb water from the chyme and to process it into feces for elimination. Most nutrients and about 90 percent of water are absorbed in the small intestine. When it reaches the large intestine, chyme still contains some electrolytes (sodium, magnesium, and chloride) and indigestible food components, such as fiber.

An abundant and varied bacterial population colonizes the human colon shortly after birth and resides in the large intestine for life. Bacteria digest fiber and produce short-chain fatty acids (acetate, propionate, and butyrate). Short-chain fatty acids promote the integrity of the colonic epithelial cells, prevent inflammation, and provide some protection against potential pathogens.

The large intestine absorbs some vitamins (mainly vitamin K) and electrolytes but mainly water-up to five liters of water per day. Water moves passively with sodium, which is mostly absorbed in the distal colon. Water absorption is in part regulated by aldosterone, a hormone that increases the absorption of sodium in response to volume depletion. Water absorption solidifies the chyme into stools.

The motility of the colon allows for mixing the contents and retaining them for prolonged periods. Periodically, the colon is swept with propulsive contractions (peristalsis) that move its contents toward the rectum. The gastrocolic reflex causes mass peristalsis after a meal. The sigmoid colon and rectum serve as a reservoir and participate in defecation.

Disorders and Diseases

A number of disorders are associated with the colon. Appendicitis is the inflammation of the vermiform appendix. It requires surgery. Constipation is the failure to empty the bowels regularly and easily. It can be linked to diet, stress, and a variety of conditions and medications. It is treated with dietary fiber and laxatives. Diarrhea involves frequent loose or liquid bowel movements. It may have many different causes and is treated mainly with loperamide or bismuth salicilate.

Diverticulitis refers to the development of outpouchings in the colon. A low-fiber diet and age are risk factors. Symptoms are linked to inflammation (diverticulosis) and are mostly treated with antibiotics. Complications may require surgical removal of the outpouchings. Hirschsprung disease (congenital aganglionic megacolon) involves the complete absence of neuronal ganglion cells (which make the intestinal muscles contract, so the stool is pushed forward) from a segment of the intestine, usually the distal colon. It requires surgery.

Inflammatory bowel disease (IBD) is a general name for diseases that cause intestinal swelling. They include ulcerative colitis (inflammation and ulcers in the top layer of the lining of the large intestine) and Crohn's disease (all layers of the intestine may be involved; healthy bowel segments alternate with affected segments). Treatment varies widely, but the condition will recur. Irritable bowel syndrome (IBS) is a functional disorder of the colon of unknown cause. Its symptoms are abdominal pain, abnormal bowel habit, bloating, and either constipation, diarrhea, or both alternating. It is worsened by stress. IBS may be linked to hypersensitivity of intestinal muscles and nerves. Its treatment varies according to symptoms.

Colorectal polyps are growths on the lining of the colon or rectum. In time, they can develop into colorectal cancer. They are removed with endoscopic microsurgery. Colorectal cancer refers to cancerous growths in the colon, rectum, and appendix, mostly thought to arise from adenomatous polyps in the colon. It requires surgery.

Perspective and Prospects

The intuition that the colon is associated with waste accumulation and release dates to antiquity. Ancient Egyptian physicians also viewed "intestinal putrefaction" as the basic cause of disease, a concept later incorporated into the humoral doctrine of disease by ancient Greeks. This concept of autointoxication lasted throughout the centuries with few adaptations. In the nineteenth century, early studies showed the presence and activity of bacteria in the colon. It was then thought that colonic bacteria generate toxic amines that shorten life span. This theory was finally abandoned by the 1920s. Later research has focused on the molecular mechanisms of water and electrolyte movements and their regulation, as well as on the pathways that modulate the secretory and absorptive functions of the colon. Recent developments in genetics and immunology have allowed a deeper understanding of inflammatory diseases of the colon. The advent of endoscopic techniques has vastly improved microsurgery and cancer prevention.

—*Donatella M. Casirola, Ph.D.*

See also Abdomen; Abdominal disorders; Anus; Appendicitis; Colitis; Colonoscopy and sigmoidoscopy; Colorectal cancer; Colorectal polyp removal; Colorectal surgery; Constipation; Crohn's disease; Diarrhea; Digestion; Diverticulitis and diverticulosis; Endoscopy; Enemas; Gastroenterology; Gastroenterology, pediatric; Gastrointestinal disorders; Gastrointestinal system; Hirschsprung's disease; Internal medicine; Intestinal disorders; Intestines; Irritable bowel syndrome (IBS); Laparoscopy; Nutrition; Obstruction; Peristalsis; Proctology; Rectum; Small intestine.

For Further Information:
Bäckhed, Fredrik, et al. "Host-Bacterial Mutualism in the Human Intestine." *Science* 307 (March 25, 2005): 1915-1920.
Barrett, Kim E. "Functional Anatomy of the GI Tract and Organs Draining into It." In *Gastrointestinal Physiology.* New York: McGraw-Hill, 2006.
"Digestive System." *MedlinePlus,* January 14, 2013.
Mahnke, Daus. "Colonoscopy." *Health Library,* February 6, 2013.
Sherwood, Lauralee. "The Digestive System." In *Human Physiology: From Cells to Systems.* 8th ed. Belmont, Calif.: Brooks/Cole/Cengage Learning, 2013.
"Your Digestive System and How It Works." *National Digestive Diseases Information Clearinghouse (NDDIC),* April 23, 2013.

Colon therapy

Treatment

Also known as: Colonic irrigation, colon hydrotherapy

Anatomy or system affected: Abdomen, anus, gastrointestinal system, intestines

Specialties and related fields: Alternative medicine

Definition: Irrigation of the colon, or large intestine, with water in order to detoxify it.

Indications and Procedures

Colon therapy involves washing out the entire approximately five-foot length of the colon with pure water in order to dislodge any impacted fecal material. Some practitioners believe that the colon may not function properly because of poor dietary habits, insufficient fluid intake, and physical or emotional stress or illness. Such malfunction can lead to a buildup of hardened, impacted fecal material, which may stagnate and decay in the colon. Bacterial decomposition of the material may create toxins that are absorbed into the bloodstream. This in turn could cause other body organs to overwork themselves as they attempt to detoxify the waste materials and could lead to a variety of illnesses, from colds to cardiovascular disease.

During this procedure, a flexible tube is inserted into the rectum and water is slowly pumped into the intestine. The pressure is regulated in order to avoid injury. Alternation of warm and cool water leads to contraction and relaxation of the intestinal walls, which helps to remove impacted pieces of dry feces from the walls. Feces, gas, mucus, and bacteria exit through the same tube. A cleaner internal surface of the colon provides more surface area for the absorption of nutrients and water. Approximately twenty gallons of water are used in the procedure, which lasts about one hour.

Uses and Complications

Irrigation of the entire colon came into prominence during the late nineteenth century in Russia. In the United States, John Harvey Kellogg espoused colonic irrigation along with other health and fitness regimes at his sanatorium in Battle Creek, Michigan, in the early twentieth century. The procedure fell into obscurity during the late 1940s, when medical research indicated no benefit to the procedure. Renewed interest in colonics in the late twentieth century led to the establishment of the International Association for Colon Hydrotherapy, which provides training and certification for practitioners. While colon therapy regained enthusiastic followers, mainstream physicians point out that waste products in the colon cannot "toxify" the body. They also believe that colonics may interfere with the natural balance of helpful bacteria that keep the intestines functioning normally.

After a procedure, some patients report feeling energized and lighter, while others report nausea, headaches, or flu-like symptoms. These symptoms generally subside within a few hours. Other side effects may include diarrhea and a loss of necessary intestinal bacteria.

—*Karen E. Kalumuck, Ph.D.;*
updated by LeAnna DeAngelo, Ph.D.

See also Alternative medicine; Colon; Gastrointestinal system; Hydrotherapy; Intestines; Preventive medicine.

For Further Information:
Collings, Jillie. *Principles of Colonic Irrigation: The Only Introduction You'll Ever Need*. New York: Thorsons, 1996.

Goldberg, Burton, John Anderson, and Larry Trivieri, eds. *Alternative Medicine: The Definitive Guide*. 2d ed. Berkeley, Calif.: Celestial Arts, 2002.

Jonas, Wayne, ed. *Mosby's Dictionary of Complementary and Alternative Medicine*. St. Louis, Mo.: Mosby/Elsevier, 2005.

Mayo Clinic. "Colon Cleansing: Is It Helpful or Harmful?" *Mayo Clinic*, May 19, 2012.

Colonoscopy and sigmoidoscopy

Procedures

Anatomy or system affected: Gastrointestinal system, intestines

Specialties and related fields: Gastroenterology, general surgery

Definition: The insertion of a flexible tube into the rectum to look at the inside surface of the colon.

Key terms:

biopsy: removal of a piece of tissue for examination under a microscope

colitis: inflammation of the inner surface of the colon

lumen: the space inside a tubelike structure such as the colon

mucosa: the layer of tissue that lines the inside of a tubelike structure such as the colon

polyp: a small piece of tissue that extends from the surface of the colon into the lumen

Indications and Procedures

Colonoscopy and sigmoidoscopy are common procedures to evaluate the lower part of the gastrointestinal tract. Colonoscopy refers to examination of the entire large bowel, whereas sigmoidoscopy examines only the part closest to the rectum (known as the sigmoid colon). The advantage of sigmoidoscopy is that it is less time-consuming and can be performed without sedation. Since sigmoidoscopy evaluates only part of the colon, however, full colonoscopy is often preferred. The most common reason for having a colonoscopy is to screen for colon cancer. If sigmoidoscopy is used for this purpose, it must be combined with a barium enema and an x-ray to evaluate the upper part of the colon.

Prior to colonoscopy, the bowel must be cleaned of stool to enable the physician to see the underlying mucosa. Patients are often asked to go on a diet of clear liquids (such as chicken broth, gelatin, and juice) for one to three days prior to the procedure. The night before the procedure, patients ingest a purgative to clear out any residual stool. The two most common preparations are polyethylene glycol (GoLytely) and a sodium phosphate mix (Fleet Phospho-Soda). Following ingestion of these solutions, patients should have clear or very light-colored liquid bowel movements. Regular medications that may cause excessive bleeding from biopsy sites, such as aspirin, warfarin, and nonsteroidal anti-inflammatory drugs (NSAIDs), are often discontinued prior to the procedure. Patients should also discontinue iron supplements, since they may create a black coating that makes it difficult for the physician to see the mucosa.

When patients enter the colonoscopy suite, they are given an intravenous (IV) catheter to administer fluids, as

---

In the News:
Risks of Flat Lesions in Intestinal Lining

Approximately 0.3 percent to 0.9 percent of patients develop colon cancer a few years after having a successful colonoscopy or sigmoidoscopy. Doctors, once puzzled by this response, now attribute at least some cancer occurrence to undetected or inadequately removed flat or depressed lesions in the intestinal lining. These lesions were previously thought to be harmless. However, a study published in March, 2008, in the *Journal of the American Medical Association* cautioned that flat or depressed growths are five times more likely to be cancerous than other more easily identified lesions such as polyps.

Flat or depressed lesions are often smaller than polyps and the same color as the colon. Consequently, they innocently blend right into the surrounding healthy colon tissue. These growths also occur infrequently, comprising only 15 percent of the total lesions detected in males. They occur even less often in the female population. The danger of flat or depressed lesions makes it even more imperative that patients follow the pretest cleansing routine carefully. Remaining waste, no matter how small, may cover and hide a serious growth.

To detect flat or depressed lesions, physicians must be trained to do the test slowly, carefully look for the growths, and inject a blue dye into the colon to define the lesion. Doctors must also learn new techniques to ensure that the growths are completely removed. Physicians are encouraged to track their own success rate in detecting these difficult lesions.

Increasingly popular virtual or relatively noninvasive colonoscopies use computed tomography (CT) to detect polyps that rise from the colon wall. However, CT is not sensitive enough to detect flat or depressed lesions. Promising new techniques to readily identify these growths include narrow-band imaging, a novel illumination technology, zoom magnification, and high-definition processor technology.

—*Renée Euchner, R.N.*

---

well as sedative and analgesic medications. Patients are asked not to eat or drink anything the day of the procedure. Sedative medications sometimes cause nausea, and any food that is present in the stomach may be vomited. Blood pressure, pulse, and oxygen saturation are monitored throughout the procedure. The patient is positioned on his or her left side, and a colonoscope is inserted through the rectum into the colon. The colonoscope is a long, flexible tube with a fiber-optic channel connected to a camera. The image of the inside of the colon is transmitted to a television screen. The colonoscope also has channels to administer air or water, as well as a suction channel. Air is introduced to expand the walls of the colon, enabling better viewing. Water is used to remove residual stool that may obstruct the view of the colon. The colonoscope is advanced to the cecum (the first part of the large bowel) or even the terminal ileum (the last part of the small bowel). The instrument is then slowly withdrawn while any abnormalities in the mucosa are noted. Following the procedure, patients are often observed for a period of time to make sure that no complications occur. If sedative medications were used, patients should not drive or operate machinery for the rest of the day.

Uses and Complications

In addition to screening for colon cancer, colonoscopy and sigmoidoscopy can be used to evaluate blood in the stool, chronic diarrhea or other changes in bowel habits, and unexplained abdominal pain. Common findings include polyps, which may be biopsied. It is common practice to remove a polyp completely, in case it turns out to be the precancerous type (known as an adenomatous polyp). Other findings include diverticula, small outpouchings of the colon which have very thin walls and are prone to spontaneous bleeding. They may also become infected, resulting in a condition known as diverticulitis. Other findings during colonoscopy may be useful in establishing the presence of a particular disease. Yellowish pseudo-membranes line the gut in colitis associated with the bacterium *Clostridium difficile*. A dusky hue is often seen in cases of ischemic colitis caused by diminished blood supply to the colon. Characteristic findings are also seen in inflammatory bowel disease.

Colonoscopy is a very safe procedure. One common aftereffect is abdominal discomfort as a result of the air used to distend the colon. This condition usually resolves over a few hours as the air is passed. The most serious complications of colonoscopy are perforation and bleeding. Perforation refers to a hole in the colon. It is an extremely rare occurrence, but it can be deadly. Patients with perforations often have severe abdominal pain and a rigid abdomen. If it is large and results in free air in the abdomen, a perforation requires emergency surgery. Rarely, very small perforations can be treated with observation and antibiotics. Bleeding is a risk if a biopsy is taken during the procedure. Most of the time, the bleeding stops by itself, but in some cases a repeat colonoscopy may be required to control the bleeding. Rarely, bleeding may occur a few hours to several days after colonoscopy, so patients should report these symptoms to their physician. Whenever sedation is used, there is a risk of too much being given, which can lead to respiratory or cardiac arrest. Other possible complications include pain and inflammation at the site of the catheter and allergic reactions to sedative or analgesic medications.

—*Ahmad Kamal, M.D.*

See also Colon; Colorectal cancer; Colorectal polyp removal; Colorectal surgery; Diverticulitis and diverticulosis; Endoscopy; Enemas; Gastroenterology; Gastrointestinal system; Intestines; Invasive tests; Oncology; Proctology; Screening; Tumor removal; Tumors.

For Further Information:
Church, James M. *Endoscopy of the Colon, Rectum, and Anus*. New York: Igaku-Shoin, 1995.

Drossman, Douglas A., et al., eds. *Handbook of Gastroenterologic Procedures*. 4th ed. Philadelphia: Lippincott Williams & Wilkins, 2005.

HealthDay. "Prepping for a Colonoscopy: Why It's a Necessary Evil." *MedlinePlus*, May 30, 2013.

Health Library. "Colonoscopy." *Health Library*, February 6, 2013.

Health Library. "Flexible Sigmoidoscopy." *Health Library*, September 10, 2012.

Longstreth, George F. "Sigmoidoscopy." *MedlinePlus*, October 8, 2012.

MedlinePlus. "Colonoscopy." *MedlinePlus*, June 7, 2013.

Waye, Jerome D., Douglas K. Rex, and Christopher B. Williams, eds. *Colonoscopy: Principles and Practice*. 2d ed. Malden, Mass.: Blackwell, 2009.

Color blindness

Disease/Disorder

Anatomy or system affected: Eyes

Specialties and related fields: Brain, optometry

Definition: An inability to distinguish certain colors resulting from an inherited defect in the light receptor cells in the retina of the eye.

Information on Color Blindness

Causes: Genetic defect resulting in photoreceptor deficiency

Symptoms: Inability to distinguish between certain colors (red, orange, yellow, green)

Duration: Lifelong

Treatments: None

Causes and Symptoms

The retina of the eye is a thin, fragile membrane that contains millions of photoreceptor cells. They convert light energy into an electrical signal, which is transmitted to the brain via the optic nerve. On a microscopic scale, the structure of the retina is like a carpet with its many fibers sticking upward. There are two types of photoreceptor cells, called rods and cones because of their distinctive shapes. Only the cones are important for color vision. There are three varieties of cones with peak sensitivities for red, green, and blue, respectively. The shades and tints of all other colors are mixtures of these three.

Color blindness involves a deficiency in these photoreceptor cells. A deficiency of green photoreceptor cells is much more common than a deficiency of red photoreceptors. Some people are totally color-blind, which means that they are completely unable to distinguish among red, orange, yellow, and green. Color blindness is quite rare in females (less than 1 percent of the population) but is more prevalent in males (about 8 percent).

Diagnostic tests are available to determine the extent of color blindness. The Ishihara color test, named after a Japanese ophthalmologist, consists of a mosaic of colored dots containing a letter of the alphabet made up of dots of a different color-for example, yellow dots in a background of green ones. Color-blind individuals would be unable to distinguish the letter because yellow and green look the same to them.

A more precise diagnostic test makes use of the Nagel anomaloscope, which has two colored light sources whose brightness can be adjusted. The patient tries to match a given color by superimposing the two light beams while varying their intensities. For normal eyes, red and green lights of similar intensities can be superimposed to create yellow. However, a patient who requires a considerably larger green component to create yellow evidently has a deficiency of green photoreceptor cells.

Treatment and Therapy

Color blindness is a genetic defect from birth, not a disease. No procedure is known by which it can be corrected. Color-blind people must find ways to counter the effects of their condition. For example, they can obtain driver's licenses because they learn that stoplights are always red on top, yellow in the middle, and green on the bottom. Color-blind individuals may need help, however, with tasks such as clothing selection. Good color discrimination is required for some occupations, such as interior decorating, graphic design, advertising, or airplane piloting. Fortunately, color blindness is not a deterrent for most jobs.

—*Hans G. Graetzer, Ph.D.*

See also Eye infections and disorders; Eyes; Genetic diseases; Vision; Vision disorders.

For Further Information:

Cameron, John R., James G. Skofronick, and Roderick M. Grant. *Medical Physics: Physics of the Body*. Madison, Wis.: Medical Physics, 1992.

"Color Blindness." *MedlinePlus*, June 1, 2011.

Kasper, Dennis L., et al., eds. *Harrison's Principles of Internal Medicine*. 18th ed. New York: McGraw-Hill, 2012.

Stresing, Diane. "Color Blindness." *Health Library*, March 15, 2013.

"Vision." In *Encyclopaedia Brittanica*. 15th ed. Chicago: Encyclopaedia Britannica, 2002.

Colorectal cancer

Disease/Disorder

Also known as: Large bowel cancer

Anatomy or system affected: Abdomen,,, gastrointestinal system, intestines, lymphatic system

Specialties and related fields: Gastroenterology, genetics, immunology, oncology, proctology, colorectal surgery

Definition: Cancer occurring in the large intestine.

Key terms:

polyp: an abnormal tissue growth that forms on the lining of the colon; may be benign or malignant

colonoscopy: a method of visualizing the colon using a camera attached to a flexible tube

hematochezia: bright red blood in stool, suggestive of a lower gastrointestinal bleed

melena: dark, black blood in stool suggestive of an upper gastrointestinal bleed or blood that has passed slowly through the GI system

Causes and Symptoms

With an estimated 51,000 deaths per year in the United States, cancer of the colon and rectum is the second most deadly cancer for both men and women, ranking only behind lung cancer. While mortality from colorectal cancer (CRC) has been declining, incidence among people less than 50 years old has been increasing over the last decade.

About 90 percent of colorectal cancers arise from the glandular epithelium lining the inner surface of the large bowel and are termed adenocarcinomas. The cells of the epithelial layer are constantly being replaced by new cells.

This fairly rapid cell division, along with the relatively hostile environment within the bowel, promotes internal cellular errors that lead to the formation of aberrant cells. These cells can become disordered and produce abnormal growths or tumors. Often, colorectal tumors protrude into the lumen (the spaces within the bowel), forming growths called polyps. Some polyps are benign and do not spread to other parts of the body, but they may still disturb normal bowel functions. Other polyps become malignant by forming more aggressive cell types, which allows them to grow larger and spread to other organs. The cancer can grow through the layers of the colon wall and extend into the body cavity and nearby organs such as the urinary bladder. Cancer cells can also break away from the main tumor and spread (metastasize) through the blood or lymphatic vessels to other organs, such as the lungs or liver. If not controlled, the spreading cancer eventually causes death by impairment of organ and system functions.

The tendency to develop colorectal polyps and cancer can be inherited; this genetic predisposition may be responsible for about 5 to 7 percent of all colorectal cancers. One example is an inherited disorder called familial adenomatous polyposis (FAP), in which hundreds of polyps develop in the colon; it often leads to colorectal cancer. Some of the defective genes that cause this and other types of colorectal cancers have been identified and are being studied to determine their pathogenic role. Inflammatory bowel disease (IBD) and exposure to certain carcinogens, such as tobacco, as well as modifiable factors such as obesity and excessive alcohol consumption are also known to increase the risk of CRC.

Symptoms of CRC can be highly variable. Many patients may be asymptomatic in early stages, with cancer being detected only through screening methods. Some of the most frequent signs and symptoms include hematochezia, melena, change in bowel habits, and shortness of breath or fatigue suggestive of iron-deficiency anemia. Of note, an iron-deficiency anemia in an older patient is suspect for a GI bleed until proven otherwise. Right-sided colon cancers typically present with bleeding and anemia while left-sided colon cancers typically present with obstructive symptoms including changes in bowel habits and abdominal pain.

Treatment and Therapy

The chances for survival are greatly increased when colorectal cancer is detected and treated at an early stage. The decline in mortality from CRC is attributed to early screening and detection. Early detection in the general population is possible with a number of methods:

Digital rectal examination, in which the physician checks the inner surface of the rectal wall with a gloved finger for abnormal growths; fecal occult blood test, in which a stool sample is tested for hidden blood that may have emanated from a cancerous growth; sigmoidoscopy, in which the physician examines the rectal and lower-colon inner lining with a narrow tubular optical instrument inserted through the anus; colonoscopy, in which an optical instrument, inserted through the anus, assesses more of the colon

---

> ### Information on Colorectal Cancer
> **Causes:** Hereditary and/or environmental factors, dietary habits, colon polyps, long-standing ulcerative colitis
> **Symptoms:** Fatigue, weakness, shortness of breath, change in bowel habits, narrow stools, diarrhea or constipation, red or dark blood in stool, weight loss, abdominal pain, cramps, bloating
> **Duration:** Chronic
> **Treatments:** Surgery, chemotherapy, radiation

---

and can remove tissue for pathological examination; virtual colonoscopy, which is a noninvasive test to assess the colon through use of X-rays; and double contrast barium enema, in which X-rays are taken after a liquid containing barium is put into the rectum. Newer screening tests, called fecal DNA testing, continue to be under study. These tests look for early genetic changes in the colon cells that are sloughed off into the stool.

Once cancer is suspected, further tests will be done to arrive at a diagnosis. These tests may include a computed tomography (CT) scan, double-contrast barium enema X-ray series, and colonoscopy. The CT scan and contrast X-rays reveal abnormal growths, and colonoscopy is similar to sigmoidoscopy but uses a longer, flexible tube in order to inspect the entire colon. During sigmoidoscopy and colonoscopy, the physician can remove polyps and obtain tissue samples for biopsy. A tissue sample is necessary to make the diagnosis of CRC. Microscopic examination of the tissue samples by a pathologist can determine the stage or extent of growth of the cancer. This is important because it helps with assessing the type of treatment needed. In one type of staging, the following criteria are used: stage 0 (cancer confined to epithelium lining of the bowel), stage 1 (cancer confined to the bowel wall), stage 2 (cancer penetrating through all layers of the bowel wall and possibly invading adjacent tissues), stage 3 (cancer invading lymph nodes and/or adjacent tissues), and stage 4 (cancer spreading to distant sites, forming metastases).

Surgery is the primary treatment for colorectal cancer. Very small tumors in stage 0 can be removed surgically with the colonoscope. Tumors in more advanced stages require abdominal surgery in which the tumor is removed along with a portion of the bowel and possibly some lymph nodes. For cases in which the bowel cannot be reconnected, an opening is created through the abdominal wall (colostomy). This is usually a temporary procedure, and the hole will be closed when the bowel can be rejoined. Some advanced cancers cannot be cured by surgery alone. Adjuvant therapies-chemotherapy, radiation therapy, and biological therapy-may be used in combination with surgery. Chemotherapy drugs kill spreading cancer cells. The most common is 5-fluorouracil (5-FU), a chemical that interferes with the production of deoxyribonucleic acid (DNA) in dividing cells. 5-FU is more effective when given together with leucovorin (a compound similar to folic acid) and levamisole (an immune system stimulant).

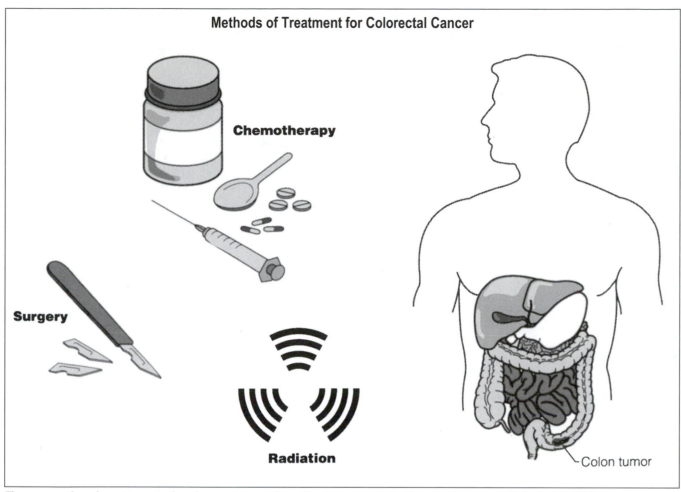

Methods of Treatment for Colorectal Cancer

Chemotherapy

Surgery

Radiation

Colon tumor

The presence of a malignant tumor in the colon requires some form of treatment or a combination of treatments, usually beginning with its surgical removal and followed by radiation therapy and/or chemotherapy (the use of anticancer drugs).

In 2004, the Food and Drug Administration (FDA) approved the use of the Eloxatin injection in combination with 5-FU and leucovorin for the treatment of patients whose cancer has recurred or become worse following initial drug therapy. This approach was shown to shrink tumors in some patients and delay resumed tumor growth. Levamisole and other treatments that reinforce the immune system are forms of biological therapy. Radiation therapy, given either before or after surgery, is helpful in killing undetected cancer cells near the site of the tumor.

Perspective and Prospects

More than 608,000 people worldwide die of colorectal cancer each year, or roughly 8 percent of all cancer deaths. The incidence of colorectal cancer is lower among women than men and rises dramatically after the age of fifty. Colorectal cancer is more common in developed countries and in densely populated, industrialized regions. Populations moving from low-risk parts of the world for developing colorectal cancer, such as Asia or Africa, to high-risk areas, such as the United States or Europe, take on the higher risk within a generation or two, and vice versa.

Research is ongoing to determine the risk factors of colorectal cancers. Recent epidemiological evidence has supported the use of nonsteroidal anti-inflammatory drugs (NSAIDs) as a means of reducing the risk of cancers of the colon and rectum, as well as the risk of intestinal cancers resulting from exposure to carcinogens. The studies focused only on the daily use of aspirin, but similar results have been reported following long-term use of sulindac and indomethacin. Sulindac and celecoxib have shown an ability to induce regression of colon polyps in patients with familial adenomatous polyposis. Researchers are still working on finding the right balance in dose and frequency since NSAIDs have potentially severe side effects and aspirin may induce bleeding if high doses are maintained on a daily basis. Regular cardiovascular exercise and a healthy diet high in fruits and vegetables have also been shown to reduce the risk of developing colorectal cancer.

—*Rodney C. Mowbray, PhD;*
updated by Connie Rizzo, MD, PhD, and Ananya Anand, MSc

See also: Biopsy; Cancer; Chemotherapy; Colon; Colon therapy; Colonoscopy and sigmoidoscopy; Colorectal polyp removal; Colorectal surgery; Ileostomy and colostomy; Intestinal disorders; Intestines; Malignancy and metastasis; National Cancer Institute (NCI); Oncology; Radiation therapy; Rectum; Stomach, intestinal, and pancreatic cancers; Tumor removal; Tumors.

For Further Information:

Adrouny, Richard. *Understanding ColonCancer*. Jackson: University Press of Mississippi, 2002.

Bub, David S., et al. *One Hundred Questions and Answers About Colorectal Cancer*. 2d ed. Sudbury, Mass.: Jones and Bartlett, 2008.

De Vita, Vincent T., Jr., Samuel Hellman, and Steven A. Rosenberg, eds. *Cancer: Principles and Practice of Oncology*. 9th ed. Philadelphia: Lippincott Williams & Wilkins, 2011.

Dollinger, Malin, et al. *Everyone's Guide to CancerTherapy*. 5th ed. Kansas City, Mo.: Andrews McMeel, 2008.

Eyre, Harmon J., Dianne Partie Lange, and Lois B. Morris. *Informed Decisions: The Complete Book of CancerDiagnosis, Treatment, and Recovery*. 2d ed. Atlanta: American Cancer Society, 2002.

Goldman, Lee, and Dennis Ausiello, eds. *Cecil Textbook of Medicine*. 23d ed. Philadelphia: Saunders/Elsevier, 2007.

LaRusso, Laurie. "Colon Cancer." *Health Library*, February 28, 2013.

Levin, Bernard, et al., eds. *American CancerSociety's Complete Guide to Colorectal Cancer*. Atlanta: American Cancer Society, 2006.

Miskovitz, Paul, and Marian Betancourt. *What to Do If You Get ColonCancer: A Specialist Helps You Take Charge and Make Informed Choices*. New York: Wiley, 1997.

Parker, James N., and Philip M. Parker, eds. *The Official Patient's Sourcebook on ColonCancer*. San Diego, Calif.: Icon Health, 2002.

"What Is Colorectal Cancer?" *American CancerSociety*, January 17, 2013.

Colorectal polyp removal

Procedure

Anatomy or system affected: Abdomen, anus, gastrointestinal system, intestines

Specialties and related fields: Gastroenterology, general surgery, proctology

Definition: The surgical removal of overgrowths of the tissue lining the rectum and colon.

Indications and Procedures

Rectal and colon polyps are growths of tissue that occur in the mucous membranes lining the colon and rectum. They are usually not malignant. Common types of colorectal polyps are juvenile polyps, Peutz-Jeghers polyps (hamartomas), hyperplasias, adenomas, and mixed hyperplastic-adenomatous polyps. Adenomas are both the most dangerous and the most common type of colon polyp.

Rectal or colon polyps are removed when they are found, even if they cause no symptoms, because identifying the kind of polyp helps doctors determine whether cancer is likely to develop. The type of polyp is determined in the laboratory after surgical removal, using microscopic techniques.

The presence of polyps does not mean that a patient has cancer, although larger polyps (greater than one centimeter) indicate a higher risk for cancer than do smaller ones. Certain types of polyps also are more likely than others to develop into cancer. Hyperplasias are polyps with no potential to develop into cancer. Juvenile polyps and Peutz-Jeghers polyps are associated with inherited disorders that indicate an increased risk for colon cancer, but they do not always develop into malignant tumors. Colorectal adenomas are particularly dangerous when they occur in conjunction with a genetic condition known as familial adenomatous polyposis (FAP). In patients with FAP, untreated colorectal adenomas develop into colon cancer virtually 100 percent of the time. Mixed hyperplastic-adenomatous polyps, although not as risky as pure adenomas, can develop into colon cancer, and patients with a diagnosis of this type of polyp should be closely monitored.

Colon polyps often cause no symptoms. They are usually detected by routine screening for colorectal cancers. The most common symptoms, when they occur, are bleeding from the anus (visible on underwear or toilet paper), constipation or diarrhea lasting more than a week, and blood in the stool, which can appear as red streaks or an overall darkening of fecal matter. The fecal occult blood test will detect blood that is not visible.

When polyps are suspected, the physician will perform a rectal examination or special tests such as barium enema x-rays, flexible sigmoidoscopy, or colonoscopy. In a rectal examination, the doctor feels the rectal tissue with his or her fingers, looking for abnormalities. Barium makes healthy intestinal tissue look white on an x-ray, and polyps appear dark against the white background. The sigmoidoscope is a flexible fiber-optic tube that can be inserted through the anus. The tube has a small video camera and a light so that the doctor can visualize the lower third of the large intestine. Colonoscopy is similar to sigmoidoscopy, but the colonoscope allows the physician to visualize the entire intestine.

Removal is most commonly accomplished using colonoscopy to visualize the polyps and specialized forceps to detach and remove the growths. Snare forceps can be used to surround a polyp and cut it from the lining of the colon or rectum. Other methods of removal include a laser beam, burning, or ultrasound, depending on the size of the polyp. Bleeding during the procedure can be controlled with electrocautery forceps, which use heat to sever the polyp from the surrounding healthy tissue and seal off blood vessels, or by pressing epinephrine-soaked gauze against the removal site.

Special precautions must be taken during surgery to remove gas from the colon so that the combustion of hydrogen or methane gas does not occur. These gases are normally produced by bacteria that inhabit the colon.

A polyp in the lower portion of the colon may be removed using similar procedures during the sigmoidoscopy. In some cases, the patient may undergo surgery to remove the polyp through the abdomen.

Uses and Complications

Since colonoscopy is somewhat uncomfortable for the patient, sedatives are usually given, but general anesthesia is usually not necessary. Rectal and colon polyp removal is typically done as an outpatient procedure.

Because of the gas that enters the intestine during the procedure, patients may experience bloating, pressure, and intestinal cramps in the twenty-four hours following removal. This discomfort subsides as the gas passes out of the intestine.

Repeat colonoscopy should be performed so that recurrent polyps can be removed and examined for malignancy. Colorectal cancer is the second leading cause of cancer deaths in the United States, and the majority of these cancers arise from colorectal polyps.

—*Matthew Berria, Ph.D.,*
and Douglas Reinhart, M.D.;
updated by Caroline M. Small

See also Biopsy; Cancer; Colon; Colonoscopy and sigmoidoscopy; Colorectal cancer; Colorectal surgery; Electrocauterization; Endoscopy; Enemas; Gastroenterology; Gastrointestinal system; Hemorrhoid banding and removal; Hemorrhoids; Intestinal disorders; Intestines; Oncology; Polyps; Proctology; Rectum; Screening.

For Further Information:

Ades, Terri, Katie Couric, and Bernard Levin. *American Cancer Society's Complete Guide to Colorectal Cancer.* Chicago: American Cancer Society, 2012.

Burke, Carol, and James Church, eds. *Hereditary Colorectal Cancer Syndromes.* New York: Blackwell, 2007.

Corman, Marvin L. *Colon and Rectal Surgery.* 5th ed. Philadelphia: Lippincott Williams & Wilkins, 2005.

Greenberger, Norton J., R. S. Blumberg, and Robert Burakoff. *Current Diagnosis & Treatment: Gastroenterology, Hepatology, & Endoscopy.* 2d ed. New York: McGraw-Hill Medical, 2012.

Health Library. "Colorectal Polyps." *Health Library,* February 8, 2013.

Longo, Walter E., and John M. A. Northover, eds. *Reoperative Colon and Rectal Surgery.* New York: Martin Dunitz, 2003.

Longstreth, George F. "Colorectal Polyps." *MedlinePlus,* October 8, 2012.

National Institutes of Health and National Cancer Institute. *Cancer of the Colon and Rectum.* Rev. ed. Bethesda, Md.: Author, 1991.

National Institutes of Health and National Cancer Institute. *What You Need to Know About Cancer of the Colon and Rectum.* Rev. ed. Bethesda, Md.: Author, 2006.

Zollinger, Robert M., Jr., Robert M. Zollinger, Sr., et al. *Zollinger's Atlas of Surgical Operations.* 9th ed. New York: McGraw-Hill, 2011.

Colorectal surgery

Procedure

Anatomy or system affected: Abdomen, anus, gastrointestinal system, intestines

Specialties and related fields: Gastroenterology, general surgery, proctology

Definition: Surgery that is required to correct pathologies of the colon, rectum, and anus.

Key terms:

abscess: a pocket of infection or inflammation

acute: referring to a short, immediate disease state

chronic: referring to an enduring disease state

ulcer: a lesion that destroys tissue

Indications and Procedures

The large intestine, or colon, is shaped like an inverted *U*. It starts at the lower right side of the pelvis, where the small intestine empties into the cecum. The colon rises from the cecum to the center of the abdomen, crosses to the left, and descends to the S-shaped sigmoid colon, the rectum, and the anus. Common disorders of the colon, rectum, and anus that require surgery are hemorrhoids, Crohn's disease, ulcerative colitis, cancer, diverticulosis, and diverticulitis.

Hemorrhoids are swollen veins in the lower part of the rectum and the anus. They protrude as nodes or lumps that can cause severe pain, itching, and inflammation. Hemorrhoids can be tied off with tiny rubber bands. After a few days, they fall off painlessly. Medications can shrink internal hemorrhoids, or hemorrhoidal tissue can be removed by photocoagulation, a process that uses electromagnetic energy to eradicate affected tissues. Sometimes, a hemorrhoidectomy is required. This procedure involves the extensive excision of hemorrhoidal tissue and can be quite painful.

Crohn's disease and ulcerative colitis are chronic inflammatory bowel diseases (IBDs) that can affect the colon. Crohn's disease usually occurs in the small intestine, although it may be limited to the colon. When Crohn's disease is severe and restricted to the colon, the surgeon may perform a colectomy and ileostomy. This procedure involves removing the entire lower intestine, rectum, and anus. The anal opening is closed, and a new opening, or stoma, is made in the abdominal wall. The ileum, the lower end of the small intestine, is then attached to the opening. A removable pouch is sealed to the opening to collect fecal matter, which must be emptied manually.

Ulcerative colitis may exist with no symptoms other than an occasional flare-up, or it can be a chronic, serious, or life-threatening disease. It is characterized by a series of ulcers on the inner wall of the colon. Bloody diarrhea, abdominal pain, and painful bowel movements are symptoms. In severe cases, there is danger of perforation of the colon wall or of swelling (toxic megacolon), either of which can be life-threatening. Ulcerative colitis may also be a precursor of colon cancer. In severe cases of ulcerative colitis, surgery is required. Colectomy and ileostomy are the surgical procedures usually performed, but recently developed is a procedure called ileoanal anastomosis. As in ileostomy, the surgeon removes the entire colon and rectum but leaves the anal sphincter muscles. The ileum is then attached to the anus. This procedure allows the patient to have natural bowel movements and avoids the necessity of the ileostomy pouch.

Cancers of the colon or rectum, called colorectal cancers, are major causes of morbidity and mortality. The possibility of colon cancer is often signaled by the presence of polyps on the lower intestinal wall. Symptoms such as mucus or blood in the stool may alert the physician to look for polyps and determine whether they are likely to become cancerous. Benign polyps are usually removed surgically.

When polyps are likely to become cancerous, and in the presence of actual colorectal cancer, surgery is usually performed to remove diseased tissue. This often requires excising part or all of the colon. Sometimes a colectomy and colostomy are performed, an operation similar to an ileostomy. In this procedure, the diseased sections of the colon, the rectum, and the anus are removed. The anal opening is sealed, and the remaining colon is brought to an opening in the abdominal wall. This opening, or stoma, is fitted with a removable colostomy bag or pouch to collect fecal matter.

Diverticula are small, sac-like pouches that develop in the colon wall, most often in the sigmoid colon. Their presence is known as diverticulosis. These sacs can collect stagnant fecal matter and become inflamed, resulting in diverticulitis. Abscesses and infection may develop. As inflammation progresses or recurs, the wall of the colon thickens, reducing the width of the passage and increasing the possibility of obstruction and distension of the colon. Perforations in the colon wall may develop and cause peritonitis (infection of the membrane that covers the abdomen).

In severe cases, it may be necessary to perform a temporary colostomy. The diseased section of colon is removed, and the rectum and anus are closed. A stoma is made in the abdominal wall and attached to the remaining colon and covered by a pouch to collect fecal matter. After the bowel has healed, the rectum and anus can be reopened and attached to the colon.

Uses and Complications

Patients with permanent ileostomies and colostomies have a hole in their abdomens that is often five or more centimeters (two or more inches) in diameter. Patients are required to wear removable pouches sealed to their stomas to collect fecal matter so that it can be eliminated. The apparatus is cumbersome, and the entire process can be unpleasant enough to cause serious depression in the patient. Patients' spouses and other family members are often involved in changing and emptying the bags, particularly with older, infirm persons. Ileoanal anastomosis solves some of these problems because it allows natural bowel movements, but it is useful only in certain conditions.

Perspective and Prospects

Current surgical procedures are often effective in serious colorectal conditions. The success rate of these surgeries for the treatment of cancer is quite high if the cancer is caught before it spreads to other parts of the body. Nevertheless, patients may have to endure the inconvenience of ostomy bags and paraphernalia for the rest of their lives. Ostomy equipment has been improved: Better sealing adhesives are now in use so that the bags do not slip or leak as they once did. The configuration of belts, bags, and other appliances has been altered to make them more convenient and easier to live with. New surgical procedures that could maintain normal bowel function for more patients, however, would be a major advancement.

—*C. Richard Falcon*

See also Abdomen; Abdominal disorders; Biopsy; Cancer; Colitis; Colon; Colonoscopy and sigmoidoscopy; Colorectal cancer; Colorectal polyp removal; Crohn's disease; Diverticulitis and diverticulosis; Electrocauterization; Endoscopy; Enemas; Fistula repair; Gastroenterology; Gastrointestinal system; Hemorrhoid banding and removal; Hemorrhoids; Hernia repair; Hernias; Ileostomy and colostomy; Intestinal disorders; Intestines; Oncology; Proctology; Rectum; Tumor removal; Tumors.

For Further Information:

Feldman, Mark, Lawrence S. Friedman, and Lawrence J. Brandt, eds. *Sleisenger and Fordtran's Gastrointestinal and Liver Disease: Pathophysiology, Diagnosis, Management*. 9th ed. 2 vols. Philadelphia: Saunders/Elsevier, 2010.

Kapadia, Cyrus R., James M. Crawford, and Caroline Taylor. *An Atlas of Gastroenterology: A Guide to Diagnosis and Differential Diagnosis*. Boca Raton, Fla.: Pantheon, 2003.

Litin, Scott C., ed. *Mayo Clinic Family Health Book*. 4th ed. New York: HarperResource, 2009.

Phillips, Robert H. *Coping with an Ostomy: A Guide to Living with an Ostomy for You and Your Family*. Wayne, N.J.: Avery, 1986.

Zollinger, Robert M., Jr., Robert M. Zollinger, Sr., et al. *Zollinger's Atlas of Surgical Operations*. 9th ed. New York: McGraw-Hill, 2011.

Coma. *See* Minimally conscious state.

Common cold

Disease/Disorder

Anatomy or system affected: Chest, lungs, nose, respiratory system

Specialties and related fields: Family medicine, internal medicine, otorhinolaryngology, public health, virology

Definition: A class of viral respiratory infections that form the world's most prevalent illnesses.

Key terms:

acute: referring to a disease process of sudden onset and short duration

chronic: referring to a disease process of long duration and frequent recurrence

coronavirus: a microorganism causing respiratory illness; one of the most prevalent causes of the common cold

pathogen: any disease-causing microorganism

rhinovirus: a microorganism causing respiratory illness; one of the most prevalent causes of the common cold

virus: an extremely small pathogen that can replicate only within a living cell

Causes and Symptoms

One of the reasons that no cure has ever been found for the common cold is that it is caused by literally hundreds of different viruses. More than two hundred distinct strains from eight genera have been identified, and no doubt more will be discovered. Infection by one of these viruses may confer immunity to it, but there will still be scores of others to which that individual is not immune. The common cold is usually restricted to the nose and surrounding areas-hence its medical name, rhinitis (*rhin* meaning "nose" and *itis* meaning "inflammation").

Children get the most colds, averaging six to eight per year until they are six years old. From that age, the number diminishes until, for adults, the rate is three to five colds per year. Colds and related respiratory diseases are the largest single cause of missed workdays and school days. Colds and related respiratory diseases are probably the world's most expensive illnesses. In the United States alone, about a million person-years are lost from work each year; this figure accounts for one-half of all absences. Worldwide, the costs of lost workdays, medications, physician's visits, and complications that may require extensive medical care are incalculable.

Among the virus types that cause the common cold are rhinovirus, coronavirus, influenza virus, parainfluenza virus, enterovirus, adenovirus, respiratory syncytial virus, and coxsackie virus. They are not all equally responsible for cold infections. Rhinoviruses and coronaviruses between them are thought to cause 25 to 60 percent of all colds. Rhinoviruses appear to be responsible for colds that occur in the peak cold seasons of late spring and early fall. Coronaviruses appear to be responsible for colds that occur when rhinovirus is less active, such as in the late fall, winter, and early spring. Enteroviruses are the most common cause of the "summer cold." During the summer months up to 20 percent of children may be shedding one of these viruses and thus are infective.

A respiratory syncytial virus can cause the common cold in adults; in children it causes much more severe diseases, including pneumonia and bronchiolitis (inflammation of the bronchioles, small air passages in the lungs). Similarly, influenza and parainfluenza viruses, adenoviruses, and enteroviruses can be responsible for rhinitis and sore throat, but they are also capable of causing more serious illnesses such as pneumonia and meningitis.

Viruses are the smallest of the invading microorganisms that cause disease, so small that they are not visible using ordinary microscopes. They can be seen, however, with an electron microscope, and their presence in the body can be detected through various laboratory tests.

Viruses vary enormously in their size and structure. Some consist of three or four proteins with a core of either deoxyribonucleic acid (DNA) or ribonucleic acid (RNA); some have more than fifty proteins and other substances.

> ### Information on Common Cold
> **Causes:** Viral infection
> **Symptoms:** Fatigue, runny or congested nose, muscle aches, sore throat, coughing, fever
> **Duration:** Typically several days
> **Treatments:** Bed rest, limiting physical stress, alleviation of symptoms via medications (antihistamines, decongestants, analgesics, cough medicines, etc.)

Viruses can replicate only within living cells. They invade the body and produce disease conditions in different ways. Some travel through the body to find their target host cells. A good example is the measles virus, which enters through the mucous membranes of the nose, throat, and mouth and then finds its way to target tissues throughout the body. Some, such as the viruses that cause the common cold, enter the body through the nasal passages and settle directly into nearby cells.

Rhinoviruses are members of the Picornaviridae family (*pico*- from "piccolo," meaning "very small"; *rna* from RNA, the genetic material that it contains; and *viridae* denoting a virus family). Coronaviruses are members of the Coronaviridae family, and they also contain RNA. Most viruses that are pathogenic to humans can thrive only at the temperature inside the human body, 37 degrees Celsius (98.6 degrees Fahrenheit). Rhinoviruses prefer the cooler temperatures found in the nasal passages, 33 to 34 degrees Celsius (91.4 to 93.2 degrees Fahrenheit). More than one hundred different rhinovirus types have been identified.

Exactly how a patient contracts a cold is better understood than it once was. Exposure to a cold environment-for example, getting a chill in winter weather-does not cause a cold unless the individual is exposed to the infecting virus at the same time. Fatigue or lack of sleep does not increase susceptibility to the cold virus, and even the direct exposure of nasal tissue to cold viruses does not guarantee infection.

A group in England, the Medical Research Council's Common Cold Unit, studied the disease from 1945 to 1990 and made many fundamental discoveries-even though the researchers never found a cure, or, for that matter, any effective methods to prevent the spread of the disease. As part of their research, they put drops containing cold virus into the noses of volunteers. Only about one-third of the subjects thus inoculated developed cold symptoms, showing that direct exposure to the infecting agent does not necessarily bring on a cold.

What appears to be essential in the spread of the disease is bodily contact, particularly handshaking or touching. The infected individual wipes his or her nose or coughs into his or her hand, getting nasal secretions on the fingers. These infected secretions are then transferred to the hand of another person who, if susceptible, can become infected by bringing the hand up to the mouth or nose. Sneezing and coughing also spread the disease. Many viral and bacterial diseases are transmissible through nasopharyngeal (nose and throat) secretions; these include measles, mumps, ru-

Sinus cavities:
frontal
maxillary
sphenoidal

The sinus cavities typically become congested with mucus as the body fights the virus that has caused the cold.

bella, pneumonia, influenza, and any number of other infections.

One or more individuals in a group become infected and bring the disease to a central place, such as a classroom, office, military base, or day care center. In the case of the common cold, transferring infected particles by touch exposes another person to the infection. In other respiratory diseases, breathing, sneezing, or coughing virus-laden particles into the air will spread the disease. The infected individual then becomes the means by which the disease is brought into the home. By far, the largest number of colds are brought into the family by children who have contracted the infection in classrooms or day care centers.

The pathogenesis of the common cold-that is, what happens when an individual is exposed to the cold virus-is not fully understood. It is believed that the virus enters the nasal passages and attaches itself to receptors on a cell of the nasal mucous membrane and then invades the cell. Viruses traveling freely in the blood or lymphatic system are subject to attack by white blood cells called phagocytes in what is part of the body's nonspecific defense system against invading pathogens.

Once inside the host cell, the virus replicates itself by stealing elements of the protoplasm of the cell and using them to build new viruses under the direction of the RNA component. These new viruses are released by the host cell to infect other cells. This process can injure or kill the host cell, activating the body's specific immune response system and starting the chain of events that will destroy the invading virus and create immunity to further infection from it.

In response to cell death or injury, certain chemicals are released that induce inflammation in the nasal passages. Blood vessels in the nasal area enlarge, increasing blood flow to the tissues and causing swelling. The openings in capillary walls enlarge and deliver lymphocytes, white blood cells that produce antibodies to fight the virus, as well as other specialized white blood cells.

Nasal mucosa swell and secretions increase, a condition medically known as rhinorrhea (-rrhea meaning "flowing," denoting the runny nose of the common cold). During the first few days of infection, these secretions are thin and watery. As the disease progresses and white blood cells are drawn to the area, the secretions become thicker and more purulent, that is, filled with pus. A sore throat is common, as is laryngitis, or inflammation of the larynx or voice box. Fever is not a usual symptom of the common cold, but a cough will often develop as excess mucus or phlegm builds up in the lungs and windpipe.

As mucus accumulates and clogs nasal passages, the body attempts to expel it by sneezing. In this process, impulses from the nose travel to the brain's "sneeze reflex center," where sneezing is triggered to help clear nasal passages. Similarly, as phlegm accumulates in the windpipe and bronchial tree of the lungs, a message is sent to the "cough reflex center" of the brain, where coughing is initiated to expel the phlegm.

The common cold is self-limiting and usually resolves within five to ten days, but there can be complications in some cases. Patients who have asthma or chronic bronchitis frequently develop bronchoconstriction (narrowing of the air passages in the lungs) as a result of a common cold. If severe purulent tracheitis and bronchitis develop, there may be a concomitant bacterial infection. In some patients, the infection may spread to other organs, such as the ears, where an infection called otitis media can develop. Sinusitis, infection of the cavities in the bone of the skull surrounding the nose, is common. If the invading organism spreads to the lungs, bronchitis or pneumonia may develop.

Other possible complications of the common cold depend on the individual virus. Rhinoviruses, usually limited to colds, may infrequently cause pneumonia in children.

In the News:
Gene Studies May Help Find a Treatment for the Common Cold

Genomic mapping has been completed for the human rhinovirus (HRV). In a collaborative effort among four research institutions, all ninety-nine strains of the common cold virus, the human rhinovirus (HRV), have been genetically sequenced. This data set provides an important baseline framework for future analysis of new HRVs that may be identified, according to the study authors Ann C. Palmenberg from the University of Wisconsin, and her colleagues at University of Maryland School of Medicine and the J. Craig Venter Institute in Rockville, Maryland. The database will help inform future research in the development of antiviral agents and vaccines.

Rhinoviruses can alter human genes. A University of Calgary study published in the *American Journal of Respiratory and Critical Care* in 2008 found that rhinoviruses causes cold symptoms not by triggering an immune response in the host, but by altering the host cellular genes that control inflammation and antiviral responses. The randomized study involved nasal scrapings from thirty-five healthy volunteers, half of whom were inoculated with rhinovirus. Changes in gene expression were analyzed for nasal scraping taken at eight and forty-eight hours after inoculation. While eight-hour samples found no differences in cellular genes between groups, the forty-eight-hour sample found more than 6,500 genes altered in the inoculation group when compared with the control group. Two affected groups of genes were genes involved in the inflammatory process and antiviral genes, according to study authors David Proud and colleagues. A faulty visperin gene, known to play a role in other viral infections such as influenza, hepatitis, and cytomegalovirus was identified. The identification of altered human genes associated with rhinovirus infection provides potential new direction for therapeutic research.

Poor sleep habits can reduce resistance to common cold. A study published in January, 2009, in the *Archives of Internal Medicine* by Sheldon Cohen and colleagues suggests there is a simple way to reduce the risk of acquiring the common cold. A study of 153 healthy men and women found that participants who got less than seven hours of sleep a night for fourteen consecutive nights were almost three times as likely to get a cold after receiving nasal drops containing rhinovirus. The researchers concluded that poor sleep habits reduce resistance to viruses such as the common cold virus.

—*Sandra Ripley Distelhorst*

Coronaviruses, also usually limited to colds, infrequently cause pneumonia and bronchiolitis. A respiratory syncytial virus causes pneumonia and bronchiolitis in children, the common cold in adults, and pneumonia in the elderly. Parainfluenza virus, which causes croup and other respiratory diseases in children, can cause sore throat and the common cold in adults and, rarely, may cause tracheobronchitis in these patients. Influenza B virus, an occasional cause of the common cold, also causes influenza and, infrequently, pneumonia.

Another condition that can closely resemble the common cold, but which is not caused by a virus, is allergic rhinitis. The major form of allergic rhinitis is hay fever. It has many of the same symptoms as the common cold: sneezing, runny nose, nasal congestion, and, sometimes, sore throat. In addition, the hay fever victim may suffer from itching in the eyes, nose, mouth, and throat. Hay fever is an allergic reaction to certain pollens. Because the pollens that cause hay fever are abundant at certain times of the year, it may be prevalent at the same times as some colds. Spring is a peak season for the common cold and also for hay fever, because of the many tree pollens that are carried in the air. In the fall, weed pollens, such as those of ragweed, affect hay-fever sufferers during another peak period for colds. Colds occur less frequently in summer, but summer is another peak season for hay fever.

Treatment and Therapy

The nose is the first barrier of defense against the bacteria and viruses that cause upper respiratory infections. The nasal cavity is lined with a thin coating of mucus, a thick liquid that is constantly replenished by the mucous glands. Inner nasal surfaces are filled with tiny hairs, or cilia. Dust, bacteria, and other foreign matter are trapped by the mucus and moved by the cilia toward the nasopharynx to be expectorated or swallowed.

The blood vessels in the nasopharyngeal bed respond automatically to stimulation from the brain. Certain stimuli cause the vessels to constrict, widening air passages and at the same time reducing the flow of mucus. Other stimuli, such as those that are sent in response to a viral infection, allergen, or other irritant, cause blood vessels to dilate and increase the flow of mucus. Nasal passages become swollen, and airways are blocked.

The mucus-covered lining of the nasal passages contains various substances that help ward off infection and irritation by allergens. Lysozyme (*lyso* meaning "dissolution" and *zyme* from "enzyme," a catalyst that promotes an activity) attacks the cell walls of certain bacteria, killing them. It also attacks pollen granules. Mucus also contains glycoproteins that temporarily inhibit the activity of viruses. Mucus has small amounts of the antibodies immunoglobulin IgA and IgC that also may inhibit the activity of invading viruses.

Bed rest is usually the first element of treatment for a common cold. Limiting physical stress may help keep the cold from worsening and may avoid secondary infections. The medications used to treat the common cold are directed at relieving individual symptoms; there is no available medication that will kill the viruses that cause it. Most cases of the common cold are treated at home with over-the-counter cold preparations. Children's colds and the complications that may arise from colds, such as bacterial and viral superinfection, may require the services of a physician.

Many medications for the common cold contain antihistamines. Histamine is a naturally occurring chemical in the body that is released in response to an allergen or an infection. It is a significant cause of the inflammation, swelling, and runny nose of hay fever. When these symptoms are seen with the common cold, however, they are probably caused by the body's inflammatory defense system rather than by histamine.

When antihistamines were first discovered, it was thought that they could inhibit the inflammatory defense against a cold. Patients were advised to take antihistamines at the first sign of a cold, in the hope of avoiding a full infection. Current thinking is that antihistamines have little value in the treatment of the common cold. They may have a minor effect on a runny nose, but there are better agents for this purpose. Antihistamines are usually highly sedative-most over-the-counter sleeping pills are antihistamines-so they may cause drowsiness. Patients taking many antihistamines are cautioned to avoid driving or operating machinery that could be dangerous.

The mainstays of therapy for the common cold are the decongestants that are applied topically (that is, directly to the mucous membranes in the nose) or taken orally. They are also called sympathomimetic agents because they mimic the effects of certain natural body chemicals that regulate many body processes. A group of these, called adrenergic stimulants, regulate vasoconstriction and vasodilation-in other words, they can narrow or widen blood vessels, respectively. Their vasoconstrictive capability is useful in managing the common cold, because it reduces the size of the blood vessels in the nose, reduces swelling and congestion, and inhibits excess secretion.

Topical decongestants are available as nasal sprays or drops. The sprays are squirted up into each nostril. The patient is usually advised to wait three to five minutes and then blow his or her nose to remove the mucus. If there is still congestion, the patient is advised to take another dose, allowing the medication to reach farther into the nasal cavity. Nose drops are taken by tilting the head back and squeezing the medication into the nostrils through the nose-dropper supplied with the medication. Clearance of nasal congestion is prompt, and the patient can breathe more easily. Nasal irritation is reduced, so there is less sneezing. Some nasal sprays and drops last longer than others, but none works around-the-clock, so applications must be repeated throughout the day.

Patients who use nasal sprays and drops are advised to follow the manufacturer's directions exactly. Applied too often or in too great a quantity, these preparations can cause unwanted problems, such as rhinitis medicamentosa, or nasal inflammation caused by a medication (also called rebound congestion). As the vasoconstrictive effect of the drugs wears down, the blood vessels dilate, the area becomes swollen, and secretions increase. This reaction may be attributable to the fact that the drug's vasoconstrictive effect has deprived the area of blood, and thus excited an increased inflammatory state, or it may simply be attributable to irritation by the drug. Use of sprays or drops should be limited to three or four days.

Oral decongestants are also effective in reducing swelling and relieving a runny nose, although they do not have as great a vasoconstrictive effect concentrated in the nasal area as sprays or drops. Because they circulate throughout the body, their vasoconstrictive effects may be seen in other vascular beds. Patients with high blood pressure; diabetes; heart disease; or who are taking certain drugs such as monoamine oxidase inhibitors (MAOIs), guanethidine, bethanidine, or debrisoquin sulfate are advised not to use oral decongestants unless they are under the care of a physician.

Three kinds of coughs may accompany colds: coughs that produce phlegm or mucus; hyperactive nagging coughs, which result from overstimulation of the cough reflex; and dry, unproductive coughs. If the phlegm or mucus collecting in the lungs is easily removed by occasional coughing, a soothing syrup, cough drop, or lozenge may be all that the patient requires. If the cough reflex center of the brain is overstimulated, there may be hyperactive or uncontrollable coughing, and a cough suppressant, such as dextromethorphan, may be needed. Dextromethorphan works in the brain to raise the level of stimulus that is required to trigger the cough reflex. Some antihistamines, such as diphenhydramine hydrochloride, are effective cough suppressants. If coughing is unproductive-that is, if the mucus has thickened and dried and is not easily removed-an expectorant should be taken. Currently, the only expectorant used in over-the-counter drugs is guaifenesin. It helps soften and liquefy mucus deposits, so that coughs become productive. When the cough of a cold is serious enough for a physician to be consulted, prescription drugs may need to be used, such as codeine to stop hyperactive coughing and potassium iodide for unproductive coughs.

For allergic rhinitis or hay fever, avoidance of allergens is recommended but is not always possible. For hay-fever outbreaks, antihistamines are the mainstays of therapy, with other agents added to relieve specific symptoms. For example, topical and oral decongestants may be required to relieve a runny nose.

Perspective and Prospects

Viruses are among the most intriguing and baffling challenges to medical science. Great progress has been made in preventing some virus diseases, such as by immunization against smallpox and hepatitis B. There has been only limited success, however, in finding agents to cure viral diseases, and so far nothing has been found to prevent or cure the common cold. Vaccines have been developed against certain rhinoviruses, and no doubt many more will be developed. Yet because the common cold is caused by so many different types of virus-more than two hundred-and vaccines against one virus are not necessarily effective against others, it is questionable whether such vaccines would ever be useful. A helpful vaccine would be one that could immunize against an entire family of viruses such as rhinoviruses or coronaviruses, the two leading causes of the common cold.

The search goes on for agents to cure the common cold. Substances, such as interferons, have been found that are effective against a wide range of viruses. One of the interferons was used by the British Medical Research Council's Common Cold Unit. Those researchers reported that interferon applied as an intranasal spray was effective in protecting subjects from cold infection. After some years, however, experimentation with interferon in the common cold was abandoned because the agent had significant side effects, nasal congestion among them.

The science of virology only began in the 1930s, so it is not surprising that viruses continue to baffle scientists. Nevertheless, many fundamental discoveries have been made and one can predict increasing success. As scientists unravel the intricacies of viral infections, they find clues that help them devise ways of interfering with virus life processes. In some cases, effective drugs have been developed, such as the interferons, acyclovir for herpes simplex, and amantadine for the influenza virus. It is likely that the cure for the common cold will continue to be elusive, unless a broad-spectrum antiviral agent could be developed that works against multiple viral infections in the way that broad-spectrum antibiotics work against multiple bacterial infections.

—*C. Richard Falcon*

See also Allergies; Antihistamines; Bronchitis; Coughing; Decongestants; Fever; Influenza; Nasopharyngeal disorders; Nausea and vomiting; Noroviruses; Otorhinolarnygology; Pneumonia; Rhinitis; Rhinoviruses; Sinusitis; Sore throat; Viral infections.

For Further Information:
Biddle, Wayne. *A Field Guide to Germs.* 2d ed. New York: Anchor Books, 2002.
Carson-DeWitt, Rosalyn. "Common Cold." *Health Library,* January 9, 2013.
"Common Cold." *National Institute of Allergy and Infectious Diseases,* February 11, 2011.
Gallo, Robert. *Virus Hunting.* New York: Basic Books, 1991.
Kimball, Chad T. *Colds, Flu, and Other Common Ailments Sourcebook.* Detroit, Mich.: Omnigraphics, 2001.
Krinsky, Daniel L., et al. *Handbook of Nonprescription Drugs.* 17th ed. Washington, D.C.:American Pharmaceutical Association, 2011.
Litin, Scott C., ed. *Mayo Clinic Family Health Book.* 4th ed. New York: HarperResource, 2009.
Woolf, Alan D., et al., eds. *The Children's Hospital Guide to Your Child's Health and Development.* Cambridge, Mass.: Perseus, 2002.
Young, Stuart H., Bruce Dobozin, and Margaret Miner. *Allergies.* Rev. ed. New York: Plume, 1999.

Computed tomography (CT) scanning
Procedure
Also known as: Computed axial tomography, CAT scan
Anatomy or system affected: Circulatory system, endocrine

system, gastrointestinal system, musculoskeletal system, nervous system, reproductive system, respiratory system

Specialties and related fields: Biotechnology, cardiology, emergency medicine, endocrinology, gastroenterology, internal medicine, oncology, preventive medicine, psychiatry, radiology, vascular medicine

Definition: The use of X rays and a computer to produce detailed cross-sectional images of most body regions to aid in diagnosis.

Key terms:

cathode: an electrode that produces electrons

cathode-ray tube (CRT): a vacuum tube whose cathode emits electrons accelerated through a high voltage anode, focused on a fluorescent image screen

slice: a CT cross section of a body part

soft tissue: tissue other than bone

tomogram: the three-dimensional image of a CT slice

X ray: high-energy electromagnetic radiation

Indications and Procedures

Computed tomography (CT) scanning collects X-ray data and uses a computer to produce three-dimensional images, called tomograms, of body cross sections, or slices. The noninvasiveness of CT scanning yields easy and safe body part analysis based on varying tissue opacity to X-rays. Bone absorbs X-rays well and appears white. Air absorbs them poorly, so the lungs are dark. Fat, blood, and muscle absorb X-rays to varying extents, yielding different shades of gray. Tumors and blood clots, for example, appear as areas of abnormal shades in normal tissue.

CT scanning is used to analyze disorders of the brain (brain CT) and most body parts (body CT), yielding tomograms that are hundreds of times more definitive than conventional X-rays. For example, conventional abdominal X-rays show bones and faintly outline the liver, kidneys, and stomach. Tomograms clearly depict all abdominal organs

In the imaging technique called computed tomography (CT) scanning (formerly known as a CAT scan), multiple X-ray pictures are taken as the scanner tilts and rotates around the patient. These images are then assembled by a computer to create a three-dimensional view of a body part, such as the head.

and large blood vessels.

Physicians call CT scanning the most valuable diagnostic method because, without it, the symptoms that patients describe may not be identified clearly as minor, serious, or life-threatening. For example, a subjective description of repeated headache does not reveal whether the cause is tension, stroke, or brain cancer. Before CT scanning, an accurate diagnosis often required complex or dangerous identification methods.

A CT patient changes into a hospital gown, removes any metal possessions, and lays on a table that can be raised, lowered, or tilted. During a scan, the patient enters a doughnut-shaped scanner that holds an X-ray source, detectors, and computer hookups. In brain CT, the patient's head is in the scanner. Some CT patients have experienced claustrophobia, which can be prevented with faster scanner speeds and less-enclosed scanners. A patient who must stay still for an extended time may be given a sedative. If small anomalies are foreseen, then contrast materials are given before or during the procedure. These materials include barium salts and iodine, X-ray blockers that allow better visualization of specific tissues. Subjects may take the materials orally, by enema, or intravenously.

The CT scanner generates a continuous, narrow X-ray beam while moving in a circle around the patient's head or body. The beam is monitored by X-ray detectors sited around the aperture through which the patient passes. Slices are produced as the scanner circles the head or body. Between slices, the table moves through the scanner. Slices become tomograms seen on a cathode-ray tube (CRT) and are stored in a computer. The procedure used to take twenty to forty minutes in a standard scanner. However, in the newer spiral CT, which is now standard in most hospitals, a patient is scanned rapidly as the X-ray tube rotates in a spiral. There are no gaps, as with slices, and tissue-volume tomograms are produced. A simple spiral scan is completed while the patient holds his or her breath, aiding the detection of small lesions and decreasing scan artifacts. Spiral CT, twenty times faster than standard CT, is useful in all patients, from restless children to the critically ill.

Uses and Complications

CT scanning detects organ abnormalities, and a major use is in diagnosing and treating brain disease. Even the earliest scanners could distinguish tumors from clots, aiding in the diagnosis of cancer, stroke, and certain birth defects. Furthermore, brain CT saves lives as physicians avoid risky methods requiring opening of the brain for pretreatment diagnosis. In addition, postsurgical scans can find recurrences or metastases.

Body CT allows for better damage appraisal of broken bones than does conventional X-ray analysis. Another use of body spiral CT is in the diagnosis of pulmonary embolism; it is safer than using pulmonary angiography, which maneuvers a catheter from the heart to the pulmonary artery. CT scans can also guide surgery, biopsy, and abscess drainage and can help fine-tune radiation therapy. Speed and excellent soft tissue elucidation make CT scanning in-

A doctor can use CT scans to detect abnormalities in brain tissue, such as tumors. (Digital Stock)

valuable for trauma detection in emergency rooms.

There are few side effects to CT scanning. Preparation for a scan may be mildly uncomfortable, but it is rarely dangerous. Before body CT, subjects often fast, take enemas to clear the bowels, and receive contrast materials through enemas or IVs. If contrast materials are used, then physicians must be told of allergies, especially to iodine. Contrast materials-enhancers of specific tissue CT-may cause hot flashes. Barium enemas for lower gastrointestinal tract scans cause full feelings and urges to defecate.

Perspective and Prospects

British engineer Godfrey Hounsfield and American physicist Allan Cormack won the 1979 Nobel Prize in Physiology or Medicine for the theory and development of computed tomography. CT scanning was first used in 1972, after Hounsfeld made a brain scanner holding an X-ray generator, a scanner rotated around a circular chamber, a computer, and a CRT. The patient laid on a gurney, head in the scanner, and emitter detectors rotated 1 degree at a time for 180 degrees. At each position, 160 readings entered the computer, so 28,800 readings were processed.

CT scanning is essential to radiology, which began in 1885 after Wilhelm Conrad Röntgen discovered X-rays. The rays soon became medical aids, and for years broad X-ray beams were sent through body parts to exit onto film, yielding conventional X-ray images. Bones absorb X-rays well, appearing white, and conventional images can show bone fractures and give some soft tissue data. However, soft tissue evaluation is poor, the tissues superimpose, and estimating their condition is difficult. CT scans allow convenient, noninvasive analysis.

CT scans and stereotaxic neurosurgery, later joined, have improved diagnosis and treatment. For example, the implantation of electrodes in a brain can be monitored using CT, enhancing accuracy. Similar techniques are used in breast biopsy. Current progress in CT scans includes thinner slices, spiral scans, and fast-operating standard scanners. Because complex scans expose patients to more radiation than do conventional X-rays, fast scans are preferred to minimize patient risk.

—*Sanford S. Singer, Ph.D.*

See also Brain; Brain disorders; Headaches; Imaging and radiology; Magnetic resonance imaging (MRI); Neuroimaging; Noninvasive tests; Nuclear medicine; Positron emission tomography (PET) scanning; Single photon emission computed tomography (SPECT); Strokes; Tumors; Ultrasonography.

For Further Information:

"CT Scans." *MedlinePlus*, June 12, 2013.

Durham, Deborah L. *Rad Tech's Guide to CT: Imaging Procedures, Patient Care, and Safety.* Malden, Mass.: Blackwell Scientific, 2002.

Hsieh, Jiang. *Computed Tomography: Principles, Design, Artifacts, and Recent Advances.* 2d ed. Bellingham, Wash.: SPIE Press, 2009.

Kalender, Willi A. *Computed Tomography: Fundamentals, System Technology, Image Quality, Applications.* 3rd ed. Weinheim, Germany: Wiley VCH, 2009.

McCoy, Krisha, and Brian Randall. "CT Scan (General)." *Health Library*, Nov. 26, 2012.

"Radiation-Emitting Products: Full-Body CT Scans" What You Need to Know." *US Food and Drug Administration*, Apr. 6, 2010.

Slone, Richard M., et al., eds. *Body CT: A Practical Approach.* New York: McGraw-Hill, 2000.

Conception

Biology

Anatomy or system affected: Cells, reproductive system, uterus

Specialties and related fields: Embryology, gynecology, obstetrics

Definition: The process of creating new life, encompassing all the events from deposition of sperm into the female to the first cell divisions of the fertilized ovum.

Key terms:

cervix: the lowest part of the uterus in contact with the vagina; contains an opening filled with mucus through which sperm can pass

ejaculation: the reflex activated by sexual stimulation that results in sperm mixed with fluid being expelled from the male's body

fertilization: the union of the sperm and the ovum, which usually occurs in the female's oviduct

menstruation: the process of shedding the lining of the uterus that occurs about once a month

oviduct: the thin tube that leads from near the ovary to the upper part of the uterus; also called the Fallopian tube

ovulation: the process by which the mature ovum is expelled from the ovary

ovum: the round cell produced by the female that carries her genetic material; also called the egg

sperm: the motile cells produced within the male that carry his genetic material

uterus: the organ above the vagina through which the sperm must pass on their way to the ovum; also called the womb

vagina: the stretchy, tube-shaped structure into which the male's penis is inserted during intercourse; the site of sperm deposition

Process and Effects

The process of conception begins with the act of intercourse. When the male's penis is inserted into the female's vagina, the stimulation of the penis by movement within the vagina triggers a reflex resulting in the ejaculation of sperm. During ejaculation, involuntary muscles in many of the male reproductive organs contract, causing semen, a mixture of sperm and fluid, to move from its sites of storage out through the urethra within the penis.

The average volume of semen in a typical human ejaculation is only 3.5 milliliters, but this small volume normally contains two hundred million to four hundred million sperm. Other constituents of semen include prostaglandins, which cause contractions of involuntary muscles in both the male and the female; the sugar fructose, which provides energy to the sperm; chemicals that adjust the activity of

the semen; and a number of enzymes and other chemicals.

In a typical act of intercourse, the semen is deposited high up in the woman's vagina. Within a minute after ejaculation, the semen begins to coagulate, or form a clot, because of the activation of chemicals within the semen. Sperm are not able to leave the vagina until the semen becomes liquid again, which occurs spontaneously fifteen to twenty minutes after ejaculation.

Once the semen liquefies, sperm begin moving through the female system. The path to the ovum (if one is present) lies through the cervix, then through the hollow cavity of the uterus, and up through the oviduct, where fertilization normally occurs. The sperm are propelled through the fluid within these organs by the swimming movements of their tails called flagella, as well as by female organ contractions that are stimulated by the act of intercourse and by prostaglandins contained in the semen. The contractions allow sperm to reach the oviduct within five minutes after leaving the vagina, a rate of movement that far exceeds their own swimming abilities.

Although some sperm can reach the oviduct quite rapidly, others never enter the oviduct at all. Of the two hundred million to four hundred million sperm deposited in the vagina, it is estimated that only one hundred to one thousand enter the oviducts. Some of the other millions of sperm may be defective, lacking the proper swimming ability. Other apparently normal sperm may become lost within the female's organs, possibly trapped in clefts between cells in the organ linings. The damaged and lost sperm will eventually be destroyed by white blood cells produced by the female.

Sperm movement through the female system is enhanced around the time of ovulation. For example, at the time of ovulation, the hormones associated with ovulation cause changes in the cervical mucus that aid sperm transport. The

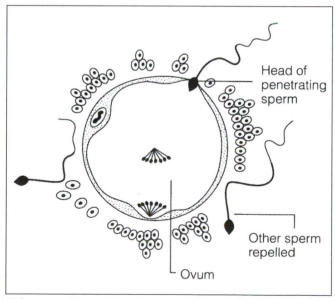

Male sperm cells propel themselves toward the ovum (female egg) by the swimming movements of their tails; fertilization occurs when a sperm cell penetrates the layers surrounding the ovum and fuses its membrane with the membrane of the ovum.

mucus at that time is extremely liquid and contains fibers that align themselves into channels, which are thought to be used by the sperm to ease their passage through the cervix. The hormones present at the time of ovulation also increase the contractions produced by the uterus and oviduct, and thus sperm transport through the structures is enhanced as well.

During transport through the female system, sperm undergo a number of important chemical changes, collectively called capacitation, that enable them to fertilize the ovum successfully. Freshly ejaculated sperm are not capable of penetrating the layers surrounding the ovum, a fact that was uncovered when scientists first began to experiment with in vitro fertilization (the joining of sperm and ovum outside the body). Capacitation apparently occurs during transport of the sperm through the uterus and possibly the oviduct, and it is presumably triggered by some secretion of the female reproductive system. With in vitro fertilization, capacitation is achieved by adding female blood serum to the dish that contains the sperm and ovum. Capacitation is not instantaneous; it has been estimated that this process requires an hour or more in humans. Even though the first sperm may arrive in the vicinity of the ovum within twenty minutes after ejaculation, fertilization cannot take place until capacitation is completed. In 2003, scientists discovered that sperm has a type of chemical sensor that causes the sperm to swim vigorously toward concentrations of a chemical attractant. While researchers long have known that chemical signals are an important component of conception, the 2003 findings were the first to demonstrate that sperm will respond in a predictable and controllable way, a fact promising for future contraception and fertility research.

The site where ovum and sperm typically come together is within the oviduct. At the time of ovulation, an ovum is released from the surface of the ovary and drawn into the upper end of the oviduct. Once within the oviduct, the ovum is propelled by contractions of the oviduct and possibly by wavelike motions of cilia, hairlike projections that line the inner surface of the oviduct. It takes about three days for the ovum to travel the entire length of the oviduct to the uterus, and since the ovum only remains fertilizable for twelve to twenty-four hours, successful fertilization must occur in the oviduct.

Upon reaching the ovum, the sperm must first penetrate two layers surrounding it. The outermost layer, called the corona radiata, consists of cells that break away from the ovary with the ovum during ovulation; the innermost layer, the zona pellucida, is a clear, jellylike substance that lies just outside the ovum cell membrane. Penetration of these two layers is accomplished by the release of enzymes carried by the sperm. Once through the zona pellucida, the sperm are ready to fertilize the ovum.

Fertilization occurs when a sperm fuses its membrane with the membrane of the ovum. This act triggers a protective change in the zona pellucida that prevents any additional sperm from reaching the ovum and providing it with extra chromosomes. Following fusion of the fertilizing

sperm and ovum, the chromosomes of each become mingled and pair up; the resulting one-celled zygote contains a complete set of chromosomes, half contributed by the mother and half by the father.

It is at the moment of fertilization that the sex of the new child is decided. Genetic sex is determined by a pair of chromosomes denoted X and Y. Female body cells contain two Xs, and each ovum produced contains only one X. Male body cells contain an X and a Y chromosome, but each sperm contains either an X or a Y chromosome. Men usually produce equal numbers of X- and Y-type sperm. The sex of the new individual is determined by which type of sperm fertilizes the ovum: If it is a Y-bearing sperm, the new individual will be male, and if it is an X-bearing sperm, the new individual will be female. Since entry of more than one sperm is prohibited, the first sperm to reach the ovum is the one that will fertilize it.

Following fertilization, the zygote or early embryo begins a series of cell divisions while it travels down the oviduct. When it arrives at the uterus about three days after ovulation, the zygote will be in the form of a hollow ball of cells called a blastocyte. Initially, this ball of cells floats in the fluid-filled cavity of the uterus, but two or three days after its arrival in the uterus (five to six days after ovulation), it will attach to the uterine lining. In 2003, researchers made an exciting discovery when they identified how embryos stop and burrow into the lining of a woman's uterus. A protein, called L-selectin, on the surface of the embryo acts like a puzzle piece when it touches and quickly locks into carbohydrate molecules found on the uterine surface. This implantation process must occur in exact synchrony during a very short time in a woman's cycle. (If it occurs outside the uterus, usually in one of the Fallopian tubes, then the result is an ectopic pregnancy, which is often a medical emergency.) In the weeks following conception, the cells of the zygote will form the fetus and the placenta, which surrounds and provides nutrients to the fetus. Over the next nine months, the fetus will increasingly take on a human form, developing muscle tissue, bone, organs, and skin. Pregnancy typically lasts for forty weeks from conception until childbirth..

Complications and Disorders

Three factors limit the time frame in which conception is possible: the fertilizable lifetime of the ovulated ovum, estimated to be between twelve and twenty-four hours; the fertilizable lifetime of ejaculated sperm in the female tract, usually assumed to be about forty-eight hours; and the time required for sperm capacitation, which is one hour or more. The combination of these factors determines the length of the fertile period, the time during which intercourse must occur if conception is to be achieved. Taking the three factors into account, the fertile period is said to extend from forty-eight hours prior to ovulation until perhaps twenty-four hours after ovulation. For example, if intercourse occurs forty-eight hours before ovulation, the sperm will be capacitated in the first few hours and will still be within their fertilizable lifetime when ovulation occurs. On the other hand, if intercourse occurs twenty-four hours after ovulation, the sperm will still require time for capacitation, but the ovum will be near the end of its viable period. Thus the later limit of the fertile period is equal to the fertilizable lifetime of the ovum, minus the time required for capacitation.

Obviously, a critical factor in conception is the timing of ovulation. In a typical twenty-eight-day menstrual cycle, ovulation occurs about halfway through the cycle, or fourteen days after the first day of menstrual bleeding. In actuality, cycle length varies widely from month to month. It appears that generally the first half of the cycle is more variable in length, with the second half more stable. Thus, no matter how long the entire menstrual cycle is, ovulation usually occurs fourteen days prior to the first day of the next episode of menstrual bleeding. Therefore, it is relatively easy to determine when ovulation occurred by counting backward, but difficult to predict the time of ovulation in advance.

Assessment of ovulation time in women is notoriously difficult. There is no easily observable outward sign of ovulation. Some women do detect slight abdominal pain about the time of ovulation; this is referred to as *Mittelschmerz*, which means, literally, pain in the middle of the cycle. This slight pain may be localized on either side of the abdomen and is thought to be caused by irritation of the abdominal organs by fluid released from the ovary during ovulation. Other signs of ovulation are an increased volume of the cervical mucus and flexibility of the cervix and a characteristic fernlike pattern of the mucus when it is dried on a glass slide. There is also a slight rise in body temperature after ovulation, which again makes it easier to determine the time of ovulation after the fact rather than in advance. It is also possible to measure the amount of luteinizing hormone (LH) in urine or blood; this hormone shows a marked increase about sixteen hours prior to ovulation. Home test kits to detect LH levels are available for urine samples. There are additional signs of the time of ovulation, such as a slight opening of the cervix and a change in the cells lining the vagina, that can be used by physicians to determine the timing and occurrence of ovulation.

Since ovulation time is so difficult to detect in most women on an ongoing basis, most physicians would counsel that, to achieve a pregnancy, couples should plan on having intercourse every two days. This frequency will ensure that sperm capable of fertilization are always present, so that the exact time of ovulation becomes unimportant. A greater frequency of intercourse is not advised, since sperm numbers are reduced when ejaculation occurs often. Approximately 85 to 90 percent of couples will achieve pregnancy within a year when intercourse occurs about three times a week.

Couples often wonder if it is possible to predetermine the sex of their child by some action taken in conjunction with intercourse. Scientists have found no consistent effect of diet, position assumed during intercourse, timing of intercourse within the menstrual cycle, or liquids that are introduced into the vagina to kill one type of sperm selectively. In the laboratory, it is possible to achieve partial separation of sperm in a semen sample by subjecting the semen to an electric current or other procedure due to the physical difference of X- and Y-containing sperm. The separated sperm can then be used for artificial insemination (the introduction of semen through a tube into the uterus). This method is not 100 percent successful in producing offspring of the desired sex and so is available only on an experimental basis.

Some couples have difficulty in conceiving a child, in a few cases as a result of some problem associated with intercourse. For example, the male may have difficulty in achieving erection or ejaculation. The vast majority of these cases are caused by psychological factors such as stress and tension rather than any physiological problem. Fortunately, therapists can teach couples how to overcome these psychological problems.

About 10 to 15 percent of couples suffer from some type of biological infertility-that is, infertility that persists for more than one year when intercourse occurs successfully. In about 10 to 20 percent of the cases of infertility, doctors are unable to establish a cause. About one-third of infertility cases are caused by the female partner's problems, while another one-third of infertility cases are caused by the male partner's problems. The remaining cases of infertility are caused by both male and female problems or are unexplained..

In men, the most commonly diagnosed cause of infertility is low sperm count. Sometimes low sperm count is caused by a treatable imbalance of hormones. If not treatable, this problem can sometimes be circumvented by the use of pooled semen samples in artificial insemination or through in vitro fertilization. In vitro fertilization may also be a solution for men who produce normal numbers of sperm but whose sperm lack swimming ability. Another cause of male infertility is blockage of the tubes that carry the semen from the body, which may be caused by a previous infection. Surgery is sometimes successful in removing such a blockage. Another problem, called varicocele, occurs when the veins on the testicle are too large or do not properly circulate blood. This causes the testicles to overheat, which may affect the number or the viability of the sperm. Varicocelectomy, the surgical correction of this problem, may be performed on an outpatient basis.

In women, a common cause of infertility is a hormonal problem that interferes with ovulation. Polycystic ovarian syndrome (PCOS) is a hormone imbalance that affects normal ovulation and is the most common cause of female infertility. Women with PCOS typically have high levels of androgens and many ovarian cysts. Treatment with one of a number of so-called fertility drugs may be successful in promoting ovulation. Clomiphene, a selective estrogen receptor modulator (SERM), is the most commonly prescribed fertility medication. Fertility drugs, however, have some disadvantages: They have a tendency to cause ovulation of more than one ovum, thus raising the possibility of multiple pregnancy, which is considered risky; and they may alter the environment of the uterus, making implantation of a resulting embryo less likely. Therefore, other causes of infertility, both male and female, should be ruled out before fertility drugs are used.

Another common cause of female infertility is blockage of the oviducts or the fallopian tubes resulting from scar tissue formation in the aftermath of some type of infection or prior surgery. Because surgery is not always successful, this condition may require the use of in vitro fertilization or the new technique of surgically introducing ova and sperm directly into the oviduct at a point below the blockage. Another cause of female infertility is an abnormally shaped uterus, which may interfere with the fertilized egg's ability to attach to the uterine wall. Uterine fibroids, noncancerous growths in the uterus, are very common among women and most often cause no symptoms; however, in certain cases, uterine fibroids can make it difficult for the fertilized egg to attach to the uterine wall. Surgery may be performed to shrink or remove the fibroids.

Finally, some cases of infertility result from biological incompatibility between the man and the woman. It may be that the sperm are unable to penetrate the cervical mucus, or perhaps that the woman's immune system treats the sperm cells as foreign, destroying them before they can reach the ovum. Techniques such as artificial insemination and in vitro fertilization offer hope for couples experiencing these problems.

Perspective and Prospects

For most of history, the events surrounding conception were poorly understood. For example, microscopic identification of sperm did not occur until 1677, and the ovum was not identified until 1827 (although the follicle in which the ovum develops was recognized in the seventeenth century). Prior to these discoveries, people held the belief espoused by early writers such as Aristotle and Galen that conception resulted from the mixing of male and female fluids during intercourse.

There was also confusion about the timing of the fertile period. Some early doctors thought that menstrual blood was involved in conception and therefore believed that the fertile period coincided with menstruation. Others recognized that menstrual bleeding was a sign that pregnancy had not occurred; they assumed that the most likely time for conception to result was immediately after the menstrual flow ceased. It was not until the 1930s that the first scientific studies on the timing of ovulation were completed.

Since there was little scientific understanding of the processes involved in conception, medical practice for most of human history was little different from magic, revolving around the use of rituals and herbal treatments to aid or prevent conception. Gradually, people rejected these practices, often because of religious teachings. By the twentieth century, conception had been established as an area of intense privacy, thought by physicians and the general public to be unsuitable for medical intervention.

In the early part of the twentieth century, the role of physicians in aiding conception was mostly limited to educating and advising couples finding difficulty in conceiving. There were few techniques, other than artificial insemination and fertility drug treatment, available to assist in conception at that time.

The situation changed with the first successful in vitro fertilization in 1978. This event ushered in an era of intense medical and public interest in assisting conception. Other methods to aid conception were soon introduced, including embryo transfer, frozen storage of embryos, and surgical placement of ova and sperm directly into the oviduct.

Paralleling the development of these techniques has been demand on the part of society for medicine to apply them. In most developed countries, infertility rates have been gradually increasing. One reason for increased infertility has been the increasing age at which couples decide to start a family, since the fertility of women appears to undergo a decline past the age of thirty-five. Another factor affecting fertility rates of both men and women has been an increased incidence of various sexually transmitted diseases, which can result in chronic inflammation of the reproductive organs and infertility caused by scar tissue formation.

People's attitudes toward medical intervention in conception have also changed. The earlier taboos against interference in conception have been somewhat relaxed, although some individuals still do not approve of certain methods of fertility management. Although there remain ethical issues to be resolved, the general public seems to have accepted the idea that medicine should provide assistance to those who wish to, but cannot, conceive children.

—Marcia Watson-Whitmyre, Ph.D.;
updated by Alexander Sandra, M.D.

See also Assisted reproductive technologies; Childbirth; Cloning; Contraception; Gamete intrafallopian transfer (GIFT); Gynecology; In vitro fertilization; Infertility, female; Infertility, male; Menstruation; Multiple births; Obstetrics; Pregnancy and gestation; Reproductive system; Sperm banks; Uterus.

For Further Information:

Doherty, C. Maud, and Melanie M. Clark. *Fertility Handbook: A Guide to Getting Pregnant.* Omaha, Nebr.: Addicus Books, 2002.

Harkness, Carla. *The Infertility Book: A Comprehensive Medical and Emotional Guide.* Rev 2d ed. Berkeley, Calif.: Celestial Arts, 1992.

"Infertility." *Medline Plus,* February 26, 2012.

"Infertility Fact Sheet." *US Department of Health and Human Services-Office on Women's Health,* July 16, 2012.

"In Vitro Fertilization (IVF)." *Medline Plus,* February 26, 2012.

Jones, Richard E., and Kristin H. Lopez. *Human Reproductive Biology.* 4th ed. Burlington, Mass.: Academic Press/Elsevier, 2013.

Kearney, Brian. *High-Tech Conception: A Comprehensive Handbook for Consumers.* New York: Bantam Books, 1998.

"Pregnancy: Condition Information." *Eunice Kennedy Shriver National Institute of Child Health and Human Development,* April 3, 2013.

Weschler, Toni. *Taking Charge of Your Fertility.* Rev. ed. New York: Collins, 2006.

Wisot, Arthur L., and David R. Meldrum. *Conceptions and Misconceptions: The Informed Consumer's Guide Through the Maze of In Vitro Fertilization and Other Assisted Reproduction Techniques.* 2d ed. Point Roberts, Wash.: Hartley & Marks, 2004.

SALEM HEALTH

MAGILL'S MEDICAL GUIDE

Entries by Anatomy or System Affected

Vitamin D deficiency
Vitamins and minerals
Well-baby examinations
Wounds
Xenotransplantation
Zoonoses

ABDOMEN
Abdominal disorders
Adrenalectomy
Amebiasis
Amniocentesis
Aneurysmectomy
Appendectomy
Appendicitis
Back pain
Bariatric surgery
Bladder removal
Bypass surgery
Campylobacter infections
Candidiasis
Cesarean section
Cholecystectomy
Cholecystitis
Colitis
Colon
Colon therapy
Colorectal cancer
Colorectal polyp removal
Colorectal surgery
Constipation
Culdocentesis
Cushing's syndrome
Diabetes mellitus
Dialysis
Diarrhea and dysentery
Digestion
Diverticulitis and diverticulosis
Eating disorders
Electrolysis
Endoscopic retrograde
   cholangiopancreatography (ERCP)
Endoscopy
Enemas
Fallopian tube
Fistula repair
Gallbladder
Gallbladder diseases
Gastrectomy
Gastroenteritis
Gastroenterology
Gastrointestinal disorders
Gastrointestinal system
Gastrostomy
Gaucher's disease
Gluten
Hernia
Hernia repair
Ileostomy and colostomy
Incontinence
Internal medicine

Intestinal disorders
Intestines
Irritable bowel syndrome (IBS)
Kidney transplantation
Kidneys
Laparoscopy
Liposuction
Lithotripsy
Liver
Liver transplantation
Mesothelioma
Nephrectomy
Nephrology
Obesity
Pancreas
Pancreatitis
Peristalsis
Peritonitis
Polyps
Pregnancy and gestation
Prostate cancer
Reproductive system
Roseola
Shunts
Small intestine
Splenectomy
Stents
Sterilization
Stevens-Johnson syndrome
Stomach
Stone removal
Stones
Tubal ligation
Tularemia
Ulcerative colitis
Ultrasonography
Urinary disorders
Urinary system
Urology
Vaginal birth after cesarean (VBAC)
Vasculitis
Virtual imaging

ANUS
Amebiasis
Anal cancer
Colon therapy
Colorectal polyp removal
Colorectal surgery
Endoscopy
Enemas
Episiotomy
Fistula repair
Hemorrhoid banding and removal
Hemorrhoids
Hirschsprung's disease
Human papillomavirus (HPV)
Intestinal disorders
Intestines
Irritable bowel syndrome (IBS)
Polyps

Rape and sexual assault
Rectum
Soiling
Sphincterectomy
Syphilis
Ulcerative colitis

ARMS
Amputation
Auras
Carpal tunnel syndrome
Casts and splints
Charcot-Marie-Tooth Disease
Cornelia de Lange syndrome
Cutis marmorata telangiectatica
   congenita
Diabetic neuropathy
Dyskinesia
Electrolysis
Fracture and dislocation
Fracture repair
Gigantism
Hand hygiene compliance
Hemiplegia
Liposuction
Muscles
Neonatal brachial plexus palsy
Phlebotomy
Pityriasis alba
Quadriplegia
Roseola
Rotator cuff surgery
Sarcoma
Skin lesion removal
Slipped disk
Spinocerebellar ataxia
Streptococcal infections
Tendinitis
Thalidomide
Tremors
Upper extremities

BACK
Ankylosing spondylitis
Back pain
Bone disorders
Bone marrow transplantation
Bones and the skeleton
Braces
Chiropractic
Cushing's syndrome
Disk removal
Dwarfism
Electrolysis
Juvenile rheumatoid arthritis
Kyphosis
Laminectomy and spinal fusion
Neuroimaging
Pityriasis alba
Pityriasis rosea
Sarcoma

Sciatica
Scoliosis
Slipped disk
Spine, vertebrae, and disks
Stevens-Johnson syndrome
Streptococcal infections
Sympathectomy
Tendon disorders

BLADDER
Abdomen
Abdominal disorders
Bed-wetting
Bladder cancer
Bladder removal
Candidiasis
Catheterization
Cystitis
Cystoscopy
Diabetic nephropathy
Diuretics
Endoscopy
Fetal surgery
Fistula repair
Hematuria
Incontinence
Internal medicine
Lithotripsy
Polyps
Pyelonephritis
Schistosomiasis
Smoking
Sphincterectomy
Stone removal
Stones
Toilet training
Ultrasonography
Uremia
Urethritis
Urinalysis
Urinary disorders
Urinary system
Urology
Williams syndrome

BLOOD
Acquired immunodeficiency syndrome
  (AIDS)
Anemia
Angiography
Antibodies
Aspergillosis
Avian influenza
Babesiosis
Biological therapies
Bleeding
Blood pressure
Blood testing
Blood vessels
Bone marrow transplantation
Bulimia

Candidiasis
Carbohydrates
Circulation
Cold agglutinin disease
Connective tissue
Cushing's syndrome
Cyanosis
Cytomegalovirus (CMV)
Deep vein thrombosis
Defibrillation
Dialysis
Dirofilaria immitis
Disseminated intravascular coagulation
  (DIC)
Diuretics
E. coli infection
Ebola virus
End-stage renal disease
Epstein-Barr virus
Ergogenic aids
Fetal surgery
Fetal tissue transplantation
Fistula repair
Fluids and electrolytes
Folate deficiency
Glycolysis
Gulf War syndrome
Heart
Hematocrit
Hematology
Hematomas
Hematuria
Hemoglobin
Hemolytic uremic syndrome
Hemophilia
Histiocytosis
Host-defense mechanisms
Hyperbaric oxygen therapy
Hypercholesterolemia
Hyperlipidemia
Hypoglycemia
Immune system
Immunization and vaccination
Jaundice
Laboratory tests
Leukemia
Liver
Lymph
Malaria
Menorrhagia
Methicillin-resistant staphylococcus
  aureus (MRSA) infection
Nephrology
Pharmacology
Phenylketonuria (PKU)
Phlebotomy
Plasma
Pulse rate
Rh factor
Salmonella infection
Schistosomiasis

Septicemia
Serology
Sickle cell disease
Single photon emission computed
  tomography (SPECT)
Snakebites
Staphylococcal infections
Sturge-Weber syndrome
Subdural hematoma
Thalassemia
Thrombocytopenia
Thrombolytic therapy and TPA
Thrombosis and thrombus
Thymus gland
Transfusion
Transplantation
Ultrasonography
Uremia
Von Willebrand's disease
Wiskott-Aldrich syndrome
Yellow fever

BLOOD VESSELS
Aneurysms
Angiography
Angioplasty
Anticoagulants
Arteriosclerosis
Avian influenza
Bedsores
Bile
Bleeding
Blood and blood disorders
Blood pressure
Blood testing
Blood vessels
Bruises
Bypass surgery
Carotid arteries
Catheterization
Cholesterol
Circulation
Claudication
Cluster headaches
Cold agglutinin disease
Cutis marmorata telangiectatica
  congenita
Deep vein thrombosis
Defibrillation
Diabetes mellitus
Disseminated intravascular coagulation
  (DIC)
Diuretics
Dizziness and fainting
Edema
Electrocauterization
Embolism
Embolization
End-stage renal disease
Endarterectomy
Erectile dysfunction

Eye infections and disorders
Facial transplantation
Hammertoe correction
Heart
Heart disease
Heat exhaustion and heatstroke
Hemangioma
Hematomas
Hemoglobin
Hemorrhoid banding and removal
Hemorrhoids
Hormone therapy
Hypercholesterolemia
Hypertension
Hypotension
Infarction
Intravenous (IV) therapy
Ischemia
Kawasaki disease
Klippel-Trenaunay syndrome
Leptospirosis
Methicillin-resistant staphylococcus
  aureus (MRSA) infection
Necrotizing fasciitis
Nephritis
Neuroimaging
Obesity
Phlebitis
Phlebotomy
Plaque
Plasma
Polycystic kidney disease
Polydactyly and syndactyly
Postural orthostatic tachycardia
  syndrome (POTS)
Pulse rate
Raynaud's Phenomenon
Rocky Mountain spotted fever
Roundworms
Schistosomiasis
Scleroderma
Scurvy
Single photon emission computed
  tomography (SPECT)
Stenosis
Stents
Strokes
Sturge-Weber syndrome
Temporal arteritis
Thalidomide
Thrombolytic therapy and TPA
Thrombosis and thrombus
Toxemia
Transient ischemic attacks (TIAs)
Umbilical cord
Varicose vein removal
Varicose veins
Vascular medicine
Vascular system
Vasculitis
Von Willebrand's disease

BONES
Amputation
Ankylosing spondylitis
Arthritis
Aspergillosis
Back pain
Bone cancer
Bone disorders
Bone grafting
Bone marrow transplantation
Bowlegs
Braces
Bunions
Casts and splints
Cells
Chiropractic
Cleft lip and palate
Cleft lip and palate repair
Connective tissue
Craniosynostosis
Cushing's syndrome
Cystic fibrosis
Dengue fever
Disk removal
Dwarfism
Ear surgery
Ears
Eating disorders
Ewing's sarcoma
Facial transplantation
Failure to thrive
Feet
Folate deficiency
Foot disorders
Fracture and dislocation
Fracture repair
Gaucher's disease
Gigantism
Hammertoe correction
Head and neck disorders
Hearing
Heel spur removal
Hip fracture repair
Hip replacement
Histiocytosis
Hormone therapy
Insulin-like growth factors
Jaw wiring
Joints
Kneecap removal
Knock-knees
Kyphosis
Leishmaniasis
Ligaments
Lower extremities
Marfan syndrome
Mesenchymal stem cells
Methicillin-resistant staphylococcus
  aureus (MRSA) infection
Motor skill development
Necrosis

Neurofibromatosis
Neurosurgery
Niemann-Pick disease
Nuclear medicine
Nuclear radiology
Orthopedic surgery
Orthopedics
Osteochondritis juvenilis
Osteoclast
Osteomyelitis
Osteonecrosis
Osteopathic medicine
Osteoporosis
Paget's disease
Periodontitis
Physical rehabilitation
Pigeon toes
Podiatry
Polydactyly and syndactyly
Prader-Willi syndrome
Rheumatology
Rickets
Rubinstein-Taybi syndrome
Sarcoma
Scoliosis
Spina bifida
Spinal cord disorders
Spine, vertebrae, and disks
Sports medicine
Syphilis
Teeth
Temporomandibular joint (TMJ)
  syndrome
Tendon disorders
Tendon repair
Upper extremities

BRAIN
Abscess drainage
Acidosis
Acquired immunodeficiency syndrome
  (AIDS)
Addiction
Adrenoleukodystrophy
Agnosia
Alcoholism
Altitude sickness
Alzheimer's disease
Amnesia
Anesthesia
Anesthesiology
Aneurysmectomy
Aneurysms
Angelman syndrome
Angiography
Anorexia nervosa
Anosmia
Antianxiety drugs
Anticoagulants
Antidepressants
Antipsychotic drugs

Gender reassignment surgery
Glands
Gynecology
Gynecomastia
Hormone therapy
Hypogonadism
Klinefelter syndrome
Mammography
Mastectomy and lumpectomy
Mastitis
Premenstrual syndrome (PMS)
Raynaud's Phenomenon
Stevens-Johnson syndrome
Tumor removal

CARDIOVASCULAR SYSTEM
Aortic stenosis
Atrial fibrillation
Diabetic nephropathy
Extracorporeal membrane oxygenation
  (ECMO)
Gluten
Hemoglobin
Hemolysis
Hyperbaric chamber
Hypokalemia
Osteogenesis imperfecta
Patent ductus arteriosus
Postural orthostatic tachycardia
  syndrome (POTS)
Statins

CELLS
Acid-base chemistry
Alzheimer's disease
Antibodies
Bacteriology
Batten's disease
Biological therapies
Biopsy
Breast cancer
Cholesterol
Cloning
Conception
Cytology
Cytomegalovirus (CMV)
Cytopathology
Defibrillation
Dehydration
Diuretics
Electrocauterization
Epstein-Barr virus
Erectile dysfunction
Ergogenic aids
Eye infections and disorders
Fatty acid
Fluids and electrolytes
Food biochemistry
Gaucher's disease
Gene therapy
Genetic counseling

Glycolysis
Gram staining
Gulf War syndrome
Hearing
Host-defense mechanisms
Hyperplasia
Immune system
Immunization and vaccination
In vitro fertilization
Karyotyping
Kinesiology
Laboratory tests
Lipids
Magnetic field therapy
Microbiology
Microscopy
Mutation
Necrosis
Osteoclast
Pharmacology
Phlebotomy
Plasma
Rhinoviruses
Sarcoma
Sickle cell disease
Sleep
Thymus gland
Turner syndrome

CENTRAL NERVOUS SYSTEM
Amphetamine
Antipsychotic drugs
Brain disorders
Caffeine
Deep brain stimulation
Delirium
Hippocampus
Minimally conscious state
Nicotine

CHEST
Achalasia
Aneurysmectomy
Antihistamines
Asthma
Bacillus Calmette-Guérin (BCG)
Bronchiolitis
Bronchitis
Bypass surgery
Cardiac rehabilitation
Cardiology
Choking
Cold agglutinin disease
Common cold
Congenital heart disease
Coughing
Defibrillation
Diaphragm
Electrocardiography (ECG or EKG)
Electrolysis
Emphysema

Gulf War syndrome
Gynecomastia
Heart
Heart transplantation
Heart valve replacement
Heimlich maneuver
Hiccups
Legionnaires' disease
Lung cancer
Lungs
Oxygen therapy
Pacemaker implantation
Palpitations
Pityriasis rosea
Pleurisy
Pneumocystis jirovecii
Pneumothorax
Pulmonary diseases
Pulmonary medicine
Respiration
Resuscitation
Rhinoviruses
Sarcoidosis
Streptococcal infections
Thoracic surgery
Trachea
Tuberculosis
Vasculitis
Virtual imaging
Whooping cough

CIRCULATORY SYSTEM
Acute respiratory distress syndrome
  (ARDS)
Aneurysms
Angina
Angiography
Angioplasty
Antibodies
Antihistamines
Apgar score
Arteriosclerosis
Autoimmune disorders
Avian influenza
Bilirubin
Biofeedback
Bleeding
Blood and blood disorders
Blood pressure
Blood testing
Blood vessels
Blue baby syndrome
Bypass surgery
Cardiac arrest
Cardiac rehabilitation
Cardiac surgery
Cardiology
Cardiopulmonary resuscitation (CPR)
Carotid arteries
Catheterization
Chest

Cholera
Cholesterol
Circulation
Claudication
Cold agglutinin disease
Computed tomography (CT) scanning
Congenital heart disease
Coronary artery bypass graft
Cutis marmorata telangiectatica
    congenita
Decongestants
Deep vein thrombosis
Defibrillation
Dehydration
Diabetes mellitus
Dialysis
Disseminated intravascular coagulation
    (DIC)
Diuretics
Dizziness and fainting
Drowning
Ebola virus
Echocardiography
Edema
Electrocardiography (ECG or EKG)
Electrocauterization
Embolism
Encephalitis
End-stage renal disease
Endarterectomy
Endocarditis
Ergogenic aids
Exercise physiology
Facial transplantation
Folate deficiency
Food allergies
Gigantism
Heart
Heart attack
Heart disease
Heart failure
Heart transplantation
Heart valve replacement
Heat exhaustion and heatstroke
Hematology
Hemolysis
Hemolytic disease of the newborn
Hemolytic uremic syndrome
Hemorrhoid banding and removal
Hemorrhoids
Hormone therapy
Hormones
Hyperbaric oxygen therapy
Hypercholesterolemia
Hypertension
Hypotension
Immune system
Intravenous (IV) therapy
Ischemia
Juvenile rheumatoid arthritis
Kawasaki disease

Kidneys
Kinesiology
Klippel-Trenaunay syndrome
Lead poisoning
Leukemia
Liver
Lymph
Lymphatic system
Marijuana
Methicillin-resistant staphylococcus
    aureus (MRSA) infection
Mitral valve prolapse
Motor skill development
Myoglobin
Neutrophil
Obesity
Osteochondritis juvenilis
Oxygen therapy
Pacemaker implantation
Palpitations
Patent ductus arteriosus
Phlebitis
Phlebotomy
Placenta
Plaque
Plasma
Postural orthostatic tachycardia
    syndrome (POTS)
Preeclampsia and eclampsia
Pulmonary heart disease
Pulmonary edema
Pulse rate
Resuscitation
Reye's syndrome
Rocky Mountain spotted fever
Roundworms
Sarcoidosis
Schistosomiasis
Scleroderma
Septicemia
Shunts
Single photon emission computed
    tomography (SPECT)
Smoking
Snakebites
Sports medicine
Staphylococcal infections
Stenosis
Stents
Steroid abuse
Streptococcal infections
Strokes
Sturge-Weber syndrome
Temporal arteritis
Testicular torsion
Thrombocytopenia
Thrombolytic therapy and TPA
Thrombosis and thrombus
Toxemia
Transfusion
Transient ischemic attacks (TIAs)

Transplantation
Typhoid fever
Typhus
Uremia
Varicose vein removal
Varicose veins
Vascular medicine
Vascular system
Vasculitis
Yellow fever

DIGESTIVE SYSTEM
Amylase
Bilirubin
Fecal bacteriotherapy
Pellagra

EARS
Adenoids
Adrenoleukodystrophy
Agnosia
Altitude sickness
Antihistamines
Aspergillosis
Audiology
Auras
Bell's palsy
Charcot-Marie-Tooth Disease
Cold agglutinin disease
Cornelia de Lange syndrome
Cytomegalovirus (CMV)
Deafness
Decongestants
Dyslexia
Ear infections and disorders
Ear surgery
Earwax
Facial transplantation
Fetal alcohol syndrome
Fragile X syndrome
Hearing
Hearing aids
Hearing loss
Hearing tests
Histiocytosis
Leukodystrophy
Lice, mites, and ticks
Measles
Motion sickness
Myringotomy
Nervous system
Neurology
Otoplasty
Otorhinolaryngology
Pharynx
Raynaud's Phenomenon
Rubinstein-Taybi syndrome
Sense organs
Speech disorders
Streptococcal infections
Tinnitus

Tonsillitis
Vasculitis
Vertigo
Williams syndrome
Wiskott-Aldrich syndrome

ELBOW

Arthroplasty
Hand hygiene compliance

ENDOCRINE SYSTEM

Addison's disease
Adrenalectomy
Adrenoleukodystrophy
Amenorrhea
Anorexia nervosa
Assisted reproductive technologies
Bariatric surgery
Biofeedback
Brain death
Breasts
Carbohydrates
Computed tomography (CT) scanning
Congenital adrenal hyperplasia
Congenital hypothyroidism
Corticosteroids
Cushing's syndrome
Diabetes mellitus
Dwarfism
End-stage renal disease
Endocrine disorders
Endocrine glands
Endocrinology
Ergogenic aids
Failure to thrive
Fibrocystic breast condition
Galactorrhea
Gender reassignment surgery
Gestational diabetes
Gigantism
Glands
Glucose tolerance test
Goiter
Gynecomastia
Hashimoto's thyroiditis
Health impact of sugar
Hormones
Hyperparathyroidism and hypoparathyroidism
Hypoglycemia
Hypothalamus
Insulin
Klinefelter syndrome
Lead poisoning
Liver
Melatonin
Nonalcoholic steatohepatitis (NASH)
Obesity
Overtraining syndrome
Pancreas
Pancreatitis

Parathyroidectomy
Pituitary gland
Placenta
Plasma
Polycystic ovary syndrome
Postpartum depression
Prader-Willi syndrome
Preeclampsia and eclampsia
Prostate gland
Prostate gland removal
Sexual differentiation
Small intestine
Steroid abuse
Steroids
Testicular cancer
Testicular surgery
Thymus gland
Thyroid disorders
Thyroid gland
Thyroidectomy
Turner syndrome
Weight loss medications
Williams syndrome

EYES

Acquired immunodeficiency syndrome (AIDS)
Adenoviruses
Adrenoleukodystrophy
Agnosia
Angelman syndrome
Ankylosing spondylitis
Antihistamines
Aspergillosis
Astigmatism
Auras
Batten's disease
Behçet's disease
Bell's palsy
Blindness
Blurred vision
Botox
Cataract surgery
Cataracts
Chlamydia
Color blindness
Conjunctivitis
Corneal transplantation
Cornelia de Lange syndrome
Cutis marmorata telangiectatica congenita
Cytomegalovirus (CMV)
Dengue fever
Diabetes mellitus
Diabetic nephropathy
Dyslexia
Electrolysis
Enteroviruses
Eye infections and disorders
Eye surgery
Face lift and blepharoplasty

Facial transplantation
Fetal alcohol syndrome
Fetal tissue transplantation
Galactosemia
Gigantism
Glaucoma
Gonorrhea
Gulf War syndrome
Hay fever
Juvenile rheumatoid arthritis
Keratitis
Kluver-Bucy syndrome
Laser use in surgery
Leptospirosis
Leukodystrophy
Lyme disease
Macular degeneration
Marfan syndrome
Marijuana
Microscopy
Motor skill development
Multiple chemical sensitivity syndrome
Myopia
Ophthalmology
Optometry
Pigmentation
Presbyopia
Pterygium/Pinguecula
Ptosis
Refractive eye surgery
Reiter's syndrome
Retina
Rubinstein-Taybi syndrome
Sarcoidosis
Scurvy
Sense organs
Sjögren's syndrome
Sphincterectomy
Spinocerebellar ataxia
Stevens-Johnson syndrome
Strabismus
Sturge-Weber syndrome
Styes
Syphilis
Tears and tear ducts
Trachoma
Transplantation
Vasculitis
Vision
Vision disorders
Williams syndrome

FEET

Athlete's foot
Bone disorders
Bones and the skeleton
Bowlegs
Bunions
Charcot-Marie-Tooth Disease
Cold agglutinin disease
Cornelia de Lange syndrome

Pancreatitis
Peristalsis
Peritonitis
Pharynx
Pinworms
Poisoning
Polycystic kidney disease
Polyps
Proctology
Protozoan diseases
Pyloric stenosis
Radiation sickness
Rectum
Reiter's syndrome
Rotavirus
Roundworms
Salmonella infection
Scleroderma
Sense organs
Shigellosis
Shunts
Small intestine
Smallpox
Smoking
Soiling
Staphylococcal infections
Stenosis
Stevens-Johnson syndrome
Stomach
Tapeworms
Taste
Teeth
Toilet training
Toxoplasmosis
Trichinosis
Tumor removal
Typhoid fever
Ulcer surgery
Ulcerative colitis
Ulcers
Vagotomy
Vasculitis
Weaning
Weight loss and gain

GENITALS
Adrenoleukodystrophy
Aphrodisiacs
Assisted reproductive technologies
Behçet's disease
Candidiasis
Catheterization
Cervical, ovarian, and uterine cancers
Cervical procedures
Chlamydia
Circumcision, female and genital
    mutilation
Circumcision
Congenital adrenal hyperplasia
Contraception
Cyst removal

Embolization
Endometrial biopsy
Episiotomy
Erectile dysfunction
Ergogenic aids
Fragile X syndrome
Gender reassignment surgery
Genital disorders
Glands
Gonorrhea
Gynecology
Hemochromatosis
Hermaphroditism and
    pseudohermaphroditism
Herpes
Hormone therapy
Human papillomavirus (HPV)
Hydroceles
Hyperplasia
Hypospadias repair and urethroplasty
Infertility
Klinefelter syndrome
Kluver-Bucy syndrome
Lice, mites, and ticks
Masturbation
Mumps
Orchitis
Pap test
Pelvic inflammatory disease (PID)
Penile implant surgery
Prader-Willi syndrome
Rape and sexual assault
Reproductive system
Rubinstein-Taybi syndrome
Semen
Sexual differentiation
Sexual dysfunction
Sexuality
Sexually transmitted diseases (STDs)
Sperm banks
Sterilization
Stevens-Johnson syndrome
Streptococcal infections
Syphilis
Testicles
Testicular cancer
Testicular surgery
Testicular torsion
Toilet training
Trichomoniasis
Urethritis
Urology
Uterus
Vas deferens
Vasectomy

GLANDS
Abscess drainage
Addison's disease
Adrenalectomy
Adrenoleukodystrophy

Assisted reproductive technologies
Biofeedback
Breast cancer
Breast disorders
Breast-feeding
Breast surgery
Breasts
Cushing's syndrome
Cyst removal
Dengue fever
Diabetes mellitus
DiGeorge syndrome
Dwarfism
Endocrine disorders
Endocrine glands
Endocrinology
Epstein-Barr virus
Ergogenic aids
Eye infections and disorders
Gender reassignment surgery
Goiter
Gynecomastia
Hashimoto's thyroiditis
Hormones
Hyperhidrosis
Hyperparathyroidism and
    hypoparathyroidism
Hypoglycemia
Hypothalamus
Immune system
Internal medicine
Liver
Mastitis
Mumps
Neurosurgery
Nuclear medicine
Nuclear radiology
Pancreas
Parathyroidectomy
Pituitary gland
Prader-Willi syndrome
Prostate gland
Prostate gland removal
Quinsy
Semen
Sexual differentiation
Sleep
Steroids
Sweating
Testicular cancer
Testicular surgery
Thymus gland
Thyroid disorders
Thyroid gland
Thyroidectomy

GUMS
Abscess drainage
Bulimia
Cavities
Dengue fever

Dental diseases
Dentistry
Dentures
Fluoride treatments
Gingivitis
Gulf War syndrome
Gum disease
Jaw wiring
Mouth and throat cancer
Oral and maxillofacial surgery
Orthodontics
Periodontal surgery
Periodontitis
Root canal treatment
Scurvy
Teeth
Teething
Tooth extraction
Wisdom teeth

HAIR
Alopecia
Angelman syndrome
Anorexia nervosa
Collodion baby
Cornelia de Lange syndrome
Cushing's syndrome
Dermatitis
Dermatology
Gigantism
Gulf War syndrome
Hair
Hair transplantation
Hyperthyroidism and hypothyroidism
Klinefelter syndrome
Lice, mites, and ticks
Pigmentation
Radiation sickness

HANDS
Amputation
Arthritis
Arthroplasty
Bone disorders
Bursitis
Carpal tunnel syndrome
Casts and splints
Charcot-Marie-Tooth Disease
Cold agglutinin disease
Cornelia de Lange syndrome
Corns and calluses
Diabetic neuropathy
Dyskinesia
Fetal alcohol syndrome
Fracture and dislocation
Fragile X syndrome
Frostbite
Ganglion removal
Gigantism
Hand hygiene compliance
Methicillin-resistant staphylococcus

aureus (MRSA) infection
Nail removal
Nails
Neurology
Orthopedic surgery
Orthopedics
Polydactyly and syndactyly
Raynaud's Phenomenon
Rheumatology
Rubinstein-Taybi syndrome
Scleroderma
Skin lesion removal
Spinocerebellar ataxia
Sports medicine
Stevens-Johnson syndrome
Streptococcal infections
Tendinitis
Tendon repair
Thalidomide
Tremors
Upper extremities
Vasculitis

HEAD
Alopecia
Altitude sickness
Aneurysms
Angelman syndrome
Angiography
Antihistamines
Bell's palsy
Botox
Brain
Brain disorders
Brain tumors
Cluster headaches
Concussion
Cornelia de Lange syndrome
Craniosynostosis
Craniotomy
Deep brain stimulation
Dengue fever
Dizziness and fainting
Dyskinesia
Electroencephalography (EEG)
Epilepsy
Eye infections and disorders
Facial transplantation
Fetal alcohol syndrome
Fibromyalgia
Functional magnetic imaging (fMRI)
Hair transplantation
Head and neck disorders
Headaches
Hemiplegia
Hydrocephalus
Meningitis
Motion sickness
Nasal polyp removal
Neuroimaging
Neurology

Neurosurgery
Oral and maxillofacial surgery
Paget's disease
Pharynx
Phrenology
Rubinstein-Taybi syndrome
Seizures
Shunts
Single photon emission computed
  tomography (SPECT)
Spinocerebellar ataxia
Sports medicine
Stevens-Johnson syndrome
Strokes
Sturge-Weber syndrome
Tears and tear ducts
Temporomandibular joint (TMJ)
  syndrome
Thrombosis and thrombus
Tinnitus
Transcranial magnetic stimulation
  (TMS)
Tremors
Whiplash

HEART
Acidosis
Anemia
Aneurysmectomy
Aneurysms
Angina
Angiography
Angioplasty
Anorexia nervosa
Anticoagulants
Anxiety
Aortic stenosis
Apgar score
Arrhythmias
Arteriosclerosis
Aspergillosis
Atrial fibrillation
Avian influenza
Beriberi
Biofeedback
Bites and stings
Blood pressure
Blood vessels
Blue baby syndrome
Brucellosis
Bulimia
Bypass surgery
Cardiac arrest
Cardiac rehabilitation
Cardiac surgery
Cardiology
Cardiopulmonary resuscitation (CPR)
Carotid arteries
Catheterization
Congenital heart disease
Cornelia de Lange syndrome

Impetigo
Juvenile rheumatoid arthritis
Kawasaki disease
Leishmaniasis
Leprosy
Lymph
Lymphatic system
Magnetic field therapy
Malaria
Marburg virus
Mesenchymal stem cells
Microbiology
Mold and mildew
Monkeypox
Multiple chemical sensitivity syndrome
Mutation
Myasthenia gravis
Nephritis
Neutrophil
Noroviruses
Pancreas
Pharmacology
Pharynx
Plasma
Poisoning
Polymyalgia rheumatica
Pulmonary diseases
Pulmonary medicine
Renal failure
Rh factor
Rheumatoid arthritis
Rheumatology
Roseola
Sarcoidosis
Scarlet fever
Scleroderma
Serology
Severe acute respiratory syndrome (SARS)
Severe combined immunodeficiency syndrome (SCID)
Sjögren's syndrome
Small intestine
Stevens-Johnson syndrome
Temporal arteritis
Thalidomide
Thymus gland
Tonsils
Toxoplasmosis
Transfusion
Transplantation
Ulcerative colitis
Vasculitis
Vitiligo
Wiskott-Aldrich syndrome

INTESTINES
Abdomen
Abdominal disorders
Acidosis
Acquired immunodeficiency syndrome

(AIDS)
Adenoviruses
Amebiasis
Anus
Appendectomy
Appendicitis
Avian influenza
Bacterial infections
Bariatric surgery
Bulimia
Bypass surgery
Campylobacter infections
Carbohydrates
Celiac sprue
Cholera
Chyme
Colic
Colitis
Colon
Colon therapy
Colonoscopy and sigmoidoscopy
Colorectal cancer
Colorectal polyp removal
Colorectal surgery
Constipation
Crohn's disease
Cystic fibrosis
Diarrhea and dysentery
Digestion
Diverticulitis and diverticulosis
E. coli infection
Eating disorders
Endoscopy
Enemas
Enterocolitis
Fiber
Fistula repair
Food poisoning
Fructosemia
Gastroenteritis
Gastroenterology
Gastrointestinal disorders
Gastrointestinal system
Gluten
Hemorrhoid banding and removal
Hemorrhoids
Hernia
Hernia repair
Hirschsprung's disease
Ileostomy and colostomy
Infarction
Internal medicine
Intestinal disorders
Irritable bowel syndrome (IBS)
Kaposi's sarcoma
Lactose intolerance
Laparoscopy
Malabsorption
Malnutrition
Meckel's diverticulum
Metabolism

Obesity
Peristalsis
Peritonitis
Pinworms
Polyps
Proctology
Rectum
Roundworms
Small intestine
Soiling
Sphincterectomy
Stomach
Tapeworms
Toilet training
Trichinosis
Tumor removal
Typhoid fever
Ulcer surgery
Ulcerative colitis
Vasculitis

JOINTS
Amputation
Angelman syndrome
Ankylosing spondylitis
Arthritis
Arthroscopy
Back pain
Bowlegs
Braces
Brucellosis
Bursitis
Carpal tunnel syndrome
Casts and splints
Celiac sprue
Charcot-Marie-Tooth Disease
Cyst removal
Electrocauterization
Endoscopy
Ergogenic aids
Exercise physiology
Fracture and dislocation
Fragile X syndrome
Gout
Gulf War syndrome
Hemiplegia
Hip fracture repair
Hyaluronic acid injections
Juvenile rheumatoid arthritis
Klippel-Trenaunay syndrome
Kneecap removal
Knock-knees
Ligaments
Lyme disease
Methicillin-resistant staphylococcus aureus (MRSA) infection
Motor skill development
Obesity
Orthopedic surgery
Orthopedics
Osteoarthritis

Osteochondritis juvenilis
Osteomyelitis
Osteonecrosis
Physical rehabilitation
Pigeon toes
Polymyalgia rheumatica
Reiter's syndrome
Rheumatology
Rotator cuff surgery
Rubella
Sarcoidosis
Sarcoma
Scleroderma
Spondylitis
Sports medicine
Streptococcal infections
Syphilis
Temporomandibular joint (TMJ)
  syndrome
Tendinitis
Tendon repair
Tularemia
Von Willebrand's disease

KIDNEYS
Abdomen
Abdominal disorders
Abscess drainage
Addison's disease
Adrenalectomy
Anemia
Anorexia nervosa
Aspergillosis
Avian influenza
Babesiosis
Carbohydrates
Cholera
Cystic fibrosis
Diabetes mellitus
Diabetic nephropathy
Dialysis
Diuretics
Drowning
End-stage renal disease
Ergogenic aids
Fructosemia
Hantavirus
Hematuria
Hemolysis
Hemolytic uremic syndrome
Hypertension
Hypotension
Infarction
Insulin-like growth factors
Internal medicine
Intravenous (IV) therapy
Kidney cancer
Kidney disorders
Kidney transplantation
Laparoscopy
Leptospirosis

Lithotripsy
Metabolism
Methicillin-resistant staphylococcus
  aureus (MRSA) infection
Nephrectomy
Nephritis
Nephrology
Nuclear medicine
Nuclear radiology
Polycystic kidney disease
Polyps
Preeclampsia and eclampsia
Proteinuria
Pyelonephritis
Renal failure
Reye's syndrome
Rocky Mountain spotted fever
Sarcoidosis
Scleroderma
Scurvy
Sickle cell disease
Stone removal
Stones
Syphilis
Toilet training
Transplantation
Typhoid fever
Typhus
Ultrasonography
Uremia
Urinalysis
Urinary disorders
Urinary system
Urology
Vasculitis
Williams syndrome
Wilms tumor

KNEES
Amputation
Angelman syndrome
Arthritis
Arthroplasty
Arthroscopy
Bowlegs
Braces
Bursitis
Carticel®
Casts and splints
Endoscopy
Exercise physiology
Fracture and dislocation
Hyaluronic acid injections
Joints
Kneecap removal
Knock-knees
Liposuction
Lower extremities
Lyme disease
Orthopedic surgery
Orthopedics

Osgood-Schlatter disease
Osteonecrosis
Patellofemoral pain syndrome
Physical rehabilitation
Pigeon toes
Rheumatology
Sports medicine
Stevens-Johnson syndrome
Tendinitis
Tendon repair

LEGS
Amputation
Arthritis
Arthroscopy
Auras
Back pain
Bone disorders
Bones and the skeleton
Bowlegs
Bursitis
Bypass surgery
Casts and splints
Charcot-Marie-Tooth Disease
Claudication
Cornelia de Lange syndrome
Cutis marmorata telangiectatica
  congenita
Deep vein thrombosis
Diabetic neuropathy
Dwarfism
Dyskinesia
Electrolysis
Fracture and dislocation
Fracture repair
Gigantism
Hemiplegia
Hip fracture repair
Knee
Kneecap removal
Knock-knees
Liposuction
Lower extremities
Methicillin-resistant staphylococcus
  aureus (MRSA) infection
Muscle sprains, spasms, and disorders
Muscles
Muscular dystrophy
Numbness and tingling
Orthopedic surgery
Orthopedics
Paget's disease
Paralysis
Paraplegia
Physical rehabilitation
Pigeon toes
Poliomyelitis
Quadriplegia
Rheumatology
Roseola
Sarcoma

Sciatica
Slipped disk
Spinocerebellar ataxia
Sports medicine
Stevens-Johnson syndrome
Streptococcal infections
Tendinitis
Tendon disorders
Tendon repair
Thalidomide
Tremors
Varicose vein removal
Vascular system
Vasculitis
Venous insufficiency

LIGAMENTS
Ankylosing spondylitis
Astym® therapy
Back pain
Bowlegs
Casts and splints
Collagen
Connective tissue
Electrocauterization
Eye infections and disorders
Flat feet
Flexibility
Joints
Knock-knees
Muscle sprains, spasms, and disorders
Muscles
Orthopedic surgery
Orthopedics
Patent ductus arteriosus
Physical rehabilitation
Pigeon toes
Sports medicine
Tendon disorders
Tendon repair
Whiplash

LIVER
Abdomen
Abdominal disorders
Abscess drainage
Acquired immunodeficiency syndrome
  (AIDS)
Alcoholism
Amebiasis
Aspergillosis
Babesiosis
Bile
Bilirubin
Blood and blood disorders
Brucellosis
Cholecystitis
Chyme
Circulation
Cirrhosis
Cold agglutinin disease

Cystic fibrosis
Cytomegalovirus (CMV)
Edema
Embolization
Endoscopic retrograde
  cholangiopancreatography (ERCP)
Ergogenic aids
Fatty acid oxidation disorders
Fetal surgery
Fructosemia
Galactosemia
Gastroenterology
Gastrointestinal system
Gaucher's disease
Glucose tolerance test
Glycogen storage diseases
Hematology
Hemochromatosis
Hemoglobin
Hemolysis
Hepatitis
Histiocytosis
Hypercholesterolemia
Immune system
Insulin
Insulin-like growth factors
Internal medicine
Jaundice
Kaposi's sarcoma
Ketogenic diet
Leptospirosis
Liver cancer
Liver disorders
Liver transplantation
Malabsorption
Malaria
Mesenchymal stem cells
Metabolism
Methicillin-resistant staphylococcus
  aureus (MRSA) infection
Niemann-Pick disease
Nonalcoholic steatohepatitis (NASH)
Phenylketonuria (PKU)
Polycystic kidney disease
Reye's syndrome
Shunts
Thrombocytopenia
Transplantation
Typhoid fever
Wilson's disease
Yellow fever

LUNGS
Abscess drainage
Acquired immunodeficiency syndrome
  (AIDS)
Acute respiratory distress syndrome
  (ARDS)
Adenoviruses
Allergies
Altitude sickness

Antihistamines
Apgar score
Apnea
Asbestos exposure
Aspergillosis
Asphyxiation
Asthma
Avian influenza
Bacterial infections
Bronchi
Bronchiolitis
Bronchitis
Cardiopulmonary resuscitation (CPR)
Chest
Childhood infectious diseases
Chlamydia
Choking
Chronic obstructive pulmonary disease
  (COPD)
Cold agglutinin disease
Common cold
Coronaviruses
Coughing
Croup
Cystic fibrosis
Cytomegalovirus (CMV)
Diaphragm
Drowning
Edema
Embolism
Emphysema
Endoscopy
Exercise physiology
Fetal surgery
Hantavirus
Hay fever
Heart transplantation
Heimlich maneuver
Hiccups
Histiocytosis
H1N1 influenza
Human respiratory system
Hyperbaric oxygen therapy
Hyperventilation
Hypoxia
Infarction
Influenza
Internal medicine
Interstitial pulmonary fibrosis (IPF)
Intravenous (IV) therapy
Kaposi's sarcoma
Kinesiology
Legionnaires' disease
Leptospirosis
Lung cancer
Lung surgery
Marijuana
Measles
Mesothelioma
Mold and mildew
Multiple chemical sensitivity syndrome

Nicotine
Niemann-Pick disease
Oxygen therapy
Patent ductus arteriosus
Plague
Pleurisy
Pneumocystis jirovecii
Pneumonia
Pneumothorax
Pulmonary heart disease
Pulmonary diseases
Pulmonary edema
Pulmonary hypertension
Pulmonary medicine
Quinsy
Respiration
Respiratory distress syndrome
Resuscitation
Rhinoviruses
Roundworms
Sarcoidosis
Schistosomiasis
Scleroderma
Severe acute respiratory syndrome
    (SARS)
Sickle cell disease
Stevens-Johnson syndrome
Thoracic surgery
Thrombolytic therapy and TPA
Thrombosis and thrombus
Transplantation
Tuberculosis
Tumor removal
Vasculitis
Wiskott-Aldrich syndrome

LYMPHATIC SYSTEM
Acquired immunodeficiency syndrome
    (AIDS)
Adenoids
Antibodies
Autoimmune disorders
Bacillus Calmette-Guérin (BCG)
Bacterial infections
Biological therapies
Blood and blood disorders
Blood vessels
Breast cancer
Breast disorders
Bruises
Cervical, ovarian, and uterine cancers
Chlamydia
Cold agglutinin disease
Colorectal cancer
Coronaviruses
DiGeorge syndrome
Edema
Elephantiasis
Embolism
Epstein-Barr virus
Gaucher's disease

Hay fever
Hodgkin's disease
Immune system
Kawasaki disease
Klippel-Trenaunay syndrome
Leishmaniasis
Leptospirosis
Leukemia
Lower extremities
Lung cancer
Lymph
Lymphadenopathy and lymphoma
Mononucleosis
Overtraining syndrome
Prostate cancer
Roundworms
Rubella
Sarcoidosis
Skin cancer
Sleeping sickness
Small intestine
Splenectomy
Thymus gland
Tonsillectomy and adenoid removal
Tonsillitis
Tonsils
Tularemia
Upper extremities
Vascular medicine

MOUTH
Acid reflux disease
Acquired immunodeficiency syndrome
    (AIDS)
Adenoids
Angelman syndrome
Auras
Behçet's disease
Bell's palsy
Braces
Candidiasis
Canker sores
Chickenpox
Cold sores
Cornelia de Lange syndrome
Crowns and bridges
Dengue fever
Dental diseases
Dentistry
Dentures
DiGeorge syndrome
Dyskinesia
Eating disorders
Endodontic disease
Epstein-Barr virus
Esophagus
Facial transplantation
Fetal alcohol syndrome
Fluoride treatments
Gingivitis
Gum disease

Hand-foot-and-mouth disease
Heimlich maneuver
Herpes
Jaw wiring
Kawasaki disease
Lisping
Measles
Mouth and throat cancer
Oral and maxillofacial surgery
Orthodontics
Periodontal surgery
Pharynx
Plaque
Quinsy
Rape and sexual assault
Raynaud's Phenomenon
Reiter's syndrome
Root canal treatment
Rubinstein-Taybi syndrome
Sense organs
Sjögren's syndrome
Taste
Teething
Temporomandibular joint (TMJ)
    syndrome
Thumb sucking
Tooth extraction
Ulcers
Wisdom teeth

MUSCLES
Acidosis
Acupressure
Aerobics
Amputation
Anesthesia
Anesthesiology
Apgar score
Astym® therapy
Avian influenza
Back pain
Bed-wetting
Bedsores
Bell's palsy
Beriberi
Bile
Biofeedback
Botox
Bowlegs
Breasts
Carbohydrates
Charcot-Marie-Tooth Disease
Chest
Chiari malformations
Childhood infectious diseases
Chronic fatigue syndrome
Cushing's syndrome
Cystic fibrosis
Diaphragm
Ebola virus
Electrocauterization

Patellofemoral pain syndrome
Physical rehabilitation
Poisoning
Poliomyelitis
Prader-Willi syndrome
Precocious puberty
Rabies
Radiculopathy
Respiration
Restless legs syndrome
Rheumatoid arthritis
Rheumatology
Rickets
Rotator cuff surgery
Scoliosis
Seizures
Sleepwalking
Slipped disk
Speech disorders
Sphincterectomy
Spinal cord disorders
Spine, vertebrae, and disks
Spinocerebellar ataxia
Sports medicine
Staphylococcal infections
Strength training
Teeth
Tendinitis
Tendon disorders
Tendon repair
Tetanus
Tics
Tourette's syndrome
Trichinosis
Upper extremities
Walking
Weight loss and gain

NAILS
Anorexia nervosa
Athlete's foot
Collodion baby
Dermatology
Fungal infections
Malnutrition
Nail removal
Podiatry

NECK
Botox
Braces
Carotid arteries
Casts and splints
Chiari malformations
Choking
Congenital hypothyroidism
Dyskinesia
Encephalitis
Endarterectomy
Facial transplantation
Goiter

Hashimoto's thyroiditis
Head and neck disorders
Heimlich maneuver
Hyperparathyroidism and
  hypoparathyroidism
Laminectomy and spinal fusion
Mouth and throat cancer
Neuroimaging
Paralysis
Parathyroidectomy
Pharynx
Pityriasis alba
Slipped disk
Stevens-Johnson syndrome
Streptococcal infections
Sympathectomy
Thyroid disorders
Thyroid gland
Thyroidectomy
Torticollis
Trachea
Tracheostomy
Vagus nerve
Whiplash
Whooping cough

NERVES
Agnosia
Alzheimer's disease
Anesthesia
Anesthesiology
Angelman syndrome
Avian influenza
Back pain
Bell's palsy
Biofeedback
Brain
Bulimia
Carpal tunnel syndrome
Cells
Cluster headaches
Concussion
Dyskinesia
Electromyography
Encephalitis
Epilepsy
Eye infections and disorders
Facial transplantation
Fibromyalgia
Guillain-Barré syndrome
Hearing
Herpes
Hirschsprung's disease
Huntington's disease
Leprosy
Leukodystrophy
Listeria infections
Local anesthesia
Lower extremities
Lumbar puncture
Lyme disease

Marijuana
Motor neuron diseases
Motor skill development
Multiple chemical sensitivity syndrome
Multiple sclerosis
Neonatal brachial plexus palsy
Nervous system
Neuralgia, neuritis, and neuropathy
Neuroimaging
Neurology
Neurosis
Neurosurgery
Numbness and tingling
Palsy
Paralysis
Physical rehabilitation
Poliomyelitis
Postherpetic neuralgia
Ptosis
Radiculopathy
Sarcoidosis
Sciatica
Seizures
Sense organs
Shock therapy
Skin
Slipped disk
Spinal cord disorders
Spine, vertebrae, and disks
Spinocerebellar ataxia
Sturge-Weber syndrome
Sympathectomy
Tics
Tinnitus
Touch
Tourette's syndrome
Tremors
Upper extremities
Vagotomy
Vasculitis

NERVOUS SYSTEM
Abscess drainage
Acetaminophen
Acupressure
Addiction
Adenoviruses
Adrenoleukodystrophy
Agnosia
Alcoholism
Altitude sickness
Alzheimer's disease
Amnesia
Amputation
Amyotrophic lateral sclerosis (ALS)
Anesthesia
Anesthesiology
Aneurysms
Angelman syndrome
Anorexia nervosa
Anosmia

Sympathectomy
Synesthesia
Syphilis
Taste
Tay-Sachs disease
Teeth
Tetanus
Thrombolytic therapy and TPA
Tics
Tinnitus
Touch
Tourette's syndrome
Toxoplasmosis
Tremors
Typhus
Upper extremities
Vagotomy
Vertigo
Vision
Walking
West Nile virus
Wilson's disease
Yoga

NOSE
Adenoids
Allergies
Anosmia
Antihistamines
Aromatherapy
Auras
Avian influenza
Casts and splints
Chickenpox
Childhood infectious diseases
Cold agglutinin disease
Common cold
Cornelia de Lange syndrome
Decongestants
Dengue fever
Epstein-Barr virus
Facial transplantation
Fifth disease
Hay fever
H1N1 influenza
Influenza
Methicillin-resistant staphylococcus
  aureus (MRSA) infection
Mold and mildew
Nasal polyp removal
Nasopharyngeal disorders
Otorhinolaryngology
Pharynx
Polyps
Pulmonary medicine
Respiration
Rhinitis
Rhinoplasty and submucous resection
Rhinoviruses
Rosacea
Rubinstein-Taybi syndrome

Sense organs
Sinusitis
Skin lesion removal
Smell
Sore throat
Stevens-Johnson syndrome
Taste
Tears and tear ducts
Vasculitis

PANCREAS
Abscess drainage
Alcoholism
Carbohydrates
Cholecystitis
Chyme
Cystic fibrosis
Diabetes mellitus
Digestion
Endocrine glands
Endocrinology
Endoscopic retrograde
  cholangiopancreatography (ERCP)
Fetal tissue transplantation
Food biochemistry
Gastroenterology
Gastrointestinal system
Glands
Glucose tolerance test
Hemochromatosis
Insulin
Internal medicine
Malabsorption
Metabolism
Mumps
Pancreatitis
Polycystic kidney disease
Polycystic ovary syndrome
Stomach
Transplantation

PSYCHIC-EMOTIONAL SYSTEM
Acquired immunodeficiency syndrome
  (AIDS)
Addiction
Adrenoleukodystrophy
Alcoholism
Alzheimer's disease
Amnesia
Anesthesia
Anesthesiology
Angelman syndrome
Anorexia nervosa
Antianxiety drugs
Antidepressants
Antihistamines
Anxiety
Aphrodisiacs
Aromatherapy
Asperger syndrome
Attention-deficit disorder (ADD)

Auras
Autism
Bariatric surgery
Biofeedback
Bipolar disorders
Body dysmorphic disorder
Bonding
Brain
Bulimia
Chronic fatigue syndrome
Cognitive development
Colic
Death and dying
Dementias
Depression
Developmental disorders
Developmental stages
Dizziness and fainting
Down syndrome
Dyskinesia
Dyslexia
Eating disorders
Electroencephalography (EEG)
Encephalitis
Endocrinology
Factitious disorders
Failure to thrive
Fibromyalgia
Frontotemporal dementia (FTD)
Gulf War syndrome
Headaches
Hormone therapy
Hormones
Hydrocephalus
Hypnosis
Hypochondriasis
Hypothalamus
Interpartner violence
Kinesiology
Klinefelter syndrome
Learning disabilities
Light therapy
Marijuana
Memory loss
Menopause
Miscarriage
Morgellons disease
Motor skill development
Narcolepsy
Neurology
Neurosis
Neurosurgery
Obesity
Obsessive-compulsive disorder
Overtraining syndrome
Paranoia
Pharmacology
Phobias
Pick's disease
Postpartum depression
Post-traumatic stress disorder

Prader-Willi syndrome
Precocious puberty
Premenstrual syndrome (PMS)
Psychiatric disorders
Psychoanalysis
Psychosis
Rabies
Rape and sexual assault
Restless legs syndrome
Schizophrenia
Seasonal affective disorder
Separation anxiety
Sexual dysfunction
Sexuality
Shock therapy
Sleep
Sleep disorders
Sleeping sickness
Sleepwalking
Speech disorders
Sperm banks
Steroid abuse
Strokes
Suicide
Synesthesia
Tics
Tinnitus
Toilet training
Tourette's syndrome
Weight loss and gain
Wilson's disease

REPRODUCTIVE SYSTEM
Abdomen
Abortion
Acquired immunodeficiency syndrome
  (AIDS)
Adrenoleukodystrophy
Amenorrhea
Amniocentesis
Anorexia nervosa
Assisted reproductive technologies
Avian influenza
Breast-feeding
Breasts
Brucellosis
Candidiasis
Catheterization
Cervical, ovarian, and uterine cancers
Cervical procedures
Cesarean section
Childbirth
Childbirth complications
Chlamydia
Chorionic villus sampling
Circumcision, female and genital
  mutilation
Circumcision
Computed tomography (CT) scanning
Conception
Congenital adrenal hyperplasia

Contraception
Culdocentesis
Cyst removal
Cystic fibrosis
Cystoscopy
Dysmenorrhea
Eating disorders
Ectopic pregnancy
Endocrine glands
Endocrinology
Endometrial biopsy
Endometriosis
Episiotomy
Erectile dysfunction
Fallopian tube
Fetus
Fistula repair
Gamete intrafallopian transfer (GIFT)
Gender reassignment surgery
Genetic counseling
Genital disorders
Gestational diabetes
Gigantism
Glands
Gonorrhea
Gynecology
Hermaphroditism and
  pseudohermaphroditism
Hernia
Herpes
Hormone therapy
Human papillomavirus (HPV)
Hydroceles
Hypogonadism
Hypospadias repair and urethroplasty
Hysterectomy
In vitro fertilization
Infertility
Internal medicine
Klinefelter syndrome
Laparoscopy
Lead poisoning
Menopause
Menorrhagia
Menstruation
Miscarriage
Myomectomy
Obstetrics
Orchiectomy
Orchitis
Ovarian cysts
Pap test
Pelvic inflammatory disease (PID)
Penile implant surgery
Placenta
Polycystic ovary syndrome
Polyps
Precocious puberty
Preeclampsia and eclampsia
Pregnancy and gestation
Pregnancy test

Premature birth
Premenstrual syndrome (PMS)
Prostate cancer
Prostate enlargement
Prostate gland
Semen
Sexual differentiation
Sexual dysfunction
Sexuality
Sexually transmitted diseases (STDs)
Sperm banks
Sterilization
Steroid abuse
Stevens-Johnson syndrome
Stillbirth
Syphilis
Testicles
Testicular surgery
Testicular torsion
Toxemia
Trichomoniasis
Tubal ligation
Turner syndrome
Ultrasonography
Urology
Uterus
Vas deferens
Vasectomy
Von Willebrand's disease

RESPIRATORY SYSTEM
Abscess drainage
Acidosis
Acquired immunodeficiency syndrome
  (AIDS)
Acute respiratory distress syndrome
  (ARDS)
Adenoviruses
Adrenoleukodystrophy
Altitude sickness
Amyotrophic lateral sclerosis (ALS)
Anthrax
Antihistamines
Apgar score
Apnea
Asbestos exposure
Asphyxiation
Asthma
Avian influenza
Babesiosis
Bacterial infections
Bronchi
Bronchiolitis
Bronchitis
Cardiopulmonary resuscitation (CPR)
Cartilage
Chest
Childhood infectious diseases
Choking
Chronic obstructive pulmonary disease
  (COPD)

Cold agglutinin disease
Common cold
Computed tomography (CT) scanning
Coronaviruses
Coughing
Croup
Cystic fibrosis
Decongestants
Defibrillation
Diaphragm
Drowning
Dwarfism
Edema
Emphysema
Epiglottitis
Exercise physiology
Fetal surgery
Fluids and electrolytes
Food allergies
Fungal infections
Hantavirus
Hay fever
Head and neck disorders
Heart transplantation
Heimlich maneuver
Hiccups
H1N1 influenza
Human respiratory system
Hyperbaric chamber
Hyperbaric oxygen therapy
Hyperventilation
Hypoxia
Influenza
Internal medicine
Kinesiology
Laryngectomy
Legionnaires' disease
Lung cancer
Lung surgery
Lungs
Marijuana
Measles
Mesothelioma
Methicillin-resistant staphylococcus
  aureus (MRSA) infection
Mold and mildew
Monkeypox
Multiple chemical sensitivity syndrome
Nasopharyngeal disorders
Niemann-Pick disease
Obesity
Otorhinolaryngology
Oxygen therapy
Pharynx
Plague
Plasma
Pneumocystis jirovecii
Pneumonia
Pneumothorax
Poisoning
Pulmonary diseases

Pulmonary edema
Pulmonary heart disease
Pulmonary hypertension
Pulmonary medicine
Respiration
Resuscitation
Rheumatoid arthritis
Rhinitis
Rhinoviruses
Sarcoidosis
Severe acute respiratory syndrome
  (SARS)
Sinusitis
Sleep apnea
Smoking
Sore throat
Staphylococcal infections
Stevens-Johnson syndrome
Thoracic surgery
Thrombolytic therapy and TPA
Thrombosis and thrombus
Tonsillectomy and adenoid removal
Trachea
Tracheostomy
Transplantation
Tuberculosis
Tularemia
Typhus
Vasculitis
Voice and vocal cord disorders
Whooping cough

SKIN
Abscess drainage
Acne
Acquired immunodeficiency syndrome
  (AIDS)
Acupressure
Adenoviruses
Adrenoleukodystrophy
Allergies
Amputation
Anesthesia
Anesthesiology
Angelman syndrome
Anorexia nervosa
Anthrax
Antihistamines
Anxiety
Athlete's foot
Auras
Bacillus Calmette-Guérin (BCG)
Bariatric surgery
Batten's disease
Bedsores
Behçet's disease
Bites and stings
Blisters
Blood testing
Body dysmorphic disorder
Bruises

Burns and scalds
Candidiasis
Canker sores
Casts and splints
Cells
Chagas' disease
Chickenpox
Cleft lip and palate repair
Cold agglutinin disease
Cold sores
Collagen
Collodion baby
Corns and calluses
Cushing's syndrome
Cutis marmorata telangiectatica
  congenita
Cyanosis
Cyst removal
Dengue fever
Dermatitis
Dermatology
Dermatopathology
Diabetic neuropathy
Ebola virus
Eczema
Edema
Electrical shock
Electrocauterization
Electrolysis
Enteroviruses
Face lift and blepharoplasty
Facial transplantation
Fibrocystic breast condition
Fifth disease
Folate deficiency
Food allergies
Frostbite
Fungal infections
Gangrene
Glands
Gluten intolerance
Gulf War syndrome
Hair
Hair transplantation
Hand-foot-and-mouth disease
Hand hygiene compliance
Heat exhaustion and heatstroke
Hemangioma
Hematomas
Herpes
Histiocytosis
Hives
Hormone therapy
Host-defense mechanisms
Human papillomavirus (HPV)
Hyperbaric chamber
Hyperhidrosis
Hyperthyroidism and hypothyroidism
Impetigo
Intravenous (IV) therapy
Jaundice

Kaposi's sarcoma
Kawasaki disease
Kwashiorkor
Laceration repair
Laser use in surgery
Leishmaniasis
Leprosy
Lice, mites, and ticks
Light therapy
Lower extremities
Lyme disease
Measles
Melanoma
Mesenchymal stem cells
Methicillin-resistant staphylococcus aureus (MRSA) infection
Mold and mildew
Moles
Monkeypox
Morgellons disease
Multiple chemical sensitivity syndrome
Nails
Necrotizing fasciitis
Neurofibromatosis
Numbness and tingling
Otoplasty
Pellagra
Pigmentation
Pinworms
Pityriasis alba
Pityriasis rosea
Polycystic ovary syndrome
Polydactyly and syndactyly
Porphyria
Psoriasis
Radiation sickness
Reiter's syndrome
Ringworm
Rocky Mountain spotted fever
Rosacea
Roseola
Rubella
Sarcoidosis
Scabies
Scarlet fever
Sense organs
Shingles
Skin cancer
Skin disorders
Skin lesion removal
Smallpox
Streptococcal infections
Sturge-Weber syndrome
Styes
Sweating
Tattoo removal
Tattoos and body piercing
Touch
Toxoplasmosis
Tularemia
Typhoid fever

Typhus
Umbilical cord
Upper extremities
Vasculitis
Vitiligo
Von Willebrand's disease
Williams syndrome
Wiskott-Aldrich syndrome

SPINE
Anesthesia
Anesthesiology
Ankylosing spondylitis
Atrophy
Back pain
Brain tumors
Brucellosis
Charcot-Marie-Tooth Disease
Chiari malformations
Chiropractic
Diaphragm
Disk removal
Fetal tissue transplantation
Flexibility
Head and neck disorders
Kinesiology
Laminectomy and spinal fusion
Lumbar puncture
Marfan syndrome
Meningitis
Methicillin-resistant staphylococcus aureus (MRSA) infection
Motor neuron diseases
Multiple sclerosis
Narcotics
Nervous system
Neuralgia, neuritis, and neuropathy
Neuroimaging
Neurology
Neurosurgery
Orthopedic surgery
Orthopedics
Paget's disease
Paralysis
Paraplegia
Physical rehabilitation
Poliomyelitis
Quadriplegia
Radiculopathy
Sciatica
Scoliosis
Slipped disk
Spina bifida
Spinal cord disorders
Spondylitis
Sports medicine
Stenosis
Sympathectomy
Whiplash
Williams syndrome

SPLEEN
Abscess drainage
Aspergillosis
Brucellosis
Cold agglutinin disease
Gaucher's disease
Hematology
Hemoglobin
Hemolysis
Immune system
Internal medicine
Leptospirosis
Leukemia
Lymph
Lymphatic system
Malaria
Metabolism
Methicillin-resistant staphylococcus aureus (MRSA) infection
Mononucleosis
Niemann-Pick disease
Sarcoidosis
Sickle cell disease
Splenectomy
Thrombocytopenia
Transplantation
Typhoid fever

STOMACH
Abdomen
Abdominal disorders
Abscess drainage
Acid reflux disease
Adenoviruses
Allergies
Avian influenza
Bariatric surgery
Campylobacter infections
Chyme
Colitis
Digestion
Drowning
Eating disorders
Endoscopic retrograde cholangiopancreatography (ERCP)
Endoscopy
Esophagus
Food biochemistry
Food poisoning
Gastrectomy
Gastroenteritis
Gastroenterology
Gastrointestinal disorders
Gastrointestinal system
Gastrostomy
Hernia
Hernia repair
Internal medicine
Lactose intolerance
Malabsorption
Malnutrition

Metabolism
Motion sickness
Nausea and vomiting
Obesity
Peristalsis
Poisoning
Polyps
Pyloric stenosis
Radiation sickness
Stomach
Ulcer surgery
Ulcers
Vagotomy
Weaning
Weight loss and gain

TEETH
Angelman syndrome
Braces
Bulimia
Cavities
Cleft lip and palate repair
Cornelia de Lange syndrome
Crowns and bridges
Dental diseases
Dentistry
Dentures
Dysphagia
Eating disorders
Enamel
Endodontic disease
Fluoride treatments
Fracture repair
Gastrointestinal system
Gingivitis
Gum disease
Jaw wiring
Lisping
Mouth and throat cancer
Oral and maxillofacial surgery
Orthodontics
Periodontal surgery
Periodontitis
Plaque
Prader-Willi syndrome
Rickets
Root canal treatment
Rubinstein-Taybi syndrome
Scurvy
Teething
Temporomandibular joint (TMJ)
  syndrome
Thumb sucking
Tooth extraction
Wisdom teeth

TENDONS
Ankylosing spondylitis
Astym® therapy
Carpal tunnel syndrome
Casts and splints

Collagen
Connective tissue
Exercise physiology
Flexibility
Ganglion removal
Hammertoe correction
Hemiplegia
Joints
Kneecap removal
Orthopedic surgery
Orthopedics
Osgood-Schlatter disease
Physical rehabilitation
Rotator cuff surgery
Sports medicine
Tendinitis
Tendon disorders
Tendon repair

THROAT
Acid reflux disease
Acquired immunodeficiency syndrome
  (AIDS)
Adenoids
Antihistamines
Auras
Avian influenza
Catheterization
Choking
Croup
Decongestants
Diphtheria
Drowning
Eating disorders
Epiglottitis
Epstein-Barr virus
Esophagus
Fifth disease
Gastroenterology
Gastrointestinal system
Gonorrhea
Hay fever
Head and neck disorders
Heimlich maneuver
Hiccups
Histiocytosis
H1N1 influenza
Human papillomavirus (HPV)
Influenza
Laryngectomy
Laryngitis
Mononucleosis
Mouth and throat cancer
Nasopharyngeal disorders
Otorhinolaryngology
Pharyngitis
Pharynx
Polyps
Pulmonary medicine
Quinsy
Respiration

Rhinitis
Rhinoviruses
Smoking
Sore throat
Streptococcal infections
Tonsillectomy and adenoid removal
Tonsillitis
Tracheostomy
Tremors
Voice and vocal cord disorders
Whooping cough

TONGUE
Dysphagia
Folate deficiency
Taste
Vagus nerve

URINARY SYSTEM
Abdomen
Abdominal disorders
Abscess drainage
Adenoviruses
Adrenalectomy
Avian influenza
Bed-wetting
Bladder cancer
Bladder removal
Candidiasis
Catheterization
Chlamydia
Cold agglutinin disease
Cystic fibrosis
Cystitis
Cystoscopy
Dialysis
Diuretics
E. coli infection
End-stage renal disease
Endoscopy
Fetal surgery
Fistula repair
Gonorrhea
Hematuria
Hemolytic uremic syndrome
Hermaphroditism and
  pseudohermaphroditism
Hormone therapy
Host-defense mechanisms
Hyperplasia
Hypertension
Hypokalemia
Incontinence
Internal medicine
Kidney cancer
Kidney disorders
Kidney transplantation
Kidneys
Laparoscopy
Leptospirosis
Lithotripsy

Entries by Specialties and Related Fields

ALL
Abscesses
Accidents
Acupuncture
Adrenal glands
Aging
Aging: Extended care
Alternative medicine
Anatomy
Antibiotic resistance
Antibiotics
Antihypertensives
Anti-inflammatory drugs
Antioxidants
Autopsy
Biomarker
Bionics and biotechnology
Birth defects
Burkitt's lymphoma
Cancer
Carcinogens
Carcinoma
Chemotherapy
Chronic granulomatous disease
Clinical trials
Club drugs
Coccidioidomycosis
Cockayne disease
Collagen
Congenital disorders
Critical care
Cryosurgery
Cysts
Death and dying
Diagnosis
Dietary reference intakes (DRIs)
Disease
Embryology
Emergency medicine
Emergency rooms
Emerging infectious diseases
Environmental diseases
Enzyme therapy
Epidemics and pandemics
Epidemiology
Epidermal nevus syndromes
Essential nutrients
Family-centered care
Family medicine
Fascia
Fatigue
Fever
First aid
First responder
Food guide plate
Forensic pathology
Genetic diseases

Genetic engineering
Genetic imprinting
Genetics and inheritance
Genomics
Geriatric assessment
Geriatrics and gerontology
Grafts and grafting
Growth
Healing
Health
Herbal medicine
Histology
Homeopathy
Hospital readmission
Hydrotherapy
Hyperadiposis
Hyperthermia and hypothermia
Hypertrophy
Hypochondriasis
Iatrogenic disorders
Imaging and radiology
Immunopathology
Infection
Infection control
Inflammation
Insect-borne diseases
Internet medicine
Invasive tests
Leptin
Lesions
Longevity
Macronutrients
Magnetic resonance imaging (MRI)
Malignancy and metastasis
Malnutrition
Massage
Medical home
Meditation
Men's health
Mental hygiene
Metabolic disorders
Metabolic syndrome
Mucopolysaccharidosis (MPS)
Multiple births
Münchausen syndrome by proxy
Neonatology
Niacin
Noninvasive tests
Nursing
Nutrition
Occupational health
Oncology
Opportunistic infections
Orthorexia nervosa
Ovaries
Over-the-counter medications
Pain

Pain management
Palliative care
Palliative medicine
Paramedics
Parasitic diseases
Pathology
Pediatrics
Perinatology
Physical examination
Physician assistants
Physiology
Phytochemicals
Plastic surgery
Positron emission tomography (PET)
    scanning
Preventive medicine
Progeria
Prognosis
Prostheses
Protein
Proteomics
Psychiatry
Psychosomatic disorders
Puberty and adolescence
Radiation therapy
Radiopharmaceuticals
Reflexes
Retroviruses
Safety issues for children
Safety issues for the elderly
Screening
Self-medication
Shock
Signs and symptoms
Stem cells
Stress
Stress reduction
Substance abuse
Sudden infant death syndrome (SIDS)
Supplements
Surgery
Surgical procedures
Surgical technologists
Syndrome
Systemic lupus erythematosus (SLE)
Systemic sclerosis
Systems and organs
Teratogens
Terminally ill: Extended care
Tissue engineering
Toxic shock syndrome
Toxicology
Transitional care
Tumor removal
Tumors
Viral hemorrhagic fevers
Viral infections

Collagen
Colon
Connective tissue
Corticosteroids
CRISPR
Cystic fibrosis
Digestion
Endocrine glands
Endocrinology
Enzyme therapy
Ergogenic aids
Fatty acid
Fatty acid oxidation disorders
Fluids and electrolytes
Fluoride treatments
Food biochemistry
Food guide plate
Fructosemia
Galactosemia
Gaucher's disease
Genetic engineering
Genomics
Gigantism
Gingivitis
Glands
Glucagon
Glycerol
Glycogen storage diseases
Glycolysis
Gram staining
Gulf War syndrome
Hemoglobin
Histology
Hormones
Hyperadiposis
Hypothalamus
Insect-borne diseases
Insulin-like growth factors
Leptin
Leukodystrophy
Lipids
Lumbar puncture
Macronutrients
Malabsorption
Malaria
Melatonin
Mesenchymal stem cells
Metabolic disorders
Metabolism
Myoglobin
Nephrology
Neuroethics
Niemann-Pick disease
Nutrition
Ovaries
Pathology
Pharmacology
Phenylketonuria (PKU)
Pituitary gland
Plasma
Protein

Respiration
Retroviruses
Rhinoviruses
Serotonin
Sleep
Small intestine
Statins
Steroids
Thymus gland
Tourette's syndrome
Urinalysis
Wilson's disease

BIOTECHNOLOGY
Antibodies
Assisted reproductive technologies
Biological therapies
Bionics and biotechnology
Cloning
Computed tomography (CT) scanning
Defibrillation
Dialysis
Electrocardiography (ECG or EKG)
Electroencephalography (EEG)
Fatty acid oxidation disorders
Gene therapy
Genetic engineering
Genomics
Glycogen storage diseases
Huntington's disease
Hyperbaric oxygen therapy
Insect-borne diseases
Magnetic resonance imaging (MRI)
Malabsorption
Nephrology
Pacemaker implantation
Positron emission tomography (PET)
  scanning
Prostheses
Rhinoviruses
Severe combined immunodeficiency
  syndrome (SCID)
Sperm banks
Xenotransplantation

CARDIOLOGY
Acute respiratory distress syndrome
  (ARDS)
Aging: Extended care
Anemia
Aneurysms
Angina
Angiography
Angioplasty
Antihypertensives
Anxiety
Aortic aneurysm
Aortic stenosis
Arrhythmias
Arteriosclerosis
Aspergillosis

Atrial fibrillation
Biofeedback
Blood pressure
Blood vessels
Blue baby syndrome
Brucellosis
Bypass surgery
Cardiac arrest
Cardiac rehabilitation
Cardiac surgery
Cardiopulmonary resuscitation (CPR)
Carotid arteries
Catheterization
Chest
Circulation
Computed tomography (CT) scanning
Congenital heart disease
Coronary artery bypass graft
Critical care
Defibrillation
DiGeorge syndrome
Diphtheria
Dirofilaria immitis
Diuretics
Dizziness and fainting
Echocardiography
Electrocardiography (ECG or EKG)
Electrocauterization
Embolism
Emergency medicine
End-stage renal disease
Endocarditis
Enteroviruses
Exercise physiology
Extracorporeal membrane oxygenation
  (ECMO)
Fetal surgery
Gigantism
Heart
Heart attack
Heart disease
Heart failure
Heart transplantation
Heart valve replacement
Hematology
Hemochromatosis
Hemoglobin
Hormone therapy
Hypercholesterolemia
Hypertension
Hyperthyroidism and hypothyroidism
Hypokalemia
Hypotension
Infarction
Internal medicine
Ischemia
Kawasaki disease
Kinesiology
Leptin
Lesions
Lyme disease

Marfan syndrome
Mesenchymal stem cells
Metabolic syndrome
Methicillin-resistant staphylococcus
  aureus (MRSA) infection
Mitral valve prolapse
Mucopolysaccharidosis (MPS)
Muscles
Neonatology
Noninvasive tests
Nuclear medicine
Osteogenesis imperfecta
Oxygen therapy
Pacemaker implantation
Palliative care
Palpitations
Paramedics
Patent ductus arteriosus
Pellagra
Plaque
Plasma
Polycystic kidney disease
Postural orthostatic tachycardia
  syndrome (POTS)
Prader-Willi syndrome
Progeria
Prostheses
Pulmonary heart disease
Pulmonary edema
Pulmonary hypertension
Pulse pressure
Pulse rate
Rheumatic fever
Rubinstein-Taybi syndrome
Sarcoidosis
Single photon emission computed
  tomography (SPECT)
Spondylitis
Sports medicine
Staphylococcal infections
Stenosis
Stents
Systemic lupus erythematosus (SLE)
Thoracic surgery
Thrombolytic therapy and TPA
Thrombosis and thrombus
Tissue engineering
Transplantation
Ultrasonography
Uremia
Varicose veins
Vascular medicine
Vascular system
Vasculitis
Williams syndrome

CRITICAL CARE
Acidosis
Aging: Extended care
Amputation
Anesthesia

Anesthesiology
Aneurysmectomy
Anthrax
Apgar score
Botulism
Burns and scalds
Carotid arteries
Catheterization
Chronic granulomatous disease
Club drugs
Concussion
Craniotomy
Defibrillation
Diuretics
Drowning
Echocardiography
Electrical shock
Electrocardiography (ECG or EKG)
Electrocauterization
Electroencephalography (EEG)
Embolization
Emergency medicine
Epidemics and pandemics
Grafts and grafting
Hantavirus
Heart attack
Heart transplantation
Heat exhaustion and heatstroke
Hydrocephalus
Hyperbaric oxygen therapy
Hyperthermia and hypothermia
Hypotension
Hypoxia
Infarction
Insect-borne diseases
Intravenous (IV) therapy
Ischemia
Lumbar puncture
Methicillin-resistant staphylococcus
  aureus (MRSA) infection
Necrotizing fasciitis
Neonatology
Nursing
Oncology
Osteopathic medicine
Oxygen therapy
Pain management
Palliative care
Paramedics
Peritonitis
Psychiatry
Pulmonary medicine
Pulse rate
Radiation sickness
Resuscitation
Safety issues for children
Safety issues for the elderly
Severe acute respiratory syndrome
  (SARS)
Shock
Stevens-Johnson syndrome

Streptococcal infections
Thrombolytic therapy and TPA
Toxic shock syndrome
Tracheostomy
Transfusion
Whooping cough
Wounds

CYTOLOGY
Acid-base chemistry
Bionics and biotechnology
Biopsy
Blood testing
Breast disorders
Cancer
Carcinoma
Cells
Cholesterol
Cytopathology
Dermatology
Dermatopathology
Epstein-Barr virus
Eye infections and disorders
Fluids and electrolytes
Food biochemistry
Gaucher's disease
Gene therapy
Genetic counseling
Genomics
Glycolysis
Gram staining
Healing
Hematocrit
Hematology
Hirschsprung's disease
Histology
Hyperplasia
Immune system
Karyotyping
Laboratory tests
Lipids
Metabolism
Microscopy
Mutation
Neutrophil
Oncology
Pathology
Pharmacology
Plasma
Rhinoviruses
Sarcoma
Serology

DENTISTRY
Aging: Extended care
Anesthesia
Anesthesiology
Braces
Canker sores
Cavities
Cerebral palsy

Cockayne disease
Crowns and bridges
Dental diseases
Dentures
Eating disorders
Enamel
Endodontic disease
Fluoride treatments
Forensic pathology
Fracture repair
Gastrointestinal system
Gingivitis
Gum disease
Head and neck disorders
Jaw wiring
Lisping
Local anesthesia
Mouth and throat cancer
Oral and maxillofacial surgery
Orthodontics
Osteogenesis imperfecta
Periodontal surgery
Periodontitis
Plaque
Prader-Willi syndrome
Prostheses
Root canal treatment
Rubinstein-Taybi syndrome
Sense organs
Sjögren's syndrome
Teeth
Teething
Temporomandibular joint (TMJ) syndrome
Thumb sucking
Tooth extraction
Von Willebrand's disease
Wisdom teeth

DERMATOLOGY
Abscess drainage
Acne
Acquired immunodeficiency syndrome (AIDS)
Adrenoleukodystrophy
Allergies
Alopecia
Angelman syndrome
Anthrax
Anti-inflammatory drugs
Athlete's foot
Bedsores
Bile
Biopsy
Blisters
Body dysmorphic disorder
Burns and scalds
Carcinoma
Chickenpox
Chronic granulomatous disease
Coccidioidomycosis

Cockayne disease
Collodion baby
Corns and calluses
Cryosurgery
Cutis marmorata telangiectatica congenita
Cyst removal
Dermatitis
Dermatopathology
Dirofilaria immitis
Eczema
Electrocauterization
Electrolysis
Enteroviruses
Facial transplantation
Folate deficiency
Fungal infections
Ganglion removal
Gangrene
Gender dysphoria
Genetic engineering
Glands
Gluten intolerance
Grafts and grafting
Hair
Hair transplantation
Hand-foot-and-mouth disease
Healing
Hemangioma
Herpes
Histology
Hives
Hyaluronic acid injections
Hyperbaric chamber
Hyperhidrosis
Hyperthyroidism and hypothyroidism
Immunopathology
Impetigo
Laser use in surgery
Lesions
Lice, mites, and ticks
Light therapy
Local anesthesia
Lyme disease
Melanoma
Mesenchymal stem cells
Methicillin-resistant staphylococcus aureus (MRSA) infection
Moles
Monkeypox
Morgellons disease
Multiple chemical sensitivity syndrome
Nails
Necrotizing fasciitis
Neurofibromatosis
Pellagra
Pigmentation
Pinworms
Pityriasis alba
Pityriasis rosea
Plastic surgery

Podiatry
Polycystic ovary syndrome
Postherpetic neuralgia
Prostheses
Psoriasis
Puberty and adolescence
Reiter's syndrome
Ringworm
Rocky Mountain spotted fever
Rosacea
Sarcoidosis
Scabies
Scleroderma
Sense organs
Shingles
Skin
Skin cancer
Skin disorders
Skin lesion removal
Smallpox
Staphylococcal infections
Stevens-Johnson syndrome
Streptococcal infections
Stress
Sturge-Weber syndrome
Styes
Sweating
Systemic lupus erythematosus (SLE)
Tattoo removal
Tattoos and body piercing
Tissue engineering
Touch
Vasculitis
Vitiligo
Von Willebrand's disease
Wiskott-Aldrich syndrome

DIETETICS
Essential nutrients
Fasting
Folate deficiency
Glycerol
Health impact of sugar
Pellagra

EMBRYOLOGY
Amniocentesis
Assisted reproductive technologies
Birth defects
Blue baby syndrome
Chorionic villus sampling
Cloning
Conception
Down syndrome
Ectopic pregnancy
Fetal tissue transplantation
Fetus
Gamete intrafallopian transfer (GIFT)
Genetic counseling
Genetic diseases
Genetic engineering

Genetic imprinting
Genetics and inheritance
Genomics
Growth
Hermaphroditism and
  pseudohermaphroditism
In vitro fertilization
Karyotyping
Klinefelter syndrome
Meckel's diverticulum
Miscarriage
Mucopolysaccharidosis (MPS)
Multiple births
Neonatology
Obstetrics
Ovaries
Perinatology
Phenylketonuria (PKU)
Placenta
Pregnancy and gestation
Premature birth
Reproductive system
Rh factor
Sexual differentiation
Spina bifida
Syphilis
Teratogens
Ultrasonography
Uterus

EMERGENCY MEDICINE
Abdominal disorders
Abscess drainage
Acidosis
Adrenoleukodystrophy
Advance directives
Altitude sickness
Amputation
Anesthesia
Anesthesiology
Aneurysmectomy
Aneurysms
Angiography
Anthrax
Appendectomy
Appendicitis
Asphyxiation
Atrial fibrillation
Back pain
Bites and stings
Bleeding
Blurred vision
Botulism
Bruises
Burns and scalds
Cardiac arrest
Cardiology
Cardiopulmonary resuscitation (CPR)
Carotid arteries
Casts and splints
Catheterization

Cesarean section
Choking
Cholecystitis
Chronic granulomatous disease
Club drugs
Cold agglutinin disease
Computed tomography (CT) scanning
Concussion
Critical care
Croup
Defibrillation
Dizziness and fainting
Drowning
Echocardiography
Electrical shock
Electrocardiography (ECG or EKG)
Electrocauterization
Electroencephalography (EEG)
Embolization
Epiglottitis
First responder
Fracture and dislocation
Frostbite
Gangrene
Grafts and grafting
Head and neck disorders
Heart attack
Heart transplantation
Heat exhaustion and heatstroke
Heimlich maneuver
H1N1 influenza
Hyperbaric oxygen therapy
Hyperthermia and hypothermia
Hyperventilation
Hypotension
Hypoxia
Impetigo
Infarction
Influenza
Insulin
Interpartner violence
Interstitial pulmonary fibrosis (IPF)
Intravenous (IV) therapy
Jaw wiring
Laceration repair
Local anesthesia
Lung surgery
Meningitis
Mental status exam
Monkeypox
Nail removal
Necrotizing fasciitis
Noninvasive tests
Nursing
Osteopathic medicine
Oxygen therapy
Pain management
Palliative medicine
Paramedics
Peritonitis
Physician assistants

Plague
Plastic surgery
Pleurisy
Pneumonia
Pneumothorax
Poisoning
Pulmonary medicine
Pulse rate
Pyelonephritis
Radiation sickness
Rape and sexual assault
Resuscitation
Reye's syndrome
Rocky Mountain spotted fever
Safety issues for children
Safety issues for the elderly
Severe acute respiratory syndrome
  (SARS)
Shock
Snakebites
Spinal cord disorders
Splenectomy
Sports medicine
Stevens-Johnson syndrome
Streptococcal infections
Strokes
Surgical technologists
Thrombolytic therapy and TPA
Toxic shock syndrome
Tracheostomy
Transfusion
Transplantation
Tularemia
Wounds

ENDOCRINOLOGY
Addison's disease
Adolescent sexuality
Adrenalectomy
Adrenoleukodystrophy
Amenorrhea
Anorexia nervosa
Assisted reproductive technologies
Bariatric surgery
Biofeedback
Brain death
Breasts
Carbohydrates
Computed tomography (CT) scanning
Congenital adrenal hyperplasia
Congenital hypothyroidism
Corticosteroids
Cushing's syndrome
Diabetes mellitus
Dwarfism
End-stage renal disease
Endocrine disorders
Endocrine glands
Endocrinology
Ergogenic aids
Failure to thrive

Fibrocystic breast condition
Galactorrhea
Gender reassignment surgery
Gestational diabetes
Gigantism
Glands
Glucose tolerance test
Goiter
Gynecomastia
Hashimoto's thyroiditis
Health impact of sugar
Hormones
Hyperparathyroidism and
  hypoparathyroidism
Hypoglycemia
Hypothalamus
Insulin
Klinefelter syndrome
Lead poisoning
Liver
Melatonin
Nonalcoholic steatohepatitis (NASH)
Obesity
Overtraining syndrome
Pancreas
Pancreatitis
Parathyroidectomy
Pituitary gland
Placenta
Plasma
Polycystic ovary syndrome
Postpartum depression
Prader-Willi syndrome
Preeclampsia and eclampsia
Prostate gland
Prostate gland removal
Sexual differentiation
Small intestine
Statins
Steroid abuse
Steroids
Testicular cancer
Testicular surgery
Thymus gland
Thyroid disorders
Thyroid gland
Thyroidectomy
Turner syndrome
Weight loss medications
Williams syndrome

ENVIRONMENTAL HEALTH
Acidosis
Asbestos exposure
Asthma
Babesiosis
Blurred vision
Cholera
Cognitive development
Coronaviruses
Creutzfeldt-Jakob disease (CJD)

Drowning
Elephantiasis
Enteroviruses
Food poisoning
Frostbite
Gastroenteritis
Gulf War syndrome
Hantavirus
Hyperthermia and hypothermia
Insect-borne diseases
Lead poisoning
Legionnaires' disease
Lung cancer
Lungs
Mercury poisoning
Microbiology
Mold and mildew
Multiple chemical sensitivity syndrome
Occupational health
Parasitic diseases
Pigmentation
Plague
Poisoning
Pulmonary diseases
Pulmonary medicine
Roundworms
Schistosomiasis
Skin cancer
Sleeping sickness
Smallpox
Stress
Stress reduction
Trachoma
Tularemia
Typhoid fever
Typhus
West Nile virus
Yellow fever

EPIDEMIOLOGY
Acquired immunodeficiency syndrome
  (AIDS)
Adolescent sexuality
Amebiasis
Avian influenza
Bacillus Calmette-Guérin (BCG)
Bacterial infections
Bacteriology
Brucellosis
Candidiasis
Cerebral palsy
Chickenpox
Childhood infectious diseases
Cholera
Coronaviruses
Creutzfeldt-Jakob disease (CJD)
Diphtheria
E. coli infection
Ebola virus
Elephantiasis
Encephalitis

Epidemics and pandemics
Food poisoning
Forensic pathology
Gulf War syndrome
Hantavirus
Hepatitis
Herd immunity
H1N1 influenza
Human papillomavirus (HPV)
Influenza
Insect-borne diseases
Laboratory tests
Legionnaires' disease
Leprosy
Leptospirosis
Lyme disease
Marburg virus
Mercury poisoning
Methicillin-resistant staphylococcus
  aureus (MRSA) infection
Microbiology
Multiple chemical sensitivity syndrome
Necrotizing fasciitis
Occupational health
Parasitic diseases
Phenylketonuria (PKU)
Plague
Pneumonia
Poisoning
Poliomyelitis
Prion diseases
Pulmonary diseases
Rabies
Rhinoviruses
Rocky Mountain spotted fever
Rotavirus
Roundworms
Screening
Severe acute respiratory syndrome
  (SARS)
Sexually transmitted diseases (STDs)
Shigellosis
Sleeping sickness
Smallpox
Staphylococcal infections
Stress
Syphilis
Trichomoniasis
Tularemia
Typhoid fever
Typhus
Viral hemorrhagic fevers
Viral infections
West Nile virus
Yellow fever
Zoonoses

ETHICS
Abortion
Advance directives
Assisted reproductive technologies

Influenza
Interpartner violence
Intestinal disorders
Juvenile rheumatoid arthritis
Kawasaki disease
Keratitis
Kluver-Bucy syndrome
Kwashiorkor
Leishmaniasis
Leukodystrophy
Malabsorption
Maple syrup urine disease (MSUD)
Mastitis
Measles
Methicillin-resistant staphylococcus
    aureus (MRSA) infection
Mitral valve prolapse
Moles
Mononucleosis
Motion sickness
Mumps
Münchausen syndrome by proxy
Muscle sprains, spasms, and disorders
Myringotomy
Nail removal
Nasal polyp removal
Nasopharyngeal disorders
Neurosis
Niemann-Pick disease
Nonalcoholic steatohepatitis (NASH)
Non-steroidal anti-inflammatory drugs
    (NSAIDs)
Obesity
Orchitis
Osteopathic medicine
Otoplasty
Over-the-counter medications
Palliative medicine
Parasitic diseases
Patient-centered medical home
Pediatrics
Pharmacology
Physician assistants
Pick's disease
Pinworms
Pituitary gland
Pityriasis alba
Pityriasis rosea
Pleurisy
Pneumonia
Polycystic ovary syndrome
Polyps
Prader-Willi syndrome
Precocious puberty
Pregnancy test
Premenstrual syndrome (PMS)
Psychiatry
Ptosis
Puberty and adolescence
Pulse rate
Pyelonephritis

Reflexes
Reiter's syndrome
Rheumatic fever
Rhinitis
Ringworm
Rocky Mountain spotted fever
Roseola
Rubella
Safety issues for children
Safety issues for the elderly
Salmonella infection
Scabies
Scarlet fever
Sciatica
Sexuality
Shingles
Shock
Sinusitis
Sjögren's syndrome
Skin disorders
Sleep
Slipped disk
Sore throat
Sports medicine
Sterilization
Stevens-Johnson syndrome
Streptococcal infections
Stress
Stuttering
Styes
Supplements
Systemic lupus erythematosus (SLE)
Temporomandibular joint (TMJ)
    syndrome
Tendinitis
Testicular torsion
Tetanus
Thalassemia
Tinnitus
Toilet training
Tonsillitis
Tonsils
Tourette's syndrome
Toxoplasmosis
Trachoma
Ulcers
Urethritis
Urology
Vascular medicine
Vasectomy
Viral infections
Vitamins and minerals
Von Willebrand's disease
Weaning
Weight loss medications
Whooping cough
Wounds

FORENSIC MEDICINE
Antianxiety drugs
Autopsy

Blood testing
Cytopathology
Defibrillation
Dermatopathology
Genetic engineering
Genetics and inheritance
Hematology
Laboratory tests
Pathology

GASTROENTEROLOGY
Abdomen
Abdominal disorders
Achalasia
Acid reflux disease
Acidosis
Acquired immunodeficiency syndrome
    (AIDS)
Adenoviruses
Amebiasis
Amylase
Amyotrophic lateral sclerosis (ALS)
Anal cancer
Anus
Appendicitis
Bariatric surgery
Bile
Bilirubin
Bulimia
Bypass surgery
Campylobacter infections
Celiac sprue
Cholecystitis
Cholera
Chronic granulomatous disease
Chyme
Colic
Colitis
Colon
Colonoscopy and sigmoidoscopy
Colorectal cancer
Colorectal polyp removal
Colorectal surgery
Computed tomography (CT) scanning
Constipation
Critical care
Crohn's disease
Cystic fibrosis
Cytomegalovirus (CMV)
Diarrhea and dysentery
Digestion
Diverticulitis and diverticulosis
Dysarthria
Dysphagia
E. coli infection
Emergency medicine
Endoscopic retrograde
    cholangiopancreatography (ERCP)
Endoscopy
Enterocolitis
Epidemics and pandemics

Esophagus
Essential nutrients
Failure to thrive
Fecal bacteriotherapy
Fiber
Fistula repair
Folate deficiency
Food allergies
Food biochemistry
Food poisoning
Gallbladder
Gallbladder cancer
Gallbladder diseases
Gastrectomy
Gastroenteritis
Gastrointestinal disorders
Gastrointestinal system
Gastrostomy
Giardiasis
Glands
Gluten
Gluten intolerance
Hemochromatosis
Hemolysis
Hemolytic uremic syndrome
Hemorrhoid banding and removal
Hemorrhoids
Hernia
Hernia repair
Hiccups
Ileostomy and colostomy
Infarction
Internal medicine
Intestinal disorders
Intestines
Irritable bowel syndrome (IBS)
Jaundice
Lactose intolerance
Laparoscopy
Leaky gut syndrome
Lesions
Liver
Liver cancer
Liver disorders
Liver transplantation
Malabsorption
Malnutrition
Meckel's diverticulum
Metabolism
Nausea and vomiting
Nonalcoholic steatohepatitis (NASH)
Noroviruses
Pancreas
Pancreatitis
Pellagra
Peristalsis
Peritonitis
Polycystic kidney disease
Polyps
Proctology
Pyloric stenosis

Rectum
Rotavirus
Salmonella infection
Scleroderma
Shigellosis
Small intestine
Soiling
Stenosis
Stevens-Johnson syndrome
Stomach
Stone removal
Stones
Systemic lupus erythematosus (SLE)
Tapeworms
Taste
Tissue engineering
Toilet training
Ulcer surgery
Ulcerative colitis
Ulcers
Vagotomy
Vagus nerve
Vasculitis
Von Willebrand's disease
Weight loss and gain
Wilson's disease

GENERAL SURGERY
Abscess drainage
Achalasia
Adenoids
Adrenalectomy
Amputation
Anesthesia
Anesthesiology
Aneurysms
Appendectomy
Arthroplasty
Back pain
Bariatric surgery
Biopsy
Bladder removal
Bone marrow transplantation
Brain tumors
Breast biopsy
Breast cancer
Breast disorders
Breast surgery
Bunions
Bypass surgery
Casts and splints
Catheterization
Cesarean section
Cholecystectomy
Chronic granulomatous disease
Circumcision, female, and genital
  mutilation
Circumcision
Coccidioidomycosis
Colon
Colonoscopy and sigmoidoscopy

Colorectal polyp removal
Colorectal surgery
Corneal transplantation
Cryosurgery
Culdocentesis
Cyst removal
Defibrillation
Disk removal
Ear surgery
Electrocauterization
Endarterectomy
Eye infections and disorders
Eye surgery
Face lift and blepharoplasty
Fistula repair
Gallbladder cancer
Ganglion removal
Gastrectomy
Gender dysphoria
Gender reassignment surgery
Gigantism
Grafts and grafting
Hair transplantation
Hammertoe correction
Heart transplantation
Heart valve replacement
Heel spur removal
Hemorrhoid banding and removal
Hernia repair
Hydroceles
Hydrocephalus
Hypospadias repair and urethroplasty
Hypoxia
Hysterectomy
Infarction
Intravenous (IV) therapy
Kidney transplantation
Kneecap removal
Laceration repair
Laparoscopy
Laryngectomy
Lesions
Liposuction
Liver transplantation
Lumbar puncture
Lung surgery
Mastectomy and lumpectomy
Meckel's diverticulum
Mesothelioma
Methicillin-resistant staphylococcus
  aureus (MRSA) infection
Mouth and throat cancer
Nasal polyp removal
Nephrectomy
Neurosurgery
Oncology
Ophthalmology
Orthopedic surgery
Otoplasty
Pain
Parathyroidectomy

Aging
Aging: Extended care
Alzheimer's disease
Arthroplasty
Assisted living facilities
Ataxia
Atrophy
Back pain
Blindness
Blood pressure
Blurred vision
Bone disorders
Brain disorders
Cartilage
Cataracts
Chronic obstructive pulmonary disease
 (COPD)
Critical care
Deafness
Death and dying
Dementias
Depression
Dyskinesia
Emergency medicine
End-stage renal disease
Eye infections and disorders
Eye surgery
Family-centered care
Family medicine
Fatigue
Fiber
Hip fracture repair
Hormone therapy
Hypotension
Incontinence
Interpartner violence
Joints
Massage
Memory loss
Neuroscience
Nursing
Osteoclast
Osteopathic medicine
Osteoporosis
Pain management
Palliative care
Paramedics
Parkinson's Disease
Physician assistants
Pick's disease
Psychiatry
Radiculopathy
Rheumatoid arthritis
Rheumatology
Safety issues for the elderly
Sleep disorders
Spine
Suicide
Temporal arteritis
Tremors
Vision disorders

GYNECOLOGY
Abdomen
Abortion
Acquired immunodeficiency syndrome
 (AIDS)
Amenorrhea
Assisted reproductive technologies
Biopsy
Bladder removal
Blurred vision
Breast biopsy
Breast cancer
Breast disorders
Breast-feeding
Breasts
Cervical, ovarian, and uterine cancers
Cervical procedures
Cesarean section
Childbirth
Childbirth complications
Chlamydia
Circumcision, female, and genital
 mutilation
Conception
Contraception
Cryosurgery
Culdocentesis
Cyst removal
Cystitis
Cystoscopy
Dysmenorrhea
Ectopic pregnancy
Electrocauterization
Embolization
Endocrinology
Endometrial biopsy
Endometriosis
Endoscopy
Episiotomy
Fibrocystic breast condition
Galactorrhea
Gender reassignment surgery
Genital disorders
Glands
Gonorrhea
Hermaphroditism and
 pseudohermaphroditism
Herpes
Hormone therapy
Human papillomavirus (HPV)
Hyperplasia
Hysterectomy
In vitro fertilization
Incontinence
Infertility
Internal medicine
Laparoscopy
Leptin
Lesions
Mammography
Mastitis

Menopause
Menorrhagia
Menstruation
Miscarriage
Myomectomy
Obstetrics
Ovarian cysts
Ovaries
Oxytocin
Pap test
Pelvic inflammatory disease (PID)
Polycystic ovary syndrome
Polyps
Postpartum depression
Preeclampsia and eclampsia
Pregnancy and gestation
Pregnancy test
Premenstrual syndrome (PMS)
Rape and sexual assault
Reiter's syndrome
Reproductive system
Sexual differentiation
Sexual dysfunction
Sexuality
Sexually transmitted diseases (STDs)
Sterilization
Syphilis
Toxic shock syndrome
Trichomoniasis
Tubal ligation
Turner syndrome
Ultrasonography
Urinary disorders
Urology
Uterus
Von Willebrand's disease

HEMATOLOGY
Acid-base chemistry
Acidosis
Acquired immunodeficiency syndrome
 (AIDS)
Anemia
Anticoagulants
Babesiosis
Biological therapies
Bleeding
Blood and blood disorders
Blood testing
Blood vessels
Bone grafting
Bone Marrow
Bone marrow transplantation
Bruises
Burkitt's lymphoma
Chronic fatigue syndrome
Circulation
Cold agglutinin disease
Connective tissue
Cyanosis
Cytology

Influenza
Insulin
Interpartner violence
Interstitial pulmonary fibrosis (IPF)
Intestinal disorders
Intestines
Jaundice
Kaposi's sarcoma
Kidney disorders
Klippel-Trenaunay syndrome
Legionnaires' disease
Leprosy
Leptospirosis
Lesions
Leukemia
Liver
Liver disorders
Lymph
Lymphadenopathy and lymphoma
Malaria
Malignancy and metastasis
Measles
Melanoma
Metabolic syndrome
Methicillin-resistant staphylococcus
  aureus (MRSA) infection
Mitral valve prolapse
Monkeypox
Multiple sclerosis
Nail removal
Nephritis
Nephrology
Niemann-Pick disease
Nonalcoholic steatohepatitis (NASH)
Non-steroidal anti-inflammatory drugs
  (NSAIDs)
Nuclear medicine
Obesity
Occupational health
Opportunistic infections
Osteopathic medicine
Pain
Palliative care
Palliative medicine
Pancreas
Pancreatitis
Parasitic diseases
Parkinson's Disease
Peristalsis
Peritonitis
Pharynx
Phlebitis
Physician assistants
Pick's disease
Plaque
Plasma
Pleurisy
Pneumonia
Polymyalgia rheumatica
Polyps
Postherpetic neuralgia

Proctology
Psoriasis
Puberty and adolescence
Pulmonary edema
Pulmonary medicine
Pulse rate
Pyelonephritis
Radiopharmaceuticals
Rectum
Renal failure
Reye's syndrome
Rocky Mountain spotted fever
Sarcoidosis
Scarlet fever
Schistosomiasis
Sciatica
Septicemia
Severe acute respiratory syndrome
  (SARS)
Sexuality
Sexually transmitted diseases (STDs)
Shingles
Shock
Sinusitis
Sleep
Sleeping sickness
Small intestine
Sports medicine
Staphylococcal infections
Stevens-Johnson syndrome
Stones
Streptococcal infections
Stress
Supplements
Syphilis
Systemic lupus erythematosus (SLE)
Tetanus
Thrombosis and thrombus
Toxic shock syndrome
Tremors
Tumors
Typhoid fever
Typhus
Ulcers
Ultrasonography
Urethritis
Viral infections
Vitamins and minerals
Weight loss medications
Wilson's disease
Wounds

MICROBIOLOGY
Acquired immunodeficiency syndrome
  (AIDS)
Amebiasis
Anthrax
Antibiotic resistance
Antibiotics
Antibodies
Autopsy

Bacillus Calmette-Guérin (BCG)
Bacterial infections
Bacteriology
Bionics and biotechnology
Brucellosis
Campylobacter infections
Chemotherapy
Chlamydia
Cholera
Chronic granulomatous disease
Coccidioidomycosis
Conjunctivitis
Creutzfeldt-Jakob disease (CJD)
Dengue fever
Diphtheria
E. coli infection
Enteroviruses
Epidemics and pandemics
Epstein-Barr virus
Fecal bacteriotherapy
Fluoride treatments
Fungal infections
Gastroenteritis
Gastroenterology
Gastrointestinal disorders
Genomics
Gonorrhea
Gram staining
Hematuria
Human immunodeficiency virus (HIV)
Immune system
Immunization and vaccination
Impetigo
Insect-borne diseases
Laboratory tests
Leptospirosis
Methicillin-resistant staphylococcus
  aureus (MRSA) infection
Microscopy
Mold and mildew
Opportunistic infections
Pathology
Pelvic inflammatory disease (PID)
Peritonitis
Pharmacology
Plasma
Pneumocystis jirovecii
Protozoan diseases
Serology
Severe acute respiratory syndrome
  (SARS)
Sleeping sickness
Staphylococcal infections
Streptococcal infections
Syphilis
Toxic shock syndrome
Trichinosis
Tuberculosis
Urinalysis
Urology

NEONATOLOGY

Amniotic fluid
Angelman syndrome
Apgar score
Apnea
Birth defects
Blue baby syndrome
Bonding
Breast disorders
Cesarean section
Childbirth
Childbirth complications
Cleft lip and palate
Cleft lip and palate repair
Collodion baby
Congenital disorders
Congenital heart disease
Cutis marmorata telangiectatica
  congenita
Disseminated intravascular coagulation
  (DIC)
E. coli infection
Embryology
Endocrinology
Extracorporeal membrane oxygenation
  (ECMO)
Failure to thrive
Fetal surgery
Genetic diseases
Hemolytic disease of the newborn
Hydrocephalus
Intraventricular hemorrhage
Karyotyping
Malabsorption
Maple syrup urine disease (MSUD)
Motor skill development
Multiple births
Neonatal brachial plexus palsy
Neurology
Nursing
Obstetrics
Patent ductus arteriosus
Pediatrics
Perinatology
Phenylketonuria (PKU)
Physician assistants
Premature birth
Pulse rate
Respiratory distress syndrome
Rh factor
Shunts
Spina bifida
Sudden infant death syndrome (SIDS)
Surgery
Syphilis
Tay-Sachs disease
Transfusion
Trichomoniasis
Umbilical cord
Well-baby examinations

NEPHROLOGY

Abdomen
Addison's disease
Anemia
Chronic granulomatous disease
Diabetes mellitus
Diabetic nephropathy
Dialysis
Diuretics
E. coli infection
Edema
End-stage renal disease
Ergogenic aids
Hematuria
Hemolysis
Hemolytic uremic syndrome
Hypokalemia
Internal medicine
Kidney cancer
Kidney disorders
Kidney transplantation
Kidneys
Leptospirosis
Lesions
Lithotripsy
Nephrectomy
Nephritis
Nuclear medicine
Palliative care
Polycystic kidney disease
Polyps
Preeclampsia and eclampsia
Proteinuria
Pyelonephritis
Renal failure
Sarcoidosis
Stenosis
Stone removal
Stones
Systemic lupus erythematosus (SLE)
Transplantation
Uremia
Urinalysis
Urinary disorders
Urinary system
Urology
Vasculitis
Wilms tumor
Williams syndrome

NEUROLOGY

Acquired immunodeficiency syndrome
  (AIDS)
Adrenoleukodystrophy
Aging: Extended care
Agnosia
Altitude sickness
Alzheimer's disease
Amnesia
Amyotrophic lateral sclerosis (ALS)
Anesthesia

Anesthesiology
Aneurysms
Angelman syndrome
Anorexia nervosa
Anosmia
Antidepressants
Antipsychotic drugs
Aphasia and dysphasia
Apnea
Asperger syndrome
Ataxia
Atrophy
Attention-deficit disorder (ADD)
Audiology
Auras
Back pain
Balance disorders
Batten's disease
Bell's palsy
Biofeedback
Blindsight
Botox
Brain
Brain damage
Brain death
Brain disorders
Brain tumors
Brucellosis
Capgras syndrome
Carotid arteries
Carpal tunnel syndrome
Cerebral palsy
Charcot-Marie-Tooth Disease
Chiari malformations
Chiropractic
Chronic wasting disease (CWD)
Cluster headaches
Cockayne disease
Cognitive enhancement
Concussion
Cornelia de Lange syndrome
Craniotomy
Creutzfeldt-Jakob disease (CJD)
Critical care
Cryosurgery
Cutis marmorata telangiectatica
  congenita
Deep brain stimulation
Delirium
Dementias
Depression
Developmental stages
Diabetes mellitus
Diabetic neuropathy
Disk removal
Dizziness and fainting
Dysarthria
Dyskinesia
Dyslexia
Dysphagia
Ear infections and disorders

Ears
Electrical shock
Electroencephalography (EEG)
Electromyography
Embolism
Emergency medicine
Encephalitis
Enteroviruses
Epilepsy
Eye infections and disorders
Fascia
Fetal tissue transplantation
Folate deficiency
Frontal lobe syndrome
Frontotemporal dementia (FTD)
Functional magnetic imaging (fMRI)
Gigantism
Glasgow coma scale
Glioma
Grafts and grafting
Guillain-Barré syndrome
Head and neck disorders
Headaches
Hearing
Hearing tests
Hematomas
Hemiplegia
Hiccups
Hippocampus
Huntington's disease
Hydrocephalus
Hyperhidrosis
Hypothalamus
Hypoxia
Infarction
Insulin-like growth factors
Intraventricular hemorrhage
Ischemia
Korsakoff's syndrome
Leaky gut syndrome
Learning disabilities
Lesions
Leukodystrophy
Lower extremities
Lumbar puncture
Lyme disease
Marijuana
Melatonin
Memory erasure
Memory loss
Meningitis
Mercury poisoning
Mesenchymal stem cells
Minimally conscious state
Morgellons disease
Motion sickness
Motor neuron diseases
Motor skill development
Multiple chemical sensitivity syndrome
Multiple sclerosis
Myasthenia gravis

Narcolepsy
Neonatal brachial plexus palsy
Nervous system
Neuralgia, neuritis, and neuropathy
Neurofibromatosis
Neuropsychology
Neurorehabilitation
Neuroscience
Neurosis
Neurosurgery
Niemann-Pick disease
Nuclear medicine
Numbness and tingling
Osteopetrosis
Otorhinolaryngology
Pain
Palsy
Paralysis
Paraplegia
Parkinson's Disease
Pellagra
Phenylketonuria (PKU)
Phrenology
Pick's disease
Poliomyelitis
Porphyria
Postherpetic neuralgia
Postural orthostatic tachycardia
  syndrome (POTS)
Prader-Willi syndrome
Precocious puberty
Preeclampsia and eclampsia
Prion diseases
Psychiatry
Quadriplegia
Rabies
Radiculopathy
Restless legs syndrome
Reye's syndrome
Rubinstein-Taybi syndrome
Sarcoidosis
Sciatica
Seizures
Sense organs
Serotonin
Shingles
Shock therapy
Skin
Sleep
Sleep disorders
Sleeping sickness
Sleepwalking
Smell
Spinal cord disorders
Spine
Split-brain
Stenosis
Strokes
Sturge-Weber syndrome
Stuttering
Subdural hematoma

Sympathectomy
Synesthesia
Syphilis
Tardive dyskinesia
Taste
Tay-Sachs disease
Tetanus
Tics
Tinnitus
Torticollis
Touch
Tourette's syndrome
Transcranial magnetic stimulation
  (TMS)
Transient ischemic attacks (TIAs)
Traumatic brain injury
Tremors
Upper extremities
Vagotomy
Vagus nerve
Vasculitis
Vertigo
Vision
Wernicke's aphasia
West Nile virus
Williams syndrome
Wilson's disease

NEUROPSYCHOLOGY

Brain disorders
Capgras syndrome
Frontal lobe syndrome
Minimally conscious state
Neuroscience
Synesthesia
Traumatic brain injury
Wernicke's aphasia
Williams syndrome

NEUROSCIENCE

Antipsychotic drugs
Blindsight
Deep brain stimulation
Frontal lobe syndrome
Functional magnetic imaging (fMRI)
Glasgow coma scale
Memory erasure
Mirror neurons
Neuroethics
Neuropsychology
Neurorehabilitation
Phrenology
Psychiatry
Split-brain
Transcranial magnetic stimulation
  (TMS)
Traumatic brain injury
Wernicke's aphasia

NEUROSURGERY

Chiari malformations

Gestational diabetes
Growth
Gynecology
Hirschsprung's disease
Incontinence
Intravenous (IV) therapy
Karyotyping
Listeria infections
Mastitis
Miscarriage
Multiple births
Neonatal brachial plexus palsy
Neonatology
Noninvasive tests
Ovaries
Perinatology
Pituitary gland
Placenta
Polycystic ovary syndrome
Postpartum depression
Preeclampsia and eclampsia
Pregnancy and gestation
Pregnancy test
Premature birth
Pyelonephritis
Reproductive system
Rh factor
Sexuality
Sperm banks
Stillbirth
Streptococcal infections
Teratogens
Toxemia
Trichomoniasis
Tubal ligation
Turner syndrome
Ultrasonography
Urology
Uterus
Vaginal birth after cesarean (VBAC)

OCCUPATIONAL HEALTH
Acidosis
Agnosia
Altitude sickness
Angelman syndrome
Asbestos exposure
Asphyxiation
Ataxia
Bacillus Calmette-Guérin (BCG)
Back pain
Biofeedback
Blurred vision
Brucellosis
Cardiac rehabilitation
Carpal tunnel syndrome
Charcot-Marie-Tooth Disease
Defibrillation
Gulf War syndrome
Hearing tests
Leptospirosis

Leukodystrophy
Lung cancer
Mercury poisoning
Mesothelioma
Multiple chemical sensitivity syndrome
Nasopharyngeal disorders
Pneumonia
Prostheses
Pulmonary diseases
Pulmonary medicine
Radiation sickness
Skin disorders
Slipped disk
Spinocerebellar ataxia
Stress reduction
Tendinitis
Tendon disorders
Tendon repair

OCCUPATIONAL THERAPY
Astym® therapy
Flexibility
Home care
Minimally conscious state
Williams syndrome

ONCOLOGY
Mesenchymal stem cells
Acquired immunodeficiency syndrome
  (AIDS)
Aging: Extended care
Amputation
Anal cancer
Analgesic
Anemia
Antibodies
Antioxidants
Anus
Asbestos exposure
Assisted suicide
Biological therapies
Biopsy
Bladder cancer
Bone cancer
Bone disorders
Bone Marrow
Bone marrow transplantation
Brain tumors
Breast cancer
Breasts
Burkitt's lymphoma
Cancer
Carcinoma
Cervical, ovarian, and uterine cancers
Chemotherapy
Cold agglutinin disease
Colon
Colorectal cancer
Computed tomography (CT) scanning
Cryosurgery
Cystoscopy

Cytology
Cytopathology
Dermatology
Dermatopathology
Disseminated intravascular coagulation
  (DIC)
Embolization
Epstein-Barr virus
Ewing's sarcoma
Family-centered care
Fibrocystic breast condition
Galactorrhea
Gallbladder cancer
Gastrectomy
Gastroenterology
Gastrointestinal system
Gastrostomy
Genetic imprinting
Genital disorders
Glioma
Gynecology
Hematology
Histology
Hodgkin's disease
Hormone therapy
Human papillomavirus (HPV)
Hyperbaric chamber
Hysterectomy
Intravenous (IV) therapy
Kaposi's sarcoma
Karyotyping
Kidney cancer
Laboratory tests
Laryngectomy
Laser use in surgery
Lesions
Leukemia
Light therapy
Liver cancer
Lumbar puncture
Lung cancer
Lungs
Lymph
Lymphadenopathy and lymphoma
Malignancy and metastasis
Mammography
Massage
Mastectomy and lumpectomy
Meckel's diverticulum
Mesothelioma
Mouth and throat cancer
Necrosis
Nephrectomy
Nuclear medicine
Nursing
Oral and maxillofacial surgery
Pain
Pain management
Palliative care
Pap test
Pathology

Pharmacology
Plastic surgery
Proctology
Prostate cancer
Prostate gland
Prostate gland removal
Prostheses
Pulmonary diseases
Radiation sickness
Radiation therapy
Radiopharmaceuticals
Rectum
Retroviruses
Sarcoma
Serology
Skin
Skin cancer
Skin lesion removal
Small intestine
Smoking
Stenosis
Stomach
Stress
Testicular cancer
Thalidomide
Thymus gland
Tonsils
Transplantation
Tumor removal
Tumors
Uterus
Wilms tumor
Wiskott-Aldrich syndrome

OPHTHALMOLOGY
Acquired immunodeficiency syndrome
　(AIDS)
Adenoviruses
Adrenoleukodystrophy
Aging: Extended care
Anesthesia
Anesthesiology
Anti-inflammatory drugs
Astigmatism
Batten's disease
Behçet's disease
Blindness
Blindsight
Blurred vision
Botox
Cataract surgery
Cataracts
Cockayne disease
Conjunctivitis
Corneal transplantation
Cutis marmorata telangiectatica
　congenita
Diabetic nephropathy
Dry eye
Eye infections and disorders
Eye surgery

Eyes
Glaucoma
Glycerol
Hyperbaric chamber
Juvenile rheumatoid arthritis
Keratitis
Kluver-Bucy syndrome
Laser use in surgery
Lesions
Light therapy
Lyme disease
Macular degeneration
Marfan syndrome
Microscopy
Myopia
Optometry
Osteogenesis imperfecta
Osteopetrosis
Presbyopia
Prostheses
Pterygium/Pinguecula
Ptosis
Refractive eye surgery
Reiter's syndrome
Retina
Rubinstein-Taybi syndrome
Sarcoidosis
Sense organs
Sphincterectomy
Spinocerebellar ataxia
Spondylitis
Stevens-Johnson syndrome
Strabismus
Sturge-Weber syndrome
Subdural hematoma
Tears and tear ducts
Trachoma
Vasculitis
Vision
Vision disorders

OPTOMETRY
Aging: Extended care
Astigmatism
Blindsight
Blurred vision
Cataract surgery
Cataracts
Cockayne disease
Color blindness
Conjunctivitis
Eye infections and disorders
Eye surgery
Eyes
Glaucoma
Keratitis
Myopia
Ophthalmology
Presbyopia
Pterygium/Pinguecula
Ptosis

Sarcoidosis
Sense organs
Spinocerebellar ataxia
Tears and tear ducts
Vision disorders
Williams syndrome

ORTHODONTICS
Bones and the skeleton
Braces
Cleft lip and palate repair
Dentistry
Jaw wiring
Periodontal surgery
Periodontitis
Teeth
Teething
Tooth extraction
Williams syndrome

ORTHOPEDICS
Amputation
Anti-inflammatory drugs
Arthritis
Arthroplasty
Arthroscopy
Ataxia
Atrophy
Back pain
Bariatric surgery
Bone cancer
Bone disorders
Bone grafting
Bones and the skeleton
Bowlegs
Braces
Bunions
Cancer
Carticel®
Cartilage
Casts and splints
Cerebral palsy
Charcot-Marie-Tooth Disease
Chiropractic
Connective tissue
Contracture
Craniosynostosis
Cutis marmorata telangiectatica
　congenita
Disk removal
Dwarfism
Endoscopy
Ergogenic aids
Ewing's sarcoma
Fascia
Feet
Flat feet
Flexibility
Foot disorders
Fracture and dislocation
Fracture repair

Growth
Hammertoe correction
Hammertoes
Heel spur removal
Hemiplegia
Hip fracture repair
Hip replacement
Hormone therapy
Hyaluronic acid injections
Insulin-like growth factors
Joints
Juvenile rheumatoid arthritis
Kinesiology
Knee
Kneecap removal
Knock-knees
Kyphosis
Laminectomy and spinal fusion
Lower extremities
Marfan syndrome
Methicillin-resistant staphylococcus aureus (MRSA) infection
Motor skill development
Muscles
Necrosis
Neonatal brachial plexus palsy
Neurofibromatosis
Non-steroidal anti-inflammatory drugs (NSAIDs)
Orthopedic surgery
Osgood-Schlatter disease
Osteoarthritis
Osteochondritis juvenilis
Osteoclast
Osteogenesis imperfecta
Osteomyelitis
Osteonecrosis
Osteopetrosis
Osteoporosis
Paget's disease
Patellofemoral pain syndrome
Physical rehabilitation
Pigeon toes
Podiatry
Prostheses
Radiculopathy
Reiter's syndrome
Rheumatology
Rickets
Rotator cuff surgery
Rubinstein-Taybi syndrome
Scoliosis
Slipped disk
Spine
Spondylitis
Sports medicine
Staphylococcal infections
Stenosis
Systemic lupus erythematosus (SLE)
Tendinitis
Tendon disorders

Tendon repair
Tissue engineering
Upper extremities
Virtual imaging
Walking
Whiplash

OSTEOPATHIC MEDICINE
Acidosis
Acquired immunodeficiency syndrome (AIDS)
Alternative medicine
Atrophy
Back pain
Bones and the skeleton
Colon
Family-centered care
Family medicine
Fascia
Muscle sprains, spasms, and disorders
Muscles
Physical rehabilitation
Pituitary gland
Radiculopathy
Rickets
Slipped disk
Small intestine

OTORHINOLARYNGOLOGY
Acquired immunodeficiency syndrome (AIDS)
Adenoids
Allergies
Anosmia
Antihistamines
Anti-inflammatory drugs
Aromatherapy
Cleft lip and palate
Cockayne disease
Common cold
Croup
Cryosurgery
Cystic fibrosis
Decongestants
Dysarthria
Dysphagia
Ear infections and disorders
Ear surgery
Ears
Earwax
Esophagus
Gastrointestinal system
Hearing tests
Laryngectomy
Laryngitis
Lesions
Motion sickness
Myringotomy
Nasal polyp removal
Nasopharyngeal disorders
Nausea and vomiting

Oral and maxillofacial surgery
Pharyngitis
Pharynx
Polyps
Pulmonary medicine
Quinsy
Respiration
Rhinitis
Rhinoplasty and submucous resection
Rhinoviruses
Sense organs
Sinusitis
Sleep apnea
Smell
Sore throat
Taste
Tinnitus
Tonsillectomy and adenoid removal
Tonsillitis
Tonsils
Trachea
Vertigo
Voice and vocal cord disorders
Whooping cough

PANCREAS
Abscess drainage
Alcoholism
Carbohydrates
Cholecystitis
Chyme
Cystic fibrosis
Diabetes mellitus
Digestion
Endocrine glands
Endocrinology
Endoscopic retrograde cholangiopancreatography (ERCP)
Fetal tissue transplantation
Food biochemistry
Gastroenterology
Gastrointestinal system
Glands
Glucose tolerance test
Hemochromatosis
Insulin
Internal medicine
Malabsorption
Metabolism
Mumps
Pancreatitis
Polycystic kidney disease
Polycystic ovary syndrome
Stomach
Transplantation

PATHOLOGY
Acquired immunodeficiency syndrome (AIDS)
Adrenoleukodystrophy
Anthrax

Astym® therapy
Ataxia
Atrophy
Back pain
Biofeedback
Bowlegs
Burns and scalds
Cardiac rehabilitation
Casts and splints
Cerebral palsy
Charcot-Marie-Tooth Disease
Cornelia de Lange syndrome
Disk removal
Dyskinesia
Electromyography
Exercise physiology
Facial transplantation
Fascia
Flexibility
Grafts and grafting
Hemiplegia
Home care
Hydrotherapy
Kinesiology
Knock-knees
Leukodystrophy
Lower extremities
Massage
Minimally conscious state
Motor skill development
Muscle sprains, spasms, and disorders
Muscles
Muscular dystrophy
Neonatal brachial plexus palsy
Neurology
Numbness and tingling
Orthopedic surgery
Orthopedics
Osteopathic medicine
Pain
Pain management
Palsy
Paralysis
Parkinson's Disease
Patellofemoral pain syndrome
Physical rehabilitation
Pigeon toes
Plastic surgery
Prostheses
Pulse rate
Radiculopathy
Rotator cuff surgery
Scoliosis
Slipped disk
Spinal cord disorders
Spine
Spinocerebellar ataxia
Sports medicine
Systemic lupus erythematosus (SLE)
Tendinitis
Tendon disorders

Torticollis
Upper extremities
Whiplash
Williams syndrome

PLASTIC SURGERY
Amputation
Bariatric surgery
Body dysmorphic disorder
Botox
Breast surgery
Breasts
Burns and scalds
Circumcision, female, and genital mutilation
Cleft lip and palate
Cleft lip and palate repair
Craniosynostosis
Cyst removal
DiGeorge syndrome
Face lift and blepharoplasty
Facial transplantation
Gender reassignment surgery
Grafts and grafting
Hair transplantation
Healing
Hyaluronic acid injections
Jaw wiring
Laceration repair
Liposuction
Malignancy and metastasis
Mastectomy and lumpectomy
Mesenchymal stem cells
Moles
Necrotizing fasciitis
Neonatal brachial plexus palsy
Neurofibromatosis
Oral and maxillofacial surgery
Otoplasty
Otorhinolaryngology
Prostheses
Ptosis
Rhinoplasty and submucous resection
Skin
Skin lesion removal
Spina bifida
Sturge-Weber syndrome
Surgical procedures
Tattoos and body piercing
Varicose vein removal
Varicose veins
Vision

PODIATRY
Athlete's foot
Bones and the skeleton
Bunions
Cerebral palsy
Corns and calluses
Diabetic neuropathy
Feet

Flat feet
Foot disorders
Gout
Hammertoe correction
Hammertoes
Heel spur removal
Joints
Lesions
Lower extremities
Methicillin-resistant staphylococcus aureus (MRSA) infection
Nail removal
Orthopedic surgery
Orthopedics
Polydactyly and syndactyly
Tendon disorders
Tendon repair
Acidosis
Acupressure
Acupuncture
Alternative medicine
Anemia
Aneurysmectomy
Antibodies
Antihistamines
Antihypertensives
Aromatherapy
Assisted living facilities
Bacillus Calmette-Guérin (BCG)
Back pain
Biofeedback
Blurred vision
Breast cancer
Brucellosis
Cardiac surgery
Cardiology
Cerebral palsy
Chemotherapy
Chiropractic
Cholesterol
Club drugs
Computed tomography (CT) scanning
Croup
Electrocardiography (ECG or EKG)
Endometrial biopsy
Exercise physiology
Family-centered care
Family medicine
Fiber
Food guide plate
Genetic counseling
Genetic engineering
Hormone therapy
Host-defense mechanisms
Immune system
Immunization and vaccination
Insect-borne diseases
Lead poisoning
Mammography
Massage
Meditation

Tardive dyskinesia
Tinnitus
Toilet training
Tourette's syndrome
Transcranial magnetic stimulation (TMS)
Traumatic brain injury
Tremors

PSYCHOLOGY
Abuse of the elderly
Abusive relationships
Addiction
Aging
Aging: Extended care
Alcoholism
Amnesia
Amyotrophic lateral sclerosis (ALS)
Angelman syndrome
Anorexia nervosa
Antidepressants
Antipsychotic drugs
Anxiety
Aromatherapy
Asperger syndrome
Attention-deficit disorder (ADD)
Auras
Bariatric surgery
Bed-wetting
Biofeedback
Bipolar disorders
Blindsight
Bonding
Brain
Brain damage
Bulimia
Capgras syndrome
Cardiac rehabilitation
Cerebral palsy
Cirrhosis
Club drugs
Cognitive development
Death and dying
Deep brain stimulation
Depression
Developmental disorders
Developmental stages
Dyslexia
Eating disorders
Electroencephalography (EEG)
Ergogenic aids
Facial transplantation
Factitious disorders
Failure to thrive
Family-centered care
Family medicine
Forensic pathology
Frontal lobe syndrome
Functional magnetic imaging (fMRI)
Gender dysphoria
Gender reassignment surgery

Genetic counseling
Gulf War syndrome
Gynecology
Hippocampus
Huntington's disease
Hypnosis
Hypochondriasis
Hypothalamus
Intellectual disability
Interpartner violence
Juvenile rheumatoid arthritis
Kinesiology
Klinefelter syndrome
Kluver-Bucy syndrome
Korsakoff's syndrome
Learning disabilities
Lesbian, gay, bisexual, transgender, and queer (LGBTQ)
Light therapy
Marijuana
Memory erasure
Memory loss
Mental status exam
Mirror neurons
Miscarriage
Motor skill development
Münchausen syndrome by proxy
Neonatal brachial plexus palsy
Neuropsychology
Neurorehabilitation
Neurosis
Obesity
Obsessive-compulsive disorder
Occupational health
Overtraining syndrome
Pain management
Palliative care
Paranoia
Phobias
Phrenology
Pick's disease
Plastic surgery
Polycystic ovary syndrome
Postpartum depression
Post-traumatic stress disorder
Premenstrual syndrome (PMS)
Psychosomatic disorders
Puberty and adolescence
Relaxation
Reminiscence therapy
Restless legs syndrome
Separation anxiety
Serotonin
Sexual dysfunction
Sexuality
Sleep
Sleep disorders
Sleepwalking
Speech disorders
Split-brain
Sports medicine

Steroid abuse
Stress
Stress reduction
Sturge-Weber syndrome
Sudden infant death syndrome (SIDS)
Suicide
Synesthesia
Systemic lupus erythematosus (SLE)
Temporomandibular joint (TMJ) syndrome
Tics
Toilet training
Tourette's syndrome
Transcranial magnetic stimulation (TMS)
Traumatic brain injury
Weight loss and gain
Wernicke's aphasia

PUBLIC HEALTH
Acquired immunodeficiency syndrome (AIDS)
Acute respiratory distress syndrome (ARDS)
Adenoviruses
Advance directives
Aging: Extended care
Amebiasis
Antibodies
Assisted living facilities
Babesiosis
Bacillus Calmette-Guérin (BCG)
Bacteriology
Blood testing
Brucellosis
Cerebral palsy
Chagas' disease
Chickenpox
Childhood infectious diseases
Cholera
Chronic obstructive pulmonary disease (COPD)
Club drugs
Common cold
Coronaviruses
Creutzfeldt-Jakob disease (CJD)
Dengue fever
Dermatology
Diarrhea and dysentery
E. coli infection
Ebola virus
Elephantiasis
Emergency medicine
Encephalitis
Epidemics and pandemics
Epidemiology
Food guide plate
Food poisoning
Forensic pathology
Gulf War syndrome
Hantavirus

Endoscopic retrograde cholangiopancreatography (ERCP)
Ewing's sarcoma
Eye infections and disorders
Gallbladder cancer
Imaging and radiology
Joints
Liver cancer
Lung cancer
Magnetic resonance imaging (MRI)
Mammography
Mastectomy and lumpectomy
Meckel's diverticulum
Mesothelioma
Methicillin-resistant staphylococcus aureus (MRSA) infection
Mouth and throat cancer
Neonatal brachial plexus palsy
Noninvasive tests
Nuclear medicine
Nuclear radiology
Oncology
Palliative care
Pneumocystis jirovecii
Positron emission tomography (PET) scanning
Prostate cancer
Radiation sickness
Radiation therapy
Radiculopathy
Radiopharmaceuticals
Sarcoidosis
Single photon emission computed tomography (SPECT)
Stents
Surgery
Testicular cancer
Ultrasonography
Virtual imaging

REHABILITATION
Astym® therapy
Neuropsychology
Neurorehabilitation
Nicotine
Traumatic brain injury

RHEUMATOLOGY
Aging: Extended care
Ankylosing spondylitis
Anti-inflammatory drugs
Arthritis
Arthroplasty
Arthroscopy
Atrophy
Back pain
Behçet's disease
Bone disorders
Brucellosis
Bursitis
Cartilage

Cold agglutinin disease
Collagen
Connective tissue
Fibromyalgia
Gout
Hip replacement
Hydrotherapy
Inflammation
Joints
Lyme disease
Mesenchymal stem cells
Methicillin-resistant staphylococcus aureus (MRSA) infection
Non-steroidal anti-inflammatory drugs (NSAIDs)
Orthopedic surgery
Orthopedics
Osteonecrosis
Paget's disease
Pain
Polymyalgia rheumatica
Polymyositis
Radiculopathy
Rheumatoid arthritis
Rotator cuff surgery
Sarcoidosis
Scleroderma
Sjögren's syndrome
Sports medicine
Syphilis
Systemic lupus erythematosus (SLE)
Temporal arteritis
Vasculitis

SEROLOGY
Babesiosis
Blood and blood disorders
Blood testing
Chronic granulomatous disease
Cold agglutinin disease
Cytology
Cytopathology
Dialysis
Epidemics and pandemics
Fluids and electrolytes
Forensic pathology
Hematology
Hemophilia
Hodgkin's disease
Host-defense mechanisms
Hyperbaric oxygen therapy
Hyperlipidemia
Hypoglycemia
Immune system
Immunopathology
Laboratory tests
Leukemia
Lymph
Plasma
Rh factor
Rhinoviruses

Sarcoidosis
Septicemia
Snakebites
Transfusion
Tremors

SPEECH PATHOLOGY
Adenoids
Agnosia
Amyotrophic lateral sclerosis (ALS)
Angelman syndrome
Aphasia and dysphasia
Ataxia
Audiology
Autism
Cerebral palsy
Cleft lip and palate
Deafness
Dyslexia
Ear surgery
Ears
Electroencephalography (EEG)
Hearing loss
Hearing tests
Jaw wiring
Laryngitis
Lisping
Pharynx
Rubinstein-Taybi syndrome
Speech disorders
Spinocerebellar ataxia
Strokes
Stuttering
Subdural hematoma
Thumb sucking
Voice and vocal cord disorders
Wernicke's aphasia

SPORTS MEDICINE
Acidosis
Acupressure
Aerobics
Arthroplasty
Atrophy
Back pain
Biofeedback
Blurred vision
Bones and the skeleton
Braces
Casts and splints
Concussion
Critical care
Defibrillation
Dehydration
Emergency medicine
Ergogenic aids
Exercise physiology
Fiber
Flexibility
Fracture and dislocation
Glycolysis

Head and neck disorders
Heat exhaustion and heatstroke
Hematomas
Hydrotherapy
Hyperbaric chamber
Impetigo
Joints
Kinesiology
Macronutrients
Massage
Methicillin-resistant staphylococcus
　aureus (MRSA) infection
Motor skill development
Muscle sprains, spasms, and disorders
Muscles
Nail removal
Orthopedic surgery
Orthopedics
Overtraining syndrome
Pain
Patellofemoral pain syndrome
Physical rehabilitation
Pigeon toes
Pulse rate
Radiculopathy
Rotator cuff surgery
Safety issues for children
Slipped disk
Spine
Steroid abuse
Steroids
Tendinitis
Tendon disorders
Tendon repair

TOXICOLOGY
Acidosis
Bites and stings
Blood testing
Chemotherapy
Club drugs
Critical care
Cyanosis
Defibrillation
Diphtheria
Emergency medicine
Ergogenic aids
Food poisoning
Forensic pathology
Gaucher's disease
Hepatitis
Laboratory tests
Lead poisoning
Leukemia
Liver
Mold and mildew
Multiple chemical sensitivity syndrome
Neuroscience
Occupational health
Pharmacology
Poisoning

Sarcoidosis
Tremors
Urinalysis

UROLOGY
Abdomen
Adenoviruses
Bed-wetting
Bladder removal
Catheterization
Chronic granulomatous disease
Circumcision
Cold agglutinin disease
Congenital adrenal hyperplasia
Contraception
Cryosurgery
Cushing's syndrome
Cystic fibrosis
Cystitis
Cystoscopy
Diabetic nephropathy
Dialysis
Diuretics
E. coli infection
Endoscopy
Erectile dysfunction
Fetal surgery
Fluids and electrolytes
Gender reassignment surgery
Genital disorders
Hemolysis
Hemolytic uremic syndrome
Hermaphroditism and
　pseudohermaphroditism
Herpes
Hydroceles
Hyperplasia
Hypogonadism
Hypospadias repair and urethroplasty
Incontinence
Infertility
Kidney cancer
Kidney disorders
Kidneys
Laser use in surgery
Leptospirosis
Lesions
Lithotripsy
Nephrectomy
Nephrology
Nuclear medicine
Orchiectomy
Pediatrics
Penile implant surgery
Polycystic kidney disease
Polyps
Prostate cancer
Prostate enlargement
Prostate gland
Prostate gland removal
Proteinuria

Pyelonephritis
Reiter's syndrome
Reproductive system
Semen
Sexual differentiation
Sexual dysfunction
Sexually transmitted diseases (STDs)
Sperm banks
Staphylococcal infections
Sterilization
Stevens-Johnson syndrome
Stone removal
Stones
Testicles
Testicular cancer
Testicular surgery
Testicular torsion
Tissue engineering
Toilet training
Transplantation
Trichomoniasis
Ultrasonography
Uremia
Urethritis
Urinalysis
Urinary disorders
Urinary system
Vas deferens
Vasectomy
Wilms tumor

VASCULAR MEDICINE
Acidosis
Amputation
Aneurysms
Angiography
Angioplasty
Antihypertensives
Arteriosclerosis
Biofeedback
Bleeding
Blood pressure
Blood vessels
Bruises
Cardiac surgery
Cardiology
Carotid arteries
Cholesterol
Circulation
Claudication
Cold agglutinin disease
Computed tomography (CT) scanning
Congenital heart disease
Cutis marmorata telangiectatica
　congenita
Defibrillation
Dehydration
Diabetes mellitus
Electrocauterization
Embolism
Embolization

VIROLOGY